Governors State University
Library Hours:
Monday thru Thursday 8:00 to 10:30
Friday 8:00 to 5:00
Saturday 8:30 to 5:00
Sunday 1:00 to 5:00 (Fall
and Winter Trimester Only)

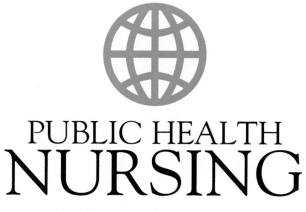

PUBLIC HEALTH
NURSING
Leadership, Policy & Practice

L. Louise Ivanov RN, DNS

Associate Professor and Chair

Community Practice Department

School of Nursing

The University of North Carolina

Greenboro, North Carolina

Carolyn L. Blue, RN, PhD, CHES

Professor

School of Nursing

The University of North Carolina

Greenboro, North Carolina

DELMAR
CENGAGE Learning·   Australia   Brazil   Canada   Mexico   Singapore   Spain   United Kingdom   United States

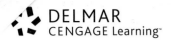

**Public Health Nursing:
Leadership, Policy & Practice**

L. Louise Ivanov

Carolyn L. Blue

Vice President, Career and
Professional Editoral:
Dave Garza

Director of Learning Solutions:
Matthew Kane

Acquisitions Editor:
Tamara Caruso

Senior Product Manager:
Elisabeth F. Williams

Editorial Assistant:
Jennifer Waters

Vice President, Career and
Professional Marketing:
Jennifer McAvey

Marketing Channel Manager:
Michele McTighe

Marketing Coordinator:
Chelsey Iaquinta

Director of Technology:
Laurie K. Davis

Director of Production:
Carolyn Miller

Content Project Manager:
Jessica McNavitch

Senior Art Director:
Jack Pendelton

For product information and technology assistance, contact us at
Professional & Career Group Customer Support, 1-800-648-7450

For permission to use material from this text or product, submit all requests online at **www.cengage.com/permissions**
Further permissions questions can be emailed to
permissionrequest@cengage.com

ExamView® and ExamView Pro® are registered trademarks of FSCreations, Inc. Windows is a registered trademark of the Microsoft Corporation used herein under license. Macintosh and Power Macintosh are registered trademarks of Apple Computer, Inc. Used herein under license.

Library of Congress Control Number: 2007942029

ISBN-10 1-4018-3965-7

ISBN-13 978-14018-3965-9

Delmar Cengage Learning
5 Maxwell Drive
Clifton Park, NY 12065-2919
USA

Cengage Learning products are represented in Canada by Nelson Education, Ltd.

For your lifelong learning solutions, visit **delmar.cengage.com**

Visit our corporate website at **www.cengage.com**

Notice to the Reader

Printed in the United States of America
1 2 3 4 5 6 7   11 10 09 08 07

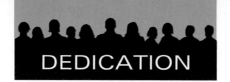

DEDICATION

We wish to dedicate this book to Dr. Beverly Flynn, a public health nursing champion who nurtured us in public health nursing as our teacher, mentor, colleague, and friend. She was a scholar, teacher, community builder, mentor, and friend to not only the editors of this book but to scores of public health nurses who were fortunate enough to have known her and worked with her. Her legacy is recognized worldwide by future generations of public health nurses.

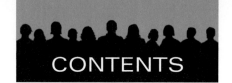

CONTENTS

Dedication   iii

Contributors   xiii

Reviewers   xvii

Preface   xix

About the Editors   xxi

Acknowledgments   xxiii

PART 1

Public Health Basics   1

Chapter 1   History of Public Health and Public Health Nursing   2

Establishing the Science of Public Health   3
Early Public Health Nursing   7
Middle Twentieth-Century Public Health Nursing   14
Public Health Nursing Today   20

Chapter 2   Core Functions of Public Health Nursing   27

Public Health and the IOM Reports   28
Public Health in America: Linking Core
Functions and Essential Public Health Services   32
The Core Public Health Functions, Essential Public Health Services,
and Workforce Competency   37
Challenges to Advancing the Public's Health Through Improving the Public
Health Infrastructure   47

Chapter 3   Practice Settings in Public Health Nursing   57

Historical Practice Perspectives   58
Practice Settings in Governmental or Official Agencies   59
Practice Settings Associated with Nongovernmental,
Community Agencies   63

	Models of Public Health Nursing Practice	71
	Issues and Challenges	73
Chapter 4	**Epidemiology and Public Health Nursing**	**86**
	Epidemiology Defined	87
	Epidemiologic Models	87
	Uses of Epidemiology in Public Health Nursing	88
	Epidemiologic Rates	91
	Types of Epidemiologic Studies	96
	Sources of Epidemiologic Data	99
	Conclusion	101
Chapter 5	**Healthy People 2010 Objectives**	**104**
	Leading Health Indicators	106
	Healthy People 2010 and Public Health Nurses	112

PART 2

Health Care Delivery and Financing   117

Chapter 6	**Law, Health Policy, and Public Health Nursing**	**118**
	Politics and Health Policy	119
	Models of Policy Formulation	120
	Political Development of Nursing	121
	Considerations for Public Health Nurses in Varied Settings	126
	Public Health Nurses as Advocates and Activists	127
Chapter 7	**Health Care Organization and Financing**	**134**
	Historical Development of the Organization of Health Care	135
	Health Care Financing	136
	Challenges for Public Health Nurses	145
Chapter 8	**Economics of Public Health Nursing**	**153**
	What Is Economics?	154
	Profit Maximization and Cost Minimization	155
	For-Profit and Not-for-Profit Organizations	157
	Individual Investment in Health	159
	Externalities	160

Decisions Under Uncertainty 162

Economic Evaluation 163

Economics of the Labor Market 166

Chapter 9   Challenges of Global Health 172

Global Health Defined 173

Challenges for Public Health Nurses in the Global Arena 174

Global Efforts in Providing Health Care 176

Public Health Nurses' Response to Challenges in Global Health 180

PART 3

Public Health Nursing Practice   187

Chapter 10   Environmental Health Risk 188

Environmental Health Challenges 189

Environmental Health Assessment 190

Vulnerable Populations 208

Environmental Justice 209

Advocacy 209

Risk Communication 210

Chemical Policies and the Precautionary Principle 211

Environmental and Public Health Infrastructure 212

Accessing Information and the "Right to Know" 213

Environmental Health and Public Nursing 213

Chapter 11   Community and Population Assessment 220

Community and Population Assessment 221

Theoretical Foundations for Community Assessment 221

Methods for Community Assessment 227

Assessment of Culturally Diverse Communities 234

Chapter 12   Health Risk Appraisal 240

History of Health Risk Appraisal 241

Purpose, Development, and Use of Health Risk Appraisals 241

Validity, Reliability, and Effectiveness of Health Risk Appraisals 243

Appropriate and Inappropriate Uses of Health Risk Appraisals 244

Social Influences and Culture's Impact 244

Selection of Appropriate Health Risk Appraisal Tools 244

Implications for Public Health Nursing   246

Chapter 13   Principles of Health Promotion   253

Holistic Concept of Health   254
Health Promotion   255
Theoretical Foundations of Health Promotion   255
Focus on Population Health   263
Ethical Issues in Health Promotion   269

Chapter 14   Principles of Health Education   278

Health Education Defined   279
Healthy People 2010 Objectives Relevant to Public Health Education   279
Fundamentals of Teaching and Learning   282
Steps of Teaching-Learning Process   283

Chapter 15   Program Development and Evaluation   303

Program Development   304
Planning as a Component of Program Development   304
Frameworks in Program Development   304
Framework for Planning Process in Program Development   306
Role of Economic Analysis in Decision Making for Program Development   308
Types of Economic Analysis   308
Program Evaluation   312
Theoretical Foundations of Program Evaluation   317
Decision Making in Evaluation   319

Chapter 16   Community Development for Health Promotion   324

Community Development Theories   325
The Healthy Cities Model   326
Choosing Programs for Health Promotion after Needs Identification   328
Linking Healthy Cities and Healthy Families   336

Chapter 17   Health Care Management   342

Management and Public Health Nurses   343
Healthy People 2010   345
Administration and Leadership   346
Basics of Internal Management   348
Basics of External Management   354

Keys to Improvement   355
Future Orientation   355

Chapter 18   Ethics and Human Rights   359

History of Ethics in Public Health, Nursing, and Public Health Nursing   360
Human Rights   361
The Intersection of Ethics and Human Rights   362
Ethics   364
Cross-Cultural Ethical Perspectives   371
Nursing and Other Ethical Codes and Principles   371
Public Health as Social Justice: Poverty and Health   378
Ethical Decision Making in Public Health Nursing   378
Selected Issues in Public Health Nursing Ethics   380

Chapter 19   Public Health Nursing Research   390

Research in Public Health Nursing: A Pioneer Who Made a Difference   391
The Role of the Public Health Nurse in Research   392
Research, Nursing Process, Epidemiology, and Quality Assurance   393
Research Priorities in Public Health Nursing   395
Types of Research Studies in Public Health Nursing   396
Outcomes Research Related to Public Health Nursing Practice   399
Evaluating Research for Evidence-Based Practice   401

PART 4

Provision of Public Health Nursing to Vulnerable Populations   405

Chapter 20   Populations with Infectious and Communicable Disease   406

Factors that Lead to the Emergence and Reemergence of Infectious
and Communicable Disease   407
Models of Transmission of Infectious and Communicable Disease   409
Levels of Prevention   413
Common Infectious and Communicable Diseases   423
Infectious and Communicable Disease in the Global Community   431
The Spectre of Bioterrorism   432
Strategies for Nurses Working with Infectious and Communicable
Disease in the Community   435
Infectious and Communicable Disease Resources   436

Chapter 21   Populations with Chronic Diseases   445

                   Causes of Morbidity and Mortality   446
                   Shift from Acute to Chronic Disease   448
                   Increasing Prevalence of Type 2 Diabetes   456
                   Diseases of the Cardiovascular System   457
                   Contextual Risk Factors for Chronic Diseases   462
                   Caregiver Burden   465
                   Disease Trajectory   466
                   Public Health Nursing Consideration for Screening
                   for and Managment of Chronic Diseases   466

Chapter 22   Maternal and Child Populations   478

                   Reduce the Rate of Maternal Deaths   479
                   Reduce the Rate of Fetal and Infant Deaths   481
                   Reduce the Rate of Child Deaths   481
                   Reduce the Rate of Adolescent and Young Adult Deaths   483
                   Reduce the Rate of Pregnancies among Adolescent Females   484
                   Reduce Obesity and Improve Nutrition in Children and Adolescents   486
                   Education and Community-Based Programs to Address Maternal
                   and Child Health Issues   488
                   Maternal and Child Health Services and Public Health Nursing   489

Chapter 23   The Elder Population   495

                   Theories of Aging   497
                   Culture and Elder Health   497
                   Family as Caregivers   498
                   Health Assessment of Older Adults   499
                   Health Promotion for Older Adults   504

Chapter 24   Rural and Migrant Populations   511

                   Rural Defined   512
                   Historical Context   513
                   Demographics and Health Status Indicators   515
                   Cultural Characteristics of Rural Populations   516
                   Migrant Rural Farmworkers   516
                   Public Health Nursing Practice in Rural Communities   518
                   Health Policy in Rural Settings   522
                   Research in Rural Settings   524

Chapter 25   Racial and Ethnic Disparities   529
              Morbidity and Mortality Trends in Racial/Ethnic Minorities   531
              Theoretical Framework of Factors Influencing Racial/Ethnic
              Minority Disparities   536
              National Studies, Reports, Initiatives, and Policies to Guide Nursing Interventions   539
              Strategies to Reduce Racial/Ethnic Health Disparities   541

Chapter 26   Immigrant and Refugee Populations   553
              Global Migration Patterns   554
              Premigration Factors That Affect Health in Immigrants   556
              Postmigration Factors That Affect Health in Immigrants   556
              Health Problems with Special Implications for Immigrants and Refugees 561
              Planning and Implementing Health Care for Immigrants and Refugees   562

Chapter 27   The Homeless Population   572
              Health of the Homeless   574
              Special Populations   576
              Overall Prevention and Policy Recommendations for the Homeless   583

Chapter 28   Populations with Substance Abuse   591
              Alcohol Use   592
              Marijuana Use   593
              Tobacco Use   594
              Populations Most At Risk for Alcohol, Marijuana, and Tobacco Abuse   597

PART 5
Public Health Nursing in the Twenty-First Century   609

Chapter 29   Disaster Preparedness and Public Health Nursing   610
              Disasters   611
              Weapons of Mass Destruction   614
              Effects of Disasters   623
              Disease Surveillance   625
              Strategic National Stockpile   626
              Disaster Preparedness   627

Chapter 30   The Future of Public Health Nursing   638
              Health Trends in the Twenty-First Century   639

Futures Thinking 644
Public Heatlh Systems Issues 646
Quality Improvement 647
Public Health Workforce 647
Building Capacity for Community Health Promotion 650
Research and Evidence Based Practice 651

Resources 660

Glossary 696

Appendices

A. Core Competencies for Public Health
Nursing Practice 713

B. Scope and Standards of Public Health
Nursing Practice 722

C. American Public Health Association Principles
on Public Health and Human Rights 736

D. Determinants of Health 737

E. Healthy People 2010 Goals 738

F. Professional Associations, Organizations,
and Institutes 764

G. Abbreviations 767

Index 771

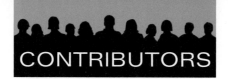
CONTRIBUTORS

CHAPTER 1

History of Public Health and Public Health Nursing

Betty Bekemeier, RN, MPH, PhD
Assistant Professor,
Psychosocial and Community Health
School of Nursing
University of Washington
Seattle, Washington

CHAPTER 2

Core Functions of Public Health Nursing

Jeanne Matthews, RN, PhD

Public Health Program Specialist
Arlington County Department of Human Services,
Public Health Division
Arlington, Virginia
and
Assistant Clinical Professor
Georgetown University
School of Nursing and Health Studies
Washington, DC

CHAPTER 3

Practice Settings in Public Health Nursing

Sonda Oppewal, RN, PhD
Associate Dean for Community Partnerships & Practice
Clinical Associate Professor
The University of North Carolina at Chapel Hill
School of Nursing
Chapel Hill, North Carolina

CHAPTER 4

Epidemiology and Public Health Nursing

R. Craig Stotts, RN, DrPH
Professor, College of Nursing
University of Tennessee Health Science Center
Memphis, Tennessee

CHAPTER 5

Healthy People 2010 Objectives

Susan Letvak, RN, PhD
Associate Professor
Community Practice Department
The University of North Carolina at Greensboro
Greensboro, North Carolina

CHAPTER 6

Law, Health Policy, and Public Health Nursing

L. Louise Ivanov, RN, DNS
Associate Professor and Chair,
Community Practice Department
School of Nursing
The University of North Carolina at Greensboro
Greensboro, North Carolina

Eileen Kohlendberg, RN, PhD
Associate Professor and
Associate Dean for Graduate Studies
School of Nursing
The University of North Carolina at Greensboro
Greensboro, North Carolina

CHAPTER 7

Health Care Organization and Financing

L. Louise Ivanov, RN, DNS
   Associate Professor and Chair,
   Community Practice Department
   School of Nursing
   The University of North Carolina at Greensboro
   Greensboro, North Carolina

CHAPTER 8

Economics of Public Health Nursing

Kevin D. Frick, PhD
   Associate Professor
   Johns Hopkins Bloomberg School of Public Health
   Departments of Health Policy and Management,
   Economics, International Health and Ophthalmology,
   and School of Nursing
   Baltimore, Maryland

Kathleen M. White, RN, PhD, CNAA, BC
   Associate Professor
   Johns Hopkins University School of Nursing
   Baltimore, Maryland

CHAPTER 9

Challenges of Global Health

Janet Gottschalk, RN, DrPH, FAAN
   Visiting Professor
   Canseco School of Nursing
   Texas A & M International University
   Laredo, Texas
   and
   Director: Alliance for Justice, Medical Mission Sisters
   Washington, DC

CHAPTER 10

Environmental Health Risk

Barbara Sattler, RN, DrPH, FAAN
   Associate Professor and Director, Environmental Health
   Education Center
   University of Maryland School of Nursing
   Baltimore, Maryland

CHAPTER 11

Community and Population Assessment

Jie Hu, RN, PhD
   Associate Professor
   Department of Community Practice
   The University of North Carolina at Greensboro
   Greensboro, North Carolina

CHAPTER 12

Health Risk Appraisal

Linda J. Hulton, RN, PhD
   Associate Professor of Nursing
   James Madison University
   Harrisonburg, Virginia

CHAPTER 13

Principles of Health Promotion

Carolyn L. Blue, RN, PhD, CHES
   Professor, School of Nursing
   Department of Community Practice
   The University of North Carolina at Greensboro
   Greensboro, North Carolina

David R. Black, PhD, HSPP, MPH, CHES, CPPE,
FASHA, FSBM, FAAHB
   Professor of Health Promotion; Health Sciences; Foods &
   Nutrition; Nursing Department of Health and Kinesiology
   Purdue University
   West Lafayette, Indiana

CHAPTER 14

Principles of Health Education

Carolyn L. Blue, RN, PhD, CHES
   Professor, School of Nursing
   Department of Community Practice
   The University of North Carolina at Greensboro
   Greensboro, North Carolina

David R. Black, PhD, HSPP, MPH, CHES, CPPE,
FASHA, FSBM, FAAHB
   Professor of Health Promotion; Health Sciences; Foods &
   Nutrition; Nursing Department of Health and Kinesiology
   Purdue University
   West Lafayette, Indiana

CHAPTER 15

Program Development and Evaluation

Carolyn K. Lewis, RN, PhD, CNAA, BC
   Assistant Dean and Associate Professor Nursing Division
   Bluegrass Community and Technical College
   Lexington, Kentucky

Christine Elnitsky, RN, PhD, CHNS
   Senior Program Analyst
   Headquarters for the Department of Veterans Affairs
   Office of the Assistant Secretary for Policy, Planning
   and Preparedness
   Department of Veterans Affairs
   Washington, DC

Joanne Martin, DrPH, FAAN
Assistant Professor, Environments for Health
Indiana University, School of Nursing
Director, Healthy Families Indiana Training & Technical
Assistance Project
Director, MOM Project
Director of the Institute for Action Research in
Community Health
Indianapolis, Indiana

CHAPTER 16

Community Development for Health Promotion

Joanne Martin, DrPH, FAAN, RN
Assistant Professor, Environments for Health
Indiana University, School of Nursing
Director, Healthy Families Indiana Training & Technical
Assistance Project
Director, MOM Project
Director of the Institute for Action Research in
Community Health
Indianapolis, Indiana

Joanne Raines Warner, RN, DNS,
Associate Dean and Professor
University of Portland, School of Nursing
Portland, Oregon

CHAPTER 17

Health Care Management

Katherine K. Kinsey, RN, PhD, FAAN
Collaborative Principal Investigator and Administrator,
Nurse-Family Partnership (NFP) sponsored by the National
Nursing Centers Consortium for Philadelphia County
Philadelphia, Pennsylvania
Director, NFP at Lutheran Children and Family Services
Philadelphia, Pennsylvania
President, Kingsley Family Foundation
Philadelphia, Pennsylvania

CHAPTER 18

Ethics and Human Rights

Carol Easley Allen, RN, PhD
Professor and Chair
Department of Nursing
Oakwood College
Huntsville, Alabama

Cheryl E. Easley, RN, PhD
Dean and Professor
College of Health & Social Welfare
University of Alaska Anchorage
Anchorage, Alaska

CHAPTER 19

Public Health Nursing Research

Martha Keehner Engelke, RN, PhD
Professor/Associate Dean for Research and Scholarship
East Carolina University School of Nursing
Greenville, North Carolina

CHAPTER 20

Populations with Infectious and Communicable Disease

Catherine Salveson, RN, MS, PhD
Associate Professor
School of Nursing
Oregon Health & Science University
Portland, Oregon

Shelley L. Jones, RN, MS, COHN-S, FAAOHN
Professor Emeritus
School of Nursing
Oregon Health & Science University
Portland, Oregon

CHAPTER 21

Populations with Chronic Diseases

Susan J. Appel, CCRN, APRN-BC (ACNP & FNP), PhD
Associate Professor
Division of Graduate Studies
School of Nursing
University of Alabama at Birmingham
Birmingham, Alabama

CHAPTER 22

Maternal and Child Populations

Anne S. Belcher, RN, DNS, PNP
Associate Professor
Indiana University
School of Nursing
Indianapolis, Indiana

CHAPTER 23

The Elder Population

Eileen K. Rossen, RN, PhD
Assistant Professor
Department of Community Practice, School of Nursing
The University of North Carolina at Greensboro
Greensboro, North Carolina

Ellen Jones ND, APRN-BC
    Associate Professor
    Department of Community Practice, School of Nursing
    The University of North Carolina at Greensboro
    Greensboro, North Carolina

CHAPTER 24

Rural and Migrant Populations

Joyce Splann Krothe, RN, DNS
    Associate Professor, Environments for Health Department
    Director, Bloomington Campus
    Fellow, Indiana University School of Nursing, Institute for
    Action Research for Community Health and the WHO
    Collaborating Center in Healthy Cities
    School of Nursing
    Indiana University
    Bloomington, Indiana

CHAPTER 25

Racial and Ethnic Health Disparities

Janie Canty-Mitchell, RN, PhD
    Professor and Associate Dean for Research and
    Community Partnerships
    School of Nursing
    University of North Carolina, Wilmington
    Wilmington, North Carolina

Barbara Battin Little, RN, MPH, DNS
    University of South Florida, Sarasota-Manatee Campus
    Sarasota, Florida

Sabrina Robinson, RN, MS
    PhD Student
    College of Nursing
    University of South Florida
    Tampa, Florida

Rasheeta Chandler, RN, MS
    PhD Candidate
    College of Nursing
    University of South Florida
    Tampa, Florida

CHAPTER 26

Immigrant and Refugee Populations

Arlene Michaels Miller, RN, FAAN, PhD
    Professor and Department Head
    Department of Public Health, Mental Health, and
    Administrative Nursing
    University of Illinois at Chicago, College of Nursing
    Chicago, Illinois

CHAPTER 27

The Homeless Population

Debra Gay Anderson, RN, BC, PhD
    Associate Professor
    College of Nursing
    University of Kentucky
    Lexington, Kentucky

Peggy Riley, RN, MSN
    Instructor
    College of Nursing
    University of Kentucky
    Lexington, Kentucky

CHAPTER 28

Populations with Substance Abuse

Martha S. Tingen, APRN, BC, PhD
    Associate Professor
    Medical College of Georgia
    Georgia Prevention Institute
    School of Medicine, Department of Pediatrics
    Augusta, Georgia

CHAPTER 29

Disaster Preparedness and Public Health Nursing

Kathleen Eid-Heberle, RN, MSN, CCRN
    Lecturer
    School of Nursing
    University of North Carolina, Charlotte
    Charlotte, North Carolina

CHAPTER 30

The Future of Public Health Nursing

Mary E. Riner, RN, DNS
    Associate Professor and
    Co-Director, World Health Organization Collaborating
    Center for Healthy Cities, and
    Fellow of the Institute for Action Research in Community
    Health
    Indiana University School of Nursing
    Department of Environments for Health
    Indianapolis, Indiana

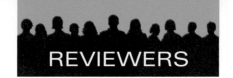

REVIEWERS

Lin Drury, RN, DNSc
Associate Professor, Lienhard School of Nursing
Pace University
Pleasantville, New York

Michelle Ficca, RN, DNSc
Associate Professor, Department of Nursing
Bloomsburg University
Bloomsburg, Pennsylvania

Beth Furlong, RN, PhD, JD
Associate Professor, School of Nursing
Faculty Associate, Center for Health Policy and Ethics
Creighton University
Omaha, Nebraska

Jackie S. Gillespie, RN, MN
Senior Lecturer, School of Nursing
Clemson University
Seneca, South Carolina

Sharon Guillet, RN, PhD
Associate Professor and Chair, BSN Program
Marymount University
Arlington, Virginia

Sara L. Groves, DrPH, MPH, MS, RN, CS
Instructor, School of Nursing
The Johns Hopkins University
Baltimore, Maryland

Janet S. Hickman, RN, EdD
Professor of Nursing
Interim Assistant Graduate Dean
West Chester University
West Chester, Pennsylvania

Dana M. L. Hinds, RN, MSN, FNP, ARNP
Nursing Instructor, Family Nurse Practitioner
Central Maine Medical Center School of Nursing
Lewiston, Maine

Barbara Holder, RN, PhD, FAAN
Senior Lecturer, School of Nursing
Clemson University
Seneca, South Carolina

Janet T. Ihlenfeld, RN, PhD
Professor, Department of Nursing
D'Youville College
Buffalo, New York

Susan Kendig, RNC, WHCNP, FAANP
Assistant Professor
Barnes-Jewish College of Nursing
St. Louis, Missouri

Linda E. Moore, RN, PhD
Former Assistant Professor, Department of Health Policy
Management
School of Public Health, College of Public Service
Jackson State University
Jackson, Mississippi

Elizabeth O'Connor Swanson, MN, MPH, APRN, BC
Board Certified Family Nurse Practitioner
Board Certified Clinical Nurse Specialist, Community
Health Nursing
Lecturer in School of Nursing, Clemson University
Nurse Practitioner/Clinical Nurse Specialist,
South Carolina Department of Juvenile Justice
Seneca, South Carolina

Donna A. Peters RN, PhD, FAAN
Professor, RN to BSN Program
St. Petersburg College of Nursing
St. Petersburg, Florida

Olive Santavenere, RN, BS, MSN, MSOB, PhD
Associate Professor, Department of Nursing
Southern Connecticut State University
New Haven, Connecticut

Jeanne Sorrell, RN, PhD
George Mason University
Winchester, Virginia

Marie Truglio-Londrigan, RN, PhD, GNP
Professor and Chair, Graduate Department of Nursing
Lienhard School of Nursing
Pace University
Pleasantville, New York

Pamela Waynick-Rogers, RNC, CNM, MSN
Instructor, School of Nursing
Vanderbilt University
Nashville, Tennessee

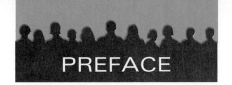

PREFACE

Public health nurses have been in the forefront of the public's health since the late 1800s. Initially, public health nurses focused on prevention of diseases. Today, with the threat of new diseases, environmental disasters, and terrorism, the focus of public health nurses is on health promotion, disease prevention, public safety, and leadership in health policy. This book includes cutting-edge public health nursing content that concentrates on high risk populations and aggregates, social justice and human rights, the political process, public health nursing activism, and leadership in health policy development and implementation, all to improve the health and quality of life for the public.

The primary audience for this book is students in advanced practice public and community health nursing programs and graduate nursing practice programs, as well as students in innovative baccalaureate public health courses. In addition, this book can be a reference book for practicing public health nurses in leadership and administrative positions in state and local health departments, home health care agencies, and other local, state, or national public positions.

CONCEPTUAL APPROACH

The current scenery for public health nurses, rather than being stable, is an ever-changing patchwork of social mobility, cultural dynamics, sectarian tensions, new diseases and hazards, environments at risk, and the seemingly always under-seige health care system. These are the realities facing nurses today. *Public Health Nursing: Leadership, Policy & Practice* takes all of these issues into account and offers a framework predicated on several fundamental principles:

- Public health nursing is caring for populations and aggregates.
- Nurses can have an impact on the overall health of society through politics, health policy, and public health nursing activism.

- Health promotion and wellness are core responsibilities of the public health nurse.
- Health disparities for various minority and ethnic groups are real, and they need to be addressed.
- *Healthy People 2010 Objectives* must be integrated into the public health context.
- Public health nurses must be prepared to address aspects of terrorism and disaster preparedness.
- Ethics, human rights, and social justice must be embraced in all aspects of care, from the national scene to the global health stage.
- Responsible nursing includes an understanding of health care financing and the economics of health care management.
- Public health nursing research is indispensable to sound nursing practice.
- Program development and evaluation can benefit from the wisdom of the informed public health nurse.

ORGANIZATION

Public Health Nursing: Leadership, Policy & Practice is organized into five major parts.

Part 1 describes the basics of public health, and offers a solid framework for the remainder of the text. Included are a history of public health and public health nursing, core functions of public health nursing, public health nursing practice settings, epidemiology, and *Healthy People 2010 Objectives*.

Part 2 gives readers a foundation in health care delivery and financing. Crucial topics such as law, health policy, health care organization and financing, economics, and global health are covered in detail, all with an eye to their importance to the public health nurse.

Part 3 introduces the many facets of public health nursing practice. Assessment of the environment, populations, and health risk is outlined in detail, as are health promotion and health education. Public health nursing's broader role in program development and evaluation and health care management is discussed. Fundamental issues such as ethics and human rights, as well as the role of public health nursing research, underscore the critical role of public health nursing in the present and future health care arena.

Part 4 offers an in-depth view of the populations for which public health nurses are responsible. Provision of care to vulnerable populations includes those with infectious, communicable, and chronic diseases, and those within vulnerable age groups. Underserved populations, the unique responsibility of the public health nurse, are discussed with compassion and depth: rural and migrant populations, minority and ethnic populations, immigrant and refugee populations, homeless populations, and populations with substance abuse.

Part 5 focuses on public health nursing in the 21st century. Real-world issues impacting the health care field, such as disaster preparedness and terrorism, are thoroughly debated. The final chapter offers a glimpse into the future of public health nursing

Numerous **appendices** include Competencies for Public Health Nursing Practice, Scope and Standards of Public Health Nursing Practice, American Public Health Association Principles on Public Health and Human Rights, Determinants of Health, and *Healthy People 2010* Goals. Also included are a list of Professional Associations, Organizations, and Institutes and a list of abbreviations useful to the public health nurse.

TEXT FEATURES

The chapter template of features and pedagogical tools was developed with the reader and instructor in mind:

- **Chapter outlines** offer an at-a-glance view of the core content to be covered in each chapter.
- **Learning Objectives** set the stage for new knowledge and highlight competencies that are targeted for mastery in each chapter.

- **Research Application** boxes highlight current research and suggest how the public health nurse can incorporate these findings into practice.
- **Practice Application** features focus on specific areas of practice and how public health principles impact daily nursing practice.
- **Critical Thinking Activities** include open-ended, discussion-style questions and activities which invite readers to critically analyze what they have learned and apply it to real-life situations. Suggested Responses to the Critical Thinking Activities are included in the online companion.
- **Policy Highlights** offer insight into how certain policies and practices can affect aggregates and the public health nurses who care for them.
- **Key Terms** are boldfaced within text and defined in the glossary.
- **Key Concepts** summarize chapter conclusions and serve as an excellent study and review tool.
- **References** include all sources cited within the chapters, underscoring the research-based nature of the text.
- **Bibliography** lists additional readings, encouraging further research and study.
- **Resources** is an invaluable list of organizations and institutions, with contact information and a brief description, supporting the chapter topic.

SUPPLEMENTAL RESOURCES

An innovative online resource, available at **www .delmarlearning.com/companions**, will supplement study and facilitate classroom lecture. Chapter Objectives, Resources, and Glossary are included from the text for easy reference. Suggested responses to the critical thinking activities are offered, to stimulate classroom discussion, debate, and problem solving. A short chapter summary offers a succinct yet pointed overview of the main ideas on each topic. Classroom presentations and student studying will be facilitated with the included PowerPoint slides. Finally, a test bank of approximately 750 questions is also available to instructors.

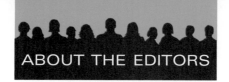
L. Louise Ivanov is Associate Professor and Chair of the Community Practice Department at the University of North Carolina—Greensboro, School of Nursing. From 1979 to 1998, she was a faculty member at the Purdue University School of Nursing, and from 1998 to 2002, she was a faculty member at the University of Virginia School of Nursing. She taught Public Health Nursing while at Purdue University, and Community Health Nursing and Health Policy at the University of Virginia. She is currently teaching Law, Policy, and Economics of Health Care in the Master's program and Health Promotion Models and Interventions in the PhD program.

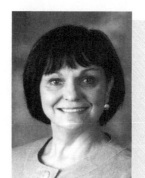

Dr. Ivanov received her BS degree in Nursing (1972) from the State University of New York at Buffalo (SUNY Buffalo) and her MSN degree in Community Health Nursing (1984) from Indiana University. She received her Doctorate of Nursing Science (DNS) in Health Policy and the Health of the Community from Indiana University. She also received a minor in Public Management from the Indiana University School of Public and Environmental Affairs. Dr. Ivanov completed an internship with the World Health Organization, Healthy Cities Project, in Russia through the Copenhagen, Denmark, office (1992) and received a Fulbright Fellowship Award to teach Public Health Nursing and Health Policy at the Department of Nursing of the St. Petersburg, Russia, Medical Academy of Post-Graduate Studies (2000–2001). In addition to teaching at the Medical Academy, she provided expertise in development of a Public Health Nursing Certificate course for nurses seeking certification and upgrading of their skills in public health nursing.

Dr. Ivanov's research interests have been focused on the effects of migration on access and quality of health care services for Russian-speaking immigrant women in the United States. She has also conducted research in Russia on the prevalence of the metabolic syndrome, as well as interventions to improve and promote cardiovascular health.

Dr. Ivanov is a member of the American Public Health Association, Public Health Nursing Section, and the Refugee and Immigrant Caucus; the Southern Nursing Research Society; and Sigma Theta Tau International, Gamma Zeta Chapter. She is active in the Public Health Nursing Section of the American Public Health Association as liaison to the global Consortium and the Trade and Health Forum; additionally, she is deployed to the International Human Rights Committee from the Public Health Nursing Section. She is also on the Global Health Committee, Membership Committee, and the Policy Committee of the Public Health Nursing Section. Dr. Ivanov has been a research grant reviewer and site visitor for the NIH Fogarty International Study Section. She is on the editorial board of the *Journal of Ataturk*, at Turkey University School of Nursing, and the *International Nurses Review Journal*. Dr. Ivanov is a peer reviewer for a number of journals, including *Public Health Nursing*, *Health Care for Women International*, and *Nursing Outlook*, and serves as a book reviewer for various publishers.

Carolyn L. Blue is Professor of Nursing in the Community Practice Department at the University of North Carolina—Greensboro, School of Nursing. From 1985 to 2004, she was a faculty member at the Purdue University School of Nursing. She taught Public Health Nursing and Health Promotion Behavior courses while at Purdue University and is currently teaching Research Methods in Nursing in the Master's program and Health Promotion Models and Interventions in the PhD program.

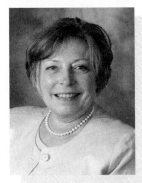

Dr. Blue received her BSN degree (1969) from Ball State University, her MS degree in Health Education/Health Promotion (1978) from Purdue University, and a MSN degree in Community Health Nursing (1985) from Indiana University. She received her PhD in Nursing Science (1996) from the University of Illinois at Chicago, with major areas of study in health promotion behaviors and occupational health nursing. She was a postdoctoral fellow at Indiana University School of Nursing from 2002 to 2004, developing her intervention program of research and participating in the Diabetes Prevention Program Outcome Study intervention in the School of Medicine.

Dr. Blue's research interests have been in the area of health promotion and illness prevention, primarily using the theory of planned behavior and the health belief model as study frameworks. Her current research is focused on improving physical activity and dietary behaviors of adults at risk for diabetes.

Dr. Blue is a member of the American Public Health Association, Public Health Nursing Section; the American Academy of Health Behavior; American Diabetes Association; American Association of Occupational Health Nurses; the Southern Nursing Research Society; and Sigma Theta Tau International, Gamma Zeta Chapter. She is an active member of the Public Health Nursing Section as past co-chair and Chair of Program Planning for the Annual Meeting, and she is also on the Research Committee. She is on the editorial board for *Diabetes Care* and is a peer reviewer for a number of journals, including *Public Health Nursing, Nursing Research, Journal of Holistic Nursing, American Journal of Health Behavior, Health Education & Behavior,* and *Health Education Research.*

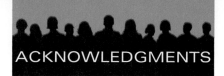

ACKNOWLEDGMENTS

We are deeply grateful to all the contributors who worked conscientiously to produce this innovative public health book. Their expertise and depth of knowledge added new insight into the practice of public health nursing as leaders in public health and health policy. We sincerely appreciate the thoughtful critiques from the reviewers of the chapters. Our editor at Cengage Delmar Learning, Beth Williams, provided expert leadership and assistance throughout the development and production of this project. We greatly appreciate her attentive guidance and could not have completed this project without her support.

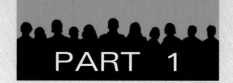

PART 1

PUBLIC HEALTH BASICS

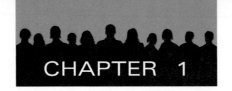

CHAPTER 1

History of Public Health and Public Health Nursing

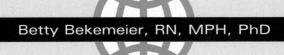

Betty Bekemeier, RN, MPH, PhD

Chapter Outline

⊕ **Establishing the Science of Public Health**
  Early Sanitation
  The Growing Science of Public Health
  Administering a Response
  Historical Antecedents of Public Health Nursing
  Major Social Changes

⊕ **Early Public Health Nursing**
  Charitable Care and District Nursing
  Lillian Wald on Henry Street
  Financing Early Public Health Nursing Activities
  A Progressive Movement
  The Risks of Reform
  Public Health Nursing in the Context of the Broader Nursing
    Profession
  Expanding Public Health Nursing Services

⊕ **Middle Twentieth-Century Public Health Nursing**
  Hospitals—The New Focus for Improving Health
  Changes in Funding for Public Health Nursing
  A Changing Profession
  Nursing Avoidance of Social Reform and Feminism
  Professionalism

⊕ **Public Health Nursing Today**
  Unresolved Controversies
  The Spirit of Our Foremothers

Learning Objectives

Upon completion of this chapter, the reader will be able to:

1. Describe social factors that influenced the early development and formalization of the field of public health.

2. Analyze the relationship between early home nursing and the subsequent development of public health nursing.

3. Describe the social context of public health nursing in the early twentieth century in the United States and its influence on the philosophies and actions of public health nurses.

4. Analyze the political and financial risks and barriers that public health nurses in history encountered.

5. Analyze the influence that the broader nursing profession had on the development of public health nursing in the twentieth century.

6. Critically appraise ways in which public health nursing today is similar or different in philosophy and practice to public health nursing of the early twentieth century.

Today we define public health as what "we as a society do collectively to assure the conditions in which people can be healthy" (Institute of Medicine, 1988). Public health nurses employ knowledge from nursing, social, and public health sciences to promote the health of populations (APHA Public Health Nursing Section, 1996). The science of public health and the profession of public health nursing are, by their nature, civic enterprises that are inseparable from social and environmental forces. As a result, the history of public health and public health nursing is marked with progressive social reformers who challenged social norms and common beliefs to improve the public's health.

The historical figures in public health history responded to epidemics, poverty, social revolutions, and international events not only as opportunities to prevent further suffering among populations but also to learn lessons about the nature of infectious disease and the policies and social changes that can be made to prevent suffering before it starts. Public health heroes in history emphasized social justice, broad system change, and political action as a way of improving the health of whole populations, not just the health of the individuals with whom they came into contact. historical public health leaders also maintained a broad conception of their responsibility to improve the health of others and emphasized an obligation to address the conditions that underlie health problems. Public health nursing reformers viewed social justice as central to nursing and inseparable from nursing work. Lillian Wald and Lavinia Dock are among those who make up nursing's "distinguished history of concern . . . for social justice" referenced in the 2001 Code of Ethics for Nurses with Interpretive Statements (ANA, 2001). Wald, Dock, and others grew indignant from witnessing the destructive outcomes of institutionalized poverty and of gender and ethnic inequalities. Each of these nurses harnessed her indignation to work toward the creation of progressive health policies.

ESTABLISHING THE SCIENCE OF PUBLIC HEALTH

Long before the science of public health began to emerge, ancient civilizations recognized a connection between hygiene and disease. Over time this connection grew from the development of structures to promote sanitation to the investigation of sources of disease and the isolation of infectious agents. Ultimately, the connection between infectious disease and poverty began to be understood as well.

Early Sanitation

"In the history of public health, epidemics occupy a prominent place among the situations that precipitated action in the interest of the community's health" (Rosen, 1993, p. 196). Rosen's classic *History of Public Health* (1993) states that ancient civilizations from both India and Egypt and as far back as 1 to 2000 years B.C. have shown evidence that attention was paid to a relationship between sanitation and better living (Figure 1-1). Rosen, one of the world's leading historians on the development of the public health movement in Western civilization, describes excavations and landscapes still showing evidence of sewers, well-drained cities, bathing facilities, and complex water supply systems that were in use by ancient civilizations (Rosen, 1993). The transmissibility of disease was recognized, long before the causes of disease were understood, as populations experienced diphtheria, malaria, small pox and many other disorders still well known today. *Airs, Waters, and Places,* written by a Greek health care provider in the fifth century B.C., was the first known description of the relationship between environment and disease (Rosen, 1993).

Later the Romans made their mark on public health history with their attention to water purity through extensive water and sanitation systems. Monasteries during the Middle Ages were particular models for ideal urban planning (and later models for hospitals), focusing on airy rooms and buildings, clean facilities, and personal hygiene. It did not go without notice that residents and frequent visitors to monasteries were healthier than the general public (Rosen, 1993). Markets, the center of Roman community life, were also seemingly well tended; care was taken by residents to keep them clean as spoiled food was known to be associated with disease.

The Growing Science of Public Health

The period 1500–1750 was an era of scientific development, particularly in anatomy and physiology. During this period, for example, the concept of the circulation of the blood began to be understood. The miasma theory,

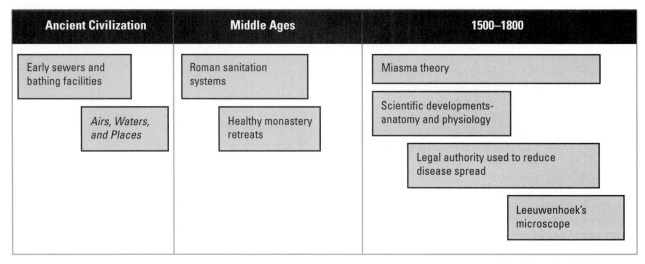

Ancient Civilization	Middle Ages	1500–1800

Early sewers and bathing facilities

Roman sanitation systems

Miasma theory

Scientific developments- anatomy and physiology

Airs, Waters, and Places

Healthy monastery retreats

Legal authority used to reduce disease spread

Leeuwenhoek's microscope

Figure 1-1 Historical timeline of early disease theories and public health advances.

developed during this time to describe the sources of disease, suggested that gases emanating from the organic matter often associated with unsanitary conditions are what cause illness. Toward the end of the 1700s, Antony van Leeuwenhoek of the Netherlands discovered bacteria through his early microscope, but for another century, "bad air" and filth were largely thought to be the underlying causes of disease (Rosen, 1993).

John Snow, considered by Rosen (1993) to have been one of the world's greatest epidemiologists, was among those who, in the early nineteenth century, began recognizing the presence of living organisms in what appeared to be sources of infection (Figure 1-2). Without ever isolating or detecting the actual bacillus that causes cholera, Snow traced the 1854 London cholera epidemic to the now famous Broad Street pump where the greatest distribution of deaths correlated to the nature of the pollution in that part of the Thames River from which the Broad Street pump obtained its water supply.

The Enlightenment and the Revolutionary era, during the latter half of the eighteenth century and the first half of the nineteenth century, were a time of tremendous change and increasing scientific discovery, but these changes are considered by Rosen to have largely been a "middle class movement" from which those in poverty gained little (Rosen, 1993, p. 157). The Victorian period of the early 1800s brought the beginnings

of the major Industrial Revolution and a rapid increase in population to urban centers. As people flocked toward industry and jobs, cities became more crowded. Ultimately the urban infant mortality rate grew very high among the poor, upsetting what had been a declining death rate in the late eighteenth century. The high infant mortality rate was perceived to be due to an increase in alcohol consumption, unwanted pregnancies and related neglect, improper infant care, and poor nutrition (Rosen, 1993). Those who benefited from the scientific discoveries of the Enlightenment were eager to translate these new ideas to the poor, but instead demonstrated the growing distance between those with ample personal and social resources and those without. Residents living in poverty, for example, were unlikely to have the resources or opportunity to adapt their unhealthy living environments when told that scientific evidence suggested they should live in well-ventilated homes rather than damp cellars and crowded tenements (Rosen, 1993).

Administering a Response

Experience with responding to disease outbreaks further informed a growing understanding of the disease process, prompting officials to respond to disease in their communities with an increasing attention to prevention.

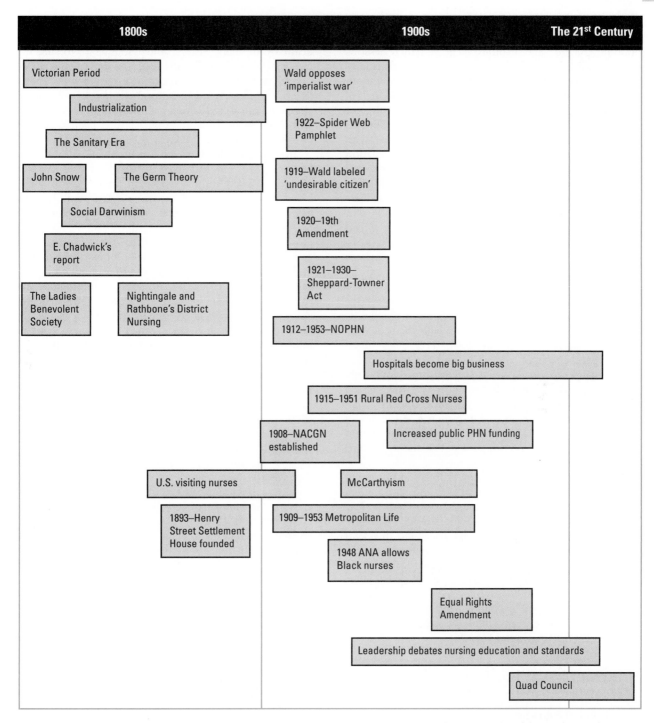

1800s   **1900s**   **The 21st Century**

Victorian Period

Industrialization

The Sanitary Era

John Snow   The Germ Theory

Social Darwinism

E. Chadwick's report

The Ladies Benevolent Society

Nightingale and Rathbone's District Nursing

Wald opposes 'imperialist war'

1922–Spider Web Pamphlet

1919–Wald labeled 'undesirable citizen'

1920–19th Amendment

1921–1930–Sheppard-Towner Act

1912–1953–NOPHN

Hospitals become big business

1915–1951 Rural Red Cross Nurses

1908–NACGN established

Increased public PHN funding

U.S. visiting nurses

McCarthyism

1893–Henry Street Settlement House founded

1909–1953 Metropolitan Life

1948 ANA allows Black nurses

Equal Rights Amendment

Leadership debates nursing education and standards

Quad Council

Figure 1-2 Timeline of modern transformations and social contexts in public health and nursing.

Despite the fact that the mechanism of disease transmission was still unknown, diseases such as leprosy, bubonic plague, and syphilis each provided lessons in containing the spread of infection. As particularly dreaded infectious diseases, leprosy and plague both have distinguished places in Medieval public health history, and both caused terror in the sixteenth and seventeenth centuries. Written accounts of outbreaks of leprosy show evidence of isolation of those with the disease and efforts to contain its spread. Isolation efforts were severe and devastating to families affected by leprosy as the separation amounted to the lifetime banishment of afflicted individuals to a separate location away from all community life. These efforts did, however, have the desired effect of reducing the spread of the disease. Measures taken to contain the transmission of leprosy show evidence of the first prophylaxis conducted through reporting disease to officials and the establishment of subsequent isolation.

The bubonic plague was not a chronic infectious condition, but it was often fatal. Victims of plague, as well as anyone who came in contact with them or traveled from plague-ravaged locations, were quarantined for varying periods of time. This laid the groundwork for the concept of using legal authority to temporarily sequester selected community members for the sake of the health of others. These legal advancements were also put into use when small pox was endemic in Europe by the early 1700s (and before the new notion of vaccination was developed by England's Edward Jenner) (Rosen, 1993).

Syphilis also became a growing problem in Europe in the sixteenth and seventeenth centuries and was a much more virulent form of the disease than we know today. Early on it was recognized as being sexually transmitted. Few intolerances regarding the discussion of sexual matters, however, existed at that time, and, as a result, there was an open and vocal campaign regarding the disease and how to avoid it. This had a noticeable effect on the spread of the disease until social stigma regarding syphilis developed as "middle class morality" began to flourish and open campaigns to control the disease were hindered (Rosen, 1993, p. 74).

Historical Antecedents of Public Health Nursing

Long before nursing began to be formalized in the nineteenth century through the development of training and related structures, the families that fell victim to these epidemics were most often nursed to health or comforted in death by mothers, sisters, and daughters. Nursing the sick has been, throughout history, a traditional part of "female apprenticeship," integral to one's role in a family and community and a natural element of a woman's character and duty (Reverby, 1987a, p. 5). Nursing the sick throughout a community has also been described as a fundamental role of early religious orders.

In the Middle Ages, municipalities were clearly beginning to see the need to tend to and oversee duties of health and hygiene in their communities. Local health care providers were often supported by a tax on townspeople; those who were religious clerics, educated as healers, were supported by their religious order and considered their work a charitable endeavor (Rosen, 1993). Similarly, nuns, deaconesses, and women of various religious orders fulfilled a critical community service by providing comfort and care to the sick in their homes. In England, public health administration remained largely under local control until the nineteenth century, when the human costs of industrialization and urbanization became a national concern. These issues were made more difficult to contend with, however, because of the lack of national health policies and the parochial nature by which most public health measures were enforced and encouraged (Rosen, 1993). Statistics were kept via surveys, demography, health care provider reports of certain diseases, and birth and death records in religious institutions. This large variety of different statistical sources meant that records were being kept in countless ways among religious, scientific, and municipal authorities. Officials in Germany, conversely, modeled public health administration after their own law enforcement and created a well-structured national model that regarded public health officials as the "medical police" (Rosen, 1993, p. 137). Germany's Johann Peter Frank was an influential public health leader in the early nineteenth century and wrote of "enlightened despotism" as an authoritarian approach to maintaining the public's health. He was one of the first on record to suggest that the "health of the people is a responsibility of the state" (Rosen, 1993, p. 138).

Major Social Changes

Poverty in rural areas, a high rate of immigration, and the introduction of industrialization to urban centers drew many residents throughout Europe to cities in the early nineteenth century. The steam engine and other new means of manufacturing meant that production could occur with speeds never before known to entrepreneurs. Factory jobs in cities became plentiful; housing, however, was not. Health conditions of families and communities deteriorated as cheap and inadequate housing was built in close proximity to the factories in which residents worked. There was no profit in building quality into these homes, but property owners found that it did pay to fit as many workers and their families into the smallest space possible as housing quickly came into short supply. Ultimately, workers were so densely packed into tenement housing that many families lived in rooms with only interior walls, no windows, and "barely room for access to their doors" (Rosen, 1993, p. 180). Bars, alcoholism, disease, and despair thrived in this atmosphere.

Along with social changes such as industrialization and immigration came changes in the theories of disease. By the mid-nineteenth century, the **sanitary era**, which proposed that disease was a direct consequence of filth and poor hygiene, was being increasingly challenged by the growing notion of the **germ theory**. For many, the mental shift between disease being a consequence of low standards, ignorance, and immorality to the notion that disease is caused by a "morally neutral" germ was too great a challenge (Reverby, 1987a, p. 7). As the concept of the existence of germs grew, **Edwin Chadwick** reinforced and advanced the relationship between dirt and disease through his adherence to the miasma theory in his seminal 1842 London "Report into the Sanitary Conditions of the Labouring Population of Great Britain." Chadwick's famous report described strong epidemiological evidence detailing plausible support for reorienting public health efforts toward public policy and engineering techniques for removing urban waste in order to raise the health status of the public as a whole, by reducing the disease-causing vapors (Rosen, 1993). **Florence Nightingale**, like many other lay and medical people in her and Chadwick's day, also refused to fully accept the germ theory of disease and, in relation to this, particularly stressed the nurse's good character, discipline, honorable morals, and model of cleanliness as some of her biggest assets in positively influencing the behavior of her charges.

The germ theory also came in conflict with notions of **social Darwinism** that were common at the time. Social Darwinists believed that poverty and its consequences were the result of laziness and weakness of character, thereby legitimizing the inequity of resources across societies and among the classes. Those who felt sympathy for the poor sought to reform them. Charitable organizations influenced by social Darwinism in the nineteenth century tended to focus their attention on the character of the individual living in poverty and used a one-way relationship to role model, educate, and provide "moral uplift" to bring about healthy personal change and to halt the transmission of the unfortunate state of the poor and sick to the next generation (Shopsis, 1993).

EARLY PUBLIC HEALTH NURSING

Providing comfort, care, and healing to individuals at home in their communities has been an informal duty, sacrifice, expectation, or act of love by women in families and religious orders throughout history. As nursing work began to formalize, trained nurses were often expected to be virtuous and disciplined as they brought moral and physical cleanliness to the "worthy" poor and sick. As the scientific basis for disease was being widely understood by the beginning of the twentieth century, visiting nurses in the United States were serving the poor through social- and health-based organizations and were drawn into advocating for broader social change that would address the underlying causes of disease. In this context, public health nursing in the United States was born at the **Henry Street Settlement** in New York City, through strong female networks with a social justice philosophy, training in health, and often a religious grounding in service.

Charitable Care and District Nursing

Even though individually focused home nursing had been practiced for millennia, many examples of the early formalization of philanthropic, systematic care to the sick poor plays a part in the evolution of public health nursing. Nursing services provided by groups other than religious orders, for example, were generally managed by a local board, often of wealthy philanthropic "ladies" who wanted to bring relief to the poor, but who would not themselves have provided the service. Philanthropic services developed independently from one another throughout the United States; as an early

1800s example of a charitable effort to serve the sick poor in their homes, Buhler-Wilkerson tells the story of the "Ladies Benevolent Society" in Charleston, South Carolina. A "visiting committee" of women, supported by the Ladies Benevolent Society, was instructed to visit the select "worthy" poor, bringing them simple staples of food, lamp oil, and blankets. Untrained nurses, or a relative of the client who was paid by the society to act as a "nurse," provided comfort, nourishment, and medications as ordered by a health care provider when specific illness or acuity called for nursing care. Even when restricted to caring only for those with no history of drunkenness, "disorderly conduct," or perceived laziness, the visiting committee eventually could not keep up with the magnitude of need for their services and the obvious chronic health needs of those who were particularly destitute (Buhler-Wilkerson, 2001, p. 6).

Later in the nineteenth century, district nursing in England became the immediate precursor to what was to eventually become public health nursing. As William Rathbone, an English Quaker and businessman, watched his wife painfully die in their home, he marveled at the comfort that both he and his wife received from the services of her home nurse Mary Robinson. After the death of his wife, the wealthy Rathbone wanted to extend the same kind of comfort to the ill poor in his home city of Liverpool. He sought to conduct an "experiment" in offering organized and regular nursing services to the poor. These services were first provided by Robinson and then by additional nurses that Rathbone hired and supported. Considering his experiment successful, Rathbone proclaimed that "the hopeless were restored to health, breadwinners and mothers were restored to independence, and the spread of weakness and disease was halted" (quoted in Buhler-Wilkerson, 2001, p. 20). By 1861, Rathbone enlisted the consultation of Nightingale to assist him in training more nurses. Subsequently, Nightingale introduced the public to the concept of district nursing.

Nightingale's influence grew, and nursing leaders in the United States reviewed her writings and theories on nursing with interest. As nurses became familiar with her concept of district nursing, an interest in applying a similar practice in the United States grew. Nightingale's district nursing was given a broader interpretation in the United States, however, where theories of the spread of disease and the existence of "germs" were more widely accepted, and increasingly nurses were seen as providing more than the promotion of cleanliness and

comfort. The English concept of district nursing grew into "visiting nurses" in the United States where nurses were generally expected to apply notions of contagion to the prevention of disease transmission, and in particular, to keep the "dangerously ill" from infecting the wealthy (Buhler-Wilkerson, 2001, p. 23). While still focusing on changing behaviors considered unclean, the American visiting nurses integrated the germ theory into their practice, recognizing that the threat of infectious disease was as much of a danger to the public's health as the character and practices of the poor. They worked hard to bring the message of cleanliness, personal hygiene, and moral uplift along with the treatment of disease and expected to reform the families they visited into habits of healthier living, raising the standard of life in their household and thereby preventing the spread of disease. Promoting strong physical and moral well-being became a popular strategy used by nurses in attempting to improve health in impoverished communities through instruction in appropriate cleanliness, childcare, diet, and lifestyle as they perceived these (Buhler-Wilkerson, 2001).

Visiting nurse services continued to grow dramatically in the United States, particularly in the 1870s and 1880s with the growing support of religious and philanthropic charities and wealthy "lady managers" who often provided oversight and supervision (Buhler-Wilkerson, 1989, p 48). By the beginning of the twentieth century, visiting nurses in Boston, Philadelphia, Chicago, Washington, Baltimore, Los Angeles, and other U.S. cities were providing this service through these charitable agencies as well as through some health departments (Buhler-Wilkerson, 1989).

Lillian Wald on Henry Street

Lillian Wald read about the growing concepts of district nursing and visiting nurses and was eager herself to work among those who were sick and living in poverty (Figure 1-3). In 1893, she enlisted Mary Brewster, a classmate and fellow graduate of the New York Bellevue School of Nursing, to move with her to the Lower East Side of New York City's Manhattan Island, where industrialization and overcrowding mimicked similar problems in Europe. With the help of a wealthy friend and patron willing to support their endeavor, Wald and Brewster moved into an apartment among the new immigrants and the working poor of the Lower East Side and quickly became well known in the com-

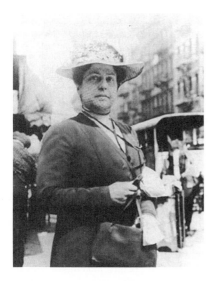

Figure 1-3 Lillian Wald at the height of her career circa 1910.

Courtesy of the Visiting Nurse Service of New York.

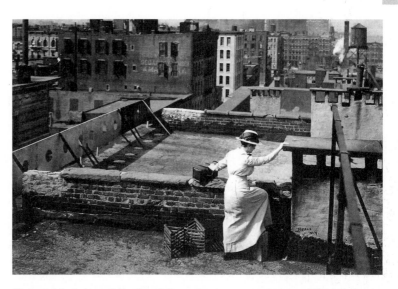

Figure 1-4 A public health nurse saves steps while visiting families by crossing over roofs and avoiding tenement stairs.

Courtesy of the Visiting Nurse Service of New York.

munity for their willingness and ability to bring valuable nursing services into the homes of residents, where the chronic and infectious diseases of cramped, overcrowded, and untended living conditions made illness and disability extremely common (Figure 1-4).

As Wald, Brewster, and then others attracted more nurses to their "Nurses Settlement," the limitations of treating illness and offering health education in these individual homes, without attention to the social and environmental barriers that seemed to underlie and perpetuate disease among whole communities and populations, became a growing frustration for them. A large family living in one windowless room of a crowded tenement could not be expected to heed advice for improving ventilation and maintaining strict standards of hygiene and cleanliness. A pregnant woman with a difficult eighth pregnancy was not likely to improve her nutritional standards while her family ate bread and a few meager vegetables. Visiting nurses among Wald's Nurses Settlement concluded that reforming the existing conditions that create and perpetuate disease was the only hope for supporting relief in their communities. Ultimately nursing organizations in other cities such as Baltimore and Boston began reaching similar

conclusions as discussions were held more widely at conferences and in the public health literature (Buhler-Wilkerson, 1989). Buhler-Wilkerson describes Wald as suggesting that "impressing upon the poor the latest findings of science without simultaneously urging reform in housing, child protection and wages was 'cruelly sardonic on the part of the nurse'" (Buhler-Wilkerson, 1989, p. 97). Charitable nursing merely as a form of service to those living in poverty avoided class conflict and brought temporary relief to people without creating change, thereby perpetuating the notion that weak individuals, not an unjust society, created unhealthy conditions. Service without participating in reform ignored the consequences of industrialization and urbanization and reinforced inequalities (Reisch & Andrews, 2001). Annie Brainard in her 1922 book *The Evolution of Public Health Nursing* describes the difference between the district nursing of "early deaconesses" and their early twentieth-century counterparts, saying that the latter combined "charity, plus science" rather than the charitable "gentle ways and tender touch" of these religious foremothers (Brainard, 1922, p. 103).

Ultimately the Nurses Settlement on Henry Street became known as the Henry Street Settlement House and was modeled after other settlement houses of that period, such as that of Wald's friend and colleague Jane Addams at Hull House in Chicago. Henry Street not only supported visiting nurses interested in social reform but also fostered what became an atmosphere for radical intellectuals. Leaders within the settlement movement tended to have a personally strong social justice philosophy, a religious background, and an orientation toward taking action. They were also often influenced by socialist movements and feminist discussions of the period (Reisch & Andrews, 2001). Wald and the nurses of Henry Street were no exception to this and acted as opinion leaders among many of their nursing colleagues across the country.

Financing Early Public Health Nursing Activities

Visiting nurse services were sponsored by a mix of philanthropic charities, religious groups, and local governments by the beginning of the twentieth century in the United States. As knowledge of the scientific basis for disease grew, the proportion of church-based support declined, and U.S. philanthropists seeking "order in the city" provided greater support (Buhler-Wilkerson, 2001, p. 25). For a time, hospitals also supported visiting nurse services to the poor, hoping to reduce their costly inpatient care and teach the poor to stay healthy, thereby reducing their costs among those less likely to pay for hospital services. By 1909, hundreds of visiting nurse associations, led by boards, directed by lay or nurse "lady managers," and funded by philanthropic individual fundraising, existed across the United States. It was in this atmosphere of lay support and philanthropy by the wealthy that the well-connected Wald obtained sponsorship for her endeavors at Henry Street. Jacob Schiff, a personal friend and one of her primary and ultimately most long-term supporters, had been the first to pay her rent and underwrite her activities at Henry Street. Soon after this, he bought Wald and her colleagues their first house on Henry Street. Wald kept close contact with her wealthy friends throughout her career as she kept them informed of the activities of the Settlement House, and they maintained their financial commitments.

A Progressive Movement

The tumultuous period of the late nineteenth century in the United States and Europe brought massive change through large-scale immigration and industrialization, transforming once predominately agricultural nations into industrialized countries with huge urban centers that were attempting to rapidly accommodate large numbers of immigrant workers. Between 1820 and 1910, 30 million new arrivals to the United States moved into American cities; at the same time, regions were shifting from largely rural to mostly urban centers where deplorable living and employment conditions for workers and families accompanied urban industrialization and the growth of big business. During this same period, African Americans struggled through the change from slavery to a troubled freedom dominated by poverty and discrimination. The nurses and community of the Henry Street Settlement sought to jointly find social solutions to effect more healthy change by acting on the unhealthy environment rather than the behavior of the individual. The rhetoric of social Darwinism, moral uplift, and traditional charity work still influenced their discussions as they considered social justice approaches to alleviating the suffering in their communities. These debates were also fueled by new research and epidemiological data that illuminated links between low wages, inadequate working conditions, and poor health.

Privileged white women were also experiencing extraordinary change during this period. Fertility rates among white American women in the United States were decreasing, and they were increasingly entering into higher education—as a result, new opportunities became increasingly available to them (Roberts & Group, 1995). This permitted many women to pursue careers outside of the home and get involved in political issues. The settlement movement provided an environment where women could gather autonomously and mobilize around issues of significance to them and to the unheard communities in which they were living and serving. The Henry Street Settlement, in particular, facilitated new roles for women and for nurses to provide leadership and influence in areas that had previously been available only to men. Public health nursing was born during this extraordinary transition from a Victorian period of suppression of opportunity for women into an atmosphere where women found they could begin to challenge structures and systems (Figure 1-5).

By the late 1800s and early 1900s, poverty, not morality or personal cleanliness, was increasingly seen by social reformers as a cause of social problems and poor health in communities (Reisch & Andrews, 2001).

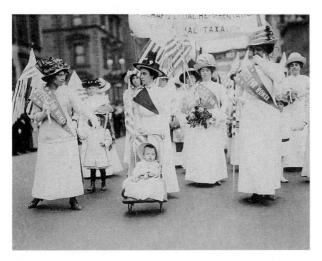

Figure 1-5 Suffrage parade, New York City, May 6, 1912.
Courtesy of Library of Congress, Prints and Photographs Division [Digital ID cph 3a52079].

Wald, her colleague Lavinia Dock, and others at Henry Street did not separate the need for social reform, as a means to meet health needs for those living in poverty, from their responsibilities as nurses. Suffrage for women, civil rights for minorities and women, and the prevention of war were perceived as integral to improving and protecting the health of whole populations. As a result, they became part of a progressive social movement to change the current social environment and to create opportunities for women and nurses to take part in reform. Prevention, mobilization of community support for health promotion, and the activities that support and sustain the health message and need for reform were the primary tools of the public health nurse. Conducting their practice outside the medical hierarchy and away from hospital structures meant that they needed broad-based lay support that recognized the value of prevention and the part that public health nurses played in promoting community health improvement. Their resulting visibility in communities made public health nurses more accessible and accountable among the communities they served and functioned to expand their scope of work, producing new consumers of the "gospel" of health and prevention (Melosh, 1982, p. 133).

The public health nurses at the Henry Street Settlement House, like their social work counterparts at the Hull House settlement in Chicago, used the strong base of support from their community and from their wealthy contributors to influence public policy in favor of improvements in population-level health and social welfare. For Wald, this meant opposing social issues that impact health such as war, child labor, unsafe working conditions, and the Ku Klux Klan and using public health principles of research and data gathering to expose social problems and promote solutions. Michael Reisch and Janice Andrews (2001) describe the Henry Street Settlement as a "focal point for pacifist activity" that began before the start of World War I. It was the "linchpin between religious pacifists, antiwar intellectuals, upper-class reformers, and radical opponents of an 'imperialist war'" (Reisch & Andrews, 2001, p. 43). For Wald, pacifism was a natural outgrowth of discussions she and others had regarding a social analysis of the causes of war. In her mind, war and militarism grew out of imperialism and were a threat to democracy and against efforts toward social and health reform (Reisch & Andrews, 2001). Her activities included mobilizing with others in the Women's Peace Party and founding the American Union Against Militarism, which lobbied Congress against actions of war (Coss, 1989; Reisch & Andrews, 2001).

Appalled by the spectacle of unregulated child labor in the cottage industries and the factories, Wald and other public health reformers also agitated for legislation to restrict the employment of children in manufacturing. Wald was ultimately successful in influencing the development of the federal Children's Bureau which was founded in 1912 to fund and support child welfare services. In an effort to improve the working conditions for women and the working class, Wald and her colleagues were also strong supporters of unions and workplace protections (Reisch & Andrews, 2001). But there were risks involved for those engaged in social reform in the early twentieth century.

The Risks of Reform

By engaging in social activism Wald, Dock, and like-minded reformers gained influence against the status quo, but engendered distrust against themselves by many of those in power (Reisch & Andrews, 2001). In the early 1900s, social reform was perceived to be an attack on institutionalized ideas and structures and required courage, boldness, and a complete departure from what had been traditional expectations for women. For Wald and others, this was treacherous ground as they risked losing government support for reforms and the financing of some private sponsors. They also risked the constructive reputations they had developed through generating political capitol by serving those in poverty. Wald, in particular, risked the wide respect she had gained in political circles for her "cautious international approach" that resisted confrontation and leveraged international connections (Reisch & Andrews, 2001, p. 43).

As social reformers became distrusted by conservatives because of their advocacy for reform and protection of civil liberties, peace activism became linked by conservatives to Bolshevism and ultimately to communism (Reisch & Andrews, 2001). An early example of this link made between reform and international "threats" came in the form of the 1922 Spider Web Pamphlet. This document, written by a librarian working for a brigadier general in the U.S. War Department, drew lines between 15 women's organizations and 25 women leaders (including Wald's friend Jane Addams), depicting the claim that this network of interrelated groups and individuals was behind a plot to subvert American institutions and support a Bolshevik coup (Reisch & Andrews, 2001). Wald, who was later to be commended to New York University's Hall of Fame for Great Americans, was in 1919 named along with others as an "undesirable citizen" by a committee of the U.S. Congress, which served as a precursor to the House Un-American Activities Committee (Reisch & Andrews, 2001, p. 47).

Promoting civil liberties meant that many of these public health reformers were also advocates of women's suffrage. When the Nineteenth Amendment was added to the U.S. Constitution in 1920 and women were given the right to vote, the nurses of the Henry Street Settlement immediately made this an opportunity to support and provide education for women regarding the activities and responsibilities of government to ensure the health and safety of the public (Roberts & Group, 1995). Eager to pursue long-neglected policy issues that had not been of interest to men, Wald and others encouraged women activists to contribute to policy issues of specific importance to women and children. Evidence of their success came with the 1921 passage of the Sheppard-Towner Act, which provided federal funds for maternal and infant health care. It did not take long for conservative forces to attack this success;

the short-lived Sheppard-Towner Act was not renewed in 1930 when it came up for reappropriation. At the time of its proposed renewal, male politicians claimed "it was fundamentally a 'woman's measure' that forced states to take responsibility for welfare and increased public health nursing responsibilities for educating the public about maternal and child care" (Roberts & Group, 1995, p. 169). Some health care providers in particular saw it as a "feminist-socialist-communist conspiracy" (quoted in Roberts & Group, 1995, p. 169).

Public Health Nursing in the Context of the Broader Nursing Profession

By 1909, there was a confusing mix of visiting nurse associations and public health nurses under the leadership of an assortment of organizations, having a variety of roles and different levels of training. New York City had one of the biggest and most confusing collections with 372 nurses sponsored by eight different organizations and working in communities around the city (Buhler-Wilkerson, 2001). Hospitals and home care agencies in the United States also employed nurses from all levels of training and experience with the more elite nurses having been trained at schools such as The Johns Hopkins Hospital School of Nursing. Others received less comprehensive training at other hospital training schools, in shorter programs, in often less-advantaged programs where only black nurses were trained, or they received no formal training at all and took to providing untrained "nursing care" when they were widowed or became impoverished. This broad range of training and personal circumstances among nurses represented a wide range of class backgrounds for nurses as a whole, but most training programs in the late 1800s and early 1900s sought to recruit and train students who were to be disciplined, self-sacrificing, well-kempt, "morally upright," hard working, and unmarried. Susan Reverby (1987b) included a description of the insistence that one not appear to be seen as an "untrained nurse," displaying crude manners, exhibiting "sexual interest," or demonstrating "comradeship with the 'help'" from other occupational categories (p. 6).

It was from these boundaried and classist environments that Lillian Wald, Mary Brewster, Lavinia Dock, and others among the first public health nurses came. While the nursing contemporaries of Wald and Dock who worked in hospital environments were positioned for subordinate service in a rigid hospital hierarchy where nursing had no separate "power base" beyond the hospital, public health nurses were creating a fully independent institution controlled by women (Reverby, 1987b, p. 75). As a result, public health nurses within the settlement house movement had a greater level of autonomy and were perceived, at the time, as having a more prestigious position than their nursing counterparts in hospitals. In the intellectual and reform-minded atmosphere of the settlement house, public health nurses were also more likely to be social reformers than their hospital sisters.

This practical and ideological spirit of reform and independence was fostered by the extent to which public health nurses had little association with the growing significance and influence of health care providers, biomedicine, and clinical science. Few health care providers sat on the boards of private sponsoring groups that backed public health nursing activity and seldom did public health nurses perceive their practice to require the consultation of a health care provider. In fact, health care providers as a whole tended to be "hostile" to the field of public health and the broad promotion of prevention, perceiving prevention as a threat to their private businesses and fee-for-service practice (Melosh, 1982; Wiley, 1995).

As national nursing organizations began to form in the late 1800s, including the National Association of Nursing Alumnae, the precursor to what was to become the *American Nurses Association (ANA)* in 1911, they focused heavily on the professionalization of nursing through state registration laws and educational reform in nursing schools. The effort toward professionalization splintered nurses differentiated by ideology and social position. Cultural clashes occurred in a context of powerful ideological differences, class distinctions, and scattered work sites. Many nurses put a strong cultural and religious importance on values of "womanly sacrifice and self–abnegation," but were perceived as (and perceived themselves as) different from those wanting "professional autonomy" (Reverby, 1987b, p. 122). The "'traditionalist'" nurse was considered to be "a good nurse defined by her innate character and devotion to service" as the core of her nursing practice and was expected to exhibit this to those with and for whom she served (Reverby, 1987b, p. 139).

In 1912, the *National Organization of Public Health Nurses (NOPHN)* was formed with the expectation that the organization could promote and coordinate public health nursing nationwide, particularly in U.S. cities (Melosh, 1982, p. 121; Roberts & Group, 1995). Supported by wealthy contributors, the organization included lay members on its board and advisory council, in keeping with the actual practice of public health work and the tradition among visiting nurse associations. Soon after its inception, a committee of the NOPHN began establishing uniform standards and record keeping for public health nursing practice. Another NOPHN committee began developing a "program of study" specific to public health nursing so that nursing students could be schooled in the relationship between the social environment and disease (Buhler-Wilkerson, 2001, p. 147).

Despite their efforts to educate others (and themselves) on social and environmental factors related to poor health, to reduce health inequalities, and to advocate for civil liberties among those who had been socially disenfranchised, public health nurses and public health structures also contributed to institutional racism. As public health nursing grew, education and training were used among many in this popular, elite discipline of nurses as a proxy for class and racial or ethnic distinctions. "Foreign born nurses," for example, were excluded from some public health nursing positions because they were described as lacking the background and training of their prestigious counterparts. Nurses of African American ancestry were considered not to be appropriate for working in communities other than "their own" communities of color. Nor were public health nurses immune from the ethnocentricity that often comes with class distinction. Many well-intentioned public health nurses working with immigrants sought to improve the living conditions of those in poverty by helping them achieve greater "Americanization" and take on approaches to cleanliness, diet, and health behavior that were more familiar to the nurses themselves (Melosh, 1982, p. 135).

Segregated schools trained many African American nurses from the 1890s until well into the twentieth century. These schools had far fewer resources and opportunities for their students than the nursing schools of their white counterparts. Nonetheless, by the 1920s and 1930s, African American public health nurses were considered in high demand, in particular to serve and work with communities of African American residents (Hine, 1985). A national survey conducted in 1924 by the Hospital Library Service Bureau described surveyed health officers as stating that black nurses were effective in providing public health services and home visits in black communities but were hampered by their inadequate training (Hine, 1985). In instances where black nurses were employed as visiting or public health nurses to serve white residents it did not go well—"the white people not receiving their services graciously" (Hine, 1985, p. 51). A study by the NOPHN in 1930 provided evidence that, when public health nurses who were African American had the opportunity to receive an adequate nursing education, they were perceived as more effective in black communities than their white counterparts. Fostering "race solidarity" was seen in this study as a solution to expand opportunity for black nurses, as social pressure and "Negro nurse clubs" were expected to encourage departments of health to provide advancement opportunities for black public health nurses (Hine, 1985, p. 70). The NOPHN also worked closely with the National Association of Colored Graduate Nurses (NACGN), established in 1908 by Martha Franklin, to advance public health training in nursing schools where African Americans were trained (Hine, 1985).

As public health nurses wrestled with the reform of systems within their profession as well as outside it, they received little support for their social reform efforts from larger nursing circles. Lavinia Dock, for example, who helped establish the structure for the National Association of Nursing Alumnae, was later very disappointed that the Association (ultimately the ANA) chose to be silent and neutral on the issue of suffrage (Roberts & Group, 1995). In 1908, Dock proposed a "reasonably and temperately expressed suffrage resolution" to the National Association of Nursing Alumnae and it was voted down by a "large majority" (Dock, 1908, p. 925). Dock had perceived a strong relationship between nursing and the women's movement and received strong backing from people such as Julia Howe. Howe (1909) supported Dock's belief in suffrage as integral to nursing, health, and the position of women in her *American Journal of Nursing* article that defended women's suffrage as important to nurses. Howe stated that the "fundamental argument for woman suffrage, of course, is its justice" and that this belief alone made it worthy of their efforts (Howe, 1909, p. 560). Ultimately, the ANA voted in favor of suffrage in 1913 (prior to its 1920 adoption as the Nineteenth Amendment to the Constitution), but not before Dock had already urged the National Association of Nursing Alumnae in 1907 to "look beyond the bounds of their professional organization to emphasize and encompass the social movements and needs of the day" (quoted in Roberts & Group, 1995, p. 152).

Expanding Public Health Nursing Services

Wald solicited the Red Cross in 1912 to extend public health nursing services widely beyond urban areas and establish them in rural settings across the United States. The American Red Cross worked through its local chapters to supply and provide administration for public health nurses to bring community-based care, disease prevention, and coordination of services to these rural areas, with local communities covering the nurse's salary. The Red Cross was intending to provide for rural areas in the United States, something similar to the nationwide structure, coordination, and promotion of public health nursing that the NOPHN was attempting to provide for the cities. Soon after the initial Red Cross mobilization of nurses, the 40–50 rural public health nurses deployed by 1915 had increased to 1,300 by 1921 (Melosh, 1982).

Yet another innovation undertaken by Wald to expand public health nursing services came in the form of an entrepreneurial arrangement she made with the Metropolitan Life Insurance Company. Metropolitan Life's initial "experiment" in 1909 sent public health nurses to homes where agents collecting premiums had found policy holders receiving inadequate medical care. That experiment was a tremendous success. Public health nurses reduced illness and pregnancy costs to the company and were a success with the policy holders, making it easier for agents to collect premiums and to sell insurance. For Wald, the subsidies that public health nurses received for visiting Metropolitan Life customers helped to defray the costs of other nonreimbursable and population-based public health nursing activity. The program was a remarkable success, and by 1924 the service was being operated in 4,000 cities and towns in the United States with nurses making 2.5 million visits a year (Rothstein, 2003).

MIDDLE TWENTIETH-CENTURY PUBLIC HEALTH NURSING

The growth of hospitals and hospital-based care, the decline in acute infectious disease rates, and changes in funding had a tremendous impact on the roles and

⊕ RESEARCH APPLICATION

Trumpets of Attack: Collaborative Efforts Between Nursing and Philanthropies to Care for the Child Crippled with Polio 1930 to 1959

Study Purpose

To explore the nature of the relationship between nursing and philanthropic organizations that focused on polio during the polio epidemic in the United States from 1930 to 1959.

Methods

Historical inquiry was conducted; it drew on original and secondary sources including personal communication with families who benefited from the philanthropic and nursing services of the period and historical research into the writings of public health nursing leaders and others who were leaders in the field of service delivery to children affected by polio and in establishing systems to respond effectively to a national epidemic.

Findings

Particular middle- and upper-class fears of polio provided the impetus for the development of philanthropic support to a treatment and prevention approach to the polio epidemic of the early part of the twentieth century. Philanthropic partnerships with institutions and groups such as hospitals, state health departments, and the National Organization

of Public Health Nurses enhanced nursing education and provided services and consultation to communities devastated by the disease. Unfortunately, these partnerships disproportionately favored white, middle-class communities and nursing education in schools for predominately white nurses.

Implications

Examination of the polio epidemic in the 1930s through the 1950s in the United States offers lessons in the significance of philanthropic partnerships to reducing disease in communities. It also provides insight into how differential health access and disparities in nursing education have been exacerbated in history, pointing to important considerations for partnerships, planning, and policies to inform public health nursing and public health practice leaders of today.

Reference

Carter, K. F. (2001). Trumpets of Attack: Collaborative Efforts Between Nursing and Philanthropies to Care for the Child Crippled with Polio 1930 to 1959. *Public Health Nursing, 18*(4), 253–261.

---

opportunities of public health nurses during the middle part of the twentieth century. At the same time, tensions and changes within the nursing profession itself focused nurses more on their differences than on their strength as a collective social force for improving health in communities and influencing healthy policy.

Hospitals—The New Focus for Improving Health

The incidence of many acute infectious diseases had been dramatically reduced through sanitation, isolation, and (to a much lesser degree) immunization by the 1930s and 1940s. Infant mortality in the United States was also again declining by the 1930s, despite the fact that the scientific evidence for the relationship between sanitation, nutrition, child welfare, and disease reduction was not well developed (Melosh, 1982). Public

health efforts by nurses, health care providers, sanitarians, boards of health, and other workers in the public health system had demonstrated the power of prevention. Meanwhile the business of medicine, hospitals, and a profit-making medical profession was maturing. By the end of the 1930s most nurses in the United States were practicing in hospitals, where, by this time, most client care was occurring. Despite reductions in infectious disease and improvements in mortality and acute morbidity rates, hospitals flourished. Hospitals were increasingly marketing themselves as the best place for health care, modern technology, and elective services, while they also promoted complicated new diagnostic procedures and hospital nurses as an integral part of the ideal health care package (Sandelowski, 2000).

As hospitals grew in number and acceptance, they became the common setting for people to receive care, and bedside hospital nursing was becoming increasingly perceived as the most effective role for nurses. The influence of early public health nurses, who had been considered the elite among the nursing profession for their generally higher level of education (Melosh, 1982) and their autonomous work environment, began to wane within the health sector. At the same time, the increasing chronic disease burden on the public's health was not yet recognized as a public health issue and as a role for public health nursing prevention activities within communities (Melosh, 1982).

Hospitals had become big business by the 1940s and had grown dramatically in number and in size, at the same time that medical specialization and complex procedures became the norm in treatment of the sick (Reverby, 1987b). Health care providers in the United States at the early part of the century were almost entirely general practitioners; by the 1940s over half of them were describing themselves as specialists (Reverby, 1987b). Hospitals were already launching sophisticated public relations campaigns to draw customers into hospital-based and specialized care. Increasingly, providers in public health were perceived by the medical community as being out of step with the business of modern medicine that promoted private practice and hospital-based treatment. As public health providers focused on prevention and on policy-related protections for the public's health in Europe, the United States, Australia, and elsewhere, they were variously perceived as competitors, "communists," and outside of the flourishing medical marketplace in the "backwater" of medicine (Wiley, 1995; Reverby, 1987b; Keleher, 2000).

Changes in Funding for Public Health Nursing

The Great Depression in the United States and the years that followed World War II brought reductions in private public health funding, due to the financial constraints of philanthropists and the decreased morbidity and mortality rates from infectious disease, implying a reduced need for public health surveillance and follow-up. Conservative postwar periods also suppressed activism in social service and hampered entrepreneurs who had long been public health supporters. The world wars of the early twentieth century, however, had focused people in government on public health, as attention was paid to the need for a fit and healthy public that could be called up for effective active duty. As a result, even though private funding for public health nursing was on the decline, government support of public health activity grew (Melosh, 1982). After the Depression and the world wars, federal and state programs in the United States hired public health nurses for relief work and temporary public health projects around the country. Other governmental subsidies underwrote dental care, immunization campaigns, nutrition programs, and the development of entire new rural health agencies. Public health nursing leaders feared that these temporary projects and funding would divert public health nurses from their previously autonomous practice and opportunity for independent, innovative social reform activity for the long term, but the funds and infrastructure were also a welcome source of immediate support (Melosh, 1982).

In the 15 years following the Great Depression in the United States, private public health nursing agencies lost 23 percent of their nurses, and the staffs of government-funded health departments doubled. During the same period, boards of education hired 50 percent more school nurses (Melosh, 1982, p. 146). Public health nurses had moved from independent, privately funded organizational settings to that of controlled state and county departmental structures. Public health nurses also found themselves increasingly dealing with less acute infectious disease prevention and treatment, rather than attending to the less quickly reversible needs of chronically ill members of the community and conducting less visible general prevention activities.

Within this transforming political, public health, and health care environment, the 1950s brought additional upheaval for public health nursing in the United States. Even though the American Red Cross and the Metropolitan Life Insurance Company had been major private employers and supporters of public health nursing services, their interest waned after World War II. What Wald had envisioned—a standardized and centralized mode of public health nursing practice through the main offices of the Red Cross—never materialized. Public health nurses, who were often from urban homes but had been placed in rural settings, were disconnected from their families and from one another and supported by vastly differing local Red Cross chapters. They and their employers struggled against a lack of consistent structure and support. By 1951, the American Red Cross withdrew its financial support and infrastructure from 40 years of privately funded rural public health nursing services. Similarly, in 1953 the Metropolitan Life Insurance Company stopped covering public health nurse home visits and discontinued nursing payments to its remaining 741 nursing services across the country (Melosh, 1982). By this time, Metropolitan Life was no longer experiencing a significant savings in insurance payouts by bearing the costs of public health nursing services. Life expectancy had increased, customers had hospitals they wanted to go to when sick or injured, and those customers in need of home services, such as the chronically ill who required long-term home care, were costly for Metropolitan Life. Home visits by public health nurses at this point did not tend to produce immediate, significant health improvements for their customers nor did they create significant cost savings to the insurance agency.

A Changing Profession

As the number of hospitals and medical procedures grew faster than nursing schools, there were dramatic shortages of nurses after World War II. Auxiliary workers were trained and hired to share nursing duties in the community, at health departments, and in hospitals (Melosh, 1982). Other workers took on some of the teaching and social service role of public health nurses, when nutritionists, social workers, and others began to work in health departments and community settings (Melosh, 1982). Rather than collaborating around their varied areas of expertise and the additional capacity they brought to working with the public, many

nurses clashed with these other workers. Some saw the increasing division of labor among public health workers acting in communities as an infringement on the public health nurse's broader role and decision-making authority among the clients and communities with whom she interacted. Younger generations of nurses, however, often viewed the impatient, negative response to this "threat" as noncollegial "elitism" (Melosh, 1982, p. 151). Division of labor among nurses and other workers was also considered an economic cost-saving measure by the organizations now managing nursing work (Lynaugh & Reverby, 1987).

Ultimately, overall reductions in financial support of public health nursing and the divisions among public health nurses and within the nursing profession led many public health nurses to seek positions within hospitals or to conduct home visits subsidized by hospitals and for the specific follow-up care of hospital clients. In some cases, public health nursing agencies or health departments could only afford a nurse part-time and so shared the nurse's services with a hospital (Melosh, 1982). The lines of practice between clinical nursing and population-level health promotion, prevention, and related policy development began to blur.

Public health nursing, as it moved closer in relationship to the medical community, adapted itself to the new spirit of specialization and division of labor that

⊕ PRACTICE APPLICATION

The Los Angeles County Department of Health Services Public Health Nursing Practice Model

Pioneers in public health nursing history are frequently invoked for their accomplishments and leadership in focusing on the root causes of poor health among populations, their engagement of community members as partners, and their attention to social reforms and public policy. As director of the Los Angeles County Public Health Nursing Department, Margaret Avilla and the staff in her department blended the contemporary articulation of public health principles and nationally recognized public health nursing standards to give direction to staff and agency leadership in returning their public health nursing programs to their roots in addressing the underlying conditions that impact health. The model they have developed

assumes that members of the communities in which they work are active participants with them in all that they do and that principles such as considering the broad determinates of health and creating healthy environmental, social, and economic conditions are vital to improving the health of their populations (Smith & Bazini-Barakat, 2003).

Author

Smith, K., & Bazini-Barakat, N. (2003). The public health nursing practice model: Melding public health principals with the nursing process. *Public Health Nursing, 20*(1), 42–48.

was the movement within health care (Melosh, 1982). The generalist public health nurse, whose mix of client care, community mobilization, and social advocacy had fostered tremendous lay support and a deep understanding of the human impact of inadequate social policies, was being transformed into a programmatic specialist in highly structured institutions. Visiting the sick at home became strictly the work of home health agencies. Prevention and health promotion activities remained the purview of public health, and public health nurses were assigned to areas such as tuberculosis programs, "venereal disease clinics," and health education classes. The close, personal relationships and the influence that public health nurses had with a broad spectrum of residents in their local communities was seemingly being lost, along with their related ability to mobilize with community members in support of broader social change.

In 1953, the NOPHN disbanded, intending to join together with and improve coordination across multiple nursing organizations (Melosh, 1982; Rosen, 1993). Although it merged with the "prestigious" National League of Nursing Education and the Association of Collegiate Schools of Nursing, this dissolution marked a significant turning point in public health nursing's autonomous relationship from the rest of the nursing profession (Melosh, 1982, p. 155). This merged relationship was conceived to bring public health nurses closer to their nursing colleagues, but in so doing public health nurses also lost their strong, independent voice for public health reform. The NOPHN was ultimately subsumed within these nursing organizations and not given specific representation on significant committee matters (Melosh, 1982).

Nursing Avoidance of Social Reform and Feminism

The roots of nursing as a profession developed from gender ideology, religious duty, moralism, and subordinate service work. These roots were a challenge for public health nursing. Elements of them lingered (and still linger today) as public health nurses attempted to stay focused on their roles as activist nurses. While conservative postwar periods had increased the level of risk that outspoken progressive public health nurses had taken in the past, the era of "McCarthyism" in the United States (from approximately 1945 to 1960) exacerbated the suppression of political expression among these advocates. Named for U.S. Senator Joseph McCarthy who fueled the hysteria, "McCarthyism" strongly associated American liberalism with communism among fearful anti-communists opposed to Franklin D. Roosevelt's New Deal and the growth of social welfare that followed World War II and the Great Depression. Reisch and Andrews (2001) describe this period as consistent with historical themes of opposition to radical reformist movements in the U.S., particularly those movements that have promoted egalitarian principles focused on human rights rather than on specific, individual needs (Reisch & Andrews, 2001). The era posed an enormous threat to public health nurses who may have wanted to emulate the vocal social stances of the previous generation of public health nurse reformers.

Some public health nurses, however, did take a stand on the Equal Rights Amendment (ERA), which first came before the U.S. Congress in 1923 but failed that year and every subsequent year until it was passed in 1972 (ultimately, to never have been ratified by enough states to put it into effect). The Equal Rights Amendment that guaranteed equal rights under the law for Americans of both genders was, like suffrage and reproductive rights earlier, a feminist issue that proved divisive within the broad nursing profession. Public health nurses tended to be more radical than their other nursing sisters and were often the most supportive of these issues, but they were less often making the connection, as their foremothers did, between their roles as social reformers, nurses, protectors of the public's health, and women requiring equal status with men. Lavinia Dock had made these connections clear in the early part of the century, but nursing authors in the middle part of the century who gave historical attention to Dock's work did not initially note her feminism. At the same time, authors writing about the women's movement did not talk about feminist nursing leaders or make any connections between nursing and feminism. With the occasional exception of nurses such as Ruth Greenberg Edelstein and Wilma Scott Heide, the profession had backed away from feminism and related reforms in the context of nursing, while the feminist movement had seemingly backed away from nursing as a source of support (Roberts & Group, 1995). Aside from issues specific to feminism, nurses gave their support to social reforms such as civil rights and the war on poverty in the 1960s, but there was little discussion of this activity in the nursing literature of that period (Roberts & Group, 1995).

Professionalism

Eventually, as the prestige of science, technology, and hospital medicine grew, the public health nurse, as independent social reformer and community advocate, could not stand up against "medical dominance" and the "pull of professional ideology" (Melosh, 1982, p. 143). Reverby describes the steps toward the professionalization of nursing as a sacrifice of nursing autonomy for altruism. Social norms and nurses' attention to duty and personal sacrifice that make up their legacy as women and family caregivers led to an "attempt to professionalize altruism without demanding autonomy" (Reverby, 1987a, p. 8).

Reverby and others suggest that the professionalization of public health nursing was a significant factor in its transition from a field of elite, influential, independent social reformers, to community specialists with varying roles in bureaucratic structures in which nurses practiced individually focused care in community according to their disease or programmatic specialty. But seemingly disparate operational definitions of and opinions about professionalization make this suggestion something for debate. Lavinia Dock, for example, epitomized the bold public health nurse social reformer and feminist at the same time that she sought the professionalization of nursing. She perceived professionalization as a mechanism for formalizing nursing independence from male-dominated institutions and the strict medical hierarchy. For others, professionalization amounted to having a recognizable framework of standards, training, registration, and leadership for nursing that would give the profession a consistently favorable image to the public and to medicine, putting nursing on a respectable trajectory for further development. For still others, professionalization was an elitist attempt to measure a nurse by her education rather than her skill, experience, or character.

Nursing leaders had for decades challenged one another over the appropriate level of training and proper background for a nurse, and public health nurses participated fully in these deliberations. Efforts toward the professionalization of nursing were intended to standardize training for public health nurses and for the nursing profession more broadly and to provide a more consistent image of nursing for the public and the medical community. These efforts were stymied by conflict within the nursing profession itself, particularly for public health nurses who tended to be among those in the profession who were better educated. Working-class private duty nurses, for example, resisted efforts toward the registration and standardization of nursing and the educational reforms of professionalization. They were less organized than the nursing leaders of the early and middle twentieth century; nevertheless, they sought to thwart these reforms (Reverby, 1987b). According to Reverby (1987b), many who opposed formal professionalism, equated it negatively with unionism and condemned political activism, hospital nursing strikes, and organizing efforts as out of place for the profession. Denial of professional reform was based on a doctrine of individualism within nursing that was resistant to collective action and of the widely held belief in the nurses' submissive role to health care provider authority and to client needs (Reverby, 1987b). The ANA, similarly, resisted supporting the notion of the unionization of nurses during this period in the middle twentieth century.

While nurses and nursing organizations grew divisive, African American nurses organized themselves and established their own objectives. The National Association of Colored Graduate Nurses had become a vital resource for nurses who were African American and found little support or influence in the American Nurses Association. Mabel Staupers and other African American nursing leaders at the middle of the century similarly sought not only to advance nursing education but to also break down discrimination against black nurses within the profession and to develop leadership within their ranks. This had not been possible through other means available to white nurses, since black nurses were not allowed membership into the ANA until 1948. Even after 1948, African American nurses needed special direct access into membership in the national organization because traditional entry through one's state affiliate was not available to black nurses in all states until 1961 (Hine, 1985). In 1951, the NACGN was dissolved as Mabel Staupers, the last president of the association, declared their full integration with ANA complete and access to integrated participation achieved. By the early 1970s, however, disillusioned African American ANA members, experiencing limited opportunities, "persistent tokenism," and a loss of identity within the ANA, created the National Black Nurses Association (NBNA; Hine, 1985, p. 158). The objectives of the NBNA were not only to advance opportunities for nurses who were African American but also to "act as a change agent in restructuring existing institutions" in order to meet the

⊕ POLICY HIGHLIGHT

Guiding Population-Level Practice

The American Nurses Association (ANA) regularly reviews and updates its Standards of Nursing Practice documents for the whole nursing profession and for many nursing specialties. In 2004, the ANA convened a national committee of public health nursing stakeholders to review and revise the *1999 Scope and Standards of Public Health Nursing Practice*. The nursing stakeholders involved in this 2-year process agreed that they should make a conscious effort to have the revised document more accurately reflect the strong and historic roles and responsibilities of public health nurses in policy development and social justice.

The *2004 Scope and Standards of Nursing*, directed toward the nursing profession as a whole, continues to describe nursing practice as largely focused on the individual and delivered in the context of the medical model. Public health nurses themselves continue to debate the conflicts between practice constraints and financial insecurities that tend to limit the scope of what public health nurses do to improve the health of populations. Despite this, the ANA committee of public health nurses working on the *2007 Scope and Standards of Public Health Nursing Practice* used the nursing profession's respect for the work of Lillian Wald and her collaborators as a model in support of language that would guide nurses toward a practice that ultimately addresses social conditions that impact the health of whole populations.

---

needs of African American populations and to "influence legislation and policies that affect black people" (Hine, 1985, p. 159).

PUBLIC HEALTH NURSING TODAY

Lillian Wald and other nurse reformers practiced in an autonomous environment, apart from the medical establishment. In the decades since the peak of public health nursing and the subsequent post–World War II decline of their numbers and prestige, public health nurses have become more a part of an institutional framework that represents government or medicine and do not have the professional independence of practice that their foremothers enjoyed. Most public health nurses today work in governmental and academic settings and continue to define their practice as promoting and protecting the health of populations. Controversy continues over the scope of that practice, how it should be funded, and what an appropriate level of minimal training for the public health nurse ought to be; however, public health nurses have the potential for political influence that their public health nursing sisters, who could not even cast a vote, only dreamed of.

Unresolved Controversies

National direction, support, and promotion of public health nursing in the United States ultimately came in the structure of the Quad Council of Public Health Nursing Organizations, represented by the leadership of the four national nursing organizations that address issues specific to public health nursing, namely, the Association of Community Health Nurse Educators (ACHNE), the American Nurses Association's Congress on Nursing Practice and Economics (ANA), the American Public Health Association—Public Health Nursing Section (APHA), and the Association of State and Territorial Directors of Nursing (ASTDN). The Quad Council was formed in the early 1980s and, in part, fulfills the role originally sought by the NOPHN when it merged with the National League of Nursing Education and the Association of Collegiate Schools of Nursing to better coordinate nursing activities across organizations. Today the Quad Council has some influence on the development of broad public health strategies, but to date it has lacked significant influence on the nursing profession as a whole or on larger health care policies.

The medical care environment, however, greatly influenced public health nursing and public health. The medicalization of public health through the pressures of division of labor, specialization, fee-for-service direct care, and dominating medical interests continued through the end of the twentieth century (and continues today) within an increasingly market-based health care environment. In applying a medical model within public health, it is often only the client or community that is acted on, cared for, or asked to change. Dreher wrote in 1982 that a tendency to narrow the scope of public health nursing to that which can clearly be accomplished with the limits of existing systems had "insidiously invaded the ranks of public health nursing since World War II" (Dreher, 1982, p. 504). Dreher called this the "think small" position as it implies a focus of nursing practice limited to that which is less complex and more manageable—attending to the behaviors of the individual client or community rather than the system that has compromised their potential for good health.

In the decades that have followed Dreher's description, the *Definition of Public Health Nursing* (APHA Public Health Nursing Section, 1996), the *Scope and Standards of Public Health Nursing* (ANA, 2006), and the *Public Health Nursing Competencies* (Quad Council, 2003) have been developed or modified regularly to better articulate and clarify the public health nurse's role in improving health at the level of the population and the environmental or social system. Nonetheless, the constraints and financial insecurities of practice have made it difficult for public health nurses to widen their scope of practice. Late in the twentieth century and indeed into the twenty-first century, funding for public health nursing work has remained unstable, varied, and controversial. The vast majority of public health nurses in the United States work in government agencies, but they have faced numerous changes in sources of funding and have had to assert and reassert their value to the public, policy makers, and within their own institutions. States and counties that supported population-based and home visiting activities among public health nurses through their general, tax-supported funds, have seen these general funds shrink dramatically in recent decades relative to inflation and their population size. As a result, public health nursing funding sources often become increasingly restrictive as fee-for-service activity is used to pay for individual public health nursing home visits and block grants or programmatic dollars fund nurses in specific, narrowly defined activities. Frequently, the rural public health nurse who is stretched across several programmatic areas is the only one able to have a comprehensive role

and maintain a broad view of health and the actions needed, through his or her varied activities. Public health nurses in many settings, however, have become forced to respond to and work with their communities through the dictates of funding rather than through dynamic partnerships with those impacted by issues that are barriers to good health.

Unresolved controversies within the field of public health nursing continue. One of these is the debate regarding public health nursing's primary role as a direct service provider or as a community mobilizer and social reformer. Another related and lingering controversy is over the nature of radicalism versus professionalism. Modern nursing scholars debate the relationship between the "caring" nature of nursing and one's duty to the client and our responsibilities to social justice and reforming systems that exacerbate health inequities among whole populations (Liaschenko, 1999; Schroeder, 2003). Fundamental documents, including the *Code of Ethics for Nurses*, published by the ANA and distributed to nurses for application in all fields of the profession, provoke this debate by giving strong direction to nurses that they consider their "duty" to their client to be one's ultimate priority and "primary commitment" in nursing (ANA, 2001, p. 9). Much weaker language in the same document says nurses "can" take action on issues of social change (Bekemeier & Butterfield, 2005). At the same time, the *Code of Ethics* invokes Lillian Wald and her public health nursing sisters as the epitome of nursing's "distinguished history" of concern for social justice and system reform. In describing Hull House's Jane Addams as one of the most celebrated of social workers in American history, Reisch and Andrews (2003) describe the social work profession as having "historical amnesia" in having overlooked how radical she and her contemporaries were, inclusive of Wald and Dock (Reich & Andrews, 2003, p. 14). Similarly, the nursing profession and the systems that support public health nursing, have at times lost sight of what the expectations had been for the profession among the very people who are held up as nursing role models.

Reverby claims that nursing was "undermined by duty" and that the underlying characteristics of nurses as traditionally subservient and submissive, ultimately meant that nurses did not assert their rights and independent roles in a developing medical structure. Instead, they were "undermined" by their own duty to care for others (Reverby, 1987a, p. 8). Public health nurses were among the most vocal and assertive within the broader profession of nurses, but they have nonetheless been repeatedly silenced by dominating social forces and ultimately by the bureaucratic and hierarchical structures in which they found themselves later in the twentieth century. Differences from within the larger nursing profession also kept a collective voice from being heard or developed in support of public health nursing autonomy and their role in social change. Nonetheless, public health nurses continue to practice, lead, and influence health policy throughout the United States and elsewhere, while internal nursing debates continue regarding required educational levels among public health nurses, credentialing, appropriate funding levels, and public health nursing's significance.

The Spirit of Our Foremothers

Public health nursing practice is not the same today as it was when it began in the early part of the twentieth century. In the first three decades of public health nursing, innovative, spirited women organized themselves and worked in and with communities to heal, partner, mobilize, support, and bring about change among the disadvantaged populations in which they lived and worked. They did this independently of the medical community and of formal structures that might have otherwise restricted their abilities to engage in overt acts of social justice and system reform. At the same time, they functioned against many odds in a highly repressive

atmosphere where people who were women, minorities, nonconformist, and unmarried faced daunting limitations that restricted even voting and political participation. Perhaps the odds against these social reformers were too great, and public health nursing practice was not able to withstand the financial, political, and professional pressures that weighed upon the activism of nurses.

Increasingly, as the middle and latter part of the twentieth century unfolded, public health nurses found themselves ever more distant from the independence and influence of their early years. At the same time, the modern public health nurse, while likely finding herself or himself in a highly structured bureaucracy or organization and perhaps well-entrenched in the medical model, has the opportunity for personal and collective political participation that our foremothers only dreamed of. Public health nurses, for instance, can maximize their roles within bureaucracies by exerting influence and addressing policy reforms from within governmental systems themselves. Collective action by public health nurses today is also more likely to include representation from a variety of racial and ethnic groups and nurses from around the world, than a gathering of nurses could draw in Wald and Dock's day. The potential exists for public health nurses to capitalize on the respect with which they are held in their communities and the knowledge and skills they have in understanding populations, to reinvigorate the spirits of our foremothers, and to boldly act on social structures to seek justice and eliminate socially constructed inequities in health.

CRITICAL THINKING ACTIVITIES

1. Experience with epidemics, developments in science, and changes in health priorities helped to establish the field of public health. Discuss the key time periods that shaped the development of public health systems and influenced public health nursing.

2. Compare the role of historical social reformers in the development of home nursing and public health nursing. Analyze the influence of these historical social reformers on current expectations and roles of public health nurses.

3. Numerous social factors influenced the development and formalization of public health nursing into a broadly reform-minded, social justice–

oriented form of nursing. Debate the social and philosophical influences that shaped public health nursing practice in the twentieth century and how and why public health nursing changed over time.

4. Analyze the influence of political barriers to advocacy and public health improvement that public health nurses encountered in their efforts to improve social conditions that impacted health in their communities.

5. Efforts in nursing professionalization played a significant role in the relationship between public health nurses and the broader nursing profession. What impact did this have on the development of public health nursing?

6. Nurses today assume the legacy of early public health nursing reformers, still encountering the same barriers, but still defining the public health nursing role in terms of improving the health of populations. Debate the similarities between public health nurses of today and those in history.

KEY TERMS

American Red Cross

district nursing

Edwin Chadwick (1780–1890)

Florence Nightingale (1820–1910)

germ theory

Great Depression

Henry Street Settlement

Hull House

Jane Addams (1860–1935)

John Snow (1813–1858)

Lavinia Dock (1858–1956)

Lillian Wald (1867–1940)

McCarthyism

New Deal

Nineteenth Amendment

public health

public health nursing

Quad Council of Public Health Nursing Organizations

sanitary era

Sheppard-Towner Act

social Darwinism

suffrage

KEY CONCEPTS

⊕ Infectious diseases and related epidemics were the primary killers until recent history. During the Enlightenment, scholars began to understand the scientific basis for disease, ultimately having an impact on infectious disease. By the late 1800s, improving health began to be understood as an effort in prevention, education, and improving conditions, particularly for the poor, who bore the neg-ative health burdens of the Industrial Revolution.

⊕ Nursing work began as an extension of a woman's role within her family and community as well as a demonstration of her religious duty. Even after nurses began to formalize the profession through specific education and standards, religious charities were commonly the supporters and dispensers of nursing services to individuals at home, bringing moral and physical cleanliness to the "worthy" poor and sick.

⊕ Public health nursing was born at the Henry Street Settlement in New York City through the strong female networks of Lillian Wald, Lavinia Dock, and others who mixed feminism, the suffrage movement, and improved health and living conditions for women, children, and the poor.

Nurses came to public health with a social justice philosophy, training in health, and often a religious grounding in service.

⊕ As the numbers and influence of public health nurses quickly grew in the United States during the early part of the twentieth century, they became increasingly involved in social change efforts such as seeking to end unsafe labor practices, supporting unions, increasing the civil liberties of women and African Americans, and promoting peaceful alternatives to war. Socially repressive periods after both World War I and World War II, however, left public health nurses wary of the risks they could and should take in bringing about social change that would improve the public's health.

⊕ As nursing began to formalize efforts to standardize training, roles, and registration of nurses, conflicts arose. Strong distinctions were made among nurses in terms of their social class and training, as well as a nurse's ideology. Professionalization of nursing was intended to promote a more consistent image of nursing, but it did not ultimately serve to promote a nursing role in social activism and broad system reform.

⊕ Reminiscent of the early days of public health nursing, the collective voice of the broader nursing community (of which public health nursing is just a part) is vocal about issues specific to nursing practice and employment but tends to be silent on broader issues of social change, giving little support or direction to all nurses (not just public health nurses) with regard to social reform.

⊕ Nurses, and women in particular, have more options and opportunities for participation in the political system for policy reform than those of Wald and her Victorian sisters. Primary function for social change has been muted from 100 years.

REFERENCES

American Nurses Association. (2001). *Code of ethics for nurses with interpretive statements.* Washington, DC: American Nurses Publishing.

American Nurses Association. (2007). *Public health nursing: Scope and standards.* Silver Spring, MD: nursebooks.org.

Bekemeier, B., & Butterfield, P. (2005). Unreconciled inconsistencies: A critical review of the concept of social justice in 3 national nursing documents. *Advances in Nursing Science, 28*(2), 152–162.

Brainard, A.M. (1922). *The evolution of public health nursing.* Philadelphia: W.B. Saunders Company.

Buhler-Wilkerson, K. (1989). *The rise and decline of public health nursing, 1900–1930.* New York: Garland Publishing.

Buhler-Wilkerson, K. (2001). *No place like home: A history of nursing and home care in the United States.* Baltimore: The Johns Hopkins University Press.

Carter, K. F. (2001). Trumpets of Attack: Collaborative Efforts Between Nursing and Philanthropies to Care for the Child Crippled with Polio 1930 to 1959. *Public Health Nursing, 18*(4), 253–261.

Coss, C. (1989). *Lillian D. Wald: Progressive activist.* New York: The Feminist Press.

Dock, L.L. (1908). The suffrage question. *American Journal of Nursing, 8,* 925–926.

Dreher, M.C. (1982). The conflict of conservativism in public health nursing education. *Nursing Outlook, 30,* 504–509.

Hine, D.C. (Ed.). (1985). *Black women in the nursing profession: A documentary history.* New York: Garland Publishing.

Howe, J.W. (1909). Woman and the suffrage: The case for woman suffrage. *The American Journal of Nursing, 9,* 559–566.

Institute of Medicine. (1988). *The future of public health.* Washington, DC: National Academy Press.

Keleher, H. (2000). Repeating history? Public and community health nursing in Australia. *Nursing Inquiry, 7,* 258–265.

Liaschenko, J. (1999). Can justice coexist with the supremacy of personal values in nursing practice? *Western Journal of Nursing Research, 21*(1), 35–50.

Lynaugh, J., & Reverby, S. (1987). Thoughts on the nature of history. *Nursing Research, 36*(1), 4 and 69.

Melosh, B. (1982*). The physician's hand: Work culture and conflict in American nursing.* Philadelphia: Temple University Press.

Quad Council. (2003). *Public health nursing competencies.* Retrieved December 10, 2004, from the Association of Community Health Nurse Educators Web site http://www.uncc.edu/achne/.

Reisch, M., & Andrews, J. (2001). *The road not taken: A history of radical social work in the United States.* Philadelphia: Brunner-Routledge.

Reverby, S. (1987a). A caring dilemma: Womanhood and nursing in historical perspective. *Nursing Research, 36*(1), 5–11.

Reverby, S. (1987b). *Ordered to care.* New York: Cambridge University Press.

Roberts, J.I., & Group, T.M. (1995). *Feminism and nursing: An historical perspective on power, status, and political activism in the nursing profession.* Westport, CT: Praeger.

Rosen, G. (1993). *The history of public health.* Baltimore: The Johns Hopkins University Press.

Rothstein, W.G. (2003). *Public health and the risk factor: A history of an uneven medical revolution.* Rochester, NY: University of Rochester Press

Sandelowski, M. (2000). *Devices and desires: Gender, technology, and American nursing.* Chapel Hill: The University of North Carolina Press.

Schroeder, C. (2003). The tyranny of profit: Concentration of wealth, corporate globalization, and the failed US health care system. *Advances in Nursing Science, 25*(3), 173–184.

Shopsis, M. (1993). The settlement house workers, 1890–1914: Were they motivated by a desire for social justice? *Culturefront: A magazine of the humanities. 2*(3), 42–47.

Smith, K., & Bazini-Barakat, N. (2003). The public health nursing practice model: Melding public health principals with the nursing process. *Public Health Nursing, 20*(1), 42–48.

Wiley, E.A.K. (1995). The transformation of nursing practice and the emergence of a new professional: *Public health nursing* 1900–1940. Masters thesis, University of Washington.

BIBLIOGRAPHY

Awofeso, N. (2004). What's new about the "New Public Health"? *American Journal of Public Health, 94*(5) 705–709.

Backer, B.A. (1993). Lillian Wald: Connecting caring with activism. *Nursing and Health Care, 14*(3), 122–129.

Brush, B.L., & Lynaugh, J.E. (1999) (Eds.). *Nurses of all nations: A history of the International Council of Nurses, 1899–1999.* Philadelphia: Lippincott.

Carter, K.F. (2001). Trumpets of attack: Collaborative efforts between nursing and philanthropies to care for the child crippled with polio 1930 to 1959. *Public Health Nursing, 18*(4), 253–261.

D'Antonio, P. (2004). Women, nursing, and baccalaureate education in 20th century America. *Journal of Nursing Scholarship, 36*(4), 379–384.

Duncan, S.M., Leipert, B.D., & Mill, J.E. (1999). "Nurses as health evangelists"?: The evolution of public health nursing in Canada, 1918–1939. *Advances in Nursing Science, 22*(1), 40–51.

Fee, E., & Krieger, N. (Eds.). (1994). *Women's health, politics, and power: Essays on sex/gender, medicine, and public health.* Amityville, NY: Baywood Publishing Company.

Francis, K. (2001). Service to the poor: The foundations of community nursing in England, Ireland and New South Wales. *International Journal of Nursing Practice, 7*(3), 169–176.

Kirby, S. (2004). Diaspora, dispute and diffusion: Bringing professional values to the punitive culture of the Poor Law. *Nursing Inquiry, 11*(3), 185–191.

Lewenson, S.B. (1990). The relationship among the four professional nursing organizations and woman suffrage: 1893–1920. Doctoral dissertation, Columbia University Teachers College, 1989. *Dissertation Abstracts International, 50/08,* 4302.

Melchior, F. (2004). Feminist approaches to nursing history. *Western Journal of Nursing Research, 26*(3), 340–355.

Smith, K., & Bazini-Barakat, N. (2003). The public health nursing practice model: Melding public health principals with the nursing process. *Public Health Nursing, 20*(1), 42–48.

Snodgrass, M.E. (2003). *World epidemics: A cultural chronology of diseases from prehistory to the era of SARS.* Jefferson, NC: McFarland & Company.

Spratt, M. (1997). Beyond Hull House: New interpretations of the settlement movement in America. *Journal of Urban History, 23*(6), 770–777.

Wald, L.D. (1915). *The house on Henry Street.* New Brunswick, CT: Transaction Publishers.

RESOURCES

American Nurses Association

8515 Georgia Avenue, Suite 400
Silver Springs, Maryland 20910
1-800- 274-4ANA
Web: http://www.nursingworld.org
The American Nurses Association was started as the Association of Nursing Alumnae. It later became the American Nurses Association's Congress on Nursing Practice and Economics representing all nurses. The Web site provides information on ANA activities and access to online nursing journals.

American Public Health Association–Public Health Nursing Section (APHA)

800 "I" Street NW
Washington, D.C. 20001-3710
202-777- APHA (2752)
FAX: 202-777-2534
Email: comments@APHA.org
Web: http://www.apha.org
This association of public health nurse educators and practitioners operates within the American Public Health Association. The Web site provides information and opportunities for involvement in nationwide PHN issues.

Association of Community Health Nurse Educators (ACHNE)

10200 W. 44th Avenue, #304
Wheat Ridge, Colorado 80033
303-422-0679
FAX: 303-422-9904
Email: ACHNE@resourcenter.com
Web: http://www.achne.org
ACHNE is an association of educators that teaches community health and public health nursing at universities and colleges. ACHNE provides a meeting ground for those

committed to excellence in community and public health nursing education, research, and practice. ACHNE was established in 1978 and is run by elected volunteer leaders who guide the organization in providing networking through the quarterly newsletter and membership directory, and providing educational opportunities through publications and the annual Spring Institute. ACHNE's mission is to promote the public's health by ensuring leadership and excellence in community and public health nursing education, research, and practice. The Web site provides information on workforce issues, PHN/CHN certification, career opportunities, public health nursing graduate education, and links to other Quad Council organizations.

Association of State and Territorial Directors of Nursing (ASTDN)

1275 K Street NW, Suite 800
Washington, D.C. 20005-4006
202-371-9090
FAX: 202-371-9797
Email: dianakp@health.ok.gov
Web: http://www.astdn.org

The Association of State and Territorial Directors of Nursing began in 1935 as an advisory group of state health department nurses. ASTDN continues today as an active association of public health nursing leaders from across the United States and its territories. ASTDN is an affiliate of the Association of State and Territorial Health Officials (ASTHO). The ASTDN mission is to provide a collegial forum to advance the public health nursing leadership role in protecting and promoting the health of the pub-

lic. The Web site provides information on publications, population-focused practice, Quad Council competencies, Partnership Project (CDC and ASTDN), newsletter, and featured state public health nursing profile.

National Association of Colored Graduate Nurses (NACGN)

8630 Fenton Street, Suite 330
Silver Springs, Maryland 20910-3803
Web: http://www.aaregistry.com

The National Association of Colored Graduate Nurses was established in 1908 by Martha Franklin to advance public health training in nursing schools where African Americans were trained.

National Black Nurses Association (NBNA)

8630 Fenton Street, Suite 330
Silver Spring, Maryland 20910-3803
FAX: 301-589-3223
Web: http://www.nbna.com

The National Black Nurses Association was organized in 1971 under the leadership of Dr. Lauranne Sams, former dean and professor of nursing, School of Nursing, Tuskegee University, Tuskegee, Alabama. NBNA is a nonprofit organization incorporated on September 2, 1972, in the state of Ohio. The NBNA represents approximately 150,000 African American nurses to "investigate, define and determine what the health care needs of African Americans are and to implement change to make available to African Americans and other minorities health care commensurate with that of the larger society."

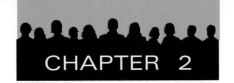

CHAPTER 2

Core Functions of Public Health Nursing

Jeanne Matthews, RN, PhD

Chapter Outline

- **Public Health and the IOM Reports**
  Defining the Core Functions
  The Core Public Health Functions and Governmental
    Public Health

- **Public Health in America: Linking Core
  Functions and Essential Public Health Services**
  The Public Health System and the Essential Public Health
    Services

- **The Core Public Health Functions, Essential
  Public Health Services, and Workforce
  Competency**
  The Public Health Nursing Competencies
  Public Health Nursing Competency: Setting the Standard for
    Education and Practice
  Making the Connections: Linking the Core Functions, Essential
    Services, and Public Health Nursing Competencies

- **Challenges to Advancing the Public's Health
  through Improving the Public Health
  Infrastructure**
  Information/Communication Systems Capacity
  Workforce Capacity
  Organizational and Systems Capacity

Learning Objectives

Upon completion of this chapter, the reader will be able to:

1. Evaluate the core public health functions.

2. Examine the federal, state, and local roles in meeting core public health functions.

3. Synthesize the relationships among the core functions, essential services, and public health nursing competencies.

4. Analyze the role of public health system partnerships in meeting the Healthy People 2010 vision of healthy people in healthy communities.

5. Analyze the role of generalist and specialist public health nurses in providing essential public health services.

6. Evaluate the challenges to meeting the recommendations of the Institute of Medicine Reports on public health.

Great changes and accomplishments have marked the history of modern public health. During the past century, the dramatic impact of death and disability from widespread communicable diseases like influenza and polio, the development of antibiotics and vaccines for immunization against serious childhood diseases such as measles, and the more recent effect of emerging infectious diseases such as AIDS and SARS have all contributed significantly to the special concerns and work of public health. Ongoing struggles in the organization and financing of health care, such as the escalating costs of care, the imbalance between dollars spent for treatment versus those spent for prevention, and the continuing increase in the numbers of the uninsured, plague the system. Compounded by the demands of emergency preparedness following the terrorist attacks of September 11, 2001, and the challenges of Hurricane Katrina in 2005, public health has struggled to find a way to meet local, state, and national health needs.

The Institute of Medicine (IOM) Report (1988) reinvigorated public health by providing a fresh view of the governmental role in meeting the health needs of the nation. Demanding a reconceptualization of the vision, mission, goals, and activities of public health, the report and its follow-up volumes have served as the impetus for a renewed focus on the health of populations. The IOM recommendations, most notably the identification of the core public health functions, began a sea change in public health, influencing how it accomplishes its goals. This chapter will provide a foundation for understanding the role of the core functions and essential public health services in promoting and protecting the health of the nation, as well as for identifying how public health nursing's professional competency in the core functions and essential services will advance the health of local, state, and national communities. As most public health nurses practice at the local level, particular attention will be paid to their involvement in local communities. Lastly, challenges to implementing the IOM goals will be addressed, along with recommendations for the future role of public health nursing.

PUBLIC HEALTH AND THE IOM REPORTS

Great public health achievements are responsible for 25 of the 30 years of increased life expectancy in the twentieth century, evidence of the importance of public health prevention.

Even though the major health achievements of the twentieth century (Box 2-1) and the accompanying increase in life expectancy are the result of public health gains, one of the notable challenges throughout the years has been the widespread lack of understanding of what public health is and does. This challenge and the implications for the direction of public health served as the clarion call to the IOM's Committee for the Study of the Future of Public Health. Its landmark study and report,

---

BOX 2-1: The 10 Great Public Health Achievements in the United States, 1900–1999

Vaccination

Motor-vehicle safety

Safer workplaces

Control of infectious diseases

Decline in deaths from coronary heart disease and stroke

Safer and healthier foods

Healthier mothers and babies

Family planning

Fluoridation of drinking water

Recognition of tobacco use as a health hazard

SOURCE: CDC (1999), *Ten Great Public Health Achievements—United States, 1900–1999, MMWR, 48,* 243–248.

The Future of Public Health, occurred during a time when the nation was assaulted by escalating rates of HIV and AIDS. Additionally, inadequate chronic disease prevention and the failure of the health system to deal with the needs of the uninsured weighed heavily on the system. At the time of the report, governmental public health was poorly financed, resulting in a system in "disarray." Public health was in need of clarity and direction (IOM, 1988).

In the mid-twentieth century, public health was an amalgam of personal health services, provider of last resort activities for the poor and underserved, and traditional population-focused activities (Turnock, 2004; Fallon & Zgodzinski, 2005). Defining public health as "what we, as a society, do collectively to assure the conditions in which people can be healthy," the Committee for the Study of the Future of Public Health began a systematic review of public health in America (IOM, 1988, p. 1). For two years, the committee analyzed epidemiological data, spoke with key stakeholders across the nation and Canada, held public meetings and worked closely with groups critical to public health organization, practice, and education. The product of this comprehensive study was a landmark report, the recommendations of which have influenced public health goals since their publication.

The report described a system in disarray and detailed a lack of consensus about the mission of public health beyond the broad vision that public health serves everyone (IOM, 1988). It also pointed out wide variation in structure and function among state and local public health agencies. From a small cadre of services in one state to a more comprehensive array in another, there appeared to be no general agreement about the appropriate mix of services, whether traditional public health functions or not. The same discrepancies were also found in localities, as were differences in the level of skill among public health agency staff.

The IOM committee recommendations have greatly influenced public health during the past 25 years and are organized around the following elements:

1. The mission of public health

2. The governmental role in fulfilling the mission

3. The responsibilities unique to each level of government

4. Those elements necessary to implement the first three recommendations (IOM, 1988, p. 7)

The committee defined the mission of public health as "fulfilling society's interest in assuring conditions in which people can be healthy" (IOM, 1988, p.7). This conceptualization of public health provided the foundation for the ecological model of health, that is, a broad, multideterminant model examining the contributions of many and varied factors supporting public health, some of which are illustrated in Figure 2-1 (IOM, 2003b). It is clear that governmental public health agencies cannot accomplish this task in isolation because it entails a significant undertaking, far broader than the work of any one organization (Mays, 2002). Yet at each level of government, the committee did identify the "unique" role of governmental public health and addressed the core functions of public health agencies as assessment, policy development, and assurance.

Defining the Core Functions

To determine the needs of its constituent community, each public health agency must perform assessment, described by the IOM as the "basic function of public health . . . which cannot be delegated" (IOM, 1988, p. 7). The assessment core function requires the public health agency to "regularly and systematically collect, assemble, analyze, and make available information on the health of the community" (IOM, 1988, p. 7).

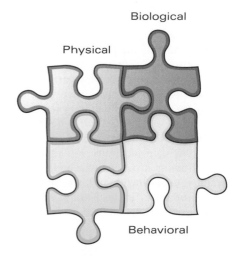

Figure 2-1 The ecological model of health: An interconnection of domains.

In order for needs to be identified, community strengths to be employed, priorities to be set, and programs to be implemented, the right questions must be asked and the appropriate data must be obtained. The resource cost in human and financial terms may be too great for every public health agency to conduct the assessment on its own; nevertheless, the responsibility still resides within the government. In discussing this public role, the IOM addressed the importance of impartiality. The public sector, it contended, is obligated to examine data without self-interest, unlike the private sector, which is likely to be driven by market incentives (IOM, 1988).

The core function of policy development integrates the wide-ranging community development and partnership elements of public health with evidence-based decision making aimed at improving the health of the community. The public health agency, acting in the public interest, plays a leadership role in developing and promoting policy that supports health promotion and protection. This leadership role, enacted in concert with many participants within the public health system, may involve a variety of functions, such as convening a public meeting and facilitating relationships among service providers (IOM, 1988).

In addition to assessment and policy development, the IOM identified assurance as a core public health function. Assurance by governmental agencies involves enforcing laws that support health and safety, linking people to needed services, making certain that the workforce is competent, and evaluating the quality of services. It may support the private sector in providing needed services to the community through a variety of actions, such as funding the service partially or in full, facilitating an environment supportive to the service, or enacting a legal mandate requiring that the service be provided. In order to carry out the assurance function, the public sector must have been effective in each of the other two core functions. Government cannot assure services unless it has knowledge of the needs of the community (assessment) and has been successful in planning, promoting, implementing, and evaluating policy that will support community needs (policy development; IOM, 1988).

The Core Public Health Functions and Governmental Public Health

The structure of government in the United States provides a division of responsibility to promote and protect the public health. Each level of government has interdependent as well as independent functions, creating opportunities for collaboration as well as potential conflict within the structure of federal, state, and local authority. The nature of each of the governmental roles gives direction to public health and may be examined broadly using the core functions framework. Each level of the public sector conducts a number of activities related to the core functions, though the way in which each does so varies greatly.

The federal government promotes and protects public health through its ability to "tax, spend and regulate interstate commerce" (Gostin, 2000, p. 2979) leading to the ability to make national policy, set standards, allocate resources, deliver services to special populations, and use its bully pulpit, or position of power, to influence health activities. In making its recommendations, the IOM identified the following federal public health "obligations":

1. Support of knowledge development and dissemination through data gathering, research, and information exchange;

2. Establishment of nationwide health objectives and priorities, and stimulation of debate on interstate and national public health issues;

3. Provision of technical assistance to help states and localities determine their own objectives and to carry out action on national and regional objectives;

4. Provision of funds to states to strengthen state capacity for services, especially to achieve an adequate minimum capacity, and to achieve national objectives; and

5. Assurance of actions and services that are in the public interest of the entire nation such as control of AIDS and similar communicable diseases, interstate environmental actions, and food and drug inspection. (IOM, 1988, pp. 143–144)

In order to meet these obligations, the federal government collects and analyzes data to examine national health status and evaluate health needs of the U.S. population in general, as well as that of special populations (assessment). It sets priorities (assessment) and legislates policy for a national health agenda (policy development).

Lastly, it assures health care for special populations, such as Native Americans and the military (assurance).

As the primary governmental body responsible for the health and welfare of citizens, the state level government's statutory authority is drawn from the Constitution, which provides that the states retain functions not delegated to the federal government (IOM, 1988; Turnock, 2004). The IOM recommended that state level public health core responsibilities include:

1. Assessment of health needs within the state based on statewide data collection;

2. Assurance of an adequate statutory base for health activities in the state;

3. Establishment of statewide health objectives, delegating power to localities as appropriate and holding them accountable;

4. Assurance of appropriate organized statewide effort to develop and maintain requisite personal, educational, and environmental health services; provision of access to necessary services; and solution of problems inimical to health;

5. Guarantee of a minimum set of essential health services; and

6. Support of local service capacity, especially when disparities in local ability to raise revenues and/or administer programs require subsidies, technical assistance, or direct action by the state to achieve adequate service levels. (IOM, 1988, p. 1\43)

Consistent with that broad perspective, states conduct a wide range of public health activities, including technical assistance to local public health agencies (assessment, policy development, and assurance); disease surveillance and monitoring (assessment); environmental regulation (policy development); workforce and organizational licensure (policy development and assurance); and administration and oversight of federal programs, such as Women, Infants and Children (WIC; assessment and assurance).

Even though the state government is the primary agent for public health, most public health services are delivered at the local level. The structure of local public health agencies (LPHAs) varies, falling into five major agency types (Box 2-2). The work of Hajat, Brown,

BOX 2-2: The Five Types of Local Public Health Agencies

1. County-based	(60%)
2. Town/township	(15%)
3. City/municipal	(10%)
4. Multi/county/district/regional	(8%)
5. City-county	(7%)

SOURCE: Retrieved February 1, 2005, p. 9 from: www.naccho.org/ files/documents/chartbook-introduction 3-17.pdf.

and Fraser (2001) documented the variety in structure within local public health agencies in the United States. Governance also varies among local agencies, with some LPHAs being part of the state governance system, some being either locally administered, reporting to local boards of health or governed by state-local cooperative agreements, and others belonging to a variation of these models.

Along with the difference in structure and governance among local public health agencies, there is a significant variability in the type and nature of services delivered. Communicable disease, environmental health and child health are most commonly identified as local service priorities, according to a large study conducted by the National Association of City and County Health Officials (NACCHO; Hajat, Brown, & Fraser, 2001). NACCHO discovered that the choice of priorities varied between metropolitan and nonmetropolitan agencies, and agencies differed in the amount of core services delivered versus primary care and chronic disease services. When considering the role of local public health agencies, the IOM recommended:

1. Assessment, monitoring, and surveillance of local health problems and needs and of resources for dealing with them;

2. Policy development and leadership that foster local involvement and a sense of ownership, that emphasize local needs, and that advocate equitable distribution of public resources and complementary private activities commensurate with community needs; and

3. Assurance that high-quality services, including personal health services, needed for the protection of public health in the community are available and accessible to all persons; that the community receives proper consideration in the allocation of federal and state as well as local resources for public health, and that the community is informed about how to obtain public health, including personal health, services, or how to comply with public health requirements (IOM, 1988, p 145).

Consistent with the core function approach to public health and the goals of Healthy People 2010, more LPHAs have moved from direct primary care and chronic disease services provided to individuals to a more population-focused service delivery. The emphasis on populations and the relationship to other targets of health services is illustrated by the health services pyramid (Figure 2-2). Serving as the foundation, the population focus establishes overall goals, and the essential services, which are fundamental to public health and safety, are implemented, laying the groundwork for clin-

ical preventive services and primary, secondary, and tertiary health care. If the foundation crumbles, the integrity of the other tiers is threatened (Turnock, 2004)

Assessment functions are likely to be associated with many of the traditional public health services provided by local agencies. Disease surveillance and investigation activities, for example, have long been linked with communicable disease control, just as immunization programs have tracked the level of vaccine-preventable disease protection in the community. Public health at the local level participates in policy development functions through education of legislative bodies at the state level, as well as advocacy work within communities. The assurance function in localities generally takes the form of one of the following approaches: developing local ordinances to protect the health of the public, linking services to those who need them, or providing services when no other organization will provide them.

PUBLIC HEALTH IN AMERICA: LINKING CORE FUNCTIONS AND ESSENTIAL PUBLIC HEALTH SERVICES

While the core functions of assessment, policy development and assurance are accepted today as the rightful place of public health, there was much early confusion about how these functions fit with public health activities of the time. Many public health organizations delivered primary care and chronic disease services when the IOM released its report in 1988. In the aftermath of the report, a renewed emphasis on health care reform provided an impetus to reaffirming the role of public health, as well as clarifying the importance of the core functions. Organizations, such as NACCHO and the Centers for Disease Control and Prevention (CDC), developed a variety of materials to inform policy makers about public health. Subsequently, the Public Health Functions Steering Committee (Box 2-3), a widely representative group of public and private partners, was charged with examining existing lists of basic public health practices and services and with establishing a consensus list of the essential services (APHA, 2005b). This list of 10 essential public health services clarifies the role of public health and continues to serve as a useful framework for most public health activities.

The essential services document, Public Health in America (Public Health Functions Steering Committee,

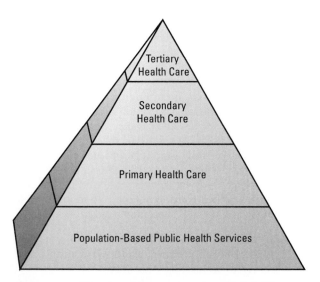

Figure 2-2 The health services pyramid. The pyramid provides a picture of the relationship of population health services to other services within the U.S. health care system.

From Department of Health and Human Services, Public Health Service (1995) *For a healthy nation: Return on investments in public health*, p. 5.

BOX 2-3: The Organizations of the Public Health Functions Steering Committee

Agency for Health Care Policy and Research

American Public Health Association

Association of Schools of Public Health

Association of State and Territorial Health Officials

Centers for Disease Control and Prevention

Environmental Council of the States

Food and Drug Administration

Health Resources and Services Administration

Indian Health Service

National Association of County and City Health Officials

National Association of State Alcohol and Drug Abuse Directors

National Association of State Mental Health Program Directors

National Institutes of Health

Public Health Foundation

Office of the Assistant Secretary for Health

Substance Abuse and Mental Health Services Administration

U.S. Public Health Service

SOURCE: Nelson, J., Essien, J., Loudermilk, R., & Cohen, D. (2002). *The public health competency handbook.* Atlanta: Affiliated Graphics /KITS.

1994), seen in Figure 2-3, provides the blueprint for local, state, and national health goals and activities. Not to be confused with traditional clinical services, the essential services translate the core functions into user-friendly and measurable practices (Turnock, 2004, p.183). Using the core functions/essential services framework, public health organizations can structure their goals and activities, as well as evaluate and improve their performance. Such a template assists in examining activities, both within and across programs, providing a means of looking at public health in its entirety.

Identifying what public health does and how it meets its goals, Public Health in America's vision of "healthy people in healthy communities" set the stage for a broad-based approach to public health. The mission to "promote physical and mental health and prevent disease, injury, and disability" embraces health promotion and all levels of disease prevention (Public Health Functions Steering Committee, 1994). It is comprehensive in its scope, envisioning linkages among all segments of the public health system to meet this challenging goal.

The Public Health System and the Essential Public Health Services

Some may see the essential services as pertaining only to governmental public health, but this limited view is likely to impede implementing the vision of healthy people in healthy communities. A broader view, one that the IOM (2003b) pictured as including all organizations participating in the support of a healthy society, is needed to provide an environment that promotes and sustains health. The CDC model of the public health system (Figure 2-4) illustrates the social connections forming this community web (CDC, 2006). No longer can we afford to look at these social organizations as independent of one another, if we are to meet the goals of the ecological model. Although governmental public health is likely to play a leadership role in ensuring that the essential services are provided in a community, it is only with an identified shared mission and a reinvigorated sense of community that the goal of health will be realized.

Community Collaboration to Ensure Public Health

Societal organizations have the opportunity to work together for a common goal, that is, a vibrant community that produces and supports health. Examples of these potential collaborators include schools, faith-based groups, health departments, businesses, hospitals, HMOs and other providers, police and fire departments, social services providers, universities, the media, and government officials. Healthy people in an effec-

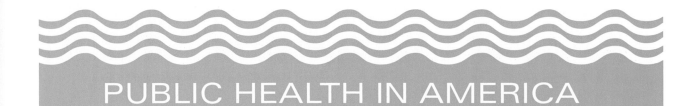

PUBLIC HEALTH IN AMERICA

Vision:
Healthy People in Healthy Communities

Mission:
Promote Physical and Mental Health and Prevent Disease, Injury, and Disability

Public Health

* Prevents epidemics and the spread of disease
* Protects against environmental hazards
* Prevents injuries
* Promotes and encourages healthy behaviors
* Responds to disasters and assists communities in recovery
* Assures the quality and accessibility of health services

Essential Public Health Services

* Monitor health status to identify community health problems
* Diagnose and investigate health problems and health hazards in the community
* Inform, educate, and empower people about health issues
* Mobilize community partnerships to identify and solve health problems
* Develop policies and plans that support individual and community health efforts
* Enforce laws and regulations that protect health and ensure safety
* Link people to needed personal health services and assure the provision of health care when otherwise unavailable
* Assure a competent public health and personal health care workforce
* Evaluate effectiveness, accessibility, and quality of personal and population-based health services
* Research for new insights and innovative solutions to health problems

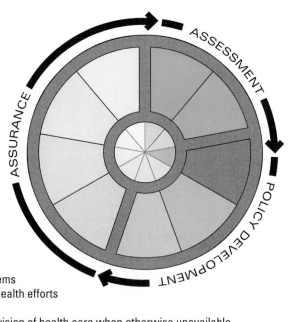

Figure 2-3 Public Health in America. Integrating the vision of healthy people in healthy communities through the work of the core public health functions and the essential public health services.

From Text adapted from http://www.health.gov/phfunctions/public.htm, accessed January 29, 2005. Graphic adapted from Public Health Steering Committee, Members (July 1995): American Public Health Association, Association of Schools of Public Health, Association of State and Territorial Health Officials, Environmental Council of the States, National Association of County and City Health Officials, National Association of State Alcohol and Drug Abuse Directors, National Association of State Mental Health Program Directors, Public Health Foundation, U.S. Public Health Service–Agency for Health Care Policy and Research, Centers for Disease Control and Prevention, Food and Drug Administration, Health Resources and Services Administration, Indian Health Service, National Institutes of Health, Office of the Assistant Secretary for Health, Substance Abuse and Mental Health Services Administration

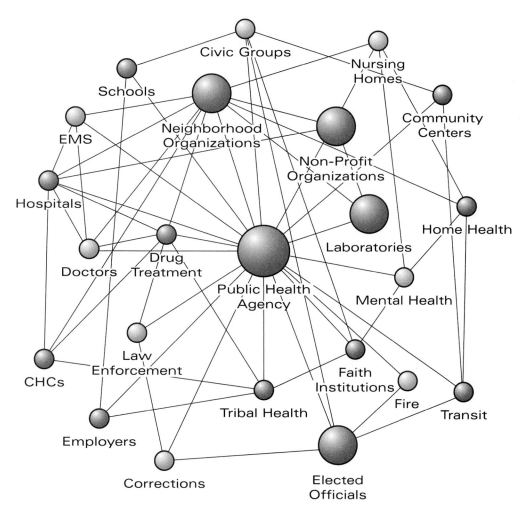

Figure 2-4 The Public Health System. A public health system includes all public, private, and voluntary entities that contribute to public health activities within a given area. By focusing on the public health system, the contributions of all entities are recognized in assessing the provision of EPHS. Entities within a public health system can include hospitals, physicians, managed care organizations, environmental agencies, social service organizations, educational systems, community-based organizations, religious institutions and many others. All of these organizations play a role in working to improve the public's health.

tive community system make informed decisions about health in an environment that respects collaboration, diversity, and the active engagement of its members. In an atmosphere that contributes to and supports health, both society and the community are likely to benefit,

in that citizens are able to participate fully in activities that grow the community.

Establishing and nurturing partnerships within the system creates the collaborative environment necessary to produce health and other societal benefits (Lasker &

🌐 RESEARCH APPLICATION

Building Sustainable Public Health Systems Change at the State Level

Study Purpose

To examine the Turning Point partnership strategies used to sustain public health system improvements.

Methods

This descriptive study included qualitative data collected from primary sources, including Turning Point site visits, online documentation of systems change, and participant input from focus groups, discussions and interviews, during 2001–2003. Secondary data were collected from the National Excellence Collaboratives' and state partner planning and progress reports. Emergent-inductive and theory-directed approaches were used to analyze the data. Analysis was completed by the research team and content experts.

Findings

Turning Point state partnerships used five strategies to sustain program change. Two of those related to the structure of the initiative: institutionalizing goals and activity among state and local government agencies and using nonprofit organizations as the new home for innovative

programs. The other three strategies were found in both types of structure: linking other program funds to Turning Point goals; strengthening strategic relationships; and using creativity to enhance communication and visibility of public health.

Implications

Sustaining the work of a time- or resource-limited activity is a common challenge during periods of fiscal constraint. In addition, multisector partnerships may complicate efforts to foster change within the public health system. Turning Point has provided a solid foundation for system-wide communication and collaboration in many states and localities. By providing a template for Turning Point partner success, the analysis of this initiative has laid the groundwork for replication and evaluation in other communities.

Reference

Padgett, S., Bekemeier, B., & Berkowitz, B. (2005). Building sustainable public health systems change at the state level. *Journal of Public Health Management and Practice, 11*(2), 109–115.

Weiss, 2003; Mays, 2002). The capacity for supporting broad growth in the community is created over time, as communities develop opportunities to work together. The links among partner organizations garner strength during the partnership process. Additionally, effective working relationships foster mutual trust over time (Zahner & Corrado, 2004). Rather than develop connections that come and go as needs are identified, healthy communities find a way to engage citizens and organizations in ongoing and varied ways, so that the strengths of the partnership are maximized as partners work together. In addition to assessing needs, partners also collaborate to develop solutions, implement strategies, and evaluate outcomes (Hausman et al., 2005).

The opportunity for successful collaboration exists at each level of the public health system. At the fed-

eral level, policy directs national priorities and provides funding to collaboratives that may ignite the partnership spark that is present in state and local communities. Perhaps the most influential national initiative today is Healthy People 2010 (Department of Health and Human Services, 2000). Through Healthy People 2010, national health objectives have been identified and leading indicators set to provide direction to the services needed to ensure health.

In addition to Healthy People 2010, national initiatives, such as Turning Point, serve a variety of functions, all of which promote the Essential Public Health Services. This multiorganizational initiative funded by The Robert Wood Johnson and Kellogg Foundations, works to "transform and strengthen the public health system in the United States by making it more community-based and collaborative" (Turning Point, 2005). To that end, Turning Point offers funding and technical assistance to promote systems change by developing and promoting partnerships in the community (Berkowitz & Nicola, 2003). These collaborations link health providers to one another and to other social sector organizations. State and local Turning Point partnerships are founded on the premise that health is a part of the social fabric of our communities, determined by a complex interaction among many factors. To enhance wellness and prevent poor health, therefore, requires an approach that is far broader than a disease prevention model (Turning Point, 2005). The work of initiatives, such as Turning Point, strengthen the public health infrastructure and position state and local communities for current and future collaborative activities, such as those listed in Box 2-4.

Like other successful partnerships, state and local communities that participate in programs such as Turning Point meet goals that are more comprehensive than the goals of any one organization. The partners share power in a balanced, synergistic way so that the organizations benefit individually, as well as collectively, from the arrangement (Lasker & Weiss, 2003). At the state level, involvement mainly takes the form of policy development and technical assistance. Much of Turning Point partner involvement at the local level deals with the day-to-day work of health planning and delivery to provide public health services for the good of the community.

Besides the Turning Point initiative, collaborative efforts such as community-based participatory research (CBPR) and the Healthy Cities Model for Health Promotion have also stimulated community partnerships and engagement. The path to successful collaboration is not always a smooth one because interorganizational priorities may be in conflict with one another. It is through active involvement in CBPR, however, that trust may be enhanced among academic, practice and community members, paving the way for future successful interactions (Box 2-5). Unlike situations where one party identifies a problem or designs research and then seeks out the buy-in of other organizations at a later stage in the process, all CBPR partners take an active role during the entire process (Agency for Healthcare Research and Quality, 2002; 2003). Ownership exists among all participants, ensuring that the work is grounded in reality, that it draws strength from all partners, and that the results are quickly disseminated throughout the community in a way that community members are able to receive the information (Singleton, 2003).

THE CORE PUBLIC HEALTH FUNCTIONS, ESSENTIAL PUBLIC HEALTH SERVICES, AND WORKFORCE COMPETENCY

In addition to its utility at an organizational level, the essential services model serves as a structure for guiding and understanding the practice of the public health workforce. This workforce was defined by the Public Health Functions Project as including "all those providing essential public health services, regardless of the nature of the employing agency" (DHHS,1997). Just as the IOM Report of 1988 changed the direction of public health, its recommendations have had a significant impact on the public health workforce in general, and the nursing profession in particular. This impact may be seen throughout the public health system as organizations and nursing professionals have increased their work around prevention and populations. Nowhere is this more powerful, however, than in the governmental public health sector, where a redirected focus on core functions demanded that public health nursing examine its role.

Much of the public health nursing discussion of its changing role and related competency is a product of the public health workforce conversation. Following the IOM report, the Council on Linkages Between Academia and Public Health Practices (COL) addressed the need to develop a set of core competencies for public health professionals (COL, 2001). The core competencies have implications for education and practice and represent a decade of work among public health stakeholders, including professional organizations, educational institutions, and governmental agencies. This extraordinary effort included the integration of content and behaviors from many source documents, a crosswalk with the Essential Public Health Services, and a review by more than 1,000 health professionals. The resulting consensus set of core competencies is categorized by domain and enumerates knowledge, skills, and attitudes required for public health practice (Box 2-6). The broad transdisciplinary public health focus of the COL competencies was not meant to direct the practice of any one discipline. Public health nursing has used the core competencies for defining public health nursing practice (Quad Council, 2003).

BOX 2-4: THE COLLABORATIVE EFFORTS OF THE TURNING POINT INITIATIVE

Turning Point is based on the commonsense idea that everyone has a stake in public health. Turning Point's underlying philosophy is that public health agencies and their partners can be strengthened by linking to other sectors (not just the private health care sector but education, criminal justice, faith communities, business, and others) because the underlying causes of poor health and quality of life are tied closely to social issues that are too complex to be approached by disease models of intervention.

Turning Point created a network of 23 public health partners across the country to

- Define and assess health, prioritize health issues, and take collective action
- Promote education to decrease the risk of infectious and chronic disease
- Strengthen environmental health services for clean air and water and safe food
- Gain access to health care for everyone
- Improve health status for minority groups

Turning Point brought health-conscious people and organizations to the table to collaborate on improving the public's health. Local-level Turning Point partners collaborated to

- Gather data to get a picture of the health status, resources, values, and priorities of community members
- Develop consensus about priority health issues in their community
- Mobilize local resources to develop action plans to address health priorities
- Develop consensus about priority health issues using a broad definition of healthy communities
- Communicate local needs, priorities, and approaches to elected officials and state agencies to assist in the development of effective health policy

State-level Turning Point partners collaborated to

- Influence good public health policy
- Expand information technology so data are available to local communities for addressing health concerns
- Stimulate state agencies and organizations to develop comprehensive state health plans

Turning Point also formed five National Excellence Collaboratives that worked to:

- Modernize public health statutes
- Create accountable systems to measure performance
- Utilize information technology
- Invest in social marketing
- Develop leadership

SOURCE: Reprinted with the permission of the Turning Point National Program Office.

> **BOX 2-5:** The Path to Overcoming Challenges to Community-Based Participatory Research
>
> - Replace community mistrust of research and researchers with trust.
> - Include typically marginalized populations and organizations as partners.
> - Ensure resource-sharing between and among partners.
> - Develop university incentives to conduct CBPR.
> - Enhance partner knowledge of CBPR process and skill to conduct CBPR.
>
> ---
>
> SOURCE: *Community-Based Participatory Research.* Conference Summary. July 2002. Agency for Healthcare Research and Quality, Rockville, MD. http://www.ahrq.gov/about/cpcr/cbpr/; and *Creating Partnerships, Improving Health: The Role of Community-Based Participatory Research.* June 2003. Agency for Healthcare Research and Quality, Rockville, MD. http://www.ahrq.gov/research/cbprrole.pdf

> **BOX 2-6:** The Eight Domains of Core Competencies for Public Health Professionals
>
> 1. Analysis and assessment
> 2. Policy development and program planning
> 3. Communication
> 4. Cultural competency
> 5. Community dimensions of practice
> 6. Basic public health sciences
> 7. Financial planning and management
> 8. Leadership and systems thinking
>
> ---
>
> SOURCE: Council on Linkages Between Academia and Public Health Practice. (2001). *Core competencies for public health professionals.* Retrieved January 29, 2005, from http://www.trainingfinder.org/competencies/list.htm.

The Public Health Nursing Competencies

The COL work provided a starting point for the development of public health nursing competencies. The Quad Council of Public Health Nursing Organizations took up the task of integrating professional nursing documents and the COL behaviors. The Quad Council, comprised of members from the Public Health Nursing (PHN) Section of the American Public Health Association (APHA), the American Nurses Association (ANA), the Association of State and Territorial Directors of Nursing (ASTDN), and the Association of Community Health Nursing Educators (ACHNE), represents all segments of public health nursing. As the organization was not permitted to change the COL competencies, the Quad Council set its sights on determining how public health nursing would "apply those competencies and the expected level of performance for each competency statement" (Quad Council, 2003, p. 2). The PHN

competencies are limited somewhat by those boundaries, and as a result, they do not include competencies that are discipline specific, that is performed by public health nurses and no other public health professionals.

Public health nurses must recognize that their practice standard is an integration of the Definition of Public Health Nursing (APHA, PHN Section, 1996), the Public Health Nursing Scope and Standards (Quad Council, 1999), and the Core Competencies of Public Health (COL, 2001), as delineated in the PHN competencies. Shaped as well by individual state practice acts and the Code of Ethics for Nurses (ANA, 2001), public health nursing practice was conceptualized by the Quad Council as having two levels of competency (Quad Council, 2003). The generalist level is consistent with expectations of the baccalaureate-prepared nurse, who must possess the broad knowledge, skills, and attitudes of baccalaureate graduates, as well as those specific to public health. These public health nurses are likely to hold a variety of roles in public health, such as working with local community groups and organizations and providing direct services to individuals and families in homes, schools, the workplace, health maintenance organizations, and other ambulatory settings. The PHN acts in each of these instances with the goal of carrying out the essential public health services to advance the health of populations.

Specialist public health nurses are prepared at the masters level in public/community health nursing and/or public health. Like generalist nurses, they may provide direct services or population-focused services. The specialist public health nurse is also involved in program management, as a result of her advanced practice knowledge and skill. Specialist public health nurses are likely to be found in the advanced practice roles of manager, consultant, advocate, clinical nurse specialist, program specialist, educator, or researcher, and in a wide variety of settings (Quad Council, 2003).

Public health nursing has been defined as "the practice of promoting and protecting the health of populations using knowledge from nursing, social and public health sciences" (APHA, PHN Section, 1996, p. 1). Guided by its professional definition, public health nursing's primary focus is advancing population health outcomes through the essential public health services. The tenets of public health nursing (Box 2-7) shed additional light on this professional practice link to populations. With a mission to promote health and prevent disease in entire population groups, this goal may be met through partnership with individuals and families, in addition to practice with populations. It is important to remember that when public health nurses practice with individuals and families, they do so within the framework of population-focused practice (Quad Council, 2003; Porche, 2004). Using the complementary strategies of individual and population practice is a hallmark of public health (Novick, 2001). This focus, and not the setting within which practice takes place, delineates public health nursing from other nursing practice (Ripke et al., 2001; Quad Council, 2003).

Public health nursing has also been described as the "synthesis of the art and science of public health and nursing" (Minnesota Department of Health, Center for Public Health Nursing, 2004, p. 2). Linking the essential elements of both disciplines, the cornerstones of public health nursing (Box 2-8) highlight the unique perspective of public health nursing practice. The accompanying public health intervention model is illustrated in the Minnesota Wheel (Figure 2-5), which integrates the individual, community, and systems-focused levels of population-based practice (Ripke et al., 2001).

BOX 2-7: Principles of Public Health Nursing

1. The client or unit of care is the population.

2. The primary obligation is to achieve the greatest good for the greatest number of people or the population as a whole.

3. The processes used by public health nurses include working with the client as an equal partner.

4. Primary prevention is the priority in selecting appropriate activities.

5. Public health nursing focuses on strategies that create healthy environmental, social, and economic conditions in which populations may thrive.

6. A public health nurse is obligated to actively identify and reach out to all who might benefit from a specific activity or service.

7. Optimal use of available resources to assure the best overall improvement in the health of the population is a key element of the practice.

8. Collaboration with a variety of other professions, populations, organizations, and other stakeholder groups is the most effective way to promote and protect the health of the people.

The Principles of Public Health Nursing set the tone for population-focused practice.

SOURCE: American Nurses Association (2006) *Public Health Nursing: Scope and Standards of Practice.* Silver Spring, MD: Nursesbooks.org.

Public Health Nursing Competency: Setting the Standard for Education and Practice

The PHN competencies, in combination with the other key nursing practice documents, were designed to provide a standard for practice. Some of the practice standards may differ from actual workforce preparation and practice. One of the areas where this is evident is in educational preparation. The Quad Council (2003) has identified baccalaureate preparation as the minimum standard for practice as a public health nurse. Despite this standard, and the fact that both the core

BOX 2-8: The Cornerstones of Public Health Nursing

Public health nursing practice:

- Focuses on entire populations
- Reflects community priorities and needs
- Establishes caring relationships with communities, families, individuals, and systems that comprise the populations PHNs serve
- Is grounded in social justice, compassion, sensitivity to diversity, and respect for the worth of all people, especially the vulnerable
- Encompasses mental, physical, emotional, social, spiritual and environmental aspects of health
- Promotes health through strategies driven by epidemiological evidence
- Collaborates with community resources to achieve those strategies but can and will work alone if necessary
- Derives its authority for independent action from the Nurse Practice Act

SOURCE: Courtesy of Minnesota Department of Health/Office of Public Health Practice.

functions and essential public health services are population-focused, most states do not require baccalaureate preparation for practice (HRSA, 2005). Public health content and a broad physical, biological, and social science base included in baccalaureate nursing programs are critical to the preparation of competent public health nurses. Additionally, skill in the liberal arts, essential for effective communication, is an integral part of baccalaureate programs. If nurses are not prepared at the baccalaureate level, some other mechanism for continuing education must be in place to ensure that PHNs are competent to practice nursing of populations.

In articulating the discrepancy between what should be and the reality of the workforce, the Quad Council identified the vital role of training and continuing education in advancing public health nursing competency (Quad Council, 2003). In their most recent study of the public health workforce, the HRSA/Bureau of Health Professions (2005) acknowledged that, despite the consensus about the need for baccalaureate preparation, there are limited opportunities for public health nurses to obtain the degree through Bachelor of Science in Nursing (BSN) completion and distance learning programs. While some free or low-cost options are available through resources like the Public Health Training Center Network (HRSA, 1998), PHNs may view appropriate preparation as too costly without financial incentives for advanced education. Coupled with noncompetitive salaries in public health, these barriers may pose a significant threat to recruiting competent public health nurses.

Aside from addressing the necessary educational preparation for public health nurses, the Quad Council document provides a roadmap for public health nursing competency by applying the nursing perspective within the COL competency domains. In considering the broad range of public health functions, there are many opportunities within each essential service to examine the impact of professional competency. The Quad Council PHN competency list has identified each level of practice, as well as the individual and family, or population and systems focus. In addition, it has applied the standard of awareness, knowledge or proficiency within each practice category. The Quad Council described the levels of awareness, knowledge and proficiency as operating on a continuum, without specific boundaries between the categories. The Quad Council defined these levels as:

> *Awareness:* a basic level of mastery of the competency. Individuals may be able to identify the concept or skill but have limited ability to perform the skill.

> *Knowledge:* an intermediate level of mastery of the competency. Individuals are able to apply and describe the skill.

> *Proficiency:* an advanced level of mastery of the competency. Individuals are able to synthesize, critique or teach the skill. (Quad Council, 2003, p. 5)

Each of the competency domains (Box 2-6) has relevance for both the generalist and specialist levels of public health nursing practice. Additionally, most of

PUBLIC HEALTH INTERVENTIONS

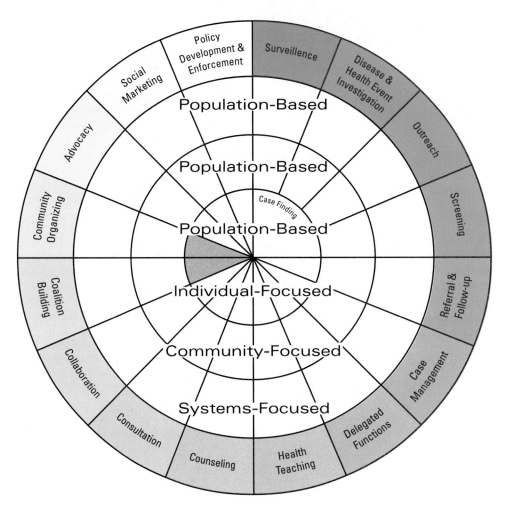

Figure 2-5 The Minnesota Wheel.
From Minnesota Department of Health/Office of Public Health Practice.

the domains can be applied to the populations and systems perspective, as well as the individual and families perspective. The three domains, which can *only* be applied to the populations and systems perspective, are those of community dimensions of practice (domain 5), financial planning and management skills (domain 7), and leadership and systems thinking skills (domain 8). The language of these domains specifically describes a populations or systems focus and is not applicable to public health nursing when it targets individuals and families. The Quad Council also articulated that the "group format" should be considered an extension of the individual and family perspective. This strategy, often used in educational interventions, is really a method of delivering information to individuals or families convened for this purpose. By definition, this individual/family public health nursing experience takes place within the context of an overall population focus, but the target is the individual, not the population (Quad Council, 2003).

⊕ PRACTICE APPLICATION

Engaging the Community to Identify Public Health Priorities: The Community Environmental Health Assessment

Arlington County, Virginia, an urban community of 190,000 people, served as one of 10 pilot sites for the National Association of County and City Health Officials (NAC-CHO)/National Center for Environmental Health (CDC) project, Protocol for Assessing Community Excellence in Environmental Health (PACE-EH). Designed to use a community collaborative approach, the Arlington team viewed the PACE-EH process as an opportunity to improve the environmental health status of the community. A steering committee was formed to guide the process. Members included state and local experts in environmental and public health, university, business, and citizen partners. Surveys were developed by the committee, piloted, and distributed among community groups, representing county residents by zip code, and education, as well as race and ethnicity. Existing groups, particularly those who did not ordinarily participate in the community comment process, were used. Among the groups chosen were civic associations, the Animal Welfare League, WIC program participants, a weight-lifting club for teens, a substance abuse treatment program, the Arlington Free Clinic and local jury pools. Participants chose environmental health concerns from among a list of 17 categories. Available morbidity and mortality data were analyzed, in addition to ambient air quality and radon levels. Scientific data were juxtaposed with survey results, and environmental health priorities were set. The top four priorities formed the basis for the county environmental health action plan. The assessment served as a means to build a constituency for environmental health; share power among community members, some of whom had a limited voice in the policy process; and match resources to needs identified by the community. Challenges during the process included time constraints, balancing the scientific view and public perceptions, and dealing with the occurrence of a well-published environmental issue during data collection.

SOURCES:

Matthews, J., & Downing, D. (2000). Community environmental health assessment: A strategy for public health policy. Presented at the International Academic Nursing Congress, Fairfax, VA.

NACCHO. (2002). PACE EH in practice: A compendium of 10 pilot communities. Retrieved July 20, 2006, from http://www.pace.naccho.org/Demonstration-Report/Arlington-Department-of-Human-Services.pdf.

Making the Connections: Linking the Core Functions, Essential Services, and Public Health Nursing Competencies

The core public health functions and essential services provide the public health system, its public health agencies and partners, with a framework for the planning, implementation, and evaluation of public health in the United States. In addition, public health professional competencies have been structured to fit within this framework. Understanding the connections between and among these component parts is integral to examining the role of the public health nurse within the public health system.

Assessment

As illustrated in Figure 2-3, each of the essential services has a primary connection with one of the core public health functions. The essential public health services, in conjunction with the public health nursing competencies, provide direction to public health nursing practice. In carrying out the assessment core function, the public health nurse incorporates a variety of competency domains to identify, diagnose, and investigate health problems and hazards in the community (essential services 1 and 2). Relying on advanced practice skills, the specialist public health nurse engages transdisciplinary and community partners in a collaborative relationship, setting the stage for determining community strengths, needs, and resources (community dimensions domain).

This partnership framework values the diversity of people and talent available in all communities. By tapping into this resource, partners bring to the table complementary strengths, which facilitate the participative environment conducive to creative and effective problem solving.

Communication skills are a critical part of the assessment process, as the nurse promotes communication methods that enable full participation by all partners (communication domain). Knowledgeable about the varied ways in which people learn, public health nurses play a key role in interpreting the technical and health information that is often part of the assessment process. Lastly, the attitude of the nurse toward the contributions of all partners is a critical element of communication that may facilitate or impede the ability of diverse groups to engage in the assessment process.

The specialist may contribute to the assessment function by providing leadership as the community assessment is designed and conducted or by serving as a content expert in the analysis of available data (analytic and basic public health domains). In both circumstances, the public health nurse works with the partnership to facilitate assessment and analysis. Subsequently, partners set community priorities (policy development/program planning domain), laying the foundation for a systems approach to meeting community needs. Mastery of data collection methods and issues, as well as knowledge of ethical principles, social justice, community culture, and the political environment serve to inform the methods used in community assessment (cultural domain). Depending on the strengths of the participants, the PHN may play a role as member and facilitator or take a more active role as leader. In addition, during the assessment process, the specialist mentors the generalist public health nurse, whose skill in defining population and systems problems is less well developed. With a basic awareness of community assessment strategies, the generalist gains experience, as the specialist models competent public health nursing practice that is population-focused. Although less experienced in population-focused practice, the generalist is proficient in defining problems at the individual and family level (analytic domain). With the help of the specialist, the generalist public health nurse will develop an understanding of the relationship between the individual/family problems and population health (leadership/systems thinking domain).

Policy Development

Policy development, as a core public health function, involves many primary roles of the public health nurse at the specialist and generalist levels. Incorporating three essential public health services, this function directs many day-to-day activities of public health agencies. As an advocate for the community, the nurse works tirelessly to educate and empower people about health issues (essential service #3). From assisting partners in the framing of a health issue to facilitating skill development in communication and advocacy, the specialist public health nurse serves as leader, and the generalist as participant, in policy development. Knowing how a wide range of determinants influences health (basic public health; analytic/assessment domains), the nurse presents information accurately and in a form that enables all partners to receive it in a meaningful way. The inherent complexity of this information may challenge the health literacy of some partners, whereas others may be comfortable with the use of more complicated terminology and concepts. The public health nurse uses knowledge of health communication skills to provide culturally, linguistically, and conceptually appropriate information to the partnership, as well as the community at large (Potter & Martin, 2003; Singleton, 2003). The nurse also uses advocacy skills when encouraging and facilitating the use of clear communication (Pfizer, 2003; cultural competency; communication domains).

Integral to health promotion and protection in the community, policy development includes a nursing role in mobilizing community partnerships (essential service #4). Using team building and negotiation skills, the public health nurse supports the effectiveness of community partnerships (community dimensions). The nurse's knowledge and skill in navigating the policy process facilitate linkages among policy makers and community partners (leadership/systems thinking; policy development). The specialist public health nurse assists the community in defining the impact of policy on health (financial planning/management) and then works with partners to develop a relevant action plan for the community (policy development). Using knowledge of change theory, the specialist educates the generalist public health nurse and empowers community partners to affect change in the community. Such linkages are fundamental to partners being able to communicate information to key policy makers, media, and other influential stakeholders, another step in developing policies that support efforts to promote and protect health (essential service #5).

Assurance

The core function of assurance integrates four essential public health services and provides a significant role for both specialist and generalist public health nurses. Key players in assurance, public health nurses are critical to the enforcement of laws and regulations that protect health and ensure safety in the community (essential service #6). Implementing the policy development and program planning domain, the nurse interprets public health law for community partners and engages collaborators in implementing public health regulations. For example, the public health nurse ensures that children are immunized prior to beginning school, promoting compliance with state law. Required immunization schedules are shared with parents, as well as information about where immunizations can be obtained, facilitating linkages with needed services (essential service #7). Public health nursing knowledge of cultural practices provides the foundation for assisting parents and school staff to understand the relevance of public health regulations and their role in safeguarding the children and the school community (cultural competency and communication). If the nurse has worked effectively with this community from the outset, the process results in a culture that supports standards for health within the school community (leadership/systems thinking domain).

In addition to linking the community with services, the public health nurse may assist in the process of establishing services that are needed, yet are unavailable or inaccessible. Collaboration during the assessment and policy processes lays the groundwork for this activity, where the specialist public health nurse is a key player. Assuming a leadership role, the specialist public health nurse works with partners to convene a forum, addressing the issue of access to services (communication; community dimensions). With knowledge of systems level resources, quality measures/indicators, key stakeholders, strategic planning, and the change process, the specialist nurse may serve as facilitator or content expert during the process (financial planning/management; leadership/ systems thinking domains). As coach to the generalist nurse during the community forum, knowledge

and skills are shared, and the generalist public health nurse learns and practices a new role, expanding her skill set, and in time, developing competency in this area (Porter & Baker, 2004).

Strategies at the local public health system level, like those involving the educational and developmental collaboration between the specialist and generalist public health nurses, are important components of assuring a competent public health workforce (essential service #8). Recognizing that meeting health needs of the community requires specialized skills, the public health nurse participates in organizational committees to identify needed workforce skills and assists in procuring the expertise to develop the skills within the workforce (analytic and leadership/systems thinking domains). Specialist mentoring of the generalist nurse may include facilitating involvement in organizational activities, such as the quality improvement committee, research activities, journal clubs, and participation in organizational recruitment and retention activities to assure a diverse and competent workforce. It is imperative that the PHN recognizes that these functions, as well as those previously discussed, may occur between and among segments of the public health system.

A crucial element of assurance is that of evaluation (essential service #9). Public health nurses actively participate in the ongoing evaluation of service delivery through monitoring of data at both the organizational and community levels (analytic and policy/program planning). Evaluating the quality of an organization's disease control program, for example, is relevant to PHN practice within and across settings. The specialist nurse may serve as a leader in the evaluation process, from design of organizational tools to the effective analysis of community-wide health data. All public health nurses, however, must have at least a knowledge-level competency in collecting and analyzing data for evaluation, an integral component of determining the need and value of health services delivery.

Besides the actual mechanics of the evaluation process, nurses at both levels serve as a vital link between the data and the community. To the extent possible, the public health nurse engages community partners in the development of evaluation measures, as well as the collection, analysis, and interpretation of data. Partner involvement is essential to ensuring representation of community groups in the decision-making process. Additional concerns about cultural, linguistic, and conceptual appropriateness of instruments, methods, and

⊕ POLICY HIGHLIGHT

Strengthening the Public Health Infrastructure—The Public Health Security and Bioterrorism Preparedness and Response Act (PL 107-188)

Signed into law in June 2002, the law directs the Secretary of Health and Human Services to "further develop and implement a coordinated strategy, building on core public health capabilities . . . for carrying out health-related activities to prepare for and respond effectively to bioterrorism and other public health emergencies," and to ensure that these activities are coordinated with state and local governments. The law also established the Strategic National Stockpile (SNS) of drugs, vaccines, biologicals, and other supplies to be available in case of a bioterrorism attack or other public health emergency. Additionally, federal funds would be directed to states for developing state and community-wide public health emergency plans, conducting exercises to test the plans, providing workforce training, overseeing surveillance and response activities, providing control over biological agents, and making available enhanced protection of the drug, food, and water supply.

Public Health Security and Bioterrorism Preparedness and Response Act of 2002, P. L. 107-188, 116 Stat. 595 (2002). Retrieved March 24, 2006, from http://frwebgate.access .gpo.gov/cgi-bin/getdoc.cgi?dbname=107_cong_public_ laws&docid=f:pub/188.107.pdf.

interpretation are best answered by the partnership. Execution of the evaluation may be enhanced through outside funding. Securing and managing outside funding is another initiative where the nurse and community collaborate for a more effective result (financial planning and management).

Evaluation and Partnership

While community partners develop project-appropriate assessment and evaluation tools, the public health system of the local community may be evaluated by using the framework and tools of the National Public Health Performance Standards Program (NPHPSP; CDC, 2006). This national initiative was developed to promote and evaluate public health system quality, at both state and local levels (Box 2-9). Designed around the framework of the Essential Public Health Services, systems use specific state and local instruments to assess optimum performance according to model standards. As a key player in both the local public health agency and the community partnership, the specialist public health nurse may initiate and facilitate use of this partnership-focused tool (leadership/systems thinking). Identification of steering committee members to guide the process is an essential element during the early phases of evaluation. Since the PHN has worked closely with community partners, this is likely to be viewed as an extension of community work. Community partners meet and come to consensus about whether and how the system has met the essential service. A significant time commitment is needed, as estimates suggest that 1.5–2 hours is likely for the assessment of each essential public health service (CDC, 2006). Specific guidance is available to the group and will assist in moving the process from start to finish. Data are submitted electronically, and analysis is completed by CDC program support. Once results of the evaluation data are obtained, the nurse communicates findings to the partners, assisting with the discussion of system performance improvement (communication; cultural competency). Challenges and opportunities are addressed, and the partners develop an action plan to guide their systems improvement activities.

The final essential service, research to address new ways of looking at and solving public health problems, is intrinsically linked to all of the core public health functions. With methodological expertise and knowledge of how the community works, the specialist public health nurse, with the generalist nurse as partner, is in a strong position to assist the community in identifying appropriate research questions (analytic/assessment domain). University collaborations provide additional expertise to the local system, facilitating the development of a strong and relevant partnership for research innovation, conduct, and application of findings (community dimensions; basic public health science). The

BOX 2-9: National Public Health Performance Standards Program

Vision:

Excellence in public health practice defined by recognized performance standards.

Mission:

To improve the quality of public health practice and performance of public health systems.

Goals:

- Provide performance standards for public health systems and encouraging their widespread use.
- Encourage and leverage national, state, and local partnerships to build a stronger foundation for public health preparedness.
- Promote continuous quality improvement of public health systems.
- Strengthen the science base for public health practice improvement.

SOURCE: Centers for Disease Control and Prevention. (2006). *National Public Health Performance Standards Program User Guide.* Retrieved July 20, 2006, from http://www.cdc.gov/od/ocphp/nphpsp/Documents/NPHPSuserguide.pdf.

securing of outside resources for the research provides an opportunity to fund community partners to attend and participate in local, state, and national dissemination conferences. Additionally, through participation in this scientific process, the generalist public health nurse will develop knowledge of the application of research to practice, as well as experience in preparing research findings for dissemination (analytic/assessment and communication domains).

Ultimately, the core function of assurance is concerned with whether or not health needs are being met. The process requires that continuous assessment and evaluation is on target and that resources are directed to meet the needs of the community. Where a broad-based health determinant framework, such as the eco-logical model, is used, the resources may be any that contribute to the community environment supportive of health. Depending on the specific needs identified, educational, political, economic, social, behavioral, or traditional health services may be required. When the public health nurse and community partners share this broad vision of health, the foundation for a successful collaboration is likely to be established. Moreover, community partners engaged in this effort are positioned to work together to arrive at a solution. Complementary skills of community participants may enhance the ability of all to contribute in a substantive way. It is the strength of such partnerships that serve the community well over time, assuring the process of promoting and protecting the public's health.

CHALLENGES TO ADVANCING THE PUBLIC'S HEALTH THROUGH IMPROVING THE PUBLIC HEALTH INFRASTRUCTURE

Even though effective partnerships within the public health system set the stage for meeting community needs, challenges to the advancement of public health prevail. Not surprisingly, many of the challenges relate to the issue of resources and the infrastructure, the roads and bridges of the public health system. CDC's conceptualization of the core public health infrastructure contains the three components of information/communication capacity, workforce capacity and organizational/systems capacity (CDC, 2001a). We have made progress in each of the three elements, but much work remains.

Information/Communication Systems Capacity

In considering **information/communication systems capacity**, the Public Health Data Standards Consortium (PHDSC; 2004), the CDC, and others have identified the potential of data standards and electronic mechanisms in surveillance, reporting, and partner communication through broadcast facsimile and other means to enhance public health system effectiveness through collecting, monitoring, and reporting health data (CDC, 2006; Gostin, Hodge, & Valdiserri, 2001). CDC's (2002) own Health Alert Network (HAN) and National Electronic Disease Surveillance System (NEDSS) serve

⊕ PRACTICE APPLICATION

Practice Strategies to Build Capacity in Public Health: The Epi Response Team

The Washington, D.C., National Capital Region conducted a variety of emergency preparedness activities as part of the 2001 Presidential Inauguration. Public Health Nurses (PHN) from the Communicable Disease Bureau, Arlington County Department of Human Services, Public Health Division (PHD) examined the chief complaint logs in local hospital emergency rooms to detect unusual syndromes that might identify emerging health problems in the community. A 365-day/year activity, the syndromic surveillance became a challenge for the small staff and a core of division PHNs. When other public health events, such as the anthrax crisis and response of November 2001, the Mock Smallpox Clinic to test the CDC model, and the PHD employee Smallpox Immunization Clinic demanded attention, new strategies were developed. As a result, the DHS Epi Response Team was created. The PHD emergency planner and epidemiologist put out a call for nurses throughout the

department to support their peers and participate in this ready-response group. Many answered this call to action. Over time, the interdisciplinary team has grown to nearly 70 employees, both managers and staff, from three departmental divisions, as well as the Employee Assistance Program. Staff members were used to participating in interdivisional meetings, but functional activities that crossed division lines were unusual. The Epi Team, now known as the Public Health Response Team, provided a model for this collaboration. The team has responded to a number of challenges to the health and safety of the Arlington community and continues to meet monthly for training. With a broad range of skills, members are prepared to respond to local public health emergencies, a successful example of one local agency's efforts to build capacity in public health.

as examples of electronic communication systems that have been used to enhance real time public health information data collection and dissemination. There is more to be done in this area, however, as wide variations are found in capacity among national, state, and local systems.

While the nation is establishing effective means of information management, Public Health Nursing is engaged in the related activity of identifying a standardized means of describing population-focused practice, consistent with other nursing practice classification systems (APHA, PHN Section 2005a). If we are to attain health goals throughout the public health system, we must have a useful set of information standards, data-sharing capability that protects confidentiality and privacy, and a public health vocabulary to show how practice, in concert with our public health and community partners, advances both core functions and essential public health services.

Workforce Capacity

Another challenge to meeting Healthy People 2010 goals through the core functions and essential services

is that of workforce capacity. Capacity includes not only the size of the workforce but also its competency. Part of the challenge of the workforce issue is determining how to measure these variables. National efforts have measured both overall public health and public health nursing workforce size, but questions remain about the adequacy of these measurements (Gebbie, 2002; Gebbie et al., 2003; Baker et al., 2005; HRSA 2000, 2005). As we continue to face a widespread nursing shortage, we must address issues of capacity in public health. Public health has been successful in its ability to retain nurses who choose this specialty, but evidence points out that PHN positions still go unfilled, that they are converted from nursing to other positions, and that PHNs may not be adequately prepared for the practice challenges of the twenty-first century (Quad Council, 2001; Greiner and Oppewal, 2003; IOM, 2003c). Though baccalaureate preparation remains the standard, it is unlikely that, in the short term, we will be able to meet this target. It is imperative, then, that states and localities with a high proportion of nonbaccalaureate programs and graduates collaborate with academic, Public Health Training Center, and practice partners to make available appropriate on-

BOX 2-10: Activities to Reduce the Public Health Nursing Shortage

- Identifying ways to make salaries in public health agencies more competitive with those for nurses with comparable preparation in other settings;

- Assuring that all faculty teaching in baccalaureate programs understand the concepts of population-focused care and their importance for the nursing curriculum as a whole;

- Improving the benefits package for PHNs, including increased annual leave, employer paid insurance, educational benefits, reimbursement of relocation expenses, etc.

- Finding ways to assure that baccalaureate nursing programs, in collaboration with public health agencies, provide students with realistic, positive clinical experiences in public health nursing;

- Assuring that faculty who teach public health nursing content and supervise clinical practice for students in this area have current expertise in the field;

- Identifying ways of providing greater incentives to PHNs to return to school to pursue a BSN and providing flexible and creative options for accessing baccalaureate nursing education for both initial education and degree completion students;

- Actively recruiting men and women from traditionally underserved populations into nursing and then public health nursing so that the workforce and service provision more closely matches the needs of the populations served by public health nurses;

- Creating rewards and incentives for those who come into public health nursing with a baccalaureate degree or who achieve this educational level while employed, including options for significant career mobility within the practice;

- Creating options for PHN employment such as job sharing, home-basing, joint appointments, faculty practice, etc. which are attractive to the population of current PHNs;

- Including service in a public health agency as a way to achieve "debt forgiveness" of loans accrued in pursuit of baccalaureate nursing education;

- Working with groups that collect data on the nursing and public health workforce to obtain data on retention of public health nurses;

- Establishing an internship program in public health nursing to provide for a better transition from education to practice; and

- Capitalizing on the autonomy of public health nursing as a way of recruiting young people into nursing and then into public health.

SOURCE: Quad Council. (2001). The impact of the nursing shortage on public health nursing. Retrieved January 29, 2005. from http://www.astdn.org/publication_impact_nursing_shortage.htm.

site and distance-learning opportunities for training in public health competencies (IOM, 2003c).

If left unchecked, significant nursing shortages in all sectors of the public health system threaten the health and safety of the nation. Innovative employment strategies and position structuring may engage nurses who are unable or not interested in holding traditional full-time positions (Box 2-10). Opportunities to share a full-time position, where nurses also share in the benefit package, may appeal to those with family or other responsibilities, including nurses enrolled in baccalaureate and masters program. The ability to work from a home base, or to combine a practice appointment with that at a university, may encourage masters and doctorally prepared profes-

sionals to continue in a practice setting. Enhanced funding of baccalaureate, masters, and doctoral programs is essential if the expertise of public health nursing is to grow. Additionally, continuing education initiatives must be used for current and future PHN workforce to ensure that PHN competencies are met (Spears & Richmond, 2002). Both broad and targeted recruitment strategies are also critical to meet the diverse workforce needs of a public health system that expects and encourages partnerships within diverse communities (IOM, 2003a; COL, 2005). Lastly, the evidence base is critical to assist in determining and evaluating adequate workforce capacity, the effectiveness of recruitment and retention strategies, and the impact of public health competencies on improving health status (CDC, 2001b; Gebbie, 2002; Beaulieu, Scutchfield, & Kelly, 2003; Lichtveld & Cioffi, 2003; Cioffi, Lichtveld, & Tilson, 2004; Mays, Halverson, & Scutchfield, 2003).

Organizational and Systems Capacity

In addition to information and workforce strength, it is essential that the public health system develop organizational and systems capacity to move communities toward improved health through the essential services. Since the September 11 attacks, emergency preparedness activities have remained a constant throughout communities. Actual and potential threats to safety and health have raised awareness of the need for ongoing communication and collaboration, as well as the need to find new ways to build capacity. National efforts, such as Project Public Health Ready, provide structure and support for localities to enhance both workforce and organizational capacity (NACCHO, 2005). Organizational and community concerns that preparedness functions may draw the workforce away from other essential activities exist. In many local public health agencies, the same employees are used for day-to-day operations and emergency planning and response. With developing concerns about a potential flu pandemic, the same staff members participate in planning for a possible pandemic, a very labor-intensive activity. Estimates that 25–50% of the health care workforce will be ill as a result of pandemic flu illustrate the future challenge, if the pandemic materializes (Trust for America's Health, 2005). Government must find a way to enhance capacity in creative ways, such as developing volunteer resources to assist during a crisis (Arlington County Department of Human Services, Public Health Division, 2005). While the local public health agency uses work in preparedness as a means to strengthen partnerships among local organizations, a way must be found to use the funding streams and activities to shore up the overall public health system.

In addition to meeting the challenges of preparedness, organizational capacity is affected by the lack of adequate funding for public health services, particularly at the population level. It has been said that the "common good of a solid public health infrastructure depends on sustained consistent Federal, State, and local investments" (CDC, 2001b). For example, as rates of TB declined in the mid-1980s, funds for TB also declined, reducing capacity for prevention (Simone & Poppe, 2000). It wasn't until 1992, in the face of escalating TB rates and multidrug-resistant TB that funds for TB increased substantially. It has been estimated that the cost of inadequate control of TB in New York City alone was more than $1 billion (IOM, 2000). Clearly, the costs of inadequate public health are far too great to bear. Shortsighted funding decisions and program-specific funding streams impede allocation for broad core functions (IOM, 2003b). Local and state public health agency workforce placement decisions are likely to be made according to categorical funding priorities, and services have been found to be particularly sensitive to local spending levels (Mays et al., 2004). Any funding changes may add significantly to the administrative burden of shifting and tracking workforce activities. Innovative approaches to funding must be developed that move organizations from thinking and acting in silos to a systems approach to public health (Public Health Foundation, 2003). Finally, organizations must meet the leadership challenge by developing capacity through such programs as the National Public Health Leadership Developmental Network, extending organizational capacity by reconceptualizing the boundaries of the organization through community collaboration and assessing effectiveness through programs such as the National Public Health Performance Standards (Wright et al., 2000; Mays et al., 2004). In times such as today, where fiscal and human resources are strained, the challenges are great. Judicious use of the resources must occur if public health nurses are to make a difference in the health of the public.

CRITICAL THINKING ACTIVITIES

1. How would you decide if the organizations in your community work together as a public health system? How would you identify what untapped resources could be mobilized to enhance the community's health status?

2. How would using the ecological model of health shape your approach to assuring the conditions in which people can be healthy?

3. Your agency has received $50,000 from a local philanthropic group to fund a teen clinic. How will you decide what services to provide? What process will you use?

4. While studying for an exam, a student peer questions the value of the core public health functions, which he thinks are too broad to be useful to public health nurses. How will you respond?

5. In a time of constrained resources, how will you justify the resources needed to develop and sustain community partnerships within the public health system?

6. A community liaison to the state legislature is meeting with your state delegate to discuss health issues and has asked you to develop talking points about the public health nursing shortage in your state. He would also like you to include potential solutions in your points. What will you address and why?

KEY TERMS

assessment

assurance

core competencies

core functions of public health

ecological model

essential public health services

health services pyramid

information/communication systems capacity

organizational and systems capacity

policy development

public health nursing competencies

workforce capacity

KEY CONCEPTS

- The 1988 IOM Report, *The Future of Public Health*, provided the impetus to reexamine and reorganize the vision, mission, and goals of public health.

- The ecological model of health, a broad framework of multiple and varied health determinants, provides a means for understanding public health's mission of assuring conditions in which people can be healthy.

- The core public health functions serve as a template for federal, state, and local public health agencies.

- The assessment function incorporates the regular and systematic collection, analysis, and communication of data about the health of the community.

- Policy development uses assessment data to make community decisions that promote and protect health.

- Public health supports the assurance function by providing, facilitating, or funding essential public health services.

- The health services pyramid illustrates the relationship among population-based public health services and primary, secondary, and tertiary health care. Public health services form the strong foundation upon which the other types of health care rest.

- The federal government promotes public health through its authority to levy and spend taxes and to regulate interstate commerce.

- The state is the governmental body with primary responsibility for the health and welfare of citizens.

- Most public health services are delivered by local public health agencies.

- The 10 essential public health services are linked to the core functions and provide a framework for understanding the role of the public health system in promoting health.

- Community partners are critical to meeting complex health needs of local, state, and national communities.

- Effective strategies, such as community-based participatory research, engage partners in all phases of community assessment, planning, implementation, and evaluation.

KEY CONCEPTS (CONT'D)

- The public health nursing competencies detail the awareness of, knowledge about and proficiency in the eight core domains that help shape public health practice. They demonstrate the intersection of public health and nursing practice, are applicable to population/systems or individual/family as the recipient of service, and provide a framework for understanding population-focused nursing practice.

- The primary goal of public health nursing practice is advancing population health outcomes through the essential public health services.

- The population focus is what differentiates public health nursing from other nursing practice specialties.

- Infrastructure capacity presents a significant challenge to effectively meeting the goals of Public Health in America.

REFERENCES

Agency for Healthcare Research and Quality. (2002). *Community-based participatory research*. Conference summary. Retrieved January 29, 2005, from http://www.ahrq.gov/about/cpcr/cbpr/.

Agency for Healthcare Research and Quality. (2003). *Creating partnerships, improving health: The role of community-based participatory research*. Retrieved February 23, 2005, from http://www.ahrq.gov/research/cbprrole.pdf.

American Nurses Association (2006) *Public Health Nursing: Scope and Standards of Practice*. Silver Spring, MD: Nursesbooks.org.

American Nurses Association. (2001). *Code of ethics for nurses with interpretive statements*. Washington, DC: Author.

American Public Health Association, Public Health Nursing Section. (1996). *The definition and role of public health nursing: A statement of APHA Public Health Nursing Section*. Washington, DC: APHA.

American Public Health Association, Public Health Nursing Section (2005). *Annual spring meeting minutes*. February.

American Public Health Association. (2005). *The essential services of public health*. Retrieved January 29, 2005, from http://www.apha.org/ppp/science/10ES.htm#bkgrnd.

Arlington County Department of Human Services, Public Health Division. (2005). *Arlington County Public Health Volunteer Management System*. Retrieved July 20, 2006, from http://www.gwu.edu/~icdrm/projects/VMS/index.htm.

Baker, E., Potter, M., Jones, D., Mercer, S., Cioffi, J., Green, L., Halverson, P., Lichtveld, M., & Fleming, D. (2005). The public health infrastructure and our nation's health. *Annual Review of Public Health, 26*, 303–318.

Beaulieu, J., Scutchfield, F.D., & Kelly, A. (2003). Recommendations from testing of the National Public Health Performance Standards instruments. *Journal of Public Health Management and Practice, 9*(3), 188–198.

Berkowitz, B., & Nicola, R. (2003). Public health infrastructure system change: Outcomes from the Turning Point initiative. *Journal of Public Health Management and Practice, 9*(3), 224–227.

Centers for Disease Control and Prevention. (1999). Ten great public health achievements—United States, 1900–1999. *Morbidity and Mortality Weekly Report, 48*, 241–243.

Centers for Disease Control and Prevention. (2001a). *Public health's infrastructure: A status report*. Prepared for the Appropriations Committee of the United States Senate. Retrieved January 29, 2005, from http://www.phppo.cdc.gov/documents/phireport2_16.pdf

Centers for Disease Control and Prevention. (2001b). *Public health workforce development implementation plan. A global life-long learning system: Building a stronger frontline against health threats, phase I*. Washington, DC: author.

Centers for Disease Control and Prevention. (2002). *Health Alert Network*. Retrieved April 7, 2005, from http://www.phppo.cdc.gov/han.

Centers for Disease Control and Prevention. (2006). *National Public Health Performance Standards Program User Guide*. Retrieved July 20, 2006, from http://www.cdc.gov/od/ocphp/nphpsp/Documents/NPHPSuserguide.pdf.

Cioffi, J., Lichtveld, M., & Tilson, H. (2004). A research agenda for public health workforce development. *Journal of Public Health Management and Practice, 10*(3), 186–192.

Council on Linkages Between Academia and Public Health Practice. (2001). *Core competencies for public health pro-*

fessionals. Retrieved January 29, 2005, from http://www
.trainingfinder.org/competencies/list.htm.

Council on Linkages Between Academia and Public Health
Practice. (2005). *Evidence-based forum on effective recruitment and retention.* Retrieved February 16, 2005, from
http://www.phf.org/Link/forum_background012505.pdf.

Department of Health and Human Services, Public Health
Service. (1997). *Public health workforce: An agenda for the
21st century. A report of the Public Health Functions Project.* Retrieved January 29, 2005, from http://www.health
.gov/phfunctions/pubhlth.pdf.

Department of Health and Human Services. (2000). *Healthy
people 2010: Understanding and improving health.* Washington, DC: author.

Fallon, L.F., & Zgodzinski, E. (2005). History of public
health. In L.F. Fallon & E. Zgodzinski (Eds.), *Essentials of
public health management* (pp. 7–17). Sudbury, MA:
Jones and Bartlett.

Gebbie, K. (2002). Holding society and nursing together.
American Journal of Nursing, 102(9), 73.

Gebbie, K., Merrill, J., Hwang, I., Gebbie, E., Gupta, M.
(2003). The public health workforce in the year 2000.
*Journal of Public Health Management and Practice,
9*(1), 79–86.

Gostin, L. (2000). Public health law in a new century: Part II:
Public health powers and limits. *Journal of the American
Medical Association, 283*(22), 2979–2984.

Gostin, L. Hodge, J., & Valdiserri, R. (2001). Informational
privacy and the public's health: The Model State Public
Health Privacy Act. *American Journal of Public Health,
91*(9), 1388–1392.

Greiner, P., & Oppewal, S. (2003). *Testimony before the Institute of Medicine Committee on the Work Environment for
Nurses and Patient Safety.* Retrieved on April 7, 2005, from
http://www.csuchico.edu/~horst/about/shortage.html#A.

Hajat, A., Brown, C., & Fraser, M. (2001). *LPHA infrastructure. A chartbook.* Retrieved February 1, 2005, from
http://archive.naccho.org/documents/chartbook_
programs18-48.pdf.

Hausman, A., Brawer, R., Becker, J., Foster-Drain, D., Sudler,
C., Wilcox, R., & Terry, B. (2005). The value template
process: A participatory evaluation method for community
health partnerships. *Journal of Public Health Management
and Practice, 11*(1), 65–71.

Health Resources and Services Administration, Bureau of
Health Professions. (1998). *Public Health Training
Centers.* Retrieved on April 7, 2005, from http://bhpr
.hrsa.gov/publichealth/phtc.htm.

Health Resources and Services Administration, Bureau of
Health Professions. (2000). *The registered nurse population. Findings from the national sample survey of registered
nurses.* Washington, DC: author.

Health Resources and Services Administration, Bureau of
Health Professions. (2005). *Public health workforce.* Washington, DC: author.

Institute of Medicine. (1988). *The future of public health.*
Washington, DC: National Academy Press.

Institute of Medicine. (2000). *Ending neglect: The elimination
of tuberculosis in the United States.* Washington, DC:
National Academy Press.

Institute of Medicine. (2003a). *In the nation's compelling
interest: Ensuring diversity in the health care workforce.*
Washington, DC: National Academies Press.

Institute of Medicine. (2003b). *The future of the public's health.*
Washington, DC: National Academies Press.

Institute of Medicine. (2003c). *Who will keep the public
healthy? Educating public health professionals for the 21st
century.* Washington, DC: National Academies Press.

Lasker, R., & Weiss, E. (2003). Broadening participation in
community problem-solving: A multidisciplinary model
to support collaborative practice and research. *Journal of
Urban Health, 80*(1), 14–47. Retrieved January 29, 2005,
from http://www.cacsh.org/pdf/modelpaper.pdf.

Lichtveld, M., & Cioffi, J. (2003). Public health workforce
development: Progress, challenges, and opportunities.
Journal of Public Health Management and Practice, 9(6),
443–450.

Matthews, J.A., & Downing, D.V. (2000). *Community environmental health assessment: A strategy for public health
policy.* Presented at the International Academic Nursing
Congress, Fairfax, VA.

Mays, G. (2002). From collaboration to coevolution: New
structures for public health improvement. *Journal of Public
Health Management and Practice, 8*(1), 95–97.

Mays, G., Halverson, P., & Scutchfield, F.D. (2003). Behind
the curve? What we know and need to learn from public
health systems research. *Journal of Public Health Management and Practice, 9*(3), 79–82.

Mays, G., Halverson, P., Baker, E., & Stevens, R. (2004).
Availability and perceived effectiveness of public health
activities in the nation's most populous communities.
Journal of Public Health Management and Practice, 94(6),
1019–1026.

Mays, G., McHugh, M., Shirin, K., Lenaway, D., Halverson,
P., Moonesinghe, R., & Honore, L. (2004). Getting what
you pay for: Public health spending and the performance
of essential public health services. *Journal of Public Health
Management and Practice, 10*(5), 435–443.

Minnesota Department of Health, Center for Public Health Nursing. (2004). Cornerstones of Public Health Nursing, Retrieved July 20, 2006, from http://www.health.state.mn.us/divs/cfh/ophp.resources/docs/cornerstones_definition_revised2004.pdf.

National Association of County and City Health Officials. (2002). *PACE EH in practice: A compendium of 10 pilot communities.* Retrieved July 20, 2006, from http://pace.naccho.org/Demonstration-Report/Arlington-Department-of-Human-Services.pdf.

National Association of County and City Health Officials. (2005). *Project Public Health Ready.* Retrieved July 20, 2006, from http://www.naccho.org/topics/emergency/documents/PPHRFactSheetDecember2005Final.pdf.

Nelson, J., Essien, J., Loudermilk, R., & Cohen, D. (2002). *The public health competency handbook.* Atlanta: Affiliated Graphics /KITS.

Novick, L. (2001). Defining public health. In L. Novick & G. Mays (Eds.), *Public health administration: Principles for population-based management* (pp. 83–91). Gaithersburg, MD: Aspen.

Padgett, S., Bekemeier, B., & Berkowitz, B. (2005). Building sustainable public health systems change at the state level. *Journal of Public Health Management and Practice, 11*(2), 109–115.

Pfizer (2003). *Clear Health Communication Initiative.* New York: author.

Porche, D. (2004). *Public and community health nursing practice. A population-based approach.* Thousand Oaks, CA: Sage Publications.

Porter, J., & Baker, E. (2004). The coach in you. *Journal of Public Health Management and Practice, 10*(5), 472–474.

Potter, L., & Martin, C. (2003). *Health communication and cultural diversity.* Fact sheet. Retrieved January 29, 2005, from http://www.chcs.org/usr_doc/FS8.pdf.

Public Health Data Standards Consortium. (2004). *Electronic health record: Public health perspectives.* Baltimore: Author.

Public Health Foundation. (2003). *From silos to systems: Using performance management to improve the public's health.* Prepared for the Performance Management National Excellence Collaborative. Retrieved March 28, 2005, from http://www.phf.org/pmc_silos_systems.pdf.

Public Health Functions Steering Committee. (1994). *Public health in America.* Retrieved January 29, 2005, from http://www.health.gov/phfunctions/public.htm.

Public Health Security and Bioterrorism Preparedness and Response Act of 2002, P. L. 107-188, 116 Stat. 595 (2002). Retrieved March 24, 2006, from http://frwebgate.access.gpo.gov/cgi-in/getdoc.cgi?dbname=107_cong_public_laws&docid=f:pub/188.107.pdf.

Quad Council. (1999). *Scope and standards of public health nursing practice.* Washington, DC: American Nurses Publishing.

Quad Council. (2001). *The impact of the nursing shortage on public health nursing.* Retrieved January 29, 2005, from http://www.astdn.org/publication_impact_nursing_shortage.htm.

Quad Council. (2003). *PHN competencies.* Retrieved January 29, 2005, from http://www.csuchico.edu/~horst/about/competencies.html.

Ripke, M., Briske, L., Keller, L., & Strohschein, S. (2001). *Public health interventions. Applications for public health nursing practice.* Retrieved July 20, 2006, from http://www.health.state.mn.us/divs/cfn/ophp/resources/docs/phninterventions_manual2001.pdf.

Simone, P., & Poppe, P. (2000). *CDC funding for TB prevention and control.* Retrieved January 29, 2005, from http://www.cdc.gov/nchstp/tb/notes/TBN_1_00/TBN-2000simone.htm.

Singleton, K. (2003). *Virginia adult education health literacy toolkit.* Retrieved April 7, 2005, from http://www.aelweb.vcu.edu/publications/healthlit/.

Spears, E., & Richmond, C. (2002). Kentucky Transition Training Initiative: Refocusing on population-based public health. *Link, 16*(1), 1, 5.

Trust for America's Health. (2005). *It's not flu as usual. What health professionals need to know about pandemic flu.* Washington, DC: Trust for America's Health, the American Medical Association.

Turning Point. (2005). *About Turning Point.* Retrieved January 27, 2006, from http://www.turningpointprogram.org/Pages/about.html.

Turnock, B. (2004). *Public health: What it is and how it works.* Sudbury, MA: Jones and Bartlett.

Wright, K., Rowitz, L., Merkle, A., Reid, W.M., Robinson, G., Herzog, B. et al. (2000). Competency development in public health leadership. *American Journal of Public Health, 90*(8), 1202–1207.

Zahner, S., & Corrado, S. (2004). Local health department partnerships with faith-based organizations. *Journal of Public Health Management and Practice, 10*(3), 258–265.

BIBLIOGRAPHY

Aday, L. (2005). *Reinventing public health: Policies and practices for a healthy nation.* San Francisco: Jossey-Bass.

Hooke, W., & Rogers, P. (Eds.). (2005). *Public health risks of disasters: Communication, infrastructure and preparedness—Workshop summary.* Washington, DC: National Academies Press.

Patel, K., & Rushevsky, M. (2005). *The politics of public health in the United States.* Armonk, NY: M.E. Sharpe.

Rowitz, L. (2005) *Public health for the 21st century: The prepared leader.* Sudbury, MA: Jones and Bartlett.

RESOURCES

American Public Health Association (APHA), Public Health Nursing (PHN) Section

800 "I" Street NW
Washington, D.C. 20001-3710
202-777-APHA (2752)
FAX: 202-777-2534
Email: comments@APHA.org
Web: http://www.apha.org

This association of public health nurse educators and practitioners operates within the American Public Health Association. The Web site provides information and opportunities for involvement in nationwide PHN issues.

Association of Community Health Nurse Educators (ACHNE)

10200 W. 44th Avenue, #304
Wheat Ridge, Colorado 80033
303-422-0679
FAX: 303-422-9904
Email: ACHNE@resourcecenter.com
Web: http://www.achne.org

ACHNE is an association of educators that teach community health and public health nursing at universities and colleges. ACHNE provides a meeting ground for those committed to excellence in community and public health nursing education, research, and practice. ACHNE was established in 1978 and is run by elected volunteer leaders who guide the organization in providing networking through the quarterly newsletter and membership directory and in providing educational opportunities through publications and the annual Spring Institute. ACHNE's mission is to promote the public's health by ensuring leadership and excellence in community and public health nursing education, research, and practice. The Web site provides information on workforce issues, PHN/CHN certification, career opportunities, public health nursing graduate education, links to other Quad Council organizations.

Association of State and Territorial Directors of Nursing (ASTDN)

1275 K Street NW, Suite 800
Washington, D.C. 20005-4006
202-371-9090
FAX: 202-371-9797
Email: dianakp@health.ok.gov
Web: http://www.astdn.org

The Association of State and Territorial Directors of Nursing began in 1935 as an advisory group of state health department nurses. ASTDN continues today as an active association of public health nursing leaders from across the United States and its territories. ASTDN is an affiliate of the Association of State and Territorial Health Officials (ASTHO). The ASTDN mission is to provide a collegial forum to advance the public health nursing leadership role in protecting and promoting the health of the public. The Web site provides information on publications, population-focused practice, Quad Council competencies, Partnership Project (CDC and ASTDN), newsletter, and featured state public health nursing profile.

Association of State and Territorial Health Officials (ASTHO)

1275 K Street NW, Suite 800
Washington, D.C. 20005-4006
202-371-9090
FAX: 202-371-9797
Web: http://www.astho.org

The Association of State and Territorial Health Officials (ASTHO) is the national nonprofit organization representing the state and territorial public health agencies of the United States, the U.S. Territories, and the District of Columbia. ASTHO's members, the chief health officials of these jurisdictions, are dedicated to formulating and influencing sound public health policy, and to assuring excellence in state-based public health practice. The Web site provides resources on public health information, workforce issues, law and public health, publications, and many other current issues.

Center for Studying Health Systems Change (HSC)

600 Maryland Avenue SW, #550
Washington, D.C. 20024
202-489-5261
FAX: 202-484-5261
Web: http://www.hschange.com

The Center for Studying Health System Change is a nonpartisan policy research organization located in Washington, D.C. HSC designs and conducts studies focused on the U.S. health care system to inform the thinking and decisions of policy makers in government and private industry. In addition, HSC studies contribute more broadly to the body of health care policy research that enables decision makers to understand change and the national and local market forces driving that change. The mission of HSC is to inform policy makers and private decision makers about how local and national changes in the financing and delivery of health care affect people. HSC strives to provide high-quality, timely, and objective research and analysis that leads to sound policy decisions, with the ultimate goal of improving the health of the American public. The Web site provides resources for a variety of health policy issues, links to current publications, and subscriptions to policy topic alerts.

KaiserEDU

Web: http://www.kaiserEDU.org

KaiserEDU is an online health policy resource for faculty and students. It is designed to provide students, faculty, and others interested in learning about health policy easy access to the latest data, research, analysis, and developments in health policy. KaiserEDU.org was developed to provide a clearinghouse of introductory materials on major areas of health care policy, particularly for students and faculty in health policy and related disciplines, as well as for anyone interested in learning more about health policy. The site provides a range of resources, including narrated slide lectures and collections of background materials, including research, data, and policy analysis, on the key issues at the forefront of health policy. The site also includes concise summaries of more narrow policy debates along with links to background materials, including policy reports, articles published in the peer-reviewed literature, and key data. Other features include a library of syllabi from health policy courses across the United States, a compilation of fellowships for students and professionals interested in health policy, a summary of the major government agencies involved in health policy, and links to datasets available for further research.

Kaiser Family Foundation

2400 Sand Hill Road
Menlo Park, California 94025
650-854-9400
FAX: 650-854-4800
Web: http://www.kff.org

The Henry J. Kaiser Family Foundation is a nonprofit, private operating foundation focusing on the major health care issues facing the nation. The Foundation is an independent voice and source of facts and analysis for policy makers, the media, the health care community, and the general public. KFF develops and runs its own research and communications programs, often in partnership with outside organizations. The Foundation contracts with a wide range of outside individuals and organizations through its programs. The Foundation is not associated with Kaiser Permanente or Kaiser Industries.

National Association of County and City Health Officials (NACCHO)

1100 17th Street NW, 2nd floor
Washington, D.C. 20036
202-783-5550
FAX: 202-783-1583

Email: craysor@naccho.org
Web: http://www.naccho.org

NACCHO is the national organization representing local health departments. NACCHO works to support efforts that protect and improve the health of all people and all communities by promoting national policy, developing resources and programs, seeking health equity, and supporting effective local public health practice and systems. The Web site provides materials, discussion guides, and videos on core public health functions, environmental health primer, links to leadership training, and directory of public health Web resources for local boards of health.

National Association of Local Boards of Health (NALBOH)

1840 East Gypsy Lane Road
Bowling Green, Ohio 43462
419-353-7714
FAX: 419-352-6278
Email: nalboh@nalboh.org
Web: http://www.nalboh.org

NALBOH vision is to represent the grassroots foundation of public health in America, actively engaging and serving the public by empowering boards of health through education and training. NALBOH's mission is to prepare and strengthen boards of health, empowering them to promote and protect the health of their communities through education, training, and technical assistance. The Web site provides information and links to various health-related organizations that NALBOH works with.

Public Health Foundation (PHF)

1300 L Street NW, Suite 800
Washington, D.C. 20005
202-218-4400
FAX: 202-218-4409
Email: info@phf.org
Web: http://www.phf.org

The Public Health Foundation is dedicated to achieving healthy communities through research, training, and technical assistance. For more than 35 years, this national, nonprofit organization has been creating new information and helping health agencies and other community health organizations connect to and more effectively use information to manage and improve performance, understand and use data, and strengthen the workforce. The Web site provides a variety of resources on public health infrastructure, including links to CDC infrastructure, COL competencies, National Public Health Performance Standards, training resources through TrainingFinder Real-time Affiliated Network (TRAIN), Healthy People tools and resources, worker recruitment and retention, emergency preparedness resources, essential public health services, and public health databases.

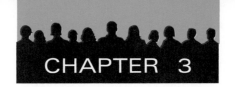

CHAPTER 3

Practice Settings in Public Health Nursing

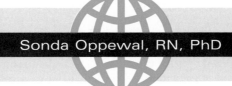

Sonda Oppewal, RN, PhD

Chapter Outline

🌐 Historical Practice Perspectives

🌐 Practice Settings in Governmental or Official Agencies
   Federal Agencies
   State and Local Public Health Agencies
   Schools

🌐 Practice Settings Associated with Nongovernmental, Community Agencies
   Community Health Centers
   Homeless Clinics
   Rural Health Clinics
   Migrant Health Centers
   Nurse-Managed Health Centers
   Faith-Based Organizations
   Workplaces
   Home Visiting
   Other Settings

🌐 Models of Public Health Nursing Practice
   Minnesota Department of Health, Public Health Nursing
       Section Intervention Wheel
   Association of State and Territorial Directors of Nursing
       Public Health Nursing Practice Model
   The Los Angeles County Public Health Nursing Practice
       Model

🌐 Issues and Challenges
   Workforce Issues and Challenges
   Educational Issues and Challenges
   Financial Issues, Rewards, and Job Satisfaction

Learning Objectives

Upon completion of this chapter, the reader will be able to:

1. Describe settings of public health nursing practice before World War I.

2. Discuss current practice opportunities for public health nurses with official agencies at local, state, and national levels.

3. Analyze similarities and differences of public health nursing practice in various settings.

4. Explain opportunities for intervening with communities and systems in various practice settings.

5. Explore issues and challenges common to public health nursing practice settings.

Public health nursing practice takes place in numerous settings within a vast network of organizations that comprise the public health system. There is no dearth of practice settings where nurses conduct activities intended to promote, protect, and improve the health of entire populations or groups of people who share a common characteristic or health concern. Often these activities take place in settings convenient for the nurse's clients such as in their homes, work settings, or various places within their neighborhoods. Public health nurses may practice in clinics, occupational settings, schools, health departments, grocery stores, faith-based organizations, correctional facilities, mobile vans, homes, department stores, and hospitals, and even from dog sleds (American Public Health Association, 1996; Minnesota Department of Health, 2001). Indeed, there is no practice setting where population-based interventions by public health nurses cannot take place, and, often nurses seek out or take services to settings most convenient for their clients.

The purpose of this chapter is to review and explore practice settings of public health nurses. A brief historical review of public health nursing practice settings is first provided because only by understanding our past can we comprehend present and future trends in public health nursing practice. A discussion of current practice settings in governmental or publicly funded agencies and nongovernmental, community agencies follows before a discussion of public health nursing issues and challenges in various practice settings.

HISTORICAL PRACTICE PERSPECTIVES

Public health nurses were first called visiting nurses in this country when visiting nursing started in 1877. Influenced by the model of district nurses in Great Britain who visited the "ailing poor" in their homes, the Women's Brand of the New York City Mission sent trained nurses to take care of poor people in their homes (Kalisch & Kalisch, 1978). Before long, other visiting nursing associations developed with funds donated primarily by female philanthropists who thought it socially unjust for poor people to not have similar access to health services as people who were more economically advantaged (Buhler-Wilkerson, 1985). These early public health nurses visited individuals and their families in their homes with the intent to restore health, promote

better health, and prevent additional disease. Nurses provided direct care services to individuals and families within the context of the community, with the notion that the entire population of people who lived in the area, immigrants and nonimmigrants, would benefit.

Lillian Wald is recognized as the founder of public health nursing. In 1893 with the help of another nurse, Mary Brewster, Wald started a visiting nursing service in a "nurse's settlement house" located in the slums of New York City to "seek out the sick and nurse them" (Kalisch & Kalisch, 1978, p. 230). They did not have to "seek out" patients for long. Soon after setting up the settlement house, numerous community members began requesting assistance. Wald and Brewster obtained additional money from philanthropists to hire more nurses and to move to a larger house they called the Henry Street Settlement House. By 1905, the Henry Street nurses had cared for 5,032 patients in their homes, and the staff had grown to 37 nurses by 1909. No patient was denied care because of inability to pay for the nursing services. Wald described the early public health nurses as the "link between families' social, economic, and health needs and the services families required to become or stay healthy" (Buhler-Wilkerson, 1993, p. 1781). Henry Street Settlement nurses developed a model of nursing practice that valued holism, community engagement, cultural sensitivity, social justice, and clinical expertise that combined acute care nursing with health promotion and disease prevention based on family needs (Kalisch & Kalisch, 1978).

With funding from philanthropists, visiting nurse associations in large cities started to multiply by the early 1900s. These voluntary organizations were "managed" cooperatively by the philanthropists with "guidance" from the nurses who envisioned improved health for the entire population and who had some authority to make decisions about the management and provision of nursing services. As the role of the visiting nurse expanded from a focus of caring for the acutely ill to a focus on disease prevention and health promotion, visiting nursing associations added specific health prevention programs that targeted specific ages and groups of people like mothers, babies, school-age children, and patients with tuberculosis (Buhler-Wilkerson, 1985). Another well-known example is the demonstration project Lillian Wald initiated with the New York City Board of Health to send a nurse to visit schools and the homes of children who were absent from school. School nursing expanded quickly after the project demonstrated with compelling evidence that school absenteeism decreased with nursing interventions that included health screenings, health classes, and home visits to children with health problems (Kalisch & Kalisch, 1978). By the early twentieth century, public health nurses practiced in various homes, settlement houses in specific communities, schools, factories, and other settings similar to ones today (Figure 3-1).

More visiting nurse associations expanded their programs to include preventive services such as tuberculosis prevention by obtaining additional funds from city coffers or other governmental agencies. These joint ventures between voluntary organizations and official agencies led to nursing practice in numerous settings such as "department stores, factories, insurance companies, boards of health and education, hospitals, settlement houses, milk and baby clinics, playgrounds, and hotels, as well as for visiting nurse associations" (Buhler-Wilkerson, 1985, p. 1158). By 1913, more and more visiting nurses were funded by official or governmental agencies or by nonofficial or voluntary agencies to practice in virtually any setting where visiting nurses were needed.

After the Great Depression, more visiting nurses took on the title of public health nurse as opportunity for employment in publicly funded agencies increased. It became more difficult for public health nursing leaders to create and maintain a comprehensive model of nursing care that combined acute care nursing services or curative services and preventive nursing services (Williams, 1977; Buhler-Wilkerson, 1985). By the end of the 1920s, the need for visiting nursing associations waned as economic conditions improved, mortality from infectious diseases declined, access to hospitals increased, and the United States accepted and received fewer immigrants (Buhler-Wilkerson, 1985). The provision of preventive nursing care by "public health nurses" and sick care by the "visiting nurses" was more noticeable as more nurses became employed by official agencies with "health officers" in leadership positions. Not only did these nurses lose their ability to maintain a strong voice in the management of their nursing practice, but they had to choose between working with a visiting nursing association, where they provided acute care services, or an official agency, where they provided preventive health services, because neither type of agency could afford a comprehensive model of care that combined both (Buhler-Wilkerson, 1985; Roberts & Heinrich, 1985; Abrams, 2004). Nursing leaders today face similar challenges with developing

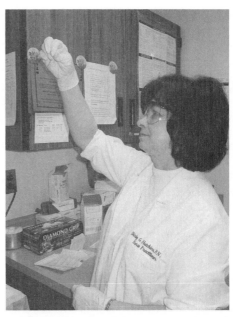

Figure 3-1 Public health nurse preparing to administer smallpox vaccine.
Courtesy of Gary Black, Mecklenburg County Health Department, Charlotte, North Carolina.

sustainable models of nurse-managed care that successfully combine preventive health services and the care of acutely ill clients.

PRACTICE SETTINGS IN GOVERNMENTAL OR OFFICIAL AGENCIES

Many laypersons and health professionals alike first consider official or governmental agencies as the main practice setting of public health nurses. The Scope and Standards of Public Health Nursing Practice (Quad Council, 2003) articulates clearly that this is not the case. The defining characteristic of public health nursing practice is not its location in the community (e.g., outside of acute care institutions) but its focus on creating conditions to improve the health of populations. Practice opportunities for nurses in governmental or official and voluntary or nonofficial organizations have held a prominent place in the history of public health nursing, and they continue to do so. Public health nurses can work with local, state and territorial, and federal agencies to apply their knowledge and skills to help achieve the core public health functions of assessment, policy development, and assurance.

Federal Agencies

The primary federal public health agency in the United States is the Public Health Service (PHS). The PHS is comprised of all agency divisions of the U.S. Department of Health and Human Services (HHS) and the Commissioned Corps, a uniformed service of more than 6,000 health professionals who serve at HHS and other federal agencies. The PHS originated in 1798 as a component of the Treasury Department with the mission to care for the nation's merchant seamen. Nurses were employed by HHS hospitals to help the sick workers regain their health. The role of the nurse expanded in the late nineteenth century to include health screenings and follow-up health care to immigrants who arrived at Ellis Island, and then expanded more around World War I to include environmental assessments and work in specific clinics such as ones designed to detect and treat venereal disease (U.S. Public Health Service, 2002).

The HHS is the main agency in the U.S. government charged with protecting the health of Americans and providing health services, especially for those who lack the resources and means to care for themselves. Federal agency employees in HHS work closely with state and local governments to protect health and prevent disease, assess and monitor national health status indicators, facilitate health services research, and work with legislators on health policies and regulations. HHS is comprised of 11 operating divisions that fall under two main program areas: Public Health Service Operating Divisions and Human Services Operating Divisions. Nurses may work in any of the divisions, but more opportunities exist in one of the eight agencies of the PHS within the Public Health Service Operating Divisions. These eight agencies are held in high esteem worldwide as leading health agencies: Agency for Healthcare Research and Quality (AHRQ), the Agency for Toxic Substances and Disease Registry (ATSDR), the Centers for Disease Control and Prevention (CDC), the Food and Drug Administration (FDA), the Health Resources and Services Administration (HRSA), the Indian Health Service (IHS), the National Institutes of Health (NIH), and the Substance Abuse and Mental Health Services Administration (SAMHSA). The Office of Public Health Preparedness (OPHP) and the Office of Public Health and Science (OPHS) sit within the Office of the Secretary (OS) of HHS, and the Office of the Surgeon General is within the OPHS (U.S. Public Health Service Overview, 2005).

Members of various disciplines work as PHS personnel to protect the public's health in numerous ways. Federal agencies provide evidence to Congress about health policies and help develop regulations in response to legislation passed. PHS personnel include Commissioned Corps (CC) officers and federal civil service employees. PHS nurses currently number approximately 6,000 and about 1,000 of these nurses are Commissioned Corps; they work in a wide variety of roles as direct care providers, supervisors, consultants, researchers, and administrators to advance the health of Americans and improve how health services are organized and delivered. U.S. PHS Commissioned Corps Nurse Officers serve in the HHS operating divisions as well as other federal agencies such as the Environmental Protection Agency, the Bureau of Prisons, the Division of Immigration Health Services, the National Oceanic and Atmospheric Administration, and the U.S. Marshals Service in the Department of Justice (U.S. Public Health Service Overview, 2005).

State and Local Public Health Agencies

State public health agencies work with local public health agencies on specific community issues of concern and use a larger pool of resources to tackle health problems that impact numerous communities (Figure 3-2). State health departments must conduct needs assessments of the population and monitor health information, identify appropriate *Healthy People 2010* national objectives when setting state objectives and program priorities, plan strategies to address needs that are unmet related to health promotion and health protection, obtain sufficient resources, set and enforce standards, and provide technical assistance to local health agencies. Public health nurses can assume a number of roles in state and local health agencies; however, a recent study found that program management and population-based services were more likely to be provided at state and district health agencies.

Local health agencies are known mainly for the direct personal services provided to community members who are usually dependent on government health coverage. Depending on how attractive reimbursement rates are by the government, private health care pro-

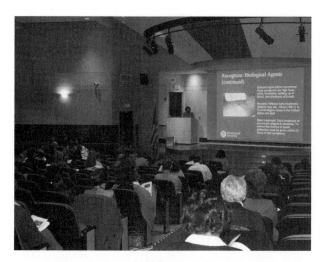

Figure 3-2 Public health nurse leading weapons of mass destruction awareness training.

Courtesy of Gary Black, Mecklenburg County Health Department, Charlotte, North Carolina.

viders may also encourage community members eligible for Medicaid to seek care at their offices or clinic settings. Public health nurses continue to provide personal direct health services at local levels to a greater extent than at the district or state levels (Bureau of Health Professions, 2005). Local public health agencies in recent years have become more grounded in providing the three core functions of public health as well as the 10 essential health services (IOM, 1988). Many public health nurses work in local health departments as direct care providers in clinic settings (such as well baby clinic or communicable disease clinic), case managers, outreach workers, and a myriad of other roles. Municipalities, cities, towns, or county governments may operate local health agencies. State public health agencies differ to some degree in their organizational relationships with local public health agencies, but most local health agencies are organized to report to state entities.

The now classic and frequently cited IOM report, *The Future of Public Health* (1988), recommended restructuring public health so that it was less reliant on federal agencies and more reliant on vibrant, energetic partnerships between local, state, and federal health agencies and nongovernmental agencies such as voluntary agencies and associations, community groups, private

businesses, health care professionals, and consumers. Public health nursing interventions related to collaboration, coalition building, and community organizing (Minnesota Department of Health, 2001) can foster this type of partnership for the purpose of improving population health.

Schools

Most schools in the United States are viewed as public agencies because they are funded by local taxes and are managed in part by local officials. Schools offer an ideal setting to provide health care services to children and youth across the nation because more than 95 percent of children and youth age 5 to 17 years attend schools (Koplan, 2001). In addition to learning academic subjects, children in schools can participate in health education programs that build capacity for healthy life skills and choices. It is widely acknowledged that children must be healthy in order to learn. This linkage provides a segue for health services in schools and the coordination of comprehensive services that can positively impact the population's health.

School nursing originated in 1902 under the direction of Lillian Wald. She proposed an experiment to decrease high absenteeism rates for children with common infectious diseases who were excluded from attending class. Wald sent a nurse, Lina Rogers, to work in four New York City public schools to screen children and obtain early treatment for health problems, and to visit homes to provide follow-up and family education. The experiment was highly successful as evidenced by a drop in the absenteeism rate by 90 percent, and school nurses increased in number quickly (Hawkins, Hayes, & Corliss, 1994; Broussard, 2004). School nurses today share some of the same challenges as they did in the early 1900s such as dealing with communicable diseases, poverty, hunger, and poor environmental home and community situations. Additional challenges that school nurses face currently include asthma, diabetes, obesity, learning disabilities, violence, sexually transmitted diseases and infections, and addiction (Figure 3-3). Today's children and youth may have complicated medical and social problems that require specialized, highly technical health procedures, close supervision by nurses, and frequent communication and teamwork with school administrators and faculty, health and social service providers, and family members (Wolfe & Selekman, 2002; Broussard, 2004).

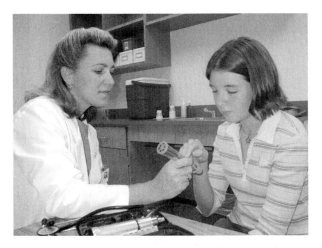

Figure 3-3 School nurse teaching student to use an inspirometer.
Courtesy of Gary Black, Mecklenburg County Health Department, Charlotte, North Carolina.

School nurses continue to help children remain healthy so they are more likely to succeed with academics. Public health nurses employed by public health departments may be the direct providers of school health services if the local education agency maintains a contract with the local public health agency for school nurse services. Whether or not school nurses are employed by public health agencies, by hospitals, or directly by the local education agency, nurses can improve the health of a "population of interest" or the entire population of children in a school, and they can improve the health of "populations-at-risk" such as groups of children that share a risk factor such as diabetes, obesity, or depression (Minnesota Department of Health, 2001). Schools provide ideal environments for nurses to intervene with individuals, families, and groups and in ways that impact healthful change within the system or structure of the school as well as the larger community (Figure 3-4).

Most school nurses use population-based approaches when caring for children in schools. In addition to screening children for problems that could impair learning, such as hearing and vision, they also assist with immunizations, medication administration, delegated medical functions, first aid and emergency procedures, health education, case management and care coordination, and advocacy. School nurses are in an ideal position to identify children most in need of health ser-

vices and to help them receive treatment and follow-up care. The school nurse often has the role of care provider, health educator, counselor, and case manager, and may also have roles including that of health promoter, collaborator, healthy policy expert, advocate, and researcher (Broussard, 2004). School nurses are well positioned to lead efforts to coordinate the eight components of the coordinated school health model program—nutrition, health services, mental health and social services, health education, school environment, physical education and activity, family and community involvement, and staff/employee wellness.

School-based health centers are primary care centers that include preventive health services and are held on school grounds. This model works well in communities where children lack access to medical care; when communities and schools are supportive of these services, which decrease barriers to accessing health services; and when the center personnel work in partnership with an advisory board of students, school administrators, faculty, parents, community leaders, business leaders, health and social service professionals, and religious and other trusted community members. Nurse practitioners serve as primary care providers on-site to diagnose and treat acute and chronic illnesses and to assist students to better learn about their health and make healthier choices. Some centers

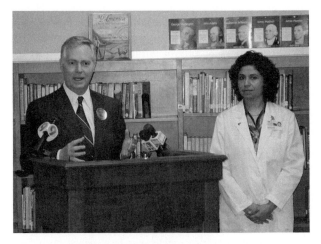

Figure 3-4 School nurse advocating for healthy children and schools with North Carolina Governor Michael F. Easley.
Courtesy of Gary Black, Mecklenburg County Health Department, Charlotte, North Carolina.

have mental health counselors who are available for individual, family or small group therapy, or dentists who may be on-site for part of the week to care for those students without access to dental care. A fact sheet entitled "School-Based Health Centers: A Blue Print for Health Learners" published by the National Association of School-Based Health Centers indicated there were approximately 1,500 school-based health centers according to a census study taken during the 2001–2002 academic year (National Association of School-Based Health Centers, 2005).

PRACTICE SETTINGS ASSOCIATED WITH NONGOVERNMENTAL, COMMUNITY AGENCIES

Public health nursing can take place in virtually any setting when nurses apply population-based approaches that focus on improving a population's health by working in partnership with community members, community groups, and other disciplines (Figure 3-5). Public health nurses have a reputation for being creative, well-known in their communities, and responsive to

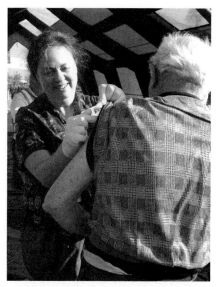

Figure 3-5 Convenient "drive through/walk through" flu immunization clinic.
Courtesy of Gary Black, Mecklenburg County Health Department, Charlotte, North Carolina.

⊕ PRACTICE APPLICATION

Establishing a Nurse-Managed Health Center

Public health nurses can lead and direct the development of comprehensive health centers that promote the health of populations at individual, community, and systems levels. In a rural county in Tennessee, two public health nurses worked in partnership with a trusted community member (the only baccalaureate-prepared nurse in the county) and other community members to conduct an in-depth community assessment. Data from the Center for Disease Control's Youth Risk Behavior Survey of the local high school students and information from the community assessment helped provide compelling evidence to secure grant funding from the Bureau of Primary Health Care to start a school-based health center at the one high school in a county with a high degree of poverty and isolation because of rural, mountainous terrain. A nurse practitioner was hired to diagnose and treat acute and chronic illnesses and provide individual health counseling and education, and a mental health counselor provided individual, family, and group behavioral health counseling. The RN health educator initiated numerous population-based interventions such as organizing school-wide assemblies to help prevent unsafe driving, conducted community-wide seatbelt screenings, led school and community health coalitions, advocated for new bleachers in the gym to replace old ones that led to minor but numerous student injuries, and taught a variety of health education sessions in classrooms and community settings to students and their parents about different health issues. Community members, school administrators and personnel, and students were highly satisfied with this nurse-managed health center.

changing health trends—characteristics that without doubt will apply to public health nurses in future years (Berkowitz et al., 2001).

The next section of this chapter discusses common practice settings for public health nurses outside of governmental agencies such as primary care settings where the focus is often on individuals and families but where community and systems level of practice interventions can successfully take place. Community health centers, homeless clinics, rural health clinics, migrant health centers, nurse-managed health centers, faith-based organizations, workplaces, and home settings will be discussed. It is outside the scope of this chapter to review every practice setting that public health nurses may work in.

Personal health care services at the local level are provided in different community settings, and professional nurses who combine their practice with principles of public health may be very involved with providing this type of nursing care. Referred to as primary care centers, the focus of care is on promoting health, preventing disease, treating episodic illnesses, and managing chronic illnesses in the context of families and communities. Primary care often takes place in clinics or private provider offices. The term primary health care normally is broader in scope than the term primary care because it includes principles of public health in its definition of services; however, these terms often are used interchangeably. A number of community-based settings provide primary care services and interventions to improve the health of the broader community or populations by providing outreach, screenings, health fairs, coalition work, and community capacity building.

Community Health Centers

Community health centers (CHCs) have increased in number in recent years as Congress has approved legislative appropriations in response to a growing number of uninsured and underinsured Americans. In the mid-1970s these centers were referred to as neighborhood health centers. As community-based nonprofit organizations, they were viewed as an innovative model of health care delivery because of their convenient location to community members who needed the services and because community members who used the clinic services helped make decisions that impacted the center's operations (Madison, 2003). CHCs are partially funded by a federal grant program under Section 330 of the Public Health Service Act with the mission of provid-

ing primary and preventive health care services in areas throughout the United States that are medically underserved. The intent of the CHC program is to improve access to health services to community members most at risk for not receiving health services because of low income, racial/ethnic diversity, language barriers, lack of health insurance, insufficient health insurance, or highly complex health problems. Furthermore, the centers improve health care access because they are located in areas where there are few health care providers.

The federal program responsible for awarding grants and working with CHCs is the Bureau of Primary Health Care, one of five bureaus in HHS's Health Resources Services Administration. The federal program requires that CHCs serve all residents without regard to insurance status by offering a sliding fee scale based on income level. Another federal requirement is that the centers to be governed by a board of members. A majority (or at least 51 percent) of the board members need to be "users" or "consumers" of the center in order to ensure active community ownership and partnership by members who can represent the center's beneficiaries and who can help resolve local health care problems (Hawkins & Proser, 2004). CHCs also strive to meet the linguistic and cultural needs of the communities they serve, and they assist their clients in accessing needed services such as transportation, translation, case management, home visitation, and health education (National Association of Community Health Centers, 2004).

In addition to benefiting from federal funds to help defray operating costs, CHCs are federally qualified health centers (FQHCs) and as such can benefit from cost-based reimbursement for Medicare and Medicaid services. CHCs may have multiple clinic sites in medically underserved areas and may apply for different types of funds from the Bureau of Primary Health Care, for example, to support a migrant health center or school-based health center. Nurses provide essential services within CHCs including direct clinical services, center management, coordination and case management services, health promotion, and health education (Figure 3-6). Advanced practice nurses who are certified as nurse practitioners in family or adult health, pediatrics, women's health, nurse midwifery, and psychiatric/mental health have numerous opportunities for practice in CHCs. In addition to CHCs that are located in medically underserved areas, additional funds may be awarded under Section 330 of the Public Health Service Act to provide similar federal support for migrant health centers, primary care centers in public housing settings, rural health clinics, school-based health centers, and homeless clinics.

Homeless Clinics

Homelessness is a significant and growing problem that pervades rural, urban, and suburban communities throughout the United States. Homeless persons and families face numerous hurdles with daily living, and health problems are especially challenging in light of limited resources and subsistence living. Homeless clinics or shelters that offer health services rely on different funding sources to provide targeted services to meet the special needs of homeless persons. Some homeless clinics receive federal funds from Section 330 funding.

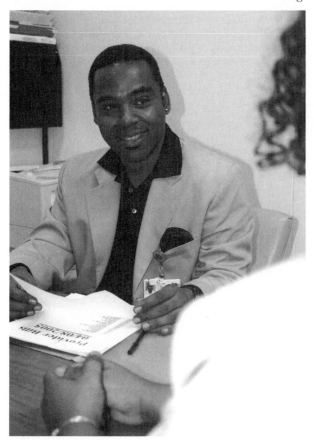

Figure 3-6 Nurse case manager.
Courtesy of Gary Black, Mecklenburg County Health Department, Charlotte, North Carolina.

Other clinics for homeless persons may be sponsored by public health agencies, hospitals, community coalitions, academic health centers, universities, or faith-based organizations. Outreach efforts and some specific primary care services may be offered on mobile vans, at shelters, or at other locations where homeless people spend time, such as camps, bus stops, and parks. Creative strategies are needed to best reach out to effectively serve the homeless given their complex social and economic situations. In addition to providing primary care, homeless clinics may provide behavioral health services, substance abuse counseling, and case management.

In 2003, the federal Health Care for the Homeless (HCH) program had 172 grantees, and during that year more than 600,000 men, women, and children from racially and ethnically diverse backgrounds received health services. Of the clients served by HCH clinics, 71 percent did not have any medical insurance and if income was known, 92 percent lived at or below the Federal Poverty Level. Interestingly, 43 percent of the clients served by the HCH sites lived in shelters, and 11 percent lived on the streets. Others reported living in transitional housing, with acquaintances or relatives, or in some other type of living arrangement (U.S. Department of Health and Human Service, n.d.).

Rural Health Clinics

Residents of rural areas in this country are more likely to experience a lower quality of health care compared to their urban or suburban counterparts. Ensuring essential health care services and a strong public health infrastructure in rural parts of the country is challenging. Approximately 20 percent of the U.S. population lives in rural parts of the country where it is very challenging to obtain accessible health care services, and it is especially difficult for rural residents who live in smaller, poorer, and more isolated communities (IOM, 2004; Young, 2004).

Rural health clinic (RHC) expansion and sustainability improved in December 1977 when Congress passed the Rural Health Clinic Services Act P.L. 95-210 to increase accessible and available primary care services to residents living in rural areas. This legislation enabled qualified RHCs to obtain cost-based Medicare and Medicaid reimbursement for core health services, and it improved Medicare and Medicaid reimbursement for nurse practitioner and physician assistant services. There were 3,477 RHCs in operation throughout the nation

⊕ RESEARCH APPLICATION

The Process of Changing Health Risk Behaviors: An Oregon Rural Clinic Experience

Study Purpose

To evaluate a counseling intervention designed to help individuals who live in rural communities change their health risk behaviors.

Methods

Participants completed an 11-item Health Status Profile developed by the investigators to ascertain whether health behavior changes were desired for tobacco use, poor diet, physical inactivity, emotional stress, or lack of knowledge about how to manage chronic illness. The intervention consisted of three counseling sessions between a nurse practitioner and participant over a period of 12 months. Quantitative data were collected using appraisal forms specific to five health risk behaviors, and qualitative data were analyzed from written comments from summaries from focus groups or from written comments from participants.

Findings

Most of the 74 participants were not successful in changing their health risk behaviors. Issues associated with barriers to changing health behaviors in rural areas were identified in the focus group discussions. In addition to an individual's lack of will to make healthful changes, participants viewed the rural community environment as a key barrier to adopting new health behaviors.

Implications

Health care providers in rural health clinics can provide important support to individuals interested in and attempting to adopt new health behaviors. Recommendations from study participants to improve the likelihood of healthful change included forming support groups that do not charge a fee; developing a peer-mentoring program; providing more education, positive reinforcement for incremental steps, and more frequent discussions about individual goals; and using strategies that build on the strengths of rural communities such as strong, close-knit community ties and close provider-client relationships.

Reference

Bowden, J.M., Shaul, M.P., & Bennett, J.A. (2004). The process of changing health risk behaviors: An Oregon rural clinic experience. *Journal of the American Academy of Nurse Practitioners, 16* (9), 411–417.

---

at the beginning of 1999. To meet the definition of a RHC, these clinics must be located in areas where the population is less than 50,000 according to the Bureau of the Census, and in areas designated by HHS as being medically underserved (Gale & Coburn, 2003).

Nurses who work in RHCs assist with the delivery of personal care services for episodic, chronic, and preventive purposes. They may make home visits to homebound clients who need nursing assessment and care. The RHC must employ a nurse practitioner or physician assistant 50 percent of the time the clinic is open (Fact Sheet Rural Health Clinic, 2004). RHCs must be certified by the Centers for Medicare & Medicaid Services (CMS) within HHS in order for the RHC to be paid for encounters that are face to face, and reimbursement is based on specific rules and regulations (National Rural Health Association, n.d.).

In addition to providing interventions that target individuals and families, nurses who work in RHCs have many opportunities to target healthful change at systems and community levels. While rural areas have strengths such as social networks and a strong sense of community, rural populations tend to have more older residents than urban settings have, and, hence, they have higher rates of chronic illness and poorer health behaviors (Young, 2004). Attracting and retaining health care professionals to serve in rural areas continues to be problematic because of isolation, limited health facilities, limited employment, and limited educational opportunities for family members.

Migrant Health Centers

Despite living and working in one of the wealthiest countries in the world, the health needs of migrant and seasonal farm workers is abysmally poor, on par with most third world nations. America's multibillion dollar agricultural industry depends on more than 3 million migrant and seasonal farm workers to provide labor for crop planting, cultivating, harvesting, and processing. The health, educational, and social needs of this group are very great due to the poor, often unsanitary living and working conditions they face, in addition to language and cultural barriers, low literacy, and frequent mobility. For example, the 1997–1998 National Agricultural Workers Survey revealed that 80 percent were men, most had a sixth grade education, 84 percent spoke Spanish, and 12 percent spoke English. Almost 75 percent of the workers earn less than $10,000 per year and three of every five families with farm workers live below the poverty level (National Center for Farmworker Health, n.d.).

Migrant workers are paid hourly and will miss wages if they are not able to work. Hence, seeking health care may not be the first priority for some migrant families, and visits to the emergency department rather than to primary care providers are likely to occur. Few legislative safeguards exist for farm laborers compared to workers in other industries (Embrey, n.d.). Migrant health centers are operated by nonprofit agencies to improve accessibility and availability of primary care services that are comprehensive in scope and culturally and linguistically competent (Bureau of Primary Health Care, n.d.). Health and social services can target individuals and families, as well as groups, communities, and the entire population of migrant and seasonal farm workers who share a number of common characteristics. Funded since 1962, the Health Resources and Services Administration Migrant Health Program has provided grants to community nonprofit organizations to provide primary, preventive, and dental health care; outreach; screenings; transportation; pharmaceuticals; and environmental and occupational health and safety. Services extend to families, and they are culturally sensitive, linguistically appropriate, and prevention oriented (Bureau of Primary Health Care, n.d.).

Public health nurses and other public health workers employed by local and state public health agencies may work in partnership with migrant health centers to improve delivery of care with partnering organizations from academic centers, area health education centers, hospitals, social service agencies, and state and regional primary care associations (Bureau of Primary Health Care, n.d.).

Nurse-Managed Health Centers

CHCs, homeless clinics, rural health clinics, and migrant health centers are considered safety net providers. In addition to these centers that receive Bureau of Primary Health Care funds, other safety net providers include federally qualified health centers (FQHCs), local health departments or agencies, and public hospitals. Nurse-managed health centers may also be considered a safety net provider if the primary mission is to provide accessible health services to vulnerable community members in partnership with those they serve. Many nurse-managed health centers can be defined as safety net providers. Some nurse-managed health centers do not target vulnerable populations and therefore do not fit the definition of a safety net provider but instead may target insured populations and offer consumers a different model of care that combines preventive services, holistic care, and primary care services (Figure 3-7) (Mundinger, 2000; Hansen-Turton et al., 2004).

Nurse-managed health centers are managed and directed by nurses who are responsible and accountable for the delivery and outcomes of health services. Sometimes referred to as nursing centers, the number of primary care centers managed by nurses in rural, underserved, and urban areas has increased in number over the past several decades as a model of renewed interest by nurse entrepreneurs and faculty members in university settings. Lillian Wald's Henry Street Settlement, initiated in 1893, represents an earlier model and prototype of nurse-managed health centers (Kennedy, 1996; Hansen-Turton et al., 2004). Nursing centers respond to the needs of community members by providing clients with access to professional nurs-

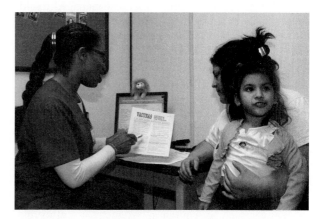

Figure 3-7 Childhood vaccines administered during a well-child visit.

Courtesy of Gary Black, Mecklenburg County Health Department, Charlotte, North Carolina.

ing services that are holistic in nature, available, and affordable. Advanced practice nurses diagnose and treat acute and chronic illnesses and integrate health promotion, health protection, disease prevention, and health education in all visits. Professional nurses in the center practice under their state's Nursing Practice Act to diagnose and treat human responses to actual and potential health problems and to promote the health of the overall community or target populations that desire nursing services. Behavioral health services may be offered concurrently with primary care services. Various organizational structures of nurse-managed health centers exist. Some nursing centers are affiliated with universities or colleges and may be referred to as academic nursing centers, or they may be freestanding and owned by individual nurses, or affiliated with other agencies (Kennedy, 1996; Edwards, Oppewal, & Logan, 2003; Hansen-Turton et al., 2004).

Nurse-managed health centers can direct services beyond individuals and families to levels that impact communities and systems. Nurses decide what services to offer, and they often incorporate and integrate population-based interventions in the practice model. Challenges that face most nurse-managed health centers include garnering sufficient resources and revenue for population-focused expenditures such as community mobilization, coalition building, outreach, and case finding, as third party reimbursement is based on individual encounters. Efforts are underway by the National Nursing Centers Consortium and other nursing organizations to focus attention on nurse-managed health centers as essential safety net providers, to advocate for cost-based reimbursement when nursing centers serve as safety net providers, and to prevent health insurers and payers from discriminating against nurse practitioners.

Faith-Based Organizations

Nursing can trace its roots to communities of faith that lent financial support to nurses to help others (Kalisch & Kalisch, 1978). Faith-based organizations are comprised of people who share a common spiritual or religious faith and who meet together in buildings designated for worship. Faith-based organizations may be in settings such as churches, synagogues, cathedrals, temples, or mosques, or other buildings used by faith communities. Authors of the IOM report, *The Future of Public Health* (1988), recognized the need for public health agencies to increase the number and type of orga-

nizations they partnered with as a strategy to improve the nation's health. The first parish nursing program in the United States was described by a Lutheran pastor, the Reverend Granger Westberg, who initiated a parish nursing program with six churches and nurses in or near Chicago (Westberg & McNamara, 1987). Parish nurses provide holistic health care with attention to the physical, emotional, and spiritual health of individuals and groups within the context of a religious community. By 1998, the American Nurses Association recognized parish nursing as a specialty practice and published specific scope and standards of practice for parish nurses (ANA, 1998).

Public-private partnerships offer public health nurses with additional opportunity for practice. Collaborative partnerships between faith-based organizations and public entities such as local health departments are viewed as an important means of improving the population's health (Zahner & Corrado, 2004). Federal support for assisting faith-based and community partnerships for needy Americans was actualized in 2001 with the development of the Center for Faith-Based & Community Initiatives within HHS (U.S. DHHS Center for Faith-based & Community Initiatives, 2005). The center can provide technical assistance through HHS programs to help strengthen the capacity of faith-based and community organizations to respond more effectively to programs that benefit vulnerable community members who may be poor, homeless, and/or socially disadvantaged.

Several studies have explored the nature of parish nursing, primarily by using descriptive research designs and qualitative methodological approaches. Research findings suggest that parish nurses are viewed positively as meaningful health care professionals, and this model can benefit the health and quality of life of congregational members and members of the larger community (Swinney et al., 2001; Wallace et al., 2002; Brudenell, 2003). Advanced practice nurses are ideally prepared for the role as parish nurses who have opportunities to promote health with a holistic perspective in community settings by working in partnership with congregational members, leaders of faith-based organizations, and faith communities to improve population health.

Workplaces

Nursing's rich history of promoting health and preventing disease, injury, and disability among groups of workers first started in the late 1900s when a nurse

⊕ POLICY HIGHLIGHT

Smallpox Vaccination and Emergency Preparedness

Different types of policies exist, such as organizational policies that can take the form of position statements or resolutions (Porche, 2004). In response to concerns of the National Smallpox Vaccination Program endorsed by the Bush administration, leaders of the Public Health Nursing Section of the American Public Health Association (APHA) drafted a position statement entitled "Statement on Smallpox Vaccination and Emergency Preparedness." The 2003 statement affirmed public health nursing's commitment to the safe and efficient implementation of the National Smallpox Vaccination Program based on scientific review and feedback of each phase. The statement emphasized the importance of public health nursing's active partnership with other agencies to develop coordinated responses to disasters, as well as the need for sufficient funding for smallpox and bioterrorism-related programs. It also stressed the importance of enhancing existing infrastructures, rather than creating additional systems that only responded to specific disease threats. Furthermore, the statement called for a national effort to provide mass public health education about smallpox immunization, accurate risk assessment prior to vaccination administration, efficient information systems, academic and practice partnerships to help with emergency preparedness, and continuing education to help providers become better prepared for emergencies.

The statement was crafted after dialogue with key leaders during a spring business meeting of the APHA Public Health Nursing Section, followed by two telephone conferences and the circulation of draft statements until consensus was reached. The statement was then shared with the American Nurses Association Congress on Nursing Practice & Economics, the Association of Community Health Nursing Educators, and the Association of State and Territorial Directors of Nursing. After minor modifications, the statement was endorsed fully by the Quad Council of Public Health Nursing Organizations. Dissemination of the position statement occurred primarily by posting it electronically on organizational Web sites for use by public health nurses in numerous settings.

Porche, D. J. (2004). *Public and community health nursing practice: A population-based approach.* Thousand Oaks, CA: Sage.

Quad Council of Public Health Nursing Organizations (2003). Statement on smallpox vaccination and emergency preparedness. Retrieved July 18, 2007 from http://www.achne.org/Documents/Smallpox_Vacc__Emerg_Preparedness_2003.pdf

---

was hired by the Vermont Marble Company and later by a group of coal miners to help take care of sick employees and family members in their homes. Other industries and companies quickly recognized the cost benefits of hiring nurses to help employees return to work settings as soon as possible following an illness. The number of nurses employed by industries increased steadily during the first few decades of the twentieth century, and by World War II there were 4,000 industrial nurses (Brown, 1981). Now referred to as occupational health nurses, this subspecialty of public health nursing evolved by focusing on improving the health of populations of workers.

Today registered nurses work in various occupational settings and clinics to improve the well-being of workers, to provide effective interventions targeted at specific aggregates at increased risk for potential health problems, and to give nursing care to individuals and families. Occupational health nursing is considered a specialty practice within work settings that focuses on health promotion; disease and injury prevention; restoration of health; and development of healthy, safe environments (AAOHN, 1999; Rogers, 2003).

Occupational health nurses may be employed, or they may contract independently to work or consult in various work settings in manufacturing, industry, service, health care, government, and a myriad of other businesses. Many occupational health nurses hold an advanced degree in nursing or public health, and they may work fairly autonomously or as members of an interdisciplinary team with other occupational health experts in areas such as medicine, social work, ergonomics, industrial hygiene, safety, environment, labor, and industry management. The American Association of Occupational Health Nurses (1997) described 10 roles appropriate for occupational health nurses. The roles include clinician, case manager, coordinator, manager, nurse practitioner, corporate director, health promotion specialist, educator, consultant, and researcher (Figure 3-8).

In addition to caring for individual workers and assessing groups of workers for health risks, occupational health nurses assess the workplace for environmental hazards, serve as advocates for workplace safety, communicate risk, and work actively for legislative changes that help protect and promote the health of workers. Nurses plan and implement programs that help prevent worker health problems by developing and conducting programs that promote physical activity, good nutrition, and stress management, for example, and by helping workers obtain needed immunizations and health and safety classes. Occupational health nurses conduct interventions designed to detect and treat disease or health problems early; these interventions include physical exams that are required before specific work assignments can be determined, screenings for hearing and vision, and blood pressure monitoring. Occupational health nurses hold an important role in conducting tertiary level of disease prevention when providing case management services for workers who qualify for worker's compensation or disability programs, or when conducting specific activities to help workers return to the work setting after injuries as soon as possible (Rogers, 2003; AAOHN, 2004).

Home Visiting

Public health nursing first started in the late nineteenth century when visiting nurses went into homes to help heal the sick, teach family members about health, and assess and help improve the family's home environment. Requests for visiting nurses expanded to activities beyond acute care needs. For example, visiting nurses increasingly were asked to help a new mother take care of her newborn baby or to help a family who recently immigrated to the United States better understand factory work and local economics. During the early twentieth century, funding sources that supported a comprehensive model of combining interventions focused on caring for ill individuals and interventions that prevented health problems eroded as agencies tended to fund one type of nursing focus or the other, but rarely both (Buhler-Wilkerson, 1985). Nurses employed by public health agencies focused on prevention, and nurses who remained with visiting nurses associations focused more on the care of acutely ill individuals. Nurses today, whether they work in official agencies or nongovernmental agencies, face similar challenges from third party payers who primarily reimburse for activities related to caring for sick individuals but do not provide reimbursement for preventive health services such as health education or counseling.

With the advent of Medicare in 1965, reimbursement for home health care increased, and numerous home health care agencies developed across the United States. Some public health departments initiated or maintained home health care agencies by garnering Medicare reimbursement for nursing services in the home. Home health care nurses provided skilled nursing care to homebound individuals, and the focus was on restorative care. Home health care nursing quickly became a subspecialty of community health nursing. Client acuity level at discharge continues to escalate,

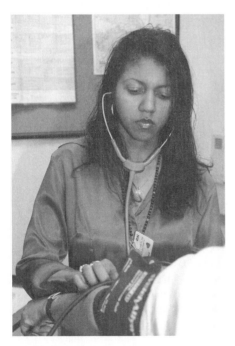

Figure 3-8 Blood pressure screening by public health nurse.

Courtesy of Gary Black, Mecklenburg County Health Department, Charlotte, North Carolina.

and more technology in home settings is needed for clients to maintain the option of staying at home rather than be hospitalized.

Public health nurses continue to offer home visiting programs if sufficient funds and resources exist in public health agencies. The home visits are conducted with the purpose of improving the health of high-risk, vulnerable community members with multiple risks and needs. Such programs have been demonstrated as highly effective for improving health and social outcomes, especially in the area of maternal child health (Olds et al., 1997; McNaughton, 2000, 2004). A recent synthesis of evaluation studies of maternal-child public health nursing visits found that an essential factor for successful intervention hinged on a long-term, consistent, well-established relationship between the nurse and client (Gomby, Culross, & Behrman, 1999; McNaughton, 2000). Other nursing research provides evidence that improved client health outcomes can exist long after the nursing interventions are completed (Olds et al., 1997; 2004).

Other Settings

In addition to the settings discussed, many other common settings for public health nursing practice cannot be discussed in the scope of this chapter. For example, population-based nursing care may be provided in correctional facilities such as federal prisons or county jails. Nurses working in community mental health centers can not only focus their care on restoring health but also on preventing adverse consequences of mental illness and promoting the health and well-being of persons at risk for debilitating mental illnesses. Senior centers and adult day health centers provide settings for nurses to care for elderly community members by encouraging wellness, promoting healthy behavioral habits, and helping clients and their caregivers to remain at home rather than in an institutionalized setting. Again, nurses can provide population-focused care in a variety of settings including large health systems, managed care organizations, and voluntary associations or organizations like the American Heart Association and the American Red Cross. Nursing knowledge and skill combined with knowledge of public health can be applied in all of these settings and many more.

Public health nurses are highly skilled at translating or interpreting essential public health activities with individuals, families, and community groups. Nurses are in unique positions to intervene at multiple levels and to apply principles of population health at individual and family levels "within the context of population-focused practice" (Quad Council, 2004).

MODELS OF PUBLIC HEALTH NURSING PRACTICE

Nursing leaders have embraced a broad vision of public health that is reflected in models of practice that serve to give structure and voice to the work of public health nurses. Three models of public health nursing practice are discussed to further our understanding of practice opportunities, issues, and challenges.

Minnesota Department of Health, Public Health Nursing Section Intervention Wheel

A model referred to as the "Intervention Wheel" or the "Wheel" helps public health nurses "refocus" attention on population-based nursing practice by strengthening their work with communities, the systems that affect the community's health, and with individuals and families that make up communities. Numerous public health nurses at local and state levels worked together to identify interventions that clearly described their work, and work that was conducted specifically beyond the level of individuals and families (Keller et al., 1998; 2004a; 2004b).

The Intervention Wheel identifies 17 interventions that cut across systems, community, and individual/family levels of care (Chapter 2, Figure 2-5). Public health nurses work in partnership with others to intervene effectively to change attitudes, health practices, behaviors, and knowledge of individuals, their families, and groups, and they work to impact communities and systems that in turn impact individuals, families, and communities. Practicing at a systems level calls for nursing interventions that target change in organizations, policies, laws, and power structures. Population-based care focused on communities includes work to change communities of people who share common characteristics in terms of community attitudes, practices, awareness and behaviors. Each intervention and practice level contributes to improving the health of populations. The model articulates the work of the public health nurses without regard to specific settings. Hence, the model does not focus on the setting of practice such as health departments, schools, correctional facilities, shelters, clinics, group homes, work sites, or hospitals.

The overarching premise of the model is that "population-based" practice focuses on entire populations, is based on community assessments with regard to numerous determinants of health, and focuses on prevention and interventions at multiple levels. The 17 interventions on the wheel are clustered into five groups that reflect their relationship to each other:

1. Surveillance, disease and other health event investigation, outreach, screening, and case finding;

2. Referral and follow-up, case management, and delegated functions;

3. Health teaching, counseling, and consultation;

4. Collaboration, coalition building, and community organization;

5. Advocacy, social marketing, and policy development and enforcement. (Keller et al., 2004a, p. 458)

The Intervention Wheel has been used in numerous public health nursing practice and academic settings as a means of giving structure to the work of public health nurses, describing the nature of the work, and helping nurses better articulate and document their work. Leaders of the Section of Public Health Nursing of the Minnesota Department of Health conducted a thorough critique of the model by examining the evidence associated with the interventions and practice levels. This critique guided some slight revisions of the model and verified that evidence did validate and confirm the interventions as encompassing the breadth and scope of public health nursing population-based practice, that all but two of the 17 interventions occurred at all three levels of practice, that there were no missing interventions, and that the interventions were distinct from each other, although some were interrelated or tended to occur sequentially or at the same time (Keller et al., 2002; 2004a; 2004b).

Association of State and Territorial Directors of Nursing Public Health Nursing Practice Model

The Association of State and Territorial Directors of Nursing (ASTDN) developed a public health nurs-

ing practice model with the intent of assisting nurses, educators, and leaders in public health nursing to conceptualize linkages between population health, nursing practice, and public health concepts. The model links the core public health functions of assessment (community diagnosis), policy development and leadership, and assurance of access to personal, environmental, and educational health services with the 10 essential public health services. The 10 essential public health services were developed and adopted in 1994 by the Public Health Functions Steering Committee as a means of articulating specific activities relevant to the work of all public health professionals and of clearly describing the core public health functions. They are reflected in the outer ring of the ASTDN Public Health Nursing Practice Model. The middle circle of the model includes the three core public health functions: assessment, policy development, and assurance. At the core of the model is the art and science of nursing practice to represent a holistic approach to health care that is grounded in the use of the nursing process and critical thinking as the basis of practice when conducting nursing interventions to fulfill the core public health functions and the essential services (ASTDN, 2003).

The Los Angeles County Public Health Nursing Practice Model

A third public health nursing practice model discussed in this chapter was developed by public health nurses who worked with the Los Angeles County (LAC) Department of Health Services (DHS). The impetus to develop this practice model was sparked by the need to have one framework that applied to public health nurses in diverse practice settings, from generalist to more specialized practice settings, and to clearly align public health nursing practice with public health nursing principles (Smith & Bazini-Barakat, 2003). The model blends several national standards and components. It helps public health nurses use the nursing process at each level of practice. The public health nurse is viewed as a critical member of an interdisciplinary team of public health professionals, and the team approach is considered essential for successful public health nursing endeavors. Other team members may include epidemiologists, nutritionists, health educators, physicians, social workers, community members, and environmental health specialists.

The LAC PHN practice model is supported by a number of tenets of population-based practice such as focusing on entire populations and being guided by population health status. It considers the broad determinants of health, community assessment, all levels of disease prevention, and all three levels of practice. It emphasizes primary prevention, reaches out to all who may benefit rather than only those people who have problems, employs principles of social justice by being concerned for the greatest good for all people, creates healthy environments, and fosters collaboration (Sakamoto & Avila, 2004). Components of the LAC PHN model include the Scope and Standards of Public Health Nursing Practice (Quad Council, 1999), the 10 essential public health services that were developed to describe the three core public health functions of assessment, assurance, and policy development (Public Health Functions Steering Committee, 1994), national and local health indicators from Healthy People 2010 (U.S. Department of Health and Human Services, 2000), and the Minnesota Department of Health, Public Health Nursing Section Intervention Wheel of the 17 interventions and the three levels of practice (Minnesota Department of Health, 2001).

These three practice models for public health nursing present several ways to help nurses conceptualize and articulate the nature of their work to the public, the nature of this nursing specialty with other nurses, and with colleagues in other disciplines.

ISSUES AND CHALLENGES

Members of the general public have more readily understood the value of strong public health and public health nursing in recent years because of attention from human-made and natural disasters. Terrorism; threats of anthrax or other biological, chemical, and radioactive agents; hurricanes like Hurricane Katrina; the tsunami in Southeast Asia; the earthquake in Pakistan and Kashmir; and emerging diseases like SARS and West Nile virus demonstrate very tangibly the need for and the importance of a strong public health workforce. Concerns about food and water safety, mercury emissions, possible human-to-human transmission of avian flu and predictions of a pandemic, and virulent strains of HIV that are resistant to current medication regimens are but a few examples of public health concerns in the American media. Ironically, in a time when more people are aware of the importance that public health plays in the global community and how public health's suc-

cesses are often "invisible," the public health workforce is shrinking in number (Columbia University School of Nursing, 2000; Government Performance Project, 2004). Nursing directors of state public health agencies reported on a survey conducted in spring 2003 that public health nursing shortages existed in 75 percent of the states (Brown & Stevens, 2003). Public health budgets have contributed to the workforce shortage. As federal funding is diverted to disaster preparedness and bioterrorism, members of the public health workforce have had insufficient funds to maintain the infrastructure needed to be prepared for any public health threat and to maintain successful preventive programs for common chronic and acute health problems (Government Performance Project, 2004). Public health workers have successfully dealt with similar challenges in the past during times of budget crises and will no doubt meet current and future problems with ingenuity, resilience, persistence, and creativity (Figure 3-9).

Workforce Issues and Challenges

Enumeration of public health nurses and other public health workers is difficult because the workforce is very diverse without clear definitions of roles or ways

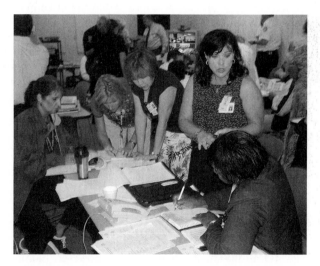

Figure 3-9 Public health nurses in emergency operations center during bioterrorism drill.

Courtesy of Gary Black & Joe Travis, Mecklenburg County Health Department, Charlotte, North Carolina.

to measure or count workers within the huge, complex array of organizations and agencies that comprise the public health system. Current numbers of public health nurses tend to reflect nurses hired by governmental agencies. Public health nurses remain the largest professional group in the public health workforce with 10.9 percent or 49,232 nurses within a total public health workforce of 448,254 (Bureau of Health Professions, 2005; Columbia University School of Nursing, 2000).

Public health nurses are best prepared to interpret public health activities with individuals and families within a community context (Quad Council, 2004). Even though the hallmark of public health nursing has always focused on improved health of populations and communities in relation to access, assurance, and quality, the work of public health nurses has often centered on individuals and families. As funding for personal health services conducted by public health agencies has increased and decreased depending on funding levels and federal allocations, nursing positions have been adversely impacted. Nursing positions may have been cut or left unfilled. Other barriers associated with recruiting and retaining public health nurses from a recent study included budget constraints, a lack of qualified candidates (especially in rural areas), noncompetitive salaries for public health nurses, and lengthy processing time for new nurse hires (Bureau of Health Professions, 2005). As the largest professional component of the public health workforce, it is essential to monitor and track public health nurse workforce shortages, disseminate best practices for recruitment and retention, develop favorable work environments, and help develop a model job description of nursing leaders to use at state levels (Brown & Stevens, 2003).

Educational Issues and Challenges

The **Quad Council of Public Health Nursing Organizations** (2001; 2004) endorses the bachelor's of science degree in nursing as the entry level required for public health nurses, and historically, the major feature distinguishing baccalaureate nursing education from diploma or associate degree programs was the required classroom and clinical experience in public health nursing (IOM, 2003). In many states, however, public health nurses without a bachelor's degree outnumber those with a bachelor's degree. Some states maintain a requirement that nurses who enter the public health

nursing workforce without a baccalaureate education must enroll in a public health course. Reasons for insufficient numbers of baccalaureate-prepared nurses in the public health workforce include trends related to a national nursing shortage, lack of funds or resources for lengthier and more expensive tuition, the loss of some public health nurse positions when health agencies shifted from a focus on core public health functions to personal health services because of available reimbursement by Medicare and Medicaid, insufficient funds for public health departments, and budget constraints that resulted in fewer nursing positions (Quad Council, 2001; Greiner & Oppewal, 2003).

Guidelines published by the Association of Community Health Nursing Educators outline the *Essentials of Baccalaureate Nursing Education for Entry Level Community Health Practice* (2000a) and *Graduate Education for Advance Practice in Community Public Health Nursing* (2000b). Nurse educators may also use the Council on Linkages core competencies for public health workers published by the Quad Council of Public Health Nursing Organizations in Public Health Nursing (2004) and the Minnesota Department of Health publication (2001), *Public Health Interventions: Application for Public Health Nursing Practice*, for curricular guidance. Regardless of the model used to organize curricular material, it is important for educators to partner actively with public health nursing practitioners and other community members to help future public health nurses achieve basic awareness or knowledge of the core competencies for public health workers and the skills needed for the 10 essential public health functions (Gebbie & Hwang, 2000).

The IOM report, *Who Will Keep the Public Health? Educating Public Health Professionals for the 21st Century* (2003), recommended that education for all public health professionals include an ecological model with an emphasis on the multiple factors that impact health. The report also specifically recommended that graduate-level public health education programs include eight areas: informatics, genomics, communication, cultural competence, community-based participatory research, global health, policy and law, and public health ethics. After completing graduate education from schools of public health or schools of nursing, public health nurses usually no longer practice as generalists but as clinical nurse specialists, managers, supervisors, or program specialists within public health agencies (IOM, 2003).

Financial Issues, Rewards, and Job Satisfaction

Most nurses who work in public health value the intrinsic reward of knowing they make a difference to numerous community members, many who have complicated issues that leave them vulnerable to numerous health problems. Even though public health nursing is challenging in various ways, the rewards that accompany it are also numerous, and dedication to the specialty often increases over time. The ability to be creative and autonomous, to work with numerous disciplines and community members on challenging issues, and to avoid shift work and instead work primarily during weekday hours are benefits that public health nurses enjoy. In addition, nurses use a wide variety of skills and knowledge while intervening at levels that extend beyond a one-to-one encounter with a client.

Most public health nurses are willing to accept less competitive salaries for their positions compared with more competitive wages available at acute care settings. Public health leaders continue to monitor gaps in salaries to make sure they do not become so wide that it will be difficult to recruit and retain a sufficient workforce. A report published in January 2005 by the Bureau of Health Professions found that newly recruited public health nurses tended to stay in their jobs in most states. Factors associated with job retention included autonomy, the favorable work hours, and benefits.

Other aspects of high job satisfaction included community member respect and trust that is bestowed on public health nurses, potentially flexible work hours, few work requirements on weekends or evenings, and relatively no shift work. Recognizing the positive differences that public health nurses and the entire public health workforce make for so many people is immensely rewarding.

Public health nursing practice takes place in numerous settings including schools, local and state health departments, federal agencies, workplaces, homes, clinics, and a myriad of other places. This specialty of nursing is not dependent on any one setting because population-based nursing care can take place virtually anywhere when the focus is to improve the health of populations by working in partnership with other community members and disciplines to foster healthful change with individuals and families, systems, and communities. Early models of public health nursing developed by Lillian Wald continue to inspire and help inform nursing practice today. The nursing process, the 10 essential functions of public health and the three core functions, indicators and goals of *Healthy People 2010*, and specific nursing interventions that can be conducted at levels of practice that target individuals and families, communities, and systems are all important components in models that inform public health nursing practice. Challenges exist financially and educationally, yet public health nursing is highly rewarding and satisfying in a wide array of practice settings.

CRITICAL THINKING ACTIVITIES

1. Many health consumers consider public health nurses as nurses hired by official agencies such as local or state health departments. Form a statement that someone with an eighth grade education could easily understand that articulates the various practice settings in which public health nurses practice.

2. Public health nursing is a highly rewarding career yet one that has challenges. Identify some of the most pressing challenges for nurses in public health settings and identify some strategies to resolve them.

3. Public health nurses typically practice in a wide variety of settings such as health departments, schools, occupational settings, and homes. The setting may focus on acute care or have a broader community mission. How are the activities of public health nurses similar when settings have these missions? How are they different?

4. Obesity in children is a prevalent health issue that poses numerous challenges, but dealing with it is essential because of the healthful benefits that controlling obesity will bring. What interventions can a school nurse make at the systems level that would help decrease the prevalence of school-age children who are obese or at risk of becoming obese? What interventions could a school nurse conduct that would be focused at a community level?

KEY TERMS

community health centers

federally qualified health centers

migrant health centers

nurse-managed health centers

occupational health nursing

population-based nursing practice

primary care

primary health care

Quad Council of Public Health Nursing Organizations

rural health clinics

safety net providers

school-based health centers

KEY CONCEPTS

- Public health nursing can take place in any setting. It is not defined by its location in the community but by its focus on creating conditions to improve the health of populations.

- Lillian Wald's model of care at the Henry Street Settlement in the early 1900s has helped inform nurse-managed health centers and other practice models today.

- Before World War I, public health nurses practiced in homes, through visiting nursing services or associations, and in numerous community sites such as schools and work sites.

- Common public health nursing practice settings today are in governmental agencies and in non-governmental, community agencies, as well as places convenient to clients.

- Practice opportunities for public health nurses at local, state, and national governmental agencies are numerous and will focus on services at the population level.

- Public health nursing roles such as clinician, case manager, health educator, advocate, coalition builder, and researcher may be similar in different practice settings.

- Nursing interventions directed toward healthful change with individuals and families, systems, and communities may be similar in different practice settings.

- Several public health nursing practice models exist as frameworks for articulating and documenting the work of public health nurses.

- Challenges related to public health and public health nursing workforce issues, educational issues, and financial issues interrelate, and they need to be addressed.

- Public health nurses generally have high job satisfaction given the intrinsic reward of knowing the positive differences they make with communities and populations.

REFERENCES

Abrams, S.E. (2004). From function to competency in public health nursing, 1931 to 2003. *Public Health Nursing, 21*(5), 507–510.

American Association of Occupational Health Nurses (AAOHN). (1997). *Guidelines for developing job descriptions in occupational and environmental health nursing.* Atlanta: Author.

American Association of Occupational Health Nurses (AAOHN). (1999). *Standards for occupational health nursing practice.* Atlanta: Author.

American Association of Occupational Health Nurses (AAOHN). (2004, August). Position statement: Delivery of occupational and environmental health services. Retrieved March 12, 2005, from the American Association of Occupational Health Nurses Inc. Web site at http://www.aaohn.org/practice/positions/index.cfm

American Nurses Association (ANA). (1998). *Scope and standards of parish nursing practice.* Washington, DC: Author and Health Ministries Association.

American Public Health Association, Public Health Nursing Section. (1996). *Definition and role of public health nursing.* Washington, DC: Author.

Association of Community Health Nursing Educators. (2000a). *Essentials of baccalaureate nursing education for entry level community health nursing practice.* Latham, NY: Author.

Association of Community Health Nursing Educators (2000b). *Graduate education for advanced practice in community public health nursing.* Latham, NY: Author.

Association of State and Territorial Directors of Nursing (ASTDN). (2003). *Public health nursing: A partner for health populations.* Washington, DC: American Nurses Publishing.

Berkowitz, B., Dahl, J., Guirl, K., Kostelecky, B.J., Mcneil, C., & Upenieks, V. (2001). *Public health nursing leadership: A guide to managing the core functions.* Washington, DC: American Nurses Association.

Bowden, J.M., Shaul, M.P., & Bennett, J.A. (2004). The process of changing health risk behaviors: An Oregon rural clinic experience. *Journal of the American Academy of Nurse Practitioners, 16* (9), 411–417.

Broussard, L. (2004). School nursing: Not just band-aids any more! *Journal for Specialists in Pediatric Nursing, 9*(3), 77–83.

Brown, A., & Stevens, R. (2003). *Public health nursing leadership, responsibilities and issues in state health departments: Results of an Association of State and Territorial Directors of Nursing (ASTDN) survey.* Retrieved January 25, 2004, from http://www.astdn.org/downloadablefiles/PHNLeadershipResponsibilitiesandIssues.pdf.

Brown, M. (1981). *Occupational health nursing.* New York: MacMillan.

Brudenell, I. (2003). Parish nursing: Nurturing body, mind, spirit, and community. *Public Health Nursing, 20*(2), 85–94.

Buhler-Wilkerson, K. (1985). Public health nursing: In sickness or in health? *American Journal of Public Health, 75*(10), 1155–1161.

Buhler-Wilkerson, K. (1993). Bringing care to the people: Lillian Wald's legacy to public health nursing. *American Journal of Public Health, 83*(12), 1778–1786.

Bureau of Health Professions, Health Resources Services & Administration (HRSA). (2005, January). *Public health workforce study.* Washington, DC: HRSA. Retrieved February 22, 2005, from http://bhpr.hrsa.gov/healthworkforce/reports/publichealth/default.htm.

Bureau of Primary Health Care. (n.d.). Migrant health program. Retrieved January 20, 2005: http://bphc.hrsa.gov/programs/MHCProgramInfo.htm.

Columbia University School of Nursing, Center for Health Policy. (*2000*). *The public health workforce: Enumeration 2000.* (HRSA/ATPM Cooperative Agreement # U76 AH 00001-03). Washington DC: U.S. Department of Health and Human Services.

Edwards, J.B., Oppewal, S., & Logan, C.L. (2003). Nurse-managed primary care: Outcomes of a faculty practice network. *Journal of the American Academy of Nurse Practitioners, 15*(12), 563–569.

Embrey, K. (n.d.). Farmworkers in the U.S.: Background for teachers. *Coming up on the season: Migrant farmworkers in the Northeast.* Retrieved April 1, 2005, from http://www.farmworkers.cornell.edu/pdf/background.pdf.

Fact Sheet: Rural Health Clinic (2004, May). Retrieved February 12, 2005, from http://www.cms.hhs.gov/medlearn/rhcfactsheet.pdf.

Gale, J.A., & Coburn, A.F. (2003). *The characteristics and roles of rural health clinics in the United States: A chartbook.* Portland, ME: University of Southern Maine. Retrieved February 1, 2005, from http://muskie.usm.maine.edu/Publications/rural/RHChartbook03.pdf.

Gebbie, K.M., & Hwang, I. (2000). Preparing currently employed public health nurses for changes in the health system. *American Journal of Public Health, 90*(5), 716–721.

Gomby, D.S., Culross, P.L., & Behrman, R.E. (1999). Home visiting: Recent program evaluations—Analysis and recommendations. *Future of Children, 9*(1), 4–26.

Government Performance Project. (2004, February). Public Health: Costs of complacency. *The Government Performance Project: A case of neglect.* Retrieved March 20, 2005 from http://governing.com/gpp/2004/public.htm.

Greiner, P.A., & Oppewal, S. (2003). *Testimony before the Institute of Medicine Study Committee on the work environment for nurses and patient safety.* (Written testimony submitted for the Public Health Nursing Section, American Public Health Association January 27, 2003.) Retrieved April 15, 2005, from http://www.csuchico.edu/~horst/about/shortage.html.

Hansen-Turton, T., Line, L., O'Connell, M., Rothman, R., & Lauby, J. (*2004, June*). *The nursing center model of health care for the underserved.* (HCFA Contract No. 18-P91720/3-01). Philadelphia: National Nursing Centers Consortium.

Hawkins, D., & Proser, M. (2004, March). A nation's health at risk: A national and state report on America's 36 million people without a regular health care provider (Special Topics Issue Brief #5). National Association of Community Health Centers, Inc. Washington, DC. Retrieved January 24, 2005, from http://www.nachc.com/piforum/files/UnservedReportSTIB5.pdf.

Hawkins, J.W., Hayes, E.R., & Corliss, C.P. (1994). School nursing in America—1902–1994: A return to public health. *Public Health Nursing, 11*(6), 416–425.

Institute of Medicine (IOM). 1988. *The future of public health.* Washington, DC: National Academy Press.

Institute of Medicine (IOM). (2003). *Who will keep the public healthy? Educating public health professionals for the 21st century.* Washington, DC: National Academies Press.

Institute of Medicine (IOM) of the National Academies, Committee on the Future of Rural Health Care, Board on Health Care Services (2004). *Quality through collaboration: The future of rural health.* Washington, DC: National Academies Press.

Kalisch, P.A., & Kalisch, B.J. (1978). *The advance of American nursing.* Boston: Little, Brown and Company.

Keller, L.O., Schaffer, M., Lia-Hoagberg, B., & Strohschein, S. (2002). Population-based practice: Community assessment, program planning and evaluation. *Journal of Public Health Management and Practice, 8*(5), 30–43.

Keller, L.O., Strohschein, S., Lia-Hoagberg, B., & Schaffer, M. (1998). Population-based public health nursing interventions: A model from practice. *Public Health Nursing, 15*(3), 207–215.

Keller, L.O., Strohschein, S., Lia-Hoagberg, B., & Schaffer, M.A. (2004a). Population-based public health interventions: Practice-based and evidence-supported. Part I. *Public Health Nursing, 21*(5), 453–468.

Keller, L.O., Strohschein, S., Lia-Hoagberg, B., & Schaffer, M.A. (2004b). Population-based public health interventions: Innovations in practice, teaching, and management. Part II. *Public Health Nursing, 21*(5), 469–487.

Kennedy, S. (1996). Nursing centers: The actualization of nurses . . . an interview with a nurse working in a nursing center. *New Jersey Nurse, 26*(10), 9, 11.

Koplan, J.P. (2001). Foreword to school health policies and programs study: A summary report. *Journal of School Health, 71*(7), 251.

Madison, D. L. (2003). Durham's exemplary health center—and its leader, Dr. Evelyn Schmidt (Special Article). *North Carolina Medical Journal, 64*(4), 161–165.

McNaughton, D.B. (2000). A synthesis of qualitative home visiting research. *Public Health Nursing, 17*(6), 405–416.

McNaughton, D.B. (2004). Nurse home visits to maternal–child clients: A review of intervention research. *Public Health Nursing, 21*(3), 207–219.

Minnesota Department of Health, Division of Community Health Services, Public Health Nursing Section. (2001). *Public health interventions: Applications for public health nursing practice.* St. Paul, MN: Author.

Mundinger, M.O. (2000). Now and future primary care. *Reflections on Nursing LEADERSHIP, 26*(1), 12–14.

National Association of Community Health Centers, Inc. (2004). *America's health centers fact sheet—August 2004* (Fact Sheet #0304). Retrieved January 30, 2005, from http://www.nachc.com/research/Files/IntrotoHealthCenters8.04.pdf.

National Association of School-Based Health Centers. (2005.). *School-based health centers: Blue print for health learners: Data from 2001–02 School-Based Health Center Census.* Retrieved April 10, 2005, from http://www.nasbhc.org/APP/2002_data_fact_sheet_blueprint.pdf.

National Center for Farmworker Health, Inc. (n.d.). *Facts about farmworkers.* Retrieved March 1, 2005, from http://www.ncfh.org/docs/fs-Facts%20about%20Farmworkers.pdf.

National Rural Health Association (n.d). *What is a rural health clinic? A RHC fact sheet.* Retrieved March 23, 2005, from http://www.nrharural.org/pdf/RHC-factsheet.pdf.

Olds, D.L., Eckenrode, J., Henderson, C.R., Kitzman, H., Powers, J., Cole, R., et al. (1997). Long-term effects of home visitation on maternal life course and child abuse and neglect. *Journal of the American Medical Association, 278*(8), 637–643.

Olds, D.L., Kitzman, H., Cole, R., Robinson, J., Sidora, K., Luckey, D.W., et al. (2004). Effects of nurse home visiting on maternal life course and child development: Age 6 follow-up results of a randomized trial. *Pediatrics, 114,* 1550–1559.

Porche, D. J. (2004). *Public and community health nursing practice: A population-based approach.* Thousand Oaks, CA: Sage.

Public Health Functions Steering Committee. (1994). *Public health in America.* Retrieved March 15, 2005, from http://www.health.gov/phfunctions/public.htm.

Quad Council of Public Health Nursing Organizations. (1999). *Scope and standards of public health nursing practice.* Washington, DC: American Nurses Association.

Quad Council of Public Health Nursing Organizations. (2001). *The impact of the nursing shortage on public health nursing.* Retrieved February 25, 2005, from http://www.astdn.org/downloadfiles/QuadCouncil-July2001-TheImpactoftheNursingsh.pdf.

Quad Council. of Public Health Nursing Organizations. (2003). *PHN competencies.* Retrieved January 29, 2005, from http://www.csuchico.edu/~horst/about/competencies.html.

Quad Council of Public Health Nursing Organizations. (2004). Public health nursing competencies: Quad Council of Public Health Nursing Organizations. *Public Health Nursing, 21*(5), 443–452.

Roberts, D.E., & Heinrich, J. (1985). Public health nursing comes of age. *American Journal of Nursing, 75*(10), 1162–1172.

Rogers, B. (*2003*). *Occupational health nursing: Concepts and practice.* St. Louis, Elsevier.

Sakamoto, S.D., & Avila, M. (2004). The public health nursing practice manual: A tool for public health nurses. *Public Health Nursing, 21*(2), 179–182.

Smith, K., & Bazini-Barakat, N. (2003). A public health nursing practice model: Melding public health principles with the nursing process. *Public Health Nursing 20*(1), 42–48.

Swinney, J., Anson-Wonkka, C., Maki, E., & Corneau, J. (2001). Community assessment: A church community and the parish nurse. *Public Health Nursing, 18*(1), 40–44.

U.S. Department of Health and Human Services. (n.d.). Bureau of primary health care: Health care for the homeless program information. Retrieved February 20, 2005, from http://bphc.hrsa.gov/programs/homelesspro-graminfo.htm#COLLABORATIVE.

U.S. Department of Health and Human Services. (2000). *Healthy people 2010.* McLean, VA: International Medical Publishing.

U.S. DHHS Center for Faith-Based & Community Initiatives. (2005). Retrieved February 5, 2005, http://www.dhhs.gov/fbci/.

U.S. Public Health Service, Nursing Professional Advisory Committee, Communications Subcommittee. (2002, July). *USPHS nurse resource manual.* Retrieved February 15, 2005, from http://phs-nurse.org/ResourceManual.htm.

U.S. Public Health Service Overview. (2005). Retrieved April 10, 2005, from http://phs-nurse.org/Overview.htm.

Wallace, D.C., Tuck, I., Boland, C.S., & Witucki, J.M. (2002). Client perceptions of parish nursing. *Public Health Nursing, 19*(2), 128–135.

Westberg, G., & McNamara, J. (1987). *The parish nurse: How to start a parish nurse program in your church.* Park Ridge, IL: Parish Nurse Resource Center.

Williams, C. (1977). Community health nursing—What is it? *Nursing Outlook, 1977*(23), 250–254.

Wolfe, L.C., & Selekman, J. (2002). School nurses: What it was and what it is. *Pediatric Nursing, 28*(4), 403–407.

Young, D. (2004). IOM sets strategy for improving rural health care quality. *American Journal of Health—System Pharmacy, 6*(24), 2618, 2623, 2627.

Zahner, S.J., & Corrado, S.M. (2004). Local health department partnerships with faith-based organizations. *Journal of Public Health Management Practice, 10*(3), 258–265.

BIBLIOGRAPHY

Anderson, D.G., Richmond, C., & Stanhope, M. (2004). Enhanced undergraduate public health nursing experience: A collaborative experience with the Kentucky Department for Public Health. *Family & Community Health, 27*(4), 291–297.

Avila, M., & Smith, K. (2003). The reinvigoration of public health nursing: Methods and innovations. *Journal of Public Health Management Practice, 9*(1), 16–24.

Barton, A. J., Clark, L., & Baramee, J. (2004). Tracking outcomes in community-based care. *Home Health Care Management & Practice, 16*(3), 171–176.

Berkowitz, B. (2002). Public Health Nursing Practice: Aftermath of September 11, 2001. *Online Journal of Issues in Nursing, 7*(3), Date: 2002-09-30. Available: http://www.nursingworld.org/ojin/topic19/tpc19_4.htm.

Berkowitz, B. (2004). Rural public health service delivery: Promising new directions. *American Journal of Public Health, 94*(10), 1678–1681.

Burgener, S.C., & Moore, S.J. (2002). The role of advanced practice nurses in community settings. *Nursing Economic$, 20*(3), 102–108, 132.

Cramer, M.E., Mueller, K.J., & Harrop, D. (2003). Comprehensive evaluation of a community coalition: A case study of environmental tobacco smoke reduction. *Public Health Nursing, 20*(6), 464–477.

dela Cruz, F.A., Brehm, C., & Harris, J. (2004). Transformation in family nurse practitioner students' attitudes toward homeless individuals after participation in a homeless outreach clinic. *Journal of the American Academy of Nurse Practitioners, 16*(12), 547–554.

DeMay, D. A. (2003). The experience of being a client in an Alaska public health nursing home visitation program. *Public Health Nursing, 20*(3), 228–236.

Drummond, J.E., Weir, A.E., & Kysela, G.M. (2002). Home visitation practice: Models, documentation, and evaluation. *Public Health Nursing, 19*(1), 21–29.

Garrett, L.H. (2005). Interdisciplinary practice, education, and research: The expanding role of the occupational health nurse. *American Association of Occupational Health Nursing Journal, 53*(4), 159–165.

Kaiser, K.L., & Rudolph, E.J. (2003). Achieving clarity in evaluation of community/public health nurse generalist competencies through development of a clinical performance evaluation tool. *Public Health Nursing, 20*(3), 216–227.

Larsson, L.S., & Butterfield, P. (2002). Mapping the future of environmental health and nursing: Strategies for integrating national competencies into nursing practice. *Public Health Nursing, 19*(9), 301–308.

Libbus, M.K., Bullock, L.F., Igoe, J., Beetem, N., & Cole, M. (2003). School nurses: Voices from the health room. *Journal of School Health, 73*(8), 322–324.

May, K.M., Phillips, L.R., Ferketich, S.L., & Verran, J. A. (2003). Public health nursing: The generalist in a specialized environment. *Public Health Nursing, 20*(4), 252–259.

McCabe, S., Macnee, C.L., & Anderson, M.K. (2001). Homeless patients' experience of satisfaction with care. *Archives of Psychiatric Nursing, 15*(2), 78–85.

McKeown, E., Barkauskas, V., Quinn, A., & Kresowaty, J. (2003). Occupational nursing service in a small manufacturing plant: Interventions and outcomes. *International Journal of Nursing Terminologies and Classifications: The Official Journal of NANDA International, 14*(4), 125–135.

Mondy, C., Cardenas, D., & Avila, M. (2003). The role of an advanced practice public health nurse in bioterrorism preparedness. *Public Health Nursing, 20*(6), 422–431.

Nies, M.A., Bickes, J.T., Schim, S.M., & Johnson, A.L. (2002). Model for community health nursing care: Application to an integrated asthma intervention program. *The Journal of School Nursing, 18* (2), 74-78.

Reifsnider, E., Hook, L, Muennink, P., & Vogt, D.J. (2004). Learning public health nursing in urban, rural, and border counties of Texas. *Family & Community Health, 27*(4), 282–290.

Robertson, J.F. (2004). Does advanced community/public health nursing practice have a future? *Public Health Nursing, 21*(5), 495–500.

Self, B., & Peters, H. (2005). Street outreach with no streets. *Canadian Nurse, 101*(1), 21–24.

Sheetz, A. H. (2003). Developing school health services in Massachusetts: A public health model. *The Journal of School Nursing, 19*(4), 204–211.

Sloand, E., & Groves, S. (2005). A community-oriented primary care nursing model in an international setting that emphasizes partnerships. *Journal of the American Academy of Nurse Practitioners, 17*(2), 47–50.

SmithBattle, L., & Diekemper, M. (2001). Promoting clinical practice knowledge in an age of taxonomies and protocols. *Public Health Nursing, 18*(6), 401–408.

SmithBattle, L., Diekemper, M., & Leander, S. (2004). Getting your feet wet: Becoming a Public Health Nurse, part 1. *Public Health Nursing, 21*(1), 3–11.

SmithBattle, L., Diekemper, M., & Leander, S. (2004). Moving upstream: Becoming a public health nurse, part 2. *Public Health Nursing, 21*(2), 95–102.

U.S. Department of Labor, Office of Program Economics (2000, March). *Findings from the National Agricultural Workers Survey (NAWS) 1997–1998: A demographic and employment profile of United States farmworkers* (Research Report no.8). Washington, DC: author.

RESOURCES

Agency for Healthcare Research and Quality (AHRQ)

540 Gaither Road
Rockville, Maryland 20850
301-427-1364
Web: http://www.ahrq.gov

AHRQ is a federal agency in the U.S. Department of Health and Human Services that conducts research on health care quality, costs, outcomes, and patient safety. It is the lead federal agency charged with improving the quality, safety, efficiency, and effectiveness of health care for all Americans. As one of 12 agencies within the Department of Health and Human Services, AHRQ supports health services research that will improve the quality of health care and promote evidence-based decision making.

Agency for Toxic Substance and Disease Registry (ATSDR)

1825 Century Blvd
Atlanta, Georgia 30345
1-800-343-5436
Web: http://www.atsdr.cdc.gov

ATSDR is a federal public health agency of the U.S. Department of Health and Human Services that uses sound scientific evidence to implement public health interventions, and provides trusted health information to prevent harmful exposures and diseases related to toxic substances.

ATSDR's Environmental Health and Nursing Initiative

Agency of Toxic Substances and Disease Registry
Division of Toxicology and Environmental Medicine
4770 Buford Hwy, NE (Mail Stop F-32)
Atlanta, Georgia 30341-3717
1-800-232-4636
FAX: 770-488-4178
Email: atsdr-nurse@cdc.gov
Web: http://www.atsdr.cdc.gov

This agency promotes and supports nurses' contributions to promoting environmental health for individuals and communities.

American Association of Occupational Health Nurses (AAOHN)

2920 Brandywine Road, Suite 100
Atlanta, Georgia 30341
770-455-7757
FAX: 770-455-7271
Email: aaohn@aaohn.org
Web: http://www.aaohn.org

AAOHN, the largest group of health care professionals serving the workplace, has a mission to ensure occupational and environmental nurses are the authority on health, safety, productivity, and disability management for worker populations. AAOHN is a principal force in furthering the profession of occupational and environmental health nursing by advancing the profession.

American Public Health Association (APHA)

800 "I" Street NW
Washington, D.C. 20001-3710
202-777-APHA (2752)
FAX: 202-777-2534
Email: comments@APHA.org

Web: http://www.apha.org

APHA is a nonprofit association of public health professionals from over 50 public health occupations working to improve the public's health and to achieve equity in health status for all. The organization strives to influence policy and set priorities in public health to help prevent disease and promote health. The organization also strives to promote the scientific and professional foundation of public health practice and policy, advocate the conditions for a healthy global society, emphasize prevention, and enhance the ability of members to promote and protect environmental and community health.

American Public Health Association— Public Health Nursing Section (APHA)

800 "I" Street NW
Washington, D.C. 20001-3710
202-777-APHA (2752)
FAX: 202-777-2534
Email: comments@APHA.org
Web: http://www.apha.org

The Association of Public Health Nurse Educators and Practitioners operates within the American Public Health Association. The Web site provides information and opportunities for involvement in nationwide PHN issues.

American School Health Association (ASHA)

7263 State Route 43
P.O. Box 708
Kent, Ohio 44240
330-678-1601
FAX: 330-768-4526
Email: asha@ashaweb.irg
Web: http://www.ashaweb.org

ASHA is a multidisciplinary association of professionals including administrators, counselors, health educators, school nurses, psychologists, health educators, physical educators, physicians, and social workers. Its mission is to protect and promote the health and well-being of school-age children and youth through coordinated school health programs.

Association of Community Health Nurse Educators (ACHNE)

10200 West 44th Avenue, #304
Wheat Ridge, Colorado 80033
303-422-0679
FAX: 303-422-9904
Email: ACHNE@resourcenter.com
Web: http://www.achne.org

ACHNE is an association of educators that teaches community health and public health nursing at universities and colleges. ACHNE provides a meeting ground for those committed to excellence in community and public health nursing education, research, and practice. ACHNE was established in 1978 and is run by elected volunteer leaders who guide the organization in providing networking through the quarterly newsletter and membership directory and in providing educational opportunities through publications and the annual Spring Institute. ACHNE's mission is to promote the public's health by ensuring leadership and excellence in community and public health nursing education, research, and practice. The Web site provides information on workforce issues, public health nursing/community health nursing certification, career opportunities, public health nursing graduate education, and links to other Quad Council organizations.

Association of Occupational and Environmental Clinics (AOEC)

1010 Vermont Avenue NW, #513
Washington, D.C. 20005
202-347-4976; 888-347-AOEC (2632)
Email: aoec@aoec.org
Web: http://www.aoec.org

AOEC is a nonprofit organization committed to improving the practice of occupational and environmental health through collaborative research and sharing of information and resources. Since its founding in 1987, the AOEC has grown to a network of more than 60 clinics and more than 250 individuals committed to improving the practice of occupational and environmental medicine through information sharing and collaborative research.

Association of State and Territorial Directors of Nursing

1275 K Street NW, Suite 800
Washington, D.C. 20005-4006
202-371-9090
FAX: 202-371-9797
Email: dianakp@health.ok.gov
Web: http://www.astdn.org

The Association of State and Territorial Directors of Nursing began in 1935 as an advisory group of state health department nurses. ASTDN continues today as an active association of public health nursing leaders from across the United States and its territories. ASTDN is an affiliate of the Association of State and Territorial Health Officials (ASTHO). The ASTDN mission is to provide a collegial forum to advance the public health nursing leadership role in protecting and promoting the health of the public. The Web site provides information on publications, population-focused practice, Quad Council competencies, Partnership Project (CDC and ASTDN), newsletter, and featured state public health nursing profile.

Association of State and Territorial Health Officials (ASTHO)

1275 K Street NW, Suite 800
Washington, D.C. 20005-4006
202-371-9090
FAX: 202-371-9797
Web: http://www.astho.org

ASTHO is the national nonprofit organization representing the state and territorial public health agencies of the United States, the U.S. territories, and the District of Columbia. ASTHO's members, the chief health officials of these jurisdictions, are dedicated to formulating and influencing sound public health policy and to assuring excellence in state-based public health practice. The Web site provides resources on public health information, workforce issues, law and public health, publications, and many other current issues.

Centers for Disease Control and Prevention (CDC)

1600 Clifton Road
Atlanta, Georgia 30333
404-639-3311 / Public Inquiries: 404-639-3534 / 1-800-311-3435
Web: http://www.cdc.gov

The CDC is one of the 13 major operating components of the Department of Health and Human Services (HHS), which is the principal agency in the U.S. government for protecting the health and safety of all Americans and for providing essential human services, especially for those people who are least able to help themselves. Since it was founded in 1946, CDC has remained at the forefront of public health efforts to prevent and control infectious and chronic diseases, injuries, workplace hazards, disabilities, and environmental health threats. Today, CDC is globally recognized for conducting research and investigations and for its action-oriented approach. CDC applies research and findings to improve people's daily lives and responds to health emergencies—something that distinguishes CDC from its peer agencies.

The Center for Health and Health Care in Schools (CHHCS)

The Center for Health and Health Care in Schools
School of Public Health and Health Services
The George Washington University Medical Center
2121 K Street NW, Suite 250
Washington, D.C. 20037
202-466-3396
FAX: 202-466-3467
Email: CHHCS@GWU.EDU
Web: http://www.healthinschools.org

CHHCS is a nonpartisan policy and program resource center located at The George Washington University School of Public Health and Health Services. CHHCS builds on a 20-year history of testing strategies to strengthen health care delivery systems for children and adolescents. For the past decade, with support from The Robert Wood Johnson Foundation, staff and consultants at the center have worked with institutional leaders, state officials, and clinical providers to maximize outcomes for children through more effective health programming in schools. Members are committed to strengthening health care delivery systems for children and adolescents through effective health programming and health care services in schools.

Centers for Medicare & Medicaid Services (CMS)

Centers for Medicare & Medicaid Services
7500 Security Boulevard
Baltimore, Maryland 21244
Web: http://new.cms.hhs.gov

CMS is the federal agency responsible for administering Medicare, Medicaid, SCHIP (State Children's Health Insurance), HIPAA (Health Insurance Portability and Accountability Act), CLIA (Clinical Laboratory Improvement Amendments), and several other health programs.

Children's Environmental Health Network

110 Maryland Avenue NE, Suite 505
Washington, D.C. 20002
202-543-4033
FAX: 202-543-8797
Email: cehn@cehn.org
Web: http://www.cehn.org

The Children's Environmental Health Network is a national organization comprised of multiple disciplines for the purpose of protecting the health of the fetus and the child from environmental health hazards and to promote a healthy environment.

DATA2010

National Center for Health Statistics
Division of Health Promotion Statistics
3311 Toledo Road
Hyattsville, Maryland 20782-2003
301-458-4013 **(Health Statistics)**
Web: http://wonder.cdc.gov

DATA2010 is an interactive database system developed by the Division of Health Promotion Statistics at the National Center for Health Statistics. It contains the most recent monitoring data for tracking Healthy People 2010 objectives.

EnviRN

Environmental Health Education Center
University of Maryland School of Nursing
655 West Lombard Street, Room 665
Baltimore, Maryland 21201
410-706-1849
Fax: 410-706-0295
Email: enviRN@son.umaryland.edu
Web: http://envirn.umaryland.edu

EnviRN is an interactive and dynamic resource with timely and accurate information on environmental health and nursing for the purpose of preventing environmental disease by improving the knowledge and skills of nurses and health professionals in preventing and intervening with environmental health problems. Based at the University of Maryland's School of Nursing, this resource is a "virtual nursing village" for sharing teaching strategies, practice guidance, information, and research on nursing and environmental health.

Food and Drug Administration (FDA)

U.S. Food and Drug Administration
5600 Fishers Lane
Rockville, Maryland 20857-0001
1-888-INFO-FDA (1-888-463-6332)
Web: http://www.fda.gov

FDA is a federal agency with the mission of promoting and protecting the public's health by helping consumers receive safe and effective products through market systems in a timely manner, monitoring the safety of products, and helping the public receive accurate, science-based information about products.

Health Care without Harm (HCWH)

HCWH—U.S. & Canada
Colleen Funkhouser
HCWH Membership Services
1901 North Moore Street, Suite 509
Arlington, Virginia 22209
703-243-0056
FAX: 866-438-5769
Email: cfunkhouser@hcwh.org
Web: http://www.noharm.org

HCWH is an international coalition of hospitals and health care organizations, community groups, health care providers, environmental and religious groups, labor unions, and health-affected constituencies who work collectively to improve health by working to reduce pollution in the health care industry.

Healthfinders

National Health Information Center
P.O. Box 1133
Washington, D.C. 20013-1133
Email: healthfinder@nhic.org
Web: http://www.healthfinder.gov

Developed by the DHHS and other federal agencies, Healthfinders is a useful and informative Web site for consumers and health professionals.

Health Resources and Services Administration (HRSA)

Health Resources & Services Administration
5600 Fishers Lane
Rockville, Maryland 20857
301-443-2216 (Elizabeth M. Duke, PhD)
Email: comments@hrsa.gov
Web: http://www.hrsa.gov

HRSA is a federal agency within the U.S. Department of Health and Human Services that provides national leadership, program resources, and services needed to improve access to health care that is culturally competent and linguistically appropriate. HRSA strives to eliminate health disparities. Information about the Bureau of Primary Health Care (BPHC), an office within HRSA, is at http://bphc.hrsa.gov/.

Healthy People 2010

U.S. Department of Health and Human Services
Office of Disease Prevention and Health Promotion
Office of Public Health and Science, Office of the Secretary
1101 Wootton Parkway, Suite LL100
Rockville, Maryland 20852
240-453-8280
FAX: 240-453-8282
Web: http://www.healthypeople.gov; http://odphp.osophs.dhhs.gov

Healthy People 2010 is a roadmap or framework for prevention and sets forward national goals and objectives to help agencies and community members prevent or reduce significant threats to health.

Healthy Schools Network, Inc. (HSN)

110 Maryland Avenue NE, Suite 505
Washington, D.C. 20002
202-543-7555
Web: http://www.healthyschools.org

HSN is a nonprofit national organization with a focus on environmental health, dedicated to ensuring that children and school employees have environmentally safe and healthy schools.

Indian Health Service (IHS)

Indian Health Service (HQ)
The Reyes Building
801 Thompson Avenue, Suite 400
Rockville, Maryland 20852-1627
301-443-1083
Email: Anna.OldElk@mail.ihs.gov
Web: http://www.ihs.gov
HIS is an agency within the U.S. Department of Health and
Human Services that is responsible for providing federal
health services to American Indians and Alaskan Natives.

Institute of Medicine (IOM)

Institute of Medicine
500 Fifth Street NW
Washington, D.C. 20001
202-334-2352
FAX: 202-334-1412
Email: iomwww@nas.edu
Web: http://www.iom.edu
IOM is part of the National Academy of Sciences that provides
science-based advice on health, medicine, and biomedical
science matters. The IOM works outside of the framework
of the government to provide expert, unbiased, evidence-
based information and advice to policy makers, professionals, and the general public.

National Area Health Education Centers (NAHECs)

109 VIP Drive, Suite 220
Wexford, Pennsylvania 15090
1-888-412-7424
FAX: 724-935-1560
Email: info@nationalahec.org
Web: http://bhpr.hrsa.gov
NAHEC is an academic-community partnership focused on
improving the supply, diversity, distribution and quality
of the health workforce. Health care providers are trained
in rural and underserved sites and are responsive to local
needs.

National Association of Community Health Centers, Inc. (NACHC)

7200 Wisconsin Avenue, Suite 210
Bethesda, Maryland 20814
301-347-0400
FAX: 301-347-0459
Web: http://www.nachc.com
Founded in 1970, NACHC is a nonprofit organization whose
mission is to enhance and expand access to quality,
community-responsive health care for America's medi-
cally underserved and uninsured. In serving its mission,
NACHC represents the nation's network of over 1,000

federally qualified health centers (FQHCs), which serve
16 million people through 5,000 sites located in all of the
50 states, Puerto Rico, the District of Columbia, the U.S.
Virgin Islands, and Guam.

National Association of School Nurses (NASN)

8484 Georgia Avenue, Suite 420
Silver Spring, Maryland 20910
240-821-1130; 1-866-627-6767
FAX: 301-585-1791
Email: nasn@nasn.org
Web: http://www.nasn.org
NASN improves the health and educational success of children
and youth by developing and providing leadership to
advance school nursing practice. It advances school nursing practice to improve the health of school-aged children
and promote their academic success.

National Association of County and City Health Officials (NACCHO)

1100 17th Street, NW, second floor
Washington, D.C. 20036
202-783-5550
Fax: 202-783-1583
Web: http://www.naccho.org
NACCHO is the national voice of local public health agencies
across the United States. It supports efforts to protect and
promote the public's health through national policies,
resources and programs, and effective public health practice and systems.

National Association of School-Based Health Centers (NASBHC)

202-638-5872, ext 200
Web: http://www.nasbhc.org
NASBHC is a national multidisciplinary group that represents
people who support, receive, and provide health care in
schools and school-connected programs. The organization
provides advocacy, leadership, resources, and technical assistance to build the capacity and sustainability of
school-based health care. School health resources are
available.

The National Center for Healthy Housing

10320 Little Pataxent Parkway, Suite 500
Columbia, Maryland 21044
410-992-0712
FAX: 443-539-415010.992.0712 / Fax: 443.539.4150
Web: http://www.centerforhealthyhousing.org
The National Center for Healthy Housing (formerly the
National Center for Lead-Safe Housing) was founded as

a nonprofit organization in October 1992, to bring the public health, housing, and environmental communities together to combat the nation's epidemic of childhood lead poisoning. It continues its important role in reducing children's risk of lead poisoning and has expanded its mission to help to decrease children's exposure to other hazards in the home including biological, physical, and chemical contaminants in and around the home. The NCHH mission is to develop and promote practical methods to protect children from environmental health hazards in their homes while preserving affordable housing.

National Institutes of Health (NIH)

9000 Rockville Pike
Bethesda, Maryland 20892
301-496-4000
Web: http://www.nih.gov

NIH is the steward of medical and behavioral research for the nation. Its mission is science in pursuit of fundamental knowledge about the nature and behavior of living systems and the application of that knowledge to extend healthy life and reduce the burdens of illness and disability.

National Nursing Centers Consortium (NNCC)

260 S Broad Street, 18th floor
Philadelphia, Pennsylvania 19102
215-731-7140
FAX: 215-731-2400
Email:Tine@nncc.us
Web: http://www.nncc.us

NNCC represents nurse-managed health centers serving vulnerable people across the country. It strengthens the capacity of its members to provide quality health care services to vulnerable populations and to eliminate health disparities in underserved communities.

National Rural Health Association (NRHA)

521 East 63rd Street
Kansas City, Missouri 64110-3329
816-756-3140
FAX: 816-756-3144
Web: http://www.nrharural.org

The NRHA is a national nonprofit membership organization with more than 10,000 members that provides leadership on rural health issues. The association's mission is to improve the health and well-being of rural Americans and to provide leadership on rural health issues through advocacy, communications, education, research, and leadership. The NRHA membership is made up of a diverse collection of individuals and organizations, all of whom share the common bond of an interest in rural health.

Office of Disease Prevention and Health Promotion

Office of Public Health and Science, Office of the Secretary
1101 Wootton Parkway, Suite LL100
Rockville, Maryland 20852
240-453-8280
FAX: 240-453-8282
Web: http://odphp.osophs.dhhs.gov

The Office of Disease Prevention and Health Promotion, Office of Public Health and Science, Office of the Secretary, U.S. Department of Health and Human Services, works to strengthen the disease prevention and health promotion priorities of the department within the collaborative framework of the HHS agencies.

Rural Assistance Center

School of Medicine and Health Sciences, Room 4520
501 North Columbia Road, Stop 9037
Grand Forks, North Dakota 58202-9037
1-800-270-1898
FAX: 1-800-270-1913
Email: info@raconline.org
Web: http://www.raconline.org

Rural Assistance Center was established in 2002 as an information conduit for rural health and human services. The center helps rural communities and other stakeholders access available programs, funding, and research that can help improve and provide quality health and human services to rural residents. The rural health clinics (RHCs) program is intended to increase primary care services for Medicaid and Medicare patients in rural communities. RHCs can be public, private, or nonprofit. The main advantage of RHC status is enhanced reimbursement rates for providing Medicaid and Medicare services in rural areas. RHCs must be located in rural, underserved areas and must use midlevel practitioners.

U.S. Department of Health and Human Services (DHHS)

The U.S. Department of Health and Human Services
200 Independence Avenue, SW
Washington, D.C. 20201
202-619-0257, 1-877-696-6775
Web: www.dhhs.gov

DHHS is the U.S. government's primary agency involved with protecting the health of all Americans and providing essential human services, especially for people with few resources. The Web site provides health related publications.

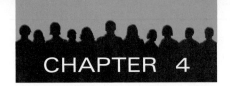

CHAPTER 4

Epidemiology and Public Health Nursing

R. Craig Stotts, RN, DrPH

Chapter Outline

🌐 Epidemiology Defined

🌐 Epidemiologic Models

🌐 Uses of Epidemiology in Public Health Nursing
   Community Assessment
   Screening
   Program Evaluation

🌐 Epidemiologic Rates
   Prevalence and Incidence
   Morbidity and Mortality
   Age-Adjusted

🌐 Types of Epidemiologic Studies
   Studies Related to Current Level of Knowledge
   Cross-Sectional Studies
   Case–Control Studies
   Cohort Studies
   Randomized Clinical Trials

🌐 Sources of Epidemiologic Data
   Census Bureau
   National Center for Health Statistics
   Centers for Disease Control and Prevention
   Surveillance, Epidemiology, and End Results

🌐 Conclusion

Learning Objectives

Upon completion of this chapter, the reader will be able to:

1. Identify the importance of epidemiology to the practice of public health nursing.

2. Analyze the definition of epidemiology vis-à-vis current real-world problems.

3. Evaluate the value and purpose of screening in public health.

4. Calculate an age-adjusted death rate.

5. Evaluate the most common epidemiologic study designs for their relevance to a given clinical problem.

6. Identify the most important sources of data useful to public health nurses.

Public health nurses need tools to do their job. Epidemiology is the most important tool any public health professional can use. It is used to collect data, analyze the problem, develop a plan, and even evaluate the results. Being astute in epidemiology can also help any nurse to be a better consumer of the scientific literature.

EPIDEMIOLOGY DEFINED

Although the term "epidemiology" sounds much like the word "epidemic," the field of epidemiology has grown far beyond a science that studies epidemics. Although even into the mid-1990s, the focus of epidemiology was indeed on infectious diseases, now the scope also encompasses chronic diseases as well as other conditions that are usually not considered diseases, such as aging.

The most commonly accepted definition of epidemiology today is the following:

> Epidemiology is the study of the distribution and determinants of health-related states and events in specified populations (Last, 1995).

This definition tells us that epidemiology tries to find the causes and risk factors of diseases and health conditions, which form the foundation of public health. Only with the knowledge that epidemiologic data give us are public health professionals able to determine what needs to be done. Is lung cancer a problem in your city? Is the rate of gunshot injuries on the rise in your state? Who is at risk for Alzheimer's? These are the kinds of questions that epidemiology can answer.

This field of science is relatively new with the first-known usage of the epidemiologic method for a public health problem occurring in the 1850s. In that instance, Dr. John Snow used what are now known as epidemiologic methods to try to stop a large outbreak of cholera. Hundreds were dying with no end in sight. Using the data he collected, he determined that one of the main public water pumps was the source of the outbreak. He convinced the city council to remove the handle from the pump and cholera deaths began to plummet. However, the local residents did not believe that the pump was the problem so they forced the city council to replace the handle. Cholera deaths immediately began occurring again and within a few days, the city council acted yet again, this time permanently removing the water pump. This pump, the Broad Street pump, is memorialized with a plaque at its former site.

Epidemiology has evolved over the years to a discipline in which its practitioners combine their knowledge of research design, biostatistics, and health to develop studies and analyze their results. Epidemiologists are valuable assets to many clinical and public health research studies. They also serve local and state health departments to identify and prevent disease outbreaks. The Centers for Disease Control provide not only epidemiologists to supplement local and state workers but also educational programs for people interested in learning more about the field.

EPIDEMIOLOGIC MODELS

Two basic models are used in epidemiology as foundations for investigations and research. The first, the Host–Agent–Reservoir Model, is the oldest and has its roots in the beginnings of epidemiology, which focused on infectious disease. The second, the Person–Place–Time Model, was derived later and is most often used with chronic disease epidemiology. Both models can be used, in different situations, to describe the characteristics of a disease or health condition that in turn enables public health professionals to address the problem more successfully.

The Host–Agent–Reservoir Model, also known as the Epidemiologic Triangle Model, exemplifies the interaction among these three elements. An example of the use of this model might be the case of malaria. The agent causing this disease is the *Plasmodium malariae* organism, which is transmitted by mosquitoes. If humans are considered the hosts, and *P. malariae*, the agent, then the reservoir (also known as the environment or vector) would be the mosquito. The main way to prevent malaria is to drain swamps. This causes the mosquitoes to occur in far fewer numbers and thus reduces the risk of humans being bit by a mosquito carrying the causative organism. If, however, normally dry areas experience unusually wet weather resulting in standing pools of water, the mosquito population can grow significantly. Humans may also be educated to use mosquito repellent, which would also result in reduced risk. The interplay of these three factors demonstrates the utility of this model.

The Person–Place–Time Model, although most often used for chronic diseases, may also be used for infectious diseases, such as in food-borne outbreaks. Although the latter is often caused by a bacterium, the Person–Place–Time Model can be used to identify whether certain people are more susceptible to the bacterium, whether the outbreak occurred more or less often in certain places, and if the occurrence of symptoms occurred in a time frame that would provide evidence as to the cause. The component of Person deals with the susceptibility of that person in terms of genetic and acquired characteristics, including age, race, gender, and socioeconomic status. Place deals with the location that may place persons at high, moderate, or low risk. This could include "cancer clusters" that may be due to a source of pollution in the neighborhood or county. It can also be much broader and be defined in terms of latitude or longitude. Multiple sclerosis, for instance, is more common in the northern United States than in the southern states. Places can also be determined by political boundaries (cities, states, countries) or by geographic characteristics (valleys versus highlands) and by rural versus urban characteristics. The component of Time may also characterize a disease. Lung cancer in men was on the increase from the 1930s until 1964 when it began a decrease that continues today, while lung cancer in women began its rise in the late 1950s and has not witnessed yet the precipitous fall seen in men. Tuberculosis can also be described in Time factors, especially in regard to the initiation of effective medications in the 1940s, the precipitous fall thereafter, and then the sudden increase when HIV/AIDS entered the scene.

With both models, it is imperative that each of the components be considered when attempting to evaluate the characteristics of a certain disease or condition. Looking back at the definition of epidemiology, the "determinants" and "distribution" are derived from a careful consideration of an epidemiological model.

Not all health-related studies are epidemiologic studies. Two particular types of studies do not rise to the level of epidemiology: case reports and case series. A case report is a report of only one individual. Some medical journals provide these reports as examples of odd things that can happen in a clinical situation. A case series involves roughly 2 to 10 clients and is an expanded version of the case study but again is not meant to be generalizable to a larger population, but rather to give anecdotal-level information about unusual situations. Epidemiologic studies are intended to be generalizable to an aggregate or population or subpopulation. The smallest sample size that is generally considered acceptable would be about 10 cases and 20 controls. A study of this size in 1970s was

able to determine that women who took diethylstilbestrol (DES) for morning sickness during pregnancy had a significantly increased risk of giving birth to daughters who would later be diagnosed with a rare form of vaginal cancer. The only reason that so few cases were chosen to be in the study was because the cancer was so rare; the study surveyed all the women in New York City who had been diagnosed with this rare cancer during a several-year time frame. Had more subjects been available, they would have been included. The authors used a case-control study design, which gave them the preliminary information they needed to recommend that pregnant women not be prescribed DES. Some epidemiologic studies are much larger, but smaller studies may be appropriate and often provide valuable information.

USES OF EPIDEMIOLOGY IN PUBLIC HEALTH NURSING

Subjective data are important in the practice of the public health nurse, but objective data are at least as important. Key decision makers and stakeholders are often more interested in objective data because they perceive this information as being more scientific. The science of epidemiology arose from the need to influence decision makers because it can often provide irrefutable "facts" as opposed to opinions. The three most important uses of epidemiology in public health nursing are community assessment, screening, and program evaluation.

Community Assessment

The community assessment process requires data collection from a number of sources. Besides interviews with community leaders and windshield surveys (Anderson & McFarlane, 2004), there is also a strong need for good epidemiologic data. Table 4-1 indicates just some of the important sources of epidemiologic data needed for a comprehensive community assessment.

Some of the data sources in Table 4-1 provide local or community-level data while others do not. Many of the incidence, mortality, and surveillance studies are conducted at the national level. There are methods, however, for extrapolating the data for use in a single community, region, or state. These extrapolations must be used with caution, however, and when used in a presentation to decision makers, it must be noted that the data are extrapolations and may not accurately

TABLE 4-1: Sources and Types of Epidemiological Data

SOURCE OF DATA	TYPE OF DATA
Vital statistics	Births, deaths
Census data	Demographics, socioeconomic status, household composition
Prevalence studies	Presence of disease within a community; an index of the burden of a disease
Incidence studies	Development of new cases of a disease; an index of the risk of acquiring a disease
Mortality studies	Disease-specific and age-specific death rates
Surveillance data	Annual monitoring of the most common diseases and health conditions

reflect the true status of the community. They can still be valuable, though, because for many diseases or conditions, there is not great variation from community to community. For instance, death rates due to lung cancer do not vary significantly from city to city or state to state because it is a very lethal disease in every case and because its treatment is nationally standardized. Other forms of data can be fairly well localized from national sources; the Youth Risk Behavioral Survey (YRBS) and the Behavioral Risk Factor Surveillance System (BRFSS), both from the Centers for Disease Control and Prevention (CDC), can provide data that are reliable at the state level and, in some cases, can even be reliable for a city, if the city is large and has provided an adequate sample size.

Convenience samples are rarely acceptable sources of data. A convenience sample is obtained by not using a scientific sampling method, such as random selection of an entire community. If a group of student nurses go to a shopping mall and interview shoppers about their health, this would be a convenience sample. The data, however, would be extremely biased, to the point of not being useful. People who are in a shopping mall may not be representative of the general population, and people who are there and willing to answer survey questions may be an even narrower demographic group of people. Epidemiologic studies use sampling techniques that reduce potential sources of bias; these methods include using random samples and control subjects or communities.

Most of the national datasets include options for selecting data specific to a given state; the Census Bureau will even provide data down to the level of a certain census tract. See the Resources section at the end of this chapter for a brief list of government Web sites providing datasets using certain criteria such as zip code.

Screening

Screening is the classification of individuals with respect to their likelihood of having a disease. The purpose of screening is not to diagnose disease but to separate the "normals" from the "abnormals" as the first step in detecting a previously undetected disease. If a person goes to a health fair where they are doing finger sticks for glucose or cholesterol and is told that his or her values are high, it does not mean that the individual can be considered a diabetic or a person with hypercholesterolemia. It merely means that he or she needs to be referred to a health care professional for a full evaluation. Only after this latter evaluation can a diagnosis be made.

Screening is primarily performed on asymptomatic persons. If they have symptoms, they should be going to their primary care provider (PCP) for evaluation; this action will yield a diagnosis, not a screening. The benefit of screening is that they are typically much cheaper and can reach more people than diagnostic tests. If a person tests positive, that person should then go for diagnostic testing. If the person tests negative, it is probably safe to not go for any further testing, at least in the near future.

Screening is heavily dependent on the natural history of the disease in question. Every disease has a different natural history, thus requiring different strategies and timetables for each disease. Two examples of very different natural histories are diabetes and hypercholesterolemia, the former being very complex and the latter being fairly simple.

Cholesterol screening is an example of a simple assessment that can often be done in the community. The American Heart Association (AHA) recommends that only adults be screened and then primarily through worksites and in low-income populations (American Heart Association, 2005). Other settings might result in screenings for many people who are at low risk, thus reducing the cost-effectiveness of the effort. The AHA also recommends that both HDL and total cholesterol should be tested for. Individuals for whom these two values are abnormal should be referred to their PCPs for repeat testing and additional testing of LDL and triglycerides. The natural history of hypercholesterolemia suggests that if this condition is untreated for many years, the risk of myocardial infarction and stroke are greatly increased.

In diabetes, the blood glucose levels change rapidly and frequently during a given day, while cholesterol levels are much more stable. If a person attends a health fair and receives a glucose screening value of 150, it would be difficult to say whether the person's value should be considered abnormal without knowing a lot more about the person. For instance, has the person eaten recently? If so, how long ago was it? If the person (let's assume it's a middle-aged woman) ate 4 hours ago, one might say that the value is abnormal because the glucose levels should have been less than 120 at that time. However, there are extenuating circumstances. If she had eaten a large meal, especially one with a lot of fat and complex carbohydrates, it might mean that she is not diabetic but rather still in the process of metabolizing the glucose. The "normal" range is 70–99, but this is for the fasting stage only. Not many people who are screened at health fairs will be fasting, thus throwing the results into doubt. Why not refer anyone who has a value over 120 to their PCP anyway? Isn't it better to be safe than sorry? No, because false positives cause two major problems: (1) unnecessary anxiety and (2) unnecessary health care utilization and expenses. The anxiety occurs because of the fear that occurs when the person is told she might have diabetes. It often takes many days to get in to see a PCP to have a definitive diagnosis made. During this time the person will suffer unnecessarily because they will read about diabetes and all its major complications and sequelae, including a potential loss of a driver's license. She may suffer from lack of sleep, nervousness, and fear, all completely avoidable had she not been screened.

The other major problem with false positives, costs to the health care system, is not insignificant. Besides the cost of an office visit, the blood tests usually cost more than $100, and if the results are not clear, which is often the case, a 5-hour glucose tolerance test must be given, which can cost almost $1,000. All these expenses then for a person who is not diabetic but had the poor luck to attend a health fair where the screening tests were being given. The American Diabetes Association has recommended, for the above reasons, that mass screenings *not* be conducted for diabetes. Rather, only people with significant risk factors should be screened for diabetes and then only if they have been fasting and are receiving the screening in a health care setting (American Diabetes Association, 2004).

Screenings depend on having a screening method that is **sensitive** (finds a large percentage of the true positives), **specific** (finds a large percentage of the true negatives), relatively inexpensive, and noninvasive (no more than a finger stick). A test that has 90 percent sensitivity and 90 percent specificity would be considered a very good test; a test with these values below 50 percent would be considered a very poor test. These values are determined by scientific studies in experimental situations and will be available by reviewing the epidemiologic literature. Health care providers should review this literature before deciding whether to use any new screening test. It is not sufficient to be told by a pharmaceutical person that their new test is "accurate." It is imperative that the health care professional review the studies on the new test to decide whether it will be cost-effective by virtue of having sensitivity/specificity values.

Other criteria important in deciding whether to mount a screening program include the following:

- The natural history of the disease is known, and a preclinical phase exists that is long enough to be detectable.

- There is a known, effective treatment for the disease that yields better health and better survival rates than if the disease is diagnosed after symptoms develop.

⊕ There is access to facilities for follow-up referral and treatment.

⊕ The disease is not rare and in fact imposes a significant health burden on society.

If all these criteria are not met, it will be either unethical or not cost-effective to conduct screening programs. Telling a person that he or she might have a certain disease without providing the follow-up diagnostic and treatment opportunities is unethical because it raises fear and anxiety without providing an opportunity to resolve those feelings. For screenings in uninsured or underinsured populations, the local health care providers must agree to provide follow-up and treatment for no or reduced costs. If this is not possible, the screening program should not be implemented. Screening programs must also be systematically implemented and not a "one-shot" opportunity. A community's expectations will be raised once a screening program is offered and they will expect to be able to be screened the next year if they were unable to be screened at the current time. Not offering screenings on at least an annual basis produces hurt feelings and distrust of the health care community.

Program Evaluation

Community programs, including disease prevention and health promotion programs, cost a lot of money. They usually also take a lot of time and energy to get them going and to maintain them. The critical question that needs to be asked is: Is this program accomplishing its goals? If it is not, then the financial and human resources being expended on it are being wasted. Some community health programs have never been formally evaluated, leaving the community with the preceding critical question being unanswered. For any program to be worthy of funding, a formal program evaluation is required.

Program evaluations have evolved over the years and are now considered very scientific, reliable ways of measuring the value of a given program. However, program evaluations must follow certain standards to be considered scientific. It no longer suffices to count the number of people attending a program to determine its value, nor does interviewing participants establish the program's credibility. Rather, a program evaluation must hew to the following set of criteria:

1. Are the program's objectives measurable? To what degree were they met?

2. Did the participants improve? Did they improve more than a comparison group?

3. What are the costs of the program? What is the cost per improved participant?

4. Did the participants value the program in terms of affordability, accessibility, acceptability?

5. Did the providers value the program in terms of relevance, efficiency, and effectiveness?

Each of these questions must be answered thoroughly and scientifically in order to arrive at valid conclusions. Evaluations may be expensive, but they often cost less than continuing a program that is ineffective or potentially harmful.

Program evaluators are currently being prepared at the doctoral level. Any program that needs a highly credible evaluation, primarily those with federal or state funding, would be best served by hiring a person with this type of expertise. Skills in this area can rarely be learned without years of formal preparation. Many books have been written on program evaluation, two of the best being those by Weiss (1998) and Grembowski (2001).

EPIDEMIOLOGIC RATES

Epidemiology uses rates in the study of disease determinants and distribution. **Rates** are measures of frequency of health events that put raw numbers into a frame of reference to the size of a population. Rates are determined by statistical adjustments to the raw data, making them useful in making comparisons or examining trends.

Prevalence and Incidence

These two terms are very different concepts and provide complementary views of the burden on society posed by a disease or condition. With some diseases, both prevalence rates and incidence rates are available and relevant, whereas one of the two rates may not be available in other diseases. The public health nurse must be aware of the definition of each type of rate, what information each rate provides, and how the rates are different.

Prevalence rates tell us what proportion of a given population has been diagnosed with a certain disease; **incidence** tells us what proportion of a given population was newly diagnosed during the year (or other time frame). Here are the formulae for calculating each:

$$\text{Prevalence rate} = \frac{\text{\# of existing cases}}{\text{Total population}}$$

$$\text{Incidence rate} = \frac{\text{\# of new cases}}{\text{Population at risk}} \quad \begin{array}{l}\text{in a given}\\\text{time frame}\end{array}$$

To conduct a study of prevalence, one would survey a population (city, state, etc.) and ask everyone if they have the disease in question. If we surveyed 1,000 people and asked them if they had osteoarthritis, we might find that 100 of them would report that they had the disease while 900 would report they did not have the disease. Putting these figures into the prevalence rate formula, would yield the following numbers:

$$\text{Prevalence rate} = \frac{\text{\# of existing cases}}{\text{Total population}}$$

$$= \frac{100}{1,000} = .1 = 10\%$$

If we had conducted this study in River City in July 2005, assuming that the 1,000 respondents were representative of the total city, we could say that the prevalence rate of osteoarthritis of River City in July 2005 is 10 percent, meaning that 10 percent of the population currently has osteoarthritis. From this datum, we would be able to draw conclusions about the burden this particular disease was placing on the citizens of this city. We could also compare this rate to previous and future prevalence rates to see if the disease's prevalence rates were increasing or decreasing (in this situation, there probably would not be much change since this disease typically has a very stable prevalence). As may be obvious, prevalence rate gives us very little information about the current threat of the disease; rather, it reflects all the people who have ever been diagnosed with the disease and are still alive. It is possible that all 100 of the cases were diagnosed in years prior to the current year and that the city has no new cases this year. If it has no new cases the following year, and no one with the disease dies, the prevalence rate will remain the same. Incidence rates, however, are much more sensitive to temporal changes in diseases.

For conducting an incidence study, we would have to take a different approach. Instead of sending out a one-time survey, we would probably need to survey PCPs in the city on a monthly basis, asking them if they had any clients who received the diagnosis of arthritis during that month. Again, assuming that 1,000 respondents were surveyed and that eight of these respondents were newly diagnosed with osteoarthritis during 2005, at the end of 2005, the incidence rate would be as follows:

$$\text{Incidence rate} = \frac{\text{\# of new cases}}{\text{Population at risk}} \quad \begin{array}{l}\text{in a given}\\\text{time frame}\end{array}$$

$$= \frac{8}{900} \quad \text{per year}$$

$$= 0.00888$$

$$= 8.88 \text{ per 1,000 per year}$$

Since those who already have osteoarthritis are no longer "at risk" of being newly diagnosed with the disease, they are subtracted from the denominator. This also assumes that the city's population is 1,000 and that everyone in this city would go to a local PCP if they were having symptoms. We would then be able to state, "During the year 2005, the incidence rate of osteoarthritis was 8.88 per 1,000."

Risk is an important concept but it can only be calculated from the incidence rate. We as humans say that we want to know our "risk" of developing a disease, but what we really want to know is, as of today, how likely we are to get Disease X. That can only be determined by data that is very time-sensitive, which is what the incidence rate provides. In the 1950s, the incidence rate of smallpox was measurable, possibly in the range of 1 per million; since 1977, when smallpox was declared by WHO to be eradicated, the incidence rate is essentially zero. Therefore, the risk of acquiring smallpox today is zero. If someone living in 1950 had asked about the chances of getting smallpox, the answer would have been, "The risk is about one in one million." Other diseases can change incidence rates much more radically. For women using tampons in 1980, the incidence of Toxic Shock Syndrome (TSS) was 9 per 100,000 women between the ages of 12 and 49, whereas the incidence had dropped to less than 1 per 100,000 by 1986. This occurred because manufacturers changed the composition of tampons, preventing most new cases of TSS. Thus, among women using tampons, their risk of TSS dropped significantly during a 6-year interval (Hajjeh et al., 1999).

Morbidity and Mortality

Morbidity is a term meaning illness or disease, whereas **mortality** refers to death. Morbidity data are reported in terms of prevalence rates and incidence rates, as noted in the previous section. Mortality rates are reported as death rates. Both morbidity and mortality data are important when evaluating a community's health. Each gives a different view; using only one type of data will not provide an accurate picture of the current health problems and strengths of a community.

Morbidity and mortality rates can be both general and very specific. For instance, one may read that "the prevalence rate of diabetes mellitus in Florida in 1998 was 48 per 1,000." That piece of information would be a good starting point for understanding the diabetes problem in Florida, but one would need to break this number down even further to better understand the true situation. Some questions that should be asked would include the following:

- What is the mean age of onset? What is the median age?
- Which decade of age has the highest rate?
- How do rates compare by gender?
- How do rates compare by race/ethnicity?
- How do rates compare by socioeconomic status?
- How do rates vary by weight or body mass index?

We can also ask these same questions of mortality data and make the data disease-specific, as we did above with diabetes. Sometimes the answers yield very unusual findings, such that they may call for brand new programs to be instituted or current programs to be shelved. For instance, the death rate due to prostate cancer is fairly high, but when we break it down by race/ethnicity, we find that African American men have a death rate that is at least 50 percent higher than among white men (Robbins et al., 2000). Certainly such a stark difference in rates bears further investigation, and possibly a program should be initiated in the African American community to screen for diabetes earlier and more extensively.

Age-Adjusted

When comparing rates, whether they are morbidity or mortality rates, be aware that some diseases are greatly influenced by age. Cancer and heart disease, for example, occur at higher rates with each advancing year of life. The chance of being diagnosed with coronary heart disease at age 3 is almost nonexistent, whereas persons in their 70s or 80s are at significant risk for receiving this diagnosis. Age is a factor in most disease and health conditions and thus must be considered in any data analysis.

Communities, states, and countries often have very different age distributions. Some states have a higher percentage of elderly residents; Florida has significantly more elderly than Alaska (Census Bureau, 2005). Alaska's population older than 65 constitutes only 5.9 percent of the population, whereas Florida's elderly constitute 17.6 percent, nearly a threefold difference. Because of these demographics, one would expect that, on a per capita basis, Florida would have a much higher rate of diseases common to the elderly such as cancer and heart disease. Indeed, this is the case, but one would be tempted to say that since cancer rates are higher in Florida than in Alaska, that there must be something dangerous in Florida's air or water or work sites causing these higher rates. This would be an erroneous assumption. One must first adjust for age before comparing cancer rates.

When we adjust for age, we are saying "what would the cancer death rates be if these two states had approximately equal age distributions?" We have a fairly simple statistical method of adjusting for age: converting the age proportions in one of the states to match that of the other state. We would then take the actual age-specific disease rate and multiply it by the new population distribution to provide an expected number of diseases, which is the number of persons with the disease we would expect if the populations had similar numbers of older and younger people.

Tables 4-2 to 4-5 provide a hypothetical example of how these rates can be age-adjusted. Table 4-2 shows the actual numbers for each state, while Tables 4-3 to 4-5 show the steps in the age-adjustment, yielding new cancer death rates that can be fairly compared.

Two new columns (Death Rate) were introduced in Table 4-3. These columns are the death rates for each state broken down to a specific age group. This was accomplished by putting into the numerator the number of deaths in that state for that age group and putting in the denominator the number of people in that age group in that state. So for Alaska, the youngest age group had 248,000 people, and of those 188 died from cancer. Putting that into the formula would yield:

TABLE 4-2: Hypothetical Number of Cancer Deaths in Two States

Age Group	ALASKA			FLORIDA	
	Population	Deaths		Population	Deaths
0–24 years	248,000	188		4,978,000	3,762
25–44 years	203,000	366		4,569,000	8,245
45–64 years	140,000	703		3,628,000	24,072
65+ years	37,000	1,451		2,807,000	127,094
Total	628,000	2,708		15,982,000	163,173

TABLE 4-3: Adjustment for Age (Step 1)

Age Group	ALASKA			FLORIDA		
	Population	# Deaths	Death Rate	Population	# Deaths	Death Rate
0–24 years	248,000	188	0.000758	4,978,000	3,762	0.000756
25–44 years	203,000	366	0.001803	4,569,000	8,245	0.001805
45–64 years	140,000	703	0.005021	3,628,000	24,072	0.006635
65+ years	37,000	1,451	0.039216	2,807,000	127,094	0.045278
Total	628,000	2,708	0.004312	15,982,000	163,173	0.010210
	4.3*			10.2*		

* per 1,000

188/248,000 = 0.000758. After using this formula for all the age groups in both states, we would have the figures indicated in Table 4-3. Notice the bottom row where it indicates that the total death rate for Alaska is 4.3 per 1,000 and that for Florida is 10.2 per 1,000. From these crude figures (crude means "before adjustment") it appears that Florida has a much more significant cancer problem than Alaska, with a rate 2.37 times greater. We know, however, that we must adjust for age before we can make truly accurate comparisons between the two states.

The first step in adjusting for age is to choose a "standard" population. Sometimes researchers choose the U.S. population (the 2000 Census figures are currently being used) or they may choose to combine the two populations to be the standard. For this example, let us use the latter method (there are other methods but these are the most common). Now we will be asking the question: If Alaska and Florida had the same age distributions, what would the expected number of cancer deaths be in each state and what would the age-adjusted cancer death rates be?

The second step is to combine the two populations by each age group to form the new standard population. Table 4-4 shows the new population figures by each age group and the total.

The last column was obtained by simply taking the numbers of people for each age group in both states, then summing to get the total. Now we will use these numbers as our base for calculating the expected

TABLE 4-4: Adjustment for Age (Step 2)

	ALASKA		FLORIDA		STANDARD POPULATION
Age Group	Population	Death Rate*	Population	Death Rate*	
0–24 years	248,000	0.000758	4,978,000	0.000756	5,226,000
25–44 years	203,000	0.001803	4,569,000	0.001805	4,772,000
45–64 years	140,000	0.005021	3,628,000	0.006635	3,768,000
65+years	37,000	0.039216	2,807,000	0.045278	2,844,000
Total	628,000		15,982,000		16,610,000

TABLE 4-5: Adjustment for Age (Step 3)

	ALASKA		FLORIDA		STANDARD POPULATION
Age Group	Population	Death Rate*	Population	Death Rate*	
0–24 years	248,000	0.000758	4,978,000	0.000756	5,226,000
25–44 years	203,000	0.001803	4,569,000	0.001805	4,772,000
45–64 years	140,000	0.005021	3,628,000	0.006635	3,768,000
65+years	37,000	0.039216	2,807,000	0.045278	2,844,000
Total	628,000		15,982,000		16,610,000

numbers of cancer deaths by age group and by state. We will need to take the death rates for each state and each age group and multiply them by the appropriate new population standard. Table 4-5 has removed the data we no longer need and includes only the data we need.

Table 4-5 shows the results of multiplying the true death rates of each state by an "artificial" or standard population in each age group. (Example: For Alaska in the 0–24 age group, multiply the actual death rate (0.00758) times the new standard population for that age group (5,226,000) to get 3,962 expected deaths). This gives us the expected numbers of deaths in each age group if the population of that age group used this new population as the base. We then sum the expected numbers of deaths in each state to arrive at the total number of expected deaths. These are our age-adjusted deaths, which can now be used to calcu-

late the final number, the age-adjusted death rate for each state. For Alaska, we divide the total expected numbers of deaths (143,017) by the total standard population (16,610,000) to get 0.00861, or 8.6 per 1,000. The comparable calculation for Florida (166,331/16,610,000) yields 0.01001 or 10.0 per 1,000. In comparing Alaska's age-adjusted death rate for cancer of 8.6 per 1,000 to Florida's 10.0, we see that they are not as different as we had first thought. Florida's rate is only 1.2 times that of Alaska's, which is very different from the 2.37 times greater rate that we obtained when using crude figures.

Age-adjusted rates are very valuable for comparing different entities, such as states and countries, especially when the disease in question varies by age. These rates can also be used when the same entity is being evaluated over time. For instance, if we were looking at cancer rates for New York City over many decades, we would want to use age-adjusted rates each time because the age distribution of the city changes from decade to decade.

TYPES OF EPIDEMIOLOGIC STUDIES

There are several main types of epidemiologic studies, all of which will be discussed in this section. The nursing and public health literature are replete with examples of each of these designs. To be a good consumer of this literature, however, requires an understanding of the strengths and weaknesses of each design. Keeping in mind that there has never been a perfect study, nor is it likely that a perfect study will ever be conducted, there are choices to be made about the quality of the research design, the data, and the conclusions. A good consumer of research literature will know when conclusions can be used in the clinical setting and when other conclusions must be put on hold for further testing. In public health, we generally do not consider any results, no matter how good the study design, ready for implementation with clients and communities until the results have been replicated several times in various populations.

Studies Related to Current Level of Knowledge

Study designs have been developed according to the need and the availability of resources. Some study designs are for very small studies and are often very cheap, whereas others require many thousands of people and are very expensive. Typically we follow a progression of small to large study designs based on our level of knowledge (i.e., the more we know about a subject, the larger the study is called for to advance our knowledge). Other facets of study design that are related to our level of knowledge are randomization and control groups. In the early stages of our knowledge, we usually do not have the luxury to randomize or to use any type of control group, but before we can reach any definitive conclusions about a problem, we must use both of these strategies. The following paragraphs will explain in detail how the most common study designs are used in epidemiology.

Cross-Sectional Studies

The cross-sectional study design is very basic but also very important. It requires neither control groups nor

hypotheses. It is an observational study because the subjects being studied are not asked to accept any new treatments or change anything about their lives; the opposite of an observational study is an experimental study. The Youth Risk Behavioral Study and the Behavioral Risk Factor Surveillance System, both conducted by CDC, are examples of cross-sectional studies. The CDC, through partnerships with the states, asks youths and adults to fill out surveys about their health habits each year. Samples can be either convenience samples or randomly chosen, but the sample size is usually large enough to be able to generalize results to an entire state.

The term "cross-sectional" means that a "slice" is taken, in that the survey is conducted over a relatively brief period of time (a month or two), which allows us to have a "snapshot" of health at a particular point in time. Statistics that come from studies like these are usually limited to frequencies. "Sixty percent of adults in Arkansas were obese in 2005" and "20 percent of high school seniors in New York report having smoked at least one cigarette in the past 7 days" are examples of possible findings. Depending on how large the sample size was, the data can often be broken down into small demographic categories, such as race/ethnicity, age, gender, and city of residence. These values can then be compared, but tests of significance (p-value, 95 percent confidence interval) must be used to determine whether differences are statistically significant (Dawson & Trapp, 2001).

Case–Control Studies

The case–control study design is very popular, mainly because it does not require large sample sizes but does provide important information that can be obtained relatively quickly. This design is also observational because the subjects are merely being asked questions about their health and not being asked to accept treatments or make lifestyle changes.

The name comes from the fact that we identify people who have the disease in question (cases) and compare them to people who do not have that disease (controls). We need at least one control for every case but to get optimal statistical power, three controls should be selected for each case.

An example of a ground-breaking case–control study will illustrate the power of this modest design. A group of health care providers in New York City in the 1970s became concerned that they had seen a few cases of a new and rare form of vaginal cancer (Herbst et al.,

1971). They canvassed all the hospitals in the city and found only 9 cases. They then randomly selected 27 controls (3 controls per case) and asked all 36 women the same questions. Remarkably, the 9 cases all had been born to mothers who had taken DES during their pregnancy, while the mothers of the controls had not taken DES. This drug was popular during the 1950s as a means for controlling nausea during pregnancy. From this small study, it was clear that in utero exposure greatly increased the risk of a rare form of vaginal cancer in daughters of pregnant women. The rarity of this condition precludes larger studies, such as cohort designs (see the next section) but was appropriately studied using the case–control design.

Case–control studies are also appropriate for common conditions if the condition is fairly new and our level of knowledge is very preliminary. If a researcher has a "hunch" about a certain factor causing a certain disease, that researcher would not get the funding necessary to commit millions of dollars and many years of work required for cohort studies. Instead, that hunch should first be tested in a smaller study, preferably the case–control design. If the results of that study were strong (i.e., showing a significantly increased risk of disease when exposed to that factor), then and only then would a cohort study be appropriate.

The statistic that is derived from case–control studies is the odds ratio. It answers the question, "If a person has Disease X, what are the odds that he or she was exposed to Factor Y?" If the odds ratio is much greater than 1.0, then it is considered significant. An extreme example is lung cancer and smoking; for people with lung cancer, the odds ratio for having smoked at least 1 pack of cigarettes for at least 10 years is about 10.0. Most odds ratios, however, are not that extreme and, instead, fall in the 1.0–3.0 range. An odds ratio of 1.7 may be considered significant if the statistical significance tests, primarily the 95 percent confidence interval, are strong (Dawson & Trapp, 2001). The 1.7 odds ratio means that a person who has the disease is 1.7 times more likely to have been exposed to the factor than people who do not have the disease; one could also say that they are "70 percent" more likely to have been exposed."

Cohort Studies

The cohort study design is the largest of observational studies. It can be used for common diseases or for rare diseases, but the sample size will vary according to how rare or common the disease is. The rarer the disease is, the more subjects are required.

Cohort means that a group of people (a cohort) are followed through time to see if they develop the disease in question. Within the cohort design framework, there are two basic approaches: prospective and retrospective. The prospective cohort means that the study begins prior to the development of the disease, whereas the retrospective cohort design begins after the disease has developed. The prospective design is usually much more expensive to conduct because of the staff time necessary to follow thousands of people for at least 3 years and often 10 or more years. The retrospective design has the luxury of having all the data already collected so that the main time requirement is that for data collectors to extract the data from existing records and statisticians to analyze the data. However, not all diseases lend themselves to a retrospective approach, and thus the prospective approach must be used.

The most common use of the retrospective cohort design is in the occupational health setting. An example would be the diagnosis of a rare form of liver cancer in the companies making a chemical called PVC. The researcher was called in to conduct a retrospective study using company records. The researcher was able to find all employees' date of hire, what part of the manufacturing process they worked in and for how long, and then compared those with liver cancer to those who did not have the disease. From this, it was determined that those workers who were exposed at the highest levels to PVC were at a significantly increased risk of this type of liver cancer.

An example of a prospective cohort study is the famous Framingham study. This study was initiated to try to determine the risk factors for cardiovascular disease. They enrolled 5,000 residents of Framingham, Massachusetts, who were free of heart disease. This is in direct contrast to both case–control and retrospective cohort designs, which begin with some subjects already having the disease. In Framingham, they regularly checked each subject's blood pressure, weight, and various blood and urine tests. They also asked about lifestyle factors such as smoking, exercise, and diet. This study began in the early 1950s and continues today with not only the surviving subjects but also their children. This study has identified new relationships and clarified other relationships about heart disease that were previously not well established. We know now, thanks to Framingham, that a dose–response relationship exists between smoking and heart disease, that control of blood pressure is important, and that weight and exercise are strong predictors of heart disease. These data sound commonplace now, but it was the Framingham study that provided us with these facts; prior to Framingham, we did not have this information.

The most important statistic that can be derived from the cohort study is relative risk (RR). Only cohort studies can provide a true relative risk. An example of how this is calculated follows. In a cohort study involving smokers and nonsmokers, lung cancer developed in 93 of every 100 smokers but in only 3 of every 100 nonsmokers. To arrive at the relative risk, divide 93 by 3 to get 31, which is the RR. This is interpreted as "smokers are 31 times more likely to get lung cancer than nonsmokers." Note that RR is based on incidence rates: the 93 cases of lung cancer per every 100 smokers means that, during this cohort study, 93 percent of smokers developed lung cancer. Incidence rates are the only way to calculate risk; prevalence rates do not provide risk information.

The Framingham study has been very expensive in one way, but it is also very cost-effective in that it has saved an untold number of lives. It builds upon knowledge gained from cross-sectional and case–control studies. These studies provided preliminary data that justified the commitment of large amounts of funds to conduct this prospective cohort study.

Randomized Clinical Trials

The randomized clinical trial (RCT) is an experimental study, not observational as the previous designs are, and is often considered the "gold standard" of epidemiological designs. There is debate about whether it truly is the gold standard, but suffice it to say that when done correctly, it provides valuable information that observational studies cannot provide. However, the experiment must be closely scrutinized to ensure that it is ethical. It would be highly unethical, for example, to require nonsmokers to take up smoking for the sake of a study; thus smoking initiation behaviors can only be studied using observational studies. Smoking cessation behaviors, on the other hand, would meet the ethical standards for a RCT.

In general, RCTs are used to study the safety and efficacy of a new drug, procedure, or lifestyle change. The disease in question must be in a very narrow area of level of knowledge (i.e., we know a little about the new treatment, but not enough to know for sure if it is effective). If too much is known about the treatment, it might be unethical to withhold it from the control group. If too little is known, it might be unethical because we might be giving the client an unsafe drug or denying the client the commonly used treatment.

The beauty of an experimental design is the fact that the researcher can often carefully control the conditions. Sample size, sample characteristics, duration of treatment, lab tests, and compliance issues are all under the control of the researcher. However, to avoid bias, the sample must be randomly chosen, using a randomization method that is fair and prevents as much selection bias as possible. In a simple study involving two groups, a pool of eligible participants will be chosen. They must all meet inclusion criteria and not match the exclusion criteria. Then they must be willing to provide consent to be randomized into either treatment or control groups. The next step is to randomize the willing, eligible subjects into one of the two groups. An additional step that makes the study design even stronger is to blind the subject as to which group they are in, and further, to blind the intervener (health care provider, educator, etc). If only the subject is blinded, it is a single-blind RCT. If both the subject and the intervener are blinded, it is a double-blind study. If the person who is analyzing the final data is blinded, it is a triple-blind study. Each level of blinding makes the findings that much stronger.

Most new drugs have to undergo multiple RCT studies before they are approved by the Federal Drug Administration. However, the sample sizes are often fairly small, and it may not be until after the drug is on the market and thousands, if not millions, of people begin using it, that adverse side effects become apparent. Efficacy also may not be clear until it is in the open market. For instance, a leading cold capsule was already on the market when a well-designed RCT found that even though 65 percent of the treatment group reported an improvement in cold symptoms, so did 55 percent of the control group. The difference in the efficacy rates between the two groups was not significant.

Many drug studies use placebos. Some controversy has arisen about the ethics of using placebos but their use for many studies is unavoidable. As long as the subjects are fully informed prior to randomization that they may be receiving a placebo and they are willing to take that risk, then most of the ethical problems are

⊕ POLICY HIGHLIGHT

Epidemiologic research plays an essential role in identifying genetic variations associated with specific diseases. HuGENet is a collaboration of individuals and organizations who are committed to the development and dissemination of population-based human genome epidemiologic information that can be used for health promotion and disease prevention. As a result of increasing information, a growing number of genetic tests have become a health care tool available for health care professionals to use to identify inherited risk for diseases. Genetic screening tests are currently available for rare diseases, but the future will hold tests for screening for inherited risk for more common diseases such as breast cancer, heart disease, and colorectal cancer. As more genetic screening tests become available, policy makers will need to make decisions about test use because of ethical, legal, and social implications of genetic tests (Burke et al., 2002). Some questions relevant to public health nurses are what counseling should be provided for recipients of test results and who should provide that guidance and how can the public be protected from *genetic discrimination*?

resolved. The full discussion of the ethics of placebos is beyond the scope of this book, but it is available in many sources elsewhere.

A randomized clinical trial requires a power analysis. This means that prior to deciding on how many subjects will be recruited, a calculation must be performed to arrive at the required number of subjects for various levels of power. Most studies aim for a power level of 80 to 90 percent, which means that at the end of the study, we will have 80 percent power to detect a significant difference. The higher the power level, the more confidence we will have in the results of the study, but more subjects will be required. Usually the minimum acceptable power is 80 percent power, but 90 to 95 percent power is even more desirable. A formula is used that takes into consideration not only the desired power level but also the estimated difference in improvement percentages between groups. The latter requires a careful review of the literature in order to predict this difference accurately. By performing the calculation, we will have the minimum number of subjects that must be recruited. Allowing for attrition, or drop-out rate, of 10 percent or more requires recruiting more subjects than the minimum in order to have sufficient power at the end of the study.

RCTs can also be used in community health promotion and disease prevention studies. In these situations, they are usually called community intervention trials, or CITs. They are identical to an RCT except that the unit of analysis may not be individuals but communities or classes. The randomization process may mean that communities are paired, and then one is randomly selected to receive the intervention. In schools, certain classes, for instance fourth graders, can be randomized to receive the intervention. The entire class would then receive the intervention while the "control" class would not. Many studies have been conducted this way, ranging from issues related to smoking to weight loss to reduction of dietary fats. Some have been successful, but others have not. A federally funded agency has been chosen to evaluate community-based intervention studies; ratings range from "model program" to "insufficient data." Anyone wishing to start a health promotion/disease prevention program may consult this Web site to see if programs that have been studied and found to be effective have already been developed (SAMSHA, 2005).

SOURCES OF EPIDEMIOLOGIC DATA

Surveillance is essentially the same as "monitoring." To monitor a client, a nurse must be continually taking vital signs, checking for skin color, and so on. Surveillance is the public health version of monitoring. Since our "client" is the public, we are obligated to monitor the public's health constantly by taking "readings" on a regular and frequent basis. If trends develop or if quick changes occur, the public health community can respond quickly and effectively to make sure the health of the community is maintained or attained.

The overall responsibility for surveillance lies with the federal and state governments. Through the governmental organizations described in this section, a wealth of surveillance data is collected on a regular basis. This surveillance, however, requires the cooperation of the health care professional community as well as the community at large. For instance, CDC relies on private practitioners to provide data on multiple diseases ("reportable" diseases) considered serious enough to pose a threat to public health should an outbreak occur. Citizens are also expected to cooperate by participating in interviews about their health and lifestyle practices so that decision makers can make more informed decisions about which programs to fund.

The following list of surveillance organizations and surveillance systems is by no means exhaustive; it merely serves as an indicator of the most commonly referred to datasets. Some are available free online, while others are only available at nominal cost to public health professionals. Some of the datasets are simple and straightforward, requiring the knowledge only of frequencies and percentages. Others, however, are more complex and require the use of software programs like SAS and SPSS to analyze.

Census Bureau

The Census Bureau provides a wide variety of information important to public health nursing. Data can be aggregated by state, county, census district, zip code, even down to a specific block. The main categories are People (which covers most of the demographic information needed for a community assessment) and Housing (which describes the number of rooms, age of the house, etc.). The Web site is highly interactive and customizable. Tables, charts, and maps are created as requested and can be downloaded, saved, and printed.

National Center for Health Statistics

The National Center for Health Statistics (NCHS) is a division of the Centers for Disease Control but is located in Maryland rather than Atlanta, where CDC is located. They have the same overall mission, protecting the public's health, but NCHS is more of the statistical and surveillance arm of CDC. Most of the datasets are available online, as are tables and figures. However, paper reports are also available at no charge. NCHS manages a number of important surveillance systems. The most important are the National Health Interview Survey (NHIS) and the National Health and Nutrition Examination Survey (NHANES).

National Health Interview Survey

This survey is conducted each year and surveys enough people (about 20,000 annually) to make the data generalizable to the entire nation. The NHIS has a set of core questions that are asked each year as well as sets of supplemental questions that are only asked every few years. One example of a supplemental survey is the Cancer Supplement, which asks more in-depth questions about tobacco use, mammography, and other cancer-related behaviors than are available through the core section. The data are used by public health professionals to track the nation's progress toward achieving Healthy People 2010 goals and other national goals. Tables and charts are available on the Web site. Datasets are also available for use in SAS or SPSS, but to calculate accurate standard errors requires the use of specialized software due to the complex sampling design.

National Health and Nutrition Examination Survey

This survey combines an interview with a physical examination. The topics of concentration include diet, children's health, and sexually transmitted diseases. In the past, this survey has provided data that helped remove lead from gasoline because of the effect it has on children. As with NHIS, the NHANES is an annual survey that provides data generalizable to the nation.

Centers for Disease Control and Prevention

CDC is the premier public health agency in the country and also plays a major role in fighting epidemics around the world. Public health nurses may call on CDC for a number of reasons, but for epidemiologic reasons, CDC is a major source of relevant and helpful data. As with the Census Bureau and NCHS, most of their surveillance data is available online. People who prefer data on CDs may purchase them at a very low cost from CDC, NCHS, and most other governmental agencies.

Behavioral Risk Factor Surveillance Survey

This is purportedly the world's largest telephone survey. Its primary purpose is to provide states with the information to make health program decisions. All states have been involved since 1994 with a smaller number of states being involved prior to that year. The data are collected by state health departments using methods designed by CDC and with technical assistance from CDC. The data are also shared with CDC, which provides these data through their Web site. The main focus of the survey is to identify in each state behavior patterns that either promote or endanger health due to chronic illness, injury, or infectious disease.

Surveillance, Epidemiology, and End Results

This branch of the National Cancer Institute collects data on new cases (incidence) of cancer. Surveillance, Epidemiology, and End Results (SEER) uses the data from 14 population-based tumor registries and three supplemental tumor registries, representing about 25 percent of the country. The data not only include the type of cancer and demographic data but also stage at diagnosis and survival rates. After signing a "public use agreement," researchers can download the data in a variety of formats. The SEER Web site provides free specialized software for analyzing the data, but the data can also be analyzed using regular statistical packages.

CONCLUSION

Epidemiology is a tool that provides the foundation for the practice of public health. Public health nurses can improve the health of their communities more effectively if they are comfortable with the use of this tool. Training in epidemiology is available through college courses at the graduate level, workshops, and online sites such as CDC and the Public Health Foundation (https://www.train.org/DesktopShell.aspx).

CRITICAL THINKING ACTIVITIES

1. How is epidemiology different from clinical research?

2. In what instances should a new screening test *not* be implemented?

3. What information does an age-adjusted death rate give that is not available from a crude death rate?

4. What are the most important strengths and limitations of the case-control study design?

5. Why is the federal government involved in collecting surveillance data?

KEY TERMS

cohort	mortality	risk
convenience sample	prevalence	screening
incidence	rates	sensitive
morbidity	relative risk	specific

KEY CONCEPTS

- Epidemiology is the foundation of public health.
- The main purpose of epidemiology is to find out who is at risk for disease and why.
- Screening is an important prevention methodology, but sensitivity and specificity of the screening test must be considered.
- Different population's disease and death rates cannot be compared until the data are adjusted for age.
- The choice of an epidemiologic research design depends on many factors; no one design is appropriate for all situations.
- Surveillance data is a valuable source of information for public health professionals.

REFERENCES

American Diabetes Association. (2004). Screening for Type 2 Diabetes. *Diabetes Care, 27*(90001), 11S–14.

American Heart Association. (2005). *Cholesterol screening (adults and children).* 7272 Greensville Avenue, Dallas, TX: Author.

Anderson, E.T., & McFarlane, J. (2004). *Community as partner: Theory & practice in nursing.* Philadelphia: Lippincott Williams & Wilkins.

Burke, W., Atkins, D., Gwinn, M., Guttmacher, A., Haddow, J., Lau, J., Palomaki, G., Press, N., Richards, C.S., Wider-off, L., & Wiesner, G.L. (2002). Genetic test evaluation: Information needs of clinicians, policy makers, and the public. *American Journal of Epidemiology, 156*(4), 311–318.

Dawson, B., & Trapp, R.G. (2001). *Basic & clinical biostatistics.* New York, NY: McGraw-Hill Medical.

Grembowski, D. (2001). *The practice of health program evaluation.* Thousand Oaks, CA: Sage.

Hajjeh, R.A., Reingold, A., Weil, A., Shutt, K., Schuchat, A. & Perkins, B.A. (1999). Toxic shock syndrome in the United States: Surveillance update, 1979–1996. *Emerging Infectious Diseases, 5*(6), 807–810.

Herbst, A.L., Ulfelder, H., & Poskanzer, D.C. (1971). Adeno-carcinoma of the vagina. Association of maternal stilbestrol therapy with tumor appearance in young women [see comment]. *New England Journal of Medicine, 284*(15), 878–881.

Last, J.M. (1995). *A dictionary of epidemiology.* New York: Oxford University Press.

Robbins, A.S., Whittemore, A.S., & Thom, D.H. (2000). Differences in socioeconomic status and survival among white and black men with prostate cancer. *American Journal of Epidemiology, 151*(4): 409–416.

SAMSHA. (2005). *SAMSHA model programs.* Substance Abuse and Mental Health Services Administration, USDHHS. Retrieved February 1, 2005, from: http://modelprograms.samhsa.gov/template.cfm?page=default.

U.S. Census Bureau. (2005). *Annual population estimates.* Retrieved June, 2005 from http://www.census.gov/.

Weiss, C.H. (1998). *Evaluation.* Upper Saddle River, NJ: Prentice Hall.

BIBLIOGRAPHY

Gordis, L. (2004). *Epidemiology* (3rd ed.). Philadelphia: Elsevier Saunders.

Weiss, C.H. (1998). *Evaluation.* Upper Saddle River, NJ, Prentice Hall.

RESOURCES

Centers for Disease Control and Prevention (CDC)

1600 Clifton Road
Atlanta, GA 30333
404-639-3311 or 1-800-311-3435
Web: http://www.cdc.gov

The CDC keeps epidemiology data, conducts epidemiologic investigations, research and public health surveillance, and offers training programs for health professionals interested in epidemiology.

National Center for Health Statistics (NCHS)

3311 Toledo Road
Hyattsville, Maryland 20782
301-458-4000, toll free data inquiries: 1-866-441-NCHS
Email: nchsquery@cdc.gov
Web: http://www.cdc.gov

The National Center for Health Statistics is a part of the CDC. NCHS provides us with information about the health status of the population and important subgroups. Statistics are used to identify disparities in health status and use of health care by race/ethnicity, socioeconomic status, region, and other important population characteristics. Health statistics from the NCHS are also used to monitor trends in health status and care delivery, identify health problems, and support biomedical and health services research. Statistical information provides information for making policy and program changes and evaluating the impact of policy and programs. *Health, United States* is an annual report on trends in health statistics. This report can be accessed at http://www.cdc.gov/nchs/hus.htm.

Public Health Foundation (PHF)

1300 L Street, N. W., Suite 800
Washington, DC 20005
202-218-4400
FAX: 202-218-4409
Email: info@phf.org
Web: http://www.phf.org

The Public Health Foundation (PHF), a national non-profit organization, devotes its support for research, training and technical assistance to promote health in every community. The PHF works to improve the public health infrastructure and performance by translating complex data for use in practice, promoting evidence-based policies and programs, producing tools and providing technical assistance, disseminating training and educational materials, and developing systems for learning management and organization. Additionally, the PHF helps diverse groups discover common solutions to public health problems and supports public health systems research and national initiatives to improve the nation's public health.

Surveillance, Epidemiology, and End Results (SEER)

Cancer Statistics Branch
Surveillance Research Program
Division of Cancer Control and Population Sciences
National Cancer Institute
Suite 504, MSC 8316
6116 Executive Boulevard
Bethesda, MD 20892-8316
301-496-8510
Web: http://www.seer.cancer.gov

The Surveillance, Epidemiology, and End Results (SEER), a program of the National Cancer Institute, provides information on cancer incidence and survival statistics in the United States. SEER is the only comprehensive source of population-based information that includes stage of cancer at the time of diagnosis and patient survival data. Data come from state registries, so SEER guides states to collect data that are compatible for pooling and improving national cancer estimates. One of SEER's efforts is a Web-based tool for public health workers, State Cancer Profiles, to find cancer statistics for specific states and counties. This effort is a joint project between the National Cancer Institute and the Centers for Disease Control and Prevention and is part of the Cancer Control P.L.A.N.E.T. Web site (http://cancercontrolplanet.cancer.gov) that provides comprehensive cancer resources for public health professionals. SEER is the most complete registry for quality cancer data being reported.

U.S. Census Bureau

4700 Silver Hill Road
Washington, D.C. 20233-0001
301-763-6440
FAX: 301-457-2654
Email: POL.Policy.Office@census.gov
Web: http://www.census.gov

The Census Bureau serves as the leading source of quality data about the nation's people and economy. The Census Bureau was established in 1790 under the responsibility of Secretary of State Thomas Jefferson. That census, taken by U.S. marshals on horseback, counted 3.9 million inhabitants. Today, in addition to taking a census of the population every 10 years, the Census Bureau conducts censuses of economic activity and state and local governments every 5 years and conducts more than 100 other surveys every year. In addition, the Census Bureau publishes notices informing the public of our collections of information and other activities in the Federal Register and offers international programs and fellowships.

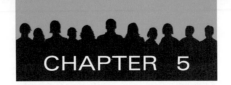

CHAPTER 5

Healthy People 2010 Objectives

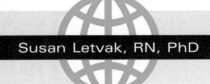

Susan Letvak, RN, PhD

Chapter Outline

- Leading Health Indicators
  - Physical Activity
  - Overweight and Obesity
  - Tobacco Use
  - Substance Abuse
  - Responsible Sexual Behavior
  - Mental Health
  - Injury and Violence
  - Environmental Quality
  - Immunization
  - Access to Health Care
- Healthy People 2010 and Public Health Nurses

Learning Objectives

Upon completion of this chapter, the reader will be able to:

1. Examine the historical development of Healthy People 2010.

2. Define the purpose of Healthy People 2010 for approving the health of the nation.

3. Describe the ten Leading Health Indicators and provide examples of specific focus areas under each.

4. Analyze the role of the public health nurse in meeting Healthy People 2010 goals and objectives.

n January 2000, the U.S. Department of Health and Human Services released *Healthy People 2010,* the nation's health goals for this decade. Healthy People 2010 is the third set of 10-year national goals. In 1979, *Healthy People: The Surgeon General's Report on Health Promotion and Disease Prevention* was produced with five goals to be achieved by 1990. Four of the goals focused on reducing premature death among infants, children, adolescents, and adults, and the fifth goal aimed to preserve independence in older adults (USDHEW, 1979). This report was quickly followed in 1980 by the document, *Promoting Health/Preventing Disease: Objectives for the Nation,* which outlined 15 focus areas and 226 health objectives for the United States to achieve in 10 years. The focus areas ranged from family planning, fluoridation and dental health, and immunizations to toxic agents and radiation control (USDHHS, 1980). In 1990, *Healthy People 2000: National Health Promotion and Disease Prevention Objectives* was released, which established health goals and objectives in 22 priority areas (USDHHS, 1991).

Healthy People 2010 was developed by the Healthy People Consortium, an alliance of 350 national organizations and 250 state agencies, which conducted three national meetings. Individuals and other health organizations provided input on national health priorities at five regional meetings. On two occasions, the American public was given the opportunity to submit thoughts and ideas. Additionally, more than 11,000 comments on draft materials were received from individuals across the United States. The final Healthy People 2010 document was developed by a team of experts under the direction of the Department of Health and Human Services (USDHHS, 2000a; 2000b).

Healthy People 2010 objectives were developed to guide organizations; governmental agencies at the local, state, and federal levels; professional associations; consumer groups; academic institutions; and policy makers to improve the health of the nation for the next 10 years. The two overriding goals of Healthy People 2010 are to

⊕ Increase quality and years of healthy life.

⊕ Eliminate health disparities.

These two goals can be monitored through 467 objectives in 28 focus areas (Table 5-1). Each objective has a target for specific improvements to be achieved

TABLE 5-1: Healthy People 2010 Focus Areas

1. Access to Quality Health Care	15. Injury and Violence Prevention
2. Arthritis, Osteoporosis, and Chronic Back Conditions	16. Maternal, Infant, and Child Health
3. Cancer	17. Medical Product Safety
4. Chronic Kidney Disease	18. Mental Health and Mental Disorders
5. Diabetes	19. Nutrition and Overweight
6. Disability and Secondary Conditions	20. Occupational Health and Safety
7. Educational and Community Based Programs	21. Oral Health
8. Environmental Health	22. Physical Activity and Fitness
9. Family Planning	23. Public Health Infrastructure
10. Food Safety	24. Respiratory Diseases
11. Health Communication	25. Sexually Transmitted Diseases
12. Heart Disease and Stroke	26. Substance Abuse
13. HIV	27. Tobacco Use
14. Immunization and Infections Diseases	28. Vision and Hearing

Note. From U.S. Department of Health and Human Services (USDHHS) (2000a). *Healthy People 2010, understanding and improving health,* p. 17. Washington, DC: Author.

by the year 2010. Public health nurses must be familiar with Healthy People 2010 objectives as they strive to improve the health of the communities they serve.

LEADING HEALTH INDICATORS

In order to provide a less complex set of criteria to guide practice and evaluation, a list of 10 Leading Health Indicators, which reflect the major public health concerns in the United States, was developed. They were chosen based on their ability to motivate action and provide access to data to measure progress, and their overall relevance as broad public health issues. Each of the 10 health indicators has specific objectives, which are used to track progress in meeting federal and state level goals. The health indicators also provide a link to the 467 objectives of Healthy People 2010 and serve as the foundation for community health initiatives with the overall goal of creating healthy people in healthy communities.

⊕ RESEARCH APPLICATION

Physical Activity, Social Support, and Health-Related Quality of Life among Persons with HIV Disease

Study Purpose

To identify and explore relations among physical activity, social support, and health-related quality of life in persons with HIV disease (HIVD) living in community settings. The study was significant because up to 900,000 Americans currently live with HIVD and 40,000 become infected annually. Advances in health care have led to fewer deaths, and HIVD is now recognized as a chronic illness. Public health nurses face new and complex challenges caring for people with HIVD, and research on this population has not emphasized health promotion. Research has demonstrated that physical activity and social support are important for maintaining and improving health-related quality of life.

Methods

The research study was guided by a health-related quality of life (HRQOL) model because the model emphasizes the person and the environment and is composed of modifiable factors, which may allow for nursing interventions. A convenience sample of 70 men and 8 women ($N = 78$) between the ages of 23 and 70 ($M = 40.4$, $SD = 8.33$) who received primary care at an infectious disease clinic or community support at a local agency were recruited to participate. Inclusion criteria included being without cognitive impairment, being able to read and write English, and having not been hospitalized for an HIV- or AIDS-related illness within a previous 4-week period. The average length of time living with HIVD was 7.9 years, and the sample was ethnically diverse (51.3 percent African American, 33.3 percent Caucasian, 5.1 percent other).

Findings

Participants completed a questionnaire that included the Medical Outcomes Survey, the Physical Activity Questionnaire, the Norbeck Social Support Survey, and a Demographic Data Tool. Study findings demonstrated that the participants viewed their quality of life in the midrange. The most common leisure time physical activity was walking (85.9 percent), but few (28.2 percent) identified meeting Healthy People 2010 recommendations for moderate physical activity, and only 7.7 reported meeting Healthy People 2010 guidelines for vigorous physical activity. Correlations between study variables indicated significant negative correlation ($p < .05$) between HRQOL and meeting Healthy People 2010 recommendations for moderate ($r = -.23$) or vigorous ($r = -.27$) physical activity. Social support was also correlated with health-related quality of life.

Implications

This study supports the importance of health promotion activities for those with HIVD, including physical activity and use of supportive networks. Public health nurses must partner with local government, faith, community and professional organizations in building environments and networks that encourage health-related quality of life for those with HIVD.

Reference

Clingerman, E. (2004). Physical activity, social support, and health-related quality of life among persons with HIV disease. *Journal of Community Health Nursing 21*(3), 179–197.

Physical Activity

The Healthy People 2010 goal for the nation's health is to improve health, fitness, and quality of life through daily physical activity. Physical activity includes any form of exercise or movement produced by skeletal muscles that result in an expenditure of energy. Research has demonstrated the importance of physical activity for all individuals. Regular physical activity substantially reduces the risk of dying of coronary heart disease, the nation's leading cause of death, and decreases the risk for stroke, colon cancer, diabetes, and high blood pressure. It also helps to control weight; contributes to healthy bones, muscles, and joints; reduces falls among older adults; helps to relieve the pain of arthritis; reduces symptoms of anxiety and depression; and is associated with fewer hospitalizations, health care provider visits, and medications (CDC, 2004c). However, more than 50 percent of American adults do not get enough physical activity to provide health benefits (CDC, 2003a; USDHHS, 1996). Physical activity decreases with age and is less common among women than men and among those with lower income and less education. Additionally, there are racial and ethnic differences in physical activity rates, particularly among women.

Public health nurses must work to ensure that physical activity and fitness become part of regular, healthy behavior patterns. Young people are at particular risk for becoming sedentary as they grow older; therefore, moderate to vigorous exercise must be especially encouraged in children and adolescents. Public health nurses must recognize that the major barriers people face when trying to increase physical activity are time, access to convenient facilities, and safe environments in which to exercise (USDHHS, 2000b). An example of a specific objective (22-6) is to have 30 percent of all adolescents engage in moderate physical activity for at least 30 minutes on 5 or more days per week.

Overweight and Obesity

The Healthy People 2010 goal for the nation's health is to promote health and reduce chronic disease associated with diet and weight. Research has demonstrated that overweight and obesity are risk factors for high blood pressure, diabetes, heart disease, stroke, gallbladder disease, arthritis, musculoskeletal disorders, and cancers (McGee, 2004). Additionally, those who are obese suffer from social stigmatization, discrimination, and poor self-esteem. Overweight is being too heavy for one's height, defined as a body mass index of 25 up to 30 kg/m^2, while obesity is having a high amount of body fat (CDC, 2006). A person is considered to be obese if he or she has a body mass index of 30 kg/m^2 or greater. In 2001, the prevalence of obesity among U.S. adults was 20.9 percent, a 61 percent increase since 1991 (Mokdad et al., 2003). Being overweight and obese is more prevalent among women with low incomes and less education. Additionally, obesity is more common in African American and Hispanic women than among white women.

Overweight and obesity is also epidemic among children and adolescents in the United States, affecting 10 to 15 percent of children, a fourfold increase between 1963 and 2000 (Hardy, Harrell, & Bell, 2004). With the exception of non-Hispanic Black girls, boys have a higher incidence of overweight than girls. American Indian, Hispanic, and African American children have higher prevalence rates than white children. Children who are overweight are at risk for Type 2 diabetes, orthopedic and psychosocial problems. Additionally, 50 percent of obese children become obese adults (Pearson et al., 2003).

Public health nurses must work to establish healthy dietary and physical activity behaviors beginning in childhood. School-age children must be educated about proper nutrition to help establish healthy eating habits early in life. Adults must be educated about the long-term consequences and risks associated with overweight and how to achieve and maintain a healthy weight. Specific objectives include (19-1) increasing the proportion of adults who are at a healthy weight from a baseline of 42 to 60 percent by 2010 and (19-3) reducing the proportion of children and adolescents who are overweight or obese from a baseline of 10 to 11 percent to 5 percent by 2010.

Tobacco Use

The Healthy People 2010 goal for the nation's health is to reduce illness, disability, and death related to tobacco use and exposure to secondhand smoke. Cigarette smoking is the single most preventable cause of disease and death in the United States (USDHHS, 2000b). Smoking is a major risk factor for heart disease, stroke, lung cancer, lung disease, premature delivery, and sudden infant death syndrome. In 2003, approximately 45.4 million (21.6 percent) of adult Americans were smokers; however, smoking rates have declined by 47 percent since 1965 (CDC, 2004a; 2005). Men have higher smoking prevalence rates (24.1 percent) than women (19.2 percent). Smoking rates are highest among Native Americans (39.7 percent) and lowest among Hispanics (16.4 percent) and Asians (11.7 percent) (CDC, 2005).

Public health nurses must target populations with high rates of smoking, especially adolescents. Approximately 90 percent of smokers begin before the age of 21 (Mowery, Brick, & Farrelly, 2000). In 2003, 22 percent of high school students and 10 percent of middle school students were smokers (CDC, 2004b). Additionally, smoking in adolescents is associated with other health-compromising behaviors, including being involved in fights, carrying weapons, engaging in high-risk sexual behavior, and using alcohol and other illicit drugs (American Lung Association, 2003). An example of a specific objective (27-2) is to reduce tobacco use by adolescents from 43 to 21 percent by 2010.

Substance Abuse

The Healthy People 2010 goal for the nation's health is to reduce substance abuse to protect the health, safety, and quality of life for all, especially children. The 2003 National Survey on Drug Use and Health (SAMHSA, 2004) reported that 19.5 million Americans, or 8.2 percent of the population aged 12 or older, were current illicit drug users. Marijuana is the most commonly used illicit drug, with a rate of 6.2 percent (14.6 million). Substance abuse rates were highest among American Indians or Alaska Natives (12.1 percent), persons reporting two or more races (12.0 percent), and Native Hawaiians or Other Pacific Islanders (11.1 percent). Rates were 8.7 percent for blacks, 8.3 percent for whites, and 8.0 percent for Hispanics. Asians had the lowest rate at 3.8 percent. An estimated 119 million Americans aged 12 or older were current drinkers of alcohol in 2003 (50.1 percent). About 54 million (22.6 percent) participated in binge drinking at least once in the 30 days prior to the survey, and 16.1 million (6.8 percent) were heavy drinkers (SAMHSA, 2004).

To meet Healthy People 2010 objectives for reducing substance abuse, public health nurses must intervene at the individual, community, state, and federal level. Education and treatment programs must be pro-

vided at the individual level. At the community level, education programs must be provided at schools and for community organizations. Television and radio public service announcements must be made concerning the risks of substance abuse and avenues for treatment. Public health nurses must advocate at the state and federal level for legislation to improve substance abuse treatment and rehabilitation. An example of a specific objective (26-10c) is to reduce the proportion of adults using any illicit drug during the past 30 days from 5.8 percent to 3.0 percent by 2010.

Responsible Sexual Behavior

The Healthy People 2010 goal for the nation's health is to promote responsible sexual behaviors, strengthen community capacity, and increase access to quality services to prevent sexually transmitted diseases (STDs) and their complications. Almost half of all pregnancies in the United States are unintended (Henshaw, 1998). Additionally, 15 million Americans become infected with an STD each year (CDC, 2000). STDs refer to the more than 25 infectious organisms transmitted primarily through sexual activity. Women suffer more serious STD complications than men, including pelvic inflammatory disease, ectopic pregnancy, infertility, chronic pelvic pain, and cervical cancer from human papilloma virus.

It is estimated that between 850,000 and 950,000 persons in the United States are living with human immunodeficiency virus (HIV), including 180,000 to 280,000 individuals (one in four) who do not know they are infected. There are an estimated 40,000 new infections each year. There has been a recent increase in high-risk sexual behaviors, especially among homosexual men, which has increased incidence rates of HIV and other STDs (del Rio, 2003). These increases are thought to be due to optimism about new therapies to treat HIV and difficulties maintaining safe sex behaviors over a lifetime.

All racial, cultural, economic, and religious groups are affected by STDs. Public health nurses must be aware of the groups disproportionately at risk, including women, adolescents and young adults, and African Americans and Hispanics. Primary prevention requires effective population-level and individual-level interventions. Behavioral interventions should focus on exposure, transmission, and duration factors (the time period during which an infected person remains infectious and able to spread the disease to others). Correct and consistent condom usage must be taught. There must be early identification and treatment of persons with STDs to break the chain of transmission. Additionally, partner notification and treatment must be effective. Public health nurses can best approach these sensitive topics by having a relaxed, matter of fact style, asking questions in a routine manner, and being non-judgmental. An example of a specific objective (13-4) is to increase the proportion of sexually active persons who use condoms from 23 to 50 percent by 2010.

Mental Health

The Healthy People 2010 goal for the nation's health is to improve mental health and ensure access to appropriate, quality mental health services. The National Institute of Mental Health (2001) estimates that 22.1 percent of Americans over age 18 (one in five) suffer from a diagnosable mental disorder in any year. Four of the ten leading causes of disability in the United States are mental disorders, including major depression, bipolar disorder, schizophrenia, and obsessive-compulsive disorder. **Mental health** is defined as a state of successful mental functioning, resulting in productive activities, fulfilling relationships, and the ability to adapt to change and cope with adversity (USDHHS, 2000b). Mental illness is the term that refers to all diagnosable mental disorders. Mental disorders are health conditions that are characterized by alterations in thinking, mood, or behavior which are associated with distress or impaired functioning.

Mental disorders occur across the life span and affect persons of all races, ethnic groups, sexes, and socioeconomic groups. Mental disorders vary in severity and their impact on people's lives. Mental illness, including suicide, accounts for over 15 percent of the burden of disease in established market economies, such as the United States. This is more than the disease burden caused by all cancers (NIMH, 2001). Additionally, there is increasing awareness and concern regarding the impact of stress, its prevention and treatment, and the need for enhanced coping skills.

Public health nurses should be involved in all aspects of improving mental health in populations. Challenges include increasing numbers of clients with fewer resources. Public health nurses must seek to dispel

myths while providing accurate education about mental illness. Additionally, there must be increased advocacy for both the rights of those who are mentally ill as well as for increased health care resources. An example of a specific objective (18-2) is to reduce the rate of suicide attempts by adolescents from 2.6 percent to 1 percent by 2010.

Injury and Violence

The Healthy People 2010 goal for the nation's health is to reduce injuries, disabilities, and deaths due to unintentional injuries and violence. Almost all people will suffer an injury at some time in their lives; however, most injuries are predictable and preventable. The National Center for Injury Prevention and Control (2002) estimates that one in 10 Americans experience an injury serious enough to require an emergency room visit each year. Motor vehicle crashes continue to be the leading cause of injury death in the United States. Falls are the leading cause of injury death and nonfatal injury in older Americans. Violence is pervasive in the United States. Homicide is the second leading cause of death for persons aged 15 to 34 and is the leading cause of death for African Americans in this age group (CDC, 2003b).

Even though every person is at risk for injury, there are disparities in which injuries affect which groups. American Indians and Alaska Natives have higher death rates from motor vehicle crashes, residential fires, and drownings. African Americans have higher deaths rates from unintentional injury. African American, Hispanic, and American Indian children are at higher risk for home fire deaths. Drowning rates are two to four times greater in males than females. Homicide deaths are also greater among African American and Hispanic youths.

To reduce the number and severity of injuries, public health nurses must have an understanding of injuries in populations so that effective primary prevention interventions can be planned. Poverty, discrimination, lower education levels, and unemployment are all risk factors for violence. Strategies for reducing violence must begin in childhood, before violent beliefs and behaviors are adopted. Specific interventions include parent training, mentoring, home visitation, and community awareness programs. An example of a specific objective (15-33) is to reduce maltreatment and maltreatment fatalities of children from 13.9 victims per 1,000 children to 11.1 per 1,000 children by 2010.

Environmental Quality

The Healthy People 2010 goal for the nation's health is to promote health for all through a healthy environment. The World Health Organization (1997) defines environmental health as those aspects of human health, disease, and injury that are determined or influenced by factors in the environment. Human exposures to toxic agents in the air, water, soil, and food are major contributors to illness, disability, and death.

Air pollution continues to be a widespread public health and environmental health problem in the United States, causing health problems as well as damage to crops, buildings, forests, and our water supply. Preservation of water quality is of concern. Efficient health-outcome measures and monitoring of toxins and wastes are needed. Healthy environments also include homes, schools, and offices. Potential risks include indoor air pollution, inadequate heating and cooling systems, lead-based paint hazards, and molds. Public health nurses must be alert to potential environmental hazards, educate the public on the relationship between the environment and health, and ensure that laws, regulations, and practices protect the public and environment from hazardous agents. Public health nurses provide direct assessment of communities to detect health hazards and must partner with community groups and environmental health coalitions to advocate for healthy communities. A specific objective (8-23) is to reduce the proportion of occupied housing units that are substandard from 6.2 percent to 3 percent by 2010.

Immunization

The Healthy People 2010 goal for the nation's health is to prevent disease, disability, and death from infectious diseases, including vaccine preventable diseases. Infectious diseases remain major causes of illness, death, and disability in the United States. New infectious agents and diseases are continually being detected and antimicrobial resistance is developing for many once treatable infectious diseases. Vaccines are effective in preventing many infectious diseases. High vaccination rates protect society as a whole because even those ⁓e unvaccinated are protected because of group immunity. Vaccination rates are at near record highs; nevertheless, disparities exist on certain emerging disease issues and in vaccination rates (National Center for Health Statistics, 2000).

Public health nurses must ensure that all children born in the United States receive 12 to 16 doses of vaccine by age 2 years to be protected against 10 vaccine-preventable childhood diseases. Efforts must be made to increase vaccination coverage for children living in poverty and those of immigrant parents. Adults older than age 65 must be encouraged to receive yearly immunization against the flu as well as a one-time immunization against pneumococcal disease. Major strategies to protect people against vaccine-preventable diseases include improving the quality and quantity of vaccination delivery services; minimizing financial burdens for needy persons; increasing community participation, education, and partnerships; improving monitoring of disease and vaccination coverage; developing new or improved vaccines; and improving vaccine use. An example of a specific objective (14-11) is to reduce new cases of tuberculosis from 6.8 new cases per 100,000 persons to 1.0 new case per 100,000 persons by 2010.

Having an understanding of the importance of vaccination, and recognizing potential barriers, the public health nurse is now ready to begin a systematic plan for ensuring that the Healthy People 2010 targets are met for immunizing at risk older adults for influenza and pneumococcal diseases. The strategy involves both health care providers in the community as well as the planning and implementation of vaccination clinics at times convenient for the community.

For health care providers, request that standing orders be written to cover all clinic clients admitted to hospitals and nursing homes to receive yearly influenza vaccinations and the pneumococcal vaccine. These orders should include administering the pneumococcal vaccination if confirmation of prior immunization cannot be obtained. The nurse should also develop a recall/reminder system for all clinic clients at the health department. Post cards will be sent two weeks in advance and phone call reminders will also be given with dates of immunization clinics. Develop education brochures to inform community residents of the benefits of immunization and to dispel any misconceptions or false beliefs. Finally, organize multiple immunization clinics at convenient times and places. Locations include places of worship, the senior citizen center, the local grocery store, and recreation centers. Home visits

⊕ PRACTICE APPLICATION

Improving Influenza and Pneumococcal Immunization Among High-Risk Adults

Public health nurses are responsible for assuring that high-risk adults are properly immunized against influenza and pneumococcal diseases. The nurse is responsible for several large neighborhood communities, which have a large percentage of low-income elderly and minorities. The public health department provides health care to a majority of these elderly residents. The public health nurse is aware that vaccine-preventable diseases, including influenza and pneumococcal diseases, are responsible for significant morbidity and 50,000 to 80,000 deaths annually in the United States among high-risk populations and the elderly (Thompson et al., 2003). Baseline data from 1997 demonstrates that 63 percent of older adults received the influenza vaccine and 43 percent received the pneumococcal vaccine. In high-risk adults, the percentages are much lower with only 25 percent receiving the influenza vaccine and 11 percent having received the pneumococcal vaccine. The Healthy People 2010 goal (14-29) is to increase the proportion of adults who are vaccinated annually against influenza and who have ever been vaccinated against pneumococcal disease. The 2010 target percentages for elderly Americans are 90 percent for influenza and 60 percent for pneumococcal disease, and for high-risk adults, 60 percent for both influenza and pneumococcal disease (USDHHS, 2000a).

In developing a plan to improve immunization rates, the first thing the nurse must understand is which adults are considered to be at high risk for complications of influenza and/or pneumococcal disease. This includes those with diseases or other conditions that increase their risk, such as

- Diabetes mellitus
- Chronic liver disease
- Chronic renal disease
- Chronic lung disease
- Chronic cardiac disease/heart failure
- HIV infection
- Cancer
- Organ transplant recipient
- Recipients of immunosuppressant therapies
- The elderly (> 65 years of age)

Others at risk for complications, not because of underlying disease, but because of underimmunization, include

- Minorities
- Those with low socioeconomic levels
- Those with low education levels
- Those living in inner cities
- Those lacking medical services
- Those with misperception of risk and comorbid disease

Public health nurses recognize that efforts must be targeted for minority populations in the community. Nurses understand that specific factors have been identified as the reasons for the underutilization of vaccines in minority populations, including decreased access to care related to low socioeconomic status and/or lack of insurance for immunizations, low motivation of primary care providers to recommend immunization to minorities, family factors (larger family size, poverty, frequent moves, language barriers, undocumented immigrant status, inadequate knowledge about vaccinations, and preconceived notions that vaccinations are ineffective), and missed opportunities to immunize (Hebert et al., 2005; Larson, 2003).

Planning for community education and immunization clinics, the nurse must first recognize the barriers to receiving immunization for older adults. Barriers that must be overcome include

- Skepticism about the effectiveness of the influenza and pneumococcal vaccines
- Uncertainty about side effects and adverse reactions
- Low recognition of the need for vaccination
- Lack of transportation to immunization clinics
- Concern about inability to pay for vaccinations

There are also provider barriers to adult immunization. These include uncertainty about who is at risk for disease, missed opportunities to provide vaccinations, and low health care provider incentives for providing vaccine services when reimbursement for service is low.

are scheduled for homebound clients who are unable to attend the immunization clinic.

To evaluate the effectiveness of the immunization program, influenza and pneumococcal disease rates will be monitored annually. Data on clinic visits and hospitalizations for flu and pneumococcal disease will be collected. Interviews with key informants and community residents will assist in determining the best way to educate and provide appropriate program planning for the target population.

Access to Health Care

The Healthy People 2010 goal for the nation's health is to improve access to comprehensive, high-quality health care services for all Americans. Health disparities refers to gaps in the quality of health and health care across racial and ethnic groups. The Health Resources and Service Administration (2000) defines health disparities as "population-specific differences in the presence of disease, health outcomes, and access to health care." Access to quality health care is necessary to eliminate health disparities and increase the quality and years of life. First, people must have access to clinical preventative services for primary and secondary prevention. Primary care services must be improved so all Americans have a usual source of care. The long-term care population needs access to nursing home care, adult daycare, assisted living, and hospice care.

Public health nurses must work to remove financial, structural, and personal barriers to health care. Financial barriers include not having health insurance or the financial resources to cover services outside of insurance plans. Structural barriers include a lack of primary care providers, medical specialists, and health care facilities to meet the needs of the population. Personal barriers include cultural or spiritual differences, language barriers, and concerns about confidentiality or discrimination. An example of a specific objective (1-4) is to increase the proportion of persons who have a specific source of ongoing care from 86 percent to 96 percent by 2010.

HEALTHY PEOPLE 2010 AND PUBLIC HEALTH NURSES

The health of the nation is dependent on nurses who have up-to-date knowledge, skills, and abilities to deliver health care services effectively. Research is needed to identify opportunities to improve health, strengthen information systems and organizations, and make more effective and efficient use of resources. There are 23 national data sources identified for tracking Healthy People 2010 objectives (USDHHS, 2000b), but objectives must also be tracked at the state and local levels. Public health nurses have an integral role in helping people increase their life expectancy and quality of life.

Healthy People 2010 provides a focus on disparities for health outcomes for disease. Disparities are not limited to ethnic and racial groups but extend to gender, education, income, geographical location, disability, and sexual orientation. A "better than best" target for each objective provides a challenge for public health nurses to not accept less than favorable health outcomes for individuals based on these disparities. Additionally, a diverse, highly skilled workforce must be recruited and trained to assist in the elimination of disparities.

To assure a strong public health workforce in meeting Healthy People 2010 objectives, essential public health services will be required. These include

- Monitoring the health status of communities to identify community health problems.

- Diagnosing and investigating health problems and health hazards in the community.

- Informing, educating, and empowering people about health issues.

- Mobilizing community partnerships to identify and solve health problems.

- Developing policies and plans that support individual and community health efforts.

- Enforcing laws and regulations that protect health and safety.

- Linking people to needed health care services and ensuring the provision of health when otherwise unavailable.

- Ensuring a competent public and personal health workforce.

- Evaluating the effectiveness, accessibility, and quality of population-based health services.

- Researching new insights and solutions to health problems.

⊕ RESEARCH APPLICATION

Older Ethnic Women in Faith Communities

Study Purpose

To explore how to offer culturally appropriate health programs to reduce the disparity of health status in older women of ethnic groups. The study was significant because ethnic minority older adults report poorer health than non-Hispanic whites, and the percentage of ethnic minority older adults is expected to double by 2050. Physical activity and nutrition are two focus areas of Healthy People 2010, yet differences in health concepts in diverse cultures have not been explored to facilitate the planning of appropriate health programs.

Methods

The researcher identified no specific conceptual framework. A convenience sample of 17 women who identified themselves as Vietnamese, Hispanic, or African American were recruited to participate from three senior citizen centers in economically impoverished areas. The ages of the women ranged from 62 to 86, and all described themselves as being in fairly good health. Interviews were also conducted with congregational health team members to examine factors contributing to effective or ineffective health programs.

Data were collected in semistructured interviews. Questions asked of the women included what the meaning of being healthy was to the participants, what they do to stay healthy, what is important in life, and what their lives are like now. Congregational health team members were asked for recommendations for successful health programming for ethnic groups.

Findings

Data were analyzed by first identifying the most commonly emerging classes of comments, which were then used as codes. Overriding themes and patterns were then formulated. The transcultural definition of "health" that emerged from the data was "Healthy is being able to do activities which have meaning, and these in turn keep me healthy." The most repeated phrase related to health promoting behaviors was "staying active." The similarities between the three cultures were more striking than different.

Implications

Public health nurses should seek the support of faith communities in providing health promotion for ethnic minority older adults. Nutrition programs addressing foods relevant to cultural groups combined with exercise information is a suggested start. Health promotion programs should begin with information dissemination about risks and screening recommendations. Prevention activities, such as breast self-examination, should be introduced by members of the same ethnic and cultural background because nurses who share a similar cultural heritage, ethnic identity, and use of language with their clients are apt to provide more culturally competent care, especially to minority groups (Powell & Gilliss, 2005). Additionally, public health nurses must educate health ministry teams about Healthy People 2010 objectives and assist teams to partner with local government and community agencies to support meeting these objectives.

Reference

Hahn, K. (2003). Older ethnic women in faith communities. *Journal of Gerontological Nursing, 29*(7), 5–12.

Healthy People 2010 provides public health nurses with a focus for improving the health of their communities. The entire Healthy People 2010 document, including access to Health Indicators, specific objectives, and progress toward health targets can be easily obtained by nurses at www.healthypeople.gov. By understanding and working toward set goals, nurses can improve the quality and years of healthy life while eliminating health disparities in their communities and for the nation.

CRITICAL THINKING ACTIVITIES

1. What are the major health problems in your community? Review the Healthy People 2010 objectives to determine the target goals for each of these problems. What will be necessary for you to improve health for your community? What are the anticipated barriers you will encounter?

2. A goal of Healthy People 2010 is to reduce health disparities in the United States. Choose a health problem and discuss the health disparities that may exist. What strategies will reduce disparities for this problem in your community?

3. Research on strategies for improving the nation's health is urgently needed, especially in target areas of Healthy People 2010. State a research problem for a specific Healthy People 2010 objective. How would a public health nurse conduct a research study on a problem to improve health?

KEY TERMS

environmental health

health disparity

Leading Health Indicators

mental health

obesity

overweight

physical activity

KEY CONCEPTS

⊕ Healthy People 2010 is the third national document developed to provide goals for the nation for a 10-year period.

⊕ The two overriding goals of Healthy People 2010 are to increase the quality and years of healthy life and to eliminate health disparities.

⊕ Healthy People 2010 provides 10 Leading Health Indicators to organize 467 objectives in 28 focus areas.

⊕ Public health nurses have an integral role in helping populations achieve Healthy People 2010 goals of increasing life expectancy and quality of life and decreasing health disparities in health care.

REFERENCES

American Lung Association. (2003). *Adolescent smoking statistics.* Retrieved December 30, 2004, from http://www.lungusa.org.

Centers for Disease Control (CDC). (2000). *Tracking the hidden epidemic: Trends in STDs in the United States.* Retrieved December 21, 2004 from http://www.cdc.gov/nchstp/dstd/Stats_Trends/Trends2000.pdf.

Centers for Disease Control (CDC). (2003a). Prevalence of physical activity, including lifestyle activities among adults—United States, 2000–2001. *Morbidity and Mortality Weekly Report, 52*(32), 764–769.

Centers for Disease Control (CDC). (2003b). *Web-based injury statistics query and reporting system* [Online]. National Center for Injury Prevention and Control, Centers for Disease Control and Prevention (producer). Retrieved on December 28, 2004, from http://www.cdc.gov/ncipc/wisqars.

Centers for Disease Control (CDC). (2004a). Cigarette smoking among adults—United States. *Morbidity and Mortality Weekly Report, 53*(20), 427–431.

Centers for Disease Control (CDC). (2004b). Cigarette use among high school students—U.S., 1991–2003. *Morbidity and Mortality Weekly Report, 53*(23), 499–502.

Centers for Disease Control (CDC). (2004c). The importance of physical activity. Retrieved on December 27, 2004, from http://www.cdc.gov/nccdphp/dnpa/physical.

Centers for Disease Control (CDC). (2005). Cigarette smoking among adults—United States. *Morbidity and Mortality Weekly Report, 54*(20), 509–513.

Clingerman, E. (2004). Physical activity, social support, and health-related quality of life among persons with HIV disease. *Journal of Community Health Nursing 21*(3), 179–197.

del Rio, C. (2003). New challenges in HIV care: Prevention among HIV infected patients. *Topics in HIV Medicine, 11*(4), 140–144.

Hahn, K. (2003). Older ethnic women in faith communities. *Journal of Gerontological Nursing, 29*(7), 5–12.

Hardy, L., Harrell, J., & Bell, R. (2004). Overweight in children: Definitions, measurements, confounding factors, and health consequences. *Journal of Pediatric Nursing, 19*(6), 376–384.

Hebert, P.L., Frick, K.D., Kane, R.L., & McBean, A.M. (2005). The causes of racial and ethnic differences in influenza vaccination rates among elderly Medicare beneficiaries. *Health Services Research, 40*(2), 239–243.

Henshaw, S.K. (1998). Unintended pregnancy in the United States. *Family Planning Perspectives, 30*(1), 24–29.

Larson, E. (2003). Racial and ethnic disparities in immunizations: Recommendations for clinicians. *Family Medicine, 35*(9), 655–60.

McGee, D. (2004). Body mass index and mortality: A meta-analysis based on person-level data from twenty-six observational studies. *Annals of Epidemiology, 15*(2), 87–97.

Mokdad, A.H., Ford E.S., Bowman B.A., Dietz. W.H., Vinicor, F., Bales, V.S., & Marks, J.S. (2003). Prevalence of obesity, diabetes, and obesity related health risk factors. *JAMA, 289*(1), 76–79.

Mowery, P.D., Brick, P.D., & Farrelly, M.C. (2000). *Legacy First Look Report 3. Pathways to established smoking: results from the 1999 national youth tobacco survey.* Washington, DC: American Legacy Foundation.

National Center for Health Statistics, USDHHS. (2000). *Fast stats a to z: Immunization.* Retrieved on December 30, 2004, from http://www.cdc.gov/nchs/fastats/immunize.htm.

National Center for Injury Prevention and Control, CDC. (2002). *Activity report of 2001 CDC's Unintentional Injury Prevention Program.* Atlanta: CDC.

National Institute of Mental Health. (2001). *Numbers count: Mental disorders in America.* NIH Publication: 01-4584. Washington, DC: Author.

Pearson, T.A., Bazzarre, T.L., Daniels, Fair, J. M., Fortmann, S.P., Franklin, B.A., Goldstein, L.B., Hong, Y., Mensah, G.A., Sallis, J.F., Smith, S., Stone, N.J., & Taubert, K.A. (2003). American Heart Association guide for improving cardiovascular health at the community level: A statement for public health practitioners, healthcare providers, and health policy makers from the American Heart Association Expert Panel on Population and Prevention Science. *Circulation, 107*(4), 645–651.

Powell, D.L., & Gilliss, C.L. (2005). Building capacity and competency in conducting health disparities research. *Nursing Outlook, 53*(3), 107–108.

Substance Abuse and Mental Health Services Administration (SAMHSA), USDHHS. (2004). *National survey on drug use and health.* Retrieved on December 30, 2004, from http://www.oas.samhsa.gov.

Thompson, W.W., Shay, D.K., Weintraub, E., Brammer, L., Cox, N., Anderson, L.J., & Fakuda, K. (2003). Mortality associated with influenza and respiratory syncytial virus in the United States. *Journal of the American Medical Association, 289*, 179–186.

U.S. Department of Health, Education and Welfare (USDHEW). (1979). *Healthy people: The surgeon general's report on health promotion and disease prevention.* Washington, DC: Author.

U.S. Department of Health and Human Services (USDHHS). (1980). *Promoting health/preventing disease: Objectives for the nation.* Washington, DC: Author.

U.S. Department of Health and Human Services (USDHHS). (1991). *Healthy People 2000: National health promotion and disease prevention objectives.* Washington, DC: Public Health Service.

U.S. Department of Health and Human Services (USDHHS). (1996). *Physical activity and health: A report of the surgeon general.* Washington, DC: Government Printing Office.

U.S. Department of Health and Human Services (USDHHS). (2000a). *Healthy People 2010, understanding and improving health.* Washington, DC: Author.

U.S. Department of Health and Human Services (USDHHS). (2000b). *Tracking Healthy People 2010.* Washington, DC: Government Printing Office.

World Health Organization (WHO). (1997). *Indicators for policy and decision making in environmental health.* Geneva, Switzerland: Author.

BIBLIOGRAPHY

Ahluwalia, I.B, Mack, K.A, Murphy, W., Mokdad, A.H., & Bales, V.S. (2003). State-specific prevalence of selected chronic disease-related characteristics—Behavioral risk factor surveillance system, 2001. *Morbidity and Mortality Weekly Report, 52*(SS-8), 1–80.

Kanarek, N., & Bialek, R. (2003). Community readiness to meet Healthy People 2010 targets. *Journal of Public Health Management and Practice, 9*(3), 249–254.

RESOURCES

Healthy People 2010

Web: http://www.healthypeople.gov

Healthy People 2010 provides a framework for prevention for the nation. It is a statement of national health objectives designed to identify the most significant preventable threats to health and to establish national goals to reduce these threats. The Healthy People 2010 home page includes all the national health objectives and publications and data that support them.

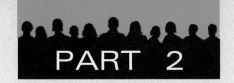

PART 2

HEALTH CARE DELIVERY AND FINANCING

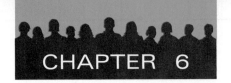

CHAPTER 6

Law, Health Policy, and Public Health Nursing

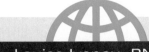

L. Louise Ivanov, RN, DNS

Eileen Kohlendberg, RN, PhD

Chapter Outline

- Politics and Health Policy
- Models of Policy Formulation
  - Kingdon Model
  - Schneider and Ingram Model
  - Cobb and Elder Model
- Political Development of Nursing
  - Legislative Process
  - Regulatory Process
  - Enforcement of Laws and Legislation
- Considerations for Public Health Nurses in Varied Settings
  - Public Health Departments
  - Home Health Care Agencies
  - Occupational Health Settings
  - School Settings
- Public Health Nurses as Advocates and Activists

Learning Objectives

Upon completion of this chapter, the reader will be able to:

1. Analyze the role of politics in health policy.

2. Analyze models of policy formulation that explain the agenda-setting process and the development of policies.

3. Evaluate the political development of nursing in the health policy arena.

4. Describe the legislative process in relation to health care bills.

5. Analyze legislation and laws that impact public health nursing practice.

6. Evaluate the legal responsibilities of a public health nurse in various work settings.

7. Analyze the role of public health nursing in health policy.

The twenty-first century has presented new challenges for public health nurses in the political arena. The increasing cost in health care services and the focus of the current health care system on payment for illness-related health care services rather than prevention or health promotion services brings new challenges for public health nurses. Nursing as an organization is beginning to be recognized as a leader in the policy arena. Understanding the dynamics of politics in the health care arena is critical if public health nurses are to have a voice in health policy. In addition, public health nurses need to understand liability issues related to their practice as they practice independently of a health care provider and in a variety of settings within the community.

POLITICS AND HEALTH POLICY

Politics is defined as the art and science of influencing the allocation of scarce resources (Leavitt, Chaffee, & Vance, 2002). Politics also denotes power. Power and influence are often viewed negatively as legislators on Capitol Hill come to mind. However, power and influence can be used to bring about positive changes in government and policy. Understanding how to use power to influence change given scarce resources in health care is needed as the health care dollar continues to shrink. Nurses are beginning to understand the role of politics in their daily lives and places of work, and their professional organizations, and are beginning to be politically active as client advocates.

The terms "public policy" and "health policy" are frequently misunderstood and used interchangeably. Public policy refers to policies formed by governmental bodies at the local, state, and federal levels that affect individual and institutional behaviors. They also refer to court rulings dealing with institutions or organizations. Examples of public policies are federal Medicare and Medicaid legislation. At the state level an example is state licensure for professional practice.

Health policy is a form of public policy. Health policies are policies that pertain to the health and the pursuit of health. They typically address the delivery of health care services to populations or groups. Health policies can be formulated by governmental bodies but the ideas or issues for the policy can come from individuals, organizations, or institutions (Block, 2004; Porsche, 2004).

The World Health Organization (WHO) coined the term "healthy public policy" in an attempt to show the interchange between public policy and health policy. The term was first described in the Ottawa Charter for Health Promotion as the means for achieving Health for All set by the WHO at the Alma Alta conference in 1977 (Ottawa Charter for Health Promotion, 1986). Healthy public policy is defined as policy whose aim is to create supportive environments that enable people to lead healthy lives (WHO Adelaide Recommendations on Healthy Public Policy, 1986). It is policy that is characterized by a focus on health, equity, and accountability for the health impact of the policy. In order to achieve equity in health and accountability, healthy public policy creates supportive environments that enable people to lead healthy lives by including all sectors of society in decisions related to health policy. Healthy public policy can be considered as public health policy because it supports policies addressing healthy personal behaviors (i.e., ban on smoking in buildings), social conditions (i.e., poverty), and environmental conditions (i.e., safe drinking water), all areas that public health addresses. It focuses on involving grassroots individuals and groups at all levels of policy decision making. It also recognizes the importance of including policy makers at all levels of decision making, encouraging them to make health-related policies a priority on their agenda and accepting responsibility for the health consequences of their decisions.

Public health nurses have historically been involved in polices related to the health of at-risk population groups and communities. In the 1800s, Lillian Wald and Mary Brewster were successful in developing the organizations that later became known as district nursing and visiting nurses (Buhler-Wilkerson, 2001). Their work started as charitable nursing but by the beginning of the twentieth century, financial support for these services was provided by philanthropic charities, religious groups, and local governments. In 1872, the American Public Health Association (APHA) was created as an organization whose purpose was to "advance sanitary science and promote the practical application of public hygiene" through involvement of health care providers at the local, state, and federal levels (Fee, 2003). Since 1872, APHA has been active in promoting public and health policies through various lobbying efforts to ensure healthy public policy for the public.

MODELS OF POLICY FORMULATION

Several models of policy formulation have been posed by researchers, political scientists, and public policy scholars. These models are used to explain the agenda-setting process and the development of policies in the political arena.

Kingdon Model

Kingdon's model answers the questions: How do issues get on the political agenda? and Once the issues are there, how are alternative solutions devised? (Furlong, 2004, p. 41). To answer these questions, Kingdon focuses on participants and the process to explain the development of the policy issue along with alternative arguments (Kingdon, 1995). In this model, participants can be individuals within government or out of government positions. In other words, a participant is any one with an idea for a policy issue. The process refers to the policy process or how policies are developed. Kingdon states that policy development follows three streams: policy streams, problem streams, and political streams. Kingdon further states that these streams are affected by a window of opportunity, which allows one or several of the streams to appear on the political agenda. He distinguishes between two types of political agenda setting that include government-formal agenda setting and nongovernmental-systematic agenda setting. The government-formal agenda includes policy issues that governmental officials are actively working on, and the nongovernmental-systemic agenda is focused on alternative solutions to the policy issue being considered. The problem stream reaches the window of opportunity and is set on the political agenda when there is a crisis such as 9/11, which saw passage of several policies related to terrorism. The policy stream is set on the political agenda when either governmental officials or nongovernmental officials are passionate about a policy and see it through until it is set on the political agenda. An example of a policy stream is the bipartisan involvement in passage of the Medicare Prescription Drug, Improvement and Modernization Act (2003). The last stream—the political stream—set policy issues on the political agenda based on "the public mood, pressure group campaigns, election results, partisan or ideological distributions in Congress, and changes of administration" (Furlong, 2004, p. 43). An example of a political stream is policies put forth during election years for legislators and presidents. In conclusion, Kingdon states that "policy windows open infrequently, and do not stay open long" (Kingdon, 1995, p. 166). For this reason, it is critical that those with policy ideas get involved in the policy process early and see the policy issue through to fruition.

Schneider and Ingram Model

The Schneider and Ingram (1991; 1993a; 1993b) model focuses on the social construction of target populations. It answers the question: Who gets what, when, and how? (Furlong, 2004, p. 55). The assumption in this model is that characteristics of certain populations influence the setting of policy agendas, the content of policies, and successful passage of policies. They state that in order to understand how policies are developed or appear on the political agenda, knowing the perception of elected officials about various target populations (social construction) is critical to successful policy development. In other words, understanding social construction will explain how and why elected officials support some policies over others. In this model, the target populations are classified as the advantaged, the contenders, the dependents, and the deviants. The model proposes that pressures are put on elected officials to work on policies that benefit populations viewed positively, whereas populations viewed negatively receive punitive policies. The populations viewed positively are the advantaged and the dependent; the populations viewed negatively are the contenders and the deviants. Examples of the advantaged populations include businesspeople and scientists, and examples of the dependent populations are children and the disabled. Examples of populations viewed negatively as contenders include the wealthy, unions, and the culturally elite; examples of deviants are criminals and drug addicts. Both groups are considered to be on a continuum of having power that fluctuates.

Cobb and Elder Model

The Cobb and Elder Model contains two main concepts that explain agenda setting in the policy process. They are systemic and formal or institutional agenda (1983). The systemic agenda items refer to policies or issues that are abstract, whereas formal or institutional agenda items are those that are seriously being considered by decision makers. One assumption of the model is that issues or policies receive serious consideration when they are specific and concrete proposals that have gained the interest of a policy maker or elected official. Cobb and Elder have identified six traits that explain why an issue gains the attention of policy makers and moves from the systemic agenda to the formal agenda. These six traits include

1. The concreteness or specificity of the issue

2. The social significance or breadth of the effect on society

3. The temporal relevance or the long-term implications of the issue

4. The complexity or the technical intricacy of the issue

5. The categorical precedence or how similar issues were previously resolved

6. The interval of time or how rapidly an issue develops public attention (Furlong, 2004, p. 56)

An example of the use of this model in agenda setting was with research conducted on the issue of Alzheimer's disease to explain why and how it reached the policy arena (Steckenrider, 1991). It was found that the policy issue of Alzheimer's reached political attention because it met the six traits especially after former President Reagan was diagnosed with Alzheimer's.

The models presented provide public health nurses with knowledge and tools for getting involved in the policy process and putting policy issues on the political agenda. Policy research has been conducted using these models, which further support understanding of the policy process.

POLITICAL DEVELOPMENT OF NURSING

The political development of nurses in the policy arena has passed through several stages (Leavitt, Chaffee, & Vance, 2002). These stages provide a framework for understanding nursing's involvement in the political arena. The first stage is "buy in." In this stage, nurses began to realize that they were excluded from the

policy arena surrounding health care issues, although they knew they had much to offer the public that would improve public health. Seeing that they were left out of the political arena, this stage provided the impetus for nurses to organize into professional groups and organizations. The second stage is "self-interest." At this stage, nurses became involved in policies related to their practice. For example, they became involved in drafting legislation for expanded practice. The third stage is "political sophistication." At this stage, policy makers recognized nursing as a profession with expertise that was useful in the development of health policies. Nurses were appointed to federal panels and campaigned for political positions at the local, state, and federal levels. The last stage is "leadership," where nursing was identified as a political entity with a recognizable agenda that guided the direction of health policy. Nursing as an organization is at the leadership stage and is recognized as a leader in health care and is sought for input on health policies. Within the American Public Health Association, the Public Health Nurse Section provides public health nurses with a forum for leadership and political action in developing and influencing health policy. At the 2004 annual meeting of APHA in Washington, public health nurses joined with other public health professionals at the meeting to lobby their legislators regarding the proposed cuts to Medicaid and organizations such as NIH. Public health nurses remain in the forefront of policy activism as advocates for at-risk populations.

Legislative Process

Understanding the legislative process for developing and passing health care bills is important for public health nurses because they use the power of influence to bring about positive changes in health care delivery. First, public health nurses need to understand that the idea for a policy or bill can come from various sources that include individual experiences with family or friends, the workplace, local agencies, coalitions and committees, and organizations that represent nurses. In other words, it can come from anywhere. One example of an issue that started with a personal experience is the development of Mothers Against Drunk Driving (MADD) and the influence they had on passage of bills related to drinking alcohol and driving. The idea for the bill came from a mother that had lost her child to a drunk driver. She organized a group of women who had similar tragedies. Through contact with their legislators they were successful in passing federal legislation on drunk driving. Once the idea has been formulated, analyzing related issues and any opposing views is important to the success of an idea becoming a policy issue. Also key to the success of an idea is the identification of key contacts such as legislators who are passionate about the policy issue. It is vital that legislators passionate about the idea or policy issue are identified early because only legislators can draft a policy issue into a bill and present it in either the House or the Senate. Once the idea or policy issue has been drafted into a bill, it follows a similar pattern through the legislative process whether it is a state or federal bill.

If a bill is drafted by a representative, it is introduced in the House. If it is drafted by a senator, it is introduced in the Senate. All bills are assigned a number and referred to a committee. It is at the committee level that bills receive the most scrutiny with expert witnesses provided. If the committee approves the bill, the bill is placed on the agenda to be presented in the chamber where it originated in (either the House or the Senate). Amendments to a bill can be made at the committee level or when it is presented in the House or the Senate. Discussion and debate of the bill proceeds with three readings, and three votes are taken after each reading. If the bill passes the first chamber (the chamber it originated in, i.e., either the House or the Senate), it proceeds to the second chamber (i.e., either the Senate or the House) where it is referred to committee. The same process occurs at this point as in the committees of the first chamber. If the bill does not make the second chamber, it is considered defeated. After consideration of the bill in committees of the second chamber, it is presented to the full second chamber. Frequently at this point, amendments are made to the bill. If the original chamber concurs with the recommended amendments, the bill is enrolled and signed into law. If the original chamber does not concur with the amendments, it is referred to a conference committee where representatives from both chambers seek to reconcile the differences. Once there is agreement between members of the two chambers on the conference committee, the bill is brought back to each house and votes are again taken on the recommended text. If either chamber rejects the conference committee's recommendation, the bill is defeated.

After a bill passes both houses it is "enrolled." In other words, a clean copy of the bill that includes all amendments is made. The presiding officers of both the House and the Senate sign the bill after which it is referred to as "ratified" and ready for signature by the president or governor at the state level. After a bill is signed into law, it still must proceed through the authorization-appropriations process prior to having funds allocated. Authorization establishes the purpose and guidelines of the bill plus sets limits on the amount that can be spent. Appropriations enable an agency or program to make spending commitments and gives permission to actually spend the money. Bills that have been enrolled and ratified at times do not make it out of this process. This is especially true of bills that require monies. If the monies are not available, the bill may not pass this process and ends up in appropriations either until monies are available or an amendment is made requesting less money. Unfortunately, many health care bills do not make it out of appropriations.

Regulatory Process

Regulation is a rule that governs individuals or agencies based on legislation that is passed into law. Regulations can be promulgated at the federal, state, or local administrative levels. Regulations are very specific in nature and outline how laws are to be implemented.

The regulatory process begins when legislation is signed into law at the federal (president) or state (governor) levels. A regulatory agency is assigned to develop specific rules and regulations that clarify definitions and outline implementation of the law (i.e., U.S. Environmental Protection Agency at the federal level). Once the assigned regulatory agency has developed a draft of the rules and regulations for the law, it is made public for 30 to 120 days. Individuals and public health nurses can provide input on the proposed draft during this time period. Comments can be made by attending board meetings and public hearings, joining an ad hoc advisory committee, and submitting a petition for rulemaking. An ad hoc advisory committee may be put together by an interested agency that includes advocacy groups and other concerned citizens to assist in drafting or amending the regulations. A petition for rulemaking refers to an agency's request to develop a new regulation or amend an existing regulation. After the 120 days, the regulatory agency reviews the comments made from interested parties and the drafts or proposed amendments. The regulatory agency has the authority to make the suggested changes or to ignore

🌐 RESEARCH APPLICATION

Strengthening the Role of Public Health Nurse Leaders in Policy Development

Study Purpose

To identify and analyze factors that affect the ability of public health nurse leaders to influence public health policy development.

Methods

A qualitative study was conducted using a semistructured interview guide based on Longest's public policy-making framework to collect the data. Subjects recruited were public health nurses in leadership positions employed by a city or county public health agency from rural, suburban, and urban areas. Data collected were arranged into categories or themes to capture a comparison of data within and between the categories.

Findings

The results of this study support Longest's model of public policy-making process. Three main themes emerged which were policy formulation, policy implementation, and policy modification. Concepts related to these themes were political competence, knowledge of the policy-making process, leadership skills, and core education in public health policy

development. These concepts are believed to directly affect the role of the public health nurse.

Implications

Findings point to the need for PHN leaders with policy development skills and staff with academic preparation in policy development. Most PHN leaders received on-the-job training in policy development through a trial-and-error process. Most descriptions for the position of PHN leader do not include policy development activities. A well-defined position description that includes policy development can provide a guide for PHN leaders and educate decision makers to the role of PHN leaders. The need for building a partnership with elected officials was identified as an important means of influencing public health policy development.

Reference

Deschaine, J.E., & Schaffer, M.A. (2003). Strengthening the role of public health nurse leaders in policy development. *Policy, Politics, & Nursing Practice, 4*(4), 266–274.

---

them. Once the regulations are approved by the regulatory agency, they are given to the executive level agency that reviews the final regulations and gives its approval. The regulations are then published and go into effect or are implemented.

Regulatory Processes for Nursing Practice

Under the U.S. Constitution, each state has the authority to regulate health care providers. Regulation of nursing practice is conducted at the state level by Boards of Nurse Examiners (BNE). In all states except for North Carolina, the BNE are appointed by the governor. In North Carolina, they are peer elected. This group develops rules and regulations to clarify the state's Nurse Practice Act and provide day-to-day regulation. Boards of nursing are separate from the BNE and have delegated authority to: "1) self govern; 2) approve or

disapprove schools of nursing; 3) examine and provide licensure to bona fide nursing applicants; 4) issue, review, grant, and inactivate licenses; 5) provide regulation for specialty practice; and 6) discipline nurses who violate aspects of licensure law" (Sportsman, Valadez, & Chater, 2001).

Role of Lobbyists

Lobbyists play a crucial role in the policy process. They represent interest groups that can be grassroots, such as MADD, or professional organizations such as the American Nurses Association (ANA), the American Public Health Association, the American Medical Association (AMA), the pharmaceutical industry, and the insurance industry to name a few. Lobbying is defined as the "art of persuasion—attempting to convince a legislator, a government official, the head of an agency, or a state official to comply with a request" (Wakefield, 2004). Lobbyists on behalf of their interest group attempt to bring pressure on legislators through various means such as attending meetings, getting their interest group involved in mailings, making phone calls, visiting legislators—meeting with legislators even during formal sessions or with the legislators' legislative assistants—and pursuing any other activity that promotes the agenda of their interest group. Lobbyists play a key role in keeping legislators abreast of their constituents' needs and desires. Nurse lobbyists for the ANA have been successful in various ways. One example is the formation of the National Institutes of Nursing Research within the National Institutes of Health (NIH) structure. Lobbyists are paid professionals, but all individuals can "lobby" their issue of interest.

The American Public Health Association's lobbying activities are focused on advocating for federal programs and policies focused on public health issues (Roper & Mays, 2003). APHA represents more than 50,000 members across 50 disciplines. Its mission at the federal level is to develop policy statements on key health issues affecting the public. This is accomplished by testifying in congressional hearings, submitting position papers, and soliciting the membership to contact legislators on key public health issues. APHA is a leading voice in providing accessible and affordable health care for all.

Role of Public Health Nurses

Public health nurses can be involved in stages of the legislative process beyond the idea stage. They can provide testimony while the bill is in committee. If they are not asked to provide testimony, a powerful avenue for influencing policy is with telegrams, phone calls, and letters to legislators and even the president. Legislators are representatives of their constituents and are open to hearing from them.

Public health nurses are an integral part of the health care system. They have a voice in the development and passage of health policy. Involvement in health policy takes time, effort, and commitment. Identifying an issue is the first step. Becoming an expert in the issue means being educated about all positions on the issue. It also means building an infrastructure of support that includes grassroots support as well as the support of at least one legislator. Staying involved in the policy process means visiting, telephoning, and writing letters to legislators who support the policy issue as well

as to those who oppose the issue. A minimum of five letters have been found to be successful in influencing the vote of legislators. When planning a visit to a legislator, it is important to send a brief letter ahead of the meeting listing concisely the issues you want to discuss. During the visit make your expertise known and state that you are available for expert testimony if needed in committees. Make sure your name becomes interchangeable with the issue. Outline a follow-up plan with the legislator visited and follow through on the plan. Involvement in the policy process is time consuming but rewarding.

Public health nurses can also be involved in the regulatory process especially at the local or state levels. They can be influential in writing Nurse Practice Acts and in making changes to them that ensure the public's safety. A number of states are in the process of defining advanced practice for nurses. Masters-prepared public health nurses' voices need to be heard at the state level in discussions regarding the regulation of advanced practice nurses.

Enforcement of Laws and Legislation

Along with understanding how to influence policy to pass health care bills, public health nurses need to understand how laws and legislation are enforced. The judicial system is responsible for enforcement of existing laws or legislation dealing with litigation, antitrust laws, liability (torts, product liability) and class action suits (Guido, 2001). Liability or tort law directly affects public health nurses. Liability or tort is defined as "a civil wrong committed against a person or the person's property" and "acts of omissions which unlawfully violate a person's rights by law and for which the appropriate remedy is a common law action for damages by the injured party" (Guido, 2001, p 78).

Liability and Tort

There are several intentional torts that public health nurses need to be familiar with since they may encounter them in practice. Intentional torts include assault, battery, false imprisonment, conversion of property, and intentional infliction of emotional distress. An example of assault is threatening to give an immunization to a child without the parent's consent, whereas battery is actually carrying out the act and administering the immunization against the parent's will. False imprison-

⊕ RESEARCH APPLICATION

A Phenomenological Approach to Political Competence: Stories of Nurse Activists

Study Purpose

To investigate the political competence skills, perspectives, and values needed for effective political involvement within nursing.

Methods

A phenomenological study was conducted using narratives from six politically expert nurse activists. The six nurses were asked to tell their stories of political activity. The interviews were transcribed, and in-depth analysis of the "conscious lived experience" of policy work and political involvement by the six subjects was conducted.

Findings

Six themes emerged that describe nursing involvement in politics and policy formation. The themes were (1) nursing

expertise as valued currency, (2) opportunities created through networking, (3) powerful persuasion, (4) commitment to collective strength, (5) strategic perspective (a view from stepping back), and (6) perseverance.

Implications

The themes that emerged inform nurses of behaviors that foster the development of greater political efficacy for individual nurses and the nursing profession.

Reference

Warner, J. (2003). A phenomenological approach to political competence: Stories of nurse activists. *Policy, Politics, & Nursing Practice, 4*(2), 135–143.

ment is restraining competent individuals against their will in a bed, chair, or wheelchair. Conversion of property can occur when a public health nurse searches an individual's belongings without permission. Intentional infliction of emotional distress may occur when a public health nurse purposefully inflicts emotional pain through dialogue or exposure to a shocking situation in an attempt to coerce the client into action.

Quasi-intentional torts also are areas of concern for public health nurses. Invasion of privacy and defamation of character are examples of this type of tort. Invasion of privacy occurs when there is public disclosure of private information. Defamation of character occurs when information that adversely affects the reputation of the person is shared with a third party. Slander refers to defamation through oral communication; libel refers to defamation through written communication.

Negligence and Malpractice

Negligence refers to deviation from the standard of care that a reasonably prudent individual would expect in a given situation. Malpractice, on the other hand, deals more with the professional standard of care as defined in state nurse practice acts. Malpractice is dif-

ferentiated from negligence in that the standard of care is used as a measure for the failure of a professional (public health nurse) to "act in accordance with the prevailing professional standards or failure to foresee consequences that a professional person, having the necessary skills and education, should foresee" (Guido, 2001, p. 79). Frequently this action results in unnecessary suffering or death. If the same action is committed by a nonprofessional, typically it is then negligence, whereas if it is committed by a professional, it then is considered as malpractice.

Elements of malpractice or negligence that generally must be proved include

- ⊕ Duty owed the person because of reliance on that relationship;
- ⊕ Breach of duty owed the person such as a deviation from the standard of care;
- ⊕ Foreseeability of events expected to cause specific results;
- ⊕ Causation of injury related to breach of duty;
- ⊕ Injury or harm which may be physical, psychological, emotional, or financial; and
- ⊕ Damages that may be compensated for injury.

Laws Related to Public Health Nurse Practice

Public health nurses need to be informed about the state laws that affect their practice working with various populations. Laws related to the health of children include, but are not limited to, minor consent; statutes of limitation; surgery on minor; immunity; communicable diseases; minor consent for treatment of venereal disease, pregnancy, substance abuse, and emotional disturbances; and child abuse and neglect. Laws related to adults include such areas as informed consent, blood alcohol level, organ procurement, Good Samaritan Laws, client rights, communicable diseases, durable power of attorney, living wills, and gunshot wounds and poisonings. These laws provide public health nurses with specific expectations for treatment and reporting at the state level.

CONSIDERATIONS FOR PUBLIC HEALTH NURSES IN VARIED SETTINGS

Public health nurses practice in a variety of settings that include clinics, schools, and occupational settings. Many work for home health care agencies. The legal responsibilities of public health nurses are different from nurses in other settings such as hospitals. The expansion of their services to include more independent work has increased the likelihood of public health nurses being sued for malpractice and negligence. Understanding the legal responsibilities of public health nurses in each setting is critical to their practice.

Public Health Departments

Public health nurses in health departments work with various populations and are exposed to situations where they are at increased risk of litigation. The populations include pregnant women, high-risk infants, elderly, and those with communicable diseases. Public health nurses work in collaboration with other health care providers at the health department such as social workers. In this role, they may encounter families where physical or sexual abuse occurs, and they may then be called to court as expert witnesses. They may also be in a position of advocating for elderly clients where neglect or financial abuse by family members or friends is occurring. In working with aggregates, public health nurses may find themselves facing both legal and ethical dilemmas as they try to find a compromise position between the demands of the public and those of the administration. Public health nurse administrators at health departments are responsible for staying abreast of laws pertaining to the practice of their public health nurses and ensuring that the nurses are kept up to date with them. These include not only nurse practice acts but also changes in Medicare and Medicaid regulation.

Home Health Care Agencies

Federal legislation such as the Omnibus Reconciliation Act (OBRA) of 1986 expanded participation of home health care agencies in the Medicare program. It provided for strict screening of clients for services, enforced client rights, and required that confidentiality forms be signed and witnessed prior to clients receiving services from home health care agencies. OBRA also provided that clients be fully informed of their care and treatment provided by the agency prior to services and that clients participate in planning their care. In 1991 the Patient Self-Determination Act was passed. This regulation requires agencies receiving federal funds (i.e., Medicare dollars) to ask all clients if a living will or power of attorney designation for health care decisions is in effect. In 1999, legislation was passed specifying that each client at a home health care agency must receive a comprehensive and specific plan of care that identifies his or her home health care, medical, nursing, rehabilitative, and social needs along with discharge planning. A final mandate was that a specific electronic data collection system be used. The system is known as the Outcome and Assessment Information Set (OASIS). The electronic system provides the basis for submission of information directly to the Centers for Medicare & Medicaid Services. Public health nurses in home health care settings need to understand and keep up with federal, state, local, and institutional regulations, as they frequently change.

Occupational Health Settings

Changes in occupational health nursing have increased the potential for liability. Federal and state laws such as workers' compensation laws, mandatory reporting laws, and occupational safety and health laws have made the work of nurses in these settings challenging. Under workman's compensation, injured employees may sue any one except employers. Nurses employed by the company are considered to be employers and are exempt from suit. However, in many cases, nurses working in occupational settings are hired by independent contractors and thus are not protected from law suits. Nurses in occupational health provide a variety of services that include disease prevention and health promotion. For their protection, they need specific guidelines to provide these services without risk of liability. In the absence of a health care provider, nurses frequently make decisions that can be life threatening such as in the case of a serious injury. They may oversee the action of nonhealth care providers who render first aid assistance. If this assistance is not properly provided, the nurse can be held liable.

School Settings

School nurses face many of the same liability issues as do occupational health nurses and state employees because the school district is under state governance in many jurisdictions. Nurses in these settings function as nurses in emergency departments but without the assistance of medical personnel and equipment. Since school nurses in many districts have a number of schools for which they are responsible, nonmedical personnel are trained in first-aid. School nurses can be held liable for actions of these nonmedical personnel if the personnel were trained by them and supervised by them.

Public health nurses working in various settings within the community need to remain current on state and federal laws that pertain to them. Their work involves independent judgment that puts them at higher risk of liability than hospital nurses. Laws pertaining to them are fluid and change frequently. Open communication with clients and families is critical to their practice. A strong and trusting nurse client relationship will reduce the risk of clients bringing lawsuits against nurses.

PUBLIC HEALTH NURSES AS ADVOCATES AND ACTIVISTS

The Scope and Standards of Public Health Nursing (ANA, 2007) outlines ways in which public health nurses function as advocates for populations and are activists in promoting health and preventing disease and disability. Eight tenets of public health nursing have been proposed to promote and protect the health of the population. The second one, "All processes must include partnering with representatives of the people" (ANA, 2007, p. 3), charges public health nurses to work with individuals and key stakeholders to develop and implement health policies that reflect "the perspectives, priorities, and values of the people" (ANA, 2007, p. 3).

Public health nursing competencies developed by the Quad Council of Public Health Nursing Organizations delineate eight domains essential to public health nursing practice (2004). A number of them directly

⊕ PRACTICE APPLICATION

School-Based Health Centers

School-based health centers were first established in the 1960s in Texas and Massachusetts. In 1994, they numbered 600 across 45 states. Recently, there has been political opposition to school-based health centers. The opposition voiced concerns that they would divert the mission of the schools from education and take away financing from educational programs. Another major opposition was to the program's focus on reproductive health issues. In Louisiana, public health nurses along with grassroots initiatives

that included phone calls, faxes, and letters of support to the governor's office resulted in Louisiana becoming one of the first states to provide funding for school-based health centers through general fund allocations.

Author
Broussard, L. (2002). School-based health centers: Politics and community support. *Policy, Politics, and Nursing Practice, 3*(3), 235–239.

⊕ POLICY HIGHLIGHT

Reacting to Budget Cuts

President Bush's 2006 budget proposal cut Medicaid by $45 billion over 10 years. The American Public Health Organization took action to protect the health of the vulnerable population of 53 million people who are covered by the Medicaid program. The association created a Medicaid Advocacy Center online at www.apha.org/legislative/legislative/medicaid.htm; it provides background on this initiative and the status of Medicaid reform. APHA members were active in Emailing and calling their legislators to inform them of their displeasure with this initiative. They were also involved in an advertising campaign voicing opposition to the cuts. An amendment was proposed and passed by the Senate that would prevent $15 billion in Medicaid cuts and create a bipartisan Medicaid commission that would oversee reforms to the Medicaid program. APHA members were once again active in contacting key legislators in support of this amendment. Public health nurses through the Public Health Nursing Section of APHA participated in this health policy initiative.

address advocacy for populations, public health programs, and resources; they also address ways in which public health nurses can be active in the health policy arena. These include working closely with community partners and the legal and political system to ensure policies that protect the health of the population. Public health nurses can use leadership skills to build community partnerships, which are necessary to effect positive change in programs and health policies. Many public health nurses are using these skills to advocate at the global level for policies such as HIV/AIDs. Chinn (2002) captures the essence of nursing as a profession that is unique, is focused on health promotion, and prepares nurses to be global citizen advocates.

In conclusion, public health nurses have traditionally been representatives for the public. Involvement in the policy process is one way to improve the public's health. This chapter has presented public health nurses with ways to get involved in the policy process. Starting small and at the local level may suit some public health nurses. Others may run for local, state, or federal positions. The twenty-first century began with challenges for all health care providers. Public health nurses can be leaders in promoting the health of the public through involvement in the policy process at all levels.

CRITICAL THINKING ACTIVITIES

1. Compare and contrast public health nursing's impact on health policy today with that of the early 1900s.

2. Select a policy issue and use one of the models of policy formulation to evaluate the possibility of its appearing on the agenda for consideration by elected officials in Congress.

3. Provide an example of nursing at the leadership stage of political development. Evaluate the success of nursing in this stage.

4. Select a policy issue and follow it through the process of becoming first a bill and then a law. Analyze the political forces and the role of public health nursing in facilitating or being a barrier to the passage of the bill.

5. Describe a situation from your work setting that was or could have been affected by tort law.

KEY TERMS

formal or institutional agenda items

health policies

healthy public policy

liability or tort

lobbying

malpractice

negligence

politics

public policy

social construction

systemic agenda items

window of opportunity

KEY CONCEPTS

- Understanding politics provides public health nurses with the knowledge and tools to be effective in the political arena.
- To be effective in the policy arena, public health nurses must understand models of policy formulation that explain the agenda-setting process and the development of policies.
- Nursing's political development in the health policy arena has progressed from the buy-in stage to one of leadership where nurses are involved directly in developing health policy.
- Understanding the legislative process for bills becoming laws is vital for public health nurses

who become involved in health policy development.

- Liability, tort law, negligence, and malpractice laws directly affect public health nursing practice in various settings. Public health nurses need to know these laws as they pertain to their practice within the state they practice.
- Public health nurses have historically represented the public in the policy arena.
- Public health nurses are an integral part of the health care system that can have a voice in the development and passage of health policy.

REFERENCES

American Nurses Association (ANA)(2007). *Public Health Nursing: Scope & Standards of Practice*. Washington, DC: Author.

Block, L.E. (2004). Health policy: What it is and how it works. In C. Harrington & C.L. Estes (Eds.), *Health policy: Crisis and Reform in the US health care delivery system* (4th ed.)(pp. 4–14). Sudbury, MA: Jones and Bartlett Publishers.

Broussard, L. (2002). School-based health centers: Politics and community support. P*olicy, Politics, and Nursing Practice, 3*(3), 235–239.

Buhler-Wilkerson, K. (2001). No place like home. *A History of nursing and home care in the United States*. Baltimore: The Johns Hopkins University Press.

Chinn, P. (2002). Living in a post-September 11 world. *Advances in Nursing Science, 24*(4), pp. v.,

Cobb, R.W., & Elder, C.D. (1983). *Participation in America: The dynamics of agenda-building* (2nd ed.). Baltimore: John Hopkins University Press.

Deschaine, J.E., & Schaffer, M.A. (2003). Strengthening the role of public health nurse leaders in policy development. *Policy, Politics, & Nursing Practice, 4*(4), 266–274.

Fee, E. (2003). History and development of public health. In F.D. Scutchfield & C.W. Keck (Eds.), *Principles of public health practice* (pp. 11–30). Clifton Park, NY: Thomson Delmar Learning.

Furlong, E.A. (2004). Agenda setting. In J.A. Milstead (Ed*.), Health policy and politics: A nurse's guide* (pp. 37–66). Boston: Jones and Bartlett Publishers.

Guido, G.W. (2001). *Legal and ethical issues in nursing* (3rd ed.). Upper Saddle River, NJ: Prentice Hall.

Kingdon, J. W. (1995). *Agendas, alternatives, and public policies.* New York: Harper Collins College Publishers.

Leavitt, J.K., Chaffee, M.W., & Vance, C. (2002). Learning the ropes of policy and politics. In D.J. Mason, J. K. Leavitt, & M.W. Chaffee (Eds.), *Policy and politics in nursing and health care.* St. Louis: Saunders.

Ottawa Charter for Health Promotion. (1986). Ottawa Charter for Health Promotion First International Conference on Health Promotion Ottawa, 21 November 1986—HO/HPR/HEP/95.1. Retrieved February 24, 2006, from http://www.who.int/en/.

Porsche, J.D. (2004). Public health policy and politics. In J.D. Porsche (Ed.), *Public and community health nursing practice: A population based approach*. Thousand Oaks, CA: Sage Publications Inc.

Quad Council of Public Health Nursing Organizations. (2004). Public health nursing competencies. *Public Health Nursing, 21*(5), 443–452.

Roper, W.L., & Mays, G.P. (2003). The federal contribution to public health. In F.D. Scutchfield & C.W. Keck (Eds.), *Principles of public health practice*. Clifton Park, NY: Thomson Delmar Learning.

Schneider, A., & Ingram, H. (1991). The social construction of target populations: Implications for citizenship and democracy. Paper presented at the annual meeting of the American Political Science Association in Washington, DC.

Schneider, A.L., & Ingram, H. (1993a). How the social construction of target populations contributes to problems in policy design. *Policy Currents 3*(1), 1–4.

Schneider, A.L., & Ingram, H. (1993b). Social construction of target populations: Implications for politics and policy. *American Political Science Review 87*(2), 334–347.

Sportsman, S., Valadez, A., & Chater, S. (2001). The legislative process. In M.E. O'Keefe (Ed.), *Nursing practice and the law* (p. 290). Philadelphia: F.A. Davis Company.

Steckenrider, J.S. (1991). *Agenda building on health issues: A focus on Alzheimer's disease*. Paper presented at the annual meeting of the American Political Science Association in Washington, DC.

Wakefield, M. (2004). Government response: Legislation. In J.A. Milstead (Ed.), *Health policy and politics: A nurses guide*. Sudbury, MA: Jones and Bartlett Publishers.

Warner, J.R. (2003). A phenomenological approach to political competence: Stories of nurse activists. *Policy, Politics, and Nursing Practice 4*(2), 135–143.

WHO Adelaide Recommendations on Healthy Public Policy. (1986). Adelaide Recommendations on Healthy Public Policy Second International Conference on Health Promotion, Adelaide, South Australia, 5–9 April 1998. Retrieved February 24, 2006, from http://www.who.int/health promotion/conferences/previous/adelaide/en/print.html.

BIBLIOGRAPHY

American Nurses Association (ANA). (1998). *Standards of clinical nursing practice* (2nd ed.). Washington DC: American Nurses Association.

American Nurses Association commends Reps. Capps, Whitfield for forming congressional nursing caucus (2003). Retrieved from http://www.nursingworld.org.G:release03/caucus_rel_319.wpd.

Cohen, S., & Milone-Nuzzo, P. (2001). Advancing health policy in nursing education through service learning. *Advances in Nursing Science, 23*(3), 28–40.

Dodd, C.J. (1997). Can meaningful health policy be developed in a political system? In C. Harrington & C. L. Estes (Eds.), *Health policy and nursing*. (pp. 415–428). Sudbury, MA: Jones and Bartlett Publishers.

Gebbie, K.M., Wakefield, M., & Kerfoot, K. (2000). Nursing and health policy. *Journal of Nursing Scholarship, 32*(3), 307–315.

Home Health Care Statistics. (2004). Statistics. Available: http://www.cdc.gov/nchs/fastats/homehealthcare.htm.

Mills, M.E. (2001). Computer-based health care data and the Health Insurance Portability and Accountability Act: Implications for informatics. *Policy, Politics, and Nursing Practice, 2*(3), 33–38.

Trotter Betts, V., & Leavitt, J.K. (2001). Nurses and political action. In K. Chitty (Ed.), *Professional nursing: Concepts and challenges* (3rd ed.). Philadelphia: W.N. Saunders.

Warner, J.R. (2003). A phenomenological approach to political competence: Stories of nurse activists. *Policy, Politics, and Nursing Practice 4*(2), 135–143.

RESOURCES

American Association of Colleges of Nursing (AACN)

One Dupont Circle NW, Suite 530
Washington, D.C. 20036
202-463-6930
FAX: 202-463-1315
Web: http://www.aacn.nche.edu

AACN is the national voice for America's baccalaureate- and higher-degree nursing education programs. AACN's educational, research, governmental advocacy, data collection, publications, and other programs work to establish quality standards for bachelor's- and graduate-degree nursing education, assist deans and directors to implement those standards, influence the nursing profession to improve health care, and promote public support of baccalaureate and graduate education, research, and practice in nursing—the nation's largest health care profession. The Web site contains government affairs link, bulletins, issue summaries, and briefings of interest to nurses.

American Health Line

The Advisory Board Company
2445 M Street NW
Washington, D.C. 20037
1-800-717-3245
FAX: 202-266-5700
Web: http://www.americanhealthline.com

American Health Line provides a concise, accurate and non-partisan synthesis of the days most important and compelling health care news, all delivered via Email by 11:30 A.M. ET. In addition to affording nurses access to the same information that the nation's health care policy makers on Capitol Hill say they can't do their jobs without, a subscription to American Health Line empowers professionals with an array of resources and expertise.

American Nurses Association (ANA)

8515 Georgia Avenue, Suite 400
Silver Spring, Maryland 20910
1-800-274-4ANA
Web: http://www.nursingworld.org

The ANA was started as the Association of Nursing Alumnae. It later became the American Nurses Association's Congress on Nursing Practice and Economics representing all nurses. The Web site provides various information on ANA activities and access to online nursing journals.

American Public Health Association (APHA)

800 "I" Street NW
Washington, D.C. 20001-3710
202-777-APHA (2752)
FAX: 202-777-2534
Email: comments@APHA.org
Web: http://www.apha.org

APHA is a nonprofit association of public health professionals from over 50 public health occupations working to improve the public's health and to achieve equity in health status for all. The organization strives to influence policy and set priorities in public health to help prevent disease and promote health. The organization also strives to promote the scientific and professional foundation of public health practice and policy, advocate the conditions for a healthy global society, emphasize prevention, and enhance the ability of members to promote and protect environmental and community health.

Bureau of National Affairs (BNA)

1231 25th Street NW
Washington, D.C. 20037
1-800-372-1033
FAX: 1-800-253-0332
Email: customercare@bna.com

Web: http://www.bna.com

BNA is a leading publisher of information and analysis products for professionals in law, tax, business, and government. The company's print and electronic products address the full range of legal, legislative, regulatory, and economic developments affecting business. Today, BNA employees in the nation's capital and around the world produce more than 350 news and information services known and valued for their unbiased reporting, including the highly respected Daily Labor Report and Daily Tax Report.

Capitol Hearings

Web: http://www.capitolhearings.org

This Web site is C-SPAN's joint production with Congressional Quarterly to provide a preview story and a daily congressional update of hearings from Capitol Hill that have been presented on C-SPAN.

Congressional Digest Corporation

4416 East West Highway, Suite 400
Bethesda, Maryland 20814-4568
1-800-637-9915
FAX: 301-634-3189
Email: info@congressionaldigest.com
Web: http://www.congressionaldigest.com

The Web site offers information on political issues from both the pro and con sides as discussed by elected officials.

Congressional E-Mail Directory

Web: http://www.webslingerz.com/jhoffman/congress-email .html

An Email directory for elected officials in Congress.

Congressional Quarterly Legislative Impact, Inc.

1255 22nd Street NW
Washington, D.C. 20037
202-419-8500; 1-800-432-2250
Web: http://www.cq.com

CQ Legislative Impact provides information on pending bills in Congress and current law, so that one can quickly decipher how legislation before Congress would affect existing public law and specific U.S. Code sections.

Constitution Facts

Oak Hill Publishing Company
Box 6473
Naperville, Illinois 60567
1-800-887-6661
FAX 630-904-2737
Web: http://www.constitutionfacts.com

In the early 1990s the first edition of "The U.S. Constitution & Fascinating Facts About It" was published as a resource for law students. Since then, the book has been used by civic organizations, school teachers and police officers, major retailers, and the U.S. armed forces. The Web site was launched in 1996 as a companion to the book to help educate those who want to learn about the Constitution.

Democratic National Committee

430 S. Capitol Street SE
Washington, D.C. 20003
Web: http://www.democrats.org
This is the official Web site for the Democratic National Committee.

Find Law

Web: http://www.findlaw.com
This is an official site for finding lawyers and legal resources.

General Accounting Office (GAO)

441 G Street NW
Washington, D.C. 20548
202-512-3000
Email: contact@gao.gov
Web: http://www.gao.gov
The U.S. Government Accountability Office (GAO) is an independent, nonpartisan agency that works for Congress. GAO is often called the "congressional watchdog" because it investigates how the federal government spends taxpayer dollars. GAO gathers information to help Congress determine how well executive branch agencies are doing their jobs. GAO's work routinely answers such basic questions as whether government programs are meeting their objectives or providing good service to the public. Ultimately, GAO ensures that government is accountable to the American people. To that end, GAO provides senators and representatives with the best information available—information that is accurate, timely, and balanced—to help them arrive at informed policy decisions.

National Center for Policy Analysis (NCPA)

601 Pennsylvania Avenue NW, Suite 900 South Building
Washington, D.C. 20004
202-220-3082
FAX: 202-220-3096
Email: govrel@ncpa.org
Web: http://www.ncpa.org
NCPA is a nonprofit, nonpartisan public policy research organization, established in 1983. The NCPA's goal is to develop and promote private alternatives to government regulation and control, solving problems by relying on the strength of the competitive, entrepreneurial private sector. Topics include reforms in health care, taxes, Social Security, welfare, criminal justice, education, and environmental regulation.

National Health Policy Forum (NHPF)

2131 K Street NW, Suite 500
Washington, D.C. 20037
202-872-1390
FAX: 202-862-9837
Email: nhpf@gwu.edu
Web: http://www.nhpf.org
NHPF was created in 1971 by senior-level congressional staff and executive agency decision makers to address their information needs and provide a safe harbor for open and frank conversations. The NHPF seeks to inform the public policy process by helping participants—federal health policy makers in the legislative and executive branches and in congressional support agencies—engage in rigorous, constructive, and respectful dialogue. NHPF is a nonpartisan organization that does not advocate particular policy positions. It provides a forum covering a broad range of health policy topics that allows for honest exchange of ideas and viewpoints.

National Republican Congressional Committee (NRCC)

320 First Street S
Washington, D.C. 20003
202-479-7000
Web: http://www.nrcc.org
This is the official Web site for the Republican Party. The NRCC's origins date back to 1866, when the Republican caucuses of the House and Senate formed a "Congressional Committee." Today, the NRCC is organized under Section 527 of the Internal Revenue Code. It supports the election of Republicans to the House through direct financial contributions to candidates and Republican Party organizations; provides technical and research assistance to Republican candidates and Party organizations; encourages voter registration, education, and turnout programs; and engages in other party-building activities.

Roll Call Newspaper Online

50F Street NW, Suite 700
Washington, D.C. 20001-1572
202-824-6800
FAX: 202-824-0475
Web: http://www.rollcall.com
This is the online version of the official newspaper of Capitol Hill. The newspaper provides information, news, and analysis of Capitol Hill proceedings.

Senate Home Page

For correspondence to U.S. Senators:
Office of Senator (Name)
United States Senate
Washington, D.C. 20510
For correspondence to Senate Committees:
(Name of Committee)
United States Senate
Washington, D.C. 20510
202-224-3121.
Web: http://www.senate.gov
This is the official Web site for the U.S. Senate. It provides
information on how to contact a senator and bills in the
Senate.

SpeakOut.com

20720 Beallsville Road
Dickerson, MD 20842
Web: http://www.speakout.com
The Web site provides a forum for political conversations
and activity.

The Hill

1625 K Street, NW Suite 900
Washington, D.C. 20006
202-628-8500
FAX: 202-628-8503
Web: http://www.hillnews.com
This Web site is an online newspaper for and about the U.S.
Congress.

The Library of Congress

Washington, D.C. 20540
202-707-5000
Web: http://www.lcweb.loc.gov
The Library of Congress is the nation's oldest federal cultural
institution and serves as the research arm of Congress. It
is also the largest library in the world, with more than 130
million items on approximately 530 miles of bookshelves.
Its mission is to make its resources available and useful to
the Congress and the American people and to sustain and
preserve a universal collection of knowledge and creativity
for future generations.

The Library of Congress THOMAS

Web: http://thomas.loc.gov
This Web site was launched in January of 1995. The leadership of the 104th Congress directed the Library of Congress to make federal legislative information freely available to the public. The Web site provides full text of laws
and bills in Congress from 1973 to currently.

Urban Institute

2100 M Street NW
Washington, D.C. 20037
202-833-7200
Web: http://www.urban.org
A nonpartisan organization focused on social policy research.
Its mission is to promote sound social policy and public
debate on national priorities. The Urban Institute gathers
and analyzes data, conducts policy research, evaluates
programs and services, and educates Americans on critical
issues and trends to improve social, civic, and economic
wellbeing. Urban Institute works in all 50 states and
abroad in over 28 countries, sharing research findings
with policy makers, program administrators, business,
academics, and the public online and through reports and
scholarly books.

U.S. Government Printing Office (GPO)

732 North Capitol Street NW
Washington, D.C. 20401
202-512-0000
Email: jbradley@gpo.gov
Web: http://www.access.gpo.gov
The U.S. Government Printing Office provides free electronic
access to important information products such as federal
documents produced by the federal government. The information provided on this site is the official, published version and the information retrieved from GPO Access can
be used without restriction, unless specifically noted. This
free service is funded by the Federal Depository Library
Program and has grown out of Public Law 103-40, known
as the Government Printing Office Electronic Information
Enhancement Act of 1993.

U.S. House of Representatives Home Page

Washington, D.C. 20515
202-224-3121(202) 225-1904
Web: http://www.house.gov
This is the official Web site of the U.S. House of
Representatives.

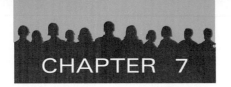

CHAPTER 7

Health Care Organization and Financing

L. Louise Ivanov, RN, DNS

Chapter Outline

- Historical Development of the Organization of Health Care
- Health Care Financing
  Insurance-Based Care
  Noninsurance-Based Models
- Challenges for Public Health Nurses

Learning Objectives

Upon completion of this chapter, the reader will be able to:

1. Analyze the ways in which social and health belief forces shape the U.S. health care system today.
2. Distinguish the differences and similarities between insurance-based care and managed care from the perspectives of the health care provider and health care consumer.
3. Distinguish eligibility and coverage under Part A, B, and D of the Medicare plan.
4. Analyze eligibility and coverage of the Medicaid plan for the elderly and the younger population.
5. Analyze Managed Competition and Universal Coverage in relation to access to health care for populations and the cost of health care.

arious external forces that include social values and health beliefs of the population, political climate, economic conditions, physical environment, and biomedical technological development define the characteristics of a health care system. Historically, in the United States there has been a distrust of "big government" and a tendency to avoid centralized control of many aspects of our lives, including health care. This has led to a decentralized form of health care delivery that is fragmented in its provision of health care to populations while at the same time providing high-quality technological care. The social values we hold are independence and fairness that at times conflict and have left populations without access to health care. Although the United States is the wealthiest country among developed countries, it is also the only one that has 45 million people without access to health care.

Public health nurses must understand the organization and financing of the U.S. health care system in order to be effective client advocates. In their work settings, they are frequently in a position to assist clients and their families maneuver through the myriad of forms that need to be filed to apply for private and public insurance coverage. This is especially true with the implementation of Medicare Part D, the new prescription drug option for Medicare recipients that many elderly found difficult to understand. In addition, public health nurses working as advanced practice nurses in some settings and states can be reimbursed for their services. Understanding the complexities of the U.S. health care system and its financing has become a required skill for public health nurses.

HISTORICAL DEVELOPMENT OF THE ORGANIZATION OF HEALTH CARE

National health insurance, also known as social insurance or social medicine, started in Germany in 1833 (Starr, 1982). At that time, the United States was decentralized, leaving health-related decisions to private and voluntary actions at the state and local levels. Lacking a national health insurance, churches were one of the local groups that became active in caring for the health needs of their congregations. It was not until 1921 that Congress passed the Shepherd-Towner Act, the first movement toward a semblance of a national health insurance program. This act gave matching funds to states that would provide prenatal care and health care to children. Lillian Wald was a strong advocate of this legislation, which provided the impetus for her establishing the Henry Street Settlement. The settlement provided prenatal care and care to children by public health nurses and was successful in decreasing the maternal and infant mortality rates in New York City. The American Medical Society in 1927 was successful in having the legislation rescinded because they considered the Sheppard-Towner Act as federal government interference in matters that should be dealt with at the local level.

As the cost of health care continued to increase, the Committee on Costs of Medical Care (CCMC) became concerned about the cost and distribution of health care. They conducted a study investigating the organization of the U.S. health care system (Starr, 1982). The report from this study described a health care system that was poorly organized with maldistributed services and no overall coordination of services. Their remedy for the situation was to endorse group practice and group payment for medical care. They strongly opposed any form of national health insurance.

It was not until 1965 and President Roosevelt's Great Society initiatives that a form of national insurance was started. He was successful in passing legislation that started the Medicare and Medicaid programs providing health care for the neediest and most vulnerable populations. One result of this legislation was the rapid growth of nursing homes in the 1960s, where more than half of their revenues came from state and federal Medicare and Medicaid dollars. This made states and the federal government accountable for the care provided at nursing homes. As the U.S. population began to live longer and more elderly were living in nursing homes, states attempted to find ways to control the growing costs of nursing homes for federal and state governments. In 1987, legislation was passed in an attempt to curb unnecessary use of nursing homes by requiring that all nursing home residents have monthly assessments and care plans that would ensure maximal health and functional status as a mechanism for determining discharge of residents (Underlich, Sloan, & Davis, 1996). However, Underlich, Sloan, and Davis (1996) note that monthly assessments and care plans were not enough to cut costs of nursing homes and to ensure quality care without ensuring adequate nursing staff. The 1960s also experienced a growth in home health care services, which were an offshoot of

⊕ RESEARCH APPLICATION

Intermittent Lack of Health Insurance Coverage and Use of Preventive Services

Study Purpose

To examine the association between intermittent lack of health insurance coverage and the use of preventive health services.

Methods

Secondary data analysis was conducted using the Health and Retirement Study for the years 1992, 1994, and 1996. The subject pool was 8309 respondents, 51 to 61 years of age.

Findings

Intermittent lack of health insurance coverage was found to be related to less use of preventive health services.

Implications

Intermittent health insurance coverage does not ensure access to needed health care services.

Reference

Sudano, J., & Baker, D. (2003). Intermittent lack of health insurance coverage and use of preventive services. *American Journal of Public Health, 98*(1), 130–137.

---

visiting nurse associations that started in the 1950s. The focus of home health care services was to provide a broad range of services by public health nurses to help maintain the public's wellness. Once diagnosis-related groups (DRGs) in the 1980s became the norm for determining length of stay in hospitals, there was a rapid growth in home health care agencies, especially for profit agencies as hospitals began to shorten the length of stay for clients.

In the 1970s, it became evident that the Medicare and Medicaid programs started in the 1960s to protect vulnerable populations were no longer ensuring a safety net for them. As a result, local communities started neighborhood health centers in an attempt to provide comprehensive health services for vulnerable populations. Migrant health centers and free health clinics were started at this time to provide health care services. However, with the high cost of health care services, many of these centers closed.

Currently, the focus of providing health care for vulnerable populations is on local communities and state governments. However, with the growing population of uninsured and the decrease in resources at the local and state levels, those in need of a safety net are left to care for themselves.

HEALTH CARE FINANCING

The main health care financing mechanisms in the U.S. health care system will be discussed in this chapter. Descriptions of private insurance such as insurance-based care and managed care will be discussed along with public insurance such as Medicaid, Medicare, and Tri Care, the health care plan for the military and their families. The discussion will also present other forms of health care financing that include managed competition and universal coverage. As client advocates, public health nurses need to understand health care financing in order to assist their clients in making health care payment decisions.

Insurance-Based Care

Insurance coverage can be classified as public and private. **Public insurance** refers to plans that are subsidized by the federal and state governments (i.e., Medicare, Medicaid, Tri Care) and will be discussed later. **Private insurance** refers to those plans purchased by employers for employees or purchased directly by individuals from insurance carriers. The definition of insurance includes the notion of risk that has been defined as "the possibility of an adverse deviation from a desired out-come that is expected or hoped for" (Whitted, 2002, p. 140). Individuals purchase health insurance to provide monies that can be used in the event of an unexpected and undesired health outcome.

Private Insurance

The Massachusetts Health Insurance Company was the first private insurance plan in the United States and was issued as a medical policy in 1847 (Finkelman, 2001). This marked the start of health insurance in the United States. The number of health insurance companies grew to 60 in the 1860s. The first company to provide benefits to employees unable to work due to illness or injury was Montgomery Ward in 1911. Other companies followed suit with employers offering health insurance instead of wage increases. In the 1920s, the health insurance industry grew substantially, marking the start of the Blue Cross/Blue Shield plans. The impetus for employers to purchase health insurance plans was the federal and state tax exemption totaling the amount paid for the plans. By the 1940s, some form of medical insurance was provided to 9 percent of the U.S. population (Whitted, 2002). In 1995, 31 percent of the population had medical insurance through employers.

A term frequently used to refer to health insurance companies is third party payer. This refers to the company or organization, either private or public, that pays or underwrites health care coverage for a business or individual. The first party is the insured individual, and the second party is the business or company the insured works for. Most health insurance companies are commercial or for-profit. The larger percentage of the U.S. population who has insurance is covered through group coverage as a benefit at their place of employment.

Reimbursement for services has changed dramatically over the past decades. Prior to the 1980s, reimbursement for services was based on a retrospective payment system. This refers to full payment to providers based on the actual care and services provided with cost of services set after they are delivered. The cost of services is based on charges set by an organization that represents cost per unit of service, treatment, or care. The cost of services may include agreed upon allowable costs such as depreciation of equipment and administrative costs. As the payment costs to health insurance companies (third party payers) increased, these com-

panies began to limit the services reimbursed. Health care costs continued to spiral upward forcing a change in reimbursement of health care services. In 1982 with passage of the Tax Equity and Fiscal Responsibility Act (TEFRA), the government began to reimburse for services under their Medicare and Medicaid plans based on a prospective payment system. Under this system, charges are based on prices predetermined by a third party payer, such as the government, rather than the provider as under the retrospective payment system. For hospital care, the predetermined prices are based on a statistical system known as diagnosis-related. The statistical system classifies medical diagnoses into groups that are then used to identify payment rates for the entire episode of care. In other words, the third party reimburses based on predictions or averages of the cost to deliver a service. For reimbursement under a prospective payment system, insurance companies frequently require preapprovals before clients can receive certain services such as hospitalization. Currently, a prospective payment system is used by all health insurance companies to reimburse for health care services. The following discussion is in reference to the prospective payment system.

A charge billed for services received is referred to as fee-for-service. The provider determines the fee or charge, and the insured pays through a third party payer (insurance company). The charge is paid in three ways: premiums, deductibles, and copayments. Premiums are the calculated amount that the insured pays per month for the health insurance plan. The third party payer determines the charge for the premium. Deductibles are the amount the insured must pay before the third party payer will pay for health care services. Copayment, also known as coinsurance, is the fixed payment that the insured must pay for each health care provider visit, procedure, treatment, or prescription. It is a copayment because of payment sharing between the third party payer and the insured.

The cost of health insurance plans today, for both employers and employees, has continued to increase in response to the increased cost in health care. Employees are paying higher premiums, deductibles, and copayments for the same services they received at a lower cost only a few years ago. As a result, employees, especially those with lower wages, have refused health coverage. Premiums increased 90 percent between the years of 1987 and 1997, and the number of employees refusing coverage doubled to six million (Cooper & Schone,

1997). The increases in premiums continued to outpace inflation increasing annually at rates at or above 20 percent (Enthoven, 2003). Others without health insurance include those working for small companies that do not offer insurance, the self-employed, and part-time and seasonal workers. This group of employees is known as the **working poor** and the **uninsured** and is continually increasing. In 2001, about 40 million people were uninsured; the number jumped to 43.6 million in 2002 and 45 million in 2003 (Employee Benefits Research Institute, 2002a; CNN Money, 2004). Reasons for the continued increase in the uninsured is the weak economy and the rising cost of providing health benefits for the working population (Employees Benefits Research Institute, 2004).

Medical Savings Accounts

Medical savings accounts (MSAs) are considered to be reforms in insurance plans. They are viewed as a positive change for the consumer as they shift in the burden of health care decision making to the consumer. MSAs are tax-exempt accounts available to individuals who have insurance plans that allow them to set aside monies to be used to cover costs not covered under insurance plans. These may include orthodontic treatment, vision treatments, copayments, and the like. The consumer is given a limit on the amount that can be contributed to an MSA. The contribution is made tax-free by the employer based on the agreed upon amount with the consumer. Any interest earned is tax-free. Unused MSA money either can be held in the account or must be used within the year based on the insurance company's stipulations. MSAs provide health care consumers with the opportunity to be more involved in health care decision making and responsible for payment of the care provided. It forces health care consumers to be knowledgeable about the care they are seeking and gives them the opportunity to "shop around" for the best care at the lowest cost since they have access to monies in MSAs accounts. For this reason, many consider MSAs as a way to control health care costs.

Managed Care Plans

Managed care is a form of private insurance. The rise in health care costs has contributed to changes in health care within the last few decades. In 2000, national health expenditure was $1.3 trillion and is projected to double by 2011 to $2.8 trillion (Chase et al., 2002).

The percentage of the gross domestic product (GDP) in 2000 spent on health care was 13.2 percent and is projected to increase to 17.0 by 2011. Private sector spending on health care mirrors the increases at the national level. For example, in 1988 total consumer payments on health care per capita were $294, in 2000 it was $638, and it is projected to double to $1,362 in 2011 (Hefler et al., 2002). Third party payments per capita also increased from $263 in 1980 to $1,394 in 2000. Projections for out-of-pocket payments on health care for 2011 are $1,295 and for third party payments, $2,763. The acceleration in third party payments and out-of-pocket spending is attributed to higher medical costs that are driven by inflation of medical prices and the increase in use of health care services (Chase et al., 2002). Inflation of medical prices is a result of wage inflation and consumer's demand for broader coverage of health care services. Managed care was considered to be one way to provide equitable distribution of health care while reigning in health care cost. It is not a new concept but rather one first introduced in the 1930s (Heinrich & Thompson, 2002). However, it was not broadly used during that time period because it lacked the support of the American Medical Association, which feared losing independent practice, relinquishing the right to independently set fees, and being forced to work for large corporations. In the 1960s, as health care costs began to increase, there was renewed interest in managed care. In 1973 the Health Maintenance Organization Act was passed in an attempt to control costs in the federal Medicare program. This was the forerunner of managed care plans, as they exist today.

Managed care has been defined in numerous ways. One definition is an organized effort by health insurance plans and providers to use financial incentives and organizational arrangements to alter provider and patient behavior so that health care services are delivered and utilized in a more efficient and lower cost manner (Fox, 1997). The main objective of managed care is cost containment through rationing of health services, increasing administrative and clinical efficiency, and reducing duplication and unnecessary services (Torrens & Williams, 2002). To accomplish this objective, managed care plans combine aspects of health insurance plans, contract practice, and prepaid group practice. The main players in managed care are the purchasers of managed care plans (employers, the federal government), health insurance plans, health care providers, and consumers of health care.

The managed care system is put into motion when the purchasers decide on the health plan, the extent of coverage, and the amount they will pay for the plan. Included in this decision is the range of choice in providers, services, and the cost to the beneficiary of the health plan. Health care providers play an important role in managed care plans as "gatekeepers" also known as primary care providers (PCP). A PCP is considered to be responsible for providing primary care to the client and for referrals to specialists. Defining the PCP as a gatekeeper includes the notion that they will control the client's use of expensive services, such as seeing specialists, or undergoing unnecessary expensive tests, and in this way control health care cost. Under managed care, consumers have less choice in health care services and providers. This is considered to be one important way to control cost.

There are two main types of managed care health plans. They are preferred provider organizations (PPOs) and HMOs. A **PPO** is a form of a fee-for-service health plan. The consumer chooses health care providers from a select group. When the health care provider from the select group is utilized, the health care consumer pays less for the health care received. The health plan has typically negotiated a discounted rate for the health care provider's services and the health care provider is guaranteed seeing more health care consumers since they are on a "preferred provider" list. In this way, there is cost savings for health care consumers, providers, and health insurance plans. If the health care consumer visits a health care provider not in the select group, they typically will have to pay more for the services. However, under PPOs health care consumers retain their ability to choose a health care provider.

A Health Maintenance Organization (HMO) differs from a PPO in several ways. First, the **HMO** has a contract with a group of physicians, both PCPs and specialists, who have agreed to be responsible for the care provided to enrolled health care consumers. Once a consumer has agreed to receive care with an HMO, they no longer have the option to choose a health care provider outside of the HMO. Health care providers under HMOs are paid a fixed fee per client (known as per capita form of reimbursement). Second, the linkages among health care providers, health plans, and health care consumers are tighter with less flexibility than in PPOs. Health plans benefit and are able to control costs because of the agreed upon per capita form of reimbursement regardless of the amount of care the

health care provider gives the consumer. Health care providers benefit because they know they will receive a certain amount of revenue regardless of the number of consumers they see. The benefit to the health care consumer is that once the premium is paid, the copayment for services is low.

Enrollment in managed care plans had grown to 86 percent of the population in 1998 (Gentry, 2001). However, the concept of managed care has not provided the control in health care costs that was envisioned. In addition, there has been a backlash to managed care especially by health care consumers and health care providers. Questions regarding quality of care, control of health care decisions by health insurance plans, and inability to sue an HMO are only a few of those raised. Currently, health care consumers are at the mercy of the managed care plans they are affiliated with. At times the plans are considered to be cumbersome and not well understood. Denial of services has led to unanticipated health outcomes. Health care providers feel that their ability to make health care decisions and provide the care they believe the consumer deserves is controlled by health plans run by professionals not in the health field. A struggle has emerged among purchasers of health plans, health care consumers, and health care providers that will need to be addressed if managed care is to remain a viable alternative in controlling health care costs.

Public Insurance

Medicaid, Medicare, and Tri Care are examples of public insurance health plans that are funded by the federal and state governments. In 1965, Congress passed amendments to the Social Security Act that created the Medicaid and Medicare programs. The programs are separate but related. **Medicare**, also known as Title XVIII, is a federal program for the elderly. **Medicaid**, also known as Title XIX, is a program jointly funded by federal and state governments.

Medicaid

Eligibility for Medicaid is determined by income and resources and is for all ages. When compared with other Western industrialized countries, 1965 is late for the establishment of a public insurance program. For example, Great Britain had one of the earliest publicly funded health programs starting in the 1800s. In the United States, prior to 1965, only middle-class working

Well-Child Clinic

Public health nurses working in various settings can use their assessment skills to identify those who are less likely to access needed health care services and work with the community and legislators to improve services to this population. In Lafayette, Indiana, a group of public health nurses assessed the need for a well-child clinic for low-income and uninsured families. They applied for a state block grant to fund a well-child clinic. The clinic was known as the Community Health Clinic. This initiative has grown to include preventive and basic health care services for low-income and uninsured persons of all ages. Most recently, they have added Hispanic translators to work with the growing Hispanic population that is now accessing the Community Health Clinic for their health care needs.

families had private insurance as the source of payment for health care. The unemployed, elderly, and poor relied on their own resources or charity, or did not get health care.

Under the initial Medicaid program, eligibility included persons receiving Aid to Families with Dependent Children (AFDC), blind and totally disabled persons who received Supplemental Security Income (SSI), pregnant women, children born after 1983 in families with incomes at or below the federal poverty line, and elderly who were considered to be "medically needy." Today, in order for states to receive the federal matching monies, states must provide a minimum set of benefits that includes hospitalization, physician visits, prenatal care, some preventive services such as dental, certain exams such as x-ray and laboratory tests, nursing home, and home health care. Since the Medicaid program is a state and federal initiative, states can decide on the breadth of benefits offered. This resulted in differences in coverage across states.

Major changes in Medicaid occurred in 1996 with passage of the Personal Responsibility and Work Opportunities Act. AFDC as a cash program was replaced with a temporary cash program called Temporary Assistance to Needy Families (TANF), and participation in this program was no longer one of the criteria for Medicaid eligibility. States were required to redefine their eligibility criteria, especially the poverty level that would qualify participants. Eligibility includes low-income families with children (below federal poverty level), SSI recipients, pregnant women whose family income is slightly above the federal poverty level (133 percent), recipients of adoption assistance and foster care, infants up to 1 year of age, qualifying elderly, and blind and disabled adults (U.S. Department of Health and Human Services, 2006). Funding for Medicaid continued as a joint federal and state initiative with federal funds coming from a general fund allocation and states matching the funds with state revenue budget allocations. States retained their ability to establish eligibility criteria and scope of services covered, set the payment rate for services, and administer their own programs. This resulted in variation among states in the Medicaid program. In 2000, 33.7 million Americans had health care coverage under the Medicaid program. This represents only 25 percent of the population living below the federal poverty level who would qualify for Medicaid (HCFA, 2001).

Another bill influencing the Medicaid program was the 1997 Balanced Budget Act that included a Child Health Provision and was known as the State Child Health Plan (SCHP). This was a $24 billion child health block grant given to states over a 3-year period. The funding was provided to states to provide health care coverage to more children. Three options for accomplishing this were given to states. They included expansion of the Medicaid program, creation of a new state program for child health, or some combination of the two. By the end of the 3-year period, all 50 states had participated in the block grant program. However, only 3.3 million of the about 9 million uninsured children were participating in this program (Pulcinic, Neary, & Mahoney, 2002).

Enrollment of Medicaid recipients into managed care plans was considered to be one way to save money for the federal government and states. With the enactment

⊕ RESEARCH APPLICATION

Quality Care in a Medicaid Managed Care Program: Adequacy of Prenatal Care for Teens in Chicago

Study Purpose

To investigate the adequacy of care given to prenatal teens in a Medicaid managed care program with the adequacy of care given to non-Medicaid prenatal teens.

Methods

One hundred one telephone surveys of obstetricians' offices were conducted to collect data on the first prenatal visit (lab tests, physical, medical history, health promotion counseling, availability of education materials) and health care provider's practice characteristics (years in practice, gender, nationality, medical graduate, office location).

Findings

Prenatal teens in a Medicaid managed care program were less likely to receive blood and urinalysis tests than were teens at a non-Medicaid prenatal center.

Implications

Since pregnant teens are more likely to have poorer birth outcomes and not continue their prenatal visits, providing adequate care that includes lab tests is critical.

Reference

Gifford, B. (2001). Quality of care in a Medicaid managed care program: Adequacy of prenatal care for teens in Chicago. *Public Health Nursing, 18*(4), 236–242.

---

of the Omnibus Budget Reconciliation Act of 1981 states were encouraged to experiment with alternative forms of delivering health care under Medicaid. Arizona was the first state to move the Medicaid program to a managed care model. In the 1990s, more states followed suit in an attempt to control Medicaid's rapid growth and problems of access created by the low level of participation among physicians with Medicaid clients. Currently, most states have enrolled their Medicaid recipients in a managed care plan. Cost savings of 10 to 15 percent below the cost of fee-for-service providers has occurred for Medicaid (McGregor, 2001). However, the cost savings may be temporary, as states have expanded their benefit coverage to include mental health benefits and expanded Medicare eligibility to cover more of the needy population.

Medicare

Medicare was also started in 1965. It provides public insurance coverage for those 65 years of age and older and for disabled workers. Prior to 1965, about half of the elderly had no health insurance compared with 96 percent in 1998 (Federal Interagency Forum on Age-Related Statistics, 2000).

Medicare is divided into parts: Part A, Part B, and most recently to cover prescription medications, Part D. Part A covers hospital insurance, and Part B covers medical insurance (Employee Benefits Research Institute, 2002b). Part D covers prescription medications. Part A is financed from payroll deduction of the working population (1.45 percent tax rate) to the Hospital Insurance Trust Fund. Part B is funded by enrollee contributions (SMI Trust Fund) and general federal revenues. Part A covers hospital stays, post-hospital skilled nursing facilities for limited conditions and stays (i.e., rehabilitation post cardiovascular accident [CVA] and myocardial infarction [MI]), home health care (for medically necessary skilled nursing care only), hospice care, and all but the first 3 pints of blood. As of 2002, Medicare will pay the first 60 days of hospitalization in full (Employee Benefits Research Institute, 2002b). For a hospital stay that extends from 61 to 150 days, Medicare pays a portion. After 150 days, the Medicare recipient assumes all costs. Medicare will pay in full the first 20 days of a skilled nursing facility after hospitalization. For any additional 80 days, Medicare will pay a portion of the cost. After 100 days, the Medicare recipient assumes all cost. For Part B, the Medicare recipient pays a monthly premium. Part B covers most medical expenses (physician's services, diagnostic tests, inpatient and outpatient surgical services and supplies, physical and speech therapy, and durable medical equipment), clinical laboratory services, home health care (medically necessary skilled nursing care), outpatient hospital treatment, and blood. Part B also covers preventive services such as bone mass measurements, cardiovascular screenings, colorectal cancer screening, diabetes screening, flu shots, glaucoma tests, hepatitis B injections, Pap test and pelvic exam including clinical breast exam, pneumococcal injection, prostate cancer screening, and screening mammograms. Before Medicare will begin to pay under Part B, a deductible must be paid. After that, Medicare pays 80 percent of the approved amount of medical expense, 50 percent of the approved outpatient mental health services, 100 percent of approved clinical laboratory services, 100 percent of approved home health care, 80 percent of the approved amount for durable medical equipment, 80 percent of outpatient hospital treatment, and 80 percent of the approved amount of blood after the first 3 pints. The Medicare recipient is responsible for the remaining medical expenses.

To assist the elderly in paying for the costs that Medicare does not cover, many elderly purchase a Medigap policy. A **Medigap** policy is additional health insurance to cover the costs that Medicare does not cover under both Parts A and B. However, purchasing additional insurance is costly for the elderly on fixed budgets. In addition, prescription medications are not covered without a substantial increase in premium. As a result, a growing number of elderly can afford to purchase neither Medigap insurance plans nor their prescription medications.

On December 8, 2003, President Bush signed into law the Medicare Prescription Drug, Improvement and Modernization Act in an attempt to provide relief from high-cost prescriptions for the elderly and disabled (Centers for Medicare & Medicaid, 2004; 2005a; 2005b; Department of Health and Human Services, 2005a; 2005b; HHS News, 2005). Prescription coverage under Medicare is now known as Part D. Qualified elderly and disabled persons now receive discount drug cards providing them with discounts from 10 to 75 percent. Low-income elderly and those with disabilities will have access to comprehensive prescription drug coverage with no or limited premiums and deductibles and low or nominal copayments. The elderly and disabled who receive both Medicare and Medicaid will

have no premium or deductible but will have a copayment ranging from $1 to $3 per prescription. Elderly and disabled who are at 135 percent of the federal poverty level (FPL; in 2004, $12,569 for individuals and $16,862 for couples) and have limited liquid assets will pay a few dollars per prescription and Medicare will cover 96 percent of the drug costs. For elderly and disabled with incomes less than 150 percent of the FPL and assets up to $10,000 for individuals or $20,000 for couples, in 2006 Medicare will provide 15 percent of the copayment with a sliding-scale premium and cover 85 percent of the prescription drug costs. For all other elderly and disabled with incomes at or above 150 percent of the FPL and assets, Medicare will pay for 75 percent of drug costs up to a coverage limit of $2,250 after a $250 deductible is met. After Medicare has paid the $2,250 coverage limit, it will not cover prescription drugs at the same rate until the elderly and disabled have spent $3,600 out-of-pocket monies. The monthly premium was $37 in 2006.

With prescribed medications costing from $300 to $800 per month for the elderly and disabled, the new law provides some relief from the high cost of prescription medications especially for those with low incomes. However, for those with middle to higher incomes, minimal relief is provided. The law has been cited as confusing for the elderly and others to understand. Implementation and evaluation of this law will provide the Centers for Medicare & Medicaid Services with necessary information on its outcomes.

In an attempt to control federal costs in the Medicare program, the Tax Equity and Fiscal Responsibility Act (TEFRA) was passed in 1983 to authorize Medicare payments to qualified HMOs. This is referred to as Medicare+Choice. Enrollment in Medicare managed care peaked in 1999 with 6.4 million enrollees (Oberlander, 2000). It is believed that many Medicare recipients joined Medicare+Choice because of the lower copayments and prescription coverage (Rector, 2000). Since then, there has been a steady decline as Medicare recipients choose not to be in the Medicare+Choice plan and as HMOs drop the elderly from coverage because they are the most costly age group to third party payers (insurance companies). By January 1, 2000, 1.5 million Medicare recipients disenrolled from the Medicare+Choice option (Ahl & Wergin, 2000). In 1998, 750,000 Medicare recipients were dropped by insurance carriers; another 930,000 were dropped in 2000 (Etheredge, 2000).

Medicaid is an option for the elderly who are considered to be "medically needy." However, to be classified as medically needy, the elderly must **spend down** their liquid assets. This means that they must spend all their liquid assets to an amount determined by the federal government. Typically this occurs when one spouse is either admitted to a long-term care facility or has been in one for more than 30 days. With the average life span increasing, the likelihood that one or both spouses will spend time in a long-term care facility is a reality. The cost of long-term care facilities increases yearly. The average monthly cost of a long-term care facility is between $2,000 and $3,000 (Centers for Medicare and Medicaid, 2002). In 1988, Congress amended the Social Security Act to include a provision for "spousal impoverishment." This was an attempt to protect the spouse living in the community from losing all his or her financial resources when the partner is in a long-term care facility or similar facility for more than 30 days. For example, eligibility to be classified as "impoverished" in 2003 included having a maximum of $90,660 in the spousal share of liquid assets, a monthly income allowance between $1,451 and $2,232 for the spouse in the community, and a maximum of $2,000 in liquid assets for the spouse in the long-term care facility. This amount changes every few years based on the cost of living. In order to reach "impoverished" status, the process of spending down liquid assets must occur before Medicaid will pay for all costs at a long-term care facility.

The federal government is the largest purchaser of long-term care (Congressional Budget Office, 1999). In 1998, Medicaid paid for 40 percent of long-term care for the elderly (Feder, Komisar, & Niefeld, 2000). Only 23 percent of elderly living in long-term care facilities paid for their own costs. In 2000, Medicaid paid $43.3 billion for long-term care, and the number is projected to almost double to 75.4 in 2020. Currently, 13 million elderly are in long-term care facilities, and this number is expected to triple by 2030 continuing the trend of the federal government as the largest payer for long-term care (Congressional Budget Office, 1999; Feder, Komisar, & Niefeld, 2000).

Tri Care

Tri Care is the federal health care program for active duty and retired service personnel, their eligible family members, and survivors (Tri Care Health Plan, 2006). It previously was known as the Civilian Health and Medical Program of the Uniformed Services (CHAMPUS). Funded through the Department of Defense, Tri Care offers its beneficiaries a choice between a managed care option (Tri Care Prime) and a fee-for-service option (Tri Care Standard). Active-duty military are required to participate in Tri Care Prime. Both Prime and Standard offer coverage for all health care benefits including dental and prescription medications. For dental, there is a yearly maximum plus life time maximum for orthodontic care. Prescription medications are offered through both plans but with higher copayments for those in Tri Care Standard. Similar to managed care options for the civilian population, Tri Care Prime offers lower copayments when visiting a physician or purchasing medications and no deductible.

Noninsurance-Based Models

Health care in the United States remains fragmented with 45 million people who do not have access to health care coverage, although numerous attempts have been made to control cost and expand health care coverage. Two models that have been proposed to deal with these problems are Managed Competition and Universal Coverage of health care. Both of these models are used in some form in Western developed countries to provide health care to their populations.

Managed Competition

Managed competition was conceptualized by economists such as Alain Enthoven in 1978 and became the foundation of former President Clinton's 1993 health care reform initiative (Goodman & Musgrave, 1994; Gentry, 2001). It was envisioned as a health care system that avoided both socialized medicine and free markets. Instead, it was viewed as a workable middle ground to controlling health care costs while providing health care to the majority of the population. There are two main concepts in managed competition that follow the economic principles of supply and demand. First, the supply side proposes formation of a delivery system, similar to managed care plans with networks of providers, but would build in accountability and be called accountable health plans (AHPs). The AHPs would be responsible for providing all health care services while being held accountable for the quality of care delivered. The second concept of demand in economic principles would include the creation of health insurance purchasing cooperatives (HIPCs). The function of HIPCs is to purchase health plans for health care consumers. The government's role would be to sponsor the creation of HIPCs in each state by appointing a board to oversee their creation and to define a standardized package of health service benefits. Purchasers of the health care plans (employers and individual health care consumers) would pay a fixed sum of money for the health care plan. Employees would pay a premium. Plans would be offered to suit individual needs at an additional cost. Employees choosing more expensive plans would be responsible for the extra cost. This component was built into managed competition to foster price-consciousness among employees as health care consumers and to encourage the insurance carriers in the AHPs to hold down health care cost by being competitive. In other words, the insurance carriers in AHPs would compete among themselves to earn business from the HIPCs. Thus, market forces would control AHPs. Because of the built in competition among insurance carriers in the AHPs, it was believed that most health care consumers would be able to purchase at least a basic health plan either through their place of employment or directly through HIPCs.

President Bill Clinton's health care reform initiative failed for numerous reasons among which was that the plan was too complex to be understood by the average health care consumer. However, variations of the concept of managed competition are being implemented in states such as California, Florida, and Texas (Gentry, 2001).

Universal Coverage

Universal coverage, also known as the single payer system of health care, is considered by many as the only option for providing access to health care for all populations. The term "universal coverage" is used to describe the population that would be covered under such a health plan. "Single-payer system" is used to describe the funding of a health care system that would provide universal coverage. A Harris Poll conducted with all industrialized nations found that Americans are the least satisfied with their health care (Robinson, 2002). This is related to the 40+ million uninsured and underinsured, limitations put on health care consumers and providers by insurance companies and managed care plans, and the continual increase in cost of health care. In 1999, the Massachusetts Medical Society was commissioned to explore changing the state's health care system to a Canadian-style, single payer system and found a savings of $170 million to $1 billion while providing care to more of the uninsured in that state (Kong, 1999).

A single payer system would involve one agency, such as the federal government, paying for medical expenses; this stands in contrast to the multiple payers we now have in the United States. Administration of the plan would be at the state and local level (Himmelstein & Woolhandler, 1997; Gebbie, 2002). It is believed that by decreasing the number of health care insurers administrative costs would be reduced and health care could be provided to the entire population. This cost reduction would then be passed on to health care consumers. A basic package of health care benefits would be guaranteed to all. The basic coverage would include acute and rehabilitative care, long-term care, home care, mental health services, dental services, occupational health care, prescription drugs, medical supplies, and preventive and public health measures.

The major payment plan for a single payer system of health care is to have the federal government pay for medical expenses with a national tax for payment (Gebbie, 2002). This would be the simplest form of payment. The tax would be a special tax similar to that used to fund Medicare and/or some portion of the general revenue. The payment would go directly to those providing the care or managed by fiscal intermediaries in the form of a "global" budget such as an annual lump-sum payment (Himmelstein & Woolhandler, 1997). A combination of federal and private dollars subsidizing universal coverage has been proposed.

Although it is agreed that universal coverage or a single payer system is the only way to provide access to health care for all, it has met with resistance from various health care and political groups as well as health care consumers. The concept of universal coverage does not fit well with our belief of decentralized control of our lives that includes health care decisions. Many Americans believe that there is an adequate amount of public and private health care options for those who need them. The idea that the government would provide health care is met with resistance as "free services" are viewed as being paid in extended waiting time for health care, loss of choice, and loss of personal dignity. A single payer system runs against the grain of a market economy that many hold as the model for democratic societies. However, as health care costs consume more of the federal dollar and out-of-pocket expenses for consumers, a change in our health care system is inevitable.

POLICY HIGHLIGHT

Influencing Reimbursement Practices

Nurse practitioners (NP) have been seeking third party reimbursement for services over the past years. One NP in Missouri, working with her nurse colleagues at the Women's Health Care Partnership (WHCP), developed an integrated model of care that included behavioral health and nursing. The model was a nursing model of care for which they sought independent reimbursement for nursing services since their services were focused on health promotion, disease prevention, and risk-reduction counseling all within the Missouri Nurse Practice Act. Reimbursement for medical services at the WHCP was funded under a managed care organization (MCO). The MCO refused to reimburse the nursing component of care unless the services were provided at a health care provider's office that

was collaborating with the MCO. The health care provider would then pay the nurse. One of the NPs realized that making changes to reimbursement was a process that would be slow and incremental and one that would take active involvement in the MCO. The NP decided to get involved in the policy process in small steps beginning with increased visibility with those in position of power in the MCO. This led to her receiving a position within the MCO that included writing proposals for Medicaid managed care funding for a large private company. Her next policy activity was an appointment to the health care provider advisory committee of a MCO. Both of these positions provided her with the opportunity to begin influencing policies related to reimbursement of NP's working within MCOs.

Americans' satisfaction with the health care system today and their confidence in the system's future continues to decline. They rank health care to be the most critical issuing facing America even above the economy, war, education, the budget deficit, and taxes. Only terrorism and national security ranks as high as health care. In relation to health care plans, 50 percent of Americans indicated they were extremely or very satisfied with their plans, while 30 percent were somewhat satisfied. Twenty-five percent of Americans indicated that because of increased costs in health care they have had to decrease their contributions to retirement plans or savings accounts (Employee Benefits Research Institute EBRI, 2004).

CHALLENGES FOR PUBLIC HEALTH NURSES

Health care systems are a product of the ideologies and social beliefs of a country. In the United States, independence and "rugged individualism" define Americans and their ideology. These beliefs have contributed to defining the U.S. health care system as one that provides high-quality care but is available only to those who can afford it.

The complexities of the U.S. health care system with its perceived inadequacies provide numerous challenges

for public health nurses. It challenges their social values regarding the best way to provide health care to the public. Public health nurses typically work for state agencies with shrinking funds that translates into fewer services for the neediest populations. In addition, health promotion and disease prevention services, the hallmark of public health, receive minimal funding by private or public insurance carriers. The continuous increase in health care costs frequently puts public health nurses in a position of prioritizing services to a population that at least can pay on a sliding fee scale. Services provided by public health nurses working for state agencies are not paid for by private insurance carriers unless they work as nurse practitioners within a qualifying setting in a state whose Nurse Practice Act allows for such coverage.

Aside from the challenge to public health nurses' social values, another challenge is to understand and keep up with the complexities and changes in organization of the health care system at the federal and state levels. This means being aware of health care bills that are passed and changes to existing health-related bills. In working with the public, public health nurses are frequently put into a position of helping clients file the necessary forms for Medicaid and Medicare, understanding what "spend down" means, and explaining how the various forms of managed care operate. The meaning of client advocacy today has expanded to include political astuteness in relation to health care bills and policies.

Public health nurses need to remain in the forefront of ensuring that health care is accessible to all clients regardless of their ability to pay for services. The continual increase in health care costs presents challenges for the U.S. health care system. One option to controlling costs and providing health care to all in the United States is a national health insurance program.

The American Public Health Organization has been a strong supporter of legislative efforts toward a national system of health care as the only way to ensure basic health care for all. Public health nurses can be a voice for change in the health care system. As stated by Gebbie (2002, p. 217) "there is no way to achieve true universality, or a truly national system without that single national voice."

CRITICAL THINKING ACTIVITIES

1. The increase in health care cost along with the aging of the U.S. population continues to drain funds from Medicare, the only public health insurance program for the elderly. What would be one policy change that you would make to improve delivery of health care to the elderly population? Explain how this change would improve services to the elderly while holding down health care costs.

2. In most states, Medicaid is provided through managed care plans. What are the advantages and disadvantages of this model for delivery of health care to the Medicaid population? Keep in mind that previously, many of the services now provided to the Medicaid population through managed care plans were provided by public health departments.

3. There is an ongoing debate as to whether health care is a basic right for all in the United States or a right for those who can afford it. Take a position and debate this position providing convincing support using statistics and examples.

4. Managed competition was the cornerstone of President Clinton's health care reform initiative. Compare and contrast this model of maintaining health care costs with the current prospective payment system.

5. The current health care system in the United States is shaped by the social values and health beliefs of the population. As a public health nurse analyze your role in shaping these values and health beliefs.

KEY TERMS

copayment	Medicare (Title XVIII)	public insurance
deductibles	Medigap	retrospective payment system
fee-for-service	PPO (preferred provider organization)	spend down
HMO (health maintenance organization)	premium	third party payer
managed care	private insurance	Tri Care
managed competition	prospective payment system	universal coverage
Medicaid (Title XIX)		working poor or uninsured

KEY CONCEPTS

⊕ External forces such as social values and health beliefs of the population, the political climate, economic conditions, physical environment, and biomedical technological development have played a role in shaping the U.S. health care system today. More specifically, these forces include a distrust of "big government," as well as a dedication to independence and fairness. These forces are frequently in conflict and, as a result, have left 40 million without access to health care.

⊕ Insurance-based care typically refers to private insurance plans provided for employees by employers. Under these plans, employees have the most choice of health care providers and pay them under a fee-for-service base. Managed care plans are a form of private insurance provided by employers. It differs in that consumers have less choice of health care providers and payment for services is based on an agreed payment system between the employer and the insurance company.

⊕ Medicare is a public insurance plan for those over 65 years of age and disabled persons funded by the federal government. Part A covers hospitalization, post-hospital skilled nursing facilities for limited conditions and stays, home health care, hospice care, and blood. Medicare Part B covers physician's services, diagnostic tests, inpatient and outpatient surgical services and supplies, physical and speech therapy, durable medical equipment, clinical laboratory services, home health care outpatient hospital treatment, and blood. Since Medicare does not cover all health care costs, many elderly purchase a supplemental insurance plan known as Medigap to cover the additional costs.

⊕ Medicaid is a public insurance plan jointly paid for by the federal government and state revenues. Those who are eligible include low-income families with children, SSI recipients, pregnant women whose family income is slightly above the federal poverty level (133 to 185 percent), recipients of adoption assistance and foster care, infants up to 1 year of age, qualifying elderly, and blind and disabled adults. Qualifying elderly refers to those who have spent down their liquid assets to $89,280. Once eligibility has been met, Medicaid requires states to provide a minimum set of benefits that includes hospitalization, physician visits, prenatal care, some preventive services such as dental, certain exams such as x-ray and laboratory tests, nursing home, and home health care. Since states can establish eligibility criteria, scope of services covered, set the payment rate for services, and administer their own programs, it has resulted in variation in coverage among states.

⊕ Managed competition provides health care through conglomerates of health insurers from which employers can select a health insurance plan. The concept of building in competition among health insurers is considered to be a viable means of controlling health care costs. Access to health care would be provided by requiring employers to cover more employees and by expanding the Medicaid program to cover more of the uninsured.

⊕ Universal coverage involves one agency, such as the federal government, paying for a basic package of health care benefits. Savings in health care cost would occur because there would be less administrative costs while providing access to health care for the entire population.

REFERENCES

Ahl, D., & Wergin, K. (2000, October). Fee-for-service joins the Medicare+Choice product line. *Healthcare Financial Management, 54*(10), 41–43.

Centers for Medicare and Medicaid Services. (2002). *Spousal impoverishment.* Retrieved February 11, 2005, from http://hhs.gov/medical/eligibility/spousal.asp.

Centers for Medicare and Medicaid Services. (2004). *Medicare drug cards provide significant savings now for beneficiaries with chronic conditions.* Retrieved February 11, 2005, from www.cms.hhs.gov/media/press/release.asp?.

Centers for Medicare & Medicaid. (2005a, January 21). *Medicare fact sheet.* Retrieved February 11, 2005, from www.cms.hhs.gov/medicareform/.

Centers for Medicare and Medicaid Services. (2005b). *Medicare modernization act.* Retrieved February 11, 2005, from www.cms.hhs.gov/medicareform/.

Chase, C., Heffler, S., Smith, S., Won, G., Clemens, K., et al. (2002). Health spending projections for 2001–2011: The latest outlook. *Health Affairs, 21*(2), 207–219.

CNN Money. (2004, August 26). Survey: Uninsured on the rise. Retrieved February 11, 2005, from http://cnnmoney.

Congressional Budget Office. (1999). *Projections of expenditures for long-term care services for the elderly.* Retrieved October 20, 2004, from www.cbo.gov/ftpdoc.cfm?index=1123&type=1.

Cooper, P., & Schone, B. (1997). More offers, fewer takers for employment-based health insurance: 1987-1966. *Health Affairs, 16*(6), 142–149.

Department of Health and Human Services, Centers for Medicare & Medicaid (2005a, February 4). *Medicare program; E-prescribing and the prescription drug program; Proposed rule* (42 CFR Part 423).

Department of Health and Human Services, Centers for Medicare & Medicaid (2005b, January 21). *Principle changes in new Medicare: From proposed rules to final rules.* Retrieved April 14, 2006, from www.cms.hhs.gov/medicareform.

Employee Benefits Research Institute (EBRI). (2002a). *Sources of health insurance and characteristics of the uninsured: Analysis of the March 2002 Current Population Survey.* EBRI Issue Brief Executive Summary, no. 25.

Employee Benefits Research Institute. (EBRI). (2002b, August). *The basics of Medicare: Updated with the 2002 Board of Trustees report.* Retrieved September 30, 2004, from www.ebri.org/facts/0802fact.htm.

Employee Benefits Research Institute (EBRI). (2004, November 2004). *Public attitudes on the US health care system: Findings from the health confidence survey,* No. 275. Retrieved February 11, 2005, from www.ebri.org/ibex/ib275.htm.

Enthoven, A. (2003). Employment-based health insurance is failing: Now what? *Health Affairs, 3,* 237–242.

Etheredge, L. (2000). Medicare's governance and structure: A proposal. *Health Affairs, 19*(5), 60–71.

Feder, J., Komisar, H., & Niefeld, M. (2000). Long-term care in the United States: An overview. *Health Affairs, 10*(3), 40–56.

Federal Interagency Forum on Age-Related Statistics. (2000). *Older Americans 2000: Key indicators of well-being.* Hyattsville, MD: Darcy Publications.

Finkelman, A. (2001). *Managed care: A nursing perspective.* Upper Saddle River, NJ: Prentice Hall.

Fox, P. (1997). An overview of managed care. In P. Kongstvedt (Ed.), *Essentials of managed health care* (pp. 184–196). Gaithersburg, MD: Aspen.

Gebbie, K. (2002). Could a national health system work in the United States? In D. Mason, J. Leavitt, & M. Chaffee (Eds.), *Policy and politics in nursing and health care* (4th ed.) (pp. 214–217). St. Louis: Saunders.

Gentry, C. (2001). Managed care and integrated organizations. In L. Shi & D. Singh (Eds.), *Delivering health care in America: A systems approach.* Gaithersburg, MD: Aspen.

Gifford, B. (2001). Quality of care in a Medicaid managed care program: Adequacy of prenatal care for teens in Chicago. *Public Health Nursing, 18*(4), 236–242.

Goodman, J., & Musgrave, G. (1994). *A primer on managed competition: NCPA Policy Report No. 183, ISBN#1-56808-017-4.* Retrieved May 13, 2004, from www.ncpa.org/studie/s183/s183.html.

Health Care Financing Administration (HCFA), Office of the Actuary. (2001). *HCFA Data and Statistics.* Retrieved May 1, 2004, from www.hcfa.gov/stats/nhe.oact.

Hefler, S., Smith, S., Won, G., Clemens, M.K., & Zezza, M. (2002). Health spending projections for 2001–2011: The latest outlook. *Health Affairs, 21*(1), 207–218.

Heinrich, J., & Thompson, T. (2002). Organization and delivery of health care in the United States: A patchwork system. In D. Mason, J. Leavitt, & M. Chaffee (Eds.), *Policy and politics in nursing and health care* (4th ed.). St. Louis: Saunders.

HHS News, U.S. Department of Health and Human Services (January 21, 2005). *HHS Takes Major Step to Prescription Drug Benefit.* Retrieved February 11, 2005, from www.cms.hhs.gov/medicareform/

Himmelstein, D., & Woolhandler, S. (1997). A national health program for the United States: A physician's proposal. In C. Harrington & C. Estes (Eds). *Health policy and nursing.* Sudbury: Jones and Bartlett.

Kong, D. (1999). *Single-payer health plan saves money, report shows.* Retrieved March 13, 2004, from www.califnurses.org/can/news/bg1042899.html.

McGregor, D. (2001). Health policy. In L. Shi & D. Singh (Eds.), *Delivering health care in America: A systems approach.* Gaithersburg, MD : Aspen.

Oberlander, J. (2000). Is premium support the right medicine for Medicare? A challenge to the emergent conventional wisdom. *Health Affairs, 19*(5), 84–99

Pulcinic, J., Neary, S., & Mahoney, D. (2002). Health care financing. In D. Mason, J. Leavitt, & M. Chaffee (Eds.), *Policy and politics in nursing and health care* (4th ed.). St. Louis: Saunders.

Rector, T. (2000). Exhaustion of drug benefits and disenrollment of Medicare beneficiaries from managed care organizations. *Journal of the American Medical Association, 283*(16), 2163–2167.

Robinson, B. (2002). *Canada's single payer health care system—It's worth a look.* Retrieved February 5, 2004,

from http://bcn.boulder.co.us/health/healthwatch/canada
.html.

Starr, P. (1982). *The social transformation of American medicine.* New York: Basic Books.

Sudano, J., & Baker, D. (2003). Intermittent lack of health insurance coverage and use of preventive services. *American Journal of Public Health, 98*(1), 130–137.

Torrens, P., & Williams, S. (2002). Managed care: Restructuring the system. In S. Williams & P. Torrens (Eds.), *Introduction to health services* (6th ed.). Albany, NY: Delmar Thomson Learning.

Tri Care Health Plan (2006). Retrieved February 27, 2006, from http://www.tricare.osd.mil

Whitted, G. (2002). Private health insurance and employee benefits. In S. Williams & P. Torrens (Eds.), *Introduction to health services* (6th ed.). Albany, NY: Delmar Thomson Learning.

Underlich, G.S., Sloan, F.A., & Davis, C.K. (1996). *Nursing staff in hospitals and nursing homes: Is it adequate?* Washington, DC: National Academy Press.

U.S. Department of Health and Human Services. (2006). *Medicaid eligibility.* Retrieved February 26, 2006, from http://www.cms.hhs.gov.

BIBLIOGRAPHY

Abood, S., & Keepnews, D. (2000). *Understanding payment for advanced practice nursing services. Volume 1: Medicare reimbursement.* Washington, DC: American Nurses Publishing.

American Nurses Association. (2001). *Code for nurses with interpretive statements.* Washington, DC: American Nurses Publishing.

Atherly, A. (2001). Supplemental insurance: Medicare's accidental stepchild. *Medical Care Research and Review, 58*(2), 131–161.

Berk, M.L., & Monheit, A.C. (2001). The concentration of health care expenditures, revisited. *Health Affairs, 20*(2), 9–18.

Born, P.H., & Simon, C.J. (2001). Patients and profits: The relationship between HMO financial performance and quality of care. *Health Affairs, 20*(2), 167–174.

Bruen, B., & Holahan, J. (May 2000). *Acceleration of Medicaid spending reflects mounting pressure,* Pub. No. 4056. Washington, DC: Kaiser Commission.

Christensen, S. & Wagner, J. W. (2000). The costs of a Medicare prescription drug benefit. *Health Affairs, 19*(2), 212–218.

Commonwealth Fund. (June 25, 2003). *Trends in Medicare+Choice plans provide warnings for Medicare debate.* New York: The Commonwealth Fund.

Ciioerm B.S., & Vladeck, B.C. (2000). Bringing competitive pricing to Medicare. *Health Affairs, 19*(5), 49–54.

Department of Defense. (2001). Tricare. Retrieved June 1, 2005, from www.Tricare.OSD.mil.

Draper, D.R., Hurley, C., Lesser, C.S. & Strunk, B. (2002). The changing face of managed care. *Health Affairs 21*(1), 11–23.

Frank, R.. (2001). Prescription drug prices: Why some pay more than others do. *Health Affairs, 20*(2), 115–128.

Fronstin, P. (2000, August). *The working uninsured: Who they are, how they have changed, and the consequences of being uninsured,* EBRI Issue Brief, no. 224. Washington, DC: EBRI.

Institute of Medicine. (2001). *Crossing the quality chasm: A new health system for the 21st century.* Washington, DC: National Academy Press.

Kaiser Commission. (2001, February). *Medicaid enrollment and spending trends,* Pub. No. 2113b. Washington, DC: Kaiser Commission.

Kaiser Commission on Medicaid Facts. (2001, March). Medicaid's role in long-term care. Retrieved April 20, 2006, from www.kff.org/content/2001/2186.

Kaiser Commission (2001). *The Medicaid program at a glance,* Pub. No. 2004b. Washington, DC: Kaiser Commission.

Kohn, L. (2000). Organizing and managing care in a changing health system. *Health Services Research, 35,* 37–52.

Ku, L., & Guyer, J. (2001, April 20). *Medicaid spending: Rising again, but not to crisis levels.* Washington, DC: Center on Budget and Policy Priorities.

Levit, K., Smith, C., Cowan, C., Lazenby, H., & Martin, A. (2002). Inflation spurs health spending in 2000. *Health Affairs 21* (1), 172–181.

Light, D.W. (2002). A conservative call for universal access to health care. Retrieved, April 2006, from http://www.med.upenn.edu.bioethics.

Managed Care on Line. (2001). Managed care national statistics. Retrieved June 1, 2006, from http://www.healthplan.about.com/industry/health-plan/GI/dynamics?offside.htm

Medicare and Prescription Drugs. (2001). Washington, DC: Kaiser Family Foundation. Miller, R.H., & Luft, H.S. (2001). HMO plan performance update: An analysis of recently published literature (1997–2000). Prepared for the Council on the Economic Impact of Health System Change: 8th Princeton Conference: The Future of Managed Care.

National Association of State Budget Officers. (2001, June). *2000 state expenditure report.* Washington, DC: NASBO.

Nichols, L.M., & Reischauer, R.D. (2000). Who really wants price competition in Medicare managed care? *Health Affairs, 19*(5), 30–43.

Nursing's agenda for health care reform. (1992). Washington, DC: American Nurses Publishing.

Perry, M., et al. (2000, January). *Medicaid and children: Overcoming barriers to enrollment, findings from a national survey,* Pub. No. 2174. Washington, DC: Kaiser Commissions

Quad Council of Public Health Nursing Organizations. (1999). *Scope and standards of public health nursing practice.* Washington, DC: American Nurses Association.

Ray, G.T., et al. (2000, July). Comparing the medical expenses of children with Medicaid and Commercial Insurance in an HMO. *American Journal of Managed Care,* 753–760.

Scott, W.R. et al. (2000). *Institutional change and health care organizations: From professional dominance to managed care.* Chicago: University of Chicago Press.

Shaffer, E.R. (2002). The California Health Service Plan, and 8 Other Models for Universal Coverage. Retrieved, April 2006, from http://www.healthcareoptions.ca.gov.

Smith, V., & Ellis, E. (2002, October). *Medicaid budgets under stress: Survey findings for state fiscal year 2000, 2001, 2002,* Pub. No. 4020. Washington, DC: Kaiser Commission.

Stuber, J., Dallek, G., & Biles, B. (2001). *National and local factors driving health plan withdrawals from Medicare + Choice: Analysis of seven Medicare + Choice markets.* Washington, DC: Commonwealth Fund.

Tamblyn, R., Laprise, R., Hanley, J., et al. (2001). Adverse events associated with prescription drug cost-sharing among poor and elderly persons. *JAMA, 285,* 421–429.

The World Health Organization. (2000). *The world health report 2000: Healthy systems improving performance.* Geneva: The World Health Organization.

Woolhandler, S., & Himmelstein, D.U. (July/August 2002). Paying for national health insurance—and not getting it. *Health Affairs,* 88–98.

RESOURCES

Agency for Healthcare Research and Quality (AHRQ)

540 Gaither Road
Rockville, Maryland 20850
301-427-1364
Web: http://www.ahrq.gov
AHRQ is a federal agency in the U.S. Department of Health and Human Services that conducts research on health care quality, costs, outcomes, and patient safety. It is the lead federal agency charged with improving the quality, safety, efficiency, and effectiveness of health care for all Americans. As one of 12 agencies within the Department of Health and Human Services, AHRQ supports health services research that will improve the quality of health care and promote evidence-based decision making.

American's Health Insurance Association of America (AHIP)

601 Pennsylvania Avenue NW
South Building, Suite 500
Washington, D.C. 20004
202-778-3200
FAX: 202-331-7487
Email: ahip@ahip.org
Web: http://www.hiaa.org
AHIP is the national association representing nearly 1,300 member companies providing health insurance coverage to more than 200 million Americans. Member companies offer medical expense insurance, long-term care insurance, disability income insurance, dental insurance, supplemental insurance, stop-loss insurance, and reinsurance to consumers, employers, and public purchasers. AHIP goal is to provide a unified voice for the health care financing industry, to expand access to high-quality, cost-effective health care to all Americans, and to ensure Americans' financial security through robust insurance markets, product flexibility and innovation, and an abundance of consumer choice.

American Public Health Association (APHA)

800 "I" Street NW
Washington, D.C. 20001-3710
202-777-APHA (2752)
FAX: 202-777-2534
Email: comments@APHA.org
Web: http://www.apha.org
APHA is a nonprofit association of public health professionals from over 50 public health occupations working to improve the public's health and to achieve equity in health status for all. The organization strives to influence policy and set priorities in public health to help prevent disease and promote health. The organization also strives to promote the scientific and professional foundation of public health practice and policy, advocate the conditions for a healthy global society, emphasize prevention and enhance the ability of members to promote and protect environmental and community health.

Blue Cross/Blue Shield Association

Web: http://www.bluecares.com
This is the official Web site for the Blue Cross and Blue Shield Association. It features information about Blue Cross/Blue Shield, answers for consumers, and provides consumers with the opportunity to sign up for a Blue Cross/Blue Shield plan on line.

Center for Health System Change (HSC)

600 Maryland Avenue SW, #550
Washington, D.C. 20024
202-484-5261
FAX: 202-484-9258
Web: http://www.hschange.org

HSC is a nonpartisan policy research organization located in Washington, D.C. It designs and conducts studies focused on the U.S. health care system to inform the thinking and decisions of policy makers in government and private industry. In addition to this applied use, HSC studies contribute more broadly to the body of health care policy research that enables decision makers to understand change and the national and local market forces driving that change. The mission of HSC is to inform policy makers and private decision makers about how local and national changes in the financing and delivery of health care affect people. HSC strives to provide high-quality, timely, and objective research and analysis that leads to sound policy decisions, with the ultimate goal of improving the health of the American public.

Center on Budget and Policy Priorities

820 1st Street NE, #510
Washington, D.C. 20002
202-408-1080
FAX: 202-408-1056
Email: center@cbpp.org
Web: http://www.cbpp.org

The Center on Budget and Policy Priorities is one of the nation's premier policy organizations working at the federal and state levels on fiscal policy and public programs that affect low- and moderate-income families and individuals. The center conducts research and analysis to inform public debates over proposed budget and tax policies and to help ensure that the needs of low-income families and individuals are considered in these debates. The center also develops policy options to alleviate poverty, particularly among working families, and examines the short- and long-term impacts that proposed policies would have on the health of the economy and on the soundness of federal and state budgets. Among the issues explored are whether federal and state governments are fiscally sound and have sufficient revenue to address critical priorities, both for low-income populations and for the nation as a whole.

Centers for Medicare & Medicaid Services (CMS)

Centers for Medicare & Medicaid Services
7500 Security Boulevard Baltimore
MD 21244
Web: http://new.cms.hhs.gov

CMS is the federal agency responsible for administering Medicare, Medicaid, SCHIP (State Children's Health Insurance), HIPAA (Health Insurance Portability and Accountability Act), CLIA (Clinical Laboratory Improvement Amendments), and several other health programs.

Children's Defense Fund (CDF)

25 E Street NW
Washington, D.C. 20001
202-628-8787; 1-800-233-1200
Email: cdfinfo@childrensdefense.org
Web: http://www.childrensdefense.org

The Children's Defense Fund grew out of the civil rights movement under the leadership of Marian Wright Edelman. It has become the nation's strongest voice for children and families since its founding in 1973. Today, The Children's Defense Fund's Leave No Child Behind® mission is to ensure every child a Healthy Start, a Head Start, a Fair Start, a Safe Start, and a Moral Start in life and successful passage to adulthood with the help of caring families and communities. CDF provides a strong, effective voice for all the children of America who cannot vote, lobby, or speak for themselves.

Congressional Budget Office (CBO)

Ford House Office Building, 4th floor
Second and D Streets, SW
Washington, D.C. 20515-6925
202-226-2602
Web: http://www.cbo.gov

CBO was founded on July 12, 1974, with the enactment of the Congressional Budget and Impoundment Control Act (P.L. 93-344). The agency began operating on February 24, 1975. CBO issues yearly federal cost estimates and impact of unfounded mandates on state and local governments, studies, reports, briefs, Monthly Budget Reviews, letters, and background papers to Congress. CBO also testifies before the Congress as needed on a variety of issues. Finally, CBO provides up-to-date data on its Web site, including current budget and economic projections and information on the status of discretionary appropriations.

Medicare Payment Advisory Commission (MedPAC)

601 New Jersey Avenue NW, Suite 9000
Washington, D.C. 20001
202-220-3700
Email: webmaster@medpac.gov
Web: http://www.medpac.gov

The Medicare Payment Advisory Commission (MedPAC) is an independent federal body established by the Balanced Budget Act of 1997 (P.L. 105-33) to advise the U.S. Congress on issues affecting the Medicare program. The commission's statutory mandate is quite broad: In addition to advising the Congress on payments to private health plans participating in Medicare and providers in Medicare's traditional fee-for-service program, MedPAC is also tasked with analyzing access to care, quality of care, and other issues affecting Medicare.

The Brookings Institution

1775 Massachusetts Avenue NW
Washington, D.C. 20036-2188
202-797-6000
FAX: 202-797-6004
Web: http://www.brook.edu

The Brookings Institution is a private nonprofit organization devoted to independent research and innovative policy solutions. For more than 90 years, Brookings has analyzed current and emerging issues and produced new ideas for the nation and the world. For policy makers and the media, Brookings scholars provide the highest quality research, policy recommendations, and analysis on the full range of public policy issues. Research at the Brookings Institution is conducted to inform the public debate, not advance a political agenda. The scholars at the Brookings Institution are drawn from the United States and abroad—with experience in government and academia—and hold diverse points of view. Brookings's goal is to provide high-quality analysis and recommendations for decision makers in the United States and abroad on the full range of challenges facing an increasingly interdependent world.

URAC

1220 L Street NW, Suite 400
Washington, D.C. 20005
202-216-9010
FAX: 202-216-9006
Web: http://www.urac.org

URAC is an independent, nonprofit organization known as a leader in promoting health care quality through its accreditation and certification programs. URAC offers a wide range of quality benchmarking programs and services that keep pace with the rapid changes in the health care system and provides a symbol of excellence for organizations to validate their commitment to quality and accountability. Through its broad-based governance structure and an inclusive standards development process, URAC ensures that all stakeholders are represented in establishing meaningful quality measures for the entire health care industry. URAC's mission is to promote continuous improvement in the quality and efficiency of health care management through processes of accreditation and education.

U.S. Department of Health and Human Services (DHHS)

200 Independence Avenue SW
Washington, D.C. 20201
202-619-0257; 1-877-696-6775
Web: http://www.dhhs.gov

DHHS is the U.S. government's primary agency involved with protecting the health of all Americans and providing essential human services, especially for people with few resources. The Web site provides health-related publications.

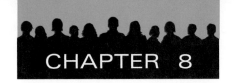

CHAPTER 8

Economics of Public Health Nursing

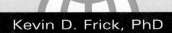

Kevin D. Frick, PhD

Kathleen White RN, PhD, CNAA, BC

Chapter Outline

What Is Economics?
Allocation of Scarce Resources
Economic Decision Making
Basic Economic Reasoning

Profit Maximization and Cost Minimization
Fixed and Variable Costs
Technical and Allocative Efficiency
Organizational Behavior and Cost Minimization

For-Profit and Not-for-Profit Organizations
Organizational Objectives
Maximizing Objectives Through Minimizing Costs

Individual Investment in Health
Motivation
Valuing the Future

Externalities
Positive Externalities
Negative Externalities

Decisions under Uncertainty

Economic Evaluation
Cost-Benefit Analysis
Cost-Effectiveness Analysis

Economics of the Labor Market
Public Health Nurse Labor Market
Reservation Wage
Individual Motivation to Work

Learning Objectives

Upon completion of this chapter, the reader will be able to:

1. Distinguish the differences and similarities between the motivations and behaviors of for-profit and not-for-profit organizations.

2. Analyze investments in health from an economic perspective.

3. Define and describe positive and negative economic externalities in public health.

4. Explain the economic concept of decisions under uncertainty in relation to health insurance.

5. Discuss the uses of cost-benefit and cost-effectiveness analysis in health care.

6. Discuss the economics of the nurse labor market.

Economics provides a logical, internally consistent paradigm for motivating public health decision making and evaluating the outcomes. Importantly, economic evaluation considers the value of the quantity of outcomes produced rather than the distribution of outcomes. Since policy makers are concerned about both the quantity and distribution of outcomes, economic reasoning should not be used in isolation. This chapter will discuss basic economic concepts relevant to public health nursing, with an example of using economic logic for each.

WHAT IS ECONOMICS?

Economics in public health nursing (and in general) is the study of how scarce resources are allocated (Nicholson, 2004). In public health, resources might be allocated to produce public health preparedness supplies or vaccines, equipment that is used by nurses (e.g., blood pressure cuffs), or services for clients like home visits. Clients use resources when adopting or changing health behaviors or using medical care. Critically, resources available are limited, and multiple possible uses of resources are considered.

The demand for goods and services is a relationship between quantities and prices that characterizes how much will be bought at each price. The supply is, in contrast, a relationship between quantities and prices that characterizes how much will be sold at each price. Figure 8-1 shows these relationships. As the price increases, the demand for goods will decrease, and the supply of goods will increase. The market reaches equilibrium when supply and demand are equal at a given price (Figure 8-1; point A on the graph).

Allocation of Scarce Resources

Individuals and organizations allocating scarce resources are making choices. Thus, economics is fundamentally about the choices that are made about the production and consumption of goods and services. Public health nurses face situations in which choices must be made about the use of scarce resources in hospitals and public health settings. Public health nurses understand that resources used for one purpose cannot be used for another, reflecting the concept of opportunity costs. The opportunity cost of using labor or supplies for one purpose is the value of what they could have produced

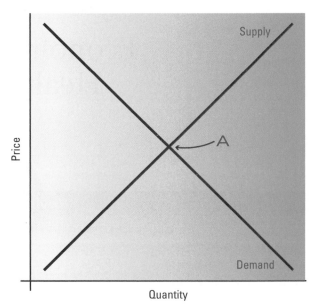

Figure 8-1 Supply and demand.

if they had been used for another purpose. The decisions about resource allocation are made based on nurses' preferences, other management preferences, and client preferences. Preferences reflect decision makers' values, wants, or needs. Decisions are often made under uncertainty about the future of an individual's or population's health. Under uncertainty, each of multiple outcomes is associated with a probability, and the expected outcome (a weighted average based on the probability of each possible outcome) is used in decision making.

Economic Decision Making

Economic logic can be used to analyze public health choices relevant to nurses:

1. Scarcity
    - An agency's choice of which services to provide with scarce resources—care for the entire family or services only for the care of children and pregnant woman
2. Preferences
    - An individual's choice of whether to become a nurse and whether to obtain a BSN, MSN, or other nursing training (Buerhaus et al., 2004; Spetz, 2002)

- An individual's choice of where to work, what hours to work (Shields, 2004), how much effort to put forth (Heyes, 2005), and when to retire (Buerhaus & Auerbach, 2000)

- A client's decision about how to use her time and money to help improve and maintain her own health and her children's health (Grossman, 1972)

3. Opportunity Costs

- An agency's decisions to use nurses in public health interventions targeted for children (Hutchins et al., 1999; e.g., what types of services will not be provided if nurses are used to treat children with asthma to prevent the need for emergency care?)

- An agency's choice about which type of labor to use (Roblin et al., 2004) in producing community health interventions (e.g., varying combinations of RNs and community health workers that need to be taken from other responsibilities)

4. Uncertainty

- A government's choice to tax cigarettes to limit second hand smoke exposure because it may cause ill health effects among some of the exposed population (Lien & Evans, 2005)

Basic Economic Reasoning

All basic economic reasoning is based on the concept of making decisions **at the margin**. Decisions at the margin focus on spending one more dollar or trying to bring about one more positive health outcome. Economic logic focuses on the cost of producing the next unit of benefit or the amount of benefit that could be obtained by spending an extra dollar. Consider a public health nursing intervention in which a nurse makes repeated visits to a client. If the client does not otherwise utilize health care, the **marginal benefit** (value) of the first visit is expected to be high. The benefit from the single visit could be due to preventive care that reduces the need for other societal expenditures or curative care that makes the individual better off and increases his **utility** (life satisfaction). If after just two visits the client is interacting regularly with the health care system and is taking better care of himself, the value of a third visit would be unclear. When the value of the visits to society or to the system paying for the visit is less than marginal cost of the visit (the public

health nurse's salary and the cost of transportation associated with that visit), then, based on strictly economic criteria, the protocol should call for the visits to end. A profit-maximizing provider would consider only the net revenue or **profit** associated with providing this type of service (i.e., the amount by which revenue exceeds costs). Another example of this type of marginal decision making would consider how far away from a central location a public health nurse should go to provide an intervention. At some point, sending public health nurses to provide an intervention further away (extending the margin) will cost more than the value of the services provided. By economic logic, there is a point at which the value of the care provided will be less than the cost to provide that care.

The remainder of the chapter will demonstrate seven examples of the use of economic reasoning in public health nursing: (1) profit maximization and cost minimization; (2) the economics of for-profit and not-for-profit organizations' behavior; (3) the economics of an individual investment in health (i.e., adopting positive or negative health behaviors); (4) the effects of one person's behavior, like smoking, on another person's health, referred to as externalities; (5) decisions under uncertainty; (6) economic evaluation using cost-benefit and cost-effectiveness analyses; and (7) the economics of the labor market, a key topic given the nursing shortage in the United States at present.

PROFIT MAXIMIZATION AND COST MINIMIZATION

Profit maximization typically refers to the total profit of a firm being as large as possible. It is assumed that this is the main objective of most firms, although there may be times that profit maximization is not the main objective. Cost minimization refers to the least costly way to produce a good without losing profit.

Fixed and Variable Costs

Costs can be divided into fixed and variable costs. **Fixed costs** are incurred regardless of the number of visits, clients, or other public health services provided, while **variable costs** depend on the quantity of visits, clients seen, or public health services provided. For example, a van to provide public health home visitation services has both fixed and variable costs. Loan or

⊕ RESEARCH APPLICATION

A Cost Comparison of Hand Hygiene Regimens

Study Purpose

To examine the comparative cost and quality of using traditional soap and water versus using an alcohol-based rub for hand hygiene.

Methods

A perspective analysis was conducted from March 2001 to January 2003 as part of a large clinical trial to examine hand hygiene practices and health care-associated infections in two Level III–IV Neonatal Intensive Care Units in New York City. Data on the use of hand hygiene products was provided monthly from the environmental services department.

Findings

Although the alcohol-based rub cost $750 more for 1,000 client days, it was found to be less costly due to shorter

application time than traditional hand washing. Traditional hand washing requires 5 seconds more time than using the alcohol-based rub.

Implications

The cost and quality of two hand hygiene regimens were compared. A waterless alcohol-based rub was significantly less costly than traditional hand washing because of reduced time required to use it and was associated with significantly better quality. The authors pointed out that the results of the study could be greater if water and paper towel usage costs had been included.

Reference

Cimiottoi, J., Stone, P.W., & Larson, E.L. (2004). A cost comparison of hand hygiene regimens. *Nursing Economics* *22*(4), 196–199, 204, 175.

---

lease payments for the van do not depend on how far the vehicle is driven. However, fuel costs will depend on the number of miles driven, a function of the number of clients visited. Total profits will be determined by the combination of fixed and variable costs, and the marginal net revenue will depend only on the variable costs that change when the quantity of services produced changes.

Technical and Allocative Efficiency

Economics considers two types of efficiency: technical and allocative efficiency. Technical efficiency simply means that the total costs of producing a quantity of a good or service are being minimized (Nicholson, 2004). Allocative efficiency requires technical efficiency and an allocation of resources across different types of production that leaves no room to reallocate resources without making someone worse off (Varian, 1992). This does not imply that there is no way to allocate resources to make some people better off; it just indicates that if some are made better off, others will be made worse off.

An example of the distinction between different types of efficiency is useful. The U.S. health care system has been described as underproducing preventive care and overproducing pharmaceutical products. Even if all preventive care services and all pharmaceutical goods are produced at the minimum cost (technical efficiency), questions regarding allocative efficiency remain. Whether resources could be reallocated to make everyone better off by producing fewer pharmaceuticals and more preventive services is an empirical question requiring economic and epidemiological data to be answered.

Consider a planner allocating resources to produce health at the minimum cost. Continuing the example introduced in the previous paragraph, we see that as fewer pharmaceuticals are produced and more preventive services are produced, the net effects on morbidity and mortality are unclear. Intuitively, the increase in morbidity associated with reducing pharmaceuticals will be small at first, while a decrease in morbidity from the first preventive measures will be large. As more resources are shifted, the increases in morbidity will become larger than the decreases in morbidity, and further resource reallocation would lead to worse aggregate health outcomes for society. When this occurs, no further resources should be shifted. Actual public health resource allocation decisions are more complex. Some empirical evidence suggests that the U.S. health care system is not technically efficient and could produce the same life expectancy with fewer inputs (Retzlaff-Roberts, Chang, & Rubin, 2004).

Organizational Behavior and Cost Minimization

Technical efficiency is applicable to an individual agency as well as the entire health care system. In a standard, market-based economic model, the assumption is that firms maximize profits. For profit-maximizing firms to achieve their objective, they must produce goods and services at a minimum cost. If the firm does not produce at the minimum cost, it could increase profits by producing the same output at a lower cost.

A concrete example of the importance of cost minimization demonstrates that the concept is important for not-for-profit agencies as well. A public health program for hypertension control may involve public health nurses, lay community health workers, transportation, and supplies. Several resource allocation decisions are necessary. First, the manager must determine how to produce each possible quantity of services at the minimum cost. Second, someone must decide how much of each service to produce.

When determining the minimum cost for each level of production, a manager will have a choice of different inputs to produce each quantity of public health services. At the simplest level, the decision maker is likely to begin with a single public health nurse, a single community health worker, and a single vehicle for transportation. Assuming that this quantity of inputs does not cover the entire community for which services are requested, the decision maker can then consider how much it would cost to add another nurse, another community health worker, or another vehicle. Using economic logic, the planner would compare the cost of each input with the change in the number of clients with hypertension in the community, controlling for the cases of hypertension associated with adding each input. The decision maker would add the input that increased the number of controlled hypertensive clients by the largest number for each dollar spent. If another input could provide more output per dollar spent, the

decision maker would not be increasing hypertension control at the minimum cost.

At complete technical efficiency, the number of additional hypertensive clients under control per dollar spent on each input should be equal across all inputs. This effectively means that the same amount is produced per dollar spent on each input, or that the "bang for the buck" is equivalent among inputs when costs are being minimized. In economic jargon, the ratio of the prices of inputs is equal to the **technical rate of substitution** (Varian, 1992).

For allocative efficiency considerations, eventually, the cost of providing more population hypertension control is larger than the value of health that is foregone by not using the agency's resources for other interventions. At that point, providing more hypertension control would not be a decision made based on economic criteria.

FOR-PROFIT AND NOT-FOR-PROFIT ORGANIZATIONS

As mentioned earlier, economists assume and empirically test motivations for individual and organizational behavior. Some consideration of what the economic motivation for behavior by for-profit and not-for-profit organizations is worthwhile as is a brief examination of empirical evidence.

Organizational Objectives

In general, producers are assumed to have maximizing profits as their primary goal, or objective. Organizational goals and objectives are referred to interchangeably.

Determining the actual objective of a not-for-profit organization is a difficult task. Sometimes this is done through qualitative research, such as when leaders of organizations are asked what their objective is (Lune, 2002). An entire branch of economics, industrial organization, focuses on organization's behavior given the economic incentives and objectives that organizations are presumed to have.

More frequently, economists develop theory consistent with organizations having a specific objective, determine the implications of the objective in terms of an organization's choices and outcomes, determine how the choices would vary under another objective, and gather data on a number of organizations to determine with which objective the behavior is most consistent. Economists prefer to observe behavior to make inferences rather than ask individuals and organizations to describe their behavior.

Basic economic theory suggests that organizations make decisions about whether to produce and how much to produce based on a combination of costs and revenues. Essentially, organizations should produce as long as the revenue they obtain from selling the goods at the price determined by the market is sufficient to cover their variable costs. If an organization paid its fixed costs, paid no variable costs, and earned no revenue, then the negative profits would equal the fixed costs. However, if the organization's revenue were more than sufficient to cover its variable costs, the organization would either make a profit or at least suffer losses smaller than the fixed costs.

This is true both for for-profit organizations and not-for-profit organizations. Consider a not-for-profit organization providing outreach care from a regional base for diabetic clients in rural Appalachia. Few not-for-profits base decisions on whether to continue particular programs based on net revenues, but suppose the program must be self-supporting. If the not-for-profit organization receives some type of reimbursement (perhaps a user fee) that at least covers the cost of the fuel and staff but still results in negative net revenues because of high program fixed costs, it should continue to provide services. If it did not, the loss would be the total fixed costs rather than something smaller in magnitude. In the long run, if the net revenue remains negative, the organization may sell the vehicles that create fixed costs and exit the market for producing services for diabetic clients.

Maximizing Objectives Through Minimizing Costs

To maximize the degree by which revenues exceed costs, not-for-profit agencies such as Public Health Departments must minimize costs, similar to for-profit organizations. For example, a not-for-profit agency with a fixed budget trying to provide prenatal care services is only able to maximize the services it provides if it minimizes the cost of the services. Ultimately, both for-profit and not-for-profit organizations need to have revenues that exceed costs (i.e., positive profits). For-profit organizations return profits to owners (shareholders or individual proprietors). Not-for-profit agencies and

organizations cannot distribute their excess revenues in the same way; instead, they have stakeholders who set the organization's objectives for which the excess revenue can be used. Multiple studies have been conducted focusing on how and whether not-for-profit hospitals' and nursing homes' behavior differs from similar for-profit organizations' behavior (Hoerger, 1991; Leone & Van Horn, 2005; Newhouse, 1970; Tuckman & Chang, 1988). The theory suggests that they exhibit different behavior, and the empirical results suggest that there are similar costs but that not-for-profit organizations have lower and less variable excess revenues (profits). Empirical studies have also suggested that not-for-profit nursing homes are more efficient and that they can make discretionary expenditures or use accounting practices to keep excess revenue low and with little variability (Farsi & Filippini, 2004; Hoerger, 1991; Leone & Van Horn, 2005). Critically, not-for-profit organizations need excess revenues (or profits) to provide free services or community outreach and could not do this without maintaining efficiency.

Not-for-profit agencies, like one that might provide outreach services for clients with diabetes, are often thought to be more concerned with the distribution of services than for-profit organizations are. One choice used by some not-for-profit organizations is to charge high-income individuals a higher price for higher quality and use the profits to provide acceptable free services to lower income individuals (Samandar et al., 2001).

In summary, there is not general agreement on the motivation for behavior of not-for-profit organizations. What is expected is that such organizations will continue to produce goods and services at the lowest cost possible in order to maximize profits or, in the case of not-for-profits, maximize output or any other objective. Understanding the objectives of not-for-profit organizations is critical in determining how the organization responds to regulations and the varying demand for the goods and services the organization produces.

In closing this section, it is important to note that even the term "for-profit" can have different implications over different time horizons. For example, for-profit organizations may appear to behave in the short-run in ways that are not perfectly consistent with maximizing profits, but their behavior may affect long-term strategic thinking. Before discussing organization's short- and long-term behavior, it is important to understand the economic logic of making comparisons between the present and future. An organization's stakeholders determine the relevant time horizon (how far in the future the organization plans). When considering the future, the difference between the weight on the present and the future (the **discount rate**) is partially a function of market forces and, also, partially determined by stakeholders. For example, loans taken out today must be repaid with interest in the future, and the interest rate partially determines the weight placed on future events. Similarly, money saved today can be used to earn interest in the future. Conversely, money spent to produce services will generate revenue in the future. All of these force an organization to make tradeoffs between the present and the future.

If any organization wants to make sure that it maximizes profits in the long run, then it may choose to forego profits at present, increase its market share, and have more complete control of the market in the future. Firms in highly competitive industries are unable to do this. Health care has never been presumed to be a perfectly competitive industry. There are a relatively small number of sellers of goods and services, entry into the market for producing and selling medical care services is highly regulated (licensing), consumers do not understand all their choices, and many consumers have limited choices. Thus, organizational behavior responds to potential market power in complex ways.

INDIVIDUAL INVESTMENT IN HEALTH

As stated earlier, individuals are assumed to maximize utility or life satisfaction. Many things can influence a person's utility such as the things they buy, the experiences they have, and their health status. Individuals have a limited amount of resources that can be used to maximize their utility. The process of maximizing utility can be considered each day, during a year, or over a lifetime. Individuals, like organizations and agencies, vary in their time horizon and how much weight they place on the future in comparison with the present (i.e., their discount rate).

Encouraging individual investment in health is an important role for public health nurses. Investments in health care take a variety of forms but are primarily related to health promotion and disease prevention. Exercise can be an investment in health as a primary prevention measure. Cancer screening can be an invest-

ment in health as a secondary prevention measure. Even careful monitoring of diabetes or hypertension can be an investment in health in order to prevent additional complications from occurring.

Motivation

Individuals must make decisions about their willingness to invest in keeping themselves healthy in the same way that they evaluate decisions on financial investments. The similarity with financial investments is in thinking about the "return" that one gets in the future on the investments one makes. Similar to other health care utilization decisions, health investment decisions are made under uncertainty. Such decisions are also made without knowing the actual price, either getting the services for free or for a reduced price by way of insurance.

While public health nurses advocate for a large number of health investments (e.g., consistent seat belt use, receiving influenza vaccinations, no smoking, moderate alcohol consumption, a suitable exercise program, recommended cancer screening, preventive dental visits every six months), many individuals do not follow these recommendations. Some public health nurses are inclined to think that individuals simply do not have or understand the information about the prevention-related behaviors. Although this may be true, the vast amount of information on health promotion and disease prevention available in the media, on the Internet, or from health care providers makes it difficult to believe that individuals do not have the information. Comprehension may be more of an issue than availability of information.

Economists have been interested in the motivation for health investments. Education has been one focal point for research. An early study collected data not only on individuals' education but also on respondents' knowledge about smoking, drinking, and exercise (Kenkel, 1991). In a multivariable analysis controlling for individuals' knowledge of positive health behaviors, the more education an individual has, the more likely he is to choose positive health behaviors. This result is consistent with education being correlated with something related to a choice of positive health behavior beyond just knowledge about the behaviors. More educated individuals may be able to translate what they are told by public health nurses into bigger changes in their individual health.

Valuing the Future

Economic logic also suggests that individuals who invest more in their education over a lifetime place a higher value on the future, or, in economic jargon, they have a lower discount rate. The economic logic is that when one is acquiring or investing in education, one is not earning money. The delay in earnings and, hence, the consumption of goods and services that can be purchased with that money, indicates that the individual places a relatively high value on the future compared with the present. In health, making the choice to forego the gratification of eating foods that taste good but that are unhealthy is consistent with having a lower discount rate and a greater preference for living longer.

Eventually public health nurses in general, and those who are concerned with government regulations in particular, must make decisions about whether to intervene at the level of mandating the use of a particular service or providing improved access as an investment in the future health of the population. This can be accomplished by requiring vaccinations before children are allowed to enter school or by increasing the availability of rural health care services, rather than by providing only more information about the services in each case. Public health nurses can play an important role in providing both the information and the services.

The policy decisions are interrelated but separate. There may be a governmental/public health role for encouraging individuals to invest more in their health. The key questions are: How much needs to be spent to encourage individuals to invest in their health? How much does this change an individual's health investment behavior? How much does this change an individual's health in the long run? This set of considerations is the basis for a cost-benefit or cost-effectiveness analysis of government programs to encourage individuals to invest more in their health, while leaving the ultimate decision to the individual. A separate policy question is whether the government should mandate that individuals invest in their health. One example of this type of policy is requiring children to have a set of vaccinations before they are allowed to attend school. This is critical because individuals who do not get vaccinations are more likely to get the conditions that the vaccinations are intended to prevent and more likely to spread the condition to other children.

The combination of these ideas can be used to motivate an economic policy analysis. Economists provide a logical interpretation of each of the complex determinants of health investments and how the set of determinants might work together. For example, individuals who care about the future more may be less responsive to changes in the out-of-pocket costs for flu vaccinations or cancer screening or time required to obtain preventive services. Economic theory can be used to generate hypotheses, suggest relevant policy interventions, and help with the interpretation. Economics is not the only lens for interpreting policy. As mentioned earlier, economics provides a consistent paradigm that can be applied to all types of prevention and all types of health care utilization in order to end up with an efficient, if not equitable, use of society's money and time, but other considerations are important.

EXTERNALITIES

As mentioned earlier, **externalities** represent outcomes or side effects of an action or behavior of an individual or firm that affect others without their consent. These side effects can be either positive or negative. Common public health-related externalities change risks. For example, positive externalities result from individuals getting flu shots that then decrease the risk of the individual getting influenza and decrease the risk of those around them getting influenza. Negative externalities often change environmental risks. Firms may produce waste that ends up in a stream or smog that ends up in the air. Individuals who smoke put others at risk through secondhand smoke. Positive and negative externalities will be discussed in turn.

Positive Externalities

As mentioned, influenza vaccinations provide an example of positive externalities. Economists expect that individuals making decisions about whether to obtain influenza vaccinations will primarily consider his or her own health. It is possible that an individual will feel that the risk of influenza is small or perceive that influenza is unlikely to be serious and decide not to get a flu shot. In spite of this, it is possible that others will benefit from a person getting a flu shot as they are less at risk.

When an individual does not perceive the benefits to others and is given no incentive to consider the benefits to others, insufficient quantities of goods and services with positive externalities will be produced or consumed. Figure 8-2 shows a situation where the demand curve (which is also a measure of the individual marginal benefit of each person consuming a flu shot) is below the societal marginal benefit curve. The point at which societal marginal benefit is equal to supply (point *B*) represents a greater quantity of flu shots than the point at which individual marginal benefit is equal to the supply (point *A*).

A policy that gives individuals an incentive to obtain goods and services that produce positive externalities can be implemented. In this case, Medicare pays for older adults to obtain influenza vaccinations. Many employers provide free flu shots for their employees. Economic analysis of these incentives provided by government and employers will focus on how many more people get flu shots with the adjusted incentives than would if they had to pay all costs themselves. Those opposed to the policy might ask if resources are being used to give flu shots to individuals who would have gotten them anyway. This would then represent a change in who pays without bringing about any extra benefit.

Negative Externalities

Smoking is a classic negative externality. The visual depiction of this negative externality would be different from that shown in Figure 8-2 because the societal marginal benefit would be below the individual marginal benefit rather than above it. In this case, the socially optimal amount of smoking is less than the individually optimal amount. This is based on the assumption that

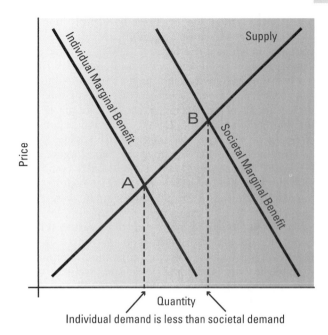

Figure 8-2 Supply and demand with positive externalities.

individuals who smoke may not consider how their behavior negatively affects others' well-being.

The government also has a role in discouraging behaviors that impose negative externalities. A common way to do this is to impose a tax. In theory, the tax should be used to provide care for those on whom the negative externality is imposed, although the end

⊕ PRACTICE APPLICATION

Cost versus Benefit

Medicare covers not only influenza vaccinations but other preventive services as well. Many older adults who are covered by Medicare were receiving these services before Medicare paid for them. Even though the life years (or quality adjusted life years) gained for the money spent may be favorable, a key question is whether the government should be paying for everyone's potential increase in health. A key question for the government is how much the health of those who were not getting the preventive services already (cancer screening in particular) will change

as a result of Medicare paying for the benefit. The impact of preventive health care services on the health of these individuals, on their families, and on society would have to be larger than the impact on the individuals who were already receiving services for the program to be just as cost-effective as covering both individuals who would pay for themselves and individuals who did not receive the services previously. Alternatively, society may simply make a choice to provide this type of care for Medicare enrollees based on other, noneconomic criteria.

result is rarely that simple. Taxes have been found to have a negative effect on smoking, particularly among younger individuals (Liang et al. 2003; Murphy et al 2003). Having public health nurses involved in smoking cessation programs might be an appropriate use of resources if the money spent on this type of intervention generates a sufficient decrease in smoking behavior, especially among adolescents and young adults, in comparison with what the nurses must be paid.

One interesting and controversial paper argued that the taxes that smokers were paying when combined with the decrease in Medicare and Social Security payments for smokers who die prematurely were high enough to offset all externalities (Viscusi, 1994). Public health nurses are likely to find this conclusion troubling, but the key is to understand that this reflects a researcher's use of the logic of economics. Economists examine incentives and behaviors and compare costs and benefits. Not all economists agree on the exact measures of costs and benefits. Public health nursing leaders who use economic analysis need to know that nearly every economic analysis includes assumptions that may or may not be realistic, and that the assumptions that are used can affect the conclusions that are drawn. For example, when assessing the impact of smoking, assumptions have to be made about the economic value of the life of the smoker and the lives of those around them. Economists make assumptions trying to develop objective measures of the values, even though others may feel that the outcomes for nonsmokers should be given more weight as they are not bringing the adverse health effects on themselves.

The first step in using the results is to understand that there are assumptions and to identify them. The second step is to know to ask an expert to help with understanding the assumptions and uncovering the assumptions that may not be noticed by nonexperts. Professional economic expertise is useful before using economic evaluation to draw conclusions about policy options that are being considered.

DECISIONS UNDER UNCERTAINTY

Most of the discussion to this point has focused on decisions not considering uncertainty. Health insurance is a topic clearly motivated by uncertainty about health in the future. It is worth considering what insurance does; how it affects the quantity of medical care demanded;

and the relationship between insurance, health care subsidies, and health care financing more generally.

A key policy of interest to public health nurses is the State Children's Health Insurance Program or S-CHIP. This program provides extended access to affordable health insurance for children with relatively low incomes who were not eligible for Medicaid (Bronstein, Adams, & Florence, Adams, & Florence, 2004). Providing children who do not have health insurance with health insurance increases the demand for medical care. Medical care includes both routine well-child visits and immunizations and unexpected services when a child comes down with an infection. This results in subsidizing care for the child. At a lower price, the child (or his parents on his behalf) will demand more care. In other words, there is movement downward along the demand curve. An economist would interpret this as increasing the quantity of care demanded, but public health experts would likely interpret it simply as ensuring access to care. This leads to the discussion of an important distinction between subsidizing care at the time of using it (which this program is doing for all types of medical care) and insurance as it was originally defined in the economic literature.

Health insurance in the United States was originally created to pay for unexpected, high-cost, or catastrophic services. Preventive services were not covered. Individuals had fairly high deductibles. Today, most of the public views catastrophic insurance as minimal insurance rather than the most appropriate type of insurance as standard economic theory would suggest.

There is a sound economic argument for catastrophic health insurance. Individuals trying to maximize their utility over time will inherently want to have as similar a level of consumption of health and nonhealth goods over time as possible. This might not occur because accidents and unexpected negative health events (i.e., heart attacks) lead to a large consumption of medical care for uninsured individuals and prevent them from paying for other goods and services they need. For insurance to function, individuals or organizations pay a premium to an insurer. The insurer spreads the risk over a population so that when a subset of the individuals suffers a loss (becomes sick), the insurer can pay for the loss (the health care in this case). Since catastrophic health care expenditures tend to occur unexpectedly (viewed over a lifetime) and tend to involve nondiscretionary spending, they can be insured in the traditional economic sense.

Many economic models of demand for health insurance assume that the insurer collects just enough premiums to pay off all the claims, but this is not exactly how the market functions. Health insurers need staff to collect claims, pay health care providers and hospitals, verify claims, and undertake the many other functions that insurers are fulfilling in the health care system. This means that the insurer needs to collect more than enough money to pay the claims. A for-profit insurer will not only collect money to staff the company but also will collect money that will end up in shareholders' pockets. Collecting more than enough money to pay off claims at a population level also implies that the insurer must collect more from each individual than his expected expenditure.

Some individuals are willing to pay more to the insurer than the average amount that a person in the population will spend. For catastrophic expenditures, this is clear. An individual may spend nothing most of the time, but the one year in which he comes down with a serious illness, he will have very little money left to spend on anything else or may go into debt if uninsured. As long as the premium is not too much higher than the expected expenditure, it will still make economic sense for the person to pay for the insurance rather than run the risk of very high medical care expenditures if he gets sick.

Other types of health care that traditional economic theory would not suggest should be insured are either predictable or discretionary. For example, dental x-rays and mammograms are services that are recommended for an individual at regular intervals. In theory, an individual or family could set aside the money to pay for the services themselves. The individual would only have to pay for the cost of the service and not the cost plus an insurer's markup.

The exclusion of preexisting conditions is also clearly economically motivated. An insurer, knowing that a client has a given condition (i.e. diabetes), knows that this client will be expected to cost much more and will either charge a higher premium, not cover services associated with that condition, or refuse to offer insurance coverage at all.

S-CHIP, and much health insurance in general in the United States, provides an insurance mechanism and subsidizes predictable, discretionary care for a segment of the population. S-CHIP is tax funded, while private insurance is often funded by premiums paid in part by the employer. One reason the government or an employer might be interested in subsidizing care as well as providing an insurance mechanism is to maximize the health of society (or employees and their families) so that the members of society (or the employees) can be as productive as possible. However, if this were the primary reason, a greater emphasis on preventive rather than curative services would be expected.

Insurance mechanisms and care subsidization are two different policy issues with two sets of economic incentives, although they are rarely discussed separately. Considering the two sets of economic incentives separately would make the discussion more transparent because individuals would better understand what is truly uncertain and can be insured against and what the society must simply decide it would like to subsidize. Public health nursing, with its focus on populations at risk, has an interest in monitoring societal decisions about health care financing through processes of subsidization or insurance.

ECONOMIC EVALUATION

This part of the chapter will deal specifically with two types of economic evaluation, cost-benefit analysis and cost-effectiveness analysis. Here, economic evaluation will refer to these two types of analyses.

Cost-Benefit Analysis

Of all the methods of economic evaluation, **cost-benefit analysis** is most closely tied to economic theory. Cost-benefit analysis compares the costs of an intervention with the dollar value of the benefits. These analyses are designed to place a monetary value on all resources being used in an intervention or to implement a policy. They also place a dollar value on all outcomes of an intervention or policy change. In health care, sometimes these analyses are disliked because they require time, preferences for health states, and an attempt to place a dollar value on life. However, cost-benefit analyses are often used in environmental health, and the technique of placing a dollar value on an individual's life is also used in legal proceedings; the technique remains preferred by some economists (Kenkel, 1997). Cost-benefit analyses can be used to evaluate policy changes, community-level interventions, or individual treatment.

An example of a nursing and public health cost-benefit analysis is the study of the net benefits that result from an intervention to increase the duration of breastfeeding among low-income mothers (Pugh et al., 2002). An intervention team consisting of a public health nurse and a peer counselor was assigned to each low-income mother. The intervention team provided in-hospital support for breast feeding, home visits, and telephone contact for up to six months. Costs included salaries, staff transportation, breast pumps and other supplies, and administrative costs to run the program. Any formula provided by Women, Infants, and Children (WIC) or purchased by anyone for the infant was also incorporated into the cost-benefit analysis, as savings on formula is an important aspect of breastfeeding. From the perspective of all society's resources, the amount of time spent by anyone involved in the feeding must also be valued. Time, as mentioned earlier, is a scarce resource that is being used to provide nutrition for the infant. Breastfeeding is likely to take a similar amount of time as formula feeding, although the distribution of the time among different individuals will certainly be different. Time is sometimes valued by using either a wage specific to the person whose time is being allocated or more often at present using an average for similar individuals (often grouped by gender and age).

The resources detailed here describe only those that are being used to educate and support the mother and provide nutrition to the child. When the intervention is implemented, the dollar value of the resources used for these purposes may be greater than the dollar value of the resources that were used prior to the intervention. The value of the public health nurse and peer counselor's time is likely to be large when they have other work-related duties.

A basic cost-benefit analysis for this study would determine whether the savings on formula and health care (perhaps for the first year of the child's life) are greater than the resources that are being spent to promote longer breastfeeding among low-income women. This analysis is limited in a number of ways. The amount of savings on formula and health care compared to a situation without the intervention will be a function of a number of parameters including the amount of time that the low-income women would have breastfed without the intervention, the number of mothers who breastfeed longer, the average change in breastfeeding duration among those who breastfeed longer, and the difference that longer breastfeeding makes in the consumption of formula and the use of the health care system. If the local low-income population were already breastfeeding for a relatively long dura-

tion, the difference that could be made by any intervention is likely to be small. If many mothers increase the duration of breastfeeding, but each mother increases by only one week, this will have a different effect on formula- and health-care-related outcomes than if a smaller number of mothers increase their breastfeeding by eight weeks. However, the average increase could be the same. For children in low-income families who do not have as healthy environmental conditions as children in higher income families, breastfeeding may be more likely to help them to remain healthy. In particular, all children who are breastfed (and especially children in low-income families) are likely to have fewer infections. This will result in fewer visits to health care providers and an associated monetary savings.

An economist analyzing the situation prior to conducting a cost-benefit analysis is likely to focus on questions regarding how the intervention involving a public health nurse and peer counselor will affect the constraints faced by the mothers. Similar to the way in which a mother must decide on whether and how much to invest in her own health, a mother must also make the same decisions about her infant's health. A mother may choose not to breastfeed because she has too many other tasks that need to be taken care of and she has no support because the only support that others are willing to provide is making formula for and feeding the infant rather than performing other household chores. A mother faced with competing demands on the scarce resource of her time has to decide how to allocate her time to maximize her health, her infant's health, and the welfare of the remainder of the household. Thus, no matter how much health benefit there is for the child, the mother may choose to stop breastfeeding sooner than is recommended because of other demands on her time that lead to outcomes that she considers at least as important for her and her family.

Cost-benefit analysis is important because there are many potential uses of resources. Society has to decide how much to invest in mothers and their children in order to promote positive outcomes that will be helpful not only for the mothers but also for others in society (i.e.. there are positive externalities associated with having healthy mothers and healthy children). Increasing breastfeeding duration is only one way to use nurses to invest in these mothers and children.

Cost-benefit analysis is limited because an analysis of one intervention for one population does not necessarily generalize to other populations of provid-

Pediatric Eye Examination

Public health pediatric ophthalmology has captured the attention of policy makers in several states as regulations are being or have been developed to require eye exams before a child can enter school. There has been some discussion of requiring gold standard exams for each child, although it is commonly recognized that this may be impossible given the relatively limited number of pediatric-focused eye care professionals. Public health nurses have an opportunity to help with this public health concern either by providing screening or directing lay individuals performing the screening. Consider the relative costs and differential benefits of having public health nurses screen or direct screening rather than having licensed eye care professionals perform the exam. What constraints and objectives should guide a decision on how to make policy and allocate resources for pediatric ophthalmology public health?

ers or clients. Placing a dollar value on outcomes like child development or maternal and child bonding or maternal satisfaction with breastfeeding as an experience is difficult. Finally, in economic valuation, results that occur in the distant future are given less value. Thus, a cost-benefit analysis helps to guide resource allocation considerations but should not be used as the only information on which to allocate resources and make policy.

Even if the initial intervention proves to have a positive net benefit (i.e., the monetary value of the benefits is higher than the monetary value of the costs), a decision maker might then ask whether the same results can be achieved by a less-expensive intervention team. This would involve asking both what role the peer counselor plays and what level of knowledge is necessary for the person accompanying the peer counselor. Public health nurse expertise should be allocated where it can increase social welfare the most, and there may be other more valued uses of the nurses' time or someone with less knowledge than a registered nurse might appropriately accompany a peer counselor.

Cost-Effectiveness Analysis

Cost-effectiveness analysis compares the costs of an intervention with the benefits that accrue from that intervention. A cost-effectiveness analysis is similar to a cost-benefit analysis except that it is not expected that outcomes will be valued in monetary terms. Emergency preparedness provides an interesting topic for a cost-effectiveness discussion. For some emergencies, any cost to prepare might seem warranted (i.e., preventing a dirty-bomb strike). However, resources, as always, are limited. Careful consideration of the resources being used in emergency preparedness, the risk of varying emergencies, and the life years that can be saved by being prepared for emergencies would guide a strictly economic evaluation of such programs. Alternative preparations for the spread of avian flu could be analyzed with a cost-effectiveness analysis focusing on how different systems including quarantine, treatment with antivirals, and administration of a vaccine in different locations would be associated with different costs and different numbers of cases and deaths. Alternatives would be compared to assess the extra spending required to achieve a lower number of deaths. Decision makers who do not place a monetary value on a case of avian flu (perhaps because they are unable to do so) will be left to make a decision based on whether they think it is worthwhile to spend a particular amount of money to avoid a particular number of cases of avian flu in humans.

Life years can be adjusted for the quality of life experienced rather than counting them all equally. A measure called a quality adjusted life year (QALY) summarizes the quantity and quality of life experienced by clients. This accounts for the fact that all life years may not be equally valuable (e.g., would a person rather be kept alive on life support for a long time or live for a shorter amount of time with more limited treatment). QALYs also make it easier to compare interventions to one another (e.g., one decreases morbidity, while another decreases mortality) as all studies can focus on the amount that is being spent to gain QALYs. QALYs assign a weight to each period a person has remaining in her life that is related to the quality of life she will experience. A client can never have more QALYs than total life years but can have substantially fewer QALYs than total life years if she is experiencing a rather adverse quality of life. For example, a blind individual who expects to experience ten more years of life will experience only six QALYs based on the quality of life that has been assigned to blindness. Her QALYs could be improved either by finding a way to increase her life expectancy even though she is blind or by finding a way to improve her quality of life or cure the condition that is making her blind.

All economic evaluations are based on principles similar to those discussed earlier. Choices must be made to produce interventions at the minimum cost and to maximize outcomes with the available money, client time, and personnel time.

ECONOMICS OF THE LABOR MARKET

A chapter on nursing and economic principles would not be complete without discussing the public health nurse labor market. Labor supply describes how wages relate to the number of hours of work that can be obtained. The hours of work is a function of the number of workers and how long each will work. The proper staffing of agencies requiring public health nurses is a key economic concept given a nursing shortage.

Public Health Nurse Labor Market

Organizations that train and hire public health nurses must consider the market labor supply for nurses. Each registered nurse (and every other worker) has a labor supply curve, representing the amount of labor a worker is willing to supply at a given wage. At each wage, a public health nurse is willing to supply a given amount of labor, and the quantity of labor available to the market is the sum of all labor individual nurses are willing to supply.

Labor supply curves are intuitively expected to indicate that an increasing number of hours of labor will be supplied as the wage increases. However, this expectation indicates nothing about the magnitude of the response to increasing wages. Empirical research on nursing labor supply suggests that wage changes are associated with little change in the services provided by nurses in the market (Chiha & Link, 2003).

The market of public health nurses available to work at present is of interest because of the time required to educate additional nurses. Higher wages are consistent with additional individuals deciding to become nurses (Chiha & Link, 2003). When a person decides to become a nurse, a certain amount of education and training is required. In the market for nursing education at present, there are programs ranging from 14 months to a typical four-year college education. This means that the supply of nurses is generally fixed for at least a one-year period and that any changes in policy designed to attract more nurses (e.g., an educational loan repayment program) can affect nursing supply in the long run but will not affect the supply immediately. The decision to be a public health nurse is based on lifetime expected earnings and individuals' preferences for different types of work, including the stressors and risks that individuals face and the flexibility available. Individuals are making lifetime utility-maximizing decisions when they make career choices. As the wage goes up, more individuals are expected to choose to become nurses. This will result in more hours of nursing time being available at a potentially lower wage as prices tend to go down when the supply of anything increases.

Reservation Wage

Not everyone works at every wage, and public health nurses are no different. This reflects the economic concept of a **reservation wage**. Public health nurses, similar to all workers, have many demands on their time and many things on which they need to spend money. A public health nurse may be in a situation with other income or have other responsibilities (like child care) that would also require resources if the public health nurse did not provide the services. In this case, at some relatively low wages, the public health nurse will not provide any labor services. However, at a high enough wage, it is expected that most public health nurses (and most workers in all markets) would be willing to provide some labor. The lowest wage at which a person is willing to enter the labor market at all is called the reservation wage.

Individual Motivation to Work

When public health nurses enter the labor market they are giving up time at home to provide child care, manage the home, or simply enjoy leisure. Child care may

⊕ RESEARCH APPLICATION

Is the Shortage of Hospital Registered Nurses Getting Better or Worse? Findings from Two Recent National Surveys of RNs

Study Purpose

To obtain RNs' perceptions of the current nursing shortage and its impact, their experiences in their work environment, and their career plans

Methods

The results of two recent national surveys of RNs that were conducted at a time when the nursing shortage in the United States was in full force (2002) and two years later (2004) were compared.

Findings

The findings provide a mixed assessment. On the one hand, there is evidence that the shortage has eased since 2002 and that there have been notable improvements in the lives of nurses. On the other hand, the shortage has had a negative impact on hospitals and nurses, and long-standing problems associated with the workplace environment remain.

Implications

Even though the findings suggest that the nursing shortage has eased since 2002, it has had negative impact on hospitals and nurses, and long-standing problems with the workplace environment remain. These results point to the urgency with which hospitals and nurses need to work together to improve the state of hospital nursing as only one-fifth of the RNs perceive that the current shortage will lead to improved working conditions or increased respect for nurses.

Reference

Buerhaus, P.I., Donelan, K., Ulraich, B.T., Norman, L., & Dittus, R. (2005). Is the shortage of hospital registered nurses getting better or worse? Findings from two recent national surveys of RNs. *Nursing Economics, 23*(2), 61–71, 96.

cost the same amount regardless of how much is purchased, but the values of housework and leisure are not necessarily constant. Suppose that a public health nurse was deciding whether to invest in further education and take one class or two. The public health nurse is an avid reader and someone for whom keeping a neat home living environment is very important. The first class might represent less reading time but all household chores would still get done. This would probably not be worth a large amount to the public health nurse and so he or she would be willing to take one course. If the public health nurse were then to sign up for a second course, only the reading would have to be given up. The second hour is expected to be worth a bit more than the first hour as the public health nurse is now losing more reading time. With each additional course the public health nurse might take, even more valuable reading time or home management time would be given up. As the time became more valuable, the public health nurse would have to obtain a higher return (more wages and benefits) from taking the class.

Wages also help to illustrate the economic concept of change at the margin. The extra amount that has to be paid to get the public health nurse to work another hour is usually more than just the wage needed to work the next hour. Most contracts pay the same amount per hour (at least up to a standard full-time work load). Consider the implications. The total that has to be paid to get a public health nurse to work 30 hours is 30 times the wage to work the last hour. If more per hour is required to get the public health nurse to work 40 hours, then the total 40 hours is equal to the amount worked the last hours times 40. The difference between the two is more than just the amount it cost to get the public health nurse to work the last hour times the difference in hours (10).

As the public health nurse earns more, more money will be available for leisure, but there will be less time to enjoy the leisure. If the wage were to continue to increase, public health nurses might eventually want to work fewer hours so that they could spend more time enjoying all of the goods and services that they are now able to purchase. The concept of a backward bending supply curve (i.e., first increase hours as the wage increases and then decrease hours as the wage increases) has been considered for health care providers who largely determine their own work schedule, and mixed evidence has been found (Gruber, Kim, & Mayzlin, 1999). Public health nurses may not have the option of determining their schedule to the point that they can choose to work fewer hours as the wage increases. Public health nurses in particular and non-hospital nurses in general have unfortunately been found to have lower salaries (Buerhaus & Staiger, 1996; Nickel et al., 1990).

Economics has tremendous implications for the public health nursing practice including the labor market. Public health nurses' wages are ultimately determined by a combination of labor supply, demand for nursing services, and resources available to public health agencies. Delivery of health promotion and disease prevention services is very much influenced by economics. It is vital that public health nurses have a basic understanding of economics and its influence on delivery of public health services.

CRITICAL THINKING ACTIVITIES

1. Individuals who are deciding whether to enter nursing consider both the money they will earn and the hours they will work. Even though it may be impossible to decrease the number of hours worked, describe a system that could be used to make nurses feel as though their time is less constrained by their work hours.

2. Public health nurses are often involved in interventions to promote health investments. Describe the costs of a public health program to increase the number of clients with diabetes who are monitoring their blood sugar properly. Discuss the benefits of such an intervention. Which benefits have obvious monetary value? For which benefits would it seem simpler to leave the results in terms of a health measure?

3. Consider a not-for-profit agency that is sponsoring a community-health visitation program with no reimbursement. What might the organization's objective be? If the organization has the money to expand, describe how it should choose which resources to employ.

4. Describe the reason that many insurers historically did not cover annual physical examinations. Why might the government want to enhance financial access to annual physicals? Why might the government choose to mandate that insurers cover such services? Would everyone necessarily benefit from a strictly economic perspective?

KEY TERMS

allocative efficiency	fixed costs	technical efficiency
at the margin	marginal benefit	technical rate of substitution
cost-benefit analysis	opportunity cost	uncertainty
cost-effectiveness analysis	preference	utility
discount rate	profit	variable costs
economics	quality adjusted life year (QALY)	
externality	reservation wage	

KEY CONCEPTS

- For-profit organizations are expected to want to maximize profits. Not-for-profit organizations may have a different set of objectives. Both types of organizations have an incentive to produce whatever they produce at minimum cost in order to achieve as much of the objective as possible.

- Investment in health can be motivated by at least two economic arguments: experiencing positive health outcomes is a desired goal by itself, or experiencing positive health outcomes is desirable because it allows the individual to produce more at home or in the workplace.

- Positive externalities provide benefits to individuals other than the buyer of service or the seller of a service; vaccinations are one example. Negative externalities impose costs on individuals other than the buyer and seller of a service; second-hand smoke is an example.

- Public health nurses must make decisions under uncertainty. The economic approach to these decisions uses a population approach that focuses on the expected likelihood of events. Decisions must be made based on what is expected to happen within a population.

- Cost-benefit and cost-effectiveness analysis can be used to help with resource allocation, providing a logically consistent and structured set of data. Cost-effectiveness analysis is most appropriate when the final outcomes are difficult to translate into quality of life or dollar figures.

- The nurse labor market is characterized by a shortage in some dimensions. The deficiency may be because the demanders for services do not pay what would be required to bring the supplies to the market to provide as much as is demanded because the suppliers of the services have other alternatives or because the suppliers of services expect more flexibility than the demands for services are willing to allow.

REFERENCES

Bronstein, J.M., Adams, E.K., & Florence, C.S. (2004). The impact of S-CHIP enrollment on physician participation in Medicaid in Alabama and Georgia. *Health Services Research, 39*(2), 301–317.

Buerhaus, P.I., Donelan, K., Ulraich, B.T., Norman, L., & Dittus, R. (2005). Is the shortage of hospital registered nurses getting better or worse? Findings from two recent national surveys of RNs. *Nursing Economics, 23*(2), 61–71, 96.

Buerhaus, P.I., & Staiger, D.O. (1996). Managed care and the nurse workforce. *JAMA, 276*(18), 1487–1493.

Buerhaus, P.I., Staiger, D.O., & Auerbach, D.I. (2000). Why are shortages of hospital RNs concentrated in specialty care units? *Nursing Economics, 18*(3), 111–116.

Buerhaus, P.I., Staiger, D.O., & Auerbach, D.I. (2004). New signs of a strengthening U.S. nurse labor market? *Health Aff (Millwood),* Suppl Web Exclusives, W4-526–533.

Chiha, Y.A., & Link, C.R. (2003). The shortage of registered nurses and some new estimates of the effects of wages on registered nurses labor supply: A look at the past and a preview of the 21st century. *Health Policy, 64*(3), 349–375.

Cimiottoi, J., Stone, P.W., & Larson, E.L. (2004). A cost comparison of hand hygiene regimens. *Nursing Economics 22*(4), 196–199, 204, 175.

Farsi, M., & Filippini, M. (2004). An empirical analysis of cost efficiency in non-profit and public nursing homes. *Annals of Public and Cooperative Economics, 75*(3), 339–365.

Grossman, M. (1972). On the concept of health capital and the demand for health. *Journal of Political Economy, 80*(2), 223–255.

Gruber, J., Kim, J., & Mayzlin, D. (1999). Physician fees and procedure intensity: The case of cesarean delivery. *Journal of Health Economics, 18*(4), 473–490.

Heyes, A. (2005). The economics of vocation or 'why is a badly paid nurse a good nurse'? *Journal of Health Economics, 24*(3), 561–569.

Hoerger, T.J. (1991). 'Profit' variability in for-profit and not-for-profit hospitals. *Journal of Health Economic, 10*(3), 259–289.

Hutchins, S.S., Rosenthal, J., Eason, P., Swint, E., Guerrero, H., & Hadler, S. (1999). Effectiveness and cost-effectiveness of linking the special supplemental program for women, infants, and children (WIC) and immunization activities. *Journal of Public Health Policy, 20*(4), 408–426.

Kenkel, D.S. (1991). Health behavior, health knowledge, and schooling. *Journal of Political Economy, 99*(2), 287–305.

Kenkel, D. (1997). On valuing morbidity, cost-effectiveness analysis, and being rude. *Journal of Health Economics, 16*(6), 749–757.

Leone, A.J., & Van Horn, R.L. (2005). How do nonprofit hospitals manage earnings? *Journal of Health Economics, 24*(4), 815–837.

Liang, L., Chaloupka, F., Nichter, M., & Clayton, R. (2003). Prices, policies and youth smoking, May 2001. *Addiction, 98* Suppl 1, 105–122.

Lien, D.S., & Evans, W.N. (2005). Estimating the impact of large cigarette tax hikes: The case of maternal smoking and infant birth weight. *Journal of Human Resources, 40*(2), 373–392.

Lune, H. (2002). Weathering the storm: Nonprofit organization survival strategies in a hostile climate. *Nonprofit and Voluntary Sector Quarterly, 31*(4), 463–483.

Murphy, J.M., Shelley, D., Repetto, P.M., Cummings, K.M., & Mahoney, M.C. (2003). Impact of economic policies on reducing tobacco use among Medicaid clients in New York. *Preventive Medicine, 37*(1), 68–70.

Newhouse, J.P. (1970). Toward a theory of nonprofit institutions: An economic model of a hospital. *American Economic Review, 60*(1), 64–74.

Nicholson, W. (2004). *Intermediate microeconomics and its applications* (5th ed.). Mason, OH: South-Western Educational Publishing.

Nickel, J.T., Thomas, G.M., Eastman, M.A., Holton, J.D., & Skuly, R.H. (1990). Public health nurse salaries: Associations with nurse, agency, and community characteristics. *Public Health Nursing. 7*(3), 181–189.

Pugh, L.C., Milligan, R.A., Frick, K.D., Spatz, D., & Bronner, Y. (2002). Breastfeeding duration, costs, and benefits of a support program for low-income breastfeeding women, *Birth, 29*(2), 95–100.

Retzlaff-Roberts, D., Chang, C.F., & Rubin, R.M. (2004). Technical efficiency in the use of health care resources: a comparison of OECD countries. *Health Policy, 69*(1), 55–72

Roblin, D.W., Howard, D.H., Becker, E.R., Adams, E.K., & Roberts, M.H. (2004). Use of midlevel practitioners to achieve labor cost savings in the primary care practice of an MCO. *Health Services Research, 39*(3), 607–626.

Samandar, R., Kleefield, S., Hammel, J., Mehta, M., & Crone, R. (2001). Privately funded quality health care in India: A sustainable and equitable model. *International Journal of Quality Health Care, 13*(4), 283–288.

Shields, M.A. (2004). Addressing nurse shortages: What can policy makers learn from the econometric evidence on nurse labour supply? *Economic Journal, 114*(499), F464–498.

Spetz, J. (2002). The value of education in a licensed profession: The choice of associate or baccalaureate degrees in nursing. *Economics of Education Review, 21*(1), 73–85.

Tuckman, H.P., & Chang, C.F. (1988). Cost convergence between for-profit and not-for-profit nursing homes: Does competition matter? *Quarterly Review of Economics & Business, 28*(4):50–65.

Varian, H.R. (1992). *Microeconomic analysis* (3rd ed.). New York: W.N. Norton & Company.

Viscusi, W.P. (1994). *Cigarette taxation and the social consequences of smoking.* National Bureau of Economic Research, BER Working Papers 4891.

BIBLIOGRAPHY

Clarke, P.M. (1998). Cost-benefit analysis and mammographic screening: A travel cost approach. *Journal of Health Economics, 17*(6), 767–787.

Folland, S., Goodman, A.C., & Stano, M. (2003). *The economics of health and healthcare* (4th ed.). Prentice Hall: Upper Saddle River, NJ.

Feldstein, P.J. (2004). *Health care economics,* Delmar Series in Health Services Administration (6th ed.). Thomson Delmar Learning: Clifton Park, NY.

Haddix, A., Teursch, S.M., & Coso, P.S. (2002). *Prevention effectiveness: A guide to decisions analysis and economic evaluation* (2nd ed.). New York: Oxford University Press.

Phelps, C.E. (2002). *Health economics* (3rd ed.). Addison Wesley: Boston, MA.

Yoo, B.K., & Frick, K. (2005). Determinants of influenza vaccination timing. *Health Economics, 14*(8), 777–791.

RESOURCES

International Health Economics Association (iHEA)

902-461-4432

Web: http://www.healtheconomics.org

This is the Web site of one of the largest international organization's specifically for health economists. This organization interprets economics quite widely, focusing both on evaluation and on using economic theory to explain individual behaviors and organizational decisions related to health. The Web site is largely aimed at health economics professionals, but it includes several items of interest to those with only an interest in health economics rather than only professionals. In particular, the Web site lists conferences, books, and educational opportunities related to health economics.

International Society for Pharmaco-economics and Outcomes Research (USA)

Email: info@ispor.org

Web: http://www.ispor.org

This Web site is the home page of one of the premier organizations supporting professionals whose business is economic evaluation. The word "Pharmacoeconomics" in the title suggests that this organization focuses largely on the evaluation of pharmaceutical products, but this is not the organization's exclusive focus. This Web site lists upcoming conferences, has links to lists of requirements for economic evaluations that have been put forward in different countries, and includes an "educator's tool kit" that lists several books that may be of interest to those learning about pharmacoeconomics and economic evaluation more generally.

Society for Medical Decision Making

100 North 20th Street, 4th floor
Philadelphia, Pennsylvania 19103
215-545-7697
FAX: 215-564-2175
Email: smdm-office@lists.smdm.org

Web: http://www.smdm.org

This is the Web site for a smaller organization focusing on medical decision making broadly. Health economics is only one aspect of medical decision making. The Web site includes education modules that are likely to be of interest to those with limited experience in the area. In particular, there is a list of academic departments with some level of interest in medical decision making. The Web site also includes educational modules, but only members of the organization can access them.

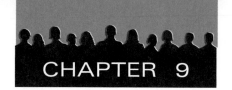

CHAPTER 9

Challenges of Global Health

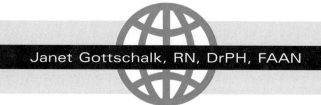

Janet Gottschalk, RN, DrPH, FAAN

Chapter Outline

⊕ Global Health Defined

⊕ Challenges for Public Health Nurses in the Global Arena
  Global Nursing Shortage
  Shortage of Public Health Nurses in the United States
  Need for a Global Perspective

⊕ Global Efforts in Providing Health Care
  "Health For All" and the World Health Organization
  The People's Health Assembly
  Corporate Globalization
  Human Rights and Public Health Nursing
  United Nations Covenants
  The World Social Forum
  The Millennium Development Goals
  The United States and the Millennium Development Goals

⊕ Public Health Nurses' Response to Challenges in Global Health

Learning Objectives

Upon completion of this chapter, the reader will be able to:

1. Understand the concept of global health and its relationship to public health nursing.

2. Analyze the human rights framework of the United Nations and its application to public health in related documents and covenants.

3. Describe the various UN and civil society organizations relevant to public health nursing with a global perspective.

4. Describe public health nursing and its challenges from a global perspective.

This chapter will present global health from the perspective of a public health nurse active in global health and human rights. The reader will be challenged to critique national and international treaties and covenants for their influence on global health. In addition, the reader will gain an understanding of the role of social justice and human rights in public health nurse practice at the local, national, and global levels.

GLOBAL HEALTH DEFINED

The terms "global" and "globalization" are often used in daily conversation, but many find it difficult to explain their exact meaning. Global, perhaps the easier term to define, immediately brings to mind the big, round globe in classrooms that identified countries and oceans. Today, with continual political and economic changes, many major boundaries have been revised, and it is almost impossible to produce globes that are not immediately out of date.

Geography, once a relatively simple subject for North American children, was taught from the perspective of persons living in the western hemisphere. As the United States became more involved in other countries, especially through wars and military alliances, U.S. citizens became familiar with the names, if not the peoples, of South East Asia: Korea, Vietnam, Indonesia, the Philippines, and perhaps even India and Pakistan.

During the 1980s, events in nearby countries such as El Salvador, Guatemala, Honduras, Nicaragua, and Cuba made Americans aware of peoples and places geographically near, but socially and culturally many miles away. With the fall of the Berlin Wall in 1989 and the almost cataclysmic transformations in Eastern Europe and the former Soviet Republics, Americans were beset with a multitude of new countries such as Kazakhstan, Uzbekistan, and Chechnya. During the 1990s, the horror of drought, famine, the HIV/AIDS epidemic, and the seemingly endless wars in sub-Saharan Africa brought nightly television reports of refugees from countries most had never heard of and probably could not locate on a map: Rwanda, Burundi, the Sudan, Ethiopia, Eritrea, Botswana, and Angola. More recently, Americans have begun to learn the names and locations of many Persian Gulf states—many little more than kingdoms of vast deserts, but kingdoms nonetheless, rich in oil and millions of citizens practicing Islam, a religion with many branches and theologies.

Such is the globe of today—a world of more than 200 nations with 6.4 billion people and growing rapidly (UN Population Fund Report, 2004). It is a world where nearly 10 million children under the age of 5 die each year from "preventable diseases," according to Carol Bellamy, the United Nations Childrens Fund's (UNICEF's) executive director (*The Baltimore Sun*, Associated Press, 12/6/04), and more than 580,000 women die each year in childbirth or from maternal health-related problems (Poplin, 2005a). It is a complex world, often frightening and puzzling; it is filled with unnecessary suffering, but also with enormous promise and hope if people can learn to live and work interdependently, with mutual respect, and seek growth, understanding, health, and happiness for all.

Until the past few decades, health was thought of biologically and quantified negatively as the absence of death, disease, and disability. While public health was for most of the twentieth century a respected subspecialty, health care predominantly focused on the individual client. In recent years, however, it has become widely accepted that social, economic, and political issues are essential determinants, not only of a person's health but also of communities' and nations' health. Today, this concept has been expanded to the point that it is possible to speak of the health of our entire globe in the same terms. One definition of health that includes a global perspective is:

> Health is a social, economic and political issue, and above all a fundamental human right (for all nations and peoples). Inequality, poverty, exploitation, violence and injustice are at the root of ill-health and the deaths of poor and marginalized people. Health for all means that powerful interests have to be challenged, that some forms of globalization have to be opposed. And that political and economic priorities have to be drastically changed. (People's Health Movement, 2000)

The term globalization describes the context in which global health takes place. Globalization is defined as the "process of increasing economic, political, and social independence and integration as capital, goods, persons, concepts, images, ideas, and values cross state boundaries" (Yach and Bettcher, 1998, p. 735).

CHALLENGES FOR PUBLIC HEALTH NURSES IN THE GLOBAL ARENA

Public health nurses are faced with numerous challenges in the global arena. These challenges are exacerbated by the shortage of nurses and especially public health nurses. An understanding of these challenges is necessary as public health nurses begin to work in the global arena.

Global Nursing Shortage

Nurses practice in this world of complex interactions between nations, intergovernmental and nongovernmental organizations and transnational corporations. One of the major challenges in global health today is the fact that in many parts of the world, there is an acute and growing shortage of nursing personnel. Areas such as sub-Saharan Africa and parts of Asia that are suffering from the ravages of HIV/AIDS, wars, drought, poor economies, and refugee dislocations are especially lacking in nurses. Even in countries such as the Philippines, which educates thousands of nurses annually, there is insufficient funding to employ the educated nurses for the country's needs. As a consequence, growing numbers of well-qualified nursing personnel are migrating to richer countries, leaving nursing positions unfilled in their home countries.

Shortage of Public Health Nurses in the United States

Similar shortages exist in the United States, and even with the many foreign-trained nurses who are now working in the United States. An Expert Panel of the American Academy of Nursing warns that the current undersupply of nurses in the United States will reach 800,000 by 2020 (AAN, 2004). In this increasingly critical situation, U.S. nurses are routinely faced with stressful work environments, greater numbers of acutely ill patients, unsafe workplace conditions, frequent mandatory overtime, and all too often, burnout.

In addition, the U.S. public health care system is in disrepair and lacks sufficient health professionals, especially well-educated public health nurses, for even routine epidemiological surveillance, let alone the ability to respond quickly to new and emerging disease and terrorist threats. Those who live in or near major cities are only too aware of how unprepared the United States is to cope with possible biochemical attacks. A few anthrax spores were able to shut down the U.S. government temporarily, terrify the residents of the Washington, D.C., metropolitan area, and close a major postal facility for more than a year. The debacle in 2004–2005, related to the U.S. shortage of flu vaccine and the government's inability to provide an adequate supply for persons at high risk raises the question: How can U.S. public health nurses be concerned about global health when local communities are so much in need?

⊕ POLICY HIGHLIGHT

Global Nursing Shortage

A global nursing shortage is having adverse affects on health care systems around the world and is challenging nursing's ability to meet clients' needs. The shortage is especially critical in countries with growing elderly populations. Nursing shortages in hospitals have been correlated with increased mortality, adverse postoperative events, and nurses' dissatisfaction with working conditions. The International Council of Nurses (ICN) organized a major initiative to address the shortage.

The initiative is organized into priority areas of policy intervention, macroeconomics and health sector funding, workforce planning and policy, positive practice environments, retention and recruitment, and nursing leadership. To meet these initiatives, nurses in the ICN have held high-level consultations with key stakeholders in government positions, are planning a positive workplace campaign across the globe, and are lobbying for safer, healthier workplaces.

⊕ PRACTICE APPLICATION

Nurses in Border Communities

Public health nurses working in border communities can practice public health nursing from a global perspective. Public health nurses in Laredo, Texas, a border town divided from its sister-city, Nuevo Laredo, Mexico, only by a bridge across the Rio Grande have to deal with multiple causes of ill health and disease. Some clients are undocumented immigrants who had to enter the United States illegally in order to earn enough to support their families. Most come from rural areas where trade agreements such as the North American Free Trade Agreement (NAFTA) have caused the destruction of their farms. Many live in colonies on the U.S. side of the river without adequate sewage or potable water. Because of their illegal status and their fear of deportation, many are afraid to use community health or educational services. Consequently, public health nurses in Laredo are frequent participants in city council meetings and need to be actively involved in immigration issues at the local, state, and national levels.

Need for a Global Perspective

Tempting as it might be to turn away from the thousands of starving and ill persons in the world to concentrate on the immediate local problems, U.S. public health nurses need to understand the concept of one world. Although U.S. public health nurses may not physically travel to other countries, the inextricable linkages through technology, banking systems, geopolitics, food, clothing, and, most especially, global systems of trade and investment cannot be ignored. The consequences of these growing linkages can be seen in every Wal-Mart and Home Depot, in every U.S. town and rural area. They can also be seen in the many manufacturing industries and businesses, long the mainstay of local growth and development, which have closed their doors completely or "outsourced" many of their operations, leaving entire areas with high unemployment, cutbacks in social and educational services, and serious questions about the future.

⊕ RESEARCH APPLICATION

Developing Political Competence: A Comparative Study across Disciplines

Study Purpose
To investigate nursing students' and political science students' understanding of political activism

Methods
Cross-sectional comparative study using qualitative data

Findings
For nursing students, several themes emerged that included public policy as a barrier and their not understanding the relationships among personal, professional, and political. Political science students were able to articulate theory and public policy.

Implications
"The data suggest a need for interdisciplinary dialogue, faculty modeling of political competence, opportunities for students to realize personal, professional, and political connections, and a concern of socialization in the context of global citizenship."

Reference
Rains, J.W., & Kriese, P.B. (2001). Developing political competence: A comparative study across disciplines. *Public Health Nursing, 18*(4), 219–224.

⊕ RESEARCH APPLICATION

Health Care Access: A Consumer Perspective

Study Purpose

To investigate factors limiting access from the consumers' perspective; to use action research as an information base for policy formulation by a collaborative partnership

Methods

Mailed surveys were sent to 475 residents. Ninety-seven participants were recruited and participated in 12 focus group sessions.

Findings

Access to numerous health care services was found to be a problem, with low-cost dental and mental health services named most frequently. The major barriers were cost of

services, length of time to get an appointment, lack of understanding from health care providers, and time off work.

Implications

The findings provide consumer input on access to health care services that provides policy makers and health care organizations with information on how to improve access.

Reference

Higgs, Z.R., Bayne, T., & Murphy, D. (2001). Health care access: A consumer perspective. *Public Health Nursing 18*(1), 3–12.

Even though some aspects of economic globalization are having negative effects on parts of the U.S. economy, they are, at the same time, providing much needed opportunities for future growth and development in other parts of the world. However, many of the people who are suffering today as a result of poverty, lack of human rights, religious fanaticism, and often the greed and lust for power of their national and tribal leaders are unwilling to wait for some future alleviation of their poverty and suffering. Should they have to wait? Do health and well-being for others mean increasing unemployment, less education, and fewer social services for Americans?

In the midst of these questions and global turmoil, can U.S. public health nurses continue to focus their practice only on those persons and institutions in their localities? Even if it were possible to close one's eyes to the suffering of the rest of the world, the multiple links among humanity on this rapidly spinning globe does not allow this to occur. What can and should U.S. public health nurses do to make their nursing practice global? How can nurses become committed to global health? Where will they find allies in the struggle for health for all? Who will help build a world of peace based on justice for all? The answers to these questions

lie in the expansion of public health nursing to include a global perspective.

GLOBAL EFFORTS IN PROVIDING HEALTH CARE

A global perspective in public health nursing includes understanding the treaties, declarations, and covenants that impact the lives of all those living in the global community. Understanding the impact of these documents will provide public health nurses with the information needed to become activists and community advocates for improving global health.

"Health For All" and the World Health Organization

Concerned public health professionals have been trying for decades to do something about the desperate plight of so many millions. More than twenty years ago, the nations of the world, called together by the World Health Organization (WHO) and UNICEF, met in Alma Ata, Russia, and issued a call for "Health For All the people of the world by the year 2000." In 1978, at the time of the declaration, such a goal seemed achievable, and primary health care (PHC) was considered to be "the key" to attaining health for all (WHO, 1978). Many nations, especially poorer nations that are today called the Global South, took the goal very seriously, and for a number of years great efforts were made. A few nations, such as the United States, unfortunately continued to develop more sophisticated and expensive health care technologies that have ultimately only made health care a commodity and not a right. Filled with optimism, many nations even spoke seriously at that time of a New International Economic Order that would eventually remedy the wealth and technology gaps between the Global North (the richer countries) and the Global South (the poorer countries).

The People's Health Assembly

As the years passed, it became clear that the World Health Assembly of the WHO was unable to hear the people's voice and a new forum was required. Such a forum would bring together individuals, groups, organizations, networks, and movements involved in the struggle for health. It took almost 15 years, but in December 2000 approximately 1,500 public health activists from 94 countries gathered in Bangladesh for an historic People's Health Assembly (PHA). Believing that health is a fundamental human right that cannot be met without a commitment to equity and social justice, the participants gathered to assess the current unjust state of affairs and to map the way forward so that health for all could in fact be achieved (People's Health Movement, 2000). Their purpose was to create a worldwide, inter- and multisectoral collective of caring people and groups that would include peoples from all classes, castes, creeds, ages, gender, abilities, ethnic origins, and nations.

The meeting was carefully planned, and several regions and nations, especially India, prepared extensively for the assembly for many months. During the actual meeting, the multifaceted diagnosis that emerged focused primarily on health care failures in developing countries. Governments had failed to invest sufficient resources and empower localities to ensure adequate nutrition, clean water, maternal and child health care, and other components of primary health care. Governmental failures were rooted in many internal problems, but they especially reflected the budgetary and policy squeeze imposed by the International Monetary Fund

(IMF), the World Bank, and foreign debt repayments, as well as the World Trade Organization (WTO). Meanwhile, multinational corporations were pushing a privatization agenda for health care that removed control of crucial health decisions and delivery systems from the public sphere, where it is subject to popular influence. Privatization also often removed access to health care from poor people.

Corporate Globalization

During the PHA, Dr. Halfdan Mahler, former director general of the WHO, indicted those forces and organizations that had contributed to the failure to achieve health for all. He emphasized that "health"—by itself—was never the end but the way to social and economic development. Speaking of the current sad state of health for many in the world, he said there is an "in-built discrimination against the poor within the UN system." He identified imperialism and the collusion between imperialists and nationals, as well as institutions such as the World Bank, for weakening PHC efforts. He further identified HIV/AIDS and the provision of arms to Africa as leading to the extinction of that continent and called it "political hypocrisy" to provide Africa with arms but not the resources to fight AIDS. Asking economists to remove barriers from people, services, and governments, he stressed that the enemies of PHC within countries must also be named. In some of his strongest words, he said people are being "betrayed by commercialized health professionals who are afraid of taking a position" in favor of the people. Almost imploring the PHA, he said, "If we do not find ways to express political and social activism, we are just dreaming" (Gottschalk, 2000). In session after session, speakers and participants stressed their commitment to Health For All, but concluded that it was unlikely to be achieved broadly in the absence of fundamental transformations in the global political economy.

A People's Charter for Health issued by the PHA asserted that health is a human right and that "health and human rights should prevail over economic and political concerns." It called for the provision of "universal and comprehensive primary health care, irrespective of people's ability to pay." But the charter also called for the cancellation of third world debt; major changes at the IMF, the World Bank, and the WTO; effective regulation to control the activities of multinational corporations; and controls on speculative international capital flows. Delegates described some of their own successes to illustrate what can be achieved, despite enormous obstacles, with determination and organization. Their success stories revealed that it is not for lack of resources or knowledge that the world has failed to deliver on the promise of the Alma Ata declaration. What is lacking is political will, from the village to the international level. "While governments have the primary responsibility for promoting a more equitable approach to health and human rights," the PHC concluded, it will require people's organizations to force them to meet this responsibility (People's Charter for Health, 2000). Few at the assembly placed much confidence in governments or international organizations. As Dr. Mahler said, it will be people's organizations—united across the world—that will bring about the much needed changes.

The **People's Health Movement (PHM)**, which grew out of a Bangladesh meeting, is an international coalition of grassroots organizations dedicated to challenging the prevailing system of health care delivery that is failing to serve most of the poor worldwide. The PHM is organized in regional and country circles. Although the North American circle is currently the smallest, it is beginning to organize various outreach activities around the topics of Health and Trade, War and Health, Environmental Health and Justice, Community-Based Primary Health Care, and U.S. Health Care Access (Gottschalk, 2001).

Human Rights and Public Health Nursing

In recent years, public health leaders have begun calling attention to health as a human right. The late Jonathan Mann and his associates at Harvard University's Francois-Xavier Bagnoud Center for Heath and Human Rights were pioneers in this effort. As early as September 2000, the Executive Committee of the American Public Health Association (APHA) approved a set of principles on public health and human rights (APHA, 2000) and encouraged its members to make them integral to their practice. They are:

1. All human beings are equal in dignity and rights.

2. All human beings are entitled to the enjoyment of all human rights without discrimination.

3. The realization of the highest standard of health requires respect for all human rights, which are indivisible, interdependent, and interrelated.

4. An essential dimension of human rights is the right to health, including conditions that promote and safeguard health and access to culturally acceptable health care.

5. Human rights must not be sacrificed to achieve public health goals, except in extraordinary circumstances, in accordance with the requirements of internationally recognized human rights standards.

6. The active collaboration of public health and human rights workers is a necessary and invaluable means of advancing their common purposes and values. (APHA, 2000)

Similar principles were developed a year earlier by the Health Caucus of the United Nation's Commission on the Status of Women, when they emphasized that "Health Is a Fundamental Human Right" and urged that all health care personnel be educated in human rights and ethics (CWS, 1999). These principles are based on a historic body of international human rights documents that were negotiated after World War II. As one of its most significant early actions, the newly established United Nations General Assembly, under the leadership of Eleanor Roosevelt, adopted the Universal Declaration of Human Rights (UDHR) on December 10, 1948. Celebrated annually on International Human Rights Day (December 10), the declaration's 30 articles have been the basis for all human rights documents since then. More importantly, they are the international basis for every person's right to equal dignity, "without distinction of any kind, such as race, color, sex, language, religion, political or other opinion, national or social origin, property, birth or other status" (UN, 1948).

Several articles within the declaration refer to each person's equality before the law; their right to freedom of thought, conscience, and religion; and their right to freedom of peaceful assembly and association. Article 22, refers to the "right to social security" and the "realization, through national effort and international cooperation in accordance with the organization and resources of each State, the economic, social and cultural rights indispensable for a person's dignity and free development of one's personality" (UDHR, 1948). The following article is the one most important for public health nurses.

Article 25 of the Universal Declaration on Human Rights:

1. All people have the right to a standard of living adequate for the health and well-being of a person and of one's family, including food, clothing, housing and medical care, necessary social services, and the right to security in the event of unemployment, sickness, disability, widowhood, old age or other lack of livelihood in circumstances beyond one's control.

2. Motherhood and childhood are entitled to special care and assistance. All children, whether born in or out of wedlock, shall enjoy the same social protection. (UN, 1948)

United Nations Covenants

Comprehensive attempts eventually set international standards for these principles, codifying them in two major covenants ratified by most nations of the world. The UN Covenant on Civil and Political Rights deals basically with persons' negative rights: what governments must not do to their citizens. On the other hand, the UN Covenant on Economic, Social, and Cultural Rights deals with positive rights: what governments must do for their citizens. Unfortunately, the United States has long refused to ratify the UN Covenant on Economic, Social, and Cultural Rights. As a result, the United States appears to be more interested in assuring democratic elections throughout the world than in caring for the economic, social, and cultural wellbeing of its own citizens and those of the global community.

The World Social Forum

Although the original goal of the Alma Ata declaration on primary health care was "Health For All by the Year 2000," it soon became obvious that this goal would never be reached, and WHO and UNICEF quietly dropped the target of the "Year 2000," simply calling for "Health For All" without specifying any time-specific target. As noted earlier, health activists around the world found WHO's efforts inadequate and began to mobilize around the implementation of the People's Health Charter. At the same time, concerned citizens from many nations began to question the economic models that are at the basis of prevailing globaliza-

tion efforts. Meeting in Porto Alegre, Brazil, at the First World Social Forum (WSF), thousands of academics, economists, and grassroots activists from across the world challenged the existing global economic system and declared that "Another World Is Possible"—one where people's human rights are respected and nations can develop in peace based on justice for all. Since then, the WSF has continued to meet annually, drawing ever larger numbers of participants. When the WSF met in Mumbai (Bombay) India in 2004, more than 10,000 people participated.

The Millennium Development Goals

In September 2000, almost simultaneously with the first WSF, the United Nations sponsored the largest ever gathering of heads of state to usher in the new millennium by evaluating global conditions and setting out a roadmap with eight specific goals to be reached by 2015. Known as the Millennium Development Goals (MDGs), they represent commitments made by 189 countries focused on reducing poverty and hunger, ill health, gender inequality, lack of education, lack of access to clean water, and environmental degradation (Millennium Development Goals). The MDGs were developed as a statement for those nations, comparatively richer in economic resources, to contribute through trade, environmental assistance, and debt relief and to provide access to essential medicines and technology transfer to the needs of other less fortunate nations.

By 2015, all 189 UN member states pledged in 2000 to:

1. Eradicate extreme poverty and hunger by reducing by half the proportion of people living on less than a dollar a day and reducing by half the proportion of people who suffer from hunger.

2. Achieve universal primary education by ensuring that all boys and girls complete a full course of primary school.

3. Promote gender equality and empower women by eliminating gender disparity in primary and secondary education preferably by 2005, and at all levels by 2015.

4. Reduce child mortality by reducing by two-thirds the mortality rate among children younger than 5.

5. Improve maternal health by reducing by three-quarters the maternal mortality ratio.

6. Combat HIV/AIDS, malaria, and other diseases by halting and beginning to reverse the spread of HIV/AIDS and halting and beginning to reverse the incidence of malaria and other major diseases.

7. Ensuring environmental sustainability by reducing by half the proportion of people without sustainable access to safe drinking water and achieving significant improvement in the lives of at least 100 million slum dwellers by 2015.

8. Develop a global partnership for development by trading and sharing financial systems, special needs of individual countries, employment, access to affordable essential drugs, and the transfer of new technologies, especially those of information and communication.

Even though eight of the MDGs refer specifically to health, improvements in health are essential if any of the MDGs are to be met by 2015. Unfortunately, when the nations of the world met at the UN in September 2005 to evaluate progress made, they had little to celebrate. Though progress had been made in some countries, many continued to fall behind, with progress especially limited in sub-Saharan Africa.

Several rich countries have failed to honor their commitments to give 0.7% of their gross national product (GNP) annually for official development assistance that could be used to meet some of these goals. The United States, for example, gives at most 0.12 percent of its gross domestic product (GDP) to economic aid.

The United States and the Millennium Development Goals

The United States is also far from meeting some of the MDGs for its own population. For example, in the industrialized world the United States ranks:

- 11th in the proportion of children living in poverty
- 16th in living standards among the poorest one-fifth of children
- 16th in efforts to lift children out of poverty
- 18th in the income gap between rich and poor children

- 21st in eighth grade math scores
- Last in protecting our children against gun violence (NETWORK, 2004)

Are public health nurses speaking out about these issues? Should these issues be a priority for public health nurses who daily see clients denied access to needed health care because of their poverty, lack of health insurance, lack of adequate public health infrastructure, and ethnic discrimination? Poverty and neglect of those made poor by unjust economic systems are global realities, and wherever public nurses live and work they are challenged to respond. Public health nurses do not need to travel to the remotest ends of the earth to see poverty and neglect. It exists in the communities where they work. What is needed is for public health nurses to join with others, wherever they live and work, in attacking the causes of so much unnecessary illness and suffering.

PUBLIC HEALTH NURSES' RESPONSE TO CHALLENGES IN GLOBAL HEALTH

In addition to excellent clinical skills that include cultural competence and sensitivity, public health nurses of the future will need to venture beyond their traditional boundaries and widen their horizons and knowledge base to include political skills, social and economic realities, and knowledge of national and international covenants, treaties, and declarations. Public health nurses with a "global" perspective need to become knowledgeable about the United Nations as well as the major global institutions such as the World Bank, IMF, and WTO, which control many of the financial realities affecting the global community. Because so many health-related problems have an economic basis, public health nurses also need to be aware of the relationships between various trade agreements and the level of local employment or development.

To be effective in the global arena, public health nurses will need to join with politicians, union organizers, and city officials to concentrate on health problems with causes in the broader society. Public health nurses can become politically active by running for local school boards, planning commissions, and elected offices at local and national levels. Public health nurses will need to develop skills required to work with alliances and coalitions, especially of nonhealth professionals' alliances and coalitions. Public health nurses are encouraged to become active members of the People's Health Movement, but they can also participate in broader social networks such as the World Social Forum, International Debt Coalitions, Anti-Sweatshop and Fair Trade Campaigns, and local migrant and labor rights groups.

Many women have been displaced to the United States because of war and other problems within their countries. Public health nurses need to be aware of the physical and sexual suffering of these women at the hands of their partners. Many U.S. communities have women who suffer as a consequence of having lived in countries torn apart by war, ethnic conflicts, environmental destruction, and desperate poverty. These women, whether they are migrants, refugees, or homeless, have been forced into prostitution or trafficked from their own countries to provide food for themselves and their families. Other women have been tortured and bear the physical and mental scars of political and ethnic unrest. Such suffering may not be immediately visible to the casual observer, but public health nurses with a global perspective need to be alert to such realities in their communities. Growing numbers of specialized centers for the treatment and counseling of women are being established across the United States. In such centers, women can receive the legal advice and support they need. As ethnic and other conflicts deepen across the world, public health nurses need to be alert to the needs of newcomers to their communities.

In many parts of the world, World Bank policies have brought increasing poverty and suffering to poor communities as they supported the increasing privatization of services such as health, education, and water. With health care in the United States increasingly becoming a commodity available only for the few, public health nurses will need to be attentive to the increasing privatization of services such as education and water. Since adequate and safe housing is also a right enshrined in Article 25 of the United Nations Declaration on Human Rights, public health nurses need to be attentive to unjust housing and welfare policies in their practice. This will require expanding knowledge beyond the purely clinical to include new political skills.

Assessing the needs of a community may be overwhelming for a public health nurse. However, assessing the needs of the world can be even more overwhelming. Yet, if one looks closely, one can see the common human-

ity in all peoples and similarities in all our problems irregardless of their community. Poverty and injustice in one area—whether it is in Ethiopia or Erie, Pennsylvania, in the Sudan or the South Bronx, New York—are all linked. Many of their causes have similar bases in political-social-economic systems. Problems caused by poverty and injustice, wherever they are located in the world, affect all and are linked one to the other.

Public health nurses with a global perspective will need to be able to see the world and its problems from the perspective of those billions of people not living in the northern and western hemispheres. Health care then will be understood to be a human right, not just for individuals but for all in the human community.

In conclusion, public health nurses are not superhuman. Typically, they concentrate on a limited number of issues or areas of concern within their communities. However, in seeking to expand their knowledge to understand the linkages among issues and areas of concern across global communities will assist public health nurses in understanding that health-related problems have broad political, social, and economic causes. Becoming activists and public health advocates will require developing political, social, and economic realities to work with concerned citizen groups, coalitions and peoples' movements in building a better world, one of peace based on justice where human rights principles are a reality, where the Millennium Development Goals are reached for all peoples, and where the principles of the Peoples' Health Charter are realized in peoples' communities and lives. Public health nurses will then truly be citizens of the world.

CRITICAL THINKING ACTIVITIES

1. Explain to a hospital-based nurse the concept of health from a global perspective.

2. Explain to this same nurse, or another specializing in critical care nursing, how political, social, and economic factors affect the health and well-being of their clients and their families.

3. Compare and contrast the principles found in the Universal Declaration on Human Rights and the Millennium Development Goals.

4. Describe the practice of a public health nurse working from a global perspective and compare it with the practice of a public health nurse working from a purely local perspective.

KEY TERMS

corporate globalization

economic globalization

global

global health

globalization

Global North

Global South

health

Health For All

Millennium Development Goals (MDGs)

People's Charter for Health

People's Health Assembly (PHA)

People's Health Movement (PHM)

UN Covenant on Civil and Political Rights

UN Covenant on Economic, Social, and Cultural Rights

Universal Declaration of Human Rights (UDHR)

World Social Forum (WSF)

KEY CONCEPTS

⊕ Global health is a social, economic, and political issue, and above all a fundamental human right. Inequality, poverty, exploitation, violence, and injustice are at the root of ill health and the deaths of poor and marginalized people. Health for all means that powerful interests have to be challenged, that some forms of globalization have to be opposed, and that political and economic priorities have to be drastically changed.

⊕ Health as a basic human right was enshrined in the Universal Declaration of Human Rights (1948) and has been applied in numerous international covenants and civil society statements.

⊕ The Millennium Development Goals were established at a United Nations summit in 2000 and the governments of the world have committed themselves to make them a reality by the year 2015.

⊕ The People's Health Movement is a worldwide movement of citizens and health professionals concerned about the health of global populations. Their broad-based commitment is to achieve health for all as outlined in the People's Health Charter. This is one example of how public health nurses can become involved in the global community.

REFERENCES

American Academy of Nursing (ANN), International Expert Panel (2004, October 10). *Draft white paper.* Washington, DC.: American Academy of Nursing

American Public Health Association (APHA). (2000). APHA's principles on public health and human rights. Retrieved October 27, 2004, from http://apha.org/private/PrincPHI.htm.

The Baltimore Sun, Associated Press, 12/6/04.

Fact Sheet: Millennium Development Goals (2004). Geneva, Switzerland: Author.

Gottschalk, J. (2000). *Private notes from People's Health Assembly.*

Gottschalk, J. (2001, February). People's health assembly. *Intercontinent* (Medical Mission Sisters) #228. Philadelphia.

Higgs, Z.R., Bayne, T., & Murphy, D. (2001). Health care access: A consumer perspective. *Public Health Nursing 18*(1), 3–12.

Millennium Development Goals (MDGs) Retrieved July 25, 2007 from http://www.un.org/millenniumgoals

NETWORK. (2004, September-October). *Connections.* Washington, DC.: Institute for Educational Leadership.

People's Health Movement. (2000). *People's charter for health.* Berkeley, CA: Hesperian Foundation.

Popline, World Population News Service (2005a, January–February). *170 million children malnourished, UNICEF reports.* Washington, DC.

Rains, J.W., & Kriese, P.B. (2001). Developing political competence: A comparative study across disciplines. *Public Health Nursing, 18*(4), 219–224.

United Nations. (1948). *Universal declaration of human rights.* New York: Hellenic Resources Network.

UN Population Fund Report, (2004) Retrieved July 3, 2007 from *http://www.unfpa.org/upload/lib_pub_file/327_file-name_en_swp04.pd*

World Health Organization (WHO). (1978, September). *Report of the international conference on primary health care, Alma Ata, USSR.* Geneva, Switzerland: Author.

Yach, D., & Bettcher, D. (1998). The globalization of public health, I: Threats and opportunities. *American Journal of Public Health,* 735–738.

BIBLIOGRAPHY

American Nurses Association. (2001). *Code of ethics for nurses with interpretive statements.* Washington, DC: author.

Canada and the North American free trade agreement. Available: http://www.dfait-maeci.gc.ca/nafta-alena/menu-en.asp

Curtin, L. (2001). Ethics and politics are not oxymorons! *Policy, Politics, & Nursing Practice, 2*(1), 6–8.

FamiliesUSA. (2002). *2 million Americans lost their health insurance in 2001: Largest one-year increase in nearly a decade.* Available: www.familiesusa.org/media/press/2002/insurnace_loss.htm.

Garrett, L. (2000). *Betrayal of trust: The collapse of global public health.* New York: Hyperion.

Gueyr, B., Smith, D.R., & Chalk, R. (2000). Calling the shots: Immunization finance policies and practices. Executive summary of the report of the Institute of Medicine. *American Journal of Preventive Medicine, 19*(35), 4-12.

Guo, G., & Phillips, L. (2006). Key informant's perceptions of health care for elders at the US-Mexico border. *Public Health Nursing, 23*(3), 224-233.

Health For All in the 21st Century–WHO. Available: http://www.who.int/archives/hfa/.

Higgs, Z., Bayne, T., & Murphy, D. (2001). Health care access: A consumer perspective. *Public Health Nursing, 18*(1), 3–12.

International Council of Nurses. (*2000*). Position statement: Participation of nurses in health services decision making and policy development. Available: www.icn.ch/pspolicydev00.htm.

International Council of Nurses. (2001). *Guidelines on shaping effective health policy.* Geneva, Switzerland: Author.

International covenant on economic, social, and cultural rights. Available: http://www.unhchr.ch/html/menu3/b/a_cescr.htm.

International Labor Organization. Commission on the Status of Women (CSW). (1999, March 11). *Health caucus statement: Health is a fundamental human right.* New York.

Lashley, E.R., & Durham, J.D. (2002). *Emerging infectious diseases: Trends and issues.* New York: Springer.

PHM advocates people's health issues at 59th WHA. Available: http://www.phmovement.org/.

Popline, World Population News Service (2005b, January–February). *Hunger kills one child every five seconds. UNICEF reports.* Washington, DC.

Schulz, W.F. (2001). *In our own best interest: How defending human rights benefits us all.* Boston: Beacon Press.

The United Nations covenant on civil and political rights. Available: http://www.hrweb.org/legal/cpr.html.

Universal declaration of human rights. Available: http://www.un.org/Overview/rights.html.

UN millennium development goals. Available: http://www.un.org/millenniumgoals/index.asp.

World social forum. Available: http://en.wikipedia.org/wiki/World_Social_Forum

RESOURCES

B'Tselem (Information Center for Human Rights in the Occupied Territories)

Web: http://www.btselem.org

The Israeli Information Center for Human Rights in the Occupied Territories was established in 1989 by a group of prominent academics, attorneys, journalists, and Knesset members. It endeavors to document and educate the Israeli public and policy makers about human rights violations in the Occupied Territories, combat the phenomenon of denial prevalent among the Israeli public, and help create a human rights culture in Israel. B'Tselem in Hebrew literally means "in the image of" and is also used as a synonym for human dignity. The word is taken from Genesis 1:27 "And God created humans in his image. In the image of God did He create him." It is in this spirit that the first article of the Universal Declaration of Human Rights states that "All human beings are born equal in dignity and rights." As an Israeli human rights organization, B'Tselem acts primarily to change Israeli policy in the Occupied Territories and ensure that its government, which rules the Occupied Territories, protects the human rights of residents there, and complies with its obligations under international law. B'Tselem is independent and is funded by contributions from private individuals in Israel and abroad and from foundations in Israel, Europe, and North America that support human rights activity worldwide.

Department of Public Information

Web: http://www.un.org

The Web site provides a daily news round-up prepared by the Central News Section of the Normal Department of Public Information. It provides international and national news. The latest update is posted daily at approximately 6:00 P.M. New York time.

Francois-Xavier Bagnoud Center for Health and Human Rights

Harvard School of Public Health
651 Huntington Avenue, 7th floor
Boston, Massachusetts 02115
617-432-0656
FAX: 1-617-432 4310
Email: fxbcenter@igc.org
Web: http://www.hsph.harvard.edu

The Center for Health and Human Rights was founded at the Harvard School of Public Health in 1993 through a gift from the Association François-Xavier Bagnoud. The François-Xavier Bagnoud Center for Health and Human Rights is the first academic center to focus exclusively on health and human rights. It combines the academic strengths of research and teaching with a strong commitment to service and policy development. Center faculty work at international and national levels through collaboration and partnerships with health and human rights practitioners, governmental and nongovernmental organizations, academic institutions, and international agencies to do the following:

⊕ Expand knowledge through scholarship, professional training, and public education

⊕ Develop domestic and international policy focusing on the relationship between health and human rights in a global perspective

⊕ Engage scholars, public health and human rights practitioners, public officials, donors, and activists in the health and human rights movement.

Office of the High Commissioner for Human Rights (OHCHR)

Web: http://www.ohchr.org

The OHCHR is a department of the United Nations Secretariat and is mandated to promote and protect the enjoyment and full realization by all people of all rights established in the Charter of the United Nations and in international human rights laws and treaties. The mandate includes preventing human rights violations, securing respect for all human rights, promoting international cooperation to protect human rights, coordinating related activities throughout the United Nations, and strengthening and streamlining the United Nations system in the field of human rights. In addition to its mandated responsibilities, it leads efforts to integrate a human rights approach within all work carried out by United Nations agencies.

People's Charter for Health

Web: http://www.phmovement.org

In the beginning, there were thousands of people across the world working very hard in big and little ways to promote the dream of a world where a healthy life is a reality for all. In the optimistic, joyous, compassionate 1970s, it seemed that this would be possible. And was not the Alma Ata declaration signed by 134 governments in 1978? Did not the declaration promise *Health For All by 2000*? When the millennium edged closer and equitable health policy was still not a reality, the optimists did not give up. They knew that the third world had been plunged into debt and that health care was in danger of complete privatization. To remind the world of the commitment made in more hopeful times, the optimists came together in solidar-

ity. People's organizations, civil society organizations, nongovernmental organizations, social activists, health professionals, academics, and researchers came together to make a strong statement against the studied indifference in this crucial area of human life. The First People's Health Assembly was organized in Savar, Bangladesh, in December 2000 to discuss the health for all challenge. In all, 1,453 participants from 75 countries came together to create and endorse a consensus document called the People's Charter for Health. The charter reflects the vision, goals, and principles that unite all the members of the PHM coalition and calls for action. It is the most widely endorsed consensus document on health since the Alma Ata declaration. The Web site provides the entire People's Charter for Health in a pdf file.

Rabbis for Human Rights

Hehovharekhavim 9
Jerusalem, Israel 93462
972-2-648-2757
FAX: 972-2-678-3611
Web: http://www.rhr.Israel.net

Rabbis for Human Rights is an international group of rabbis working toward human rights. The Web site provides information on human rights issues and activities of this group.

ReliefWeb

ReliefWeb New York
Office for the Coordination of Humanitarian Affairs
United Nations
New York, NY 10017
212-963-1234
Web: http://www.reliefweb.int

ReliefWeb is the global hub for time-critical humanitarian information on Complex Emergencies and Natural Disasters. It is founded within the United Nations Office for the Coordination of Humanitarian Affairs. The Web site provides information on the needs of the humanitarian relief community.

The Peoples' Movement for Human Rights Education (PDHRE)

526 West 111th Street, Suite 4E
New York, New York 10025
212-749-3156
FAX: 212-666-6325
Email: pdhre@igc.org
Web: http://www.pdhre.org

Founded in 1988, the People's Decade of Human Rights Education (PDHRE—International) is a nonprofit, international service organization that works directly and indirectly with its network of affiliates—primarily women's and social justice organizations—to develop and advance pedagogies for human rights education relevant to people's daily lives in the context of their struggles for social and economic justice and democracy. PDHRE's members include experienced educators, human rights experts, United Nations officials, and world renowned advocates and activists who collaborate to conceive, initiate, facilitate, and service projects on education in human rights for social and economic transformation. The organization is dedicated to publishing and disseminating demand-driven human rights training manuals and teaching materials, and otherwise servicing grassroots and community groups engaged in a creative, contextualized process of human rights learning, reflection, and action. PDHRE views human rights as a value system capable of strengthening democratic communities and nations through its emphasis on accountability, reciprocity, and people's equal and informed participation in the decisions that affect their lives.

The World Bank

1818 H Street NW
Washington, D.C. 20433
202-473-1000
FAX: 202-477-6391
Web: http://www.worldbank.org

The World Bank is a vital source of financial and technical assistance to developing countries around the world. The World Bank is a vital source of financial and technical assistance to developing countries around the world. It is not a bank in the common sense. The World Bank is made up of two unique development institutions owned by 184 member countries—the International Bank for Reconstruction and Development (IBRD) and the International Development Association (IDA). Each institution plays a different but supportive role in the mission of global poverty reduction and the improvement of living standards. The IBRD focuses on middle-income and creditworthy poor countries, while IDA focuses on the poorest countries in the world. Together they provide low-interest loans, interest-free credit, and grants to developing countries for education, health, infrastructure, communications and many other purposes.

United Nations

Web: http://www.un.org

This is the official Web site for the United Nations. The information provided on this Web site includes but is not limited to daily briefings, press releases, documents, publications, and databases.

United Nations Economic and Social Development

Web: http://www.un.org

One of the UN's central mandates is the promotion of higher standards of living, full employment, and conditions of economic and social progress and development. The UN has unique strengths in promoting development. Its presence is global and its comprehensive mandate spans social, economic and emergency needs. The UN does not represent any particular national or commercial interest. When major policy decisions are taken, all countries, rich and poor, have a voice. This Website provides information on UN's progress in these areas.

United Nations Association of the United States of America (UNA–USA)

801 Second Avenue, 2nd floor
New York, New York 10017
212-907-1300
FAX: 212-682-9185
Email: unahq@unausa.org
Web: http://unausa.org

UNA–USA is part of the World Federation of UNAs. It is a center for innovative programs to engage Americans in issues of global concern, from education and HIV/AIDS to peace, security, and international law. Its educational and humanitarian campaigns, including teaching students in urban schools, clearing minefields, and providing school-based support for children living in HIV/AIDS-affected communities in Africa, allow people to make a global impact at the local level. A not-for-profit organization, UNA–USA encourages United States leadership in the United Nations.

United Nations System of Organizations

Web: http://www.unsystem.org

This Web site serves as a portal to Web sites of the United Nations, its funds, programs, and specialized agencies. It also includes links to key projects and initiatives to various joint programs of the UN.

United Nations World Food Program

Via C.G.Viola 68
Parco dei Medici
00148 - Rome - Italy
39-06-65131
FAX: 39-06-6513 2840
Email: wfpinfo@wfp.org
Web: http://www.wfp.org

The UN World Food Program was established to meet one of the Millennium Development Goals, which the United Nations set for the 21st century, halving the proportion of hungry people in the world is top of the list. This Web site provides information concerning progress toward the goal.

PART 3

PUBLIC HEALTH NURSING PRACTICE

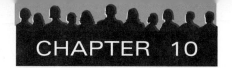

CHAPTER 10

Environmental Health Risk

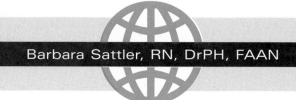

Barbara Sattler, RN, DrPH, FAAN

Chapter Outline

- Environmental Health Challenges
  - Magnitude of Environmental Health Issues
  - Multidisciplinary Approaches
- Environmental Health Assessment
  - Environmental Health Risks in the Home
  - Environmental Health Risks in Schools
  - Environmental Risks in the Community
  - Environmental Health Risks at Work
- Vulnerable Populations
- Environmental Justice
- Advocacy
- Risk Communication
- Chemical Policies and the Precautionary Principle
- Environmental and Public Health Infrastructure
  - Federal Responsibilities
  - State and Local Responsibilities
- Accessing Information and the "Right to Know"
- Environmental Health and Public Health Nursing

Learning Objectives

Upon completion of this chapter, the reader will be able to:

1. Explore the range of environmental health exposures in home, work, school, and community settings.

2. List sources of information that are critical to environmental health.

3. Articulate the four key elements in risk communication.

4. Identify the special risks of vulnerable populations to environmental exposures.

The environment is one of the primary determinants of individual and community health. **Environmental health** comprises those aspects of human health, including quality of life, that are determined by physical, chemical, biological, social, and psychological problems in the environment. It also refers to the theory and practice of assessing, correcting, controlling, and preventing those factors in the environment that can potentially adversely affect the health of present and future generations.

Nurses must understand the mechanisms and pathways of exposure to environmental health hazards, basic prevention and control strategies, the interdisciplinary nature of effective interventions, and the role of research and advocacy. Environmental protection standards in the United States are intended to be health-based and therefore health protective; however, they are often predicated on protecting the otherwise healthy, adult, white male and therefore may not provide the same protection for our most vulnerable human populations: the embryo/fetus, infants and children, those with chronic diseases, and the frail elderly. Basing standards on the adult male is substantially a decision based on economics and politics rather than sound science. Diagnosis, treatment, and prevention of environmentally related diseases are critical, as is history taking, exposure assessment, risk communication, required reporting, and an understanding of advocacy related to environmental health.

ENVIRONMENTAL HEALTH CHALLENGES

The last century may very well be remembered as the chemical century. More than 100,000 chemicals were synthesized. These are chemicals that never before existed on earth. Some of these chemicals, such as those pharmaceuticals that helped to cure and prevent diseases, were important to the progress of the last century. Other new chemicals have less positive claims to fame and have been found to create ecological and human health risks. Even though there are biological and radiological risks in our environment, the legacy of chemicals from the last century is the focus of this chapter. This includes the many layers of lead-based paint found in 52 million American homes; the hundreds of Superfund sites, which are highly contaminated waste sites found in every state in the country; and the mercury and pesticides levels sufficient to declare fish alerts in many of the country's lakes and streams.

Concurrent with the environmental pollutants in our air, water, food, and contaminated lands has been an unexplained increase in infertility, asthma, autism, Alzheimer's, cancer, and learning disabilities (Swann, 2006; Landrigan et al., 2002; Heininger, 2000; Clapp et al., 2005; Landrigan and Slutsky, 2006). Many of today's pollutants are persistent chemicals, meaning they do not break down; are found in the human body; and are associated with a range of health risks. There is a growing body of science, epidemiological and toxicological, supporting an association with the exposures to these toxic chemicals and the rise in some of the most troubling diseases that affect our population. Clearly, there are individual lifestyle choices that one can make to reduce exposures to toxic chemicals. However, population-based reductions will require policy and practice changes in energy production, transportation, agricultural production, product manufacture, and other key activities in our modern-day culture. As such, this chapter explores the role of public health nurses to reduce environmental risks in individual communities and states and reviews public health nurses' advocacy roles in helping to demand broader national and global reductions in pollution. Both levels of public health interventions are equally important.

Magnitude of Environmental Health Issues

The Centers for Disease Control and Prevention (CDC) assesses the health status of the U.S. public through the use of the National Health and Nutrition Exam Study (NHANES), an annual survey (with physical assessments) of a representative group of Americans. NHANES is a unique program conducted by CDC's National Center for Health Statistics that collects data on the health of people living in the United States through interviews, direct physical examinations, and laboratory tests (CDC, 2006).

In the past few years, the NHANES has begun to sample bodily tissues and fluids for the presence of toxic and persistent chemicals (United States Department of Health and Human Services, 2006). The results of this new study initiative are a call to action. The chemicals that now reside in human bodies reflect the pollution and toxic chemicals found in the air, water, food, and products that we all use; refer to Box 10-1.

For example, the study found that in certain geographic areas, women's breast milk contains several pesticides, including DDT, a toxic yet persistent chemical that was banned in the United States in the 1970s. The presence of DDT in the environment and in the human body 40 years after it was banned is a testament to its **persistence**, or the length of time a substance stays in the environment after it has been introduced. The implications of these discoveries are yet to be fully understood, but from a public health perspective it is important to think in terms of disease prevention and see reduction of all toxic chemicals as a step in a positive direction.

Chemical, Biological, and Radiological Risks

There are distinct chemical exposures that occur in homes, workplaces, schools, and communities, as well as exposures that are common to all of these settings. For example, air pollution is inescapable regardless of setting, whereas exposure to ethylene oxide is only likely to occur in a workplace. Pesticides are ubiquitous—found in street soot and the dust in our homes (even if we do not use pesticides) and, as noted, in every nursing mother's breast milk (CDC, 2005a). Examples of biological exposures in our environment include the pathogenic organisms associated with food poisoning, such as salmonella; the pathogenic organisms in recreational and drinking water such as cryptosporidium; and the various pathogenic microbes that are passed along from child to child in schools. Each of the exposures lends itself to public health nursing interventions such as presenting educational programs on food handling and storage; working with local media to draw attention to alerts about unhealthy recreational waters; and initiating school health programs that raise awareness about and improve handwashing.

Radiological exposures falls into two categories: ionizing and nonionizing radiation. Nonionizing radiation includes visible light, infrared radiation, microwaves, and radio frequencies. Nonionizing radiation also includes the carcinogenic ultraviolet waves of the sun. A great number of organizations and programs address sun safety and preventing one of the most common types of cancer—skin cancer. Ionizing radiation is distinguished by the fact that it can strip electrons from atoms and includes alpha, beta, and gamma rays, as well as X-rays. Radon is included in this category (see Figure 10-1).

Multidisciplinary Approaches

Public health approaches often demand interdisciplinary efforts. This is certainly true in environmental health where we may rely on a range of scientific experts like toxicologists and geologists; technical experts such as the sanitarians and industrial hygienists; and research and surveillance experts like epidemiologists and biostatisticians. Additionally, public health nurses might call upon a housing inspector or an animal control technician to help address a problem. Public health nurses play a variety of roles in environmental health situations, and they are very often called upon to field questions and to help translate technical environmental health information into language that makes sense to the communities they serve. In the context of this unique role, they are trusted conveyors of information and important observers of early warnings of environmental health issues.

ENVIRONMENTAL HEALTH ASSESSMENT

Potential environmental exposures and environmentally related diseases can be assessed individually or on

---

BOX 10-1: Body Burden Study: The National Report on Human Exposure to Environmental Chemicals

The CDC is sponsoring an ongoing assessment of the exposure of the U.S. population to environmental chemicals using biomonitoring (CDC, 2005a). The First Report on 27 chemicals was issued in March 2001. This Second Report, released in January 2003, presents blood and urine levels of 116 environmental chemicals from a sample of people that represent the noninstitutionalized, civilian U.S. population during the two-year period 1999–2000. The Third Report was released in June 2005.

SOURCE: http://www.cdc.gov/exposurereport/default.htm

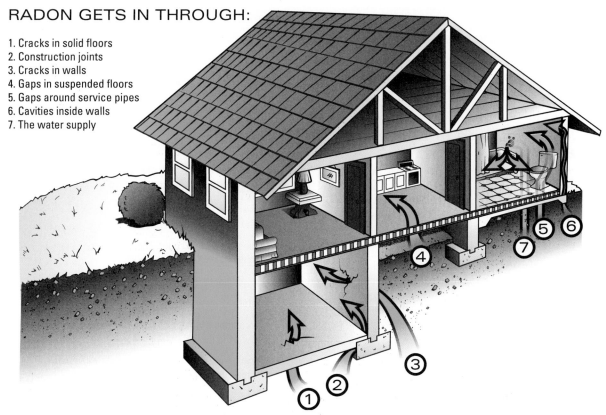

RADON GETS IN THROUGH:

1. Cracks in solid floors
2. Construction joints
3. Cracks in walls
4. Gaps in suspended floors
5. Gaps around service pipes
6. Cavities inside walls
7. The water supply

Figure 10-1 Radon in homes.
From www.epa.gov.

a community-wide basis. Assessing individual risks to potentially toxic exposures can be aided by the use of the mnemonic: I PREPARE (Box 10-2). This tool helps the public health nurse to keep information organized and consistent during the assessment of health risks to individuals and their families. Such assessments can aid in the development of individualized plans for exposure reduction and health education messaging. Aggregating such assessments at the clinic or community level can help to identify common threats that might lend themselves to community-wide approaches.

In assessing community-level exposures there are a few questions that must be asked:

- *What is the nature of the exposures?* Chemical, biological, or radiological

- *Where is the exposure coming from?* Air (indoor, outdoor), water, food, soil

- *What is the route of exposure?* Inhalation (air pollution, dusts, aerial spraying), ingestion (food and water sources), dermal (dusts, soil contamination, recreational water)

- *What are the health effects associated with the exposure?* The National Library of Medicine's online ToxNet Program is one of the best, most reliable, up-to-date, and most user-friendly sources of toxicity information. Additional sources are identified in the Resources section.

- *What are the special vulnerabilities of the population at risk?* Children, pregnant women, the elderly, the infirm (especially immunocompromised populations) may be at special health risk.

- *What are the risks or probability that a health effect will occur?* This last question requires three bits of information. (1) What is known about the

BOX 10-2: I PREPARE

I PREPARE is a mnemonic that was developed by nurses to help remember the range of occupational and environmental risks that a nurse should ask about when assessing a client's health.

I—Investigate Potential Exposures

Ask the worker if he or she has ever felt sick after coming in contact with chemicals, pesticides, dust, or other substances. If the answer is yes, ask whether the symptoms go away when he or she is away from the workplace.

P—Present Work

At your present work: Are you exposed to solvents, dust, fumes, radiation, loud noises, pesticides, or other chemicals? Do you know where to find Material Safety Data Sheets* on chemicals that you work with? Do you wear personal protective equipment? Are work clothes worn home? Do co-workers have similar health problems?

R—Residence

When was your residence built? What type of heating do you have? Have you recently remodeled your home? What chemicals are stored on your property? Where does your drinking water come from?

E—Environmental Concerns

Are there environmental concerns in your neighborhood (i.e., air, water, soil)? What types of industries or farms are near you home? Do you live near a hazardous waste site or landfill?

P—Past Work

What are your past work experiences? What is the longest job held? Have you been in the military, worked on a farm, or done volunteer or seasonal work?

A—Activities

What activities do you and your family engage in? Do you burn, solder, or melt any products? Do you garden, fish, or hunt? Do you eat what you catch or grow? Do you use pesticides? Do you engage in any alternative healing or cultural practices?

R—Referrals and Resources

Use these key referrals and resources:

- Agency for Toxic Substances & Disease Registry—www.atsdr.cdc.gov
- Association of Occupational & Environmental Clinics—www.aoec.org
- Environmental Protection Agency—www. epa.gov
- Material Safety Data Sheets—www.hazard.com/msds
- Occupational Health & Safety Administration—www.osha.gov
- Local health department, environmental agency, poison control center

E—Educate (A Checklist)

Are materials available to educate the client? Are alternatives available to minimize the risk of exposure? Have prevention strategies been discussed? What is the plan for follow-up?

* Note: Material Safety Data Sheets (MSDS) are chemical information materials that are created by the manufacturer. It is mandatory to have an MSDS for all potentially hazardous substances in workplaces, as per the OSHA Hazard Communication Standard.

SOURCE: www.atsdr.cdc.gov. For more information contact ATSDR at 1-888-42-ATSDR (1-888-422-8737), or visit ASTDR's Web site at www. Atsdr.cdc.gov.

toxicity, or the amount of injury to a living cell, of the pollutant source? (2) What is the dose, or the amount of a substance ingested or absorbed, at which it can cause damage? (3) What is the actual exposure, or quantitative contact with environmental pollutants and other agents, that the individual or community is experiencing? These three elements of information help to produce a risk assessment. Risk assessment is the process used to set environmental standards.

There are a variety of sources of information about community exposures. The two main federal agencies that provide good information are the National Library of Medicine and the U.S. Environmental Protection Agency (EPA). The National Library of Medicine's *ToxTown* provides excellent general information about hazardous risks associated with occupations as well as different locations, such as the home, hospital, and farm. The Environmental Protection Agency, through its EnviroMap and EnviroFacts sites, provides information that can be accessed by zip code and other geographic designations.

Environmental epidemiology is the study of associations between environmental exposures and human disease outcomes. Few environmental epidemiologic studies are performed other than for occupational exposures; some examples include the studies that determined the association between lung cancer and asbestos exposure and the investigations into the results of catastrophic exposure from leaks, explosions, or spills, such as the tragic 1984 incident when a Union Carbide plant caused a leak of deadly isocyanates that killed over 20,000 and has caused chronic health conditions in tens of thousands more in Bhopal, India (Lapierre and Moro, 2002). The epidemiological studies of the short- and long-term effects of accidental exposure have provided us with information that we would never have otherwise ascertained. A significant challenge in environmental epidemiology is the difficulty in finding a population that is not exposed to hazardous chemicals. For instance, when we all have evidence of exposure, who will be the "control group"? DDT is not just found in the bodies of Americans, it is also found in the breast milk of people as far away as the Inuit natives who live in the circumpolar regions of the world (Dallaire, Muckle, & Ayotte, 2003).

Other factors can also challenge environmental epidemiologists. For example, in studying indoor exposures to radon, the EPA (2006a) notes that the following factors would have to be considered:

- *Mobility:* Over time, people live in different areas; it is virtually impossible to go back and test every home where an individual has lived.

- *Housing Stock Changes:* Over time, older homes are often destroyed or remodeled so that radon measurements can be nonexistent or highly varied; a home's radon level may change, higher or lower, over time if new ventilation systems are installed, the occupancy patterns are substantially different, or the home's foundation shifts or cracks appear.

- *Inaccurate Histories:* Often a majority of the lung cancer cases (individuals) being studied are deceased or too sick to be interviewed by researchers. This requires reliance on secondhand information, which may not be as accurate. These inaccuracies primarily affect:

  - *Residence History:* A child or other relative may not be aware of all residences occupied by the client—particularly if the occupancy is distant in time or of relatively short duration. Even if the surrogate respondent is aware of a residence, he or she may not have enough additional information to allow researchers to locate the home.

  - *Smoking History:* Smoking history historically has reliability problems. Individuals may underestimate the amount they smoke. Conversely, relatives or friends may overestimate smoking history.

- *Other:* Complicating factors other than variations in smoking habits include an individual's genetics, lifestyle, exposure to other carcinogens, and home heating, venting and air conditioning preferences.

Toxicology is the science that studies poisons, or chemicals that make us sick. Toxicologists rely substantially on animal models to determine the effects of exposure to chemicals. When designing a toxicological study, the scientist can control almost everything. Genetically identical mice are often chosen because the confounding influence of genetic diversity can be eliminated. Additionally, variables that can be controlled include diet, ambient air, and exercise, among many other factors. Then the scientist can begin to give the mice varying doses of a chemical. The doses and the effects of the doses are plotted on a dose–response curve, which is a graphical representation of the relationship between the dose of a substance and the biological response to that substance. The dose–response curve is much the same as the dose–response curve that is plotted to show the effects of therapeutic drugs (see Figure 10-2). For each curve, a distinct response is plotted, such as renal failure or tumor development. In order to infer the damage that the chemical in question might cause to a human, the data from the dose–response curve is extrapolated, meaning that a best scientific guess is offered as to how a human cell, tissue, organ, or organ

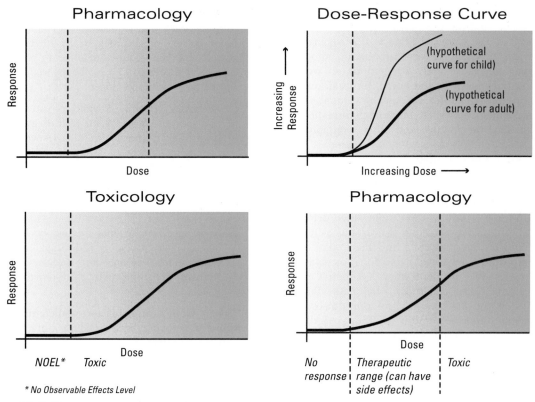

Figure 10-2 Dose–response curves.

NOTE: The dose–response curve for pharmacology indicates a dose range at which there is no therapeutic response, a therapeutic range, and a level at which there may be toxicity. In the dose–response curve for toxicology, there is a dose range that is called the No Observable Effects Level (NOEL), then there is a range at which toxicity begins and continues. The third curve shows how the dose–response curve shifts when the "host" is a child rather than an adult.

system might respond at varying doses. This information is then inserted into the risk assessment formula. The risk assessment process can be quite imprecise for predicting human health risks. In the groundbreaking 1996 Food Quality Protection Act, Congress demanded that the EPA take into consideration the special vulnerabilities of children to pesticide exposure and to consider the multiple sources that children have to pesticides, such as residues on multiple foods in their daily diet and pesticide use in homes and on lawns.

Our lack of scientific study in the area of chemical mixtures and their associated health risks is a significant issue. Rarely are mixtures of chemicals studied; yet, at any point in time, humans are always exposed to many chemicals. In those few studies that we have, we know that environmental exposures can significantly change the risk of health outcomes. For example, workers who smoke and are exposed to radon are 10 times as likely to get lung cancer as those who smoke but are not exposed to radon (Fabrikant, 1990). More research in the area of exposures to chemical mixtures is warranted in order to develop the safest exposure standards.

Environmental Health Risks in the Home

There are several common health risks in homes that can effectively be addressed with public health approaches. These include lead, radon, carbon monoxide, contaminants in drinking water, and consumer products. Common exposures are shown in Table 10-1.

Lead

Lead-based paint contributes to childhood lead poisoning. Lead is a highly toxic chemical that does not belong in the human body. Lead poisoning can cause a wide range of health risks: learning and language skill disturbances, anemia, hypertension, damage to peripheral nerves and kidneys, and a number of reproductive problems for both men and women (NLM, 2006). Adult lead poisoning is most often the result of occupational exposures and also from rehabbing and renovating areas where lead-based paint is present (CDC, 2005b).

In 1978 lead-based paint was banned for interior paints in the United States. The older the house the

TABLE 10-1: Common Chemical Exposures, Sources, and Associated Health Effects

Chemical	Chemical
Lead	Mercury
Use	**Use**
Formerly used in plumbing, paint, gasoline	Medical equipment, switches, thermometers, dental fillings
Where Found	**Where Found**
Old paint in homes older than 1975, contaminated dust, aging pipes, hazardous waste sites	Contaminated fish (especially large predatory types)
(*Note:* Lead based paint was banned for interior uses in 1978.)	Coal, health care settings, schools (labs), thermostats, homes (thermometers), junked automobiles
Major Health Effects	**Major Health Effects**
If not detected early, children with high levels of lead in their bodies can suffer from:	*Methylmercury*
_ Damage to the brain and nervous system	_ Fetuses, infants, and children: Impaired neurological development. Impacts on cognitive thinking, memory, attention, language, and fine motor and visual spatial skills have been seen in children exposed to methylmercury in the womb.
_ Behavior and learning problems (e.g., hyperactivity)	
_ Slowed growth	
_ Hearing problems	_ All ages: Symptoms of methylmercury poisoning may include impairment of the peripheral vision; disturbances in sensations ("pins and needles" feelings, usually in the hands, feet, and around the mouth); lack of coordination of movements; impairment of speech, hearing, walking; and muscle weakness.
_ Headaches	
Lead is also harmful to adults. Adults can suffer from:	
_ Difficulties during pregnancy	
_ Other reproductive problems (in both men and women)	*Elemental Mercury*
_ High blood pressure	_ Tremors; emotional changes (e.g., mood swings, irritability, nervousness, excessive shyness); insomnia; neuromuscular changes (e.g., weakness, muscle atrophy, twitching); headaches; disturbances in sensations; changes in nerve responses; performance deficits on tests of cognitive function
_ Digestive problems	
_ Nerve disorders	
_ Memory and concentration problems	
_ Muscle and joint pain	_ Higher exposures: kidney effects, respiratory failure and death. People concerned about their exposure to elemental mercury should consult their health care provider.

(continued)

TABLE 10-1: Common Chemical Exposures, Sources, and Associated Health Effects (cont'd)

Chemical

Manganese

Use

Gasoline additive, steel manufacture, pesticide, compound used in hospitals to test if a client has certain types of cancer

Where Found

Many types of rock, airborne dust particles, dissolved into water, combustion from automobiles, hazardous waste sites

Major Health Effects

Manganese is an essential trace element and is necessary for good health (about 1–10 mg manganese per day).

Neurotoxin

_ Neurological symptoms characterized by severe extrapyramidal dysfunction resembling the dystonic movements associated with Parkinson's disease, also known as "manganism." People with compromised liver function may be at greater risk than the normal population to the toxic actions of Mn.

Chemical

Environmental

Tobacco smoke

Use

N/A

Where Found

Near smoke emitted from the burning end of a cigarette, cigar, or pipe, and smoke exhaled by the smoker

Major Health Effects

Lung cancer, nasal sinus cancer, respiratory tract infections, and heart disease

Chemical

PCBs

Use

Electrical, heat transfer, and hydraulic equipment; and as plasticizers in paints, plastics and rubber products; in pigments, dyes and carbonless copy paper and many other applications

Where Found

Hazardous waste sites, incinerator releases, landfills, contaminated fish

Major Health Effects

_ Probable human carcinogens

_ May suppress the immune system

_ May have reproductive effects (low birth weight, lower live births, difficult conception)

_ May cause neurological deficits (learning deficits and changes in activity)

_ Associated with decreased thyroid hormone levels

_ Elevations in blood pressure, serum triglyceride, and serum cholesterol have also been reported

Chemical

Bisphenol A

Use

Used primarily to make polycarbonate plastic and epoxy resins. It is also used in flame retardants and rubber chemicals, and as a fungicide.

Where Found

Digital media (e.g., CDs, DVDs), electrical and electronic equipment, automobiles, sports safety equipment, reusable food and drink containers, and many other products

Major Health Effects

_ Contact can irritate or even burn the skin and eyes.

_ Bisphenol A may cause a skin allergy. If allergy develops, very low future exposures can cause itching and a skin rash.

_ There is limited evidence that Bisphenol A may damage the developing fetus and reduce fertility.

(continued)

TABLE 10-1: Common Chemical Exposures, Sources, and Associated Health Effects (cont'd)

Chemical

PERC (tetrachloroethylene)

Use

Dry cleaning and metal degreasing

Where Found

Dry cleaning operations and on clothes that have been dry cleaned, industrial emissions, water repellents, spot removers, glues, wood cleaners

Major Health Effects

_ Short term: Dizziness, headache, sleepiness, confusion, nausea, difficulty breathing, speaking, and or walking, unconsciousness, and possible death

_ Long term: Reasonably anticipated to be a human carcinogen

Chemical

Brominated flame retardants

Use

Routinely added to consumer products to reduce fire-related injury and property damage

Where Found

Computers, electronics and electrical equipment, televisions, textiles, foam furniture, insulating foams, and other building materials.

Major Health Effects

_ Limited information in humans

_ Animals: linked to thyroid hormone disruption, permanent learning and memory impairment, behavioral changes, hearing deficits, delayed puberty onset, fetal malformations, and possibly cancer. Exposure in utero or infancy leads to much more significant harm than adult exposure, and at much lower levels.

Chemical

Solvents

Use

Used to dissolve other substances

Where Found

Paints, inks, and other coatings; in cleaners, degreasers, and paint strippers; and as refrigerants and coolants; is also found in thousands of other products at work and at home

Major Health Effects

_ Have been associated with toxicity to the nervous system, reproductive damage, liver and kidney damage, respiratory impairment, cancer, and dermatitis

Chemical

Dioxin

Use

No commercial usefulness

Where Found

Formed during combustion processes (e.g., waste incineration, forest fires, and backyard trash burning) and manufacturing processes (e.g., herbicide manufacture and paper manufacture)

Major Health Effects

_ High-level exposures can lead to cancer, reproductive and developmental problems, increased heart disease, and increased risk for diabetes

_ Long-term low-level exposure: cancer, endometriosis

more likely it will be to have some lead-based paint. For example, homes built before the 1950s are quite likely to have some lead-based paint and the most common areas in which the paint was used are the kitchen and bathrooms, windows, porches, stair rails, doors, and trim. If a home has lead-based paint in the undersurfaces of paint, it is critical to keep the outermost surface intact. This will prevent exposures. Any chipping and peeling paint must be attended to immediately. The culprit is lead-based paint *dust*. This dust is created by abrading paint that results from opening and closing doors, double-hung windows, and banging into trim railings. The most critical way in which young children get the lead into their bodies is during their normal, exploratory hand-to-mouth activities.

Checking for lead-based paint dust is a very simple test. Any public health nurse can do it or teach community members to do it. While the results may not be admissible evidence in a legal situation, a parent's sampling can help to determine whether their children are at risk, which can result in actions to decrease exposures. Pregnant women should be encouraged to do lead dust sampling of their homes. The "equipment" for dust sampling is simple: a zip lock baggy, a pen that will write on a plastic bag, a baby wipe (without aloe), and something with which to measure a 12-inch square. The baby wipe is swiped in one direction and then the other on a 12″ area of floor, placed in the baggie, marked with the location within the home and date, as well as the name and address of the home owner or tenant. This sample is then sent to an environmental lab which will analyze it (for a very modest fee) and return the results indicating whether the EPA's lead dust standards have been exceeded.

If the lead dust sample exceeds acceptable levels and the person living in the home is a renter, an inquiry should be made to the local health department to determine the lead-based paint laws and processes to protect renters. Homeowners are responsible for all activities to reduce the exposure, such as ensuring that all painted surfaces are intact. Replacing windows that have been painted with lead-based paints is extremely helpful.

Replacement may be recommended or insertion of plastic sleeves that can be placed on the friction points

⊕ PRACTICE APPLICATION

Needleman's Lead Poisoning Studies over the Decades

While Dr. Herbert Needleman was a resident in Boston, from 1975 to 1978, he was interested in the effects of lead poisoning on young children. He designed a study by which he collected children's baby teeth when they lost them at age 6–7 years. The moms brought the children and the children's liberated teeth to Dr. Needleman. The moms received a modest incentive and the children received a silver dollar. He then analyzed the teeth for the presence of lead. Neurobehavioral functioning was found to be inversely related to dentin (tooth) lead levels meaning that the children tested did better on a battery of tests (reading, language skill development, etc.) if they had less lead in their teeth.

To determine whether the effects of low-level lead exposure persisted, he reexamined 132 of the 270 children, who had initially been studied as primary school children, when they were young adults in 1988. As compared with those restudied, the other 138 subjects had somewhat higher lead levels on earlier analysis, as well as significantly lower IQ scores and poorer teachers' ratings of classroom behavior. When the 132 subjects were reexamined in 1988, impairment in neurobehavioral function was still found to be related to the lead content of teeth shed at the ages of 6 and 7. Lead levels were inversely related to self-report of minor delinquent activity. Needleman concluded that exposure to lead in childhood is associated with deficits in central nervous system functioning that persist into young adulthood. (Needleman, H.L., Schell, A., Bellinger, D., Leviton, A., & Allred, E.N. (1990). The long-term effects of exposure to low doses of lead in childhood. An 11-year follow-up report. *New England Journal of Medicine, 322*(2), 83–88.)

In 1990, Needleman conducted a retrospective cohort to examine the relationship between tooth lead in children and bone lead levels in young adults. Members of a cohort of young adults were reassessed 13 years after an initial examination at an ambulatory clinical research center. It was concluded that lead exposure in early life may be used to predict elevated body burden up to 13 years later. (Kim, R., Hu, H., Rotnitzky, A., Bellinger, D., & Needleman, H. (1996). Longitudinal relationship between dentin lead levels in childhood and bone lead levels in young adulthood. *Archives of Environmental Health, 51*(5), 375-382.)

Most recently, Needleman implemented a case-control study of 194 youths aged 12–18 who had been arrested and adjudicated as delinquent by the Juvenile Court of Allegheny County, Pennsylvania, and 146 nondelinquent controls from high schools in the city of Pittsburgh. Higher body lead burdens, measured by bone lead concentrations, that elevated lead levels were associated with elevated risk for adjudicated delinquency. (Needleman, H.L., McFarland, C., Ness, R.B., Fienberg, S.E., & Tobin, M.J. (2002). Bone lead levels in adjudicated delinquents. A case control study. *Neurotoxicology & Teratology, 24*(6), 711–717.)

⊕ RESEARCH APPLICATION

Bone Lead Levels in Adjudicated Delinquents: A Case Control Study

Study Purpose

To explore the effects that early childhood lead exposures may have on subsequent behaviors that result in adjudicated delinquency

Methods

Case-control epidemiological study with 194 youths aged 12–18 who were arrested (case) and 146 nondelinquent youths. Both groups were from Pennsylvania. Bone lead was measured by x-ray fluorescence in the tibia.

Findings

Cases had significantly higher mean concentrations of lead in their bones than controls (11.0 ± 32.7 vs. 1.5 ± 32.1 ppm). This was true for both whites and African Americans. The unadjusted odds ratio for a lead level ≥ 25 vs. <25 ppm was 1.9 (95% CL: 1.1–3.2). After adjustment for covariates

and interactions and removal of noninfluential covariates, adjudicated delinquents were four times more likely to have bone lead concentrations <25 ppm than controls (OR = 4.0, 95% CL: 1.4–11.1).

Implications

Elevated body lead burdens, measured by bone lead concentrations, are associated with elevated risk for adjudicated delinquency. The cost of childhood lead poisoning includes long-term costs to the individual, his or her family, and society. Lead poisoning prevention is the only approach that can reverse this tide of unfortunate, long-term sequela.

Reference

Research scientists at the University of Pittsburgh, MDs, and PhDs.

---

to reduce abrasion; carefully clean the home from top to bottom using a three bucket system of soapy, rinse, and clean water. The three bucket system, with frequent water changes, has been found to be effective, whereas cleaning with a single bucket has not been proved to be beneficial. Use of heat guns and dry scraping should never be employed in removing lead-based paint. Both of these practices create great risk for the person doing the task and can result in dangerous levels of lead in the area.

Primary prevention of lead-based paint poisoning requires the removal of the exposure. Many lead poisoning programs and laws focus on the secondary prevention strategies that encourage testing children's blood lead levels. This is obviously an important component of a public health strategy; note, however, that lead screening and surveillance programs help to identify lead poisoned children, not prevent their poisoning. Therefore, the more important focus for addressing lead poisoning is to remove the exposure. The removal of lead from gasoline, which began in the United States in 1972 and was completed in 1995, has resulted in almost fourfold reductions in median blood lead levels in U.S. children from 1976 to 1991 (Silbergeld, 1997).

The phase-out of lead in gasoline is an excellent example of a primary prevention approach for lead poisoning. Secondary prevention activities commonly found in local health departments are surveillance programs to identify children with elevated blood lead levels, which, in turn, results in an investigation of potential sources of lead in the child's environment. This then leads to tertiary prevention when the child's poisoning is medically managed, in order to minimize the harm and symptoms associated with lead poisoning.

Radon

Radon is a naturally occurring radioactive gas that is colorless and odorless, and in regions of the country where radon is in the ground, it easily seeps into and accumulates in basements and ground floor spaces. It is also a carcinogen and is the second leading cause of lung cancer in the United States (EPA, 2006a). As in the case of lead poisoning, the public health approach is to test for its presence and remediate the exposure if the testing shows an exceedence of the EPA radon standard. Radon testing kits are widely available at hardware stores and are easy to use. The solution to high radon exposures is "dilution." The space in which radon is accumulating must be adequately ventilated so the air exchange and removal occurs at a level to keep the radon levels safe. Every state has a radon program in the department that deals with environmental protection. The department can offer suggestions for experts who can assist with remediation recommendations, if radon levels are found to be high. Nurses should encourage homeowners to test for radon.

Carbon Monoxide

Carbon monoxide is another colorless, odorless gas. It is the product of combustion and results in homes when gas stoves, furnaces, and other gas-driven appliances operate. It is not uncommon to have high levels of carbon monoxide from furnaces that have not been maintained. Carbon monoxide detectors can also be purchased in hardware stores and should be set up where the furnace is and in the kitchen (if there is a gas stove). If the detector indicates high levels, the furnace or appliance should be checked. Acute carbon monoxide poisoning is life threatening. However, chronic low-level exposures are associated with headaches, drowsiness, poor cognition, flu-like symptoms, and depression (Raub et al., 2000).

Drinking Water

About half the country purchases its drinking water from a water company and the other half gets it from private wells. Of those who purchase drinking water, the water may come from surface water, such as lakes, rivers, and reservoirs, or it may come from groundwater. Both groundwater (from which well water comes) and surface waters can be contaminated by environmental pollutants. The EPA's Safe Drinking Water Act requires water companies to test their water, communicate the results of the tests to their consuming public on an annual basis, and sound an immediate alert if the water poses a public health threat (Box 10-3). In most states, there is no requirement to test private wells except when they are first put in. It is therefore important to encourage people to periodically test their well water. It's also important that we protect our ground- and surface waters from industrial, agricultural, and street runoff contamination. We all live in a watershed—the area that drains to a common waterway, such as a stream, lake, estuary, wetland, or even the ocean—and our individual and collective actions can directly affect it. Every watershed is required to have a watershed pro-

tection plan. To obtain the plan for a given community, contact the state agency that is responsible for environmental protection. This agency has different names in different states. For example, in Maryland it is called the Maryland Department of the Environment, in Pennsylvania it is called the Department of Environmental Protection, and in Delaware it is called the Department of Natural Resources and Environmental Control.

Many people will ask about water treatment devices, such as filters for their kitchen faucets. This is what they need to know. What's in the water? If they cannot answer this question, then they cannot determine which device or filter is best suited for their needs. As a public health nurse, recommend that they have the water tested to see if there is, in fact, something that needs to be taken out. There are often trace elements and minerals in water that are important to human health that should not be removed, if possible. Once the water has been tested, then the right device must be chosen to address the problem chemical. For people who are immunosuppressed and concerned about pathogenic organisms, a HEPA filter (similar to the ones on IV tubing) can be used to filter out microbes. If there are volatile compounds that give the water an unpleasant odor and/or are present health risks, then a charcoal filter may be the best choice. However, it is important to note that most volatile organic compounds (VOCs) can also enter the body through the skin—such that exposures can occur when bathing. Therefore, the solution may be to place a charcoal treatment device at the point at which the water enters the home, thereby preventing all water-related exposures to VOCs.

BOX 10-3: Challenges to Safe Drinking Water

Categories of Drinking Water Contaminants

- ⊕ Microbial
  - Bacterial
  - Viral
  - Parasites
- ⊕ Chemicals
  - Inorganic
  - Organic

- ⊕ Radionuclides
  - Gross alpha radiation
  - Radon

Consumer Products

In the last few years, much more information is available regarding the chemical makeup of consumer products, which include cleaning solutions, personal care products, lawn products, and hobby materials. The National Library of Medicine recently initiated a Web site that has information about such products and their associated health risks. Chemicals can be searched by brand name. The site notes the chemicals that are revealed on the product labels and provides independent, peer-reviewed information about the health risks associated with the chemicals that the product manufacturer lists.

Note that not all ingredients are always listed. For example, in the case of pesticide (insecticide and herbicide) labels, there are "active ingredients" and "inerts." An active ingredient is one that prevents, destroys, repels, or mitigates a pest or is a plant regulator, defoliant, desiccant, or nitrogen stabilizer. By law, the active ingredient must be identified by name on the label together with its percentage by weight. An inert ingredient refers to any substance, other than an active ingredient, that is intentionally included in a pesticide product. For example, inert ingredients may serve as a solvent, allowing the pesticide's active ingredient to penetrate a plant's outer surface. In some instances, inert ingredients are added to extend the pesticide product's shelf life or to protect the pesticide from degradation due to exposure to sunlight. Pesticide products can contain more than one inert ingredient, but federal law does not require that these ingredients be identified by name or percentage on the label. Only the total percentage of inert ingredients is required to be on the pesticide product label. This is despite the fact that inerts may make up 80 or 90 percent of the ingredients and, in fact, may be associated with health risks. Instead, the active ingredients are listed.

Additionally, chemicals that the producer considers "trade secret" may not be listed. Comprehensive and accurate product labeling is a critical element of our right-to-know, and it is important for nurses to advocate for the most comprehensive labeling possible for all products. In 2006, the American Nurses Association (ANA) passed a chemical policy resolution calling for full disclosure of chemical ingredients on labels to facilitate informed decision making when purchasing products (ANA, 2006). This resolution provides the underpinning for nurses to engage in state and national legislative and regulatory advocacy.

When addressing any and all environmental health problems, it is important to understand the type and amount of exposure. This sometimes requires some form of testing, as was described for lead, CO, radon, and drinking water. For home assessments, there are a number of test kits available or environmental services that can be hired to do the testing. When we look at community-level exposures, such as air and recreational water or foods, we must rely on the environmental and public health agencies to do sampling and report the results. Information regarding such results is now often available on Web-based resources or can be obtained by simple request or a request based on the Freedom of Information Act (FOIA) (Box 10-4). Since the terrorist attacks on September 11, 2001, access to many of the previously available sources of information have been threatened.

Environmental Health Risks in Schools

On any given school day, one-sixth of the U.S. population can be found in a school building, and many of these people are children. Over the last few years, three high visibility issues associated with environmental health risks in schools have developed: indoor air quality, pesticide use, and the location of the schools.

Indoor Air Quality

A number of phrases have been coined in the last decade or so to describe problems with indoor air—sick building syndrome and tight buildings. The names reflect some of the problems. During the energy crisis of the 1970s, many buildings were weatherized and "tightened up" to prevent cool air from getting

---

BOX 10-4: Freedom of Information Act (FOIA)

All federal agencies are required under the FOIA to disclose records requested by the public. Under the provisions of the FOIA, federal agencies are to make their records available to the greatest extent possible, based on the principle of openness in government. Agencies may, however, withhold information pursuant to certain exemptions and exclusions in the statute.

SOURCE: From U.S. Department of Justice (2004)

in and hot air from escaping. At the same time, and also in the name of energy conservation, many schools decreased the number of air exchanges in the building. Air exchanges help to keep the air "fresh" by diluting the pollutants that accumulate in an occupied room, like carbon dioxide (which humans exhale); fumes from cleaning solutions, art supplies, and home economics and shop rooms, and the fumes that are emitted from furnishings and carpets. (It's extremely important to have a CO monitor in the auto shop area of schools.) In older buildings, the ventilation system may have been intended for fewer pupils per room. In addition, deferred maintenance of school buildings often results in water leaks and moisture problems that create the perfect conditions for mold growth. Given the increasing rates of asthma in children (and adults) it has become very important to make sure there are as few chemicals and biologicals as possible that might cause an asthma event.

To improve the air quality in schools, several commonsense approaches are prevalent: (1) Maintain the buildings and quickly report and respond to water/moisture-related problems, (2) make sure the heating, ventilation, and air conditioning systems are clean/maintained and operating at a level to properly ventilate for the number of occupants in the room, and (3) choose products that do not or minimally emit potentially hazardous or sensitizing chemicals. The first two on this list are not the responsibility of a public health or school nurse, but it's important to know that it should be done. The last item is something that school and public health nurses can influence. For instance, when furnishings are needed, there should be a preference for products that will not "out gas" or give off chemicals that may be harmful. There are many "green" cleaning products that do not emit VOCs, and these should also be selected. This guidance is appropriate for any type of commercial building, including the ones that house health departments, which are also often old buildings. The EPA has a program called IAQ/Tools for Schools and many nurses have participated in it. To obtain this toolbox with several excellent reference and decision-making materials that nurses will find very helpful, call the federal EPA office.

Pesticides

Pesticides can be found in our schools, but also in our homes, workplaces, and out of doors. In 2003, there were 97,677 pesticide poisonings reported in the United States, of which 50,938 were children under 6 years old (Watson et al., 2004). Because of the special vulnerabilities of children and pregnant women to pesticide exposures, control of pesticide use in schools and daycare settings is particularly important.

The term "pesticide" encompasses several types of chemicals, all of which were formulated to either kill something or prevent its reproduction. Included in the list of pesticides are insecticides, fungicides, rodenticides, biocides, and antimicrobials (this includes antimicrobial soaps, commonly used by nurses). All pesticides must be registered with the EPA, and their specific use must be stated. For example, some pesticides are registered for agricultural use on a particular crop, like tomatoes. Unless they were also registered for in-home use, they should not be used inside a home. Given the widespread use and misuse of pesticides and the fact that people suffer from pesticide poisoning on a regular basis, it is critical for public health nurses to understand the health risks associated with pesticides and to encourage reduction/elimination of use whenever possible, especially around vulnerable populations. Use of herbicides on athletic fields should be strongly discouraged.

Some schools around the country have banned the use of pesticides in schools and still others have demanded that integrated pest management (IPM) be implemented. IPM is an approach to pest identification and reduction/elimination that relies on first removing the pests' necessities—water, food, and a nesting place. By removing this part of their hierarchy of needs, it becomes difficult for them to survive. However, if they persist, the next thing to do is use nontoxic solutions, including traps and chemicals that are nontoxic to humans. There are examples of schools around the country that have successfully become pesticide and pest free. The nonprofit organization Beyond Pesticides (2006a; 2006b) provides excellent materials on toxic-free pest management, as well as providing up-to-date fact sheets on many pesticides that could be used in public health education programs.

School Locations

School locations can have a significant influence on health. Placing schools in areas where there is heavy industry, aerial spraying of agricultural chemicals, or major highways creates greater risk for air pollutants that are breathed in the schools, as well as when the children are on the playing fields. Determining a site for a school may present limited choices. Typically, school

⊕ POLICY HIGHLIGHT

Integrated Pest Management (IPM)

We often think about policy in terms of legislative and regulatory changes, but sometimes nurses can make important changes in other ways. When a nurse and soccer mom in Georgia discovered that they regularly sprayed herbicides on the soccer field where her young children play, she went into action. She found out the names of the chemicals that were being used, discovered that there were known health threats associated with the chemicals, organized other soccer moms, and met with a representative from the local Department of Recreation,

which was responsible for maintaining the fields. Together they learned about integrated pest management (IPM) and made a departmental policy decision to adopt IPM as the strategy of choice in maintaining all recreational fields and building grounds. The nurse employed several important elements of environmental health nursing practice as she helped to develop a sound primary prevention policy and strategy. She made an assessment that included learning the relevant science, she helped develop a coalition, helped to build consensus, and advocated for change.

---

districts have few resources, and so they may choose a site that has previously been used for a factory or gas station. When a site has been used previously and is considered to present possible environmental risks, this is called a brownfield site. Such sites should be carefully evaluated before making plans for development; however, in most states, school boards are not required to do in-depth evaluations of prospective building sites for schools. Public health and school nurses can advocate for such evaluations by working with the school board or equivalent in the school district, thus helping to prevent future exposures from toxic chemicals that may be in the soil.

Noise—from inside and outside sources—is another factor that should be considered. Noise is measured in decibels and is recorded with a sound meter. The presence of noise can have a significant negative effect on reading ability, test scores, and behavior. It has an even more significant effect on learning in children with English as a second language. Additionally, the following health effects are associated with noise pollution: high blood pressure, ulcers, and indigestion (Stansfeld & Matheson, 2003). For teachers, undue voice strain may also be caused by noise pollution. The primary sources of noise pollution in schools are heating and ventilation and air conditioning systems, and transportation sources account for most of the noise outside of schools. Cafeterias are notoriously loud. Noise is recognized as a controllable pollutant that can be improved by interventions. Both the EPA and the Occupational Safety and Health Administration (OSHA) set noise

standards, for the general environment and workplaces, respectively.

Environmental Health Risks in the Community

Community-wide environmental health risks include air and water pollution, soil contamination, contaminated waste sites, and risks associated with agricultural production.

Water Quality

Approximately 70% of the human body is water. Therefore, it is critical that our drinking and recreational waters be as free of contaminants as possible. Millions of Americans drink water that exceeds drinking water standards for fecal matter, parasites, pathogenic microbes, radiation, heavy metals, and/or other toxic chemicals. Knowledge about what is in community drinking and recreational waters, the associated health risks, the sources of the contaminants, and how to protect drinking water sources are all part of the public health nurses' environmental health armament.

Drinking water is derived from one of two sources: groundwater (aquifers) or surface water (streams, reservoirs, rivers). Well water is drawn from groundwater. Both groundwater and surface water are vulnerable to contamination from a wide variety of sources. Water contamination is divided into two large categories: (1) "Point source" pollutants come from a single, identifiable source such as a factory's wastewater (which may include permitted and/or nonpermitted chemicals) or sewer overflow pipe and (2) "non-point source" pollutants are from a great range of more diffuse sources, such as agricultural runoff of pesticides or fertilizers or from air pollutants that land on the surfaces of great bodies of water. Point source pollution is often regulated by the Environmental Protection Agency. If an industry or municipal public works entity such as a wastewater treatment facility discharges a pollutant into a body of water, they must have a permit from the state regulatory agency. As a society, we have decided that it is acceptable to discharge a certain amount of hazardous chemicals into our waterways, as long as it is within limits. The permitting process is the way in which the government gives permission to pollute. All permits should be publicly accessible for review. The permitting process should be a public process in which citizens can learn about the permit, including its limits.

There are hundreds of thousands of underground storage tanks in the United States, a significant number of which are storing gasoline at gas stations or fuel oil for residential use. A new contaminant has joined the ranks of water pollutants. Several years ago, methyl tertiary butyl ether (MTBE) was added to gasoline to increase gas efficiency and "decrease pollution." Unfortunately, it is a human carcinogen (known to cause liver and kidney tumors in mice) and has been detected in groundwater in every state from leaking underground storage tanks (EPA, 2006b). MTBE is no longer being added to gasoline but the pollution remains in many communities' groundwater, from which many communities draw their water. The case of MTBE raises a broader question about U.S. chemical policies, and it will be discussed later in this chapter.

Non-point sources of water pollution are sometimes more difficult to identify and control. Rain carries the oil, as well as the salt that we place on our icy roads, to the nearest surface water via the storm management system. Rain similarly carries lawn and agricultural chemicals to our surface waters. In addition, chemicals that are water-soluble may be absorbed into the earth and leach into the aquifers. Leaching is the gradual removal of contaminants, such as pesticides or fertilizers, from the soil by water trickling through. The U.S. Geologic Survey estimates that 42 million American wells are contaminated with VOCs derived from gasoline, solvents, paints, and MTBE (American Chemical Society, 1999).

The U.S. Geological Survey regularly surveys the aquifers and surface waters. The chemicals that we use in our everyday lives are being found in measurable amounts in our nation's water: acetaminophen, caffeine, codeine, cotamine (a metabolite of nicotine, spilled in the urine), 17b-estradiol (estrogen), and sulfamethoxazole (and other antibiotics, particularly in areas where large-scale farming occurs). There are also many naturally occurring chemicals in our water that may create health risks. Arsenic, radon, radium, and heavy metals can be naturally occurring contaminants in water.

Air Pollution

The 1990 Clean Air Act is the primary statute addressing outdoor air pollution. The EPA has designated a set of regulated pollutants as "criteria pollutants" that include the six most common air pollutants in the United States and help to define air quality within the National Ambient Air Quality Standards (Box 10-5). Criteria air pollutants are responsible for many adverse effects on human health, causing thousands of cases of premature mortality and tens of thousands of emergency room visits annually.

Health effects associated with air pollution include asthma and other respiratory diseases, cardiovascular diseases (including hypertension), cancer, immunologic effects, reproductive health problems (including birth defects), and neurological problems (Brunekreef and Holgate, 2002). Air pollution standards are based on protecting the health of healthy, middle-aged white males, but it should be noted that adverse health effects have been found at levels below the EPA air quality standards. The elderly and those with chronic pulmonary and/or vascular diseases appear to be at increased risk for mortality from short-term increases in both indoor and outdoor air pollution.

There are a range of **persistent, bioaccumulative, and toxic chemicals (PBTs)**. These chemicals typically have long molecular chains and do not break down in nature. They typically are the result of agricultural use (pesticides, chemical fertilizers), industrial processes, energy production, incineration, and automobile exhaust. **Fate and transport** refers to the process by which a pollutant moves through (and sometimes back and forth from) the air, soil, surface water, and groundwater. **Media** is the word for the different environments—air, water, and soil. Environmental laws and regulations are most often directed to a specific medium, such as the Clean Air Act, the Clean Water

BOX 10-5: Criteria Air Pollutants under the EPA's National Ambient Air Quality Standards

Sulfur dioxide is produced during combustion and industrial processes.

⊕ Sulfur dioxide is a major contributor to acid rain.

⊕ It is associated with respiratory illness, alterations in pulmonary function, aggravation of existing cardiovascular disease, and asthma.

Nitrous dioxide is produced during combustion; it affects the lungs, immune function, and asthma.

Carbon monoxide is produce during the burning of fossil fuel.

⊕ Carbon monoxide is substantially produced by motor vehicles.

⊕ Carbon monoxide binds very effectively with hemoglobin, precluding the binding of oxygen, resulting in anoxia; the most sensitive populations are those with cardiovascular diseases.

Particulate matter (PM) consists of liquid and solid aerosols from fuel combustion, motor vehicle exhaust, high-temperature industrial processes, and incineration.

⊕ Particulate matter includes dust, dirt, soot, smoke, and liquid droplets.

⊕ The lungs are a prime site for damage and exacerbation of underlying disease; the size of the particle determines the deposition in the lungs.

Lead in the aerosolized particulate matter is from industrial processes and incineration; lead is toxic to the nervous, immune, cardiovascular, reproductive systems, as well as damaging to heme synthesis and to the kidneys.

Ozone is an odorless, colorless gas composed of three atoms of oxygen. Ozone occurs both in the earth's upper atmosphere and at ground level. Ozone can be good or bad, depending on where it is found.

⊕ The "good" ozone occurs at a layer in the stratosphere about 10–25 miles above the earth; it serves to protect us from the most damaging ultraviolet rays. It has been significantly damaged by chlorofluorocarbons (CFCs).

⊕ The "bad" ozone is ground-level ozone that is created by reaction of hydrocarbons, which include VOCs, and nitrogen oxides in the presence of sunlight.

⊕ The VOCs are emitted from a wide range of sources: dry cleaners, cars, chemical manufacturers, paint shops, and many others.

⊕ The prime target organ for ozone is the lungs where it causes damage, diminishes lung function, and sensitizes the lungs to other irritants.

⊕ The burning of fossil fuel (e.g., in diesels, industrial boilers, and power plants) and waste incineration are two other major contributors.

⊕ Bad, ground-level (man-made) ozone can irritate the respiratory system, aggravate asthma, reduce lung function, and inflame and damage the lung epithelium.

SOURCE: Adapted from EPA sources by B. Sattler.

Act, or Brownfields Legislation. Multimedia implies a chemical pollutant that contaminates two or more media. The fate and transport of mercury illustrates multimedia occurrences and the need for multimedia control strategies: Mercury that is emitted from a coal-fired power plant travels as an air pollutant and deposits on a body of water where it migrates to the bottom; it is digested by the bottom-dwelling microorganisms during which process it is converted to methyl mercury, is eaten by fish and then eaten by larger fish, and eventually is eaten by mammals (including humans). The environmental protection/public health approaches to these multimedia exposures include air pollution standards, water pollution standards, fishing alerts for fisherman, and health education for women of childbearing ages regarding safe consumption of fish that may contain mercury.

The United Nations has identified 12 particularly toxic chemicals in its Stockholm Convention calling for their ban or calling for ways in which to diminish their occurrence. The Stockholm Convention addresses PBTs, chemicals that not only are highly toxic but also persist in our environment and the human body. Ten of the 12 toxic chemicals are pesticides: aldrin, chlordane, DDT, dieldrin, endrin, heptachlor, hexachlorobenzene, and mirex. The other two listings are a form of dioxins and a form of furans, which are the unintended by-products of combustion from chlorinated compounds resulting from industrial processes (e.g., the production of vinyl chloride—the key component in PVCs, polyvinyl chloride plastics) and waste incineration (including medical waste incineration). Incinerated hospital waste is a major source of dioxin in the United States because of the heavy reliance on PVCs in the health care industry.

Soil Contamination

Soil becomes contaminated from a variety of ways. Air pollutants ultimately fall to earth, contaminating either soil or water. Previous uses of land—factories, nuclear weapons production sites, and other past uses—have left a significant legacy of contaminated land around the country. Brownfields are abandoned, idled, or underused industrial and commercial facilities/lands where expansion or redevelopment is complicated by real or perceived environmental contamination (EPA definition). The EPA has regulations addressing brownfields, but many players are often involved in the redevelopment of brownfields: local planning departments, local development agencies, state departments of environmental quality, among others.

Highly contaminated land may be designated **Superfund** sites by the EPA. Administered by the U.S. Environmental Protection Agency, this program investigates and cleans up the largest and most contaminated sites in the United States. The National Priorities List (NPL) is a compilation of the most serious sites that are targeted for cleanup under Superfund. The presence of Superfund sites in the community can be searched on the EPA's Web site. Under both Superfund and brownfields law community members have the right to know and the right to be involved in the assessment phase, selection of remediation, and involvement in reuse decision, as well as any long-term monitoring for the site. Land use choices can have a significant effect on a community's health and well-being. Consider the different impact that a park versus a sewage treatment plant would have on a community.

Agricultural Production

In the last half century, there have been enormous changes in agricultural production. The number of family farms has dropped precipitously at the same time that large, corporate farms have taken the main role in producing our nation's livestock and produce. Some of the practices in contemporary agriculture create health risks and/or raise concerns. Broad reliance on pesticides increases the risk of unhealthy levels of pesticides in the air, ground- and surface water, and food. Farm workers and farm families are at the greatest risks for exposure, with pregnant women and children being the most sensitive populations. Public health nurses working in rural areas should know the types of chemicals that are commonly used on the crops and the associated health effects, both for acute poisoning and for chronic low-level exposures.

More than half the U.S. supply of antibiotics is fed to cattle, chickens, and hogs, not because they are sick or for disease prevention, but rather to increase their growth rate (Shea, 2004). An animal that is fed low levels of antibiotics will gain about 5% more weight. If giving the animals antibiotics was innocuous, there would not be a problem. However, misuse of antibiotics places the effectiveness of antibiotics at risk. When organisms learn to adapt to our current armament of antibiotics, we run the risk for the development of pathogenic organisms that may create animal or human infections, for which we will have no treatment. The American Nurses Association understood the peril that this could create when they adopted their 2004 resolution calling for a ban on nontherapeutic antibiotics in animal feed (ANA, 2004).

As consumers increasingly choose food products that have been grown/raised without pesticides, bovine growth hormones, genetically modified organisms, and nontherapeutic antibiotics (U.S. Department of State, 2006), this demand, or market force, is influencing the supply side, such that an increasing number of producers are changing their practices. Though still small in relative numbers, the number of organic farms and organic farm products are increasing in the United States.

Public health nurses should be prepared to answer basic questions about these important emerging food issues. Equally important, nurses should always advocate for the most comprehensive labeling of all products, but particularly food products, so that consumers can make informed choices. Unless a product qualifies for "organic" status and is labeled as such (Box 10-6), *labeling is not required* to inform consumers when genetically engineered foods have been included, nontherapeutic antibiotics used, bovine growth hormone have been administered, or pesticides have been applied. This labeling deficiency hinders informed, health-based, consumer decision making.

BOX 10-6: Defining Certified Organic

What is certified organic food?

Organic food is produced by farmers who emphasize the use of renewable resources and the conservation of soil and water to enhance environmental quality for future generations. Organic meat, poultry, eggs, and dairy products come from animals that are given no antibiotics or growth hormones. Organic food is produced without using most conventional pesticides, fertilizers made with synthetic ingredients or sewage sludge, bioengineering, or ionizing radiation. Before a product can be labeled "organic," a government-approved certifier must inspect the farm where the food is grown to make sure the farmer is following all the rules necessary to meet USDA organic standards. Companies that handle or process organic food before it gets to your local supermarket or restaurant must be certified, too.

SOURCE: http://www.ams.usda.gov/nop/Consumers/brochure.html

Global Warming

Changes in the temperature of the earth's atmosphere raise a number of public health questions. Our current dependency on fossil fuel—coal, oil, and gas—is escalating the conditions for a "greenhouse effect," which, in turn, is resulting in a global warming trend. This rise in temperature is associated with a rise in sea level, extreme weather patterns, and heat-related changes in flora and fauna. Changes in rodent and insect patterns, in turn, increase the risk of vector-borne, infectious diseases. A rising sea level threatens coastal communities all over the world.

Staving off the global warming trends is going to take a concerted effort worldwide, with changes in individual choices, national policies, and global agreements. At the individual level, selecting energy-efficient vehicles and appliances can be effective. At the national level, energy policies must emphasize reliance on renewable resources rather than continued dependency on fossil fuels. The international Kyoto Protocols, which originated in 1997, fosters agreement among nations to reduce the production of greenhouse gases. In 2001, the United States withdrew support for the agreement stating that there was inadequate science supporting the global warming trends and the associated risks. This continues to be largely a political rather than scientific debate.

Environmental Health Risks at Work

Workplaces are host to a wide range of high-level exposures from industrial strength chemicals, deafening noises, dangerous physical hazards, heat and cold, and psychological stressors. It is critical for public health nurses to know the types of occupational hazards associated with workplaces in their communities. Workers can be affected by their exposures at work, and in the case of chemical exposures, they can bring them home on their clothes so that their whole family can be exposed. Some classic occupationally related diseases are asbestos-related asbestosis (known as White Lung disease), coal-related pneumoconiosis (known as Black Lung disease), and cotton dust-related byssinosis (known as Brown Lung disease).

As per the 1970 Occupational Safety and Health Act (OSHAct), workers in the United States have the right to a healthy and safe workplace. The workplace is regulated by OSHA (or the Mine Safety and Health Administration, MSHA, for mining). An extensive set of workplace standards has been promulgated by federal OSHA, which is responsible for enforcement in half of the states. In the other half, state-level OSHAs are responsible for enforcement where they may promulgate standards that are even more effective than the federal standards. They may not, however, have standards that are less effective than the federal ones.

Under the OSHAct, workers have the right to submit a complaint and request that an inspector come to their workplace. When OSHA inspectors come to worksites, they can inspect as much of the workplace as they wish, they are not limited to inspecting the place associated with the complaint. After the inspection is completed, citations may be issued for noncompliance with OSHA standards. A fine may be associated with the citation. A listing of a company's citations can be obtained from OSHA.

Even though it is a worker's right to request an OSHA inspection, it should be noted that many workers may not be comfortable exercising this right for fear of reprisals in their workplace. As public health nurses, there are several ways to gather information about workers' exposures: (1) Ask the workers what they know about their health and safety conditions; (2) request information directly from the company; (3) speak with the union health and safety representative, if the workers are represented by a union, or (4) request available information from OSHA (state or federal) regarding the company's history of compliance.

The health care setting poses a unique set of occupational risks that include biological exposures (pathogenic microbes, viruses); radiological exposures (x-rays, therapeutic radiological implants in clients with cancer); chemical exposures (gluteraldehyde, antichemotherapeutic drugs, industrial-strength cleaning products); as well as physical hazards from lifting, needle sticks, and workplace violence. The Center for Occupational and Environmental Health at the American Nurses Association actively addresses nurses' workplace hazards and provides a wealth of information and expertise on these issues.

VULNERABLE POPULATIONS

There are several highly sensitive times in human development when we are more susceptible to the effects of environmental pollutants. The most sensitive time is during embryonic and fetal development. During this time of rapid cell division (tissue, organ and organ system development), orchestrated biological and chemical events must all be successful for normal growth and development to occur. During this time period, toxic chemical exposures can have their most insidious effects. The placenta, once thought to be a protective barrier for the fetus, has been shown to be permeable to most toxic chemicals. Thus, the chemicals that a pregnant woman is exposed to may be passed on to the fetus. In addition, toxic chemicals are sometimes stored in a woman's body, and they can be mobilized during pregnancy. For instance, one of the places lead is stored is in bone and teeth. During pregnancy, this lead can be mobilized when bone calcium shifts to provide needed calcium for fetal bone development. (Pregnant women should take calcium supplements to prevent calcium shifts in their bones, which also will prevent lead shifts.)

Pre-conception exposures to both males and females can affect birth outcomes, as can embryonic/fetal exposure in utero. There are two excellent sources of reproductive health information specific to occupational and environmental exposures: DART (Developmental and Reproductive Toxicology) databases housed by the National Library of Medicine and REPROTOX. REPROTOX also provides information about toxicants expressed during lactation.

Breast milk was tested during the CDC's body burden studies and found to contain a similar mix of PBTs as were found in people's blood and urine. It is still extremely important to encourage breastfeeding, which continues to offer the most nutritious option for infants. However, it is disconcerting that "mother's milk" now comes with pesticides, flame retardants, DDT, and dioxins (among many others). There is no way to extract these chemicals from the milk. Primary prevention—preventing such toxic chemicals from entering the environment—is the only meaningful solution.

Early childhood presents an additional set of environmental exposure risks. Several facts about children must be noted:

- Children breathe more per body weight than do adults. Therefore their "dose" of toxicants that are in the air winds up being higher than that of adults.

- Children eat and drink more per body weight than do adults. Therefore their "dose" of toxicants that are in food (including pesticide residues) and beverages, including water, are higher than that of adults.

- Children hang out at ground level because of their relative height, and they're more likely to play on the ground, both indoors and out. Therefore, children are more likely to be exposed to those chemicals that are in dust, soot, and soil.

- Children place their hands and objects into their mouths as part of their normal exploration. Therefore, any toxic chemicals that are on their hands or the objects may be ingested.

- Children's growth and development does not stop until they are in their teens. Therefore, they continue to be especially susceptible to the effects of toxic chemicals while they are still developing.

The majority of toxicological research is done with adult animals, and human epidemiological studies are almost invariably with adult populations. Thus our knowledge of the specific effects on children has been slow to unfold. It should be noted that air and water pollution standards are established to protect adults and do not necessarily take into account the special vulnerabilities of children. Nurses' perspective about human vulnerability through the lifespan is an important addition during legislative and regulatory decisions about air, water, and other pollutants.

The aging process also creates increased susceptibility to the effects of toxic pollutants. With age, many systems become less efficient. For example, kidney and liver functions diminish, thus decreasing clearance and transformation of toxic chemicals, which in turn results in accumulation of the toxic chemicals. The elderly are more likely to suffer from chronic diseases, which may make them more susceptible to the effects of toxic chemicals. This population is more likely to suffer from diarrheal diseases associated with contaminants in their drinking water. Elderly populations are more likely to regularly take medications. Little is known about the interactions between medications and the toxic chemicals in the environment, as well as the interactions among the environmental exposures in our homes, workplaces, schools, and communities.

One other population that may be particularly vulnerable to certain types of environmental exposures includes people who are immunocompromised, such as people with HIV/AIDS, people who have received organ transplants, and people on medications that suppress immune function. These people will be at increased risk of infections from pathogens in drinking water or food. As such, they may need to take special precautions regarding their food and drinking water quality.

ENVIRONMENTAL JUSTICE

Environmental justice refers to equity in environmental quality across populations. The term evolved in the 1980s with the increasing knowledge that people of color and poor people in the United States were being disproportionately exposed to environmental health risks in the places they lived and worked. Evidence mounted about increased exposures from hazardous waste sites, dangerous jobs, substandard housing stock, and most recently disproportionately higher body burdens of toxic chemicals.

In 1992, then President Clinton's Environmental Justice Executive Order demanded that every federal agency consider the ways in which their agency's decisions (or lack of decisions) might affect environmental justice (Executive Order 12898, 1992). In half the states in the country there is now a state-level commission or task force appointed to look at issues associated with

environmental justice. Such issues are steeped in conditions that create and sustain poverty and racism and threaten civil rights. These are also the conditions that public health professionals are dedicated to addressing.

Public health nurses can bring valuable information about environmental health, as well as knowledge about navigating bureaucratic systems in order to help level the playing field in communities, especially poor communities. Additionally, nurses can make sure that information is in a form and language that is understandable and accessible. For example, signage for fishing alerts should be in a language(s) that are understood by the people who are likely to fish there. Public health nurses need to know both the government agencies, as well as the legal and advocacy organizations that address housing issues, immigration problems, and employment situations, so they can work at a systems level to help address environmental justice issues.

ADVOCACY

Advocacy is a vital element of public health practice. Advocacy can mean a number of things. One can advocate for an individual or family, as their case manager by requesting mattress covers for allergic/asthmatic children; or advocate for increased funding or policy changes for a whole community or population, such as increased lead surveillance to children or improved occupational health conditions for workers; or advocate for legislative or regulatory changes to affect a problem at a higher systems level, like requiring least toxic approaches to pest management in schools or mandating food labeling regarding the use of bovine growth hormone in dairy production. The public health community as a whole has been engaged in environmental health advocacy and recently nurses are increasingly involved. The recent passage of environmental resolutions by the ANA and the creation of an Environmental Task Force by the Public Health Nursing Section of the American Public Health Association are evidence of this increasing engagement.

Traditionally, environmentalist organizations have been the most visible advocates for environmental protection. Historically, they focused on protection of the natural world and land preservation. In the last two decades, there has been an additional focus by many of the environmentalist organizations on human health threats associated with environmental degradation. Additionally, several newer organizations have been very effective in raising awareness about environmental health issues, such as the Children's Environmental Health Network and Physicians for Social Responsibility. Nurses provide a unique and powerful voice when working in coalition with environmentalist organizations on environmental health protection. Nurses' scientific credibility and selfless interest in the public's health contribute to their designation as the most trusted professionals regarding environmental health issues.

A unique coalition of organizations, including many nursing organizations, has been working on the occupational and environmental health risks associated with the provision of health care services. This coalition, called Health Care Without Harm, has been addressing occupational health issues such as needlestick injuries and improved ergonomics and environmental health issues including advocating the 3 R's—reduction, reuse, and recycling—which translates into such activities as reduction of the amount of packing, purchasing products that can be reused versus one-time-use products, and recycling paper, plastic, electronic equipment, batteries, and other products used in health care. The coalition is also working with architects on designing health care facilities that are more environmentally sound such as hospitals that use less energy, access more natural lighting, are designed for noise control, are built with nontoxic materials, and are designed to be healthful for the employees, the clients, and the community at large. These design elements have been incorporated into the Green Guidelines for Health Care. Health Care Without Harm has also been addressing the use of mercury, pest control, cleaning products, indoor air quality, and a range of issues associated with health risks.

RISK COMMUNICATION

Risk communication is a common practice in the health care setting. When clients ask about their "chances" for a side effect from a drug or the "odds" that a problem will reoccur, they are really asking about the "risk" of something happening. Communicating about risks that are associated with the environment is an important role for public health nurses. Risk communication can occur in a variety of settings. When a community discovers a new threat, such as a leaking underground storage tank or a new regional plan to spray for West Nile virus, they will often organize a public event in which the community can learn about issue. The meetings can take place at faith-based locations, town halls, schools,

and even in community members' homes. Community members will typically have many questions, some easy and some not so easy to answer. Depending on the circumstances, these meetings can sometimes become emotional.

There are four key elements to risk communication: message, messenger, audience, and context.

- ⊕ *Message:* More often than not, there is imprecise knowledge about the risk of a health effect or other problem associated with environmental pollutants or toxic chemicals in our homes, schools, workplaces, or communities. It is essential that nurses gather as much scientific evidence as possible. This should include knowing the health risks associated with the exposure based on toxicology and/or epidemiology; knowing the routes of exposure (inhalation, ingestion, dermal via air, water, soil, food); and knowing the evidence of exposure to individuals or a whole community (based on sampling, monitoring, or estimations). This information must then be translated into language and examples that the audience can understand. An opportunity for questions and answers should be allowed.

- ⊕ *Messenger:* One of the most important attributes of successful risk communication messengers is that they are good listeners. In most communities that are hearing about an environmental health risk, it is important to allow the community members to say their piece and to ask their questions. Listening attentively and answering questions honestly and frankly is critical to productive risk communication. It is best to receive information about a health risk from someone who is trusted; the best messengers are people whom communities believe they can trust. Messengers also need to speak clearly, without technical jargon, in a manner that most community members will understand. This requires cultural and linguistic sensitivity by the messengers. When needed, translators should be arranged or recruited from the community members. This should be arranged before a risk communication effort begins. Messengers should be prepared for the possibility of emotional and/or heated discussions. Messengers with good facilitation skills can encourage open communication and make sure that everyone feels that they have been heard and acknowledged.

Audience: In any given audience, there will be people with different biases, interests, and abilities regarding their understanding of technical information. For example, a parent who is a homeowner and lives next to a hazardous waste site may want to know the potential health risks to their children but will also be concerned about how news of the contamination will affect their property values. They may or may not trust the government to do the right thing, and they may be angry that the government "let this happen" or "haven't done anything about it." Community members will want their questions answered and will easily become suspicious if they feel that information is being withheld. A "suspicious audience" will begin to suspect the worst and become distrustful of the risk communication process. Therefore, full and honest disclosure is essential. If the messenger does not know the answer to a question, he or she should say so and, when appropriate, agree to find the answer to the question.

Context: In any given risk communication situation, there will be a history of activities and an assortment of players. This history will contribute to the tone of the risk communication. Resources and capacity will affect a community's ability to respond to and cope with the news of an environmental problem. A well-educated and well-resourced community will respond to the news of a new environmental health risk quite differently from a poor community in which English is a second language. The community-based and public health nurse can make sure that community members have as good an understanding and as many resources as possible to adequately address the environmental health risks that may threaten their communities. Good risk communication processes will contribute to the success of this objective.

Public health nurses can play a vital role in organizing public forums, ensuring that as many stakeholders as possible are invited. Because of their trusted role in the community and their understanding of the culture and values in the community, they are ideal people to be involved in risk communication activities. Note that it is critical that the messengers maintain their scientific integrity and be clear about the boundaries of their knowledge. This will maintain the important covenant of trust that nurses have with their communities.

CHEMICAL POLICIES AND THE PRECAUTIONARY PRINCIPLE

In the United States, chemical policies are not consistent. The mechanism for chemicals that are developed for pharmaceutical purposes are held to the highest standards of testing. As most nurses know, manufacturers of drugs must start with animal testing, move through limited clinical trials with humans, and into more extensive, rigorous clinical trials. Any given clinical trial is for a specified therapeutic use and side effects are closely monitored. Contrast this safety-oriented process to the development of chemicals for household products or personal care products. The manufacturer does not have to do original research into the potential harm that the chemical might cause on the environment or on human health. They can bring the product to market, and anyone can buy it off the shelf—clean their children's room with it; spray it in the air to "refresh" it; or smear it on their body—without any further testing. The legacy of the U.S. chemical policies has included widespread use of products like asbestos, arsenic in pressure-treated wood, gasoline additives (MTBE), and flame retardants that have been found to be harmful after they have been in the market and have subsequently been removed from the market, banned by the government, or have required costly replacement and/or cleanup, all the while creating human health risks.

The Precautionary Principle brings to mind the adage that it is better to be safe than sorry. It is directed toward issues associated with environmental risks and speaks to the need to test products before releasing them, as well as heeding early warnings of potential harm from chemicals and other hazards in our environment. Early warnings might include new animal data indicating a chemical or product. Responses to the warnings could include removal or reduction of the exposure and finding safer alternatives. Additionally, next steps might include more research to enhance a fuller understanding of the risks; full disclosure by the chemical manufacturer about what they know; and a "right to know" about the risks for workers, consumers, community members, and health professionals. In 2006, the ANA endorsed the Precautionary Principle as a public health tool to guide its environmental health policy and advocacy work (Gilbert & Davies, 2006).

Globally, chemical policies are being developed through regional agreements and UN treaties. Three important international policies are the Kyoto Protocols (described earlier in the chapter), the Stockholm Convention on Persistent Organic Pollutants (POPs), and the European Union's Registration, Evaluation, and Authorization of Chemicals (REACH) program. The POPS Treaty calls for the reduction/elimination of 12 persistent and toxic chemicals—PCBs (polychlorinated biphenols, which were already banned in the United States), dioxins/furans, and 10 chemicals that are pesticides. The Stockholm Convention also recognizes the need to take global action on all chemicals with POP-like characteristics, such as those that are persistent in the environment, travel long distances via air and water, are toxic, and bioaccumulate in living things. The Stockholm Convention creates a worldwide, primary prevention approach to health risks associated with these 12 chemicals.

In Europe, a comprehensive approach to chemical policies has resulted in the REACH policy, which requires that chemicals be registered for use with an independent European agency; evaluated for the potential risk to the environment or humans; and authorized (or not) for a specific use. If a safer substitute exists, the REACH agency will not authorize a more toxic chemical for the same use. If no safer substitute exists, then the authorization may limit the chemicals used to specific functions. The European's forward-thinking policy is a primary prevention approach to chemical policies.

ENVIRONMENTAL AND PUBLIC HEALTH INFRASTRUCTURE

Environmental health is the responsibility of numerous governmental agencies, at the state, local, and federal levels. The agencies can have both unique and overlapping responsibilities.

Federal Responsibilities

The U.S. Environmental Protection Agency is the primary regulator of environmental health. Congress passes major environmental legislation, such as the Clean Air Act, the Safe Drinking Water Act, and the Food Quality Protection Act, which are signed into law by the president. The EPA is then tasked with the development and promulgation of the regulations associated with the individual statutes (laws). National environmental health policies can be influenced before or dur-

ing their legislative development and debates, as well as during the development of regulations.

Virtually every federal agency has some responsibility regarding environment and health. For example, the Department of Agriculture, the Federal Food and Drug Administration, and the EPA all are responsible for some aspects of food safety. The Department of Transportation regulates the transportation of hazardous materials on roads and rails, whereas the Federal Aviation Administration is responsible for hazardous materials transported by air; the Department of Energy is concerned about energy production and is engaged in environmental cleanups of its nuclear weapons production plants; and the Occupational Safety and Health Administration is responsible for workplace environments.

The U.S. Department of Health and Human Services (DHHS) is the department of the federal executive branch most concerned with the nation's human health concerns. The public health infrastructure is vital to environmental health. Within DHHS, several agencies have environmental health responsibilities:

- Within the Centers for Disease Control and Prevention is the National Center for Environmental Health, the Agency for Toxic Substances and Disease Registry (ATSDR), and the National Institute for Occupational Safety and Health (NIOSH)
- The National Institute of Environmental Health Sciences is part of the National Institute of Health

State and Local Responsibilities

In every state there is a state-level equivalent of the Environmental Protection Agency. These agencies are responsible for enforcing environmental protection laws and regulations. The state agencies may also have additional programs and policies that are state specific. At the local level (city and county) environmental programs are often found in the local health department. In rare instances there is a separate agency for environmental protection or environmental health. At the local level the following services are often provided: food safety inspections, rodent control, and activities related to lead-based paint. At some local health departments only mandatory activities occur, whereas at others a wide range of activities may be found, such as asthma education programs, green building programs, and integrated pest management resources.

Another important activity that occurs at the local level is zoning. Zoning is a policy and process by which land use is designated as residential, commercial, industrial, parks, or some combination of these. The designation can have a significant impact on health. For instance, the combined designation of industrial and residential occurs more often in poor neighborhoods, and the proximity of residential housing to polluting industries has contributed to environmental justice problems.

ACCESSING INFORMATION AND THE "RIGHT TO KNOW"

Access to information about environmental risks in our food, water, and soil is provided through a variety of agencies via an array of federal and state statutes. The overarching law that allows for citizen access to governmental information is the Freedom of Information Act (FOIA) (Box 10-4). Through FOIA requests, information can be requested from virtually any federal agency, and there is often the equivalent at the state level. States have the equivalent Freedom of Information laws. The primary manner in which information is shared about consumer products is through labeling requirements. However, there are a number of informational gaps regarding labeling, and because manufacturers of consumer products do not have to do any original testing for toxicity, the information may not be available. In the absence of data, the fact that there is no evidence of harm should not be considered evidence that there is no potential harm. In the best of situations, labeling can only be as good as the existing data.

Workers' right to information about hazardous chemical exposures is covered by the Hazard Communication Standard, which requires that potentially hazardous chemicals be labeled; that employees have access to the associated Material Safety Data Sheets (MSDSs), which are chemical information sheets created by the chemical manufactures; and that all workers be trained about proper work practices, worker protection, health effects, and other critical information to their health and safety related to the potentially hazardous chemical.

Under EPA regulations air pollution and water pollution for a set of 600 chemicals must be reported to the EPA, if a certain action level of chemicals is emitted. This information, known as the Toxic Release Inventory (TRI), is made publicly available by the EPA on their EnviroFACTS Web site. When doing environmental health assessments of a community, utilizing the worker right to know law and the TRI databases can be very helpful.

ENVIRONMENTAL HEALTH AND PUBLIC HEALTH NURSING

When the Institute of Medicine convened a committee to look at the nursing profession's ability to address environmental health issues, they discovered a serious deficit in nursing's capacity to integrate environmental health into nursing education, practice, research, and policy/advocacy. The committee's resulting 1995 report, entitled *Nursing, Health and the Environment* provided a road map for environmental health integration into the nursing profession (Box 10-7). There has been much progress on the integration of environmental health into nursing activities since the publication of the report. The country is now dotted with environmental health nursing champions in the form of educators, practitioners, researchers, and others who are engaged in legislative and policy work. In 2006, the ANA adopted a set of Principles for Environmental Health Nursing Practice to guide nurses' ventures into environmental health. This will lead to the development of best practices.

The ANA and the Public Health Nursing Section of the American Public Health Association have been leaders in the profession's reemergence into environmental health—its rediscovery of Florence Nightingale's emphasis on environmental risks and its impact on health. Nursing science is in its early stages of development regarding environmental health and there is a crucial need for work in this area. Today, environmental health risks are far more complicated than in Nightingale's time but the imperative for public health nurses to engage in environmental health issues has never been more critical.

CRITICAL THINKING ACTIVITIES

1. How can nurses who are making home visits incorporate environmental health assessments into their visit time?

2. What environmental health programs are provided by the local health department in your community? Compare and contrast the quantity and quality of programs from different local health department in the region.

3. The Department of Natural Resources has posted a fish alert on a local waterway commonly used by local fishermen. Is there a role for the local health department regarding this alert?

4. A suburban community just discovered that there has been an underground storage tank leak of gasoline in the neighborhood. The community members all have their own private wells. As a public health nurse in the local health department, you have been asked to help develop the risk communication strategy. How will you do this?

5. Mold has been discovered in a local daycare center. The public health nurse gets a call from a concerned parent. What are possible next steps for the nurse?

BOX 10-7: Institute of Medicine Report:
Nursing, Health and the Environment

Nurses' roles in environmental health

The following summarizes the recommendations from the Institute of Medicine report, *Nursing, Health and the Environment* (IOM, 1995).

General Environmental Health Competency for Nurses

All nurses should have the following competencies:

A. Understand the scientific principles and underpinnings of the relationship between individuals or populations and the environment, including the following:

1. The basic mechanisms and pathways of exposure to environmental health hazards
2. Basic prevention and control strategies
3. The interdisciplinary nature of effective interventions
4. The role of research

B. Assess and refer, using the following strategies:

1. Successfully completing an environmental health history
2. Recognizing potential environmental hazards and sentinel illnesses
3. Making appropriate referrals for conditions with probable environmental etiologies
4. Accessing and providing information to clients and communities, and locating referral sources

C. Demonstrate knowledge of the role of advocacy (case and class), ethics, and risk communication in patient care and community intervention with respect to the potential adverse effects of the environment on health.

D. Understand the policy framework and major pieces of legislation and regulations related to environmental health.

(continued)

BOX 10-7: Institute of Medicine Report: Nursing, Health and the Environment (cont'd)

IOM Recommendations on Nursing Practice, Education, Research, and Advocacy

A. Environmental health should be reemphasized in the scope of responsibilities for nursing practice.

1. Resources to support environmental health content in nursing practice should be identified and made available.

2. Nurses should participate as members and leaders in interdisciplinary teams that address environmental health problems.

3. Communication should extend beyond counseling individual patients and families to facilitating the exchange of information on environmental hazards and community responses.

4. The concept of advocacy in nursing should be expanded to include advocacy on behalf of groups and communities, in addition to advocacy on behalf of individual patients and their families.

5. Research regarding the ethical implications of occupational and environmental health hazards should be conducted and findings incorporated into curricula and practice.

B. Environmental health concepts should be incorporated into all levels of nursing education.

1. Environmental health content should be included in nursing licensure and certification examinations.

2. Expertise in various environmental health disciplines should be included in the education of nurses.

3. Environmental health content should be an integral part of lifelong learning and continuing education for nurses.

4. Professional associations, public agencies, and private organizations should provide more resources and educational opportunities to enhance environmental health awareness in nursing practice.

C. Multidisciplinary and interdisciplinary research endeavors should be developed and implemented to build the knowledge base for nursing practice in environmental health.

1. The number of nurse researchers should be increased to build the knowledge base in environmental health as it relates to the practice of nursing.

2. Research priorities for environmental health nursing should be established and used by funding agencies for resource allocation decisions and to give direction to nurse researchers.

3. Current efforts to disseminate research findings to nurses, other health care providers, and the public should be strengthened and expanded.

D. Nurses should have the skills to work with the community, environmental groups, and local government, including the following activities:

1. Legislative lobbying

2. Reporting community hazards

3. Advocating for safer environments

4. Policy implementation

KEY CONCEPTS

- Environmental risks come in the form of biological, chemical, and radiological exposures.

- The dose of the exposure is critical to determining the health outcome.

- Environmental health risks can be categorized by their form (biological, chemical, radiological), the

medium from which the exposure is derived (air, water, soil, food), the environmental location (home, work, school, community), and the effects that the risks may have on human development.

- Many governmental agencies are involved in environmental health issues. The EPA is the primary

⊕ agency for environmental protection regulations, while OSHA is primarily responsible for occupational safety and health regulations.

⊕ Environmental health advocacy and policy work is a critical part of the nursing profession.

⊕ Risk communication is an important role for public health nursing.

⊕ Nurses and their communities must have access to processes and information in order to make informed decisions regarding the occupational and environmental health and safety.

⊕ Environmental health should be integrated into all levels of nursing practice, education, research, policy, and advocacy.

KEY TERMS

brownfield site

decibel (dB)

dose

dose–response curve

environmental epidemiology

environmental health

environmental justice

fate and transport

integrated pest management (IPM)

leach

media

noise pollution

persistence

persistent, bioaccumulative, and toxic chemicals (PBTs)

risk assessment

Superfund

toxicity

toxicology

watershed

zoning

REFERENCES

American Chemical Society. (1999, October 29). *42 million Americans use groundwater vulnerable to contamination by volatile organic compounds.* Retrieved October 1, 2006, from the Science Daily Web site:

American Nurses Association. (2004). *Inappropriate use of antimicrobials in agriculture.* American Nurses Association 2004 House of Delegates Resolution. Retrieved July, 2007, from http://www.noharm.org/details.cfm?type=document&ID=1521

American Nurses Association. (2006). *Nursing practice, chemical exposure and right to know.* American Nurses Association 2006 House of Delegates Resolution. Retrieved July 19, 2007, from http://www.nursingworld.org/coeh/ChemicalExposureRes06.pdf

Beyond Pesticides. (2006a). *Integrated pest management.* Retrieved October 1, 2006, from http://www.beyondpesticides.org/.

Beyond Pesticides. (2006b). *What is integrated pest management (IPM)?* Retrieved October 1, 2006, from http://www.beyondpesticides.org/infoservices/pcos/IPM.HTM.

Brunekreef, B., & Holgate, S.T. (2002). Air pollution and health. *Lancet, 360,* 1233–1242.

Centers for Disease Control and Prevention (CDC). (2005a). *National report on human exposure to environmental chemi-*

cals. Retrieved November 21, 2006, from http://www.cdc.gov/exposurereport/default.htm

Centers for Disease Control and Prevention (CDC). (2005b). Adult blood lead epidemiology and surveillance—United States, 2003–2004. *MMWR, 55,* 876–879.

Centers for Disease Control and Prevention (CDC). (2006). *About the National Center for Health Statistics.* Retrieved July 19, 2007, from http://www.cdc.gov/nchs/nhanes.htm

Clapp, R., Howe, G.K., & Jacobs, M.M. (2005, September). *Environmental and occupational causes of cancer: A review of recent scientific literature.* Prepared by Boston University School of Public Health and Environmental Health Initiative, University of Massachusetts Lowell For the Cancer Working Group of the Collaborative on Health and the Environment.

Dallaire, F., Muckle, G., & Ayotte, P. (2003) Time trends of persistent organic pollutants and heavy metals in umbilical cord blood of Inuit infants born in Nunavik (Quebec, Canada) between 1994 and 2001. *Environmental Health Perspectives, 111,* 1660–1664.

EPA. (2006a). Answer 17, describe the radon epidemiological studies. *Radon: Frequent questions.* Retrieved October 1, 2006, from http://www.epa.gov/radon/radonqa1.html#faq2.

EPA. (2006b). *MTBE (methyl tertiary-butyl ether) and underground storage tanks.* Retrieved October 1, 2006, from http://www.epa.gov/OUST/mtbe/index.htm.

Fabrikant, J.I. (1990). Radon and lung cancer: The BEIR IV report. *Health Physiology, 59*(1), 89-97.

Gilbert, S.G., & Davies, K. (2006). Resolution 06-02: Endorsing the precautionary principle as a public health tool for preventing harm from persistent bioaccumulative toxic chemicals (PBTS). Retrieved July 19, 2007, from http://www.wspha.org/Resolution_06-02.pdf

Heininger, K. (2000). A unifying hypothesis of Alzheimer's disease. IV. Causation and sequence of events. *Reviews in the Neurosciences, 11,* Spec No. 213-328.

Institute of Medicine (IOM). (1995). *Nursing, health and the environment.* Washington, D.C.: National Academies Press.

Landrigan, P., & Slutsky, J. (2006*). Are learning disabilities linked to environmental toxins?* Retrieved October 1, 2006, from Learning Disabilities Worldwide Web site: http://www.ldam.org/ldinformation/resources/O1-04_LDToxins.html.

Landrigan, P., Schechter, C.B., Liptom, J.M., Fahs, M.C., & Schwartz, J. (2002). Environmental pollutants and disease in American children: Estimates of morbidity, mortality, and costs of lead poisoning, asthma, cancer, and developmental disease. *Environmental Health Perspectives, 110*(7), 721–728.

Lapierre, D., & Moro, J. (2002). *Five past midnight in Bhopal: The epic story of the world's deadliest industrial disaster.* New York: Warner Books.

National Library of Medicine (NLM), Medline Plus, Medical Encyclopedia. (2006). *Lead poisoning.* Retrieved October 1, 2006, from http://www.nlm.nih.gov/medlineplus/ency/article/002473.htm.

Raub, J.A., Mathieu-Nolf, M., Hampson, N.B., & Thom, S.R. (2000). Carbon monoxide poisoning—A public health perspective. *Toxicology, 145*(1), 1–14.

Sattler, B, & Clouse, R. L. (2005). Common chemical exposures, sources and associated health effects. Unpublished educational material. Author.

Shea, K.M. (2004). Nontherapeutic use of antimicrobial agents in animal agriculture: Implications for pediatrics. *Pediatrics, 114*(3), 862–868.

Silbergeld, E.K. (1997). Preventing lead poisoning in children. *Annual Review of Public Health, 18,* 187–210.

Stansfeld, S.A., & Matheson, M.P. (2003). Noise pollution: Non-auditory effects on health. *British Medical Bulletin, 68,* 243–257.

Swann, S. (2006). Does our environment affect our fertility? Some examples to help reframe the question, *Seminars in Reproductive Medicine, 24,* 142–146.

U. S. Department of Health and Human Services (DHHS). (2006). *National health and nutrition examination survey.* Retrieved October 1, 2006, from http://www.cdc.gov/nchs/nhanes.htm.

U.S. Department of Justice. (2004). *Freedom of information act.* Retrieved November 3, 2006, from http://www.usdoj.gov/oip/04_3.html.

U.S. Department of State, USINFO (2006) *U.S. consumers consider ethics, health concerns in food purchases.* Retrieved October 1, 2006, from http://usinfo.state.gov/scv/Archive/2006/Jul/07-803668.htm.

Watson, W.A., Litovitz, T.L., Klein-Schwartz, W., Rodgers, G.C., Youniss, J., Reid, N., Rouse, W. G., Rembert, R. S., & Borys, D. (2004). 2003 Annual report of the American Association of Poison Control Centers toxic exposure surveillance system. *American Journal of Emergency Medicine, 22*(5), 335–404. Retrieved May 25, 2005, from http://www.aapcc.org/Annual%20Reports/03report/Annual%20Report%202003.pdf.

BIBLIOGRAPHY

Bullard, R. (2000). *Dumping in Dixie: Race, class, and environmental quality* (3rd ed.). Boulder, CO: Westview Press.

Carson, R. (1962). *Silent spring.* New York: Houghton Mifflin Company.

Colborn, T., Dumanoski, D., & Meyers, J.P. (1997*). Our stolen future: How we are threatening our fertility, intelligence and survival—A scientific detective story.* New York: Penguin Books.

Davis, D.L. (2002). *When smoke ran like water: Tales of environmental deception and the battle against pollution.* New York: Basic Books.

Fagin, D., & Lavelle, M. (1999). *Toxic deception: How the chemical industry manipulates science, bends the law and endangers your health.* Monroe, ME: Common Courage Press.

Frumkin H., Frank L, & Jackson, R.J. (2004). *Urban sprawl and public health: Designing, planning, and building for healthy communities.* Washington, DC: Island Press.

Gibbs, L.M. (1998*). Love Canal: The story continues.* Gabriola Island, Canada: New Society Publishers.

Harr, J. (1995). *A civil action.* New York: Random House.

McCally, M. (2002). *Life support: The environment and human health.* Cambridge, MA: The MIT Press.

Pierce, J., & Jameton, A. (2001). *The ethics of environmentally responsible health care.* New York: Oxford University Press.

Pollan, M. (2001). *The botany of desire: A plant's-eye view of the world.* New York: Random House.

Pollan, M. (2006). *Omnivore's dilemma.* New York: Penguin Books.

Sattler, B., & Lipscomb, J. (2002). *Environmental health and nursing practice.* New York: Springer.

Schettler, T., Solomon, G., Valenti, M., & Huddle, A. (1999). *Generations at risk: Reproductive health and the environment.* Cambridge, MA: The MIT Press.

Schettler, T. (2005). *In harm's way: Toxic threats to child development.* Available online: http://www.mnceh.org/documents/In%20Harms%20Way.pdf.

Schlosser, E. (2001). *Fast food nation.* New York: Houghton Mifflin Company.

Steingraber, S. (1997). *Living downstream. An ecologist looks at cancer and the environment.* Cambridge, MA: Perseus Publishing.

Steingraber, S. (2001). *Having faith.* Cambridge, MA: Perseus Publishing.

RESOURCES

Center for Health, Environment, and Justice (CHEJ)

P.O. Box 6806
Falls Church, Virginia 22040-6806
703-237-2249
Email: chej@chej.org
Web: http://www.chej.org

The CHEJ is a national environmental grassroots organization that assists individuals, families, and communities facing exposures to dangerous environmental chemicals, in the air, water, and soil. CHEJ was involved in establishing some of the first national policies critical to protecting community health like the Superfund Program and Right-to-Know. CHEJ has become the preeminent national leader among grassroots groups reducing the burden of toxic substances on our environment.

EnviRN

Web: http://www.enviRN.umaryland.edu

This Web site is from the University of Maryland School of Nursing and is a virtual resource for environmental health and nursing. Information presented here includes nursing advocacy in environmental health, a spotlight of nurse environmental heroes, and activities and educational offerings in environmental health at the University of Maryland School of Nursing.

Environmental Protection Agency (EPA)

Ariel Rios Building
1200 Pennsylvania Avenue, NW
Washington, D.C. 20460
202-564-4700
Web: http://www.epa.gov

The EPA is a government agency with a mission to protect human health and the environment. The EPA has several federal offices including but not limited to Homeland Security, Children's Health Protection, Civil Rights, Cooperative Environmental Management, Environmental Appeals Board, and Environmental Education. Regional offices are located throughout the United States and are responsible for states' carrying out the mission of the EPA. The Children's Health Protection site (http://yosemite.epa.gov/ochp/ochpweb.nsf/content/homepage.htm) contains information about children's environmental hazards, health topics, and tips to protect children from environmental hazards. The EPA's aging initiative (http://www.epa.gov/aging/index.htm) will prioritize and study environmental health hazards to older persons. The Web site provides a wealth of information to protect the environmental health of older persons. IRIS (http://www.epa.gov/iris/index.html), developed by the EPA and its Office of Research and Development, National Center for Environmental Assessment, is a database of human health effects that may result from exposure to various substances found in the environment.

Institute of Medicine (IOM)

500 Fifth Street, NW
Washington, D.C. 20001
202-334-2352
FAX: 202-334-1412
Email: iomwww@nas.edu
Web: http://www.iom.edu

IOM, a nonprofit organization, provides scientifically informed advice and information concerning biomedical science, medicine, and health. Its mission is to be an adviser to the nation to improve health. One of its topics is environmental health, and it sponsors a Roundtable on Environmental Health Sciences, Research, and Medicine, established to encourage discussion and dialogue to illuminate environmental issues. An IOM report specific to nursing and the environmental is Nursing, Health, and the Environment, which can be accessed at http://www.nap.edu/books/030905298X/html/index.html.

National Center for Environmental Health, Centers for Disease Control and Prevention (NCEH)

1600 Clifton Road
Atlanta, Georgia 30333
404-639-3311; 888-232-6348
Email: cdcinfo@cdc.gov
Web: http://www.cdc.gov

The NCEH aims at promoting American's health and quality of life by preventing or controlling illness, disability, or death that results from interactions between people and their environment. NCEH is particularly committed to safeguarding the health of populations that are particularly vulnerable to certain environmental hazards—children, the elderly, and people with disabilities. The NCEH offers data, information, publications, and programs and training opportunities that relate to environmental health.

National Institutes of Environmental Health Sciences (NIEHS)

P.O. Box 12233
111 T.W. Alexander Drive
Research Triangle Park, North Carolina 27709
919-541-3345
Email: webcenter@niehs.nih.gov
Web: http://www.niehs.nih.gov

The NIEHS has a mission to reduce illness and disability by understanding how the environment influences the development and progression of human disease. The NIEHS focuses on clinical research in environmental health science; basic research to understand basic mechanisms of toxicants in human biology; environmental health research programs to address the cross-cutting problems in human biology and human disease; population-focused research; markers of environmental exposure, early (preclinical) biological response, and genetic susceptibility; and multidisciplinary training for researchers.

Physicians for Social Responsibility

1875 Connecticut Avenue, NW, Suite 1012
Washington, D.C. 20009
202-667-4260
FAX: 202-667-4201
Email: psrnatl@psr.org
Web: http://www.psr.org

Physicians for Social Responsibility represents medical and public health professions and concerned citizens, working together to protect human life from the gravest threats to human health and survival. Their focus includes toxic chemicals, global warming, air pollution, safe drinking water, nuclear disarmament, and gun violence. The national Physicians for Social Responsibility has several constituencies. One good resource for environmental health material is The Greater Boston Physicians for Social Responsibility. A particularly good publication, *In Harm's Way: Toxic Threats to Child Development*, can be accessed at http://psr.igc.org/ihwrept/frontmatter.pdf. The publication provides a thorough discussion of the relationship of toxic chemicals and child development.

Scorecard

c/o Green Media Toolshed
1212 New York Avenue NW, Suite 300
Washington, D.C. 20005
202-464-5350
FAX: 202-776-0110
Email: info@greenmediatoolshed.org
Web: http://www.scorecard.org

Scorecard is a pollution information site. Upon entering a zip code, pollution information for a particular community and who is responsible is presented. Information about geographic areas and companies that have the worst pollution records are also included in this Web site. There is also information about how to take action as an informed citizen.

ToxTown

c/o U.S. National Library of Medicine
8600 Rockville Pike
Bethesda, Maryland 20894
1-888-FIND-NLM
Email: tehip@teh.nlm.nih.gov
Web: http://toxtown.nlm.nih.gov

ToxTown is an incredibly useful site for assessing environmental health risks in our everyday lives. The site is from the National Library of Medicine and would be helpful for guiding an environmental nursing assessment. ToxTown provides information about everyday locations where toxic chemicals are found, descriptions of chemicals, Internet links to authoritative chemical information and other resources, and how the environment can impact human health.

Toxicology and Environmental Health Information Program at the National Library of Medicine

Specialized Information Services
Two Democracy Plaza, Suite 510
6707 Democracy Boulevard, MSC 5467
Bethesda, Maryland 20892-5467
301-496-1131
FAX: 301-480-3537
Email: tehip@teh.nlm.nih.gov
Web: http://www.sis.nlm.nih.gov

The Toxicology and Environmental Health Information Program has two objectives: (1) to create automated toxicology data banks and (2) to provide toxicology and environmental health information and data services. The National Library of Medicine has a free online toxicology tutorial that can be accessed at http://sis.nlm.nih.gov/Tox/ToxTutor.html. There are three tutorials: Basic principles, Toxicokinetics, and Cellular toxicology.

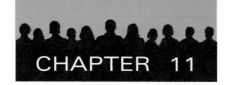

CHAPTER 11

Community and Population Assessment

Jie Hu, RN, PhD

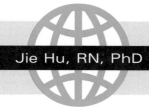

Chapter Outline

- Community and Population Assessment
- Theoretical Foundations for Community
  Assessment
  - Community-As-Partner Model
  - Epidemiologic Triangle Model
  - Roy's Adaptation Model
  - Helvie's Energy Theory
  - Health Promotion Model
- Methods for Community Assessment
  - Windshield Survey
  - Surveys
  - Secondary Data
  - Interviews
  - Focus Groups
  - Needs Assessment
- Assessment of Culturally Diverse Communities

Learning Objectives

Upon completion of this chapter, the reader will be able to:

1. Define models and nursing theories.
2. Discuss the assessment of ethnic and other cultural considerations by diverse populations.
3. Apply epidemiologic and nursing models for the assessment of communities and populations.

Community assessment requires nurses to use their knowledge and skills to assess the environment and health conditions of the client, family, and population in a community. Community assessment is the first step that nurses must take to identify risk factors, needs, strengths, resources, and other issues of a population or community. Community assessment is a nursing process that requires public health nurses to apply appropriate theoretical/conceptual models and use assessment methods relevant to the community. This chapter introduces models and theories for community assessment, discusses methods of community and population assessment, and discusses assessment of ethnic and other cultural considerations by diverse populations in the community.

COMMUNITY AND POPULATION ASSESSMENT

A community assessment is the first step in assessing the health status and health concerns of populations in the community. The community assessment process includes collecting data, analyzing the data, and planning, implementing, and evaluating interventions. A community assessment also involves assessment of ethnic characteristics and changes in the demographics of population structure. It identifies the risk factors, health problems, protective factors, assets, needs, strengths, and resources of populations in the community. The assessment focuses on the entire population in the community and includes broad health indicators. Some of these indicators are, for example, history, demographics, socioeconomic status, housing, employment and working conditions, social support networks, education, physical environment, neighborhood safety and issues related to violence and teen pregnancy, health beliefs and practices, nutrition, cultural customs, values and beliefs, and health and social services, in addition to the local economy, transportation, politics and government, communication systems, recreation, and community capacity to provide supports to growing populations (Anderson & McFarlane, 2004; Keller et al., 2002).

THEORETICAL FOUNDATIONS FOR COMMUNITY ASSESSMENT

Community assessment models provide conceptual frameworks to guide public health nurses in data collec-

tion, analysis, implementation, and evaluation. Nurses can use these models to conduct a systematic community and population assessment. Conceptual models of nursing have four central concepts: person, environment, health, and nursing (Fawcett, 1995). The following models are commonly used by public health nurses for assessment.

Community-As-Partner Model

The Community-As-Partner Model uses a community assessment wheel as the overall framework for assessment (Anderson & McFarlane, 2004). The model was developed based on Betty Neuman's systems model in which a person is surrounded by three lines of defense and nursing functions as three levels of prevention. The Community-As-Partner Model focuses on the nursing process and consists of three parts: the community core, the community subsystems, and perceptions. The community core has been defined as people in the community and includes their history, demographics, ethnicity, and values and beliefs. The components of the community core also include household types; marital status; vital statistics such as births, deaths by age, and leading causes of death; and religion. Community is represented by the normal line of defense or the level of health. For example, immunizations and infant mortality are the major characteristics of the normal line of defense or level of health of the community. The flexible line of defense is a buffer zone that protects the community from stressors, such as flooding. The lines of resistance are internal mechanisms that defend against stressors, for example, a free clinic to provide education and checkups for clients with sexually transmitted diseases or a program to teach teenage mothers how to take care of their babies.

Community subsystems include the physical environment, health and social services, economy, transportation and safety, politics and government, communication, education, and recreation. Perceptions consist of the perceptions of both the residents in the community and the nurse's perception of the community (Anderson & McFarlane, 2004). This model provides a comprehensive conceptual framework for public health nurses to conduct a holistic assessment. The model consists of the following components of the community assessment.

Community Core:

1. *History:* History of the area and the community

2. *Demographics:* Types of people and families who live in the community

3. *Ethnicity:* Different ethnic and cultural groups in the community

4. *Values and beliefs:* Culture, art, religion, and values of the people in the community

Subsystem:

1. *Physical environment:* Community surroundings, including housing, zoning, space, and people

2. *Health and social services:* Availability of health and social services in the community, for example, clinics, hospitals, and public health and social services

3. *Economics:* Opportunities for employment in the community, which include industries, stores, and places

4. *Transportation and safety:* Availability and types of public and private transportations and protective services in the community

5. *Politics and government:* Political activity, party affiliation, and governmental jurisdiction of the community

6. *Communication:* Means of communication in the community, for example, newspaper, TV, and formal and informal communication

7. *Education:* Schools, libraries, and school health services in the community

8. *Recreation:* Major recreation for adults and children in the community

Perceptions:

1. *Residents' perceptions:* Assess residents' perception of the community, strength and weakness residents identified about their community

2. *Nurse's perceptions:* Identify strengths and potential issues of the community and summarize the health of the community

Epidemiologic Triangle Model

The Epidemiologic Triangle Model, discussed in Chapter 4, provides a conceptual framework for community assessment. Data collection on the disease agent includes identifying risk factors that cause disease, such as infectious disease agents like tuberculosis that spread to individuals or populations. Populations at risk for TB include persons with HIV/AIDS, persons who are homeless, and persons who are victims of substance abuse. Assessment of the host (individuals, families, or populations) may involve data collection about physiological, economic, social, spiritual, and cultural factors, such as health condition, age, gender, level of education, ethnicity, income, religion, and cultural norms and values. For example, when nurses assess a population with tuberculosis or a population at risk for TB, they focus on characteristics of the population, such as homelessness, poverty, drug use, and status of new immigrants. This information is important for nurses to plan interventions to prevent the transmission of tuberculosis. Environment is an important part of the model because it influences both agent and host. Nurses assess how the physical, biological, and social environment

⊕ PRACTICE APPLICATION

Community as Partner

Shellman (2000) used Anderson and McFarlane's Community-As-Partner Model as a theoretical framework for the development and implementation of a community-based blood pressure clinic for elders in a rural community. A community assessment was conducted using Anderson and McFarlane's model prior to the opening of the elder wellness program. Community health nurses assessed eight community subsystems according to

Anderson and McFarlane's model. Assessment data of eight subsystems were analyzed and a community health diagnosis and subsequent planning of appropriate community interventions were developed. Public health nurses use the Community-As-Partner Model as a guide. The Community-As-Partner Model played an important role in nursing practice for the development of an elder wellness clinic.

may influence populations and cause disease to occur. For example, housing and socioeconomic status may be considered parts of environment for people with tuberculosis. Other environmental conditions that may also be considered when evaluating tuberculosis and its spread within a community include community resources, health and social services, and politics.

Roy's Adaptation Model

Roy's Adaptation Model is a systems model that has been used to guide community assessment and nursing practice. In Roy's Adaptation Model, individuals or populations receive stimuli from the environment. A changing environment may stimulate a person or a population to use coping mechanisms to make an adaptive response.

Adaptation consists of individuals' or the population's ability to positively interact with the environment (Roy & Andrews, 2005). In the adaptation model, an individual, family, population, community, or society is viewed as a holistic and open system that uses two coping mechanisms, referred to as the cognator and the regulator when applied to individuals, and as the stabilizer and innovator when applied to groups or communities. These coping mechanisms can be observed in four adaptive modes: physical, group identity, role function, and interdependence mode. Health is defined as a state and process of being and becoming an integrated and whole person. The environment is defined as conditions or circumstances that influence the development and behavior of persons and groups. The environment consists of all the conditions, circumstances, and influences that affect persons' and groups' adaptation level; these influences are categorized as focal (immediately confronting the person), contextual (other contributing factors), and residual (other unknown factors, such as beliefs, attitudes, experiences, and expectations) (Roy & Andrews, 2005). Roy defined focal, contextual, and residual stimuli as the zone of adaptation. Adaptation is the process of coping with a stressor. The stimuli and adaptive levels serve as inputs to the person responding as an adaptive system. An individual's or group's behavioral response or reaction to a situation is output, which could be viewed as either adaptive or ineffective (Roy & Andrews, 2005).

Roy's Adaptation Model provides public health nurses with a conceptual framework for assessment and data collection. Table 11-1 is a community assessment guide using Roy's model. The assessment guide can help public health nurses identify ineffective community behaviors in the four adaptive modes—physical, group identity, role function, and interdependence (Dixon, 1999). Assessment of community behavior in the physical mode includes examining positive adaptations, described as resource adequacy, participants, physical facilities, monetary resources, and availability of physical facilities and operational resources. Assessment of the community in group identity mode includes interpersonal relationships, group self-image, social milieu, and culture. Role function mode refers to the roles of group members that work together to achieve goals and mission (Roy & Andrews, 2005). Assessment of role function in the community would include evaluation of community resources such as hospitals, the fire department, social service agencies (Dixon, 1999). Assessment of a community in the interdependence mode includes relationships among community members (Dixon, 1999), demographic and social changes such as the growing aging population, family structure, cultural integration, and changes in the community (Roy & Andrews, 2005). Stimuli assessment requires community health nurses to identify the problems and causes of behaviors that might affect adaptive response (Dixon, 1999). Common stimuli include culture, integrity of the adaptive modes, innovator effectiveness, and environmental considerations (Roy & Andrews, 2005). Dixon (1999) applied Roy's Adaptation Model to develop a community health assessment guide that provides guidance for community health nurses.

Helvie's Energy Theory

Helvie's energy theory views community as an open system and the population as changing energy of three types: bound, kinetic, and potential. Bound energy refers to the population in the community that consists of families, individuals, neighborhoods, and community. Kinetic energy refers to role functions and patterns of behavior of community members and organizations. Potential energy refers to community organizations' and community populations' knowledge, skills, attitudes, and values. In Helvie's energy theory, community populations exchange energies through interactions within the environment. The community has both internal and external environments. The internal environment consists of community resources and services, such as

TABLE 11-1: Community Health Assessment Guide

I. PHYSICAL MODE: The manner in which the collective adaptive system manifests adaptation relative to basic operating resources includes participants, physical facilities, and fiscal resources.

COMPONENT	DEFINITION OF COMPONENT	STIMULI (POSSIBLE)
Participants		
Knowledge	Awareness of community resources for health and prevention of potential health problems	Innovator ineffectiveness Access to and availability of health services and resources including information and health education
Skills	Performance of preventive health behaviors	
Health	Health status and problems of community members	High incidence of chronic or communicable disease Behavioral choices regarding such issues as smoking, exercise, eating habits, etc.
Commitments	Behavioral choices related to health	
Facilities and Operational Resources		
Physical environment	Potential health threats present in environment (water, pollution, etc.)	Innovator ineffectiveness
Housing	Adequacy and affordability of housing	Governmental policies and support to community
Food	Affordability and quality of food	
Health services facilities	Availability of and access to health services	Fiscal resources and capacities of community members
Political/governmental systems	Presence of political and governmental systems to govern community	Urban or rural characteristics of the community
Transportation	Adequacy and affordability of transportation	
Educational systems	Adequacy of educational systems	
Social service systems	Availability of social service agencies	
Communication systems	Adequacy of communication systems	
Public health systems	Availability of public health agencies	
Public safety and emergency resources	Availability of police, fire, paramedics, and emergency services	
Open space	Space for recreational use	

(continued)

TABLE 11-1: Community Health Assessment Guide (cont'd)

Fiscal Resources

Capital resources	Source, stability of funding for community health services	Innovator ineffectiveness
		Government policies regarding health protection and promotion
		Tax base of the community
		Resources of community agencies that protect and promote health

II. GROUP IDENTITY MODES: The manner in which the collective human adaptive system manifests adaptation relative to group self-perception, which includes interpersonal relationships, self-image, social milieu, and culture.

COMPONENT	DEFINITION OF COMPONENT	STIMULI (POSSIBLE)
Interpersonal relationships	The nature and quality of community interpersonal relationships that influence group self-perception	Innovator ineffectiveness

Socioeconomic status |
Group self-image	Community self-perception	Availability of community support systems to promote group pride
Social milieu	The general climate of the community which either enhances or detracts from the community's self-perception	Concerns regarding personal safety
Culture	Cultural group represented in the community	Cultural integration or segregation of community members

III. ROLE FUNCTION MODE: The manner in which the collective human adaptive system manifests adaptation as it pertains to the roles humans occupy relative to each other.

COMPONENT	DEFINITION OF COMPONENT	STIMULI (POSSIBLE)
Performance of roles assumed by community members	Functioning of families, neighbors, community activists, and organizers within their role(s)	Innovator ineffectiveness

Educational level of persons within and persons serving the community |
Performance of roles assumed by persons serving the community	Functioning of police, firemen, community health nurses, social workers, governmental officials, etc.	Fiscal and/or capital constraints
Clarity of roles	Expectations of roles clearly established	Positive or negative social milieu
Commitment to roles	Roles performance demonstrates commitment to the mission and goals of associated role	
Articulation of roles	The manner in which various roles work together to serve and benefit the community	

(continued)

TABLE 11-1: Community Health Assessment Guide (cont'd)

IV. INTERDEPENDENCE MODE: The manner in which the collective human adaptive system manifests adaptation relative to the interdependence relationships of group members.

COMPONENT	DEFINITION OF COMPONENT	STIMULI (POSSIBLE)
Context	Internal and external influence that affect the relationships among community members and between the community and the larger society	Innovator ineffectiveness Availability of community support systems to promote nurturing relationships among community members
Infrastructure	Affectional, resources, and developmental processes that exist within the relationships of the community members	Fiscal constraints Stage of community's development (established versus new community)
People	Community members	Normative behavioral expectations of community members

Note. From Dixon, E. L. (1999). Community Health Nursing Practice and the Roy Adaptation Model. *Public Health Nursing, 16*(4), pp. 290–300. Reprinted with permission of Blackwell Publishing.

⊕ PRACTICE APPLICATION

Roy's Adaption Model

Roy's Adaptation Model was used as a guide when conducting an assessment of a group of young women who were in the precontemplation stage of quitting smoking (Villareal, 2003). According to Roy's model, four adaptive modes were assessed. The physiologic mode includes the clients' needs in oxygenation, nutrition, elimination, activity, and rest and protection. Clients with smoking behaviors were identified as having needs in oxygenation. The self-concept mode consists of the physical self and the personal self. Two clients were identified as having work-related stress that negatively influenced their self-concept. The role function mode refers to the primary role, which includes age, sex, and developmental state. The primary role in this study included females in their mid-twenties. The secondary role refers to complete tasks associated with developmental stage. Villareal (2003) identified the secondary role of clients as daughter, sister, and registered nurses. The tertiary role is associated with the accomplishment of the task (Roy & Andrews, 2005). This role was assumed to be caregiver and member of a gym where women are contemplating quitting smoking. The independent mode refers to the interdependent relationships of individuals (Roy & Andrews, 2005), which includes relationships with significant others and a support system. These two relationships were assessed and identified as boyfriends, family members, and friends as clients' significant others. The focal stimulus that contributes to an ineffective behavior was identified as women's addiction to nicotine, and the contextual stimulus was identified as the women's beliefs that smoking was enjoyable and provided good feelings and comfort. Residual stimuli were identified as women's beliefs and attitudes that smoking cessation may cause alteration in body image and weight gain. Nursing diagnosis based on Roy's model was identified as the lack of motivation to quit smoking related to dependency. Nursing interventions that focused on management of stimuli to promote adaptation and help women quitting smoking was implemented (Villareal, 2003).

health, education, welfare, recreation, political, cultural, social, legal communications, and economic resources. The external environment is other communities, the state, and the nation (Helvie, 1998).

A community assessment based on Helvie's energy theory includes assessment of community populations with health problems; evaluation of health indicators in the community; and comparison of data with previous data and data from other communities, states, and the nation. Evaluation of community balance includes how well the community functions; changes in demographics and population structure in the community; and future health problems (Helvie, 1998).

Health Promotion Model

Pender's Health Promotion Model describes the likelihood that an individual's healthy lifestyle patterns or health-promoting behaviors will occur. The Health Promotion Model consists of three components in which individual characteristics and experiences, behavior-specific cognitions, and affect influence behavior outcomes through immediate competing demands and commitment to a plan of action. The behavior outcome is health-promoting behavior. The model (Figure 11-1)

depicts "the multidimensional nature of persons interacting with their interpersonal and physical environment as they pursue health" (Pender, Murdaugh, & Parsons, 2002, p. 61).

METHODS FOR COMMUNITY ASSESSMENT

Community assessment involves using various methods to collect and analyze data. These methods include performing a windshield survey and a community survey, gathering secondary data, conducting interviews and focus groups, and performing the needs assessment.

Windshield Survey

A windshield survey is a commonly used method for collecting data in the community. In a windshield survey, the community nurse drives or rides a bus or walks through the community to assess the characteristics of the community. The components of a windshield survey include the dimensions of a community: housing and zoning, open space, boundaries, commons, transportation, service centers, stores, street people, signs of decay, race, ethnicity, religion, health and

---

⊕ POLICY HIGHLIGHT

Population Assessment

Community and population assessment can identify risk factors influencing health, populations at risk, health needs, and available community resources and also provide useful information and data on the health status of a community that policy makers could use for development of health policy and intervention programs. Community and population assessment provides a clear picture of the community's health to public health providers for the evaluation of the effectiveness of new policies or community intervention programs.

The population assessment data can be used for planning and prevention programs devoted to achieving the

nation's *Healthy People 2010* objectives. The Centers for Disease Control and Prevention (CDC) has provided the *Assessment Initiative* project that guides the communities for health decisions and policy development (http://www.cdc.gov/epo/dphsi/assessment.htm). CDC also provides evidence-based intervention programs based on community assessment data and research findings that can support proposed legislation or policy (http://www.thecommunity-guide.org/). Public health nurses can conduct community health assessment, provide data, and get involved in policy development and decision making.

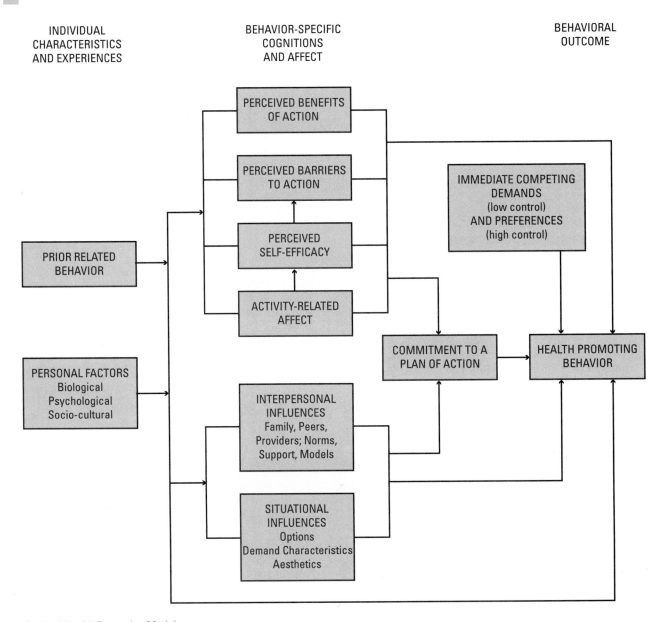

Revised Health Promotion Model

Figure 11-1 Pender's Health Promotion Model.

From PENDER, NOLA J.; MURDAUGH, CAROLYN L.; PARSONS, MARY ANN, HEALTH PROMOTION IN NURSING PRACTICE, 5th Edition, ©2006, p. 50. Reprinted by permission of Pearson Education, Inc., Upper Saddle River, NJ.

RESEARCH APPLICATION

Community Assessment: A Church Community and the Parish

Study Purpose

To determine the health status of parishioners, identify their perceived health needs and perceived barriers in meeting those needs, and to assist the church and parish nurse in developing a health program for their faith community.

Methods

Questionnaires and focus groups were used for data collection. Four hundred twenty-one questionnaires were completed, and six focus groups were held to validate the data.

Findings

Results showed that most parishioners felt they were in good health (93%), believed faith and spiritual beliefs were

important in maintaining health and well-being (91%), and thought that the church should play a role in helping parishioners meet their health needs (70%). In addition, focus group discussions revealed a need for respite care for primary caretakers of the ill and elderly, and health education programs for their teen and elderly populations.

Implications

Parishioners were positive and articulated support of the parish nurse and activities designed to address the physical, emotional, and spiritual needs of their community.

Reference

Swinney, J., Anson-Wonkka, C., Maki, E., & Corneau, J. (2001). Assessment: A church community and the parish nurse. *Public Health Nursing*, 18, 1–40.

---

morbidity, politics, and the media (Anderson & McFarlane, 2004). Anderson and McFarlane (2004) expanded a windshield survey to the community assessment wheel, which includes the community core, community subsystems, and perceptions, as discussed in the Community-As-Partner Model.

Surveys

A **survey** is self-report data collected from community residents, and it generally uses questionnaires to obtain information about demographics, knowledge, attitudes, perceptions, opinions, health beliefs, and behaviors. The purpose of a survey is usually to describe the needs and concerns of populations in the community.

The most commonly used survey methods in community assessment include self-administered questionnaires and face-to face-interviews. Surveys may also be conducted by mail or telephone. Surveys include closed-ended and open-ended questionnaires. Closed-ended questionnaires ask community members to select an answer among several possible answers to a question. This technique is often used in large community surveys

to identify community members' opinions, knowledge, attitudes, and health behaviors. Open-ended questionnaires ask community members to describe or explain their specific answers. For example, a public health nurse can ask teenage mothers to describe their concerns and needs regarding pregnancy and child care. This technique allows nurses to obtain more information since respondents are not limited to a fixed choice as on a closed-ended questionnaire.

Secondary Data

Secondary data refers to data already collected and archived. Public health nurses can use databases or secondary data to obtain information on the morbidity and mortality of populations of interest in the community. These data include statistical data and health survey results. Secondary data may be obtained from national, state, and local databases, such as the Centers for Disease Control and Prevention, National Institutes of Health, Health Resources and Services Administration, and U.S. Bureau of the Census at the national level; from state vital statistics; and from county government at the local level.

⊕ RESEARCH APPLICATION

Needs Assessment and Intervention Strategies to Reduce Lead-Poisoning Risk among Low-Income Ohio Toddlers

Study Purpose

To examine Medicaid parents of toddlers who received lead-poisoning prevention information and preferred methods of receiving this information.

Methods

A cross-sectional study design with mailed survey of parents with children 1–2 years old enrolled in Medicaid was used. This study employed the Blood Lead Education and Screening Tool.

Findings

The majority of parents received lead-poisoning prevention information, but only 28% reported receiving a reminder to have their child's blood lead level tested. Preferred information of obtaining lead-poisoning prevention includes brochures and discussion with health care providers.

Minority parents preferred receiving information via videos, billboards, and home visits. Parents identified multiple means of receiving information on lead-poisoning prevention.

Implications

Public health nurses need to implement intervention on the individual, community, and system levels for comprehensive lead-poisoning prevention education. A community assessment can provide detailed information to use for educational media.

Reference

Polivka, B. J. (2006). Needs assessment and intervention strategies to reduce lead-poisoning risk among low-income Ohio toddlers. *Public Health Nursing, 23*(1), 52–58.

Interviews

Interviews are a method of data collection in which the public health nurse asks questions about health, attitudes, beliefs, and health behaviors of community members through face-to-face or telephone interviews. Three types of interviews are generally used for data collection: structured interviews, semistructured interviews, and unstructured interviews. Structured interviews ask the same questions in the same order to all interviewees (Nieswiadomy, 2002). With this type of interview, public health nurses can analyze and compare data across all interviewees. Semistructured interviewers generally ask specific questions but encourage interviewees to explain the answers to questions (Nieswiadomy, 2002). Public health nurses can obtain in-depth data in semistructured interviews. In unstructured interviews public health nurses allow interviewees to direct the course of the interview, and the interviews are conducted in a normal conversation (Nieswiadomy, 2002). For example, a public health nurse may ask an elderly client to tell the nurse about his or her experiences with chronic illness and physical and social activities.

Focus Groups

A focus group is a group of people with similar experiences or interests who meet to discuss their perceptions and perspectives on a topic of interest (Urden, 2003). Focus groups are group interviews in which a moderator or researcher guides the interview. The data are what the group of people say during their interview. Using group interviews, researchers can learn about the experiences and opinions of the group (Morgan, 1998). Focus groups provide opportunities to explore a topic of interest. For example, public health nurses may decide that they would like to gain in-depth understanding of attitudes and behaviors in a particular area related to health from a group of community residents.

A focus group typically has six to eight participants from similar backgrounds who participate in an in-depth discussion. A researcher guides and facilitates the group discussion and encourages the expression of personal opinions. Focus group interviews can be used to identify problems and to gain insight into planning, implementation, and evaluation (Morgan, 1998). Problem identification emphasizes exploration and

⊕ PRACTICE APPLICATION

Assessment Program

Focus groups provide an effective means of communicating with community residents and gaining insight into problems that interest public health nurses. Public health nurses can use this method to involve community residents in assessment and intervention programs. For example, Clark and colleagues (2003) used focus group interviews of a comprehensive community assessment in a multicultural community of 76,000 residents in southern California. Several focus group interviews were conducted to solicit participation and opinions from residents regarding their concerns, health needs, and assets. The participants in the focus groups included minority groups, the elderly, and community youth. The interview questions in the focus groups included: "What is it like to live in this community? What could make life in this community better? What kinds of things could improve the health of people who live in this community? What could the health department do to improve the health of people who live in this community? What could you, or people you know, do to improve life

in this community?" (Clark et al., 2003, 458). Focus group interviews were conducted in English, Spanish, Hmong, Vietnamese, Chinese, and Somali, and with different age groups. Three major concerns were identified through the focus group interviews: housing, environmental, and safety issues. Other issues include access to health care, communication, economic development and employment, transportation, education, legal aid, and the availability, accessibility, and quality of local resources, such as grocery stores, recreation and child care. Five community assets are identified as geographic, residents, health and social service, business, and other (Clark et al., 2003). The findings of the focus groups were used to develop housing task forces that will work with officials and landlords to address housing issues in the community. The results of the focus groups also led to the development of Neighborhood Health Councils and ongoing community involvement in regards to health needs (Clark et al., 2003).

discovery of a problem. Interview discussions are usually unstructured and open-ended for purpose of discovering problems (Morgan, 1998). Community residents in focus groups can discuss community health problems that nurses may have little knowledge about. Planning is emphasized in listening to group participants' perspectives and suggestions. Group discussions often use unstructured interview questions. Focus groups can also provide insights into issues related to implementation, such as how plans developed by interdisciplinary groups would work out for populations in the community. Group discussions can also be guided to understand the outcome of a project and learn lessons for future planning (Morgan, 1998).

Needs Assessment

Needs assessment is used in public health to identify population-based needs, to evaluate a current target population in need of services, to identify new target populations that have unmet needs, and to provide resources available to meet those needs. Needs assessment focuses on "who is the target population and

what are the needs of that population" (Petersen & Alexander, 2001, 17). Needs assessment also identifies diversity in needs within target populations. The needs assessment process involves identification of problems or needs and ways to solve these problems or needs and integrate the solutions into policy (Petersen & Alexander, 2001).

Needs may be identified as comparative needs and expected, wanted, desired, felt, or expressed needs. States commonly use comparative needs. For example, a state may use Healthy People 2010 to compare its objectives to national objectives for health and to establish goals for health promotion and protection. Expected, wanted, desired, or felt needs are identified by the target population, the public, and policy makers. These needs are important for populations in the community but have not been met. For example, educational programs for health promotion for individuals, families, communities, and populations are expected by the public, but discrepancies may exist. When people in the community take actions such as purchasing additional or different services to meet their felt needs, these needs are considered to be expressed needs

PHASE 1 Pre-assessment (exploration)	PHASE 2 Assessment (data gathering)	PHASE 3 Post-assessment (utilization)
Set up management plan for the needs assessment Define general purpose of the needs assessment Identify major needs and/or issues Identify existing information regarding need areas Determine: 　　　　Data to collect 　　　　Sources 　　　　Methods 　　　　Potential uses of data	Determine context, scope, and boundaries of the needs assessment Gather data on needs Set preliminary priorities on needs–Level 1 Perform causal analyses at Levels 1, 2, and 3 Analyze and synthesize all data	Set priorities on needs at all applicable levels Consider alternative solutions Develop an action plan to implement solutions Evaluate the needs assessment Communicate results
Outcomes: Preliminary plan for Phases 2 and 3, and plan for evaluation of the needs assessment	**Outcomes:** Criteria for action based on high-priority needs	**Outcomes:** Action plan(s), written and oral briefings, and reports

Figure 11-2 Three-phase plan for needs assessment.

From Witkin, B. R., & Altschuld, J. W. (1995). *Planning and conducting needs assessments: A practical guide.* Thousand Oaks, CA: Sage Publications. Reprinted with permission of Sage Publications.

(Petersen & Alexander, 2001). Table 11-2 presents Petersen and Alexander's process of needs assessment.

Witkin and Altschuld (1995) proposed three levels of need: primary (level 1), secondary (level 2), and tertiary (level 3). Primary need refers to service receivers, such as clients, patients, and potential customers. Secondary need refers to service providers and policy makers, such as teachers, parents, social workers, caretakers, and health care professionals. Tertiary need refers to resources or solutions, such as buildings, facilities, equipment, programs, transportation, and program delivery system. People at the primary need level are the target of needs assessment. These needs may include identifying the learning needs of children who are disabled or developmentally delayed, the physical health needs of the elderly who live alone in the community, and the mental health needs of the homeless. Needs assessment

also can be applied to secondary and tertiary levels such as training needs for people at the secondary level and the needs of organizations or resources at the tertiary level (Witkin & Altschuld, 1995).

According to Witkin and Altschuld (1995), needs assessment consists of three phases: pre-assessment, main assessment, and post-assessment. Pre-assessment is the exploratory stage that is primarily designed to identify the needs of populations in the community, including issues and major health concerns. In the main assessment, nurses collect data, analyze information, and establish priorities for needs. In the post-assessment, nurses propose solutions and set priorities to plan for interventions based on the information collected in the assessment (Witkin & Altschuld, 1995). Witkin and Alschuld's (1995) three-phase plan for needs assessment is presented in Figure 11-2.

TABLE 11-2: Stages in the Needs Assessment Process

Start-up Planning Stage

1. Establish the organizational structure for the needs assessment
2. Identify the potential uses of the needs assessment
3. Identify the stakeholders of the needs assessment
4. Identify the overall target population
5. Identify the types of needs to be assessed

Operational Planning Stage

1. Establish who will help determine the need indicators and data sources to be considered
2. Establish who will produce the data reports on the indicators
3. Determine the method to be used to rank or prioritize needs in terms of importance
4. Determine a strategy for organizing and managing meetings
5. Determine a strategy for managing conflicts and reaching consensus
6. Determine a strategy for building ongoing coalitions

Data Stage

1. Identify indicators to characterize needs
2. Identify available data sources
3. Identify other data needed and strategies for obtaining data
4. Identify data to create a Resource Inventory
5. Assemble data

Needs Analysis Stage

1. Prioritize needs in terms of importance
2. Determine subpopulations to which specific needs apply
3. Identify workable solutions to address needs
4. Reassess needs in light of available solutions
5. Identify available resources to meet needs
6. Reach consensus among stakeholders regarding priority unmet needs and best solutions for specific subpopulations

Program and Policy Development Stage

1. Develop plans to translate need statements and related solutions into policy
2. Secure internal agency approval of policy action plans
3. Communicate results of needs analysis and policy action plans to advocacy groups, the general public, and other agencies
4. Collaborate and cooperate with advocacy groups and related agencies to foster support for program and policy proposals
5. Develop plans for monitoring and evaluating proposed programmatic and policy initiatives when implemented

Resource Allocation Stage

1. Develop criteria for selection of multiple need indicators
2. Determine basic tenets to guide the development of funding formulas
3. Research consensus among stakeholders on indicators and tenets
4. Assemble data and construct initial funding formulas
5. Present formulas to stakeholders and adjust as indicated to reach consensus and broad support

Note. From Peterson, D. J., & Alexander, G. R. (2001). *Needs assessment in public health: A practical guide for students and professionals.* New York: Kluwer Academic. Reprinted with permission of Kluwer Academic.

ASSESSMENT OF CULTURALLY DIVERSE COMMUNITIES

Each cultural group has unique ways of maintaining and promoting health (Leininger, 1995). Providing culturally competent care requires community health nurses to understand the culture and conduct culturally sensitive assessments. This section focuses on cultural assessment of diverse populations in the community, with emphasis on cultural assessment guidelines.

With growing minority populations in the United States, public health nurses must acquire cultural knowledge and assessment skills for working with diverse populations in the community. A public health nursing assessment involves data collection on populations and assessment of the characteristics of populations, such as the norms, values, beliefs, religion, health practices, and behaviors that constitute the uniqueness of each culture in the community. Clark (2003) proposed four basic principles for nurses conducting cultural assessments: "*1) All cultures must be viewed in the context in*

TABLE 11-3: Components of the Cultural Assessment

CULTURAL COMPONENT	DESCRIPTION
Family and kinship systems	Is the family nuclear, extended, or "blended"? Do family members live nearby? What are the communication patterns among family members? What is the role of family members? The status? How old are family members? What is the gender?
Social life	What is the daily routine of the group? What are the important life cycle events such as birth, marriage, and death? How are educational systems organized? What are the social problems experienced by the group? How does the social environment contribute to a sense of belonging? What are the group's social interaction patterns? What are its commonly prescribed nutritional practices?
Political systems	Which factors in the political system influence the way the group perceives its status vis-à-vis the dominant culture (i.e., laws, justice, and cultural heroes)? How does the economic system influence control of resources such as land, water, housing, jobs, and opportunities?
Language and traditions	Are there differences in the dialect or language spoken between health care professionals and the cultural group? How do major cultural traditions such as history, art, and drama influence the cultural identity of the group? What are the common language patterns in regard to verbal and nonverbal communication? How is the use of personal space related to communication?
Worldview, value orientations, and cultural norms	What are the major cultural values about the relationships of humans to nature and to one another? How can the group's ethical beliefs be described? What are the norms and standards of behavior (authority, responsibility, dependability, and competition)? What are cultural attitudes to time, work, and leisure?
Religion	What are the religious beliefs and practices of the group? How do they relate to health practices? What are the rituals and taboos surrounding major life events such as birth and death?
Health beliefs and practices	What are the group's attitudes and beliefs regarding health and illness? Does the cultural group seek care from indigenous health (or folk) practitioners? Who makes decisions about health care? Are there biologic variations that are important to the health of this group?

Note. From Boyle, J. S. (2003). Culture, family, and community. In M. M. Andrews & J. S. Boyle (Eds.), *Transcultural concepts in nursing care* (pp. 315–360). Philadelphia: Lippincott Williams & Wilkins.

which they have developed; 2) the underlying premises of behavior must be examined; 3) the meaning and purpose of a behavior must be interpreted within the context of the specific culture; and 4) there is such a phenomenon as intracultural variation" (pp. 338). Table 11-3 presents components of the cultural assessment based on Boyle (2003).

The Purnell Model for cultural competence provides a framework for assessment from a cultural perspective. The Purnell Model consists of three circles, with global society in the outlying rim, community in the second rim, and person in the inner rim (Purnell & Paulanka, 2005). Major components for assessment in the Purnell Model for cultural competence include overview and heritage, communication, family roles and organization, workforce issues, biocultural ecology, high-risk health behaviors, nutrition, pregnancy and childbearing practices, death rituals, spirituality, health care practices, and health care practitioners (Purnell & Paulanka, 2005).

Overview and heritage include assessment of the country of origin and current residence and their impacts on health, education, occupation, and reasons for migration. *Communications* includes assessment of the dominant language, and verbal and nonverbal communications, for example, eye contact, gesturing and facial expressions, touch and body language, and spatial distancing practices. *Family roles and organization* include assessment of the head of the household, gender roles, family priorities, roles of the elders in the family and extended family, social status in the community, and acceptance of different lifestyles such as divorce and single parenting. *Workforce issues* include assessment of autonomy, acculturation, gender roles, and ethnic communication styles. *Biocultural ecology* includes assessment of physical, biological, and physiological variables among ethnic and racial groups. For example, their genetic makeup may make people in certain ethnic groups vulnerable to hypertension and diabetes. Assessment of *high-risk health behaviors* include drug and alcohol use and abuse, tobacco use, physical inactivity, and risky sexual behaviors related to HIV and sexually transmitted disease. *Nutrition* includes assessment of the meaning of food, food rituals, and use of food for health promotion and disease prevention, such as cold and hot food practices in Asian cultures. *Pregnancy and childbearing practices* include assessment of "culturally sanctioned and unsanctioned fertility practices" (Purnell & Paulanka, 2005, p. 14), perceptions of pregnancy, and taboo practices related to birthing, pregnancy, and postpartum. *Death rituals* include assessment of ethnic and racial groups' perceptions of death rituals and bereavement behaviors. *Spirituality* includes assessment of religious beliefs and practices and their meaning to life. *Health-care practices* include assessment of health beliefs and health care practices, individual responsibilities for health, and views of mental illness, chronic conditions, and organ donation and transplantation. *Health-care practitioners* include assessment of people's perceptions of health-care providers and the gender of the health-care provider. For example, pregnant women may refuse to allow male obstetricians to examine or deliver their babies.

CRITICAL THINKING ACTIVITIES

1. If you were to conduct a community health assessment on your community, what would it involve?

2. How can a public health nurse apply theories/models to conduct a community assessment?

3. Use a theory to assess the needs of a community.

4. What factors would you consider when assessing individuals, families, populations, and communities?

5. What methods would a public health nurse use to conduct a community health or population assessment?

6. How would a public health nurse make an assessment of an individual, a family, a population, and a community with diverse cultural and ethnic backgrounds?

KEY TERMS

Community-As-Partner Model	interviews	Roy's Adaptation Model
community assessment	needs assessment	secondary data
focus group	Pender's Health Promotion Model	survey
Helvie's energy theory		windshield survey

KEY CONCEPTS

⊕ Community assessment is a nursing process that involves data collection on the characteristics and health status of the community.

⊕ Community assessment requires nurses to apply appropriate theoretical/conceptual models and use assessment methods relevant to the assessment of the community.

⊕ The Community-As-Partner Model focuses on community as partner and the nursing process. It consists of three parts: the community core, the community subsystems, and the community perceptions. This model provides a comprehensive conceptual framework for community health nurses to conduct a holistic assessment.

⊕ The Epidemiologic Triangle Model views health and disease from the perspective of epidemiology and consists of three elements: agent, host, and environment. Agent is an organism or event that causes disease. The host is the person or population at risk or susceptible to the disease. The environment includes physical, biologic, and social factors that influence both agent and host to make disease process occur.

⊕ In Roy's Adaptation Model, an individual or a group receives stimuli from the environment. A changing environment may stimulate a person or a group to use coping mechanisms to make an adaptive response. A community assessment using Roy's model can help community health nurses identify ineffective community behaviors in the four adaptive modes.

⊕ Helvie's energy theory views community as an open system and the population as changing energy of three types: bound, kinetic, and potential. A community assessment based on Helvie's energy theory includes assessment of community populations with health problems; evaluation of health indicators in the community; and comparison of data with previous data and data from other communities, states, and the nation.

⊕ Pender's Health Promotion Model describes an individual's likelihood to take actions for health behavior.

⊕ The windshield survey includes the dimensions of a community: housing and zoning, open space, boundaries, commons, transportation, service centers, stores, street people, signs of decay, race, ethnicity, religion, health and morbidity, politics, and the media.

⊕ A survey is self-report data collected from community residents, and it generally uses questionnaires to obtain information about demographics, knowledge, attitudes, perceptions, opinions, and health beliefs and behaviors.

⊕ Interviews are a method of data collection in which the community health nurse asks questions about health, attitudes, beliefs, and health behaviors of community members through face-to-face or telephone interviews.

⊕ A focus group is a group of people with similar experiences or interests who meet to discuss their perceptions and perspectives on a topic of interest.

- ⊕ Needs assessment is used in public health to identify population-based needs, to evaluate a current target population in need of services, and to identify new target populations that have unmet needs.

- ⊕ Major components for assessment in the Purnell Model for cultural competence include overview

and heritage, communication, family roles and organization, workforce issues, biocultural ecology, high-risk health behaviors, nutrition, pregnancy and childbearing practices, death rituals, spirituality, health care practices, and health care practitioners.

REFERENCES

Anderson, E. T., & McFarlane, J. (2004). Community assessment. In E. T. Anderson & J. McFarlane (Eds), *Community as partner: Theory and practice in nursing* (pp. 169–221). Philadelphia: Lippincott Williams & Wilkins.

Boyle, J. S. (2003). Culture, family, and community. In M. M. Andrews & J. S. Boyle (Eds.), *Transcultural concepts in nursing care* (pp. 315–360). Philadelphia: Lippincott Williams & Wilkins.

Cashaw, S. (2004). Epidemiology, demography, and community health. In E. T. Anderson & J. McFarlane (Eds.), *Community as partner: Theory and practice in nursing* (pp. 28–55). Philadelphia: Lippincott Williams & Wilkins.

Clark, M. J. (Ed.). (2003). *Nursing in the community* (4th ed.). Upper Saddle River, NJ: Prentice-Hall.

Clark, M. J., Cary, S., Diemert, G., Ceballos, R., Sifuentes, M., Atteberry, I., Vue, F., & Trieu, S. (2003). Involving communities in community assessment. *Public Health Nursing, 20*(6), 456–463.

Dixon, E. (1999). Community health nursing practice and the Roy Adaptation Model. *Public Health Nursing, 16*(4), 290–300.

Fawcett, J. (1995). *Analysis and evaluation of conceptual models of nursing* (3rd ed.). Philadelphia: F. A. Davis.

Helvie, C. O. (1998). *Advanced practice nursing in the community.* Thousand Oaks: Sage Publications.

Keller, L. O., Schaffer, M. A., Lia-Hoagberg, B., & Strobschien, S. (2002). Assessment, program planning, and evaluation in population-based public health practice. *Journal of Health Management Practice, 8*(5), 30–43.

Leininger, M. (1991). Leininger's acculturation health care assessment tool for cultural patterns in traditional and nontraditional lifeways. *Journal of Transcultural Nursing, 2*(2), 40–42.

Leininger, M. (1995). Teaching transcultural nursing in undergraduate and graduate programs. *Journal of Transcultural Nursing, 6*(2), 10–26.

Morgan, D. L. (1998). *The focus group guidebook: Focus group kit 1.* Thousand Oaks, CA: Sage Publications.

Nieswiadomy, R. M. (2002). *Foundations of nursing research* (4th ed.). Stamford, CT: Appleton & Lange.

Pender, N. J., Murdaugh, C. L., & Parsons. M. A. (2002). *Health promotion in nursing practice* (4th ed.). Upper Saddle River. NJ: Prentice Hall.

Peterson, D. J., & Alexander, G. R. (2001). *Needs assessment in public health: A practical guide for students and professionals.* New York: Kluwer Academic.

Polivka, B. J. (2006). Needs assessment and intervention strategies to reduce lead-poisoning risk among low-income Ohio toddlers. *Public Health Nursing, 23*(1), 52–58.

Purnell, L. D., & Paulanka, B. J. (2005). *Guide to culturally competent health care.* Philadelphia: F. A. Davis Company.

Roy, C., & Andrews, H. (2005). *The Roy Adaptation Model: The definitive statement.* San Mateo, CA: Appleton & Lange.

Shellman, J. (2000). Promoting elder wellness through a community-based blood pressure clinic. *Public Health Nursing, 17*(4), 257–263.

Swinney, J., Anson-Wonkka, C., Maki, E., & Corneau, J. (2001). Assessment: A church community and the parish nurse. *Public Health Nursing, 18*, 1–40.

Urden, L. D. (2003). Don't forget to ask: Using focus groups to assess outcomes. *Outcomes Management, 7*(1), 1–3.

Villareal, E. (2003). Using Roy's adaptation model when caring for a group of young women contemplating quitting smoking. *Public Health Nursing, 20*(5), 377–384.

Witkin, B. R., & Altschuld, J. W. (1995). *Planning and conducting needs assessments: A practical guide.* Thousand Oaks, CA: Sage Publications.

BIBLIOGRAPHY

Averill, J. (2003). Keys to the puzzle: Recognizing strengths in a rural community. *Public Health Nursing, 20,* 449–455.

Caley, L. M. (2004). Using geographic information systems to design population-based interventions. *Public Health Nursing, 21,* 547–554.

Clark, M. J., Cary, S., Diemert, G., Ceballos, R., Sifuentes, M., Atteberry, I., Vue, F., & Trieu, S. (2003). Involving communities in community assessment. *Public Health Nursing, 20,* 456–463.

Clark, N., & Buell, A. (2004). Community assessment: An innovative approach. *Nurse Educator, 29,* 203–207.

Davis, R., Cook, D., & Cohen, L. (2005). Race, genetics, and health disparities. A community resilience approach to reducing ethnic and racial disparities in health. *American Journal of Public Health, 95,* 2168–2173.

Eide, P. J., Hahn, L., Bayne, T., Allen, C. B., & Swain, D. (2006). The population-focused analysis project for teaching community health. *Nursing Education Perspectives, 27*(1), 22–27.

Escoffery, C., Miner, K. R., & Trowbridge, J. (2004). Conducting small-scale community assessments. *American Journal of Health Education, 35,* 237–241.

Gesler, W. M., Dougherty, M., Arcury, T. A., Skelly, A. H., & Nash, S. (2003). The importance of obtaining information from assessment of community service providers for a disease prevention program. *Journal of Multicultural Nursing & Health, 9*(2), 14–21.

Huttlinger, K., Schaller-Ayers, J., & Lawson, T. (2004). Health care in Appalachia: A population-based approach. *Public Health Nursing, 21,* 103–110.

Kelly, P. J. (2005). Practical suggestions for community interventions using participatory action research. *Public Health Nursing, 22*(1), 65–73.

Kim, S., Flaskerud, J. H., Koniak-Griffin, D., & Dixon, E. L. (2005). Using community-partnered participatory research to address health disparities in a Latino community. *Journal of Professional Nursing, 21,* 199–209.

Morgan, L. L., & Reel, S. J. (2002). Developing cultural competence in rural nursing. Online *Journal of Rural Nursing & Health Care, 3*(1), 28-37.

Reifsnider, E., Dominguez, A., Friesenhahn, J., Hodges, P., Chapin, C., & Sims, W. B. (2005). Educational innovations. Collaboration with city agencies: A winning approach to community assessment. *Journal of Nursing Education, 44,* 323–325.

Rothman, N. L., Lourie, R. J., Brian, D., & Foley, M. (2005). Temple Health Connection: A successful collaborative model of community-based primary health care *Journal of Cultural Diversity, 12,* 145–151.

Rowley, C. (2005). Health needs assessment. *Journal of Community Nursing, 19*(6), 11–12, 14.

Salem, E., Hooberman, J., & Ramirez, D. (2005). MAPP in Chicago: A model for public health systems development and community building. *Journal of Public Health Management & Practice, 11,* 393–400.

Zahner, S. J., Kaiser, B., & Kapelke-Dale, J. (2005). Local partnerships for community assessment and planning. *Journal of Public Health Management & Practice, 11,* 460–464.

RESOURCES

Community Toolbox

Work Group on Health Promotion & Community Development
4082 Dole Human Development Center
University of Kansas
1000 Sunnyside Avenue
Lawrence, Kansas 66045-7555
785-864-0533
FAX: 785-864-5281
Email: Toolbox@ku.edu
Web: http://www.ctb.ku.edu

The Community Toolbox is a Web site for a toolkit to support your work in promoting community health and development, providing examples and "how-to" information for assessing community needs and resources. The Toolbox includes practical information about skill building in assessment, strategic planning, leadership, intervention, evaluation, advocacy, marketing; planning, developing, and sustaining a program; problem solving and support; and online forums, resources, and advisers for best practices.

Free to Grow (FTG)

Mailman School of Public Health
Columbia University
722 West 168th Street, 8th Floor
New York, New York 10032
212-305-8120
FAX: 212-342-1963
Email: info@freetogrow.org
Web: http://www.freetogrow.org

The Free To Grow–Head Start partnership is a national program supported by the Robert Wood Johnson Foundation and the Doris Duke Charitable Foundation to promote substance-free communities. The site offers information on community assessment approaches and links to community assessment strategies. There are 15 Free To Grow sites in the United States collaborating with schools, law enforcement, and mental health programs using community-based efforts to strengthen the environment of young children, families, and communities to prevent substance abuse and child abuse.

Healthy Carolinians, North Carolina Health Assessment

Office of Healthy Carolinians
Division of Public Health
1916 Mail Service Center
Raleigh, North Carolina 27699-1916
919-707-5150
FAX: 919-870-4833
Email: hcinfo@ncmail.net
Web: http://www.healthycarolinians.org

Healthy Carolinians, North Carolina Health Assessment provides links to a community assessment guidebook, assessment information and partnership development, and community health opinion survey.

U.S. Department of Agriculture, Economic Research Service (ERS)

1400 Independence Avenue SW
Washington, D.C. 20250
202-694-5050
Email: InfoCenter@ers.usda.gov
Web: http://www.ers.usda.gov

The ERS is a resource for a Community Food Security Assessment Toolkit. The toolkit is useful for assessment of household food security and resources, accessibility, availability and affordability, and community production resources. It also has focus group guides and materials to use for assessment.

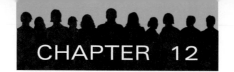

CHAPTER 12

Health Risk Appraisal

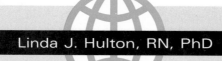

Linda J. Hulton, RN, PhD

Chapter Outline

- History of Health Risk Appraisal
- Purpose, Development, and Use of Health Risk Appraisals
- Validity, Reliability, and Effectiveness of Health Risk Appraisals
- Appropriate and Inappropriate Uses of Health Risk Appraisals
- Social Influences and Culture's Impact
- Selection of Appropriate Health Risk Appraisal Tools
- Implications for Public Health Nursing

Learning Objectives

Upon completion of this chapter, the reader will be able to:

1. Describe the history, purpose, development, and uses of health risk appraisal tools
2. Compare appropriate and inappropriate uses of health risk appraisal tools
3. Differentiate the spheres of social influence and culture's impact on health risk appraisal
4. Apply appropriate health risk appraisal tools for an array of settings
5. Examine public health surveillance and the impact on health risk appraisal for populations

A health risk appraisal (HRA) tool is an instrument that identifies specific factors in individuals that increase the risk of impairments or disabilities and then recommends behavioral modifications to minimize their impact (Breslow et al., 1997). The tool may provide an estimate of health threats to which a client may be vulnerable because of genetic makeup, family history, or lifestyle choices (Hyner et al., 1999). Nurses can use these instruments to help identify personal habits that are detrimental to health. HRAs have the potential to enhance the decision-making processes of clients with unhealthy lifestyles as they begin to understand their own susceptibility to death and disease. Unlike a screening tool, the emphasis of HRAs is on the period of time prior to the onset of disease, the period of primary prevention.

This chapter will review the (1) historical use of HRAs; (2) purpose, development, and use of HRAs; (3) validity, reliability, and effectiveness of HRAs; (4) appropriate and inappropriate uses; (5) social influences and cultural impacts; (6) an explanation of how to select appropriate HRA tools; and (7) implications for public health nursing practice.

HISTORY OF HEALTH RISK APPRAISAL

During World War II, a concern developed for troops who displayed numerous behavioral disorders. Many service recruits were found to be unfit for service due to emotional disorders, and troops were returning from the war with significant traumatic stress reactions (Kessler & Wang, 1999). Screening scales were developed to respond to these concerns.

After World War II, additional screening scales led to a number of community epidemiological studies in communities. Robbins & Hall (1970) introduced the HRA in the 1950s as a counseling tool for use by health care providers. It was used for practicing "prospective medicine," meaning health care providers could use the instrument systematically to collect epidemiological information and predict the risk of dying within a specified period (e.g., 10 years). It was hoped that clients would make behavioral changes as a result of this information (Breslow et al., 1997).

By the early 1980s, nurses began to use the tools, and approximately 12 HRA instruments were available to them. However, nurse researchers Doerr and Hutchins (1981) stated in a study appearing in *Nursing Research* that although HRAs demonstrated innovation in improving health measurement, they also cautioned that more sophisticated studies were needed in nursing to improve validity and reliability of the tools and improve research methodologies.

During the 1980s and 1990s, HRAs began to be used in home-, community-, and worksite-based health programs (Anderson & Staufacker, 1996; Deitchman & Sanderson, 1999). Since then, experts in the fields of epidemiology, biostatistics, preventive medicine, health education, behavioral medicine, and computer science have been involved in developing the instruments. HRAs vary from simplistic questionnaires about health habits to more specific appraisals of social support, emotional health, and spirituality (Christopher, Christopher, & Dunnagan, 2000). A simple internet search can reveal more than 50 vendors, many of whom offer more than one appraisal.

PURPOSE, DEVELOPMENT, AND USE OF HEALTH RISK APPRAISALS

The purpose of an HRA is to provide a client with an estimate of health threats based on genetic makeup, family history, and lifestyle. These self-reported questionnaires may address the areas of well-being, nutrition, fitness, environmental safety, stress, responsibilities, personal habits, and attitudes regarding health. Public health nurses can use these instruments to individualize assessment of risk and to recommend behavioral changes with their clients in hopes of motivating a healthier lifestyle. A systematic collection of data about the client's health status, beliefs, and behaviors is part of a nursing assessment that can enhance the development of a health promotion prevention plan (Pender, Murdaugh, & Parsons, 2006).

Based on health behavior theories (Becker, Haefner, & Kasl, 1977; Pender, 1996), an HRA can conceivably increase the client's knowledge of personal susceptibility to disease and may stimulate individuals to change their lifestyles to prevent illness and promote overall health. Using HRAs, client risk factors can be classified according to six categories of risk as shown in Figure 12-1.

Traditionally, the use of an HRA is a process that may entail (1) collecting data about an individual,

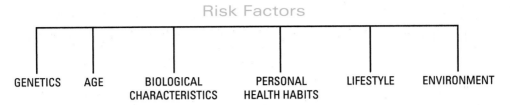

Figure 12-1 Categories of risk factors.
From "Health Promotion in Nursing Practice, 3rd ed" by Nola J. Pender, 1996, Appleton and Lange, p. 123. Reprinted with permission of the author.

(2) using a computerized algorithm to analyze the data, and (3) producing feedback designed to encourage behavioral change to improve health and avoid premature mortality (Breslow et al., 1997). HRAs were first available in paper-and-pencil format, but the computerized forms are now more popular and widely available. An HRA was the first health education tool that provided computer-tailored feedback to the user almost immediately (Strecher & Kreuter, 1999). The growth of computer technologies has certainly catapulted the popularity of electronic HRAs among both consumers and health care providers. Computerized forms of HRAs are widely available from several commercial sources and in the public domain through the World Wide Web. Most of these appraisals also provide computerized analysis of individual risk based on national mortality data for selected health problems.

Occupational health has traditionally focused on health and safety issues within the workplace. But in recent years, these worksites have begun to recognize that the health and lifestyle choices of the individual worker can impact work performance and overall health costs. Health risk appraisals are being utilized to promote wellness programs in the workplace and encourage the best practices for human resources. They have become a valuable evaluation method in analyzing the effectiveness of worksite health promotion programs (Musich et al., 2001; Ozminkowski et al., 2004; Williams & Wold, 2000; Wright, Beard, & Edington, 2002; Yen et al., 2003).

⊕ POLICY HIGHLIGHT

HRA in Action

The Worksite and Community Health Promotion/Risk Reduction Project was implemented in a rural six-county area in southwestern Virginia to help employees and residents reduce their cardiovascular and cancer risks by adopting healthy lifestyles. Results from a Centers for Disease Control and Prevention (CDC) health-risk appraisal survey revealed that 62% of persons surveyed did not exercise regularly, 53% were overweight, 51% had never had their cholesterol checked, 32% were smokers, and 20% knew they were hypertensive. The health screenings were used to design health promotion programs and promote policy changes. For example, one company established a policy to reduce environmental tobacco smoke, and another company hired a new food vendor that prepared low-fat, low-cholesterol, low-sodium foods. The program was so successful that the General Assembly in Virginia implemented resolutions requiring local health departments to assess the availability of worksite health promotion activities in their areas (CDC, 1992).

The managed care era brought new uses of HRAs into focus. Health care providers have now expanded their use from the primary purpose as a health education tool to a method of program planning and evaluation. HRAs are now used to estimate the cost of providing health care to individuals and populations while assisting to measure potential outcomes (Musich et al, 2001; Williams & Wold, 2000; Wright, Beard, & Edington, 2002). Moreover, recent work has demonstrated that a well-developed HRA that measures an individual's overall health can be significantly associated with prospective short-term medical claims costs (Yen et al., 2003).

⊕ RESEARCH APPLICATION

CVD Prevention Strategies with Urban and Rural African American Women

Study Purpose

To compare cardiovascular disease (CVD) risk factors in two groups of low-income African American women (LAAW), one rural (n = 160) and the other urban (n = 134), to national risk factor data for African American women; and to test a work site intervention designed to reduce CVD risk factors in LAAW.

Methods

Based on Pender's Health Promotion Model, individual CVD risk profiles were identified at a work site through (1) health risk appraisal, (2) blood pressure measurement, (3) body mass index calculation, (4) individual interviews about diet and exercise behaviors, and (5) total cholesterol analysis. The intervention, based on identified individual risk, focused on diet and physical activity behavior change to reduce CVD risk.

Findings

The two groups, one urban and one rural, exhibited higher or similar pretest CVD relative risk when statistically compared with a national sample of African American women. The LAAW study samples were younger and more edu-

cated. Pretest cholesterol and fat intake for rural women were higher than for the urban women ($p = <.05$). Posttest changes in cholesterol and fat intake risks were more significant in rural LAAW than in urban LAAW.

Implications

There is a need for additional research on effective interventions for rural and urban populations for CVD prevention. On pretest, rural women were less likely to have had previous CVD risk measurement, despite higher cholesterol levels and high dietary fat intake. The pretest–posttest analysis showed that the intervention was effective in rural women in the areas of reducing dietary fat intake and lowering cholesterol. This confirms the need for preventative CVD interventions with employees of small companies in rural areas. However, neither rural nor urban LAAW had significant changes in physical activity levels.

Reference

Williams, A., Wold, J., Dunkin, J., Idleman, L., & Jackson, C., (2004). CVD prevention strategies with urban and rural African American Women. *Applied Nursing Research, 17*(3), 187–194.

VALIDITY, RELIABILITY, AND EFFECTIVENESS OF HEALTH RISK APPRAISALS

Although HRAs have been widely used since the 1950s, documenting their effectiveness for actual behavior change has been challenging. One major obstacle to evaluating their usefulness has been the lack of documented reliability and validity for most of the instruments. In the early years, when HRAs were being used as an educational tool, these issues were less important. At that time, the appeal of the tools was the low cost and adaptability. However, now as these instruments are used in evaluation and research programs, the reliability, validity, and general effectiveness needs to be scrutinized (Edington, Yen, & Braunstein, 1999).

There is general agreement that when used as a tool to increase awareness and health education, the HRA is very useful if considering only face validity. However, the true validity of the HRA depends upon its application (Edington, Yen, & Braunstein, 1999). Its use as a predictor for morbidity or health care costs will still require additional research. Because the HRA is a self-reported tool and neither anonymous, confidential, nor randomly assigned, individuals may be more inclined to report acceptable health behaviors to gain social desirability.

The overall effectiveness of the HRA remains an open question. The accuracy of mortality predictions has been questioned (Pender, Murdaugh, & Parsons, 2001). An HRA alone is unlikely to result in reductions in risk. Unfortunately, in the past, most HRAs were not personalized enough to address the individual's perceived susceptibility, perceived severity, or perceived benefits. However, without addressing these components of behavioral change, there was little likelihood of increased self-efficacy or the building of skills to make changes in complex behavior (Becker & Janz, 1987).

However, in the present era, new communication technologies have the potential to allow users to engage in more powerful HRA formats that lend greater interactivity and individualized counseling for health modifications and motivations (Strecher & Krueter, 1999). A more contemporary approach to preventative services would be to collect the HRA data before a health care visit by using a mailed questionnaire or a waiting room assessment. This pre-visit planning would include interactive technologies, such as Web-based or interactive voice response technology that would assess multiple risk factors (Babor, Sciamanna, & Prink, 2004). The integrated use of HRA data may also be captured in the automated medical record and allow for discussion between the health care provider and the client, followed by a referral to an extended care team that may also include health educators, dietitians, exercise physiologists, or lifestyle counselors to support healthy behavior changes (Babor, Sciamanna, & Prink, 2004). Health care settings that require data reporting to assess quality and those benefiting from automated clinical information technology with client identification systems are more likely to routinely administer HRAs to their clients than those settings that use less technology (Halpin et al., 2005). Selecting an appropriate tool for maximum impact will be discussed later in this chapter.

APPROPRIATE AND INAPPROPRIATE USES OF HEALTH RISK APPRAISALS

Since HRAs are not meant to diagnose or screen for disease, these instruments are usually intended for persons who are free from chronic diseases such as cancer or heart disease. The appraisal is not meant to be a substitute for a complete medical history, nor is it a substitute for a medical exam. In contrast to screening, HRAs usually measure multiple risk factors along a continuum of severity of disease and combine them to produce a risk index (Babor, Sciamanna, & Prink, 2004). Moreover, it is not a health promotion program in itself. Since the development of HRAs has been founded on studies of middle-class white populations, all instruments are not appropriate for more diverse individuals (Alexander, 1999).

Public health nurses who use HRA instruments must be aware of several ethical principles that apply: confidentiality, voluntary participation, appropriateness for the population, and quality assurance. Seven general ethical guidelines have been defined by the Society of Prospective Medicine to help protect the rights and safety of clients. These guidelines appear in Box 12-1.

SOCIAL INFLUENCES AND CULTURE'S IMPACT

Culture influences the understanding of health and wellness and their effect in psychological, mental, and emotional health. The development of HRAs has been impacted by the values and assumptions of Western culture. Questions that address spiritual, psychological, mental, and emotional health may be particularly troubling when these instruments are used with diverse populations. Many cross-cultural researchers have identified two primary variants in understanding culture's influence on health: individualism and collectivism (Christopher, Christopher, & Dunnagan, 2000). The dominant cultural outlook in the West is individualism; however, many cultures espouse collectivism, which prioritizes the group over the individual and sees the group as more than the sum of its individual members. However, only 30% of the world's population adopts the individualism variant.

This fact has several implications for the use of HRAs. First of all, merely translating HRAs into different languages or dialects is insufficient to address the cultural influences (Harthorn & Oaks, 2003). Rather, HRA information should be developed by gathering information on how cultures define and understand health. More qualitative methods will be needed to accomplish this. Second, HRAs may not be appropriate within collectivist societies and in some cross-cultural settings. Not only may it be inappropriate for certain questions to be asked, but how the questions are asked and by whom needs to be addressed (Christopher, Christopher, & Dunnagan, 2000).

SELECTION OF APPROPRIATE HEALTH RISK APPRAISAL TOOLS

The most important question for nurses to ask when selecting an appropriate HRA concerns the target audience. Nurses should question whether this tool is

BOX 12-1: Seven Guidelines for Use of Health Risk Appraisals by the Society of Prospective Medicine

Health Assessment Program Planning: Each health assessment program should have a well-defined written statement detailing the goals, objectives, methodology, and requirements of participation.

Health Assessment Instrument Selection: Several factors should be examined when selecting a health assessment instrument (e.g., appropriateness for the target population, credibility of scientific basis and/or database(s) underlying its construction, and cultural and ethic sensitivity). Other key factors include the ease of use, the types of data analysis performed, and the clarity and intelligibility of reports generated.

Health Assessment Participant Orientation: Individual participants should receive an orientation, either written or oral, before completing a health assessment. This orientation describes the purpose of the assessment, the science base of or approach underlying the instrument, the time commitment for completion, who has access to the results, the information to be reported, and the use of the results.

Health Assessment Administration: Individual participants should be free to accept or decline any health assessment without fear of consequences.

Health Assessment Data Security: The data and report from health assessment are private and should not be shared with others unless expressly permitted by the individual participant. Administrators of health assessments are responsible for protecting individual data or results from unauthorized access and must respect the wishes of the individual participant. The information obtained from the health assessment should not be used to discriminate on the basis of job eligibility or insurability or render harm in any manner.

Health Assessment Report Interpretation: If the assessment generates individual reports, as with the HRAs, individuals should receive a report that is easily understood. The reporting should be accompanied by an explanation of the implications of the result for the individual's health and well-being. If possible, a competent health educator or provider should be available to explain the report and answer questions.

Health Promotion Resource Accessibility: When individuals receive personal reports as a result of the assessment process, a list of local and national resources that ameliorate risk factors of other problems identified should be made available to them. When individual reports are not returned to participants, general resource information appropriate to the characteristics of that group should be made available to the participants.

SOURCE: Hyner, G. C., Peterson, K. W., Travis, J. W., Dewey, J. E., Foerster, J. J., Framer, E. M., eds. *SPM Handbook of Health Assessment Tools.* Pittsburgh, PA: The Society of Prospective Medicine & The Institute for Health and Productivity Management. 1999.

---

appropriate in terms of its scientific base, the types of risks included, the reading level and comprehensiveness, and the type of report it generates (Alexander, 1999). The history of the development of the tool, the focus on modifiable risks, and the ease of instructions for consumers to minimize misinterpretation are necessary. Pilot testing instruments with specific populations is recommended. Safeguards for privacy and confidentiality are important considerations as well. Psychosocial and behavioral effects of HRAs as addressed by Strecher & Kreuter (1999) can be maximized if the following recommendations are addressed:

1. Provide feedback designed to correct users' inaccuracies and perceptions of their own risk

2. Provide feedback that establishes behavior change priorities when multiple risk factors exist

3. Provide feedback that enhances the user's ability to make recommended health behavior changes (Strecher & Kreuter, 1999)

Most HRA tools consist of between 40 and 80 questions designed to address multiple risk factors. These usually include lifestyle or behavioral areas including tobacco and alcohol use, nutrition or diet, physical activity or exercise, height and weight, self-care, motor vehicle use, safety, back care, preventative self-exams, and readiness to change (Babor, Sciamanna, & Prink, 2004).

IMPLICATIONS FOR PUBLIC HEALTH NURSING

Healthy People 2010 has two overarching goals: (1) to increase the quality and years of healthy life and (2) to eliminate health disparities (USDHHS, Healthy People 2010, 2000). Educational and community-based programs, including settings of schools, work sites, and health clinics, will be necessary to reach people outside traditional health care settings for improvement of health promotion and quality of life. The use of HRAs by public health nurses has a promising future as a mechanism to meet Healthy People 2010 objectives that relate to educational and community-based programs (Healthy People Objectives 7-1 through 7-12).

However, more research should be done to demonstrate the effectiveness of HRAs for behavior changes in both individuals and aggregate populations.

Public health nursing has the goal of preventing disease and injury in groups or populations of people. In contrast, the goal of clinical practitioners focuses on the disease or injury of an individual. Nurses working in public health conduct health activities in a systematic manner by recognizing a problem, defining the scope of the problem, conducting surveillance and epidemiological activities to determine its causes, designing and implementing public health interventions, and evaluating the effectiveness of those interventions. This public health surveillance involves on-going collection, analysis, and dissemination of data in order to prevent disease and injury in populations.

Public health nurses can use surveillance techniques, including HRAs to monitor the potential for infectious diseases, chronic diseases, injuries, or specialized

---

⊕ RESEARCH APPLICATION

Testicular Self-Examination in Young Adult Men

Study Purpose

To describe patterns of testicular self-examination (TSE) in a sample of young adult men and to identify factors distinguishing between men who do and do not practice TSE.

Methods

A comparative descriptive design used a convenience sample ($n = 191$) of adult men aged 18–35 recruited from a large industrial complex in the U.S. Midwest. A self-reported 75-item health risk appraisal was administered to identify health-related lifestyle habits. Data were collected during several occupational health fairs held from 1999 to 2001. Men who did and did not perform TSE regularly were compared using Mann-Whitney U statistics for discrete variables and t-tests for continuous variables. Discriminant function analysis was used to identify factors allowing prediction of frequent or infrequent TSE performance.

Findings

Sixty-four percent of the 191 participants reported rarely or never performing TSE, and 36% practiced TSE monthly or every few months. Men who infrequently performed

TSE were more often African American or Hispanic and had less than a college education. Other significant factors associated with infrequent TSE practice included less satisfaction with current job assignment; less satisfaction with life in general; greater worries interfering with daily life; more serious family problems in dealing with spouse, children, or parents; and reduced availability of people to turn to for support.

Implications

Demographic and socioeconomic variables appear related to TSE knowledge and performance. Programs of health education and promotion for men are needed. Continued research is needed to understand factors influencing TSE practice, particularly social support. Since testicular cancer is curable if detected early, the need for additional health education research and intervention testing is important.

Reference

Wynd, C. (2002). Testicular Self-Examination in Young Adult Men. *Journal of Nursing Scholarship, 34*(3), 251–255.

⊕ PRACTICE APPLICATION

Initiating a Cardiovascular Health Promotion Program for Women at a Rural Poultry Plant

Ms. K is an occupational health nurse working in a rural poultry plant. At least 60% of the employees at this work site are Hispanic women. Throughout her years at this work site, she has noted a high incidence of cardiovascular disease, including hypertension and cerebral vascular accidents among the women. She has also observed a prevalence of obesity with the women. Ms. K. has grown increasingly concerned about these issues, especially in light of the high levels of stress brought about by the multiple roles the women must play both at work and in the home. Recently, rumors around the plant speak about layoffs and the outsourcing of jobs to other countries. This has caused increased stress among the women who must provide for their families.

Assessment

Ms. K met with the plant administrators and drew up a proposal and agreement to work in partnership with her employer. She also highlighted recent research on the cost benefits of improving the health of employees to decrease absenteeism, increase worker productivity, decrease the use of medical insurance and worker's compensation claims, and improve employee morale and the company image. After some gentle persuasion, she was able to convince her employer to support her new program and was awarded a small grant to launch her efforts.

Ms. K identified the following Healthy People 2010 objectives that would have salience to her new program:

⊕ 12-11: HYPERLINK "http://www.healthypeople.gov/document/html/objectives/12-11.htm" Increase the proportion of adults with high blood pressure who are taking action (e.g., losing weight, increasing physical activity, and reducing sodium intake) to help control their blood pressure.

⊕ 12-15: HYPERLINK "http://www.healthypeople.gov/document/html/objectives/12-15.htm" Increase the proportion of adults who have had their blood cholesterol checked within the preceding 5 years.

⊕ 22-1: HYPERLINK "http://www.healthypeople.gov/document/html/objectives/22-01.htm" Reduce the proportion of adults who engage in no leisure-time physical activity.

⊕ 22-2: HYPERLINK "http://www.healthypeople.gov/document/html/objectives/22-02.htm" Increase the proportion of adults who engage regularly, preferably daily, in moderate physical activity for at least 30 minutes per day.

⊕ 22-3: HYPERLINK "http://www.healthypeople.gov/document/html/objectives/22-03.htm" Increase the proportion of adults who engage in vigorous physical activity that promotes the development and maintenance of cardiorespiratory fitness three or more days per week for 20 or more minutes per occasion.

conditions such as occupational injuries and illnesses in populations. Data can be obtained from communicable disease reporting networks and other epidemiological data often collected by the CDC and the local health departments. Managed care organizations are now using electronic medical records and other systems to standardize the collection and storage of data that would be very useful for public surveillance purposes.

Another implication for public health nurses is to expand the use of HRAs as a component of a broader health promotion intervention (Anderson & Staufaulker, 1996). The objective of an HRA is to increase the awareness of the individual's risk, which may lead to

a behavioral change. A solid theory-based intervention implemented with the HRA as the first step has the best potential for incremental changes in health behaviors. Certainly, one rationale for offering such programs by public health nurses is that they can save work sites money by reducing medical expenditures. A few studies suggest a direct relationship between improvements in health risks and consequent medical cost savings (Goetzel et al., 1998; Musich, Adams, & Edington, 2000; Musich et al., 2003; Ozminkowski et al., 2004; Wright, Beard, & Edington, 2002).

Although the use of HRAs has many limitations, if used for the proper purposes and with an understanding

⊕ PRACTICE APPLICATION

Work Site Health Promotion Plan

Ms. K decided to create a committee to plan the work site health promotion program. She included a poultry worker, a supervisor, and an administrator on the planning committee. The new health promotion program was marketed through posters, invitations in paycheck envelopes, and an article in the work site newsletter. The committee agreed that priority should be placed on addressing smoking cessation, alcohol and drug abuse, stress management, and exercise and fitness.

After careful consideration, Ms. K selected a standardized health risk appraisal instrument, the Healthier People Health Risk Appraisal 4.0. This instrument had been targeted for Hispanic populations and was available in appropriate language format. Local nursing students measured blood pressure with a calibrated aneroid blood pressure cuff, calculated body mass index (BMI) by securing height and weight measurement, and identifying the total cholesterol level through a fasting finger still sample via portable Abbott Vision Analyzer cholesterol machine analysis.

The collected data were entered into a software program and analyzed. Individual results were shared during a scheduled interview with the nursing students. Each interview included an interpretation of the employee's personal cardiovascular disease risk profile. All the data were aggregated into a work site profile. Identified risk factors of the work site women included an increased risk of morbidity and mortality based on age, family history, smoking, drug and alcohol use, stress, poor nutrition, and fitness patterns. Many individuals lacked knowledge of health promotion behaviors and their own personal risk factors. Other identified risk factors included a lack of access to affordable health promotion services and a lack of supportive social networks to encourage healthful behaviors. Based on these findings, the following nursing diagnoses were developed:

Deficient knowledge related to health promotion and risk reduction behaviors

Ineffective health maintenance related to multiple personal and environmental risks to health and lack of access to health promotion services

Planning

The objective of the proposed intervention was to reduce cholesterol levels through changes in diet and exercise behaviors. During interviews with clients, the interpretation of the participant's risk for cardiovascular disease guided the discussion of behavior changes that might reduce cholesterol values and elevated BMI and/or blood pressure.

Each participant received both written and verbal information on suggested diet and exercise behaviors that would reduce cardiovascular risk.

Under Ms. K's direction and coordination, a monthly educational session that highlighted various health promotion activities was held. Smoking cessation programs were offered during all shifts. Support groups were developed for employees to share their concerns and promote supportive social relationships. A weight loss clinic was also held once a week. Focus groups were held with workers to seek their input on how to reduce stress in the work site environment. Supervisors and administrators met to discuss ways to restructure the work environment to optimize health and enhance a healthy work environment to decrease stress. Individual follow-up interviews continued with Ms. K to recheck blood pressure and reinforce adherence to the program.

Evaluation

After the program was in existence for 6 months, the committee began to analyze data to evaluate the effectiveness of the program. Evaluation continued at 6 month intervals. Data revealed the following about the program participants:

⊕ A 25% increase in self-reported actions to reduce blood pressure (weight loss program and/or increasing physical activity)

⊕ A 30% increase in the number of adults who had their blood pressure checked in the preceding 6 months

⊕ A 15% self-reported action of increased regular physical activity

⊕ A 10% drop in cholesterol levels and weight loss for program participants

⊕ A 30% increase in reports of job satisfaction

⊕ A 10% drop in cholesterol levels and weight loss for program participants

Measurable improvements in employee health, well-being, and productivity were substantial enough to justify continued funding and expansion of the program by administrators. Nurses in the community are often untapped resources who can provide health appraisals, screenings, and health education in local work sites that can make lasting and enduring impacts on health.

of cultural sensitivity and ethical issues, these techniques have tremendous possibilities for successful use in the future. Particularly, with new emphasis being placed on the responsibility of individuals for their own health

behaviors, the use of interactive Internet Web sites has the potential to raise levels of an individual's awareness of personal susceptibility of potential disease or injury and tailor a workable plan for health improvements.

CRITICAL THINKING ACTIVITIES

1. The nurse has administered a health risk appraisal assessment to a group of employees at a work site. Upon analyzing the data, she observes a high number of smokers among the female workers. Discuss potential barriers to a behavioral change of smoking cessation for these workers.

2. Discuss how a health risk appraisal instrument might fit into a comprehensive health promotion program for obesity reduction in school age children. Study cultural differences for this aggregate and then develop a plan of client care for African American school-age children.

3. Interview an occupational health nurse who has been involved in establishing a new health promotion program. Discuss who was involved in the assessment, how long the process took, and what the sources of money, equipment, and space were. Ask why the program was proposed and how successful it was. Ask what might have been done differently.

4. Explore the concepts of wellness and illness among persons from different socioeconomic,

occupational, or cultural groups. What similarities and differences might exist among these persons and how might that affect the use of an HRA?

5. Take a health risk appraisal yourself. What risks to health are you able to identify in your own attitudes and behaviors? Choose one personal behavior that you routinely engage in that you would like to modify. Attempt to make a change for one week. What was this experience like for you? What factors were barriers to your behavior change? What factors were helpful to your behavioral change?

6. Collect data from the CDC Web site (http://www.cdc.gov) and your local health department on reportable diseases in your community. Identify the major disease that may cause high levels of mortality and morbidity. Now search for an appropriate health risk appraisal tool that would be appropriate to use to raise awareness in individuals who may be at risk of developing this disease in your community.

KEY TERMS

health risk appraisal (HRA) tool

nursing assessment

KEY CONCEPTS

⊕ Public health nurses can use health risk appraisal instruments to individualize assessment of risk and to recommend behavioral change for their clients in hopes of motivating a healthier lifestyle. They can be administered to large groups and can be generated and calculated by computers and/or using the World Wide Web.

⊕ Elements that should be part of a health risk appraisal are assessment, estimation, and education.

⊕ Health risk appraisals can be used to enhance program planning and evaluation, to identify those in need of secondary prevention activities (e.g., screening), to help recruit participants into health promotion programs, and to provide information to clients that hopefully will motivate and facilitate a behavioral change.

⊕ Public health nurses who use HRA instruments must be aware of several ethical principles that apply: confidentiality, voluntary participation, appropriateness for the population, and quality assurance. HRAs may not be appropriate for use in some cross-cultural settings since they have been developed based on Western cultures.

⊕ Combining HRAs used with a theory-based comprehensive health promotion program has been shown to demonstrate better outcomes for behavioral change.

⊕ Public health nurses can use surveillance techniques, including HRAs, to monitor potential for infectious diseases, chronic diseases, injuries, or specialized conditions such as occupational injuries and illnesses in special populations.

REFERENCES

Alexander, G. (1999). Health risk appraisal. In G. C. Hyner, K. W. Peterson, J. W. Travis, J. E. Dewey, J. J. Foerster, & E. M. Framer (Eds.), *SPM handbook of health assessment tools* (pp. 5–8). Pittsburgh: The Society of Prospective Medicine and the Institute for Health and Productivity Management.

Anderson, D., & Staufacker, M. (1996). The impact of worksite-based health risk appraisal on health related outcomes: A review of the literature. *American Journal of Public Health, 10,* 499–508.

Babor, T. F., Sciamanna, C. N., & Prink, N. P. (2004). Assessing multiple risk behaviors in primary care: Screening issues and related concepts. *American Journal of Preventative Medicine, 27*(2S), 42–53.

Becker, M. H., Haefner, D. P., & Kasl, S. V. (1977). Selected psychosocial models and correlates of individual health-related behaviors. *Medical Care, 15,* 27–46.

Becker, M., & Janz, N. (1987). On the effectiveness and utility of health hazard/health risk appraisal in clinical and non-clinical settings. *Health Services Research, 22,* 537–551.

Breslow, L., Beck, J. Morgenstern, H., Fielding, J., Moore, A., Carmel, M. & Higa, J. (1997). Development of a Health Risk Appraisal for the Elderly (HRA-E*). American Journal of Health Promotion, 11*(5), 337–343.

Centers for Disease Control and Prevention. (1992). Worksite and community health promotion/risk reduction project—Virginia, 1987–1991. *Morbidity and Mortality Weekly Report, 41*(4), 55–57.

Christopher, S., Christopher, J., & Dunnagan, T. (2000). Culture's Impact on Health Risk Appraisal Psychological Well-being Questions. *American Journal of Health Promotion, 24*(5), 338–348.

Deitchman, S., & Sanderson, L. (1999). Public health surveillance: Health appraisal for populations. In G. C. Hyner, K. W. Peterson, J. W. Travis, J. E. Dewey, J. J. Foerster, & E. M. Framer (Eds*.), SPM handbook of health assessment tools* (pp. 63–71). Pittsburgh: The Society of Prospective Medicine and the Institute for Health and Productivity Management.

Doerr, B. T. & Hutchins, E. B. (1981). Health risk appraisal: Process, problems, and prospects for nursing practice and research. *Nursing Research, 30*(5), 299–306.

Edington, D., Yen, L, & Braunstein, A. (1999). The reliability and validity of HRAs. In G. C. Hyner, K. W. Peterson, J. W. Travis, J. E. Dewey, J. J. Foerster, & E. M. Framer (Eds.), *SPM handbook of health assessment tools* (pp. 135–142). Pittsburgh: The Society of Prospective Medicine and the Institute for Health and Productivity Management.

Goetzel, R. Z., Jacobson, B. H., Aldana, S. G., Vardell, K., & Yee, L. (1998). Costs of worksite health promotion participants and nonparticipants. *Journal of Occupational and Environmental Medicine, 40*(4), 341–346.

Halpin, H. A., McMenamin, S.G., Schmittdiel, J., Gillies, R., Shortell, S., Rundall, T., & Casalino, L. (2005). The routine use of health risk appraisal: Results from a national study of physician organization. *American Journal of Health Promotion, 20*(1), 34–38.

Harthorn, B. H., & Oaks, L. (2003). *Risk, culture, and health inequality: Shifting perceptions of danger and blame.* Westport, CO: Praeger.

Hyner, G. C., Peterson, K. W., Travis, J. W., Dewey, J. E., Foerster, J. J., & Framer, E. M. (Eds.). (1999). *SPM handbook of health assessment tools.* Pittsburgh: The Society of Prospective Medicine and the Institute for Health and Productivity Management.

Kessler, R. C., & Wang, P. (1999). Screening measures for behavioral health assessment. In G. C. Hyner, K. W. Peterson, J. W. Travis, J. E. Dewey, J. J. Foerster, & E. M. Framer (Eds.), *SPM handbook of health assessment tools* (pp. 33–40). Pittsburgh: The Society of Prospective Medicine and the Institute for Health and Productivity Management.

Musich, S., Adams, L., DeWolf, G., & Edington, D. W. (2001). A case study of 10-year health risk appraisal: Participation patterns in a comprehensive health promotion program. *American Journal of Health Promotion, 15*(4), 237–240.

Musich, S. A., Adams, L., & Edington, D. W. (2000). Effectiveness of health promotion programs in moderating medical costs in the USA. *Health Promotion International, 15*(1), 5–15.

Musich, S., Hook, D., Barnett, T., & Edington, D. W. (2003). The association between health risk status and health care costs among the membership of an Australian health plan. *Health Promotion International, 18*(1), 57–65.

Ozminkowski, R. J., Goetzel, R. Z., Santoro, J., Saenz, B. J., Eley, C., & Gorsky, B. (2004). Estimating risk reduction required to break even in a health promotion program. *American Journal of Health Promotion, 18*(4), 316–325.

Pender, N. J. (1996). *Health promotion in nursing practice* (3rd ed.). Stamford, CT: Appleton & Lange.

Pender, N. J., Murdaugh, C. L., & Parsons, M. A. (2001). *Health promotion in nursing practice* (4th ed.). Upper Saddle River, NJ: Prentice-Hall.

Pender, N. J., Murdaugh, C. L., & Parsons, M. A. (2006). *Health promotion in nursing practice* (5th edition). Upper Saddle River, NJ: Prentice-Hall.

Robbins, L., & Hall, J. (1970). *How to practice prospective medicine.* Indianapolis: Methodist Hospitals of Indiana.

Society of Prospective Medicine. (1999). Ethical guidelines for the development and use of health assessment. In K. W. Peterson, J. W. Travis, J. E. Dewey, E. M. Framer, J. J. Foerster, & G. C. Hyner (Eds.). *SPM handbook of health assessment tools* (4th ed.). Pittsburgh: The Society of Prospective Medicine.

Strecher, V. J., & Kreuter, M. W. (1999). Health risk appraisal from a behavioral perspective: Present and future. In G. C. Hyner, K. W. Peterson, J. W. Travis, J. E. Dewey, J. J. Foerster, & E. M. Framer (Eds.), *SPM handbook of health assessment tools* (pp. 75–82). Pittsburgh: The Society of Prospective Medicine and the Institute for Health and Productivity Management.

U.S. Department of Healthy and Human Services (USDHHS). (2000, November). *Healthy people 2010: Understanding and improving health* (2nd ed.). Washington, D.C.: U.S. Government Printing Office.

Williams, A., & Wold, J. (2000). Nurses, cholesterol, and small work sites: Innovative community intervention comparisons. *Family and Community Health, 23*(3), 59–75.

Williams, A., Wold, J., Dunkin, J., Idleman, L., & Jackson, C., (2004). CVD prevention strategies with urban and rural African American Women. *Applied Nursing Research, 17*(3), 187–194

Wright, D., Beard, M. J., & Edington, D. W. (2002). Association of health risks with the cost of time away from work. *Journal of Occupational and Environmental Medicine, 44:* 1126–1134.

Wynd, C. (2002). Testicular Self-Examination in Young Adult Men. *Journal of Nursing Scholarship, 34*(3), 251–255.

Yen, L., McDonald, T., Hirschland, D., & Edington, D. (2003). Association between wellness score from a health risk appraisal and prospective medical claims costs. *Journal of Occupational Environmental Medicine, 45,* 1049–1057.

BIBLIOGRAPHY

Alexander, G. (2000). Health risk appraisal. *International Electronic Journal of Health Education, 3,* 133–137. Available at http://www.aahperd.org/iejhe/index.html

Burton, W. N., Chen, C., Conti, D. J., Schultz, A. B., Pransky, G., & Edington, D. W. (2005). The association of health risks with on-the-job productivity. *Journal of Occupational & Environmental Medicine, 47*(8), 769–777.

Christopher, S., Christopher, J. C., & Dunnagan, T. (2000). Culture's impact on health risk appraisal psychological well-being questions. *American Journal of Health Behavior, 24*(5), 338–348.

Kashima, S. R. (2006). Transitioning from a pen-and-paper health risk appraisal to an online health risk appraisal at a petroleum company. *Health Promotion Practice, 7*(4), 450–458.

Strecher, V. J., & Krueter, M. W. (2000). Health risk appraisal from a behavioral perspective: Present and future. *International Electronic Journal of Health Education, 3,* 169–179. Available at http://www.aahperd.org/iejhe/index.html.

Williams, A., Mason, A., & Wold, J. (2001). Cultural sensitivity and day care workers: Examination of a worksite based cardiovascular disease prevention project. *AAOHN Journal, 49*(1), 35–43.

Williams, A., & Wold, J. (2000). Nurses, cholesterol, and small worksites: Innovative community intervention comparisons. *Family & Community Health, 23*(3), 59–75.

Williams, A., Wold, J., Dunkin, J., Idleman, L., & Jackson, C. (2004). CVD prevention strategies with urban and rural African American women. *Applied Nursing Research, 17*(3), 187–194.

Witte, K., Meyer, G., & Martell, D. (2006). *Effective health risk messages: A step-by-step guide.* Thousand Oaks, CA: Sage.

Yen, L., Schultz, A., Schnueringer, E., & Edington, D. W. (2006). Financial costs due to excess health risks among active employees of a utility company. *Journal of Occupational & Environmental Medicine, 48*(9), 896–905.

RESOURCES

Employer Health Register

Web: http://www.employerhealth.com

The Employer Health Register is a link to direct employee health specialists with products and services, including health risk appraisals. Published from the Work Loss Data Institute.

Guide for Wellness Professionals

Web: http://www.bsu.edu

This Web site provides the reader with history, benefits, limitations, uses, and recommendation for using health risk appraisals. The goal is to help wellness professionals make informed choices from available instruments and vendors.

Healthier Students Health Risk Appraisals

Web: http://www.csupomona.edu

The Health Risk Appraisals Web site, developed by Jim Grizzell (Student Health Services, California State Polytechnic University, Pomona, CA), provides a slide presentation and other resources from Healthy People 2010 National College Health Objectives. The Web site topics include injury prevention, alcohol abuse, tobacco use, sexual behaviors, dietary behaviors, and physical activity.

Healthier Worksite Initiative, Centers for Disease Control and Prevention

1600 Clifton Road
Atlanta, Georgia 30333
404-639-3311
Web: http://www.cdc.gov

The Healthier Worksite Initiative addresses worksite health promotion. The Web site summarizes how to use a health risk appraisal, important considerations for implementation, and ethical considerations. The content source is the Division of Nutrition and Physical Activity, National Center for Chronic Disease Prevention and Health Promotion.

Mayo Clinic Health Solutions

Mayo Clinic Health Management Resources
Centerplace 4, 200 First Street SW
Rochester, Minnesota 55905
1-800-430-9699
FAX: 507-284-5410
Email: MayoClinicHealthManagementResources@mayo.edu
Web: http://mayoclinichealthmanagementresources.com

This health risk appraisal has a unique emphasis on health education and behavior change. The tool is designed to identify risks within a population, deliver follow-up interventions for those at risk, and track and analyze population health trends over time.

Protocol Driven Healthcare

Web: http://www.pdhi.com

The Web site provides a comprehensive assessment from self-reported health status information. It is available in both English and Spanish.

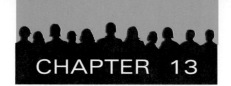

CHAPTER 13

Principles of Health Promotion

Carolyn L. Blue, RN, PhD, CHES

David R. Black, PhD, HSPP, MPH, CHES, CPPE, FASHA, FSBM, FAAHB

Chapter Outline

- Holistic Concept of Health
- Health Promotion
- Theoretical Foundations of Health Promotion
  - Behavioral Models
  - Ecological Models
- Focus on Population Health
  - Making Health Communication Programs Work
  - PRECEDE-PROCEED Model
  - Social Marketing
- Ethical Issues in Health Promotion

Learning Objectives

Upon completion of this chapter, the reader will be able to:

1. Differentiate meanings of health.
2. Examine principles of health promotion as applied to public health nursing practice.
3. Explore the range of health promotion activities.
4. Compare health promotion models and theories.
5. Compare stages of the health communication program process with the nursing process.
6. Describe social marketing as a strategy to develop health promotion programs.

There are several ways to define health. The World Health Organization (WHO) defined health globally as "a state of complete physical, mental, and social well-being and not merely the absence of disease or infirmity" (1948, p. 1). The definition in the WHO's preamble to the Constitution continues with emphasis on health as a human right that is fundamental to peace and security, healthy child development, living harmoniously in a healthy environment, social participation in health, and governmental responsibilities for adequate health and social measures. Clearly, the World Health Organization defines health as a social responsibility, and in 1977, the Thirtieth World Health Assembly decided that the main social targets of governments and the WHO in the coming decades should be "the attainment of all citizens of the world by the year 2000 of a level of health that would permit them to lead socially and economically productive lives" (WHO, 1977). This statement is important in that it specifies both the level of health needed and the accomplishment at that level. In 1985, the WHO defined health as "the extent to which an individual or group is able, on the one hand, to realize aspirations and satisfy needs; and, on the other hand, to change or cope with the environment"; it is "seen as a resource for everyday life, not the objective of living; it is a positive concept emphasizing social and personal resources, as well as physical capacities." In their *Health Promotion Glossary,* health is defined holistically to include physical, social, mental, and spiritual well-being (WHO, 1998).

Health is defined in Healthy People 2010 as the health of the total population and the consequences of the determinants of health—biology, behavior, social environment, physical environment, and policies and interventions that promote health (USDHHS, 2000). Monitoring the health of whole populations includes using information about mortality, morbidity, use of health facilities, and other information such as injury data and health surveillance surveys. The U.S. Department of Health and Human Services (USDHHS) also recognizes that the health of individuals where they live, work, and play is essential to the health of communities and health of the nation.

HOLISTIC CONCEPT OF HEALTH

Nursing and public health specialists define health and wellness as a holistic concept encompassing physical, psychological, social, and spiritual dimensions (Insel & Roth, 2002; Pender, Murdaugh, & Parsons, 2002). According to them, effective physical health refers to the ability of the body's anatomical and biological structures to adapt in ways that result in positive health status. Psychological health encompasses not only the ability to think clearly and coherently but also high self-esteem, inner-directedness, creativity, and the ability to effectively adapt to and cope with challenging situations. Social health means the ability to make and maintain relationships with other individuals, groups, and communities. Spiritual health is a relationship with a higher power and inner peace essential to maintaining health and well-being.

Smith (1981) described individual differences in various conceptualizations of health. Her four health concepts included (1) clinical health, in which health is the absence of illness or symptoms; (2) role-performance health, or the ability to effectively perform one's role in society; (3) adaptive health, meaning one's ability to engage in effective interaction with the physical and social environment; and (4) eudaemonistic health, meaning general well-being and realization of one's human potential. Laffrey (1985) supported this multidimensional conception of health by finding a relationship between Smith's (1981) definitions of health and health-promoting behavior choices and demonstrated nursing's promotion of health in all four dimensions. However, Laffrey's (1985) and others' (Pender et al., 1990) research supported only two dimensions of health—clinical health and wellness.

Pender defined health "as the actualization of inherent and acquired human potential through goal-directed behavior, competent self-care, and satisfying relationships with others, while adjustments are made as needed to maintain structural integrity and harmony with relevant environments" (Pender, Murdaugh, & Parsons, 2002, p. 22). This definition is very broad, holistic, and humanistic, encompassing, actualizing, and stabilizing dispositions. The definition resulted in a classification of affect, attitudes, activities, aspirations, and accomplishments consistent with health.

Green and Krueter (1999) described outcomes of health as improved quality of life, efficient functioning, the capacity to perform at more productive and satisfying levels, and the opportunity to live out the life span with vigor and stamina. Many definitions of health focus on the individual, but health outcomes can be inferred for families, communities, and populations, as the health of these larger groups depends on the health of the members.

HEALTH PROMOTION

The WHO defined health promotion in the Ottawa Charter as "the process of enabling people to increase control over, and to improve their health . . . and reducing differences in current health status and ensuring equal opportunities and resources to enable all people to achieve their fullest health potential" (1986, p. 1). The Ottawa Charter included enabling people to reach a level of well-being by advocating healthy public policy, creating supportive environments, strengthening community actions, developing personal skills, reorienting health services, and moving into a future where health is created where people learn, work, play, and love.

Green and Kreuter (1999) defined health promotion as the "combination of health educational and ecological supports for actions and conditions of living conducive to health" (1999, p. 27). These authors focus on both ends of the health illness continuum. Pender, Murdaugh, and Parsons (2002) differentiate between health promotion and health protection. They state that health protection focuses on the avoidance of illness or injury, while health promotion focuses on efforts to increase the level of well-being and self-actualization of an individual or group. While there is some disagreement among health care professionals about definitions of health promotion, it includes both practices aimed at preventing disease and those aimed at promoting positive health. Approaches to health promotion include advocacy and policy together with concrete resources necessary to increase control over and improve a state of health and well-being for individuals, communities, and populations.

Health promotion is a multi- and transdisciplinary practice to improve and maintain the health of individuals, families, communities, and populations. The promotion of the health of individuals, families, and communities has been an integral part of nursing practice throughout history. Nursing has traditionally practiced within a framework of promoting health. Florence Nightingale (1859/1992) believed in health as a wellness–illness continuum, and she promoted health through the education of individuals and families, social reform, and nursing care that included education in personal living and healthful environments. Nursing's meta-paradigm of person, environment, health, and nursing interacting dynamically has continued since Nightingale's influ-

ence. Although health promotion was overshadowed by illness care in the United States in the mid-twentieth century, the economic crisis in health care in the latter part of the twentieth century has placed a renewed emphasis on the health-person-environment connection. By the early 1970s, health promotion was gaining value in keeping individuals, families, communities, and populations healthy. In 1973, the American Nurses Association's (ANA) Standards of Nursing Practice identified health promotion as a major goal of nursing (ANA, 1973). Donaldson and Crowley (1978) noted a consensus among nurse leaders that nursing is concerned with the promotion of health. In 1979, the U.S. Public Health Service published Healthy People: Surgeon General's Report on Health Promotion and Disease Prevention outlining strategies for keeping people healthy. The report identified nursing and other health professionals' obligation in providing disease prevention and health promotion services. One year later, the U.S. Public Health Service (1980) published Promoting Health/ Preventing Disease: Objectives for the Nation, the first of three decades of national health objectives aimed at preventing disease and promoting health. These objectives placed disease prevention and health promotion firmly in the health policy picture and provided specific direction and goals for public health nurses and other health promotion professionals to protect and promote the health as well as to reduce health risks.

Nurses have a unique opportunity to promote health for individuals, families, and communities globally because of their biophysical-psychosocial expertise, because they provide continuous care and contact with people, and because of the level of societal trust nurses have achieved. The WHO proposed that nurses have the potential to lead the health promotion movement (WHO, 1989). However, it is clear that collaboration with other health care professionals is a basic premise for providing health promotion services. Because health promotion must be delivered holistically, it is essential to be able to work in a complementary atmosphere with health educators, health promotion specialists, nutritionists, sociologists, environmentalists, and others.

THEORETICAL FOUNDATIONS OF HEALTH PROMOTION

Because health behavior is so complex, theoretical models are needed to help explain and guide health behavior (Glanz, Rimer, & Lewis, 2002). Theory can also be used to provide the guiding framework for health-promoting and health-protecting interventions that optimize behavior change (Glanz, Rimer, & Lewis, 2002). Numerous models and theories developed by nurses and other health care professionals explain and predict healthy behaviors of individuals, families, and communities. It is important to recognize the reciprocal nature of individual, family, and community health behaviors. Community health behaviors influence individuals and families, and health behaviors of individuals influence the collective health behavior of communities. Models and theories presented in this chapter include those with concepts affecting health behaviors within individuals, models including interpersonal and environmental concepts, and models examining health behaviors at a community level.

Behavioral Models

Any community, whether it is a work site, school, community, state, or nation, is composed of individuals whose behavior influences health. Within each level of community, public health nurses and other health professionals work with individuals and groups of individuals to help people make healthy behavioral choices. The models presented can be used by public health nurses to better understand the health behaviors of their clients and to help them identify a focus and strategy of intervention. The public health nurse's ability to apply theories of health behavior is one of the most essential skills needed in designing, implementing, and evaluating programs to address health behavior change.

All the models presented are based on the premise that people regulate their own behavior through cognitive activity and that, specifically, behavior is a function of a rational decision-making process. Lewin (1951) was the first to recognize the importance of expectancies and values in human motivation. Lewin (1951) postulated that behavior is determined by the interaction of an individual with his or her meaningful, present environment and that it is a function of the interaction between the person and his life space as perceived by the person. People have a positive valence (being attracted to), a negative valence (being repulsed by), or a neutral valence to certain objects in their environments. They are drawn to objects of positive valence and try to attain those things that are of value to them. In this frame of reference, people select a behavior with the greatest likelihood of reaching their most valued goals. Theories with this premise are called value-expectancy theories. Behavior is a function of the subjective *value* of an outcome and the subjective *expectation* that a particular action will achieve that outcome (Lewin et al., 1944).

Health Belief Model

In the 1950s, researchers at the U.S. Public Health Service began work to understand why some individuals participated and others did not in tuberculosis-screening programs. Based on value-expectancy theory, people were likely to get a chest x-ray to detect tuberculosis if they (a) desired to identify tuberculosis early (value) and (b) if they believed getting a chest x-ray would identify early tuberculosis (expectancy). Hochbaum (1958) recognized that people were more likely to get a chest x-ray if they believed they were susceptible to tuberculosis and believed in the benefits of early detection. Rosenstock (1966) added variables to the model to more fully describe whether or not an individual would undertake action to prevent, screen for, or control illness. Variables in the Health Belief Model (HBM) that explain or predict behavior include an individual's perceptions of (a) level of personal susceptibility to the illness or condition under question, (b) the degree of severity of serious consequences that might result from having the illness or condition, (c) the behavior's potential benefits in preventing or reducing susceptibility or severity, and (d) physical, psychological, financial, or other unpleasant barriers related to beginning or maintaining the behavior. The model also specifies cues to action catalysts or strategies to activate the behavior by making the individual conscious of his or her feelings about the health threat. Rosenstock, Strecher, and Becker (1988) added Bandura's (1977) self-efficacy concept to the HBM to account for a person's confidence that he or she could initiate and maintain the behavior.

Glanz, Rimer, and Lewis (2002) have reported extensive use of the HBM to explain and predict health behavior as well as to guide interventions. The HBM has been used with a variety of cultures, including African American, Native American, Hispanic, Chinese, and Asian cultures (Glanz, Rimer, & Lewis, 2002; Newell-Withrow, 2000; Plowden, 2003). Recent applications of the model have focused on dietary behaviors (Abood, Black, & Feral, 2003), influenza vaccine acceptance (Blue & Valley, 2002), Lyme disease prevention (McKenna et al., 2004), mammography screening

(Champion et al., 2003), osteoporosis prevention programs (Sedlak, Doheny, & Jones, 2000), and skin cancer prevention (Lamanna, 2004). These examples of research using the HBM support public health nursing practice. Knowledge of a person's beliefs can be used to intervene to educate the person about susceptibility and seriousness of the health threat, benefits of the behavior to reducing the threat, and ways to reduce the barriers to the behavior. In addition, cues such as postcard reminders, phone calls, or for communities, billboard and other media messages could be used to increase the likelihood of taking the recommended action.

Pender's Health Promotion Model

Pender (1982), a psychologist and nurse, modified the Health Belief Model so that it would be more appropriate for explaining and predicting health-promoting behaviors. Health-promoting behavior is any behavior that attains a positive health outcome (Pender, Murdaugh, & Parsons, 2002). The Health Promotion Model (HPM) integrates concepts from the HBM and social cognitive theory. The model is unique because it does not rely on threat or fear avoidance and because it is holistic in nature. The initial HPM included seven cognitive-perceptual factors and five modifying factors. Cognitive-perceptual factors were importance of health, perceived control of health, definition of health, perceived health status, perceived self-efficacy, perceived benefits, and perceived barriers. The modifying factors were demographic and biologic characteristics, interpersonal influences, situational influences, and behavioral factors.

The model was revised in 2002 and can be seen in Figure 13-1. The concepts in the model are grouped under three major categories: individual characteristics and experiences, behavior-specific cognitions and affect, and behavioral outcome (Pender, Murdaugh, & Parsons, 2002). Individual characteristics include prior related behavior and a person's unique personal factors including biologic, psychological, and sociocultural factors that may affect carrying out the behavior. Behavior-specific cognitions and affect reflect a person's motivation to carry out a behavior and include (a) perceived benefits or outcomes of the action; (b) perceived barriers to the action; (c) perceived self-efficacy or a judgment about one's personal capability to organize and carry out a particular action; (d) activity-related affect, which is a subjective positive or negative feeling state about the behavior; (e) interpersonal influences including social influences, social support, and model-

ing the action by others; and (f) situational influences including perceptions about behavioral options, other demands, and environmental factors that could influence action. The behavior-specific cognitions and affect factors have an effect on a person's commitment to a plan of action to initiate and sustain the behavior and reflect the following: (a) a commitment to carry out the behavior at a specific time and place and under specific conditions and (b) specific strategies for initiating and continuing the behavior. The HPM also includes an immediate competing demands and preferences concept, which reflects urgent, last-minute alternative behaviors that compete for action. The extent to which a person can resist or work around other demands can influence the health promoting behavior. Pender's HPM has been used by nurse researchers as a framework for a cardiovascular disease prevention intervention (e.g., Wold et al., 2004)

Theory of Planned Behavior

Ajzen's (1988) Theory of Planned Behavior (TPB), an extension of the Theory of Reasoned Action (Ajzen & Fishbein, 1980), has been widely used by health professionals to investigate a wide assortment of health-promoting behaviors. The TPB posits that a person's *intention* to perform a behavior (or not perform the behavior) is the immediate antecedent of the behavior; and intention to perform the behavior is determined by the person's *attitude* toward the behavior, the *subjective norm*, and *perceived behavioral control*. A person's attitude toward a behavior is formed from beliefs about perceived outcome expectancies or outcomes that would occur if the person were to perform the behavior and whether those outcomes had a positive and negative value for the person. Subjective norm is formed from a person's beliefs about social influences to perform the behavior and the person's willingness or motivation to comply with those social influences. Perceived behavioral control is formed from beliefs about factors that would facilitate or inhibit taking action and how much power those factors possess. According to the theory, a favorable attitude toward the behavior, positive social influence, and one's control over factors that facilitate or inhibit the behavior will result in a strong intention to carry out the behavior and thus will result in the behavior being completed.

The TPB holds promise for health professionals to assess the causal antecedents of behavior, and enable them to design interventions to strengthen the positive beliefs and weaken the negative beliefs about the behaviors.

INDIVIDUAL
CHARACTERISTICS
AND EXPERIENCES

BEHAVIOR-SPECIFIC
COGNITIONS
AND AFFECT

BEHAVIORAL
OUTCOME

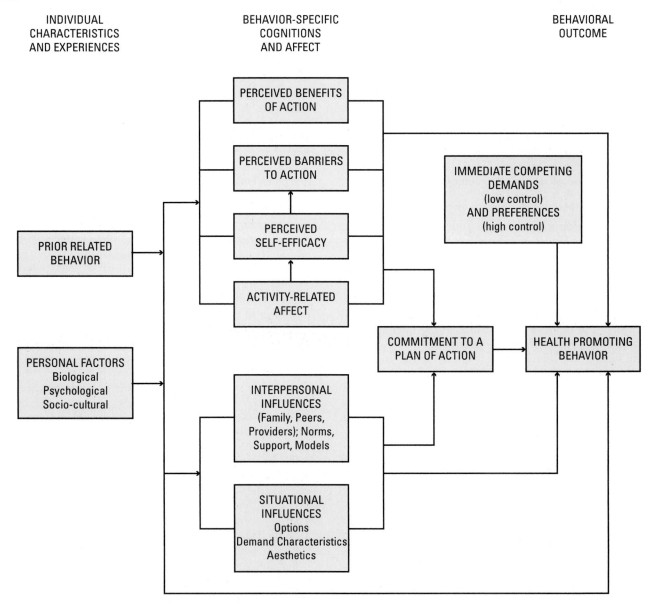

Figure 13-1 Pender's Health Promotion Model

From PENDER, NOLA J.; MURDAUGH, CAROLYN L.; PARSONS, MARY ANN, HEALTH PROMOTION IN NURSING PRACTICE, 5th Edition, ©2006, p. 50. Reprinted by permission of Pearson Education, Inc., Upper Saddle River, NJ.

By doing so, behavioral intentions will be strengthened, which will modify behavior in a positive health-promoting direction. Nurse researchers have used the TPB to investigate health-promoting behaviors among African American women (Drayton-Brooks & White, 2004) and specific health-promoting behaviors such as handwashing (O'Boyle, Henly, & Larson, 2001), physical activity among the elderly (Conn, Tripp-Reimer, & Maas, 2003), breast-feeding (Rempel, 2004), postpartum smoking (Gantt, 2001), and adolescent violence (Jemmott III et al., 2001).

Transtheoretical Model of Behavioral Change

The Transtheoretical Model (TTM) of behavior change was developed by DiClemente & Prochaska (1985) to explain or predict the extinction of problem behaviors such as addictions and in particular, initially, smoking behavior. However, it quickly became a popular model that has been useful in examining a large number of health behaviors (Prochaska, Redding, & Evers, 2002). According to the TTM, individuals progress through stages during the process of changing their behavior. People engaging in a new behavior move through a sequence of stages from precontemplation through maintenance and will relapse back to an earlier stage in the model (perhaps several times) before the person completes the change process (Prochaska & DiClemente, 1992). During precontemplation, individuals have no thoughts about behavior change; in order

to move to the next stage, precontemplators need to acknowledge that the problem is theirs, and they need to change their behavior. The second stage is contemplation where people begin to consider change and evaluate their options. They may evaluate their losses and rewards with respect to the change. In order to move to the next stage, they must decide to take action. The third stage is preparation where individuals have a plan of action, and past attempts to change may provide information for the initiation of the behavior. The fourth stage is action where overt behavioral changes are attempted. Skills are needed to interrupt habits and initiate new patterns of behavior to prevent impending resumptions of old behaviors or relapses. The fifth stage is maintenance; individuals are considered to be in this stage if the new behavior is sustained over time, generally for 6 months or longer. The behavior may not be permanent as relapse may occur. When relapse occurs, the individual begins at an earlier stage and recycles

⊕ RESEARCH APPLICATION

Promoting Participation: Evaluation of a Health Promotion Program for Low-Income Seniors

Study Purpose

To evaluate a health promotion program for low-income seniors.

Methods

Qualitative study methods were used to examine the 10-month Seniors ALIVE program, a health promotion program for older adults living in senior housing. The program was evaluated on program participation, program impacts, and program outcomes using Pender's Health Promotion Model as a framework. Twenty-three of the 90 low-income seniors aged 61 to 90 years agreed to participate in the program evaluation. Data were collected from semistructured interviews. Content analysis was used to analyze the data for consistencies and meanings.

Findings

Factors that influenced participation were perceived benefits, encouragement by others, a positive social atmosphere, and having fun. Barriers were other priorities, deteriorating health, and forgetting to come. Self-efficacy

and past exercise behavior were important to participation in physical activity. Program impacts were both positive and negative. The positive impacts were feeling better, having more strength, being more flexible, and so on. There were also positive and negative social interactions mentioned by the participants.

Implications

This study demonstrated how Pender's Health Promotion Model could be used to frame feedback from older adults about a health promotion program. Pender's model can also be used as a framework to encourage participation in health promotion activities, emphasizing, for example, the benefits of reducing barriers and creating an environment that is fun and provides positive social interactions.

Reference

Buijs, R., Ross-Kerr, J., Cousins, S. O., & Wilson, D. (2003). Promoting participation: Evaluation of a health promotion program for low-income seniors. *Journal of Community Health Nursing, 20,* 93–107.

⊕ RESEARCH APPLICATION

Comparison of Tailored Interventions to Increase Mammography Screening in Nonadherent Older Women

Study Purpose

To determine the efficacy of different combinations of health care provider recommendations and in-person or telephone counseling interventions on mammography adherence at 2, 4, and 6 months postintervention.

Methods

The experimental, randomized, prospective study of 773 women was conducted over 4 years. The women were from a large HMO and were nonadherent to having had a mammogram in the last 15 months and did not have a history of breast cancer. The study used the Health Belief Model and Transtheoretical Model to tailor an intervention aimed at increasing mammography adherence. If the woman was in the precontemplation stage, counseling emphasized susceptibility to breast cancer and benefits of mammography screening. Women in the contemplation stage were counseled based on barriers identified by the individual women.

Findings

Mammography adherence increased significantly relative to usual care. All of the intervention delivery methods were successful in increasing mammography screening. Women in the precontemplation stage increased their adherence from 13% to over 30%, and women in the contemplation stage increased their adherence from 50% to 70% during the 6 months.

Implications

Public health nurses should assess a woman's readiness to be screened for breast cancer and discuss the woman's susceptibility to breast cancer and benefits of screening as well as barriers to carrying out the activity to increase adherence.

Reference

Champion, V., Maraj, M., Hui, S., Perkins, A. J., Tierney, W., Menon, U., et al. (2003). Comparison of tailored interventions to increase mammography screening in nonadherent older women. *Preventive Medicine, 36,* 150–158.

---

through to the maintenance stage again. Relapses can offer learning experiences, which can be used to eventually complete and terminate the cycle.

The TTM also offers three constructs hypothesized to influence behavior change: processes of change, self-efficacy, and decisional balance. Processes of change are strategies people use to modify their thoughts, feelings, and environment in order to change their behavior (i.e., move to the next stage). Self-efficacy is a person's belief that he or she can accomplish a behavior or behavioral goal (Bandura, 1977). Decisional balance (Janis & Mann, 1977) is a schema people use to monitor the pros (gains or positive aspects) and cons (losses or negative aspects) resulting from any decision. A behavior will not be initiated or continued unless there is an expectation of pros exceeding cons. Researchers have found that pros and cons are an excellent indicator of a

person's progress from precontemplation to contemplation and preparation (Ma et al., 2002; Marshall & Biddle, 2001; Prochaska et al., 1994). Individuals who are in the precontemplation and contemplation stages of behavior change could best be helped by professionals emphasizing the benefits of the behavior and assisting the person to reduce or eliminate any negative barriers or perceptions about the behavior. Public health nurses have used the TTM as a framework for assessment, planning, and interventions relevant to behaviors such as using a condom (Gullette & Turner, 2004), eating a low-fat diet (Frenn, Malin, & Bansal, 2003), promoting physical activity (Clement et al., 2004), pursuing smoking cessation (Macnee & McCabe, 2004), screening for sexually transmitted diseases (Chacko, von Sternberg, & Velasquez, 2004), and preventing violence (Anderson, 2003).

Ecological Models

Some of the most successful paths to behavior change consider the interaction of the people and their environment. The ecologic perspective places people in their primary social context and observes their interaction with other important factors influencing their health-related behaviors. The social context with the most immediate effects on behavior, and with the greatest implications for intervention, is the family and other significant others. The ecologic perspective also emphasizes the importance of organizations, communities, and society as a whole. Ecological models consider the interaction between people and intrapersonal, socio-cultural, policy, and physical-environmental factors (Sallis & Owen, 2002).

Social Cognitive Theory

A tenet of Social Cognitive Theory (SCT) is that the person, environmental factors, and the behavior interact dynamically and simultaneously in triadic reciprocal determinism not only to determine the behavior but also to affect the person and environment in which the behavior occurs (Bandura, 1986). In this relationship, a person's perceptions as well as the environment can influence his or her behavior, and a person's behavior can influence perceptions about the behavior as well as how to manipulate the environment to carry out the behavior. According to SCT, behavior is a function of outcome expectations, outcome expectancies, and self-efficacy expectations. A person's outcome expectations are a belief that a particular behavior will lead to certain outcomes. When individuals expect certain things to happen when they attempt to carry out the behavior, they can develop and try strategies for dealing with any of the situations that may occur.

Outcome expectancies, or values that a person places on behavioral outcomes, can be positive or negative and can be quantified in magnitude (Bandura, 1986). Thus, a person will be more likely to carry out a behavior when the person believes the behavior maximizes positive outcomes and minimizes negative outcomes.

Bandura (1977) was the first behavioralist to introduce the notion of self-efficacy expectations. Self-efficacy expectations are a judgment about one's capability of successfully executing a particular behavior to produce the expected outcomes (Bandura, 1986). Self-efficacy expectations are developed from four sources of information: (1) enactive attainment or past performance accomplishments, (2) vicarious experiences or observing others performing the behavior in similar situations, (3) verbal persuasion or hearing about the behavior from others, and (4) physiological or emotional arousal (Bandura, 1986).

Public health nurses have used SCT as a framework for assessing interventions to modify behaviors. For example, SCT has been used with encouraging mothers to breastfeed infants (Blyth et al., 2002), promoting physical activity among older adults (Allison & Keller, 2004; Conn et al. 2003), promoting hearing protection among workers (Eakin, Brady, & Lusk, 2001), promoting healthy behaviors among adolescents (Montgomery, 2002), and teaching older adults the safe use of over-the-counter medications (Neafsey et al., 2001).

Ecological Model of Health Behavior

The Ecological Model of Health Behavior (EMHB), described by McLeroy et al. (1988), is a multilevel approach that posits five system levels—intrapersonal, interpersonal, organizational, community, and public policy. The intrapersonal level includes the following factors: self-efficacy, self-esteem, and perceived susceptibility. At the interpersonal level, factors include social-psychological variables such as social norms and social support. Organizational level factors include larger models of organizational development to promote or prevent effective or efficient goal attainment. At the community level, the model draws on community organization and development theories, including values, cultural norms, and cultural practices. Finally, the model at the public policy level describes public policy influence on socioeconomic status, poverty, human rights, and social justice. The ecological model includes an immense variety of variables that have been found to affect health behavior.

An example of an ecological approach to health behavior is the case of smoking cessation. Working with the Centers for Disease Control and Prevention (CDC, 1999), public health nurses are currently involved with other health professionals and policy makers to control tobacco use in the United States. The Tobacco Control Program (CDC, 1999) is an extensive multilevel effort targeting individual behavior, societal norms, policy initiatives, and changes in the environment that forbid smoking, decrease cigarette availability, offer financial incentives to those who do not smoke, and so on. It is likely that public health nurses are currently involved in multilevel, ecological efforts to control obesity, increase

⊕ POLICY HIGHLIGHT

Teenage Smoking Prevention

Statewide comprehensive tobacco control programs to reduce teenage smoking focus on behavior change at the population level through a variety of ecological strategies. These strategies involve public education, policies to prevent youth access to tobacco and restrict tobacco advertising, community initiatives for training and assistance to health professionals, school-based programs, and direct cessation services such as quit smoking hotlines. A review of five statewide comprehensive tobacco control programs in the United States was conducted to determine the effectiveness of these tobacco control programs in reducing teenage smoking (Wakefield & Chaloupka, 2000). The review revealed that community-wide sustained ecological programs aimed at teenage smoking are effective in reducing teenage smoking. Funding for mass media campaigns, community and school smoking prevention programs, smoke-free indoor environments, and price increases on tobacco are critical factors in teenage smoking prevention.

physical activity, improve diets, and encourage other healthy people behavioral targets.

Other Ecological Frameworks

Other ecologic frameworks for integrating individual, social, and environmental factors to effect health-promoting behaviors are the Integrative Model for Community Health Promotion (IMCHP; Laffrey & Kolbok, 1999) and the Structural Model of Health Behavior (SMHB; Cohen, Scribner, & Farley, 2000). The IMCHP was developed to assist public health nurses to plan multilevel, holistic interventions for individuals, families, aggregates, or communities (see Figure 13-2). The model depicts three foci of care: illness/disease preven-

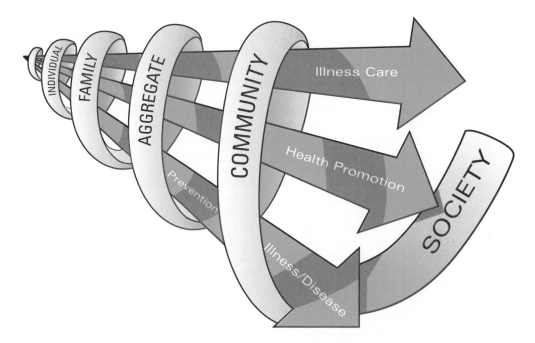

Figure 13-2 Integrative model for community health promotion.

From Laffrey & Kulbok, *Journal of Holistic Nursing* (17, 1) pp. 88–103, ©1999 by Sage Publications, Reprinted by permission of Sage Publications.

tion, health promotion, and illness care. Health promotion is at the core of the model to emphasize that all of the public health nurse's interventions are directed toward optimizing health potential. The other two foci of care—illness/disease prevention and illness care—are encompassed by health promotion efforts. The model also shows client systems including the individual, family, aggregate, and community. The systems are continuous from individual-as-client to community-as-client. Interventions can be directed toward any of the levels within the client system.

The SMHB includes four factors that influence the health at the population level and may complement each other in their impact on health. The four factors include: (a) availability/accessibility of consumer products, (b) physical structures, (c) social structures and policies, and (d) media and cultural messages. Availability or accessibility of consumer products can influence health outcomes positively (e.g., fruits and vegetables, condoms) or negatively (e.g., tobacco products, high-fat foods). Physical structures are those tangible objects that reduce or increase opportunities for healthy behaviors or outcomes. For example, well-lit neighborhoods diminish injury from violent crimes; attractive neighborhood parks promote opportunities for physical activity. Social structures pertain to laws and policies that direct or prohibit behaviors. Laws such as seat-belt and infant-seat use influence behaviors directly, while policies that promote youth after-school activities influence behaviors indirectly by providing alternatives to violence, drug use, or other crimes and creating a new social norm for teens. Media and cultural messages are those that affect social norms and individual attitudes and values in ways that positively or negatively impact health behaviors. These structural factors make important contributions to the health behaviors of communities and populations. Public health nurses can join with other health promotion professionals to address structural factors and thereby provide a means to focus on conditions that are health promoting at the community level.

There are many more models that can be useful to public health nurses to help them understand individual and community health behaviors (see, for example, DiClemente, Crosby, & Kegler, 2002, and Glanz, Rimer, & Lewis, 2002). Public health nurses can examine models of behavior to help them understand behavior as well as ways to address interventions to promote healthy behaviors or extinguish unhealthy behaviors. The health promotion professional can advance peoples'

readiness to change by making them more aware of the benefits of adopting a healthy behavior or discontinuing a health risk behavior. Health risk appraisals, blood chemistry screening, dietary assessments, fitness assessments, and other risk factor assessments can be used to show the client the consequences of the behavior relevant to chronic conditions. Awareness can also be elevated with written materials and media campaigns.

Promoting self-efficacy has very positive results in promoting healthy behaviors. Public health nurses can offer verbal persuasion or model a positive health behavior. When the client performs the behavior, praise and positive feedback on the behavior will reward the client and enhance the client's confidence to perform the behavior again. Self-efficacy can also be enhanced when the client is assisted with identifying a set of strategies to overcome any barriers or adverse conditions that could negatively affect performing the behavior. Support groups also can be helpful as individuals can learn of ways from others who have been successful in changing behavior in a positive way to overcome any personal or environmental barriers.

FOCUS ON POPULATION HEALTH

The health promotion strategies oriented to individuals and groups previously discussed may be relevant for population health promotion programs. Populations are comprised of individuals, families, and groups of individuals, so population health promotion efforts include behavior change at the individual level. At the population level, the emphasis is on lowering the average risk of all individuals in the community. There are many approaches for influencing a population's behavior change. This section will discuss three approaches: a framework for health communication programs (USDHHS, 2002), the PRECEDE-PROCEED model (Green & Krueter, 1999), and social marketing (Andreasen, 1995; Kotler, Roberto, & Lee, 2002).

Making Health Communication Programs Work

The National Cancer Institute (USDHHS, 2002) developed a systematic framework for public health nurses and other health promotion specialists to use to create health education messages and programs. (See Figure 13-3.) This framework has been widely used for promoting public health via health communication programs since it first appeared in 1989. Health communication programs are developed in collaboration with other disciplines and can be used with individuals, groups, communities, and the population as a whole. The four stages in the Health Communication Program Cycle resemble the nursing process and include the following circular process: (a) planning and strategy development; (b) developing and pretesting concepts, messages, and materials; (c) implementing the program; and (d) assessing the effectiveness and making refinements. In each of the four stages, the needs and perceptions of the intended audience are essential to guide the process. It must be remembered that needs and perceptions can change as behavior changes, so it is imperative that these changes be addressed as the program is planned, implemented, evaluated, and refined.

Stage 1

The planning and strategy development stage is used to identify a health problem and identify how health communication can effectively address the problem. The intended audience or people who have the health need is identified, and based on consumer research or assess-

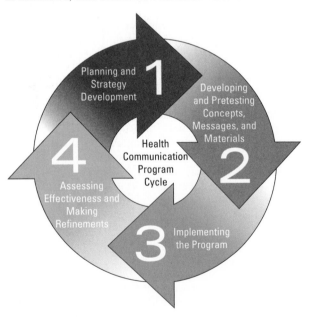

Figure 13-3 Framework for developing health communications.
From *Making Health Communication Programs Work*, by National Cancer Institute, NIH 2002, p. 11.

ment, objectives and a communication strategy are developed. A plan is articulated that includes specific activities, community partnerships, and baseline assessments for outcome evaluation. The following planning guide is a brief outline of *Making Health Communication Programs Work* (USDHHS, 2002).

Planning Steps: Assess the health issue or problem and identify all the components of a possible solution (e.g., communication as well as changes in policy, products, or services).

1. Define communication objectives.
2. Define and learn about intended audiences.
3. Explore settings, channels, and activities best suited to reach intended audiences. A channel refers to how the nurse will reach the audiences, such as via churches, community organizations, or special community programs.
4. Identify potential partners and develop partnering plans.
5. Develop a communication strategy for each intended audience; draft a communication plan.

Questions to Ask:

⊕ What health problem are we addressing?
⊕ What is occurring versus what should be occurring?
⊕ Whom does the problem affect and how?
⊕ What role can communication play in addressing the problem?
⊕ How and by whom is the problem being addressed? Are other communication programs being planned or implemented?
⊕ What approach or combination of approaches can best influence the problem? (Communication? Changes in policies, products, or services? All of these?)
⊕ What other organizations have similar goals and might be willing to work on this problem?
⊕ What measurable, reasonable objectives will we use to define success?
⊕ What types of partnerships would help achieve the objectives?
⊕ Who are our intended audiences? How will we learn about them?

⊕ What actions should we encourage our intended audiences to take?

⊕ What settings, channels, and activities are most appropriate for reaching our intended audiences and the goals of our communication objectives? (Interpersonal, organizational, mass, or computer-related media? Community? A combination?)

⊕ How can the channels be used most effectively?

⊕ How will we measure progress? What baseline information will we use to conduct our outcome evaluation?

Stage 2

Developing and pretesting concepts, messages, and materials includes the development of meaningful messages, drafted materials needed for the planned activities, and pretesting the messages and materials to assure their acceptability and effectiveness with the intended audience. The public health nurse and colleagues can draft or select materials and then test them with members from the audience for feedback.

Planning Steps:

1. Review existing materials.
2. Develop and test message concepts.
3. Decide what materials to develop.
4. Develop messages and materials.
5. Pretest messages and materials.

Questions to Ask:

⊕ What materials will fit our strategy, appeal to our intended audience, and adequately convey our message? How can we make the materials as effective as possible?

⊕ Do we need to create new materials? What types?

⊕ How do we develop culturally appropriate messages and materials?

⊕ How do we develop effective materials for low-literacy intended audiences?

⊕ How can we make sure the materials will be used?

⊕ When and how should we pretest our materials?

⊕ How can we keep pretesting costs down?

⊕ What should we do with pretest results?

⊕ How can we get the best results from creative and research professionals? From reviewers?

Stage 3

Implementing the program involves presenting the program through all channels of communication by distributing educational materials and other activities. Process evaluation assesses and documents the components of the health education program and includes distributing materials to the right people, determining whether program activities are occurring as intended, and evaluating other considerations of program integrity and fidelity. Process evaluation is essential at this stage to track intended audience exposure and reaction to the program and determine whether adjustments to the program activities are needed. If adjustments are needed, the program components are revised according to the evaluation.

Planning Steps:

1. Prepare to launch and implement your program.
2. Hold a press conference.
3. Maintain media relations after the launch.
4. Work with the media during a crisis.
5. Manage implementation: monitoring and problem solving.
6. Maintain partnerships.

Questions to Ask:

⊕ How should we launch the program?

⊕ Should we use a kickoff event?

⊕ How should we develop and sustain media coverage, partner involvement, and audience interest?

⊕ How should we manage a press conference?

⊕ How should we work with the media during a crisis?

⊕ How can we ensure that our program operates according to plan?

⊕ How can we use process evaluation?

⊕ How can we find out whether we are reaching the intended audience with our information?

⊕ How can we find out whether they are responding favorably to our message and materials?

⊕ Are we maintaining good relationships with our partners?

Stage 4

Assessing the effectiveness and making refinements is the outcome evaluation planned for in Stage 1. Outcome evaluation assesses the extent to which a program achieved its objectives. Effectiveness of the program is evaluated and refinements are made that would increase effectiveness of future programs. The stages are connected in a circle because program planning is a recurring process.

Planning Steps:

1. Determine what information the evaluation must provide.
2. Define the data to collect.
3. Decide on data collection methods.
4. Develop and pretest data collection instruments.
5. Collect data.
6. Process data.
7. Analyze data to answer the evaluation questions.
8. Write an evaluation report.
9. Disseminate the evaluation report.

Questions to Ask:

⊕ How can we use outcome evaluation to assess the effectiveness of our program?

⊕ How do we decide what outcome evaluation methods to use?

⊕ How should we use our evaluation results?

⊕ How can we determine to what degree we have achieved our communication objectives?

⊕ How can we make our communication program more effective?

PRECEDE-PROCEED Model

The PRECEDE-PROCEED Model is a nine-step assessment and planning framework for health education and health promotion interventions (see Figure 13-4). The acronym PRECEDE stands for Predisposing, Reinforcing, and Enabling factors in Educational/Environmental Diagnosis and Evaluation. The acronym PROCEED stands for Policy, Regulatory, and Organization factors for Education and Environmental Development. The two parts of the model work in tandem to provide a continuous series of steps in planning, implementing, and evaluating the health promotion process of a community (Green & Krueter, 1999). The PRECEDE framework (moving from right to left in the upper half of the model) examines factors that determine health status and provides information for targeting the intervention and developing objectives and criteria for evaluating the program. The PROCEED framework (moving from left to right in the lower half of the model) provides steps for developing policy and implementing and evaluating the program. Because the approach is systematic, interventions can be more efficiently and effectively delivered based on influencing factors and characteristics of the preferred population.

The PRECEDE-PROCEED Model has been extensively applied, and the utility of the model has been demonstrated in over 900 empirical studies (Green, 2005). The Centers for Disease Control and Prevention (CDC, 1987; Parcel, 1987) have advocated the model and supported its application. Examples of health problems where the model has been applied are HIV/AIDS (Alteneder et al., 1992; Bolan, 1986; Deren et al., 2003; Kocken et al., 2001; McCoy, Dodds, & Nolan, 1990; Walter & Vaughn, 1993), cancer (Brouse et al., 2004; Buller et al., 1998; Canto, Drury, & Horowitz, 2001; Coleman et al., 2003; Glanz, Carbone, & Song, 1999; Maxwell, Bastani, & Warda, 1997; Wismer et al., 2001), and heart disease (Bailey et al., 1994; Carlaw et al., 1984; Green, Frankish, & Wharf-Higgins, 1993; Leviton et al., 1999; Naylor et al., 2002; Taylor, Elliott, & Riley, 1998). Because the model is comprehensive, often only specific aspects of the model are empirically evaluated. For example, Chang et al. (2003) successfully applied the PRECEDE portion of the model to develop an instrument to measure predisposing, enabling, and reinforcing factors affecting food selection. Veenendaal, Grinspun, and Adriaanse (1996) applied Phase 4, behavioral and organizational assessment, to examine the educational needs of stroke survivors and their families.

Social Marketing

The term social marketing was coined by Kotler and Zaltman (1971) who discussed the application of commercial marketing principles and techniques to promote socially relevant behaviors. Social marketing is a multistage process using marketing strategies to create a competitive advantage for changing behavior in populations (Black & Blue, 2004). The process includes three concepts: (a) audience segmentation, (b) marketing

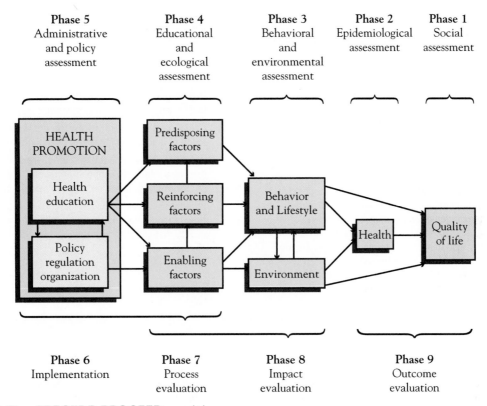

Figure 13-4 The PRECEDE-PROCEED model

From *Health Promotion Planning: An Educational and Ecological Approach*, 3rd ed., by L. W. Green & M. W. Kreuter 1999, p. 35. ©1999 by McGraw-Hill.

4 Ps, and (c) marketing mix. Audience segmentation involves subdividing a population into similar segments or "preferred audiences." Because different preferred audiences have different needs and wants, it is essential to assess each segment on a variety of factors to assist with developing strategies that appeal uniquely to a particular segment. Although a variety of strategies that appeal uniquely to multiple segments of the population could be developed, ideally one segment is chosen for the campaign. Segmentation can be based on demographic variables such as age, gender, marital status, income, race, or education, or a population can be segmented based on geographic areas such as states, counties, cities, neighborhoods, places of work, or schools. Segmentation also could divide a population based on psychological or behavioral similarities such as self-esteem levels or readiness to change behavior. In

reality, social marketers usually use many variables to segment a population rather than using just one variable. Perhaps one variable such as age will be used in an initial segmentation and then age groups will be further segmented based on other variables. This strategy of segmentation results in smaller, better defined target groups that have rich, unique, but more homogeneous profiles. Finally, segmentation could result in a number of segments that cannot possibly be reached within budget limits, necessitating eliminating segments from the program plan. Measures used to make decisions about targeted segments include (a) the greatest need, (b) most ready for behavior change, (c) easiest to reach, and (d) best match considering organizational mission, expertise, and resources (Kotler, Roberto, & Lee, 2002). The final point in the planning process is to develop program objectives and then further assess the target audience

⊕ PRACTICE APPLICATION

Lead Poisoning Prevention

Jenny, a public health nurse working for the city health department, noted a high prevalence of lead-poisoning among low-income toddlers. To assess the diffusion of information to parents of toddlers about lead-poisoning prevention, Jenny invited parents from a lead-testing clinic to five focus group sessions to explore their knowledge regarding sources of lead poisoning and their preference for receiving lead-poisoning prevention information. Most of the parents revealed that they had obtained lead-poisoning prevention information, but only 14% reported receiving a reminder to have their child's blood lead level tested. Jenny also found that brochures and a personal discussion with a health care provider when they used the Women, Infants, and Children (WIC) supplemental nutrition program were the preferred methods of obtaining lead-poisoning prevention information.

⊕ How can Jenny use this information to improve lead-level screening of low-income toddlers?

⊕ Can Jenny use this information to decrease the prevalence of lead poisoning in the community?

⊕ What should be included in a brochure that provides lead-poisoning prevention information? What other considerations should be made in developing the brochure?

⊕ How could Jenny ensure that health care providers at WIC discuss lead-poisoning prevention with their clients?

for even deeper understanding of them in terms of benefits of their current behavior and costs to their current behavior if they were to make a behavior change.

The benefits and costs can be assessed using the four Ps of marketing. The marketing 4 Ps are product, price, place, and promotion. In social marketing, the product is the behavior change and the associated benefits of the behavior we are "selling" as well as tangible objects and services that are provided as part of a campaign (Kotler, Roberto, & Lee, 2002). For example, a campaign may be aimed at increasing women's physical activity levels. The desired behavior or "actual product" is an increase in physical activity, the associated benefits or "core product" is weight loss and generally feeling better, and the "augmented products" are a tangible object of the campaign such as a free pedometer to keep track of activity and a service such as free babysitting at a local YWCA. Decisions about the product and planning are made with information from the target audience about how they think and feel about the behavior and product.

The price of social marketing is the cost that the target market associates with adopting the new behavior and perhaps extinguishing an unwanted behavior (Kotler, Roberto, & Lee, 2002). These costs can be monetary, those most often associated with tangible objects or services, or nonmonetary. Nonmonetary costs may include time, effort, and energy needed to adopt the behavior. Psychological risks and losses as well as physical discomforts are also nonmonetary costs of adopting a new behavior. For the social marketer, the benefits of the new behavior must outweigh or at least be equal to the costs to have a competitive pricing objective. Therefore, the social marketer must develop strategies that will "balance the scale" either by increasing the benefits of the behavior, decreasing the costs, or a combination of both (Kotler, Roberto, & Lee, 2002).

Place is when and where the new behavior will occur or where the client will acquire any tangible objects or receive any services associated with the behavior (Kotler, Roberto, & Lee, 2002). Place can include both personal and nonpersonal strategies. Personal strategies may include number and location of places to carry out the behavior, moving locations closer to the target audience, or providing units that are mobile and come to work sites or neighborhoods. A "place" may have a more appealing ambience or include extended hours of service or be offered via the phone, mail, or online; it can also be an offer of free parking or a reduced wait-time to be more attractive to the targeted audience. The social marketer must make the desired behavior appear more appealing and be more convenient than the competing behavior at the point of decision making while selecting the most efficient and cost-effective options.

Promotion is the created message that will persuade the target audience that the product is greater than the price (Kotler, Roberto, & Lee, 2002). Promotion involves selecting (a) the content or "best words" or images to use; (b) the benefits to highlight; (c) the communication channels such as mass communication, selective communication, or personal communication to use; (d) a spokesperson who is credible and appealing to the target audience; and (e) the timing, duration, and frequency of the campaign to sell the product (Black & Blue, 2004).

The marketing mix is the blend of strategies (4 Ps) that will be integrated in a campaign that will appeal to the preferred audience (Kotler, Roberto, & Lee, 2002). The marketing mix is essential to produce the desired behavior in the target audience. Table 13-1 shows a social marketing plan outline from beginning to program management using the marketing mix.

Social marketing is appealing to public health professionals because it is based on successful commercial marketing strategies and has shown the same success in marketing healthy behaviors. Social marketing uses a grassroots, "bottom-up" process with the program being informed by the preferred audience rather than a "top-down" approach where health professionals make the decisions about the needs and wants of the target audience (Black & Blue, 2004). Insights into the needs and wants of the target audience can only be known through extensive assessment and feedback from them. This thorough assessment approach is paying off in the success social marketing is having in changing behaviors.

ETHICAL ISSUES IN HEALTH PROMOTION

The study of ethics enables public health nurses and other health care professionals involved with health promotion of individuals, families, groups, and communities to make professional decisions based on basic principles that reflect the values and morals of a society and of the profession. Ethics that govern professional conduct typically center on five principles: (a) attaining personal freedom or autonomy, (b) doing good, (c)

avoiding harm, (d) preserving justice, and (e) adopting professional accountability. At first glance, it seems reasonable to promote education and practice of positive health behavior, a clean environment, and methods to prevent illness and injury. However, questions begin to arise about individual rights and whether health education and health promotion activities are morally, ethically, and legally appropriate in a society. Is it ethical and just to pressure individuals to change their behavior to promote their health or the health of the population? Sciacca, Dennis, and Black (2004) question the ethics of trying to change a person's behavior when the person is informed about the benefits of the new behavior and risks of the current behavior, has the skills and self-efficacy, and yet chooses not to change. For example, should overweight persons be forced to participate in weight reduction programs to maintain their health insurance? Should parents of public school children be required to have their children immunized against childhood diseases? What are the appropriate limits in regulating, promoting, or preventing behaviors that lead to premature morbidity and mortality? How much shaping, molding, and influencing of needs, wants, and behaviors of people can we realize to protect the public's health? Certainly, the 1979 Surgeon General's report *Healthy People* urging citizens to give up their pleasurable but damaging habits stirred up controversy about what role the government should play in individual behavioral rights.

The right of self-direction and self-determination of the individual is a major tenet of professional nursing practice (ANA, 2001). Nurses embrace the widely known principles of health care ethics including respect for autonomy, beneficence, non-maleficence, and concern for justice (Beauchamp & Childress, 2001). Autonomy is valued in situations where the behavior is not a threat to the health and welfare of others. John Stuart Mill (1869) in his essay "On Liberty" discusses paternalism as an attempt to impose limitations upon others for his or her own good and as being justified with children and those with cognitive limitations because they are not capable of deciding on their own behalf and when one acts in a way that may pose harm to others. This "harm principle" asserts "your freedom to swing your arm ends where my nose begins." Although we value autonomy as a nation and as a profession, this principle can create an ethical dilemma surrounding the promotion of behavior change at the individual

TABLE 13-1: Social Marketing Plan Outline

WHERE ARE WE?

Social Marketing Environment

Step 1:	Determine program focus	
	Identify campaign purpose	
	Conduct an analysis of Strengths, Weaknesses, Opportunities, and Threats (SWOT)	
	Review past and similar efforts	

WHERE DO WE WANT TO GO?

Target Audiences,
Objectives, and Goals

Step 2:	Select target audiences	
Step 3:	Set objectives and goals	
Step 4:	Analyze target audiences and the competition	

HOW WILL WE GET THERE?
Social Marketing Strategies

Step 5:	Product:	Design the market offering
	Price:	Manage costs of behavior change
	Place:	Make the product available
	Promotion:	Create messages Choose media (communication) channels

HOW WILL WE STAY ON COURSE?

Social Marketing Program Management

Step 6:	Develop a plan for evaluation and monitoring	
Step 7:	Establish budgets and find funding sources	
Step 8:	Complete an implementation plan	

Note. From Kotler, P., Roberto, N., & Lee, N. *Social Marketing: Improving the Quality of Life* (2nd ed.). Copyright 2002 by Sage Publications, Inc. Reprinted by Permission of Sage, Inc.

or group level that ultimately has an impact on the health of a society (Cribb & Duncan, 2002).

When we plan a health promotion encounter, our goal is to support the individual or community to make them feel empowered to make their own behavioral or policy choices. However, issues of ethical concerns appear when health promoters are not absolutely sure that (1) the behavior change will result in "more

health," (2) there is value in encouraging the behavior change, and (3) it is known what to do to help people change their behavior (Cribb & Duncan, 2002). Based on these concerns, public health nurses need to explain and justify interventions and ensure that the Code of Ethics for Nurses (ANA, 2001) is followed in designing and implementing health promotion encounters. It is the ethical duty of public health nurses and other health professionals to provide sound information on which individuals, families, and communities can select their behaviors and lifestyles. However, we must be aware that people will not always choose the most health-promoting behaviors, and this is their right when their behaviors do not affect others (Sciacca, Dennis, & Black, 2004).

⊕ PRACTICE APPLICATION

Occupational Health

Robert is an occupational health nurse working for a large automobile plant. He notes a rise in insurance claims for diabetes and heart disease during the past 3 years. After examining risk assessments over the 3-year period, he concludes that workers have increased their body mass index at an alarming rate and that there is a correlation between weight increase and diabetes or heart disease. Robert asks you, a public health nurse in the city health department, to assist him in planning an intervention to reduce overweight and obesity in the work site.

⊕ What other assessments are needed for planning the intervention?

⊕ Choose a behavioral model and describe how you would use it to assist in planning an intervention.

⊕ Choose an ecological model and describe its usefulness in planning an intervention.

⊕ Describe the planning steps to help Robert alleviate this health promotion problem.

CRITICAL THINKING ACTIVITIES

1. What meaning does health have for you personally?

2. What does health promotion mean, beyond health maintenance and illness prevention?

3. How can public health nurses be involved with mass media to promote health of communities and populations?

4. Do you believe laws that mandate helmet use for motorcyclists are paternalistic measures that should not be used? Provide justification for your answer.

5. What are ethical issues that may arise from using social marketing to affect health behavior change?

KEY TERMS

activity-related affect	negative valence	social marketing
ecological models	outcome expectancies	triadic reciprocal determinism
health-promoting behavior	positive valence	value-expectancy theories
health promotion	self-efficacy	

KEY CONCEPTS

⊕ Health is a holistic concept encompassing physical, psychological, social, and spiritual dimensions of well-being on a continuum.

⊕ Health promotion is the process of enabling individuals, families, and communities to increase control over and to improve their own health.

⊕ Health promotion activities can include environmental measures, healthy public policies, health education programs, and preventive health services.

- Individuals and groups can be assisted in changing their behaviors by using models of behavior change to identify areas of intervention.

- The stages of the health communication process are comparable to the nursing process, beginning with planning and strategy development and ending with assessing the effectiveness of the program and making refinements.

- Marketing and ecological models can be used to design, implement, and evaluate community health promotion programs.

REFERENCES

Abood, D. A., Black, D. R., & Feral, D. (2003). Nutrition education worksite intervention for university staff: Application of the Health Belief Model. *Journal of Nutrition Education and Behavior, 35,* 260–267.

Ajzen, I. (1988). *Attitudes, personality, and behavior.* Chicago: Dorsey Press.

Ajzen, I., & Fishbein, M. (1980). *Understanding attitudes and predicting social behavior.* Englewood Cliffs, NJ: Prentice-Hall.

Allison, M. J., & Keller, C. (2004). Self-efficacy intervention effect on physical activity in older adults. *Western Journal of Nursing Research, 26*(1), 31–58.

Alteneder, R., Price, J. H., Telljohann, S., Didion, J., & Locher, A. (1992). Using the PRECEDE model to determine junior high school students' knowledge, attitudes, and beliefs about AIDS. *Journal of School Health 62*(10), 464–470.

American Nurses Association. (1973). *Standards of nursing practice.* Kansas City, MO: author.

American Nurses Association. (2001). *Code of ethics for nurses with interpretive statements.* Retrieved January, 2005, from http://www.nursingworld.org/ethics/code/protected_nwcoe303.htm.

Anderson, C. (2003). Evolving out of violence: An application of the Transtheoretical Model of behavior change. *Research and Theory in Nursing Practice, 17,* 225–240.

Andreasen, A. R. (1995). *Marketing social change: Changing behavior to promote health, social development, and the environment.* San Francisco: Jossey-Bass.

Bailey, P. H., Rukholm, E. E., Vanderlee, R., & Hyland, J. (1994). A Heart Health Survey at the worksite: The first step to effective programming. *American Association of Occupational Health Nursing Journal, 42,* 9–14.

Bandura, A. (1977). Self-efficacy: Toward a unifying theory of behavioral change. *Psychological Review, 84,* 191–215.

Bandura, A. (1986). *Social foundations of thought and action.* Englewood Cliffs, NJ: Prentice Hall.

Beauchamp, T. L., & Childress, J. F. (2001). *Principles of biomedical ethics.* New York: Oxford University Press.

Black, D. R., & Blue, C. L. (2004). Social marketing. *Encyclopedia of Health and Behavior* (pp. 759–764). Thousand Oaks, CA: Sage.

Blue, C. L., & Valley, J. (2002). Predictors of influenza vaccine acceptance among healthy adult workers. *AAOHN Journal, 50*(5), 227–233.

Blyth, R., Creedy, D. K., Dennis, C., Moyle, W., Pratt, J., & De Vries, S. M. (2002). Effect of maternal confidence on breastfeeding duration: An application of breastfeeding self-efficacy theory. *Birth, 29,* 278–284.

Bolan, R. K. (1986). Health education planning for AIDS risk reduction in the gay/bisexual male community: Use of the PRECEDE framework. American Public Health Association, 114th Annual Meeting Abstracts, Las Vegas, p. 162.

Brouse, C. H., Basch, C. E., Wolf, R. L., & Shmukler, C. (2004). Barriers to colorectal cancer screening: An educational diagnosis. *Journal of Cancer Education, 19,* 170–173.

Buijs, R., Ross-Kerr, J., Cousins, S. O., & Wilson, D. (2003). Promoting participation: Evaluation of a health promotion program for low income seniors. *Journal of Community Health Nursing, 20,* 93–107.

Buller, D., Modiano, M. R., Guernsey de Zapien, J., Meister, J., Saltzman, S., & Hunsaker, F. (1998). Predictors of cervical cancer screening in Mexican American women of reproductive age. *Journal of Health Care for the Poor and Underserved, 9,* 76–95.

Canto, M. T., Drury, T. F., & Horowitz, A. M. (2001). Maryland dentists' knowledge of oral cancer risk factors and diagnostic procedures. *Health Promotion Practice, 2,* 255–262.

Carlaw, R. W., Mittlemark, M., Bracht, N., & Luepker, R. (1984). Organization for a community cardiovascular health program: Experiences from the Minnesota Heart Health Program. *Health Education Quarterly, 11,* 243–252.

Centers for Disease Control (CDC). (1987). *Information/education plan to prevent and control AIDS in the United States.* Washington, D.C.: U.S. Public Health Service, Department of Health and Human Service.

Centers for Disease Control and Prevention (CDC). (1999). *Best practices for comprehensive tobacco control—August 1999*. Atlanta: Office on Smoking and Health.

Chacko, M. R., von Sternberg, K., & Velasquez, M. M. (2004). Gonorrhea and Chlamydia screening in sexually active young women: The processes of change. *Journal of Adolescent Health, 34,* 424–427.

Champion, V., Maraj, M., Hui, S., Perkins, A. J., Tierney, W., Menon, U., et al. (2003). Comparison of tailored interventions to increase mammography screening in nonadherent older women. *Preventive Medicine, 36,* 150–158.

Chang, M. W., Brown, R. L., Nitzke, S., & Coifu-Baumann, L. (2003). Development of an instrument to assess predisposing, enabling, and reinforcing constructs associated with fat intake behaviors of low-income mothers. *Journal of Nutrition Education and Behavior, 36,* 27–34.

Clement, J. M., Schmidt, C. A., Bernaix, L. W., Covington, N. K., & Carr, T. R. (2004). Obesity and physical activity in college women: Implications for clinical practice. *Journal of the American Academy of Nurse Practitioners, 16,* 291–299.

Cohen, D. A., Scribner, R. A., & Farley, T. A. (2000). A structural model of health behavior: A pragmatic approach to explain and influence health behaviors at the population level. *Preventive Medicine, 30*(2), 146–154.

Coleman, E., Lord, J., Heard, J., Coon, S., Cantrell, M., Mohrmann, C., & O'Sullivan, P. (2003). The Delta Project: Increasing breast cancer screening among rural minority and older women by targeting rural healthcare providers. *Oncology Nursing Forum, 30,* 669–677.

Conn, V. S., Burks, K. J., Pomeroy, S. L., & Cochran, J. E. (2003). Are there different predictors of distinct exercise components? *Rehabilitation Nursing, 28*(3), 87–91, 97, 100.

Conn, V. S., Tripp-Reimer, T., & Maas, M. L. (2003). Older women and exercise: Theory of planned behavior beliefs. *Public Health Nursing, 20*(2), 153–163.

Cribb, A., & Duncan, P. (2002). *Health promotion and professional ethics.* Malden, MA: Blackwell Publishing.

Deren, S., Kang, S. Y., Rapkin, B., Robles, R. R., Andia, J. F., & Colon, H. M. (2003). The utility of the PRECEDE Model in predicting HIV risk behaviors among Puerto Rican injection drug users. *AIDS & Behavior, 7,* 405–412.

DiClemente, R. J., Crosby, R. A., & Kegler, M. C. (Eds.). (2002). *Emerging theories in health promotion practice and research.* San Francisco: Jossey-Bass.

DiClemente, C. C., & Prochaska, J. O. (1985). Processes and stages of self-change: Coping and competence in smoking behavior change. In S. Shiffman & T. A. Wills (Eds.), *Coping and substance abuse* (pp. 319–343). New York: Academic Press.

Donaldson, S. K., & Crowley, D. M. (1978). The discipline of nursing. *Nursing Outlook, 26,* 113–120.

Drayton-Brooks, S., & White, N. (2004). Health promoting behaviors among African American women with faith-based support. *The ABNF Journal, 15* (5), 84–90.

Eakin, B. L., Brady, J. S., & Lusk, S. L. (2001). Creating a tailored, multimedia, computer-based intervention . . . purpose to increase factory workers' use of hearing protection devices. *Computers in Nursing, 19,* 152–163.

Frenn, M., Malin, S., & Bansal, N. K. (2003). Stage-based interventions for low-fat diet with middle school students. *Journal of Pediatric Nursing, 18* (1), 36–45.

Gantt, C. J. (2001). The theory of planned behavior and postpartum smoking relapse. *Journal of Nursing Scholarship, 33,* 337–341.

Glanz, K., Carbone, E., & Song, V. (1999). Formative research for developing targeted skin cancer prevention programs for children in multiethnic Hawaii. *Health Education Research, 14,* 155–166.

Glanz, K., Rimer, B. K., & Lewis, F. M. (2002). *Health behavior and health education* (3rd ed.). San Francisco, CA: Jossey-Bass.

Green, L. (2005). Published applications of the PRECEED-PROCEDE Model. Retrieved on March 28, 2005, from http://lgreen.net/precede%20apps/preapps.htm.

Green, L. W., & Kreuter, M. W. (1999). *Health promotion planning: An educational and ecological approach* (3rd ed.). Mountain View, CA: Mayfield.

Green, L. W., Frankish, C. J., & Wharf-Higgins, J. (1993). Scientific basis for cardiovascular disease prevention and heart health promotion policy: Psychosocial and community determinants. *Canadian Journal of Cardiology 9,* 50D–51D.

Gullette, D. L., & Turner, J. G. (2004). Stages of change and condom use among an internet sample of gay and bisexual men. *Journal of the Association of Nurses in AIDS Care, 15*(2), 27–37.

Hochbaum, G. M. (1958). *Public participation in medical screening programs: A sociopsychological study* (PHS Publication No. 572). Washington, DC: U.S. Government Printing Office.

Insel, P. M., & Roth, W. T. (2002). *Core concepts in health* (9th ed.). Boston: McGraw Hill.

Janis, I. L., & Mann, M. A. (1977). *Decision making: A psychological analysis of conflict, choice, and commitment.* New York: The Free Press.

Jemmott III, J. B., Jemmott, L. S., Hines, P. M., & Fong, G. T. (2001). The Theory of Planned Behavior as a model of intentions for fighting among African American and Latino Adolescents. *Maternal and Child Health Journal, 5,* 253–263.

Kotler, P., Roberto, N., & Lee, N. (2002). *Social marketing: Improving the quality of life* (2nd ed.). Thousand Oaks, CA: Sage.

Kotler, P., & Zaltman, G. (1971). Social marketing: An approach to planned change. *Journal of Marketing, 35* (3), 3–12.

Laffrey, S. C. (1985). Health promotion: Relevance for nursing. *Topics in Clinical Research, 7*(2), 29–38.

Laffrey, S. C., & Kulbok, P. A. (1999). An integrative model for holistic community health nursing. *Journal of Holistic Nursing, 17*(1), 88–103.

Lamanna, L. M. (2004). College students' knowledge and attitudes about cancer and perceived risks of developing skin cancer. *Dermatology Nursing, 16,* 161–176.

Leviton, L. C., Finnegan, J. R., Zapka, J. G., Meischke, H., Estabrook, B., Gilliland, J., Linares, A., Weitzman, E. R., Raczynski, J., & Stone, E. (1999). Formative research methods to understand patient and provider responses to heart attack symptoms. *Evaluation and Program Planning, 22,* 385–397.

Lewin, K. (1951). *Field theory in social science: Selected theoretical papers.* Chicago: University of Chicago Press.

Lewin, K. Dembo, T., Festinger, L., & Sears, P. S. (1944). Level of aspiration. In J. Hunt (Ed.), *Personality and behavior disorders.* New York: Ronald Press.

Ma, J., Betts, N. M., Horacek, T., Georgiou, C., White, A., & Nitzke, S. (2002). The importance of decisional balance and self-efficacy in relation to stages of change for fruit and vegetable intakes by young adults. *American Journal of Health Promotion, 16,* 157–166.

Macnee, C. L., & McCabe, S. (2004). The transtheoretical model of behavior change and smokers in southern Appalachia. *Nursing Research, 53,* 243–250.

Marshall, S. J., & Biddle, S. J. H. (2001). The transtheoretical model of behavior change: A meta-analysis of applications to physical activity and exercise. *Annals of Behavioral Medicine, 23,* 229–246.

Maxwell, A. E., Bastani, R., & Warda, U. S. (1997). Breast cancer screening and related attitudes among Filipino-American women. *Cancer, Epidemiology, Biomarkers & Prevention, 6,* 719–726.

McCoy, H. V., Dodds, S. E., & Nolan, C. (1990). AIDS intervention design for program evaluation: The Miami Community Outreach Project. *Journal of Drug Issues, 20,* 22–243.

McKenna, D., Faustini, Y., Nowakowski, J., & Wormser, G. P. (2004). Factors influencing the utilization of Lyme disease—Prevention behaviors in a high-risk population. *Journal of the American Academy of Nurse Practitioners, 16*(1), 24–30.

McLeroy, K. R., Bibeau, D., Steckler, A., & Glanz, K. (1988). An ecological perspective on health promotion programs. *Health Education Quarterly, 15,* 351–377.

Mill, J. S. (1869). *On liberty.* London: Longman, Roberts, & Green; Bartleby.com, 1999. Retrieved January, 2005, from http://www.bartleby.com/130/.

Montgomery, K. S. (2002). Health promotion with adolescents: Examining theoretical perspectives to guide research. *Research and Theory for Nursing Practice, 16,* 119–134.

Naylor, P. J., Wharf-Higgins, J., Blair, L., Green, L., & O'Connor, B. (2002). Evaluating the participatory process in a community-based heart health project. *Social Science & Medicine, 55,* 1173–1187.

Neafsey, P. J., Strickler, Z., Shellman, J., & Padula, A. T. (2001). Geropharmacology. Delivering health information about self-medication to older adults: Use of touchscreen-equipped notebook computers. *Journal of Gerontological Nursing, 27*(11), 19–27.

Newell-Withrow, C. (2000). Health protecting and health promoting behaviors of African Americans living in Appalachia. *Public Health Nursing, 17,* 392–397.

Nightingale, F. (1992). *Notes on nursing: What it is and what it is not.* Philadelphia: J. B. Lippincott Company. (Original work published 1859)

O'Boyle, C. A., Henly, S. J., & Larson, E. (2001). Understanding adherence to hand hygiene recommendations: The theory of planned behavior. *American Journal of Infection Control, 29,* 352–360.

Parcel, G. S. (1987). *Smoking control among women: A CDC community intervention handbook.* Atlanta: Centers for Disease Control, Center for Health Promotion and Education, Division of Health Education.

Pender, N. J. (1982). *Health promotion in nursing practice.* Norwalk, CT: Appleton-Century-Crofts.

Pender, N. J., Murdaugh, C. L., & Parsons, M. A. (2002). *Health promotion in nursing practice* (4th ed.). Upper Saddle River, NJ: Prentice Hall.

Pender, N., Walker, S., Sechrist, K., & Frank-Stromborg, M. (1990). Predicting health-promoting lifestyles in the workplace. *Nursing Research, 39,* 326–331.

Plowden, K. O. (2003). A theoretical approach to understanding black men's health-seeking behavior. *The Journal of Theory Construction & Testing, 7*(1), 27–31.

Prochaska, J. O., & DiClemente, C. C. (1992). Stages of change in the modification of problem behaviors. *Progress in Behavioral Modification, 28,* 183–214.

Prochaska, J. O., Redding, C. A., & Evers, K. E. (2002). The transtheoretical model and stages of change. In K. Glanz, B. K. Rimer, & F. M. Lewis (Eds.), *Health behavior and health education* (3rd ed., pp. 99–120). San Francisco: Jossey-Bass.

Prochaska, J. O., Velicer, W. F., Rossi, J. S., Goldstein, M. G., Marcus, B. H., Rakowski, W., et al. (1994). Stages of change and decisional balance for 12 problem behaviors. *Health Psychology 13,* 39–46.

Rempel, L. A. (2004). Factors influencing the breastfeeding decisions of long-term breastfeeders. *Journal of Human Lactation, 20,* 306–318.

Rosenstock, I. (1966). Why people use health service. *Milbank Memorial Fund Quarterly, 44,* 94–123.

Rosenstock, I. M., Strecher, V. J., & Becker, M. H. (1988). Social learning theory and the health belief model. *Health Education Quarterly, 15*(2), 175–183.

Sallis, J. F., & Owen, N. (2002). Ecological models of health behavior. In K. Glanz, B. K. Rimer, & F. M. Lewis (Eds.). *Health behavior and health education: Theory, research, and practice* (3rd ed., pp. 462–484). San Francisco: Jossey-Bass.

Sciacca, J. P., Dennis, D. L., & Black, D. R. (2004). Are interventions for informed, efficacious pre-contemplators ethical? *American Journal of Health Education, 35,* 322–327.

Sedlak, C. A., Doheny, M. O., & Jones, S. L. (2000). Osteoporosis education programs: Changing knowledge and behaviors. *Public Health Nursing, 17,* 398–402.

Smith, J. (1981). The idea of health: A philosophical inquiry. *Advances in Nursing Science, 3*(3), 43–50.

Taylor, S. M., Elliott, S., & Riley, B. (1998). Heart health promotion: Predisposition, capacity and implementation in Ontario public health units, 1994–96. *Canadian Journal of Public Health, 89*(6), 410–414.

U.S. Department of Health and Human Services. (2000). *Healthy people 2010* (2nd ed.). With understanding and improving health and objectives for improving health, 2 vols. Washington, DC: U.S. Government Printing Office.

U. S. Department of Health and Human Services. (2002). *Making health communication programs work* (NIH Publication No. 02-5145). Bethesda, MD: National Cancer Institute, National Institutes of Health.

U. S. Public Health Service. (1979). *Healthy people: Surgeon general's report on health promotion and disease prevention.* (DHHS Publication No. 79-55071). Washington, DC: U.S. Government Printing Office.

U. S. Public Health Service. (1980). *Promoting health/preventing disease: Objectives or the nation (HE20.2:D63/4).* Washington, DC: U.S. Government Printing Office.

Veenendaal, H., Grinspun, D. R., & Adriaanse, H. P. (1996). Educational needs of stroke survivors and their family members, as perceived by themselves and by health professionals. *Patient Education and Counseling, 28,* 265–276.

Wakefield, M., & Chaloupka, F. (2000). Effectiveness of comprehensive tobacco control programmes in reducing teenage smoking in the USA. *Tobacco Control, 9,* 177–186.

Walker, S. N., Sechrist, K. R., & Pender, N. J. (1987). The health-promoting lifestyle profile: Development and psychometric characteristics. *Nursing Research, 36*(2), 76–81.

Walter, H. J., & Vaughan, R. D. (1993). AIDS risk reduction among a multiethnic sample of urban high-school students. *Journal of the American Medical Association, 270,* 725–730.

Wismer, B. A., Moskowitz, J. M., Min, K., Chen, A. M., Ahn, Y., Cho, S., Jun, S., Lew, A., Pak, Y. M., Wong, J. M., & Tager, I. B. (2001). Interim assessment of a community intervention to improve breast and cervical cancer screening among Korean American Women. *Journal of Public Health Management Practice, 7,* 61–70.

Wold, W. A., Dunkin, J., Idleman, L., & Jackson, C. (2004). CVD prevention strategies with urban and rural African American women. *Applied Nursing Research, 17,* 187–194.

World Health Organization. (1948). *Preamble to the Constitution of the World Health Organization as adopted by the International Health Conference,* New York, 19–22 June, 1946; signed on 22 July 1946 by the representatives of 61 States (Official Records of the World Health Organization, no. 2, p. 100) and entered into force on 7 April 1948.

World Health Organization. (1977, May). *Resolution WHA40.43–Technical cooperation.* Geneva: World Health Organization.

World Health Organization. (1986). *Ottawa Charter for Health Promotion.* Retrieved November 9, 2004, from http://search.yahoo.com/search?fr=slv1-&p=Ottawa+Charter+for+Health+Promotion.

World Health Organization. (1989). *Nursing leadership for health for all.* Geneva: World Health Organization Division of Health Manpower Development.

World Health Organization. (1998). *Health promotion glossary* (WHO/HPR/HEP/98.1). Geneva. Retrieved July, 2004, from www.who.int/hpr/NPH/docs/hp_glossary_en.pdf.

BIBLIOGRAPHY

Bernard, M. (2006). Health promotion/disease prevention to the rescue! Tempering the giant, geriatric tsunami. *Geriatrics, 61*(2), 5–6.

Butterfoss F. D. (2006). Process evaluation for community participation. *Annual Review of Public Health, 27,* 323–340.

Condon, L., Hek, G., & Harris, F. (2006). Public health, health promotion and the health of people in prison. *Community Practice, 79*(1), 19–22.

Cramer, M. E., Atwood, J. R., & Stoner, J. A. (2006). A conceptual model for understanding effective coalitions involved in health promotion programming. *Public Health Nursing, 23*(1), 67–73.

Evers, K. E. (2006). eHealth promotion: The use of the Internet for health promotion. *American Journal of Health Promotion, 20,* suppl., 1–7.

Green, L. W. (1999). *Health promotion planning: An educational and ecological approach* (3rd ed.). Boston: McGraw Hill.

Kickbusch I. (2006). Mapping the future of public health: Action on global health. *Canadian Journal of Public Health, 97*(1), 6–8.

Kline K. N. (2006). A decade of research on health content in the media: The focus on health challenges and sociocultural context and attendant informational and ideological problems. *Journal of Health Communications, 11*(1), 43–59.

Kreuter, M. W., Lezin, N. A., Kreuter, M. W., & Green, L. W. (2003). *Community health promotion ideas that work* (2nd ed.). Boston: Jones and Bartlett Publishers.

Naumanen, P. (2006). The health promotion of aging workers from the perspective of occupational health professionals. *Public Health Nursing, 23*(1), 37–45.

Porche, D. J. (2005). Men's health: Why is it important? Why should ANAC care? *The Journal of the Association of Nurses in AIDS Care, 16*(5), 1–2.

Tang, K. D., Beaglehole, R., & O'Byrne, D. (2005). Policy and partnership for health promotion—Addressing the determinants of health. *Bulletin of the World Health Organization, 83,* 884.

Ureda, J., & Yates, S. (2005). A systems view of health promotion. *Journal of Health and Human Services Administration, 28*(1), 5–38.

Valente, T. W. (2002). *Evaluating health promotion programs.* New York: Oxford University Press.

Whitehead, D. (2003). Evaluating health promotion: A model for nursing practice. *Journal of Advanced Nursing, 41,* 490–498.

Whitehead, D. (2004). Health promotion and health education: Advancing the concepts. *Journal of Advanced Nursing, 47,* 311–320.

Whitehead, D. (2006). The health-promoting school: What role for nursing? *Journal of Clinical Nursing, 15,* 264–271.

Young, L. E., & Hayes, V. E. (2002). *Transforming health promotion practice: Concepts, issues, and applications.* Philadelphia: F. A. Davis Company.

RESOURCES

Adult Literacy Estimates

Web: http://www.casas.org

The Web site provides literacy, education, race/ethnicity, English proficiency, and labor force statistics for any state, county, or city in the United States.

Agency for Healthcare Research and Quality (AHRQ)

Office of Communications and Knowledge Transfer
540 Gaither Road, Suite 2000
Rockville, Maryland 20850
301-427-1364
FAX: 301-594-3212
Email: info@ahrq.gov
Web: http://www.info.ahrq.gov

The mission of the AHRQ is to improve the quality, safety, efficiency, and effectiveness of health care for all Americans. The agency provides clinical and consumer health information, funding, data and surveys, research findings, quality and client safety information, and public health preparedness.

American Association of Occupational Health Nurses (AAOHN)

2920 Brandywine Road, Suite 100
Atlanta, Georgia 30341
770-455-7757
FAX: 770-455-7271
Email: aaohn@aaohn.org
Web: http://www.aaohn.org

The AAOHN, the largest group of health care professionals serving the workplace, has a mission to ensure occupational and environmental nurses are the authority on health, safety, productivity, and disability management for worker populations. AAOHN is a principal force in furthering the profession of occupational and environmental health nursing by advancing the profession, protecting the profession, guiding the profession, and promoting the profession.

American Association of Retired Persons (AARP)

601 E Street NW
Washington, D.C. 20049
202-424-3410
Web: http://www.aarp.org

The AARP, a nonprofit, nonpartisan membership organization for people age 50 and over, is dedicated to enhancing quality of life for all as we age. AARP leads positive social change and deliver value to members through information, advocacy and service.

American Diabetes Association (ADA)

1710 North Beauregard Street
Alexandria, Virginia 22311
703-439-1500; 1-800-DIABETE
FAX: 703-549-1715
Email: customerservice@diabetes.org
Web: http://www.diabetes.org

The mission of the ADA is to prevent and cure diabetes and to improve the lives of all people affected by diabetes. The

ADA is a source for health promotion programs to prevent diabetes, programs to promote health for people living with diabetes, and research and clinical information.

American Heart Association (AHA)

7272 Greenville Avenue
Dallas, Texas 75231
214-373-6300; 1-800-AHA-USA1
Web: http://www.americanheart.org
The AHA is a national voluntary health agency whose mission is to reduce disability and death from cardiovascular diseases and stroke. The AHA is a source for health promotion programs to prevent heart disease and stroke and promote healthy lifestyles. It is also a resource for health care professionals.

Dietary Guidelines for Americans 2005

Web: http://www.healthierus.gov
The Web site provides new dietary guidelines as well as brochures on how to be healthier, based on the new dietary guidelines, toolkits for health professionals, and press releases. Additional resources are listed at the end of the Web site.

Health Information

Web: http://www.health.nih.gov
This National Institutes of Health's site provides information on body location/systems, conditions/diseases, health and wellness, health newsletters, health databases, health hotlines, and federal health agencies.

Healthier US Gov

The U.S. Department of Health and Human Services
200 Independence Avenue SW
Washington, D.C. 20201
202-619-0257; 1-877-696-6775
Web: http://www.healthierus.gov
This Web site is an outline of government Web sites promoting healthy lifestyles. It provides links to physical fitness, disease/illness prevention, nutrition, making healthy choices, and many other government sites.

Medline Plus

U.S. National Library of Medicine
8600 Rockville Pike
Bethesda, Maryland 20894
Web: http://www.nlm.nih.gov
Medline Plus is a service of the U.S. National Library of Medicine and the National Institutes of Health, provides information on health topics, drugs and supplements, and current health news, and features a medical encyclopedia and health care directories.

National Cholesterol Education Program, National Heart, Lung, and Blood Institute

Health Information Center
Attention: Web Site
P.O. Box 30105
Bethesda, Maryland 20824-0105
301-592-8573
FAX: 240 629 3246
Email: nhlbiinfo@nhlbi.nih.gov
Web: http://www.nhlbi.nih.gov
The goal of the National Cholesterol Education Program is to reduce the percentage of Americans with high blood cholesterol. Links are provided to program description, roster and meeting notes of the coordinating committee, health-related information for clients as well as health care providers, and clinical practice guidelines for cholesterol management in adults.

National Diabetes Information Clearinghouse:

1 Information Way
Bethesda, Maryland 20892-3560
301-654-3333, 1-800-860-8747
FAX: 301-907-8906
Email: ndic@info.niddk.nih.gov
Web: http://www.niddk.nih.gov
The National Diabetes Information Clearinghouse, a service of the National Institute of Diabetes and Digestive and Kidney Diseases, provides educational materials and educational programs on diabetes, digestive diseases, endocrine and metabolic diseases, hematologic diseases, and kidney and urologic diseases.

Shaping America's Health—Association for Weight Management and Obesity Prevention

1701 North Beauregard Street
Alexandria, Virginia 22311
703-253-4808
Web: http://www.obesityprevention.org
Shaping America's Health is a new organization formed from the American Diabetes Association and the North American Association for the Study of Obesity, aimed at weight loss and weight management. The organization will be involved with educating the public and issuing new clinical guidelines and evidence-based initiatives.

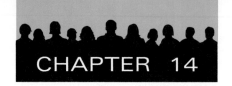

CHAPTER 14

Principles of Health Education

Carolyn L. Blue, RN, PhD, CHES

David R. Black, PhD, HSPP, MPH, CHES, CPPE, FASHA, FSBM, FAAHB

Chapter Outline

⊕ Health Education Defined

⊕ Healthy People 2010 Objectives Relevant to Public Health Education
  Priorities Based on Evidence of Need
  Priorities Based on Demographics

⊕ Fundamentals of Teaching and Learning
  Definitions of Teaching and Learning
  Domains of Learning
  Adult Learning

⊕ Steps of Teaching-Learning Process
  Assessing the Learner
  Planning and Developing the Objectives
  Implementing the Plan
  Evaluating the Plan

Learning Objectives

Upon completion of this chapter, the reader should be able to:

1. Examine critically Healthy People 2010 educational objectives that guide public health education endeavors.

2. Illustrate Knowle's assumptions of adult learning.

3. Arrange the steps in the educational process.

4. Differentiate formative, process, and outcome educational evaluations.

5. Create ways to reduce barriers to learning.

Throughout American history, health education has been a major part of the role of public health nurses. During the late nineteenth and early twentieth centuries, nurses addressed the challenges of new immigrants with communicable diseases, cared for the sick at home, and used personal hygiene and environmental sanitation measures to promote health and prevent illness. Since those early contributions to promoting the health of society, there has been progress in prevention of morbidity and premature mortality, early detection and screening, treatment of diseases, injury prevention, and disability attenuation/management. The following six great public health achievements in the United States collectively have contributed to sharp drops in mortality through the years: vaccination, motor-vehicle safety, safer workplaces, control of infectious diseases, healthier mothers and babies, and safer and healthier foods (CDC, 1999). The average life span of Americans has increased 30 years from 47.3 years in 1900 to 77.8 years in 2004 (CDC, 2007).

In the twenty-first century, nurses continue to educate to control communicable diseases, many of which are reemerging and drug resistant, and to provide care and focus on illness, injury prevention, and disability. Today, the greatest health threats include chronic diseases such as heart disease, cancer, diabetes, and AIDs; obesity; and injuries; as well as potential exposure to chemical, biological, radiological, nuclear agents, and explosives. Most of these threats require lifestyle, social, economic, political, and environmental changes to promote, restore, or maintain health. Educating to prevent or control the ill effects from these illnesses in individuals, families, and communities involves a knowledge base and skill in principles, planning, implementation, and evaluation of health education interventions.

HEALTH EDUCATION DEFINED

The World Health Organization (1998) defined health education as comprising "consciously constructed opportunities for learning involving some form of communication designed to improve health literacy, including improving knowledge, and developing life skills which are conducive to individual and community health" (p. 4). Health education is concerned with information delivery as well as fostering the motivation, skills, and confidence needed to take action to improve the social, economic, and environmental determinants of health. The United States Joint Commit-

tee on Health Education Terminology (2002) defined health education as "any combination of planned learning experiences based on sound theories that provide individuals, groups, and communities the opportunity to acquire information and the skills needed to make quality health decisions" (p. 6). The Society for Public Health Education (2005) defined health education as "a social science that draws from the biological, environmental, psychological, physical, and medical sciences to promote health and prevent disease, disability, and premature death through theory-based voluntary behavior change activities, programs, campaigns, and research" (p. 1). These definitions take into account an ecological model (i.e., those including people and their social and physical environment) of health education that considers determinants of health such as social, economic, cultural, health, environmental conditions, individual behavior, individual traits, and biological factors that impact the health of individuals, families, and communities. A primary premise is that personal choices as well as social, physical, and environmental factors can influence health behaviors.

HEALTHY PEOPLE 2010 OBJECTIVES RELEVANT TO PUBLIC HEALTH EDUCATION

Educating the public is an applied effort that is responsive to the changing social and health environment. The Healthy People 2010 goal for the Educational and Community-Based Programs focus area is to "increase the quality, availability, and effectiveness of community and education-based programs designed to prevent disease and improve health and quality of life" (USDHHS, 2000). Racial and ethnic minorities are often socioeconomically deprived, underserved by health care delivery, and have higher prevalence of preventable and/or manageable health problems (USDHHS, 2004). Thus, it is important for public health nurses and other health care professionals to prioritize health education based on public need and demographics of special populations.

Priorities Based on Evidence of Need

Chapter 5 addressed objectives presented in Healthy People 2010. To meet these objectives, public health nurses need to be active in promoting healthy lifestyles across all ages and in a variety of settings such as work-sites, schools, and in the community at large. A number of national health objectives are directed at educational and community-based programs to assist people in the community achieve health and quality of life (USDHHS, 2000). Listed in Table 14-1 are Healthy People 2010 educational and community-based program objectives with priority components. The educational objectives emphasize people working together to improve health and people living healthier lives by improving the physical and social aspects of communities. For example, components of school health education include prevention of unintentional injury, violence, suicide, tobacco use and addiction, unintended pregnancy, HIV/AIDS, and sexually transmitted infections and promotion of healthy dietary patterns, physical activity, and environmental health. There also are related objectives from other focus areas such as nutrition and overweight, arthritis and diabetes education, and medical product use that require health education efforts to meet the goals. Public health nurses collaborate with other health professionals and members of the community to create healthy communities. Public health nurses assess and identify health education needs in the community, plan, and implement health education programs that promote the national objectives and evaluate the outcomes.

In addition to the educational objectives, there is a national health goal "to use communication strategically to improve health" (USDHHS, 2000, p. 11-6). Effective health communication, which is an approach to change a set of behaviors in a target aggregate or population, is essential to health education. All the leading health indicators depend on health communication

TABLE 14-1: Healthy People 2010 Educational and Community-Based Programs

Goal: Increase the quality, availability, and effectiveness of educational and community-based programs designed to prevent disease and improve health and quality of life.

NUMBER	GOAL
School Setting	
7-1	Increase high school completion
7-2	School health education
7-3	Health-risk behavior information for college and university students
7-4	School nurse-to-student ratio
Worksite Setting	
7-5	Worksite health promotion programs
7-6	Participation in employer-sponsored health promotion activities
Health Care Setting	
7-7	Client and family education
7-8	Satisfaction with client education
7-9	Health care organization sponsorship of community health promotion activities
Community Setting and Select Populations	
7-10	Community health promotion programs
7-11	Culturally appropriate and linguistically competent community health promotion programs
7-12	Older adult participation in community health promotion activities

Note. Modified from USDHHS (2000).

for improvement whether it be educational messages in printed materials, public media campaigns, or face-to-face interactions. Box 14-1 outlines the attributes of effective health communication. Priority areas for public health education based on evidence of need and ability to measure progress are the leading health indicators (USDHHS, 2000). These priority areas include physical activity, overweight and obesity, tobacco use, substance abuse, sexual behavior, mental health, injury and violence, environmental quality, immunization, and access to health care. None of these priority areas identified as part of the Healthy People 2010 national health objectives can be achieved without appropriate and adequate health education interventions. The public health nurse's ability to collaborate with the community is key to planning, implementation, and evaluation of educational interventions that target these priority areas.

Priorities Based on Demographics

Health education needs may be different based on demographic variables such as gender, age, income, education, and ethnicity. Men and women have different health concerns, different lifestyles, and different incidence of disease. Men, for example, have higher rates of deaths from unintentional injury, suicide, and homicide than women do (CDC, 2004b; National Institute of Mental Health, 2003). Women, on the other hand, have higher rates of chronic illnesses such as arthritis and osteoporosis than men (Arthritis Foundation, 2006; National Osteoporosis Foundation, 2006). Issues involving contraception, reproductive choices, and prenatal care also may affect women, especially low-income women, more than men (USDHHS, 2000).

Consideration of age, education, and income also are factors determining health education needs. Health education for children may focus on nutritional needs, immunizations, prevention of adolescent pregnancy, and prevention of substance abuse. Community and school programs to prevent violent deaths among youth, especially those 10–24 years old, also need emphasis (CDC, 2006). Older adults may have educational needs surrounding diet or managing a chronic illness. Persons who have lower incomes and educational levels may be in need of counseling about health behaviors as well as access to health services.

Education needs also may vary by ethnic or cultural group, if certain health concerns are more prevalent in these groups. For instance, African Americans may be a

BOX 14-1: Attributes of Effective Health Communication

- **Accuracy**: The content is valid and without errors of fact, interpretation, or judgment.

- **Availability**: The content (whether targeted message or other information) is delivered or placed where the audience can access it. Placement varies according to audience, message complexity, and purpose from interpersonal and social networks to billboards and mass transit signs to primetime TV or radio, to public kiosks (print or electronic) to the Internet.

- **Balance**: Where appropriate, the content presents the benefits and risks of potential actions or recognizes different and valid perspectives on the issue.

- **Consistency**: The content remains internally consistent over time and also is consistent with information from other sources (the latter is a problem when other widely available content is not accurate or reliable).

- **Cultural competence**: The design, implementation, and evaluation process that accounts for special issues for select population groups (for example, ethnic, racial, and linguistic) and also educational levels and disability.

- **Evidence base**: Relevant scientific evidence that has undergone comprehensive review and rigorous analysis to formulate practice guidelines, performance measures, review criteria, and technology assessments for telehealth applications.

- **Reach**: The content gets to or is available to the largest possible number of people in the target population.

- **Reliability**: The source of the content is credible, and the content itself is kept up to date.

- **Repetition**: The delivery of/access to the content is continued or repeated over time, both to reinforce the impact with a given audience and to reach new generations.

- **Timeliness**: The content is provided or available when the audience is most receptive to, or in need of, the specific information.

- **Understandability**: The reading or language level and format (including multimedia) are appropriate for the specific audience. Retrieved February 1, 2005, p. 9 from: www.naccho.org/ files/documents/ chartbook-introduction3-17.pdf.

SOURCE: From USDHHS (2000).

priority population of focus for prevention and control of high blood pressure and stroke (Black Health Care, 2006). Needed too is a focus on diabetes prevention and control especially for African Americans, Hispanics, and American Indians and Alaska Natives who have the highest diabetes prevalence (CDC, 2005; National Institute of Diabetes and Digestive and Kidney Diseases, 2003).

Health education needs of population aggregates can be established by reviewing Healthy People 2010 focus areas (USDHHS, 2000). In addition, the public health nurse can identify health education needs by conducting a needs assessment as discussed in chapter 11. Communication between the public health nurse and members of the community or aggregate is essential to understanding the health information needs.

FUNDAMENTALS OF TEACHING AND LEARNING

Nurses and other health education specialists have realized they cannot make a person learn, rather they can only help them do so. Furthermore, health educators now have realized that knowledge alone is insufficient to change behavior (Egger et al., 1999). Rather, health education is about helping people make informed choices about their behavior by increasing their understanding of the health consequences of their actions or inactions, and acquiring the skills to make their choices a reality (Kemm, 2003). An understanding of adult learning is necessary to translate knowledge into the desired health behavior.

Definitions of Teaching and Learning

All learning theories view behavior change as a learning process. For example, Haggard (1963) defined learning as a change in behavior as the result of experience. Skinner (1968) included in his definition of learning that control of conditions is optimal for producing changes in behavior and that educational techniques can be used to shape behavior. Cognitive theorists focused on information recognition, processing, and organizing, and adding new information to form new understanding (Sternberg, 1996). Piaget (Wadsworth, 1996), a cognitive theorist, was influential in

describing the maturation of children's minds. The four stages he included are sensorimotor (birth to 2 years), preoperational (2 to 7 years), concrete operational (7 to 11 years), and formal operational (abstract thinking; 11 years and up). Each stage has major cognitive tasks that must be accomplished. In the sensorimotor stage, the focus of mental development is on mastery of concrete objects. The mastery of symbols takes place in the preoperational stage. In the concrete stage, children learn mastery of classes, relations, and numbers and how to reason. The last stage deals with the mastery of thought. Piaget's stages of cognitive development have been used as a basis for assessing childhood cognitive development and for scheduling school curriculum. He supported the idea that learning is much more meaningful if children are allowed to experiment on their own rather than listen to a lecture.

More recently, Fenwick and Tennant (2004) proposed that there is no single theory of learning. They make an assumption that there is a more holistic theory of learning, a process of change that links the learner to the active and dynamic context of the person's life, including cultural, political, physical, and social dynamics. They also assume that the learner and educator are connected and that "the positionality of the educator . . . affects how learners perceive, feel, behave, and remember" (p. 55). Fenwick and Tennant (2004) provide four perspectives for viewing the learning process:

- Learning as acquisition: understands knowledge as a substantive thing—a skill or competency, concept, new language, habit, expertise or wisdom—that an individual obtains through learning experiences.

- Learning as reflection: focuses on learners as active constructors of knowledge, creating new meanings and realities rather than ingesting pre-existing knowledge.

- Practice-based community process: focuses more on people's ability to participate meaningfully in everyday activities within particular communities of practice than on their mental meanings.

- Learning as embodied co-emergent process: challenges people-centered notions to portray learning as emerging in the relationships that develop among all people and everything in a particular situation, people, spatial arrangements and movements, tools, and objects (p. 56).

The point to remember is that there is no one learning theory and no one learning style. People are likely to learn using a variety of learning styles and through a variety of learning processes. As health educators, the objective is to appeal to a variety of learning styles and processes. The definition of teaching, then, is an act of behavior shaping. Knowles, Holton, and Swanson (1998) define education as "an activity undertaken or initiated by one or more agents that is designed to effect changes in the knowledge, skill, and attitudes of individuals, groups, or communities" (p. 10).

Domains of Learning

Bloom's Taxonomy of Educational Objectives is a framework for classifying learning that results from instruction (Bloom, Madaus, & Hastings, 1981). Bloom et al. divided learning into three types of domains or skills: cognitive, affective, and psychomotor. These domains were identified to describe the nature of learning. Cognitive skills are concerned with developing and increasing knowledge. If people learn that they can help to prevent a heart attack by increasing their physical activity levels, they have increased their cognitive skills. Affective skills are concerned with interests, attitudes, and values. These skills are often the most difficult to change because people are attached to existing values and beliefs. If they begin to believe that promoting their cardiovascular health is a positive thing and they can influence the outcome, then their affective skills have been increased. Finally, psychomotor skills are those that involve some kind of physical manipulation such as a client with diabetes who can manipulate drawing up insulin into a syringe and giving him- or herself an injection.

Adult Learning

Teaching has traditionally been defined and described using the principles of pedagogy (from the Greek, "to lead children"). Pedagogy is a predominantly teacher-centered educational model where the teacher decides what, how, and when content will be learned, and whether teaching content has been learned (Knowles, Holton, & Swanson, 2005). Knowles (1913–1997), a widely known and influential professor of adult education, emphasized that adult learners do best when they are involved in the learning process and are treated with respect and dignity. His andragogy (adult learning) model of learning is based on six assumptions:

- Adults need to know the benefits and value of what is to be learned as well as the negative consequences of not learning.
- Adults want to be autonomous, self-directed learners because they feel a responsibility for their own decisions, including the decision to learn.
- Adults have a variety of life experiences, creating diversity of resources and mental models within groups, and are negatively affected if these experiences are ignored or devalued.
- Adults learn better when they see an immediate need; timing education to coincide with an immediate need is more effective because the learner will see the immediate goal and be ready to learn.
- Adults are life-, task-, or problem-centered and are motivated to learn when the content is directed to real-life situations.
- Adults are highly motivated by internal pressures and less motivated by external motivators (Knowles, Holton, & Swanson, 2005, p. 162).

The process for effective adult education includes four phases (Knowles, Holton, & Swanson, 2005). In phase 1, "need," the educator determines what the individual needs to learn to achieve his or her goals, whereas in phase 2, "create," the educator creates a strategy and the resources to achieve the individual's learning goal. Phase 3, "implement," is the implementation of the learning strategy and utilization of learning resources. Phase 4, "evaluate," is the evaluation of attainment of the learning goal(s) and the process of reaching the goal(s).

STEPS OF TEACHING-LEARNING PROCESS

Nurses in all specialties use the nursing process and its problem-solving method in practice to individualize and plan approaches to care, implement interventions, and evaluate outcomes. The teaching-learning process is similar to the nursing process and includes assessing the learner, planning and developing the objectives, implementing the plan, and evaluating the teaching-learning encounter. The teaching-learning process is a systematic and strategic approach aimed at targeting appropriate messages and educational interventions to individuals, groups, and communities.

Assessing the Learner

The first step in health education is assessing the people who need and want information that will result in health knowledge that is a necessary component of a positive health outcome. We want to emphasize that health knowledge alone may not be sufficient to trigger a healthy behavior. Many other factors are necessary for motivating healthy behaviors including attitudes, beliefs, and values of the target population. Enabling factors include availability and accessibility of resources, community policies, and health related skills, and reinforcing factors are family, health professionals, and community leaders (Green & Krueter, 1999). Nevertheless, health education is an important part of improving healthy behaviors and health, and whether the health education is developed for individuals, groups, or communities, the health education process begins with an assessment of health education needs, learning styles, and readiness of the individual, family, or community to learn.

Assessment is a process of collecting data systematically from a variety of sources to accurately identify learning needs (Rankin & Stallings, 1996). It is important to consider not only the learning needs of the individual and family, but also the learning needs of the larger community. The assessment of learning needs can and should be used in conjunction with the community assessment in planning a health education encounter.

Assessment of Learner Needs

The main reason to assess learning needs is to help educational planning. Learner needs are defined as the discrepancy or gaps between knowledge, skills, and abilities or competencies needed for performance and their present level of development by the learner (Knowles, Holton, & Swanson, 2005). This includes characteristics and learning capabilities of the learner(s), health promotion and risk reduction needs, skills relevant to the health needs, motivation to change behaviors, and barriers and facilitators of behavior change (Heady & Hooper, 2002).

Characteristics of the learner include the demographic, psychographic, and geographic characteristics of the intended audience segments discussed in chapter 13. Age and developmental level, educational level, and socioeconomic level are essential demographics to evaluate for planning health education. The identification of social and cultural characteristics of the learner may be accomplished with a formal needs assessment such as personal interviews, focus groups, and surveys, but

general information also may be gleaned from existing data and statistics, literature associated with the target group, or review of prior surveys. Specific social and cultural characteristics that can be assessed include peer influence, support systems, cultural norms, meaning of health, and preferences. In addition, prior experiences and current knowledge and skills of the learner are important to assess as diverse experiences may create additional individual differences, biases that could inhibit or shape learning, a foundation for self-identity, and a resource for current learning (Knowles, Holton, & Swanson, 2005).

Assessment of Learner Styles

"One-size-fits-all" instruction does not result in learning for one and all because people have individual learning differences and preferences for different learning styles. Learning style refers to a person's or group's preferred modes and environments for learning and includes cognitive, affective, and psychomotor/physiological dimensions as well as characteristics of instruction and settings for instruction (Knowles, Holton, & Swanson, 2005). Teaching content is not altered to accommodate learning style. Rather, the delivery of the content material is altered to better serve the person's learning style and, thereby, enhance learning. Learning preferences have been found to be related to age of individuals and variation in groups (Johnson & Romanello, 2005). For example, persons born between 1925 and 1942 are the "silent generation," who remain silent learners and may have difficulty adjusting to technological advances. On the other hand, the "baby boomers," born between 1943 and 1960 have an excellent work ethic, are motivated to learn, appreciate positive reinforcement, and prefer learning through organized lecture and note taking rather than self-study methods. Generation X individuals, born between 1961 and 1981, prefer only information that will directly benefit them and that is presented in a straightforward manner in the easiest and quickest way possible; they enjoy flexible learning times. Finally, Johnson and Romanello (2005) describe the millennials, born between 1982 and 2002, as those who grew up with computers, the Internet, and other teaching technology. Growing up with this information access, they prefer using technology, experiential activities, and group collaboration.

Several assessment tools to assess learning styles are available. One assessment tool is Kolb's (1984)

⊕ PRACTICE APPLICATION

Assessing Smoker's Knowledge Level

An article in *Nicotine & Tobacco Research* (Cummings et al., 2005), cited in *The Nation's Health* in 2005, reported on a study of smokers who are grossly misinformed about many aspects of cigarettes and stop-smoking medications. Smokers were least knowledgeable about low-tar and filter cigarettes. They were most knowledgeable about the health risks of smoking. Those who were most misinformed tended to be older, smokers of ultralight cigarettes, smokers who believe they will quit before any serious health problems occur, smokers who have never used a stop-smoking medication, and those with a lower educational level. Smokers in the study indicated they wanted more information about the cigarettes they smoke.

⊕ How would you assess if the same were true for your community?

⊕ As a public health nurse, who would you target to provide information about cigarettes and stop-smoking medication in your community?

⊕ What content would you include in a health education program to address misinformation of smokers?

Learning Style Inventory, one of the most common assessment tools; it classifies experiential learners according to different processes of grasping experiences and transforming those experiences into new ways of thinking or new behaviors. This 12-item questionnaire asks the subject to rank order the endings of given sentences. Each response corresponds to one of the four types of learner. According to Smith and Kolb (1986), the "diverger" tends to prefer experiencing and internalizes the experience by reflecting (emotional and imaginative), whereas the "converger" prefers thinking about abstract ideas and internalizes learning through doing. The "assimilator" prefers reflecting and thinking about abstract conceptualization, and the "accommodator" prefers doing with concrete experiences and internalizes the experience with active experimentation (risk takers and depend on trial and error).

The Visual, Aural, Read/write, and Kinesthetic (VARK) Inventory (Fleming & Mills, 1992) assesses visual learning style or preference for pictures, posters, videos, diagrams, graphs, and flow charts and the spacing of visual materials. According to Hamilton (2005), the VARK also assesses auditory learning style including verbal presentations, interesting stories, examples, and descriptions of information; the assessment of read/write learning style includes preference to written words such as handouts, pamphlets, and Web sites; and the kinesthetic learners prefer to attach new learning to information they already possess, so they prefer case studies and real-life examples to illustrate information, samples, and photographs to present information.

The Myers-Briggs Type Indicator (Briggs-Myers & McCaulley, 1985) can be used to assess learners' preferences: where they direct their energy and how they process information, make decisions, and organize their lives. The Myers-Briggs Type Indicator is based on the theory of psychological types described by Jung (Jung & Baynes1921). His dichotomous dimensions of personality are extraversion–introversion, sensing–intuition, and thinking–feeling. Isabel Briggs Myers and her mother, Katharine Briggs, identified basic preferences of four dichotomies, adding judgment–perception, implicit in Jung's theory, and described 16 personality types that result from the interactions among the preferences (Myers & Briggs Foundation, 2006). The different combinations of these dimensions can be used to understand learner preference of processing information. For example, the extrovert may prefer learning by group discussion, while the introvert may prefer accessing the computer for information. The person who learns by sensing may prefer to have clear, concrete information; a person who learns by intuition may prefer using imagination and creating new possibilities. The person who learns by thinking prefers clear, action-oriented objectives and critical analyses, whereas the person who learns by feeling may desire consensus, popular opinions, and light-hearted humor. Finally, the person who learns by judgment may make plans in detail and use targets and dates to manage life, whereas the person who learns by perceiving may tolerate time pressure, multitask, and avoid commitments that interfere with freedom and variety.

Assessment of Learner Readiness

Learner readiness has been defined as "the time when the learner demonstrates an interest in learning the type or degree of information necessary to maintain optimal health" (Kitchie, 2003, p. 84). Learners are motivated to learn when they realize there is a gap between what they know and what they want to know (Knowles, Holton, & Swanson, 1998). Assessment of learner readiness provides information about where the individual, family, or community stands with respect to knowledge, attitudes, and skills important to health. Two main types of learner readiness should be considered: emotional and experiential readiness.

Emotional readiness refers to the need to know and the "why" behind people's actions (Knowles, Holton, & Swanson, 1998). Emotional readiness is the internal motivation toward knowledge, beliefs, and skills that will help people solve problems and concerns in their own lives. This position is consistent with value-expectancy theory where a behavior is a function of the subjective *value* of an outcome and the subjective probability, or *expectation,* that a particular effort will achieve that outcome (Lewin et al., 1944).

Experiential readiness refers to a person's ability to learn. Factors influencing experiential readiness are life experiences, whether they be positive or negative; cognitive ability or the ability to think conceptually, which is determined by educational level and sensorium (e.g., hearing, seeing, touching, and smelling); affective ability or the attitudes and values toward learning and the object to be learned; and psychomotor ability to perform skills or tasks. According to Kolb (1983), there are four steps in the experiential learning cycle that combine to create four distinct learning styles (Table 14-2):

1. Concrete experience, which requires full involvement in new here-and-now experiences

2. Observations and reflection of the learner's experiences from many perspectives (i.e., learning by observing others)

3. Abstract conceptualization and generalization, creation of concepts that integrate the learners' observations into logically sound theories

4. Testing implications of new concepts in new situations or using these theories to make decisions and solve problems

Planning and Developing the Objectives

Once learners' needs, learning styles, and learner readiness are determined, the educator focuses on planning the education. In planning a health education, the educator needs to determine what the learner is expected to accomplish as a result of the education. The educator, along with the learner, needs to determine goals and behavioral objectives. These goals and behavioral objectives are written to guide the educational process. Goals or **long-term objectives** are broad, long-term statements of expected outcomes, such as "The prevalence of teenage pregnancy will be reduced by 20% in the next 2 years." Goals set the general direction and intent of a health education encounter.

Educational or **short-term objectives** are specific, clear, and unambiguous descriptions of educational

TABLE 14-2: Kolb's Model with Suggested Learning Strategies

KOLB'S STAGE	EXAMPLE LEARNING/TEACHING STRATEGY
Concrete experience	Simulation, case study, field trip, real experience, demonstrations
Observation and reflection	Discussion, small groups, buzz groups, designated observers
Abstract conceptualization	Sharing content
Active experimentation	Laboratory experiences, on-the-job experience, internships, practice sessions

Note. From The Adult Learner: The Definitive Classic in Adult Education and Human Resource Development by M. S. Knowles, E. F. Holton III, & R. A. Swanson, 1998, Woburn, MA: Butterworth-Heinemann. Copyright by E. F. Holton III and R. A. Swanson. Reprinted with permission.

⊕ RESEARCH APPLICATION

Healthy Behaviors and Sources of Health Information among Low-Income Pregnant Women

Study Purpose

To explore sources of health information in low-income pregnant women.

Methods

Responses from open-ended questions describing healthy behaviors and sources of health information from a sample of 150 low-income pregnant women. Women who were waiting for their appointments in a public prenatal clinic were invited to participate in the study. This study, which was part of a larger study, used the following two questions: (a) "Other than coming to the clinic, what kinds of things do you do to stay healthy during pregnancy or to have a healthy baby?" and (b) "How did you know to do those things?" Qualitative content analyses were used to examine and categorize the data from the questions.

Findings

Healthy behaviors used by the women and mentioned most frequently included eating a healthy diet, followed by pursuing exercise/rest/activity; quitting or cutting down on smoking, alcohol, and other drug use; and being attentive to physical appearance and emotional needs. Sources of information for the women included female family members, health care providers, or reading about it in books, magazines, and pamphlets provided by the clinic.

Implications

Public health nurses need to support low-income women in their health behaviors. Time in the waiting room in clinics could be used for educational purposes. If women are obtaining prenatal health information from magazines and books and people other than health professionals, the nurse should assess their knowledge to ensure the information was accurate.

Reference

Lewallen, L. P. (2004). Healthy behaviors and sources of health information among low-income pregnant women. *Public Health Nursing, 21*(3), 200-206.

expectations about ways the learner is expected to be changed by the learning process (Bloom et al., 1981). They are what we intend for the learner to know (cognitive domain), think (affective domain), or do (psychomotor domain) because of the educational experience. Educational objectives are more specific, short-term statements that address each of the learning needs identified (Knowles, Holton, & Swanson, 1998). Objectives should be *SMART: S*pecific, *M*easurable, *A*chievable, *R*ealistic, and *T*imely (Piotrow et al., 1997).

When written in behavioral terms, an objective will include three components: behavior, conditions of performance, and performance criteria. The behavior component includes a knowledge or skill to be gained and the action or skill the learner is able to do. The behavior part uses specific, measurable action verbs dependent upon assessment of the client's cognitive, psychomotor, or affective ability. The conditions of performance include the circumstances or context under which the behavior will be performed. Performance criteria describe rules of acceptability or how well the

behavior is to be performed, compared to a standard. Sample educational objectives are in Table 14-3.

Bloom, Madaus, and Hastings (1981) developed a taxonomy of educational objectives. This taxonomy of hierarchical educational terminology can be classified under the three domains of learning (i.e., cognitive, affective, and psychomotor). Table 14-4 shows the educational terminology, or learning tasks, arranged in the level of complexity of skill involved in each of the three domains. For example, in the cognitive domain, it is easier for a learner to identify behaviors that would lead to heart health than to apply behaviors that lead to heart health. Similarly, it is easier for a community to recognize a need for a smokeless society than to endorse a smoke-free community. One of the difficulties in writing objectives for health education is writing them so they can be accurately measured. It is most difficult to measure objectives in the affective domain because beliefs, values, and attitudes are subjective and not readily observed. Public health nurses often write objectives that reflect changes in communities or

TABLE 14-3: Sample of Educational Objectives in the Cognitive, Affective, and Psychomotor Domains

BEHAVIOR	CONDITIONS OF PERFORMANCE	PERFORMANCE CRITERIA
Objectives in the Cognitive Domain		
Each member of the Adams family will describe	the health benefits from walking	at the end of the heart disease prevention program.
Reduce the rate of teenage pregnancies	by 50 percent	one year from the program initiation.
Objectives in the Affective Domain		
Members of the Adams family will discuss	the value of walking to heart health	within one month of the heart disease prevention program.
Objectives in the Psychomotor Domain		
Each member of the Adams family will walk	moderately for 30 minutes	three times a week for one year.

Note. Modified from USDHHS (2000). *Healthy People 2010: Understanding and improving health* (2nd ed). Washington, DC: U.S. Government Printing Office.

TABLE 14-4: Taxonomy of Educational Terminology within Domains of Learning

LEVELS	COGNITIVE DOMAIN		AFFECTIVE DOMAIN		PSYCHOMOTOR DOMAIN	
	Taxonomy	**Example of Verbs**	**Taxonomy**	**Examples of Verbs**	**Taxonomy**	**Examples of Verbs**
Level 1	Knowledge	Defines Identifies Names	Receiving	Recognizes Shares Chooses	Manipulation	Follows Places Uses
Level 2	Comprehension	Recalls Recognizes Describes	Responding	Participates Follows Approves	Precision	Performs in order Combines Maintains
Level 3	Application	Applies Discusses Organizes	Valuing	Defends Endorses Convinces	Efficiency	Performs skillfully Executes smoothly Performs spontaneously
Level 4	Synthesis	Plans Proposes Designs	Organization of values	Discusses Weighs Arranges	Adaption	Improvises Modifies Adapts
Level 5	Evaluation	Creates Formulates Validates	Characterization of values	Revises Integrates Resolves	Origination	Tests Examines Designs

Note. From Bloom, B. S., Madaus, G., & Hastings, J. T. (1981). *Evaluation to improve learning.* New York: McGraw-Hill.

community groups by using prevalence rates of a phenomenon. Examples are to reduce the prevalence rates of teenage smoking by 20 percent in 1 year, increase immunization rates in 3 year olds to 90 percent within 2 years, or increase fruits and vegetables consumption in the workplace by 40 percent within 6 months of program completion. Note that these objectives show not only a target measure to reach but a timeframe in which to reach the target.

Health education goals and behavioral objectives are used to plan the health education intervention. Many factors come into play during the planning phase of health education. First, collaboration is an essential skill for the public health nurse and is vital for achieving a health education program that is acceptable and appropriate for the individual as well as for a community (Cavanaugh & Cheney, 2002). Collaboration with the community is defined as people with various interests working together toward a common goal, whether it is a goal for an individual, family, or community. Community collaboration may involve working together with other disciplines or groups in a community, striving for a "win-win" resolution of a problem. Community participation and building coalitions in the community are essential for health education efforts within a community as well as community health-education efforts (Green & Kreuter, 1999).

Selecting the Content

Content for the educational encounter is prescribed by the learning objectives. What new information, facts, relationships, values, or skills are needed to reach the objectives? In selecting content, it is important to consider resources, both material and human, needed to accomplish each objective. In addition, it is important to consider personal and group differences in abilities, experiences, levels of knowledge, educational expectations, and cultural beliefs and practices.

Selecting the Format

Houle (1972) identified a number of components necessary to the design of the educational format to be implemented by the educator. He identified the components of a suitable format design as the following:

- Selection of learning resources
- Selection of educational leader or educator
- Methods of teaching
- Time schedule
- Sequence of events
- Provision of social reinforcement of learning
- The nature of the individual learner
- Criteria for evaluating progress
- Clarity of the educational design

There are many formats or teaching and learning methods to choose from. A sensitive educator will use a variety of them in planning a health education program. There are two types of teaching methods, teacher-centered and learner-centered methods (Corder, 2002). In teacher-centered methods, the teacher is the leader. Lectures and mass media campaigns are examples of teacher-centered learning. The teacher decides the content of the learning and emphasizes key points. In student-centered methods, the student is encouraged to take more control of his or her own learning. Examples of student-centered methods are small group discussion, real-life simulations, role-playing, experiential learning, and brainstorming.

In addition to details about the educational format, Knowles, Holton, and Swanson (1998) described a learning environment that is comfortable and conducive to interaction between the learner and teacher and, if applicable, among other learners. A healthy learning environment includes the physical environment (e.g., room temperature, noise level, lighting) as well as a safe psychological environment where the teacher demonstrates respect of a student's worth, feelings, and ideas. It is essential in an adult educational encounter that the teacher builds trusting relationships among students by encouraging cooperation and discouraging competitiveness and negative judgments.

Health Literacy

The public health nurse and members of the community who are planning a health education program also must consider literacy and all its aspects when developing educational materials and teaching strategies. Health literacy is a relatively new area of study emerging in the 1990s. Although a complete consensus of definition of health literacy has not emerged, the Joint Committee on National Health Education Standards (1995) defined **health literacy** as "the capacity of individuals to obtain, interpret, and understand basic health information and services and the competence to use such information and services in ways which enhance health" (p. 5). More recently, the U.S. Department of Health and Human Services defined health literacy as "the degree to which individuals have the capacity to obtain, process, and understand basic health information and services needed to make appropriate health decisions" (2003, p. 1). Thus, health literacy is not simply the ability to read. A complex group of reading, listening, analytical, and decision-making skills are necessary along with the ability to apply these skills to health education encounters and education-focused situations.

The public health nurse must realize that health literacy affects not only health knowledge but also health status and access to health services. Although results of the 2002 National Adult Literacy Survey are not compiled, the 1992 National Adult Literacy Survey found about 90 million American adults to have inadequate or marginal literacy skills (Kirsch et al., 1993). Low income, low levels of education, older age, and minority race or ethnic groups are increasingly associated with low literacy levels (Educational Testing Service, 2003; Kirsch et al., 1993). Literacy is associated with income level, occupation, education, housing, and access to medical care. People with low health literacy levels are more likely to report poor health and have a greater risk of hospitalization and are less likely to understand health problems and treatment (Baker et al., 1997). Higher levels of health literacy were associated with use of health care services and positive health outcomes (Berkman et al., 2004). Lower income persons are more likely to be illiterate, work under hazardous conditions, have health conditions that limit their activity, and make poor behavioral choices (National Center for Education Statistics, 1993). Fisher (1999) found that low literacy is more prevalent in the United States than is generally recognized and that public health education materials frequently require reading levels as high as an alarming 12th grade reading level. The 2003 National Assessment of Adult Literacy report is not published yet, but it will include adults' abilities to use literacy skills in reading and understanding health-related information (National Center for Education Statistics, 2006).

The public health nurse can make assessment(s) of the literacy levels of their clients informally or formally. Informally, the nurse can ask the client whether or not they can read, what they like to read, and how often they read for pleasure. Persons who like to read, read for pleasure, and read a variety of materials generally have a high literacy level. Clients also can be asked where they obtain their health information. Again, people who obtain health information in written form (e.g., pamphlets, books, and the Internet) are skilled readers. People who prefer to get health information directly from other persons or from television or radio may have lower literacy skills.

For a more formal assessment of literacy skill, there are easily administered literacy tests that public health nurses can use to assess clients for literacy skills or assess educational materials for literacy levels. Readability tests are a simple technique for measuring structural difficulty and predicting the reading grade level of written text. Most of the more than 40 different formulae count language variables and sentence length to provide a measure of reading difficulty. Most readability tests are available in foreign languages. The Rapid Estimate of Adult Literacy in Medicine (REALM; Davis, Crouch, & Long, 1993) is a screening instrument to assess an adult client's ability to read common medical words and lay terms for body parts and illnesses. The SMOG Readability Formula (McLaughlin, 1969; available at http://www.cdc.gov/od/ads/smog.htm), Fry Readability Graph (1968, 1977, available at http://www.cdc.gov/od/ads/fry.htm), and Flesch-Kincaid Formula (Flesch, 1948; Spadero, 1983) are useful in assessment of reading level of educational materials such as brochures or information sheets. Many word-processing programs have readability statistics that can be used to assess reading level and sentence length. Other factors that should be taken into account in addition to reading level are text layout, use of illustrations, and font shape and size.

Considering Cultural Influences

It is not possible for the public health nurse who is a member of one culture to know all aspects of all cultures. Even if we know some generalities about a particular cultural group, we must remember that there are variations of beliefs and values within a culture. Therefore, it is essential that the public health nurse conduct cultural assessments on individuals, families, and communities to plan appropriate content, materials, and delivery of the health education. Cultural domains to assess include culturally relevant lifestyles, cultural values and norms, expressions of the culture, cultural myths and taboos, rituals and rites, lay practices, and so forth. In addition to cultural differences between and among groups of persons, there are differences in the culture of organizations (Knowles, Holton,

⊕ POLICY HIGHLIGHT

Health Literacy at the Core of Health Education

Health literacy is concerned with more than reading ability, and studies have shown that many Americans with the greatest health care needs have the least ability to gather, process, and understand information necessary to function in the U.S. health care system, achieve higher levels of wellness, or manage health problems. Health literacy is a policy issue and is one of the nation's Healthy People 2010 objectives, and the Institute of Medicine (IOM) named health literacy as one of the priorities to transform health care in America. Health literacy is also part of the World Health Organization's new health promotion strategy. The Health Resources and Services Administration (HRSA) has taken responsibility in health literacy by educating and increasing awareness about the need to improve health literacy among health care providers and clients. Public health nurses can get involved by accessing HRSA programs through their Web site (http://www.hrsa.gov/ConsumerEd/).

& Swanson, 1998). An understanding of the norms, values, work styles, informal systems, politics, and taboos of an organization is essential to planning health education within an organization. When planning a health education program for a culture different from one's own, the nurse is prudent to include members of the learner group, as well as key persons who have an understanding of organizational culture, in the total assessment, planning, implementation, and evaluation process of the program.

Implementing the Plan

The overall plan for the health education encounter involves choosing among a variety of traditional instructional methods, including lecture, group discussion, one-to-one instruction, demonstration, as well as a number of nontraditional instructional methods such as gaming, simulation, role-playing, and role-modeling (Fitzgerald 2003). Selecting the teaching method depends on the behavioral objectives, the comfort and expertise of the educator in using the methods, the needs and abilities of the learner(s), and whether the education is aimed at the individual, family, group, or community. It is vitally important to know the audience when selecting and implementing the teaching plan. Major components of the plan include the content that is actually delivered and the organization of the content and the delivery system that is used to deliver the content. The delivery system as well as the knowledge it carries has resulted in the Information Age, a term applied to the period where there is a dramatic increase in communication channels and where movement of information became faster than physical movement as a result of advances

in information technology (Hefzallah, 2004). Public health nurses and other health care professionals need to work together to ensure that the educational content and technologies provide everyone access, understanding, and useful information to prevent injury and illness and promote and maintain health.

Organizing the Educational Content

Whether the educational program is for an individual, family, or group of people, it is essential to organize the material into a logical framework. There are several ways to organize educational content. One way to organize content is from easy to difficult. The learner may be familiar with easy content, and this may help to engage the learner. Arranging material in a natural sequence is another way to organize content. For example, telling the learner(s) what the health problem is, followed by specific and precise advice for problem solutions, and then ending with ways the learner could incorporate the solutions into his or her lifestyle is a natural sequence of educational content. The final content engages the learner into the solution of the problem. Organizing content from most to least interesting is a third way to frame an educational encounter. Although telling the learner(s) about the most interesting first may engage the learner, following with less interesting information, if lengthy, may result in losing the learner's attention.

Use of Technology

The availability of communication and information technology has fostered a rich array of learning delivery mechanisms that can be accessed nearly any time, anywhere, and on any topic. Public health nurses can reach more clients easier than ever before. One of the greatest technological advances of the twentieth century was the Internet and the technology for e-learning. E-learning is learning facilitated and enhanced through the use of information and communication technology, including methods such as personal computers, CD-ROMs, video conferencing, Internet, interactive television or satellite broadcast, e-mail, and discussion forums and may include online interaction between the learners and their teacher or peers. The new e-learning technology includes computer-mediated learning, learning networks and video conferencing, Web-based learning, technology-aided learning, online learning, and asynchronous learning networks (Ó Fathaigh, 2001).

Certainly, the potential of e-learning is to make teaching and learning more effective and efficient. The Pew Internet and American Life Project, a national survey of the 73 million people in the United States who have gone online for health information, revealed that more people get medical advice online than people who actually visit health professionals (Fox & Rainie, 2002). These people mostly use the Internet to look for information about a particular illness or condition, drug information, or alternative treatments or medications. The elderly are the fastest growing population group to use the Internet and e-mail (Kiel, 2005). Even though the desire for "connectedness" among the elderly provides an avenue for meeting the health education needs of this population, it is questionable that older adults use e-learning as a source of health information (Meischke et al., 2005; Tak & Hong, 2005). Health educators need to manage e-learning carefully so that it does not add to disparities in health education as e-learning is based on computer literacy and access (Web-based Education Commission, 2000). There should be caution about e-learning and Web sites. Many sources of online information are not regulated, managed, or screened for quality of health information. Research suggests that much of the health-related information online is incomplete or inaccurate or promotes false claims (e.g., Fricke et al., 2005; Griffin, McKenna, & Worrall, 2004; Hajjar et al., 2005).

The term "Digital Divide" has been used to describe lack of access to information technologies for racial and ethnic minorities, disabled persons, rural populations, and lower socioeconomic groups (Chang et al., 2004). The percentage of U.S. households with a computer rose from 24.1 to 56.5 percent from 1994 to 2001, but the number of households with a computer is correlated with income (U.S. Bureau of the Census, 2001). While 89.0 percent of households with income of $75,000 and over had a computer, only 25.9 percent of households with incomes of $5,000 and under had a computer. Further, whites (61.1 percent) and Asian Americans (72.7 percent) had disproportionately more households with computers than did blacks (37.1 percent) or Hispanics (40.0 percent). The aggregates with the least access to Web-based education are already at risk for health problems, have the most health disparities in the nation, and are in the most need for health education access. Public health nurses are in a position to make access to Web-based health education convenient and affordable to everyone by promoting Internet access in schools, community libraries, homeless shelters, community clinics, and other public places.

Even if there was equal access to e-learning, public health nurses need to address other issues such as computer literacy, health literacy, and the match between desired and available information. The millions of Americans who do not have the ability to read traditional written material above the ninth grade level also will have limited capacity to read and understand health information from the Internet (Gottlieb & Rogers, 2004). However, some projects have successfully reached broad populations, including the underserved. For example, the Comprehensive Health Enhancement Support System (CHESS) and Consumer Health Internet Support System (CHIS) are client-oriented interactive telephone, palm, and Internet-based programs that provide information services, library links, consumer guides to resources, and help with decisions, behavior change, and emotional support (Gustafson et al., 2002). The programs include personal stories and a video gallery in addition to services that help people make decisions about their health and treatment options. There is emerging evidence that CHESS and CHIS have had a positive health impact on underserved African Americans, the elderly, and people with HIV/AIDS (Gustafson et al., 2002).

Public health nurses are a main link for clients to connect with health information through e-learning via a community focus. This focus might include advocating accessible computers and other technology in the community; assisting clients with technology literacy needs; identifying relevant resources, support groups, and discussion groups; and educating clients about accessing reliable information. As noted earlier, there is no editorial or ethical control of information on the Internet. Therefore, one of the most important considerations in helping clients to connect with reliable health information is providing them with criteria by which to evaluate the Internet resources. Without evaluation criteria, the public can be deceived with fraudulent and inaccurate information. Public health nurses can use the Tips for Finding Accurate Internet Information in Box 14-2 to assist their clients to make personal judgments about the usefulness and reliability of information they find on the Web.

Evaluating the Plan

Three types of evaluation are discussed: formative evaluation, process evaluation, and outcome or summative evaluation. All three types of evaluation are essential to

health education to ensure that the content and presentation are appropriate and executed as planned, and the outcomes produced are the ones intended.

Formative Evaluation

Formative evaluation is an assessment of the effects of the education while it is being given. Formative evaluation may deal with one aspect of content as it relates to one or more domains. In other words, formative evaluation addresses single segments of the total health education program as independent learning units. This type of ongoing evaluation is valuable for feedback and corrective modifications to the presentation, if necessary.

Process Evaluation

Process evaluation is conducted to document and analyze the way a health education program is implemented. By conducting a process evaluation as the program is being implemented, it can serve as an early "warning system," and the public health nurse can make midprogram adjustments and revisions if some aspect of the program is not being implemented or accepted as intended. The process evaluation also can assist the nurse in interpreting educational outcomes within the context of education delivery. If there is no change in behavior at the end of the education, the process evaluation can lend insight as to whether or not the education was delivered as intended. The process evaluation also can inform future educational programs. If the educational program was successful, the process evaluation can provide operational information so it can be replicated. Unfortunately, process evaluation is not routinely done, and the result is that the relevancy and appropriateness of the content and delivery of the educational program, as well as learner satisfaction, are kept in a "black box," with emphasis on educational outcomes only rather than on reasons for their success (Blue & Black, 2005; Valente, 2002). For these reasons, it is important for the public health nurse to ensure the appropriateness of the health education message for the learner, the appropriateness of the delivery method, the "dose" or intensity of the information needed, and the possible reasons the educational outcomes were or were not achieved. Process data can be collected from direct observation, subjective feedback from comments and individual or focus group interviews, statistics such as education attendance, or organizational sources of information.

BOX 14-2: Tips for Finding Accurate Internet Information

- The author should be clearly identified with a name, credentials, and affiliation.
- Find out if the Web site is managed by government, university, or health professionals.
- The date of the information should be visible and current.
- Look for links and references to other sources of health information.
- Never use just one Internet site for information. Validate the information by comparing it with information from other sources.
- Be suspicious if only one source has the information.
- Be wary of testimonials about treatments and offerings of cures.
- Be skeptical if the Web site charges an access fee.
- Reputable health professionals do not diagnose and treat clients over the Internet.
- Read the Web site's privacy statement before providing any personal information.
- If the information seems "too good to be true," it probably is not true.

TABLE 14-5: Examples of Nonparametric (Nominal/Categorical and Ordinal) and Parametric (Interval/Ratio) Variables for Different Educational Outcome Domains

OUTCOME	VARIABLES		
	Nominal/ Categorical	Ordinal	Interval/Ratio
Cognitive Domain:			
Knowledge of the effects of tobacco use	Agree/disagree	Three common ways tobacco affects the body	Score on knowledge survey about tobacco effects
Understanding of health outcomes from from regular physical activity	Selecting moderate vigorous activities	Level of agreement with health outcomes of physical activity	Score on an outcome expectancy physical activity scale
Affective Domain:			
Willingness to receive primary care from a community clinic rather than emergency room	Agree/disagree	Level of readiness to use community clinic	Probability (on a 100-point scale) of using community clinic
Wearing helmet when riding a bicycle	Yes/no wears helmet	Frequency of wearing helmet	Percent time wearing helmet
Psychomotor Domain:			
Practice of breast self-examination	Yes/no self-examination	None, 3 to 6 times/year more 6 times/year	Number of months/ year
Uses hearing protection	Yes/no likely to wear hearing protection	Never true (1) to always true (5)	Number of observations

Note. Adapted from Health program planning and evaluation: A practical, systematic approach for community health (pp. 294–295) by M. Issel, 2004, Boston: Jones and Bartlett.

Outcome Evaluation

The definition of outcome evaluation is the degree to which the educational objectives were met (Bloom, Madaus, & Hastings, 1981). Ideally, the evaluation plan should have been formulated when the health education was conceived, along with the education planning process. Measurement of the outcomes depends on the for-

mulated objective. Table 14-5 shows different variables for different outcome domains. An educational outcome always is considered to be a measurable change in health or behavior of the individual, family, or community. In addition to being measured, consideration of sensitivity of measures is warranted because sensitivity determines whether or not minor variations and fluctuations can be detected. A sensitive measure can detect individual variations, variations over time, or the influence of factors other than the education that may be influencing the outcome. In general, parametric (interval/ratio) data are most sensitive and nonparametric (ordinal/nominal) data are least sensitive to detecting change. Of course, reliable and valid measures also are necessary to assure that the data is free of error (reliability) and has captured what it purports to measure (validity).

Health education is one of the public health nurse's most frequently used roles, yet it also can be one of the most challenging. To assist the nurse in developing a health education program that is most productive in facilitating positive outcomes, it is essential to systematically plan, execute, and evaluate an educational encounter. Public health nurses as health educators should strive for excellence as they continue this important role.

CRITICAL THINKING ACTIVITIES

1. Thinking of your own professional practice, which aggregates of population should receive health education that is guided by the national health objectives and priority areas? What would need to be considered in planning a health education program for these people?

2. What criteria should be used to evaluate or assess the credibility of information from newspaper or magazine articles? Is this criterion appropriate for making decisions about your own health?

3. Discuss possible ethical issues in health education such as the manipulation of individuals to change behaviors, the possible negative outcomes, health disparities, and cultural norms.

⊕ RESEARCH APPLICATION

Collaboration between Nurses and Agricultural Teachers to Prevent Adolescent Agricultural Injuries: The Agricultural Disability Awareness and Risk Education Model

Study Purpose

To determine whether the educational intervention could move an adolescent from thinking about safety consequences of farm work behavior to acting on the behavior in order to improve safety.

Methods

Fourteen schools from Midwest states participated in Agricultural Disability Awareness and Risk Education (AgDARE), an educational safety program to reduce agricultural injuries. Researchers used the Transtheoretical Model of Behavior Change (Prochaska, DiClemente, & Norcross, 1992) to guide the study, focusing on the contemplation and action stages of the model. The researcher-developed Farm Safety Attitude Instrument was used to measure the students' attitudes toward disabilities from farm injuries and their ability to prevent injuries to themselves. The instrument was applied to students who attended AgDARE and those in the seven schools who served as a control group.

Findings

Students in both the contemplation and action groups who participated in AgDARE thought more about farm safety and took more action to protect themselves from injury than students in the control group.

Implications

AgDARE is an example of how public health nurses can collaborate with teachers in existing classroom settings to improve attitudes and health and safety behaviors of students.

Reference

Reed, D. B., & Kidd, P. S. (2004). Collaboration between Nurses and Agricultural Teachers to Prevent Adolescent Agricultural Injuries: The Agricultural Disability Awareness and Risk Education Model. *Public Health Nursing, 21,* 323–330.

4. Do you believe that a certain degree of stress and anxiety promotes learning? Why or why not? If you believe a certain degree of stress and anxiety promotes learning, how much is good?

5. If learning objectives of a health education plan are not met, how could you determine if the problem is the identification of learning needs, learning objectives, or learner readiness?

KEY TERMS

affective skills

andragogy

cognitive skills

e-learning

emotional readiness

experiential readiness

formative evaluation

health communication

health education

health literacy

learner needs

learner readiness

learning

learning style

long-term objectives

outcome evaluation

pedagogy

process evaluation

psychomotor skills

short-term objectives

teaching

teaching-learning process

KEY CONCEPTS

- Health education is essential to addressing priorities for Healthy People 2010.

- Learning has taken place only when a behavior change results.

- Learning takes place in the cognitive, affective, and psychomotor domains. The public health nurse considers the importance of these domains in planning a health education program.

- Steps in the education process parallel the nursing process.

- Behavioral objectives are essential to planning and evaluating learning experiences.

- Knowles' assumptions of learning should be useful in planning the content and format of an educational encounter.

- The three types of educational evaluation include formative, process, and outcome evaluation.

REFERENCES

Arthritis Foundation. (2006). *The facts about arthritis.* Retrieved March 200, from http://www.arthritis.org/resources/gettingstarted/default.asp.

Baker, D. W., Parker, R. M., Williams, M. V., Clark, W. S., & Nurss, J. (1997). The relationship of patient reading ability to self-reported health and use of health services. *American Journal of Public Health, 87,* 1027–1030.

Berkman, N. D., DeWalt, D. A., Pignone, M. P., Sheridan, S. L., Lohr, K. N., Lux, L., Sutton, S. F., Swinson, T., & Bonito, A. J. (2004). *Literacy and health outcomes.* Summary, Evidence Report/Technology Assessment No. 87 (Prepared by RTI International–University of North Carolina Evidence-based Practice Center under Contract No. 290-02-0016). AHRQ Publication No. 04-E007-1. Rockville, MD: Agency for Healthcare Research and Quality.

Black Health Care. (2006). *Stroke epidemiology.* Retrieved February 2006 from http://www.bnlackhealthcare.com/BHC/Stroke/Epidemiology.asp.

Bloom, B. S., Madaus, G., & Hastings, J. T. (1981). *Evaluation to improve learning.* New York: McGraw-Hill.

Blue, C. L., & Black, D. R. (2005). Synthesis of intervention research to modify physical activity and dietary behaviors.

Research & Theory for Nursing Practice: An International Journal, 29, 25–61.

Briggs-Myers, I., & McCaulley, M. H (1985). *Manual: A guide to the development and use of the Myers Briggs type indicator.* Palo Alto, CA: Consulting Psychologists Press.

Cavanaugh, N., & Cheney, K. S. W. D. (2002). Community collaboration: A weaving. *Journal of Public Health Management Practice, 8,* 13–20.

Centers for Disease Control and Prevention. (1999). Ten great public health achievements—United States, 1900–1999. *Morbidity and Mortality Weekly Report, 48,* 241–264.

Centers for Disease Control and Prevention. (2004a). *Life expectancy at birth, at 65 years of age, and at 75 years of age, according to race and sex: United States, selected years 1900–2002.* Retrieved January 8, 2005, from http://www.cdc.gov/nchs/data/hus/hus04trend.pdf#027.

Centers for Disease Control and Prevention. (2004b). Surveillance for fatal and nonfatal Injuries—United States, 2001. *Morbidity and Mortality Weekly Report, 53*(SS07), 1–57. Retrieved March 2006 from http://www.cdc.gov/ncipc/pub-res/unintentional_activity/01_overview.htm.

Centers for Disease Control and Prevention. (2005). *National diabetes fact sheet.* Retrieved September, 2006, from http://www.cdc.gov/diabetes/pubs/factsheet05.htm.

Centers for Disease Control and Prevention. (2006). *Youth violence: Fact sheet.* National Center for Injury Prevention and Control. Retrieved February 2006 from http://www.cdc.gov/ncipc/factsheets/yvfacts.htm.

Chang, B. L., Bakken, S., Brown, S. S., Houston, T. K., Kreps, G. L., Kukafka, R., & Safran, C. (2004). Bridging the digital divide: Reaching vulnerable populations. *Journal of the American Medical Informatics Association, 11,* 448–457.

Corder, N. (2002). *Learning to teach adults: An introduction.* New York: RoutledgeFalmer.

Cummings, K. M., Hyland, A., Giovino, G. A., Hastrup, J. L., Bauer, J. L., & Bansal, M. A. (2004). Are smokers adequately informed about the health risks of smoking and medicinal nicotine? *Nicotine & Tobacco Research, 6,* 333–340.

Davis, T., Crouch, M., & Long, S. (1993). Rapid estimate of adult literacy in medicine: A shortened screening instrument. *Family Medicine, 25,* 56–57.

Education Testing Service. (2003). Reading and literacy in America. *ETS Policy Notes, 11*(2), 3–14.

Egger, G., Spark, R., Lawson, J., & Donovan, R. (1999). *Health promotion strategies & methods* (2nd ed.). New York: McGraw-Hill.

Fenwick, T., & Tennant, M. (2004). Understanding adult learners. In G. Foley (ed.), *Dimensions of adult learning: Adult education and training in a global era* (pp. 55–73). Berkshire, England: Open University Press.

Fisher, E. (1999). Low literacy levels in adults: Implications for patient education. *The Journal of Continuing Education in Nursing, 30,* 56–61.

Fitzgerald, K. (2003). Teaching methods and instructional settings. In S. Bastable. *Nurse as educator: Principles of teaching and learning for nursing practice* (2nd ed.). Boston: Jones and Bartlett.

Fleming, N. D., & Mills, C. (1992). Not another inventory, rather a catalyst for reflection. *To Improve the Academy, 11,* 137–155.

Flesch, R. (1948). A new readability yardstick. *Journal of Applied Psychology, 32,* 221–233.

Fox, S., & Rainie, L. (2002). *Pew Internet & American life.* Retrieved August 2005 from http://www.pewinternet.org/pdfs/PIP_Vital_Decisions_May2002.pdf.

Fricke, M., Fallis, D., Jones, M., & Luszko, G. M. (2005). Consumer health information on the Internet about carpal tunnel syndrome: Indicators of accuracy. *The American Journal of Medicine, 118,* 168–174.

Fry, E. (1968), A readability formula that saves time. *Journal of Reading, 11,* 265-71.

Fry, E. (1977). *Elementary reading instruction.* Boston: McGraw-Hill.

Gottlieb, R., & Rogers, J. L. (2004). Readability of health sites on the Internet. *The International Electronic Journal of Health Education, 7,* 38–42.

Green, L. W., & Kreuter, M. W. (1999). *Health promotion planning: An educational and ecological approach* (3rd ed.). Boston: McGraw-Hill.

Griffin, E., McKenna, K., & Worrall, L. (2004). Stroke education materials on the world wide web: An evaluation of their quality and suitability. *Topics in Stroke Rehabilitation, 1*(3), 29–40.

Gustafson, D. H., Hawkins, R. P., Boberg, E. W., McTavish, F., Owens, B., Wise, M., Berhe, H., & Pingree, S. (2002). CHESS: 10 years of research and development in consumer health informatics for broad populations, including the underserved. *International Journal of Medical Informatics, 65,* 169–177.

Haggard, E. A. (1963). Learning a process of change. In Crow, L. D., & Crow, A. (Eds.), *Readings in human learning* (p. 20). New York: McKay.

Hajjar, I., Gable, S. A., Jenkinson, V. P., Kane, L. T., & Riley, R. A. (2005). Quality of internet geriatric health information: The GeriatricWeb project. *Journal of the American Geriatric Society, 53,* 885–890.

Hamilton, S. (2005). How do we assess the learning style of our patients? *Rehabilitation Nursing, 30,* 129–131.

Heady, S. A., & Hooper, J. I. (2002). Health education. In C. L. Edelman & C. L.Mandle (Eds.), *Health promotion throughout the lifespan* (pp. 247–267). St. Louis: Mosby.

Hefzallah, I. M. (2004). *The new educational technologies and learning. Empowering teachers to teach and students to learn in the information age* (2nd ed.). Springfield, IL: Charles C. Thomas.

Houle, C. O. (1972). *The design of education.* San Francisco: Jossey-Bass.

Issel, M. (2004). *Health program planning and evaluation: A practical, systematic approach for community health.* Boston: Jones and Bartlett.

Johnson, S. A., & Romanello, M. L. (2005*).* Generational diversity: Teaching and learning approaches. *Nurse Educator, 30,* 212–216.

Joint Committee on National Health Education Standards. (1995). *National health education standards: Achieving health literacy.* New York, NY: American Cancer Society.

Jung, C. G., & Baynes, H. G. (1921). *Psychological types.* London: K. Paul Trench Trubner. (H. Godwyn Baynes, Trans., 1923). Retrieved March 2006 from http://psychclassics .yorku.ca/Jung/types.htm.

Kemm, J. (2003). Health education: A case for resuscitation. *Public Health, 117,* 106–111.

Kiel, J. M. (2005). The digital divide: Internet and email use by the elderly. *Medical Informatics and the Internet in Medicine, 30* (1), 19–23.

Kirsch, I. S., Jungeblut, A., Jenkins, L., & Kolstad, A. (1993). *Adult literacy in America: A first look at the findings of the national Adult Literacy Survey.* Washington, DC: National Center for Education Statistics, U.S. Department of Education.

Kitchie, S. (2003). Determinants of learning. In S. B. Bastable (Ed.), *Nurse as educator: Principles of teaching and learning for nursing practice* (pp. 75–118). Boston: Jones and Bartlett Publishers.

Knowles, M. S., Holton, E. F., & Swanson, R. A. (1998). *The adult learner: The definitive classic in adult education and human resource development* (5th ed.). Woburn, MA: Butterworth-Heinemann.

Knowles, M. S., Holton III, E. F., & Swanson, R. A. (2005). *The adult learner: The definitive classic in adult education and human resource development* (6th ed.). Boston: Elsevier.

Kolb, D. A. (1983). *Experiential learning: Experience as the source of learning and development.* Englewood Cliffs, NJ: Prentice-Hall.

Lewallen, L. P. (2004). Healthy behaviors and sources of health information among low-income pregnant women. *Public Health Nursing, 21*(3), 200-206.

Lewin, K., Dembo, T., Festinger, L., & Sears, P. S. (1944). Level of aspiration. In J. Hunt (Ed.), *Personality and behavior disorders.* New York: Ronald Press.

Lyberg, L., Biemer, P., Collins, M., de Leeuw, E., Dippo, C., Schwarz, N., & Trewin, D. (Eds.). (1997*). Survey measurement and process quality.* New York: John Wiley & Sons.

McLaughlin, G. (1969). SMOG grading: A new readability formula. *Journal of Reading, 12,* 639–646.

Meischke, H., Eisenberg, M., Rowe, S., & Cagle, A. (2005). Do older adults use the Internet for information on heart attacks? Results from a survey of seniors in King County, Washington. *Heart & Lung, 34,* 3–12.

Myers & Briggs Foundation. (2006). *MBTI basics.* Retrieved March, 2006, from http://www.myersbriggs.org/

National Center for Education Statistics, U. S. Department of Education. (1993). *Adult literacy in America: A first look at the findings of the National Adult Literacy Survey.* Retrieved January, 2005 from http://nces.ed.gov/ pubs93/93275.pdf.

National Center for Education Statistics, U.S. Department of Education. (2006). *National assessment of adult literacy: Health literacy.* Retrieved March 2006 from http://nces .ed.gov/NAAL/index.asp?file=AssessmentOf/HealthLiteracy.asp&PageId=12.

National Institute of Diabetes and Digestive and Kidney Diseases. (2003*). General information and national estimates on diabetes in the United States, 2000.* Retrieved May 2003 from http://www.niddk.nih.gov/health/diabetes/ pubs/dmstats/dmstats.htm.

National Institute of Mental Health. (2003). *In harm's way: Suicide in America.* Retrieved September 2006 from http://www.nimh.nih.gov/publicat/harmsway.cfm.

National Osteoporosis Foundation. (2006). *Fast Facts.* Retrieved March, 2006, from http://www.nof.org/ osteoporosis/diseasefacts.htm.

Ó Fathaigh, M. (2002, March). *E-learning and access: Some issues and implications.* Paper presented at the UACE Conference, University of Bath, Bath, United Kingdom. Retrieved August 3, 2007, from http://www.ucc.ie/en/ace/ Publications/DocumentFile,19890,en.pdf

Piotrow, P. T., Kincaid, D. L., Rimon, J., & Rinehart, W. (1997). *Health communication: Lessons learned for public health.* New York: Praeger.

Prochaska, J., DiClemente, C., & Norcross, J. (1992). In search of how people change: Applications to addictive behaviors. *The American Psychologist, 47,* 1102–1114.

Rankin, S. H., & Stallings, (1996*). Patient education: Issues, principles, practices.* (3rd ed.). Philadelphia: Lippincott Williams and Wilkins.

Reed, D. B., & Kidd, P. S. (2004). Collaboration between Nurses and Agricultural Teachers to Prevent Adolescent

Agricultural Injuries: The Agricultural Disability Awareness and Risk Education Model. *Public Health Nursing, 21,* 323–330.

Skinner, B. F. (1968). *The technology of teaching.* New York: Appleton-Century-Crofts.

Smith, D., & Kolb, D. (1986). *User's guide for the learning-style inventory: A manual for teachers and trainers.* Boston: Mcber & Company.

Society for Public Health Education. (2005*). Health education.* Retrieved January 19, 2005, from http://www.sophe.org

Spadero, D. C. (1983). Assessing readability of patient information materials. *Pediatric Nursing, 9,* 274–278.

Sternberg, R. J. (1996). Styles of thinking. In P. B. Baltes & U. M. Staudinger (Eds.), *Interactive minds: Life-span perspectives on the social foundation of cognition* (pp. 347–365). New York: Cambridge University Press.

Tak, S. H., & Hong, S. H. (2005). Use of the Internet for health information by older adults with arthritis. *Orthopaedic Nursing, 24,* 134–138.

U.S. Bureau of the Census. (2001). *A nation online: How Americans are expanding their use of the Internet.* Retrieved July 2005 from http://www.ntia.doc.gov/ntiahome/dn/hhs/HHScharts index.html.

U.S. Department of Health and Human Services (USDHHS). (2000). *Healthy People 2010: Understanding and improving health* (2nd ed). Washington, DC: U.S. Government Printing Office.

U.S. Department of Health and Human Services (USDHHS). (2003). Remarks of Vice Admiral Richard H. Carmona. "Health literacy: Key to improving American's health." *Proceedings of the H Pfizer Sixth National Health Literacy Conference.* Retrieved January 21, 2005 from http://www.surgeongeneral.gov/news/speeches/healthlit09192003.htm.

U. S. Department of Health and Human Services (USDHHS). (2004). *2004 National healthcare disparities report.* Rockville, MD: Agency for Healthcare Research and Quality.

U. S. Joint Committee on Health Education Terminology. (2002). Report of the 2000 Joint Committee on Health Education and Promotion Terminology. *Journal of School Health, 72,* 3–7.

Valente, T. W. (2002). *Evaluating health promotion programs.* New York: Oxford University Press.

Wadsworth, B. J. (1996). *Piaget's theory of cognitive and affective development.* White Plains, NY: Longman.

Web-based Education Commission. (2000). *Moving from promise to practice: Report of the Web-based Education Commission to the President and the Congress of the United States.* Retrieved July 2005 from http://www.ed.gov/offices/AC/WBEC/FinalReport/WBECReport.pdf

World Health Organization (WHO). (1998). *Health promotion glossary.* Geneva: author, Division of Health Promotion, Education, and Communications.

BIBLIOGRAPHY

Bastable, S. B. (2003). *Nurse as educator: Principles of teaching and learning for nursing practice.* Boston: Jones and Bartlett Publishers.

Bastable, S. B. (2006). *Essentials of patient education.* Boston: Jones and Bartlett Publishers.

Bensley, R. J., & Brookins-Fisher, J. (2003). *Community health education methods: A practical guide* (2nd ed.). Boston: Jones and Bartlett Publishers.

Burke, M. J., Sarpy, S. A., Smith-Crowe, K., Chan-Serafin, S., Salvador, R. O., & Islam, G. (2006). Relative effectiveness of worker safety and health training methods. *American Journal of Public Health, 96*(2), 315–324.

Chaney, E. H., Chaney, D., & Eddy, J. (2006). Utilizing a multilevel approach to support advocacy efforts in the advancement of health education. *American Journal of Health Education, 37*(1), 41–50.

Jackson, K. M., & Aiken, L. S. (2006). Evaluation of a multicomponent appearance-based sun-protective intervention for young women: Uncovering the mechanisms of program efficacy. *Health Psychology, 25*(1), 34–46.

Kelley, M. A. (2004). Culturally appropriate breast health educational intervention program for African-American women. *Journal of National Black Nurses' Association, 15*(1), 36–47.

Kirsch, I. S., Jungeblut, A., Jenkins, L., & Kolstad, A. (2002). *Adult literacy in America: A first look at the findings of the National Adult Literacy Survey* (3rd ed.). Washington, DC: U.S. Department of Education, Office of Educational Research and Improvement.

Luquis, R. R., & Pérez, M. A. (2003). Achieving cultural competence: The challenges for health educators. *American Journal of Health Education, 34*(3), 131–140.

Neuhauser, L., & Kreps, G. L. (2003). Rethinking communication in the E-health era. *Journal of Health Psychology, 8*(1), 7–23.

Rosales, A. (2004). Health education for nonreaders: Translating across cultures. *Migrant Health Newsline, 21*(4), 4–5.

Vallejos, Q, Strack, R. W., & Aronson, R. E. (2006). Identifying culturally appropriate strategies for educating a Mexican immigrant community about lead poisoning prevention. *Family & Community Health, 29*(2), 143–152.

Vastag, B. (2004). Low health literacy called a major problem. *Journal of the American Medical Association, 291*(18), 2181–2182.

Vezeau, T. M. (2005). Literacy and vulnerability. In M. deChesnay (Ed.). *Caring for the vulnerable: Perspectives in nursing theory, practice, and research* (pp. 407–418). Boston: Jones and Bartlett Publishers.

Watters, E. K. (2003). Literacy for health: An interdisciplinary model. *Journal of Transcultural Nursing, 14*(1), 48–54.

Whitehead, D. (2006). The health-promoting school: What role for nursing? *Journal of*

Clinical Nursing, 15(3), 264–271.

Wilson, K. E., & Beck, V. H. (2002). Entertainment outreach for women's health at CDC. *Journal of Women's Health & Gender-Based Medicine, 11*(7), 575–578.

RESOURCES

American Academy of Pediatrics (AAP)

141 Northwest Point Boulevard
Elk Grove Village, Illinois 60007
847-434-4000
FAX: 847-434-8000
Web: http://www.aap.org

The AAP is committed to the attainment of optimal, physical, mental, and social health and well-being for all infants, children, adolescents, and young adults. Their Web site is a resource for health professionals and parents. The site has publications and educational resources on a number of health topics relevant to pediatric and special populations and community health.

FirstGov for Consumers

Email: gateway@ftc.gov
Web: http://www.consumer.gov

FirstGov for Consumers is a link to a broad range of federal departments and information resources for consumers from the U.S. federal government. Information includes food, health and safety, money, transportation, children, and home and community. The site also has an "In the Spotlight" section that highlights new educational and consumer awareness campaigns such as scam alerts and identity theft.

Health Care Education Association (HCEA)

P.O. Box 388
Florissant, Missouri 63032-0388
1-888-298-3861
FAX: 314-869-5811
Email: Hcea03@cox.net
Web: http://www.hcea-info.org

HCEA is a professional organization of educators whose mission is to support and mentor health care educators to provide a learning community for professionals committed to improving health care and the organizations they serve through education. Full services require membership to the association, but there is information on educational products, programs, and publications that can be accessed without membership.

Health Education Assets Library (HEAL)

Email: info@healcentral.org
Web: http://www.healcentral.org

HEAL is a digital library that provides free and accessible digital teaching resources of the highest degree that meet the needs of health sciences educators and learners. Resources go through rigorous peer review to assure high quality materials.

Health Education Resource Exchange (HERE in Washington)

Washington State Department of Health
Office of Health Promotion
P.O. Box 47833
Olympia, Washington 98504-7833
Email: HERE@doh.wa.gov
Web: http://www.doh.wa.gov

The site provides public health education and health promotion projects, materials, and resources in the state of Washington and is designed to help community health professionals share their experience with colleagues around the state. There is a menu including community projects, educational materials, a health educator's toolbox, a link to make connections with other health professionals and organizations, a calendar of conferences and training opportunities, relevant health education literature, and links to other health Web sites.

Healthfinder®

P.O. Box 1133
Washington, D.C. 20013-1133.
Email: healthfinder@nhic.org
Web: http://www.healthfinder.gov

Healthfinder is sponsored by the Office of Disease Prevention and Health Promotion, U. S. Department of Health and Human Services. The site provides reliable health information for consumers including health news items, a health library, consumer guides, and organizations. There are also special sections in Spanish language and for children.

KidsHealth

Web: http://www.kidshealth.org

KidsHealth is a Web site by the Nemours, one of the largest children's health systems. The site is a resource of up-to-date, health care provider-approved information on growth, food and fitness, childhood infections, immunizations, and medical conditions for parents, kids, and teens. There are separate areas for kids, teens, and parents with age-appropriate content and delivery. In-depth features, articles, animations, games, and resources have been developed by experts in the health of children and teens.

National Cancer Institute Clear and Simple Program

NCI Public Inquiries Office
6116 Executive Boulevard, Room 3036A
Bethesda, Maryland 20892-8322
1-800-422-6237
Email: cancergovstaff@mail.nih.gov
Web: http://www.cancer.gov

The site provides a basis and introduction for producing health education materials, specifically for those with low literacy levels. The content was developed using the following five: (1) define the target audience, (2) conduct target audience research, (3) develop a concept for the product, (4) develop content and visuals, and (5) pretest and revise draft materials.

National Commission for Health Education Credentialing (NCHEC)

1541 Alta Drive, Suite 303
Whitehall, Pennsylvania 18052-5642
1-888-624-3248
FAX: 1-800-813-0727
Web: http://www.nchec.org

NCHEC's mission is to improve the practice of health education and to serve the public and profession of health education by certifying health education specialists, promoting professional development, and strengthening professional preparation and practice. The Web site provides information about responsibilities and competencies for health educators.

National Diabetes Education Program (NDEP)

One Diabetes Way
Bethesda, Maryland 20814-9692
301-496-3583
Email: ndep@mail.nih.gov
Web: http://www.ndep.nih.gov

NDEP is a partnership of the National Institutes of Health, the Centers for Disease Control and Prevention, and more than 200 public and private organizations. The site provides information on how to prevent or control diabetes, offering resources for health education, awareness campaigns, and partnerships.

National Eye Institute's National Eye Health Education Program (NEHEP)

2020 Vision Place
Bethesda, Maryland 20892-3655
301-496-5248
Email: 2020@nei.nih.gov
Web: http://www.nei.nih.gov

NEHEP conducts large-scale public and professional education programs in partnership with national organizations. Their goal is to ensure that vision is a health priority by translating eye and vision research into public and professional education programs. Their Web site provides information about NEHEP's education programs and free educational materials and public service announcements.

National High Blood Pressure Education Program (NHBPEP)

NHLBI Health Information Center
P.O. Box 30105
Bethesda, Maryland 20824-0105
301-592-8573
FAX: 301-592-8563
Email: nhlbiinfo@nhlbi.nih.gov
Web: http://www.nhlbi.nih.gov

The NHBPEP is a cooperative effort among professional and voluntary health agencies, state health departments, and many community groups and is coordinated by the National Heart, Lung, and Blood Institute. The goal of the NHBPEP is to reduce death and disability related to high blood pressure through programs of professional, client, and public education. The NHBPEP Web site features links to program description, roster and meeting notes of the coordinating committee, health-related information for clients and health care professionals, and a guide to lowering high blood pressure.

Partners in Information Access for the Public Health Workforce

Web: http://www.phpartners.org

Partners in Information Access for the Public Health Workforce is a collaboration of resources (U.S. government agencies, public health organizations, and health sciences libraries) for health educators and health promotion specialists. Their website contains resources for health educators and health promotion specialists including links to professional literature, health statistics, grants and funding, education and training, legislation and policy, conferences, and public health professionals and organizations.

Pfizer, Inc., Health Communication Initiative

Web: http://www.pfizerhealthliteracy.com

The Pfizer Foundation Health Literacy Community Grants Program funds community-based interventions that improve client outcomes and reduce health disparities. The Partnership for Clear Health Communication offers resources for improving communication with low-literacy persons. The Health Communication Initiative website contains information for public health professionals to ensure that health information is delivered in easy-to-understand, actionable, and culturally relevant terms.

Quackwatch

Web: http://www.quackwatch.com

Quackwatch, a nonprofit corporation, offers a guide to quackery, health fraud, and intelligent decisions. Some of Quackwatch activities include investigating questionable claims, answering inquiries about products and services, distributing reliable publications, improving the quality of health information, and attacking misleading advertising on the Internet.

Sexuality Information and Education Council of the U.S. School Health Education Clearinghouse (SIECUS)

130 West 42nd Street, Suite 350
New York, New York 10036-7802
212-819-9770
FAX: 212/819-9776
Web: http://www.siecus.org

SIECUS was developed to give professionals easy access to essential school health information. It provides information from all over the Web in one place on state and local policies, sexual health promotion programs, national guidelines, information on curricula, and links to additional information.

Society for Public Health Education (SOPHE)

750 First Street NE, Suite 910
Washington, D.C. 20002-4242
202-408-9804
FAX: 202-408-9815
Email: info@sophe.org
Web: http://www.sophe.org

SOPHE is an international professional association made up of a diverse membership of health education professionals and students. The society's primary focus on health education promotes healthy behaviors, healthy communities, and healthy environments. The Web site offers additional information about SOPHE as well as meetings and publications of interest to public health professionals.

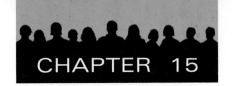

CHAPTER 15

Program Development and Evaluation

Carolyn K. Lewis, RN, PhD, CNAA, BC

Christine Elnitsky, RN, PhD, CHNS

Joanne Martin, DrPH, FAAN

Chapter Outline

◉ Program Development

◉ Planning as a Component of Program Development

◉ Frameworks in Program Development
Mission Statement Clarification
Stakeholder Analysis
Problem Identification
Strengths, Weaknesses, Opportunities, and Threats

◉ Framework for Planning Process in Program Development
Formulating
Conceptualizing
Detailing
Evaluating
Implementing

◉ Role of Economic Analysis in Decision Making for Program Development

◉ Types of Economic Analysis
Cost-Minimization Analysis
Cost-Consequence Analysis
Cost-Effectiveness Analysis
Cost-Utility Analysis
Cost-Benefit Analysis
Factors Leading to Understating or Overstating the Cost-Effectiveness of Prevention

◉ Program Evaluation
Program Components, Objectives, Outputs, and Effects
Phases and Steps in Evaluation Process

◉ Theoretical Foundations of Program Evaluation
Model One: Program Theory
Model Two: PRECEDE-PROCEED Framework
Model Three: Diffusion of Innovations Theory

◉ Decision Making in Evaluation

Learning Objectives

Upon completion of this chapter, the reader will be able to:

1. Describe program development and planning and identify the basic concepts.

2. Analyze the principles of program development to public health nursing.

3. Analyze the various cost analyses in management of health care programs.

4. Critically analyze the components of program evaluation.

5. Compare and contrast theories related to program evaluation.

The landscape of health care is dramatically changing. This transition has evolved from a profitable environment based on cost plus payment to a system with capitation and fixed reimbursement. These declining revenue streams demand more comprehensive internal analysis that determines need for new community programs and evaluation of these programs based on a rational decision-making system. Planning for new programs provides a framework and process for attaining goals and gives direction and purpose to the program. No program can be effective without planning. This chapter focuses on the historic development of public health program planning, the framework for planning, the economic analysis for decision making in program planning and the method of evaluating the impact and effectiveness of the program. More today than ever before public health nurses must be able to identify health problems and plan, design, implement, and evaluate programs that can effect positive changes in health status of defined clients using population-focused strategies.

PROGRAM DEVELOPMENT

The history of program planning as a major concept of program development has a different history than that of program evaluation. It is only within the last 10 years that this linkage between planning, development, and evaluation has begun to overlap with synergistic outcomes. Rosen (1993) believed that public health planning began approximately 4,000 years ago with the planned cities in the Indus Valley that had covered sewer systems. Blum (1981) believed planning was related to efforts that were done on behalf of the public well-being to achieve change. He further believed that planning provides a direction and strategies for proceeding with program development. Program development is the strategic alignment of activities undertaken to meet an intended purpose to ensure that an identified problem has the best possible likelihood of success with adequate resources. Planning is the core of program development; it is not a single task and can be time intensive. It is the planning, more than the plan that leads to positive outcomes in program development.

PLANNING AS A COMPONENT OF PROGRAM DEVELOPMENT

Planning is an unconscious act that occurs every day of our life; however, in the context of program develop-

ment, it becomes a conscious act. In health programs, planning is needed to identify the particular services that will produce the desired results. Planning is an organized, systematic method to conceptualize, detail, implement, and evaluate the effectiveness of a program. Today, there is a need for public health nurses to thoroughly understand program planning and development so the planning process shifts from, "What is the problem?" to "What do we need to do about this problem?" and "How do we develop a program, that when executed and evaluated will provide the desired results or stated goals?" Although there are many models in program planning and development, nurses most frequently use planning tools that closely parallel the nursing process of assessment, diagnosis, planning, implementation, and evaluation of a program. The major difference is that one set of planning tools are applied to specific populations and the other is applied to individuals, families, or communities. Further, as in the nursing process, program planning requires (1) assessing and identifying a problem or need, (2) diagnosing the problem or the need, (3) planning a strategic action plan, (4) implementing the plan to achieve a desired outcome, (5) and evaluating the plan.

FRAMEWORKS IN PROGRAM DEVELOPMENT

Pollack (1994) states that the success of new program development increases when using a four-step planning process framework known as a "pre-start up plan." The pre-start up plan includes: (1) mission statement clarification, (2) stakeholder analysis, (3) problem identification, and (4) Strengths, Weaknesses, Opportunities, and Threats (SWOT) analysis (Table 15-1). This framework is intended only as a starting point in program planning and if implemented should create a flexible planning environment. Management literature (Bryson, 1988) emphatically stresses that careful planning at the beginning point in program development will enhance any program.

Mission Statement Clarification

Mission statement clarification requires having a clear sense of direction; this will drive the activities and set the expectations of the program development. No program should occur with an unclear mission or with multiple missions. A well-developed mission statement will clearly state:

- The population served
- What is to be accomplished
- Why the service or program is provided

The mission drives the goals and objectives of the program. The goals set overall direction and are neither concrete nor quantifiable. The objectives are measurable and quantifiable and so can be used to determine whether the goals are met and further used to assess progress and possibly identify other needed programs. A program that does not expand and augment the mission will be unsuccessful.

Stakeholder Analysis

Stakeholder analysis involves identifying that group of people who have a vested interest or who may benefit from the program. Successful programs must balance the needs of the stakeholders. When developing a program, carefully consider the potential differences in the stakeholders. If the needs of the stakeholders are not addressed, the program will not be successful or survive. If a public health nurse is developing a program on middle school obesity and does not consider the students to be the critical stakeholders, they may feel degraded, intimidated, or embarrassed by the program. Thus, if this step is not completed, it is very unlikely that the identified stakeholders will participate. Pollack (1994) identified four steps in stakeholder analysis:

- Identify the target group for the program.
- Determine the criteria the stakeholders will use to assess the effectiveness of the program.
- Evaluate if the program will meet the stakeholder criteria.
- Evaluate the importance of each of the criteria.

The stakeholders and their perceptions may be the critical element that will determine the success of a program.

Problem Identification

Problem identification serves as the motivation of any new program. The gap between what is available and what is needed for the stakeholder group becomes apparent to the program planner once the problem is identified. This process may seem simple; however, data to support the identified problem must be collected. A systematic review of evidenced-based research that relates to the program topic and to the effects of an intervention needs to occur. Decisions regarding what to provide in a program as related to best practices can be made after the literature is reviewed and analyzed (Ciliska, Cullum, and Marks, 2001). In public health nursing, the best practices must come from evidence that is applicable to communities and populations, and the programs must be based on this evidence and include interventions based on proven theory and research.

Strengths, Weaknesses, Opportunities, and Threats

SWOT are valuable to the development of the program in the pre-start up planning phase. Strengths and weaknesses usually have more of an internal focus, while opportunities and threats have more of an external focus. Strengths are usually easier to identify, but if weaknesses are not identified, they will cause barriers to the success of a program. Strengths and weaknesses are often linked, and in the planning phase a weakness needs to be identified and made into a strength. Opportunities and threats, if recognized, can

TABLE 15-1: Concepts for Pre-Start Up Program Planning Framework

CONCEPTS ELEMENTS

1. Mission clarification: Statement that drives the program goals and objectives.

2. Stakeholder analysis: Individuals with a vested interest in the program.

3. Problem identification: Identifying the gap of what is needed and what is available.

4. SWOT analysis: Identifying the areas of strengths, weaknesses, opportunities, and threats.

be used to create new programs to identify opportunities that may become future threats and to use creative thinking to plan for these accordingly. These processes become powerful tools in program planning to assist in clarifying the problems and determining the program options.

FRAMEWORK FOR PLANNING PROCESS IN PROGRAM DEVELOPMENT

Nutt (1984) developed a planning process that has been useful in public health program development to identify steps in planning methodology. His process includes an organized, systematic framework of planning: (1) formulating, (2) conceptualizing, (3) detailing, (4) evaluating, and (5) implementing. Once the public health nurse defines the problem, utilizing these five steps will provide tools for successful program planning.

Formulating

This stage in program development is the most crucial; formulating consists of defining the problem based on a needs assessment of the program population. Witkin and Altschuld (1995, p. 4) define a needs assessment "as a systematic set of procedures undertaken for the purpose of setting priorities and making decisions about program or organizational improvement and allocation of resources." The priorities are based on the identified needs. A needs assessment will give information and value perceptions and can be used as a tool for program planning to identify those needs for a specific population or group of people. This will serve as a rational approach in identifying specific areas of need and will serve as a mechanism in developing programs to meet or ameliorate the identified needs of the targeted population. The program can now be formulated by considering data from the needs assessment, to assure success.

Witkin and Altschuld (1995) further delineate a three-phase plan for assessing needs. The first phase is pre-assessment, which determines what is already known about needs in the population, decisions on boundaries, sources of data, and how data will be used to determine the need. The second phase is the main assessment, or the data gathering. This involves analyzing the data and formulating opinions on the needs and priority setting. The third phase is the post-assessment phase and involves using the data to plan for the action. This phase would be the program planning phase, where the data are collected and analyzed, and the action plans are begun. The information and action plan are then communicated to the stakeholders. The evaluation of the needs assessment is also completed in phase three.

In formulating the plan, the program population must be identified and assessed, the need of this target population must be identified, and the population must be involved in the program planning. The size and geography of the population must be determined and identified if there are other programs addressing the need. The boundaries for the identified population are established by the need and the program goals that are formulated. Another important consideration when formulating the plan is the feasibility of the program, especially identifying the stakeholders, internally and externally, who agree with the need for the program and those who do not. Completion of this phase will formulate the need and demand for the program.

Conceptualizing

The second stage of Nutt's systematic framework is the conceptualizing phase, that is, the articulation of thoughts and ideas in an objective format. This involves finding solutions to the needs identified in the formulation phase and identifying those risks and potential outcomes. Frequently, to identify one's thoughts and ideas, concept mapping or decision trees are used to assist in problem solving and to aid in selecting the best solutions with the best identified outcomes. In concept mapping or decision trees, a pictorial representation of one's thinking is displayed in order to show how the ideas relate to each other. This allows for the selection of ideas or concepts that are more relevant or important to the main issue.

Detailing

In the third stage, the feasibility of moving forward with the program is assessed in relation to the solutions that have been identified in the conceptualization phase; this is termed detailing. Once stakeholders or decision makers are confident about the identified solution, additional planning will follow. Objectives that will meet the program goal(s) are formulated for the identified solution(s). These need to be measured against the activities needed to conduct the alternative solutions. Details of the program plan are outlined for the determined solution as well as the alternative solutions. Goals and objectives derived from learning needs and stakeholders' interests are assumed to have greater value than those goals and objectives derived in other ways. Objectives illuminate and guide all subsequent actions in program design and planning.

Evaluating

In this phase, those alternatives from the previously described detailing phase are evaluated related to costs, economic analysis, benefits, and how the program provider, the population, and the community may react to the alternatives. The feasibility and practicality of conducting the program to meet the desired outcomes are evaluated. Information and data are collected to assist in the evaluative phase, and changes are made based upon the analysis.

Implementing

In the final phase, implementing, the best plan is selected to meet the needs of the target population. The goals and objectives must reflect the solution that has

⊕ PRACTICE APPLICATION

Evidence-Based Practice

Evidence-based practice is now the standard of care for public health nursing programs. However, lack of sufficient resources often limits the extent to which evidence-based practice can be implemented. In making decisions, nurses need to weigh the economic evidence along with research evidence, clinical expertise, and client or community values. Therefore, nurses need to understand how to measure the economic values of different interventions (Stone, Curran, & Bakken, 2002).

the greatest value in meeting the defined problem/need. The solution chosen must be based on the data collected in the evaluating phase.

If the five planning stages in Nutt's process are followed, the desired outcomes, which are population focused and consider the well-being of the public, will be achieved. Planned programs bear a distinct advantage over unplanned ones. Planned programs are targeted for a particular population to meet a determined

⊕ RESEARCH APPLICATION

Stroke Care in the Home: The Impact of Social Support on the General Health of Family Caregivers

Study Purpose

To investigate elements of social support available to family caregivers during the first 12-weeks of home care of their family member following stroke.

Methods

This cross-sectional descriptive study used regression models to explain types of social support received and the general health of family caregivers. Characteristics of situation-specific supports were examined using open-ended questions.

Findings

Health care tasks were the most stressful for family caregivers. Tangible support and information support were

inadequate. Professional advice and feedback on home care skills were inadequate.

Implications

Social support is an important function of community nursing care. Findings of the study provide planning information and data to better coordinate community stroke care support services.

Reference

Sit, J. W., Wong, T. K., Clinton, M., Li, L. S., & Fong, Y. M. (2004). Stroke care in the home: The impact of social support on the general health of family caregivers. *Journal of Clinical Nursing, 13*(7), 816–824.

need. Research conducted by Winer and Vázquez-Abad (1995, p. 60) revealed common reasons why program planners do not perform typical steps in planning. They found that the most common reasons were:

- Program planner lacked expertise.
- Step was not supported by stakeholders.
- Decision had already been reached without taking the step.
- Step was viewed as unnecessary.
- Insufficient time existed.
- Money was not available to support taking the step.

Program planning is a comprehensive process, and the literature contains many program-planning models that have merit, usability, and practicality. The most important element to note is that effective program planning must be carefully and thoroughly completed to achieve desired outcomes.

ROLE OF ECONOMIC ANALYSIS IN DECISION MAKING FOR PROGRAM DEVELOPMENT

It is important to recognize the role economic analysis actually plays in decision making. First, it can inform the decision makers, but it is not a major deciding factor. Values such as justice, social welfare, and religious beliefs often trump economic evidence. Policy makers are loath to consider costs when saving lives is at stake. For example, the high-profile debate over end-of-life in Florida eventually reached the floor of the United States Congress in 2005. Economic analysis was not a main criterion for policy makers.

Second, economic analysis does not tell the decision maker if the increased expenditure is worthwhile. When evaluation of a new intervention demonstrates improved outcomes, economic analysis can determine how much more it would cost to achieve better outcomes. The decision makers are better informed, but they still need to judge if the improvement is worth the increased expenditure.

Third, rigorous economic analysis is not always available. It is complex, and doing a proper analysis is not easy. Yet, if not done properly, economic analysis can be misleading. Understandably, policy makers hesitate to base their decisions on results of an analysis they do not understand.

Given these caveats, why should public health nurses care about economic analysis? Efforts to improve standardization of economic analyses likely will increase its availability and utilization (Bell et al., 2001; Neumann et al., 2000; Phillips & Chen, 2002; Siegel et al., 1996; Stone et al., 2000a; Stone et al., 2000b; Weinstein et al., 1996). Public health nurses need to become astute consumers who develop a good understanding of economic analysis and know how to use it. They then will be better equipped to make good decisions

Public health nurses also need to participate in doing economic analyses. As a profession, nurses have lagged behind other disciplines in publishing economic analyses (Stone, Curran, & Bakken, 2002). Relatively few nurses have developed sufficient expertise in doing economic analysis. However, a multidisciplinary team approach makes it feasible. Public health nurses have clinical insight and expertise and health economists bring expertise in economic analysis.

Wise decisions will need to be made about allocating scarce public resources. Policy makers may come to rely more on economic analysis as pressures increase to meet the needs of an aging population. Public health nurses who broaden their expertise to include economic analysis will be prepared to contribute significantly to public policy and decision making. Policy makers can benefit from advice provided by a knowledgeable clinician who understands the implications of economic analysis.

TYPES OF ECONOMIC ANALYSIS

A full tutorial on methods and techniques used in performing an economic analysis is beyond the scope of this chapter. The intent of this section is to familiarize public health nurses with five types of economic analysis and encourage further exploration. This is a beginning step toward improving utilization of economic analysis in public health decision making and incorporating proper economic analysis into program evaluation and research.

Cost-Minimization Analysis

Cost-minimization analysis (CMA) assumes each approach has equal effects. Therefore, it compares only the costs between alternative approaches. CMA is used to determine which alternative is least costly. CMA is appropriate when alternative approaches truly are equally effective. However, this is rarely the case. Therefore, CMA usually is not an appropriate method of analysis in health care.

Cost-Consequence Analysis

Cost-consequence analysis (CCA) measures the consequences as well as the costs. The cost and outcomes for each approach are listed separately so the decision maker can interpret and weigh the findings. For example, a CCA of two home visiting programs would list the cost for each program and then list the measurable outcomes. Option 1 might cost $600,000 per year for 100 families and outcome measures would include changes in HOME scale scores in the first 6 months after birth and number of unintended subsequent pregnancies in the first 12 months after birth. Option 2 might cost $500,000 per year for 100 families and the same outcome measures would be used.

Each outcome has a different measure, thus it is harder to compare across outcomes. Compared with Option 2, Option 1 costs an average of $1,000 more per year for each family, but it is more effective in reducing unintended pregnancy and improving parent-child interaction. Is this worth the increased incremental expenditure? Would it still be a worthwhile investment if Option 1 costs an average of $1,000 more per year for each family but only improves parent-child interaction or only reduces unintended pregnancies? Although CCA can be used in health care, these are examples of questions raised rather than answered by the analysis.

Cost-Effectiveness Analysis

Cost-effectiveness analyses (CEA) measures outcomes in the same units across alternatives, typically dollars per life year. This allows the analyst to calculate a cost-effectiveness ratio. It works best when there is a single outcome of interest. The decision maker can learn how much more it would cost to get a defined amount of improved outcome. The cost-effectiveness ratio is calculated as $(C_1 - C_2)/(E_1 - E_2)$ or the difference between the cost of Option 1 and cost of Option 2 divided by the difference between the effects of Option 1 and the effects of Option 2. For example, the cost of Option 1 might be $6,000 per person and the cost of Option 2 might be $5,000 per person. If the effect of Option 1 is living 3 years and the effect of Option 2 is living 2 years, the cost-effectiveness ratio would be

$1,000/1 year. It would cost an extra $1,000 to extend life for 1 year.

Cost-Utility Analysis

Cost-utility analysis (CUA) overcomes a disadvantage inherent in CEA. The dollars per life year gained does not measure the quality of the life year gained. It does not distinguish between a person who is relatively healthy and functional and a person who has a severe disability. CUA is a variation on CEA because it measures both quality and quantity of life. The outcome measure is quality-adjusted life years or QALYs. Different methods are used to determine the quality of life, based upon individual preferences or utility. Usually perfect health is 1 on a scale of 0–1 and death is 0. QALY is calculated as the utility times the number of years. If utility is 0.7 (somewhat less than perfect health) and the person lives 30 years, it would be 21 QALYs. This level of analysis is recommended by the U.S. Office of the Assistant Secretary for Health Panel on Cost Effectiveness in Health and Medicine because use of a standardized measure allows comparison across populations and disease states (Gold et al., 1996; Russell et al., 1996; Siegel et al., 1996; Weinstein et al., 1996).

Cost-Benefit Analysis

Cost-benefit analysis (CBA) measures both costs and outcomes in dollars. This allows the analyst to calculate a single-dollar figure by subtracting benefits from costs. In health care, this can be problematic because it is difficult to assign a dollar figure to life. Even if it were possible to calculate the dollar amount, ethical issues are an important concern; therefore, CBA is not used as much as CEA.

Factors Leading to Understating or Overstating the Cost-Effectiveness of Prevention

Prevention is touted as a way to improve health status and reduce health care costs, yet prevention accounts for only 3 percent of total health expenditures. Does the use of economic analyses help or hurt the argument for spending more money on prevention? Sometimes the methods used in economic analysis help, and sometimes they hurt.

⊕ RESEARCH APPLICATION

Transitional Care of Older Adults Hospitalized with Heart Failure: A Randomized, Controlled Trial

Study Purpose

To examine the effectiveness of comprehensive transitional care directed by advance practice nurses (APN) in reducing re-hospitalizations and total health care costs and in improving quality of life, satisfaction with care, and functional status. Re-hospitalization of elder adults with heart failure is estimated to cost over $24.3 billion in direct health care expenditures each year. Older adults have high rates of preventable poor post-discharge outcomes during the transition period from hospital to home.

Methods

Eligible clients 65 and older hospitalized with heart failure were randomly assigned to a control group or intervention group. The control group (n = 121) received routine hospital care and standard care from a home care agency. The intervention group (n = 118) received care management by three masters-prepared APNs, who received 2 months of special training from a multidisciplinary team of heart failure experts. The protocol included daily visits during the index hospitalization and at least eight APN home visits (weekly during the first month and biweekly during second and third months). Research assistants (RAs) conducted structured telephone interviews periodically during the first 52 weeks after hospital discharge. Data were abstracted from client records and bills. Resource costs were estimated using Medicare reimbursement. Intervention costs were calculated from detailed logs of intervention-related efforts and representative annual salaries, plus benefits.

Findings

Control and intervention groups were similar in baseline sociodemographic and clinical characteristics and attrition due to death or withdrawal. The intervention group experienced fewer re-hospitalizations and death at 52 weeks and longer time intervals between index hospital discharge and readmission or death. Total and mean costs per client were lower in the intervention group. Adjusting for unequal follow-up, mean 52-week costs were $7,636 for the intervention group and $12,481 for the control group, resulting in a mean cost savings of $4,845 per client. Higher direct costs for the intervention group were a result of additional APN home visits, higher APN salaries, and involvement of heart failure experts. However, those costs were more than offset by reductions in other home visits, acute care visits, and re-hospitalizations. In addition, quality of life and satisfaction with care were enhanced in the intervention group. There was no difference between groups in functional status.

Implications

A nursing intervention that results in a 37.6% reduction in total health care expenditures is impressive, especially when it involves a growing population group whose health care is financed by shrinking public dollars. Promising approaches such as this have been stymied by lack of Medicare reimbursement and health care delivery systems organized around a traditional medical model. In this case, economic analysis supports adoption of a more effective, efficient, acceptable model of care. Economic analysis will not be the sole deciding factor, but it could provide policy makers with convincing evidence to change reimbursement policies. It is hard to ignore spending less money to achieve a better outcome. When public dollars are at stake and public policies are involved, tertiary prevention is an important public health issue.

Reference

Naylor, M. D., Brooten, D. A., Campbell, R. L., Maislin, G., McCauley, K. M., & Schwartz, J. S. (2004). Transitional care of older adults hospitalized with heart failure: A randomized, controlled trial. *Journal of American Geriatrics Society, 52,* 675–684.

Three methods of valuation affect the economic analysis of prevention efforts: discounting, externalities, and intangibles. Discounting values future costs and benefits. Externalities refer to the way costs and benefits are valued for people who are not the users of preventive services. Intangibles refer to how nonmonetary costs and benefits are valued.

Discounting is universally recommended. Both the costs and health benefits need to be discounted using a standard rate. Individuals vary widely in their judgment of future values. The standard rate is considered a social discount rate and is especially appropriate for population-based policies. The U.S. Office of the Assistant Secretary for Health Panel on Cost-Effectiveness in Health and Medicine recommends a discount rate of 3 percent (Gold et al., 1996). Health care evaluations commonly use 5 percent. Discounting reduces the cost-effectiveness of prevention because the cost of the intervention is present value and the benefits occur in the future when the value is discounted. At 3 percent, about half the value is discounted after 24 years. Sensitivity analyses using 0 and 5 percent can be used to examine the impact of discounting.

Using commonly accepted methods of discounting adversely affects the economic analysis of prevention efforts because of the relatively long lag time between the intervention and the benefits of improved health status. A lower discount rate might better reflect how society values prevention, and it would make prevention appear more cost-effective. However, using a different discount rate is a value judgment that might not be uniformly shared (Phillips & Holtgrave, 1997). Public health nurses need to understand how discounting affects prevention. Discounting reduces the cost-effectiveness of any intervention when costs are current and benefits occur in the future.

Compared with treatment, prevention has costs and benefits that accrue to people who are not the users of the service. These are termed externalities and should be included in the economic analysis. Costs of prevention are often paid by someone else who rarely receives the benefit. For example, insurers and employers pay for the health care that employees receive. Taxpayers pay for health care that benefits elderly, disabled, pregnant, and young Medicaid recipients. Economic analysis usually fails to include benefits to future generations. Even if benefits were included, discounting would substantially reduce the value of benefits that occur in the far future (Phillips & Holtgrave, 1997).

Tracking the costs for people who are not the direct users of the prevention intervention is challenging. Equally challenging is linking prevention to future health outcomes. If it is not feasible to include this in the analysis, potential costs and benefits to nonusers should at least be identified and discussed. If attempts are made to estimate current and future costs and benefits, underlying assumptions should be clearly stated.

When the external and future benefits are excluded from economic analysis, the cost-effectiveness of prevention will be understated. When external and future costs are excluded, the cost-effectiveness of prevention will be overstated. If prevention programs

🌐 RESEARCH APPLICATION

Cost Assessment of a School-Based Mental Health Screening and Treatment Program in New York City

Study Purpose

To estimate the cost of a school-based mental health screening and treatment program and provide a model for exploring the costs of such programs.

Methods

Students in grades 6–8 were screened for depression, anxiety, and substance use in a middle school in a low-income, largely Hispanic neighborhood in New York City. Social workers offered individual and group counseling. Costs of screening and treatment were assessed using a before and after study design with societal perspective, economic methods, and administrative data and staff interviews.

Findings

Screening cost per student ranged from $149 to $234, and treatment cost per session ranged from $90 to $115.

Implications

The process of cost analysis can generate useful estimates for decision making in school programs.

Reference

Chatterji, P., Caffray, C. M., Crowe, M., Freeman, L., & Jensen, P. (2004). Cost assessment of a school-based mental health screening and treatment program in New York City. *Mental Health Services Research, 6*(3), 155–166.

provide significant benefits or costs to nonusers, externalities should be included, and the analysis should measure both costs and benefits (Phillips & Holtgrave, 1997).

Intangibles, or nonmonetary benefits and costs, associated with prevention should be included in the analysis. Inclusion or exclusion of intangibles in the analysis affects the cost-effectiveness of prevention. One benefit of effective prevention is that nothing bad happens going forward. For example, children who are immunized against measles do not contract the disease. Proper use of seat belts prevents serious motor vehicle injuries and deaths. Intangible benefits also occur from the time preventive measures are initiated until some future date. Not worrying that their child will have complications from measles or reduced fear of motor vehicle crash is an intangible benefit. Peace of mind is an intangible benefit resulting from a normal prenatal ultrasound examination. If the ultrasound is abnormal, time to psychologically prepare for birth is an intangible benefit.

Intangible costs of prevention need to be considered and included in an economic analysis. If wearing seat belts increases reckless driving, this would be an intangible cost of prevention. Likewise, a false sense of security from improperly installed child safety seats could be considered an intangible cost of a prevention effort. Unnecessary anxiety from false-positive HIV test results would be another intangible cost of prevention. Time and effort spent on preventive behaviors to improve health is an intangible cost, especially when it detracts from other worthwhile or more enjoyable activities.

Economic analysis of prevention programs can provide useful information for deciding how to allocate scarce resources. Prevention can save money, and policy makers often hear the chant of "pay now or pay later." The role of economic analysis is expanding, and prevention advocates need to be keenly aware of its methodological pitfalls for prevention programs. Public health nurses who are interested in learning more about economic analysis can read the resources provided at the end of this chapter. Public health nurses who want to develop expertise in this area should consider enrolling in appropriate credit or continuing education courses or workshops.

PROGRAM EVALUATION

Program evaluation is the "use of scientific methods to measure the implementation and outcomes of programs, for decision-making purposes" (Rutman & Mow-bray, 1983, p. 12). Evaluation is concerned with the implementation and impact of public health programs. A public health program is defined as an intervention, or set of activities, to meet a social need. The program focus is on implementation and outcomes; understanding how the program activities are delivered informs management decisions about modifications to help achieve program objectives. Evaluation allows assessment of both the quality of administration and the value of the program. Understanding the program processes allows public health nurses to relate the activities to the outcomes.

Program evaluation may be further defined by time elements, methods, and purpose and focus. The evaluation of a public health program may be scheduled as a periodic assessment or as an on-going monitoring activity. An on-going measurement system can be incorporated into program delivery and administrative records. On-going monitoring allows continued assessment as projects are modified during their life spans and adjustments to program processes as information is provided to decision makers.

Operations, management processes, strategic planning, personnel performance appraisals, and support services, though important to program management, are not the focus in program evaluation.

To clarify concepts in program evaluation, a single program will be used for illustrative purposes in the remaining pages of this chapter. The Rural Nurse Practitioner Mobile Health Unit (RNPMHU) was an innovative health delivery system that provided primary care health services to older adults in rural communities along the eastern seaboard (funded by a national Institute of Nursing Research grant). Explanation of evaluation concepts will be based largely on this advanced practice nursing delivery system.

Program Components, Objectives, Outputs, and Effects

The evaluation focuses on **program components**, objectives, outputs, and effects. Public health programs are composed of several components. Each component of the program has specific objectives associated with it. For example, in the RNPMHU program, components included health education sessions and ambulatory care treatment.

Program objectives are the aims that the public health program is meant to achieve. The program manager directs resources and activities toward the program objectives. Objectives may be immediate, intermediate, or ultimate. Ultimate objectives are long-term benefits to the population. The intermediate aims of the RNPMHU program were to improve or maintain functional and health status, and increase health promotion behaviors of older residents in the community. The program provided services for nearly 250 residents in two rural counties.

Program outputs represent the services provided in a public health program. Such services may also be known as the program's activities. The program is accomplished according to these prespecified activities. For example, the RNPMHU outputs could be the number of educational sessions provided and number of persons receiving primary care services from nurse practitioners.

Program effects represent the consequences of the program components. Such consequences should include both those that are intended and those that are unintended. To show evidence that the program compo-nents resulted in the specific consequences requires linkages between program components, outputs, and objectives. Objectives may include both proximal and distal aims. Public health programs may evaluate knowledge, health and functional status outcomes, as well as cost-effectiveness or cost-utility outcomes.

Program evaluation serves as the mechanism to provide information on the programs' interventions and outcomes. The information is used to facilitate management and decision making about the program. The program evaluation may have dual purposes based on the external and internal stakeholder perspectives.

For external sponsors, the program evaluation informs purpose, relevance, and financial priorities. Evaluation is a tool that aids decision making, such as cutting budgets in an environment of economic constraints. The advent of the Government Performance and Results Act (GPRA) indicated an increased emphasis on performance measurement in federal, state, and local governments and public programs (Koskinen, 1997). External sponsors require evidence that programs

---

⊕ RESEARCH APPLICATION

Patterns of Utilization for the Minnesota Senior Health Options Program

Study Purpose
To compare utilization of health services covered by Minnesota Senior Health Options (MSHO; a special program designed to serve dually eligible older persons) with utilization of those covered by fee-for-service Medicare and Medicaid managed care.

Methods
Clinical trial using quasi experimental design with two control and one treatment group of dually eligible elderly in urban Minnesota community and nursing home long-term care. Control groups were non-enrollees living in the same area and another from comparable persons living in another urban area where the program was not available.

Findings
MSHO enrollees had fewer preventable hospitalizations and emergency services than the control group in the same area. MSHO nursing home enrollees had fewer hospital admissions than either control group.

Implications
The results of the evaluation favored MSHO. Lower utilization rates of MSHO enrollees suggests the MSHO program influenced the care process perhaps by providing more preventive and community-based services for residents of this community.

Reference
Kane, R. L., Homyak, P., Bershadsky, B., Flood, S., & Zhang, H. J. (2004). Patterns of utilization for the Minnesota Senior Health Options program. *American Geriatrics Society, 52*(12), 2039–2044.

have a positive impact, thus evaluation must gather such evidence.

For internal program managers, evaluation has another purpose. In this case, the evaluation facilitates continuous learning about the program, problem solving, program delivery, and program improvement throughout the life span of the program. The program manager uses evaluation as a tool for making decisions about the program. Evaluation results may facilitate program changes and improvements by providing information about:

- Design and delivery of projects
- Type and amount of resources
- Measures of program inputs, processes, outcomes
- Development of indicators and performance metrics
- How programs are being implemented
- Accomplishments, barriers, facilitators, and lessons learned
- Recommendations for program improvement

Phases and Steps in Evaluation Process

Program evaluations consist of five phases: (1) identifying program objectives, (2) selecting or creating measures of impacts, (3) collecting data, (4) interpreting data in terms of the evaluation framework and program context (Polit & Beck, 2004), and (5) disseminating the evaluation information. Steps in the evaluation process vary based on the role of the individual involved. Program evaluations may be conducted internally or externally, that is, the program manager may conduct the evaluation or employ the expertise of an external program evaluator.

Manager Steps

For the program manager, the first step in the evaluation process is to determine the purpose of the evaluation. The second step is to evaluate the pros and cons of internal versus external evaluation and to consider mixed internal and external evaluator roles. In the RNPMHU program, combined internal and external evaluator roles were used. The program manager worked directly with the external evaluator to design and implement the evaluation. Program evaluation purposes included assessment of the impacts and the cost-effectiveness of the program and its interventions.

Evaluator Steps

For the evaluator, the first step is to identify the purpose, objectives, and questions of interest in collaboration with the program manager and base these on an applicable theory. The second step is to design the most rigorous evaluation possible within the practical constraints of the situation. The evaluator considers the level of rigor necessary based on the identified purpose, feasibility, resources, timeline, and availability of data, measurement instruments, and staff. In the RNPMHU program, the evaluator consulted with the program manager, reviewed program documents, and interviewed program staff to design the model and both cross-sectional and longitudinal evaluations.

The evaluator examines the assessment of the program. Using this process, the evaluator will fully understand the program and its true purpose and the environmental context of the evaluation. The process of developing the program theory includes evaluating the assessment of the program. As the theory is developed, the evaluator often discovers that the program is not ready for a formal evaluation. Further program development and refinement of objectives or implementation activities may be indicated. The program design may be altered to be consistent with new information about what is known to work. Program implementation may be improved to increase the likelihood of affecting outcomes. In the RNPMHU Program, the external evaluator conducted an evaluation of the assessment during development of the program logic model. Program objectives were clearly stated in the grant proposal, facilitating planning and design of the program evaluation.

A formative evaluation may provide a better understanding of the program processes and effects and may lead to continuous improvement or change in program goals and objectives (Figure 15-1).

The process of developing the program theory often helps the evaluator prioritize evaluation questions and helps the manager decide how to focus the evaluation purpose and allocate evaluation resources. Logical theory or program theory, specific evaluation questions, and practical considerations inform the methodological choices. During the formative evaluation of the RNPMHU program, interviews of local community-

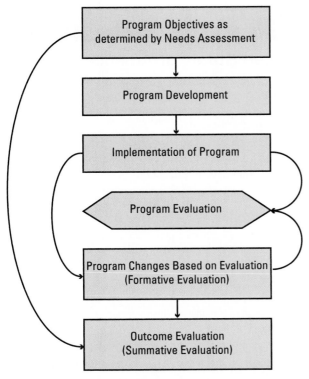

Figure 15-1 The relationship between program development and evaluation.

based collaborators and field program staff provided rich data on how to improve enrollment of community-based clients. Recommended program changes included locations for the mobile health unit (e.g., shopping center versus social services facility) and days of the week for practitioners to be present (e.g., Tuesday versus Wednesday). In addition, to meet the needs of the clients, program staff identified needed program changes such as changes to measurement instruments and educational informational handouts.

The program evaluation will follow a design established by the evaluator to appraise the program's effectiveness, efficiency, and quality objectively and without bias. Evaluation design depends upon the purpose of the evaluation, the objects of interest, and the standards of acceptability. Comparisons incorporated into the design may focus on changes over time, between groups, or both. The study design selection aims to omit errors in interpretation of results. Therefore, the evaluation will employ valid and reliable measurement tools and methods in the collection of program information. Because the RNPMHU program was implemented over multiple years and used multiple methods, the program evaluation employed prospective longitudinal as well as cross-sectional nested study designs. A participatory, theory-driven approach was used. This set of studies used qualitative interviews and quantitative data collection techniques. A basic cost-benefit analysis of the program was conducted, providing further support for program outcomes.

The Centers for Disease Control (1999) Framework for Planning and Implementing Practical Program Evaluation is used in public health. The framework is composed of steps in program evaluation practice as well as standards for effective program evaluation. The framework describes six steps taken in any evaluation. The first step is to engage stakeholders in identifying their values and information needs and to help with other steps. Stakeholders include sponsors, collaborators, administrators, staff, clients, families, neighbors, advocacy groups, institutions, organizations, professional associations, and primary users of the evaluation. In the RNPMHU program, the evaluator consulted and collaborated with all stakeholders—community organizations, staff, and program manager—throughout the project.

The second step describes the public health program, the program mission and objectives, its stage of development, and its relationship with the larger organization and community. It is important to identify expected effects of the program, activities, resources, and setting and environmental context. This step further includes the creation of the program logic model summarizing the planned changes by linking processes to ultimate effects. The RNPMHU objectives and effects were incorporated into the program logic model. Both expected and unintended effects were considered. The program expected to improve health promotion behaviors of the older adult participants and measured these effects, but it also considered the possibility of unintended hospitalization due to chronic illness and injury and measured these unintended effects as well.

In the third step, the focus is on the evaluation design. This requires identifying the evaluation's purpose and the users of evaluation findings as well as specific uses of the evaluation findings. Questions about the various aspects of the program, the scientific research methods used, and the roles and responsibilities of the stakeholders

⊕ POLICY HIGHLIGHT

Development of Aging Policy in the United States of America

Public Law 106-501 sec. 201 of the Older Americans Act Amendments of 2000 establishes the authority to convene the White House Conference on Aging (U.S. Government, 2000). The purpose of the White House Conference on Aging (WHCoA) is to develop recommendations for aging policy to guide the President, Congress, and federal agencies, state, tribes, communities, private sector, and individuals in the needs of older adults. The 2005 WHCoA sought input from a wide array of stakeholders including public health nurses to develop an agenda for the conference. Issues were identified and refined through public input received from participants in more than 400 events and from general comments received by the WHCoA involving approximately 130,000 people across the nation from August 2004 to December 2005. Independent aging events, listening sessions, solutions forums and miniconferences organized by communities, academic institutions, business and industry, national and local organizations, and public agencies were held across the country to provide public input to the 2005 WHCoA. The WHCoA Policy Committee made available for comment and adopted a broad agenda of issues facing the older adult population. Policy agenda categories identified by the WHCoA include:

⊕ Planning along the life span

⊕ The workplace of the future

⊕ Our community

⊕ Health and long-term living

⊕ Civic and social engagement

⊕ Technology and innovation in an emerging senior/boomer marketplace

Recommendations in reports and innovative solutions from public and private sectors were drafted into 73 resolutions related to each WHCoA agenda section.

On December 12, 1,200 delegates to the 2005 WHCoA selected the top 50 resolutions they believed were the most important for current and future generations of senior citizens. Groups of delegates identified and supported specific actions to implement the new policies contained in the resolutions. In addition, delegates specified policy makers and organizations responsible for accomplishing the activities. For example, actions may be recommended for implementation by federal, state, tribal, or local government, communities, nonprofit organizations, business/industry, or individuals.

The top 10 resolutions as selected and voted by the delegates are:

1. Reauthorize the Older Americans Act within the first 6 months following the 2005 White House Conference on Aging

2. Develop a coordinated, comprehensive long-term care strategy by supporting public and private sector initiatives that address financing, choice, quality, service delivery, and the paid and unpaid workforce

3. Ensure that older Americans have transportation options to retain their mobility and independence

4. Strengthen and improve the Medicaid program for seniors

5. Strengthen and improve the Medicare program

6. Support geriatric education and training for all health care professionals, paraprofessionals, health profession students, and direct care workers

7. Promote innovative models of noninstitutional long-term care

8. Improve recognition, assessment, and treatment of mental illness and depression among older Americans

9. Attain adequate numbers of health care personnel in all professions who are skilled, culturally competent, and specialized in geriatrics

10. Improve state- and local-based integrated delivery systems to meet twenty-first-century needs of seniors (WHCoA, 2005)

By statute, the final report of the 2005 WHCoA was delivered to Congress and the President of the United States in June 2006. The next steps in the evolution of aging policy promise to involve all levels of public and private partners in the community to improve the well-being of older Americans and ensure independent aging for the baby boomer population and those that follow.

are also addressed in this step. Several studies related to the RNPMHU program were conducted; these studies included methodological studies of multiple measures to identify clusters of clients based on different levels of health and functional status needs.

The fourth step is to gather credible evidence. Credible evidence meets the standards of the primary users. Furthermore, the credibility of evidence depends on the evaluation questions and the planned uses of the findings. It may be necessary to consult an external evaluator on issues of data quality, indicators, sources of evidence, or evaluation methods and protocol. Evidence collected in the RNPMHU program included health and functional status, health promotion behaviors, cost-benefit measures, and utilization of health services. These measures met the requirements of sponsors, those funding the program, and the program manager.

In the fifth step, the program evaluation conclusions are justified. At this phase, program inputs are linked to evidence and judged in light of agreed-upon values and standards. Data are collected, analyzed, synthesized, and interpreted. Finally, judgments and recommendations are made. The program manager, staff, sponsors, and those funding the program considered the conclusions reached in the RNPMHU program. As stated, the formative evaluation conclusions led to changes in program practices.

The sixth step is to ensure use of the evaluation and share the lessons learned. This step involves communicating findings with the stakeholders and providing follow-up technical and emotional support for users during and following evaluation. Dissemination or communication of procedures and lessons learned to relevant audiences is included in this step. Lessons learned and evaluation findings were disseminated in a variety of manners in the RNPMHU program. For example, findings were reported to community partners in collaborative meetings. Final reports to the sponsors and those funding the program provided substantive feedback for future planning by the sponsor. Peer-reviewed abstracts, panel discussions, and poster presentations were provided at professional public health nursing and health services research conferences. Multiple manuscripts were submitted for scientific peer review and published in professional research journals, disseminating results to readers on an international scale.

THEORETICAL FOUNDATIONS OF PROGRAM EVALUATION

This section considers the agreement of principles in models of program evaluation and provides an overview of three models. Theoretical frameworks provide conceptual models, evolving from empirical observations, to organize and guide the evaluation process and interpretation of results. The evaluation models discussed here are based on three common principles. First, each of the program evaluation models assumes populations, communities, and programs will change and grow throughout their life cycles. Second, linkages or relationships between components in the theories are based on a systems or quality approach. A systems approach would document inputs and processes of the program and measure outcomes and improvements in program performance. Third, the models emphasize the need for flexibility in programs to adapt to local community, organization context, and stakeholder priorities. Participant and stakeholder perspectives should be represented in planning, establishing objectives, implementing activities, and evaluating the programs. Local community needs and resources and organizational practices, policies, and procedures must be considered. Three evaluation models are discussed.

Model One: Program Theory

The notion of an implicit conceptual model, a theory of action for understanding how programs work and for assessing their effectiveness, emerged nearly 40 years ago (Suchman, 1967). The theory of action implies the links between program inputs and ultimate effects as specified in program components, objectives and the environment or context under which the effects are to be achieved. Today these are commonly known as logic models.

Logic models focus on developing a model of the reasoning implicit in the public health program design, a model of how the program works. The model describes the logical process by which program inputs and activities are intended to create the outcomes or effects (Donaldson, 2003). The logic model provides the basis for a plausible story for the programs' intended performance. Such theories of action, or logic models, are useful frameworks for identifying short- and long-term outcomes of programs (Funnell, 2000).

Evaluators have used logic models for at least 25 years (McLaughlin & Jordan, 1998). The logic model approach to evaluation practice is the foundation of widely used textbooks on program evaluation (Donaldson & Scriven, 2003; Rossi, Freeman, & Lipsey, 1999; Weiss, 1998). Models are developed by assessing the public health program and its purpose. The logic model is both descriptive and prescriptive; that is, manager, staff, and documents are used to explain program components and the logic of how the program works (Chen, 1990). Stakeholder perceptions of how the program works, also known as "espoused theory of action" (Patton, 1997), may be included in the logic model.

The logic model theoretical framework focuses on features of the program and its intended performance. Specific factors that must be considered are resource inputs, activities, outputs, customers, outcomes (short term, intermediate, and long term), and key contextual factors external to the program that could influence its outcomes. The activity of identifying these factors and their interrelationships helps clarify program assumptions on which performance expectations are set (Weiss, 1997).

Alexy and Elnitsky (1998) developed a logic model of the RNPMHU program. The program logic model was constructed through a collaborative process including information from community-based organization partners, clients/participants, program manager, program staff, program documents, data, and photographs. The logic model guided the collection of program evaluation data used to continually improve program effectiveness and evaluate long-term client health outcomes. Program processes identified in the program theory were explored in formative evaluations (focused on developing and improving the program) and summative evaluations (historical analysis) of the program (Alexy & Elnitsky, 1998) and facilitated exploratory methodological studies of health and functional status metrics (Elnitsky & Alexy, 1998).

Model Two: PRECEDE-PROCEED Framework

PRECEDE-PROCEED is a second framework used for program planning and evaluation. The PRECEDE-PROCEED framework helps program managers identify factors affecting public health and plan targets for intervention, specify objectives, and criteria for evalu-

ation. The PROCEED framework provides steps for policy, implementation, and evaluation (Green & Kreuter, 1991). The acronym PRECEDE stands for predisposing, reinforcing, and enabling constructs in educational/environmental diagnosis and evaluation. The acronym PROCEED stands for policy, regulatory, and organizational constructs in educational/environmental development.

The PRECEDE and PROCEED phases, together, provide a stepped approach for program planning, implementation, and evaluation. During the PRECEDE phases, priorities are identified and objectives are set and establish "objects and criteria for policy, implementation, and evaluation in the Proceed phases" (Green & Kreuter, 1991, p. 24). The PRECEDE-PROCEED framework encourages multidimensional efforts and involves multiple sectors and levels of the community to effect change.

As a model, PRECEDE-PROCEED poses a system of hypothesized relationships between public health program processes and outcomes that may be tested in evaluation. The developers of the framework define program evaluation as the "comparison of an object of interest against a standard of acceptability" (Green & Kreuter, 1991, p. 217). Objects of interest include program inputs (human, physical, and fiscal investments) described in terms of objectives that specify who will have what type of change by what timeline, implementation processes, impact or intermediate effects, and ultimate effects or outcomes. Standards of acceptability are program targets of how much and when a change is expected. Standards may be levels of improvement anticipated by program managers, scientific standards, historical performance measures, or norms such as state averages.

The PRECEDE-PROCEED Model integrates evaluation planning and program planning. It provides a process for collecting baseline data and program planning that facilitates future measurement and evaluation. The PRECEDE plan for the program will include social, behavioral, health, environmental, and educational objectives as well as program activities targeted to the objectives. Evaluation is continuous and integral to the model, incorporated from the beginning phase of the model. The PRECEDE-PROCEED Model has been used in randomized controlled trials, health program planning, review, and evaluations by multiple health and educational disciplines at local, regional, state, national, and international levels of the community (Green & Kreuter, 1991).

Model Three: Diffusion of Innovations Theory

Rogers's (1995) Diffusion of Innovations Theory, the third model, has been used to evaluate the dissemination and use of products or health services in the community. The focus of the Diffusion of Innovations Theory is on understanding the modes and processes of communication among members of social systems and how new ideas spread throughout the community. Important characteristics of diffusion include the following assumptions:

- Diffusion of innovation takes an extended period of time through interpersonal networks.

- People go through stages (knowledge, persuasion, decision, implementation, and adoption) in the process of adopting innovations.

- Some people adopt innovations right away and others may wait until later.

Characteristics of the innovation, of the target audience, and of the structure of the organization affect the rate of adoption. Characteristics of the innovation to consider are its advantage over current practice, compatibility, complexity/ease of trying, radical nature, ability to observe others adopting, and cost. Characteristics of the target audience include age, socioeconomic status, and community characteristics. Organizational structure elements to consider include centralization, complexity, formality, interconnectedness, and availability of resources or elasticity.

Diffusion of Innovations Theory has been used to assess development, dissemination, and impact of Treatment Improvement Protocols (TIPs) on substance abuse treatment practices (funded by the Center for Substance Abuse Treatment). This series of evaluation studies includes retrospective, cross-sectional, and prospective study designs (Hubbard & Hayashi, 2003; Hubbard, Huang, & Mulvey, 2003). The studies allowed investigators to assess members' awareness of and implementation of practices recommended by the TIPs, evaluate effects of TIPs on delivery of addiction treatment services; and identify methods for strengthening development, formatting, marketing, disseminating, using, and evaluating TIPs.

Results from the TIPs evaluation studies were used to improve the development of all TIPs and dissemination of further innovations. For example, the retrospective study identified barriers to the implementation of guidelines in the TIPs, identified inconsistencies with the organization, and highlighted the need to consider such factors necessary for implementation of programs. The results supported tenets of the Diffusion of Innovations Theory. For example, Hubbard, Huang, and Mulvey (2003) reported support for the tenet of attitudes helping to determine whether an individual will eventually use the innovation in practice. They were able to identify providers' specific concerns (e.g., need for culturally sensitive TIPS) surrounding the use of TIPs and later address these in the redesign of future protocols. Again, both qualitative and quantitative methods were employed in this set of studies. The use of measures identified in the Diffusion of Innovations Theory, that is, individual's knowledge, attitudes, and practices related to the new innovation or practice, made it possible for program managers and investigators to identify the rate and pattern of diffusion of innovation (in this case the TIPs) within the clinical field (Hubbard, Huang, & Mulvey, 2003).

DECISION MAKING IN EVALUATION

The theoretical approaches and frameworks provide models for public health program evaluation design. Program evaluation complements program development by gathering necessary information for documenting program effectiveness. The evaluation results provide information for program changes and improvement. The use of scientific approaches for decision making in public health programs is the basis of evidence-based practice (CDC 1999). At the services level in public health, there is concern about how the processes outlined in program development ultimately can affect the quality. Since program planning and economic analysis and evaluation are at the infrastructure level, this will be where the decisions are made on program development. Issel (2004, p. 213) states that "implementing the health program requires acquiring and overseeing adequate resources to provide the program in a manner that is consistent with the program theory and the purpose of the program."

CRITICAL THINKING ACTIVITIES

1. You are a public health nurse and attended Parent Teacher's Night at your child's middle school. While attending, you realized that many of these students are overweight. The middle school is in your public health area, and you wish to integrate into the school system an Eat Healthy Program. What information would you need to decide the feasibility of this program and what analysis would you need to conduct before deciding on the program?

2. What type of economic analysis is feasible to use in evaluating public health nursing interventions?

3. What are the greatest barriers to conducting a cost-utility analysis?

4. Consider an existing evidence-based intervention or program. How would you justify continued funding without having some level of economic analysis? Would cost-consequence analysis help or hurt the case for expanding the intervention or program?

5. Suppose you are an external evaluator, employed by the public health department to evaluate the impacts of a childhood immunization program in the county where you live. How would you involve the stakeholders in the evaluation plan? Defend your approach.

6. A school health program is working with middle school students to develop citizenship skills and the program manager is interested in evaluating the program. Explain how you might proceed if you were to use (a) the program logic model and (b) the PRECEDE-PROCEED Model. Which approach do you think would be more useful and why?

7. Imagine you are the program manager for a nurse-managed clinic supported by the city government and affiliated with the School of Nursing at the local university. Explain how you would use program evaluation methods and cost-effectiveness analysis to provide evidence of the success of the clinic.

8. Read an article in a recent issue of a community health journal in which a program evaluation only reported participants' health or functional impacts. Suggest some possibilities for how collection and analysis of cost data might have enhanced the analysis and supported the program and its continuation.

KEY TERMS

conceptualizing	evaluating	problem identification
cost-benefit analysis (CBA)	externalities	program components
cost-consequence analysis (CCA)	formative evaluation	program development
	formulating	program effects
cost-effectiveness analysis (CEA)	implementing	program evaluation
cost-minimization analysis (CMA)	intangibles	program objectives
	logic models	program outputs
cost-utility analysis (CUA)	mission statement clarification	program planning
detailing	planning	stakeholder analysis
Diffusion of Innovations Theory	PRECEDE-PROCEED framework	summative evaluations
discounting		SWOT

KEY CONCEPTS

- Program development is the strategic alignment of activities undertaken to meet an intended purpose to ensure that an identified problem has the best possible likelihood of success with the adequate resources.

- Program planning is an organized, systematic method to conceptualize, detail, implement, and evaluate the effectiveness of a program.

- SWOT analysis is identifying the areas of strengths, weaknesses, opportunities, and threats in program development and planning.

- Formulating the plan consists of defining the problem based on a needs assessment of the program population.

- Conceptualizing the plan is the articulation of thoughts and ideas in an objective format that involves finding solutions to the identified needs.

- To detail the plan, the program is assessed in terms of the solutions that have been identified and objectives are formulated that will meet the program goal.

- Implementing the best plan involves selecting the plan that meets the needs of the target population; the goals and objectives need to reflect the solution based on the data collected in the evaluating phase.

- Various cost analyses exist to conduct economic analyses of programs. They inform decision makers of the cost value of a program but may not always indicate whether the decision to implement the program is worthwhile.

- Program evaluation is the use of scientific methods to measure the implementation and outcomes of programs, for decision-making purposes, focusing on program components, objectives, outputs, and effects.

- Three theoretical frameworks that can be used in program development and evaluation are the logic model, PRECEDE-PROCEED framework, and the Diffusion of Innovations Theory. The logic model describes the logical process by which program inputs and activities are intended to create the outcomes or effects. The PRECEDE-PROCEED Model helps program managers identify factors affecting public health and plan targets for intervention, specify objectives, and criteria for evaluation and provides steps for policy, implementation, and evaluation. The Diffusion of Innovations Theory is used to evaluate the dissemination and use of products or health services in the community.

- The phases of program evaluation are (1) identifying program objectives, (2) selecting or creating measures of impacts, (3) collecting data, and (4) interpreting data in terms of the evaluation framework and program context.

- The use of scientific approaches for decision making in public health programs is the foundation of evidence-based practice.

REFERENCES

Alexy, B. A., & Elnitsky, C. A. (1998). Rural mobile health unit: Outcomes. *Public Health Nursing 15*(1), 3–11.

Bell, C. M., Chapman, M. S., Stone, P. W., Sandburg, E. A., & Neumann, P. J. (2001). An off-the-shelf help list: A comprehensive catalog of preference scores from published cost-utility analyses. *Medical Decision Making, 21*, 288–294.

Blum, H. L. (1981). *Planning for health: Generics for the eighties* (2nd ed.). New York: Human Science Press.

Bryson, J. M. (1988). *An effective strategic planning approach for public and nonprofit organizations. Strategic planning for pubic and nonprofit organizations* (pp. 46–70). San Francisco: Jossey-Bass Publishers.

Centers for Disease Control (1999, September 17). *Framework for Program Evaluation in Public Health.* MMWR Recommendations and Reports 48 (RR11); 1–40. Available at www.cdc.gov/epo/mmwr/preview/mmwrhtml/rr4811a1.htm.

Chatterji, P., Caffray, C. M., Crowe, M., Freeman, L., & Jensen, P. (2004). Cost assessment of a school-based mental health screening and treatment program in New York City. *Mental Health Services Research, 6*(3), 155–166.

Chen, H. T. (1990). *Theory-driven evaluations.* Newbury Park, CA: Sage.

Ciliska, D., Cullum, N., & Marks, B. A. (2001). Evaluation of systematic reviews of treatment or prevention interventions. *Evidenced Based Nursing, 4*(4), 100–103.

Donaldson, S. I. (2003). Theory-driven program evaluation in the new millennium. In S. I. Donaldson & M. Scriven (Eds.), *Evaluating social programs and problems: Visions for the new millennium* (pp. 109–141). Mahwah, NJ: Erlbaum.

Donaldson, S. I., & Scriven, M. (Ed.). (2003). *Evaluating social programs and problems: Visions for the new millennium* (pp. 109–141). Mahwah, NJ: Erlbaum.

Elnitsky, C. A., & Alexy, B. A. (1998). Identifying health status and health risks of older rural residents. *Journal of Community Health Nursing, 15* (2), 61–75.

Funnell, S. (2000). Developing and using a program theory matrix for program evaluation and performance monitoring. *New Directions in Evaluation, 87,* 91–102.

Gold, M. R., Siegel, J. E., Russell, L. B., & Weinstein, M. C. (1996). *Cost-effectiveness in health and medicine.* Oxford: Oxford University Press.

Green, L. W., & Kreuter, M. W. (1991). *Health promotion planning: An education and environmental approach.* Mountain Views, CA: Mayfield.

Hubbard, S. M., & Hayashi, S. W. (2003). Use of diffusion of innovations theory to drive a federal agency's program evaluation. *Evaluation and Program Planning, 26,* 49–56.

Hubbard, S. M., Huang, J. Y., & Mulvey, K. P. (2003). Application of diffusion of innovations theory to the TIPs evaluation project results and beyond. *Evaluation and Program Planning, 26,* 99–107.

Issel, M. L. (2004). *Health program planning and evaluation.* Boston: Jones and Bartlett.

Kane, R. L., Homyak, P., Bershadsky, B., Flood, S., & Zhang, H. J. (2004). Patterns of utilization for the Minnesota Senior Health Options program. *American Geriatrics Society, 52*(12), 2039–2044.

Koskinen, J. A. (February 12, 1997). Office of Management and Budget Testimony Before the House Committee on Government Reform and Oversight Hearing.

McLaughlin, J. A., & Jordan, G. B. (1998). Logic models: A tool for telling your program's performance story. *Evaluation and Program Planning, 22,* 65–72.

Neumann, P. J., Stone, P. W., Chapman, R. H., Sandberg, E. A., & Bell, C. M. (2000). The quality of reporting in published cost-utility analyses, 1976–1997. *Annals of Internal Medicine, 132,* 964–972.

Naylor, M. D., Brooten, D. A., Campbell, R. L., Maislin, G., McCauley, K. M., & Schwartz, J. S. (2004). Transitional care of older adults hospitalized with heart failure: A randomized, controlled trial. *Journal of American Geriatrics Society, 52,* 675–684.

Nutt, P. (1984). *Planning methods for health and related organizations,* New York: Wiley.

Patton, M. Q. (1997). *Utilization-focused evaluation: The new century text* (pp. 221–223). Thousand Oaks, CA: Sage.

Phillips, K. A., & Chen, J. L. (2002). Impact of the U.S. panel on cost-effectiveness in health and medicine. *American Journal of Preventive Medicine, 22*(2), 98–105.

Phillips, K. A., & Holtgrave, D. R. (1997). Using cost-effectiveness/cost-benefit analysis to allocate health resources: A level playing field for prevention? *American Journal of Preventive Medicine, 13*(1), 18–25.

Polit, D. F., & Beck, C. T. (2004). *Nursing research: Principles and methods* (7th ed.). Philadelphia: Lippincott Williams, & Wilkins.

Pollack, C. D. (1994). Planning for success: The first steps in new program development. *Journal of School Nursing, 10*(3) 11–15.

Rogers, E. M. (1995). *Diffusion of innovations* (4th ed). New York: Free Press.

Rosen, G. (1993). *A history of public health* (Expanded ed.). Baltimore: John Hopkins University Press.

Rossi, P. H., Freeman, H. E., & Lipsey, M. W. (1999). *Evaluation: A systematic approach* (6th ed.). Thousand Oaks, CA: Sage.

Russell, L. B., Gold, M. R., Siegel, J. E., & Weinstein, M. C. (1996). The role of cost-effectiveness analysis in health and medicine: Panel on cost-effectiveness in health and medicine, *JAMA, 276,* 1172–1177.

Rutman, L., & Mowbray, G. (1983). *Understanding program evaluation. Sage human services guide,* 31. Newbury Park, CA: Sage.

Siegel, J. E., Weinstein, M. C., Russell, L. B., & Gold, M. R. (1996). Recommendations for reporting cost-effectiveness analyses: Panel on cost-effectiveness in health and medicine, *JAMA, 276,* 1339–1341.

Sit, J. W., Wong, T. K., Clinton, M., Li, L. S., & Fong, Y. M. (2004). Stroke care in the home: The impact of social support on the general health of family caregivers. *Journal of Clinical Nursing, 13*(7), 816–824.

Stone, P. W., Chapman, R. H., Sandberg, E. A., Liljas, B. & Neumann, P. J. (2000a). Measuring costs in cost-utility analyses: Variations in the literature. *International Journal of Technology Assessment in Health Care, 16*(1), 111–124.

Stone, P. W., Curran, C. R., & Bakken, S. (2002). Economic evidence for evidence-based practice. *Journal of Nursing Scholarship, 34*(3), 277–282.

Stone, P. W., Teutsch, S., Chapman, R. H., Bell, C., Goldie, S. J., & Neumann, P. (2000b). Cost-utility analyses of clinical preventive services: Published ratios, 1976–1997. *American Journal of Preventive Medicine, 19*(1), 15–23.

Suchman, E. A., (1967). *Evaluative research: Principles and practice in public service and social action programs.* New York: Russell Sage Foundation.

Weinstein, M. C., Siegel, J. E., Gold, M. R., Kamlet, M., S., & Russell, L. B. (1996). Recommendations of the panel on cost-effectiveness in health and medicine. *JAMA, 276,* 1253–1258.

Weiss, C. (1997). Theory-based evaluation: Past, present, and future. In D. Rog & D. Founier (Eds.), Progress and future directions in evaluation: Perspectives on theory, practice, and methods. *New directions for program evaluation.* San Francisco: Jossey-Bass.

Weiss, C. H. (1998). *Evaluation: Methods for studying programs and policies* (2nd ed.). Upper Saddle River, NJ: Prentice Hall.

Winer, L. R., & Vázquez-Abad, F. (1995). The present and future of ID practice. *Quality Performance Improvement Quarterly, 8(*3), 55–67.

Witkin, B. R., & Altschuld, J. W. (1995). *Playing and conducting needs assessments: A practical guide.* Thousand Oaks, CA: Sage.

U.S. Government. (2000). U. S. Code Title 42: P.L. 106-501 Older Americans Act Amendments of 2000. Retrieved June 10, 2006, from http://www.access.gpo.gov/uscode/title42/chapter35_.html.

WHCoA. (December 14, 2005). News from the White House Conference on Aging. Press release. *The 2005 White House Conference on Aging Closes.* Retrieved June 10, 2006, from http://www.whcoa.gov/about/resolutions/top%2010.pdf.

BIBLIOGRAPHY

Bell, C. M., Chapman, M. S., Stone, P. W., Sandburg, E. A., & Neumann, P. J. (2001). An off-the-shelf help list: A comprehensive catalog of preference scores from published cost-utility analyses. *Medical Decision Making, 21,* 288–294.

Glick, D. F., & Kulbok, P. K. (2001). Program revision: A dynamic outcome of evaluation. *Quality Management in Health Care, 10* (1), 37–45.

Kaluzny, A., & Veney, J. (1999). Evaluating health care programs and services. In Williams, S. & Torrens, P. (Eds.), *Introduction to health services.* New York: Wiley.

Prosavac, E. J., & Carey, R. G. (2000). *Program evaluation: Methods and case studies.* Englewood Cliffs, NJ: Prentice Hall.

Stone, P. W., Teutsch, S., Chapman, R. H., Bell, C., Goldie, S. J., & Neumann, P. (2000). Cost-utility analyses of clinical preventive services: Published ratios, 1976–1997. *American Journal of Preventive Medicine, 19*(1), 15–23.

RESOURCES

Health Resources and Services Administration (HRSA)

5600 Fishers Lane
Rockville, Maryland 20857
301-443-2216
Email: comments@hrsa.gov.
Web: http://www.hrsa.gov

HRSA is a federal agency within the U.S. Department of Health and Human Services that provides national leadership, program resources, and services needed to improve access to health care that is culturally competent and linguistically appropriate. HRSA strives to eliminate health disparities.

Turning Point

Email: turnpt@u.washington.edu
Web: http://www.turningpointprogram.org

Turning Point, started in 1997, was an initiative of The Robert Wood Johnson Foundation and the W. K. Kellogg Foundation. Its mission was to transform and strengthen the public health system in the United States by making it more community-based and collaborative. The initial idea for Turning Point came from the foundations' concerns about the capacity of the public health system to respond to emerging challenges in public health, specifically the system's capacity to work with people from many sectors to improve the health status of all people in a community. Turning Point created a network of 23 public health partners across the country to:

- Define and assess health, prioritize health issues, and take collective action.
- Promote education to decrease the risk of infectious and chronic disease.
- Strengthen environmental health services for clean air and water and safe food.
- Gain access to health care for everyone.
- Improve health status for minority groups.

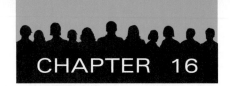

CHAPTER 16

Community Development for Health Promotion

Joanne Martin, DrPH, FAAN, RN

Joanne Raines Warner, RN, DNS

Chapter Outline

- Community Development Theories
- The Healthy Cities Model
  History of the Healthy Cities Model
  Implementing the Healthy Cities Model
- Choosing Programs for Health Promotion after Needs Identification
  One Success Story: Healthy Families America
  Effective Leadership Roles for Public Health Nurses
- Linking Healthy Cities and Healthy Families

Learning Objectives

Upon completion of this chapter, the reader will be able to:

1. Explore the possibilities of meeting local needs by integrating several community-based health promotion models.

2. Evaluate Healthy Cities as one model of community development and participatory action.

3. Examine factors in selecting a program for meeting an identified community need, for example, strengthening families.

4. Apply elements necessary for program sustainability to Healthy Families.

5. Describe leadership roles public health nurses can play at the national, state, and local level.

The attributes of community health are as complex and unique as each community; the strategies to enable each community to collectively define health, bolster assets, and address health needs can be just as complex and varied. A range of models and theoretical perspectives can guide these processes. Public health nurses in leadership positions play a pivotal role in helping communities understand options and select models and programs that accomplish desired outcomes, match local idiosyncrasies, and demonstrate the mechanism for citizen input that is increasingly mandated for federal funding.

This chapter explores community development from the perspective of the Healthy Cities Model, a social ecological approach to needs identification, capacity building, and citizen participation. A practice application of a Healthy City that has actively used the community health promotion model for over 10 years is presented to provide insights into the role of public health nursing leadership. Additionally, the chapter illustrates the process and considerations that follow the community's identification of a specific health need and how programs can be chosen and integrated into community development process. Healthy Families America is the exemplar chosen to illustrate this integration.

COMMUNITY DEVELOPMENT THEORIES

Stokols (1996) discusses three categorical approaches to community development relative to health promotion. The theoretical bases of these approaches range from social learning theory to health belief model to operant conditioning principles. The first approach is individually focused behavioral change and lifestyle modification strategies, such as smoking cessation or exercise promotion. This individual approach requires active and sustained interventions for targeted individuals.

The second category of community development for health promotion involves environmental change and restructuring, such as eliminating air pollutants or requiring tamper-proof medication bottles. The theoretical bases for these approaches include ergonomics, organizational social support theory, and the epidemiology of occupational hazards. These approaches involve passive interventions to improve environmental safety and do not require specific effort by individuals.

Finally, the social ecological approach to community development takes into account the interrelationships of diverse personal, institutional, and environmental factors inherent in health and illness and is a more comprehensive perspective. It incorporates a variety of variables from systems theory, cultural change models, and ecology of human development, to name a few; is inherently interdisciplinary; and incorporates both active and passive interventions for health.

Healthy Cities is an example of a social ecological approach. Because this chapter focuses on the Healthy Cities Model, this approach to community development and health promotion will be discussed in more detail. The social ecological approach has strengths as well as limitations. The use of a comprehensive systems perspective to integrate behavioral change and environmental alteration is a strong asset. This allows the community and public health leaders to consider health from more than one analytic level (i.e., personal, institutional, community) thereby allowing examination of both individual and collective responses to health risks and community interventions. This rich analysis can present a more complete and unifying understanding of community dynamics and influences.

Limitations of the social ecological approach include the cumbersome, time-consuming, and impractical nature of the coordination of large groups of people and divergent ideas, as well as the challenge of integrating various interdisciplinary theories. An overinclusiveness of factors in the planning, implementation, and evaluation can result in very complex processes that overwhelm the community and breed despair in leaders and citizens. The complexity and nature of multilevel analyses is also a limitation; ecological health promotion initiatives can neither be evaluated like clinical interventions nor use the rigor of experimental or quasi-experimental methods "because the units of analysis do not lend themselves to random assignment to experimental and control groups, nor to manipulation as independent variables given the interdependence of person and environments" (Green, Richard, & Potvin, 1996, p. 273).

Within this broad frame of community development, the Healthy Cities Model can be seen as one social ecological approach to community problem solving, development, and health promotion. Public health nurse leaders with strong communication and interpersonal skills can mitigate the limitations discussed earlier and assist citizens in actively engaging in their community's processes. The Pan American Health Organization (PAHO) describes its framework for community-based health promotion as participatory development, a phrase that indicates their preference for vigorous citizen participation within the collaborative process of community growth and development (PAHO, 2005).

THE HEALTHY CITIES MODEL

The classic and most-cited definition of a Healthy City is "one that is continually creating and improving those physical and social environments and strengthening those community resources which enable people to mutually support each other in performing all the functions of life and achieving their maximum potential" (Hancock & Duhl, 1988, p. 54). The PAHO description of a healthy city emphasizes the "social pact between civil society organizations, institutions from various sectors, and local political authorities" toward the goals of promoting health and improving quality of life (PAHO, 2002, p. iii). The model is process oriented, and one that values intervening with the underlying determinants of health, as well as intervening broadly through policies, legislation, and services.

Lee (2000) delineates the eight principles that characterize the model and process, noting that successful initiatives attend to all of the principles as a holistic enterprise (Box 16-1). The broad definitions of health and community allow the adaptation of the model to the local characteristics and preferences and reference again the social ecologic nature of the model. Defining health broadly requires all systems, structures, and processes in a community to consider the health implication of their actions, especially the impact the actions have on individual and collective health. Minimally, the significant influences to health as broadly defined are living and working conditions; psychosocial attributes and resources in the community; individual behaviors and habits; and genetic factors. From this perspective, "health is as much the result of our physical and social environment . . . as it is a product of the health-care system and health services" (PAHO, 2002, p. 9).

The shared vision of health and how people define health for their city springs from community values, further individualizing the projects for each locale. Equality is emphasized, as enhanced quality of life is pursued for all citizens, including and especially those

---

BOX 16-1: Eight Healthy Cities/Communities Principles

1. Broad definition of health
2. Broad definition of community
3. Shared vision from community values
4. Address quality of life for everyone
5. Diverse citizen participation and widespread community ownership
6. Focus on "system change"
7. Build capacity using local assets and resources
8. Benchmark and measure progress and outcomes.

SOURCE: Lee, P. (2000). Healthy Communities: A young movement that can revolutionize public health. *Public Health Reports, 115*(2, 3), 115.

---

whose influence and participation has been minimized by their life situation.

Healthy Cities have decentralized power and wide participation in public policy decisions. The integral role of local government in the Healthy Cities process is a distinctive characteristic of this model of community health promotion and development, highlighting the twin forces of political endorsement and citizen engagement. Citizen participation must include authentic opportunities and rights related to decisions that affect their lives. Strategies to initially mobilize and continually sustain participation involve culturally appropriate and persistent communication that links the community initiatives to their individual, family, and community well-being (Flynn, 1996; PAHO, 2002).

Healthy public policies address the determinants of health and seek a positive impact on health outcomes and quality of life. Examples include factors like transportation, housing, education, nutrition, or employment. "Healthy public policies seek to create a supportive environment that enables people to live a healthy life, make healthy choices, and transform social and physical environments" (PAHO, 2002, p. 11). A city is the level of government closest to citizens' daily lives; a city's laws and regulations can implement national policies and institutionalize change in ways consistent with local priorities.

Communities that conduct their business and design their collective life with the eight principles demonstrate particular characteristics. They are self-reflective and self-repairing in the face of challenges and change. They attend to the quality and integrity of the infrastructures that relate to their social, physical, and economic interactions (Duhl, 2000).

History of the Healthy Cities Model

Healthy Cities is a relatively young model of community development and health promotion that began in 1984 in Canada and 1986 in Europe. It has grown in credibility and visibility through local implementation, international collaboration, and World Health Organization (WHO) support.

The Canadian activities began in Toronto under Trevor Hancock's leadership and became a prevalent form of community health promotion among many Canadian cities. The initial European effort targeted six to eight cities, and grew to 35 European cities by 1991. The movement expanded beyond Europe and Canada to Australia, Central America, and several developing nations. The first International Conference on Healthy Cities and Communities in 1993 held in San Francisco drew an audience of nearly 1,400 from dozens of countries, and international collaboration and conversations continue today (Duhl, 1996; Flynn, 1996; Hancock, 1997).

Activities in the United States began in 1988 with two statewide initiatives, the California Healthy Cities Project and Healthy Cities Indiana. In 1989, the U.S. Department of Health and Human Services endorsed the Healthy Cities concept and directed the National Civic League to create a coordinating U.S. Healthy Communities Initiative. In 1991, Indiana University School of Nursing (IUSON) was designated as a WHO Collaborating Center in Healthy Cities, and continues under nursing leadership within IUSON. The Healthy Communities Initiative was bolstered by federal partners like the Office of Disease Prevention and Health Promotion at the Centers for Disease Control and Prevention, by national institutional leaders like the Health Forum and Voluntary Hospital Association, Inc., and significant foundations like the Robert Wood Johnson and W. K. Kellogg who funded early initiatives (Flynn, 1996; Hancock, 1997, Norris & Pittman, 2000).

Implementing the Healthy Cities Model

The process of community health promotion via the Healthy Cities Model can be delineated in a series of nine steps summarized in Box 16-2 (World Health Organization Collaborating Center in Healthy Cities, 2005). It begins with the community orientation to community health promotion philosophy and the principles of Healthy Cities. Community forums serve this purpose, as well as one more of an iterative process of articulating shared values, engendering a shared vision of a Healthy City, and building public commitment to improve quality of life.

Building the partnership, step 2, begins with establishing official community commitment by the public health departments and civic leaders. In Healthy Cities Indiana, a Memorandum of Understanding signed by the mayor and health officer represented official commitment, and further activities were implemented to engender the understanding and buy-in of the citizens.

Step 3, development of a community structure for health promotion, involves the creation of a multisectoral Healthy Cities Committee. Suggested sectors from which representation is important include, but are not limited to, the following: arts and culture, business and industry, dentistry, education, employment, environment, finance, health and medical care, local government media, parks and recreation, planning and housing, populations group (often those underrepresented

---

BOX 16-2: Steps in Implementing Healthy Cities/ Communities

1. Conduct community forum(s)
2. Build partnership and community commitment
3. Develop community structure for health promotion
4. Develop leadership
5. Conduct community assessment
6. Include community-wide planning for health
7. Offer community action for health
8. Advocate for healthy public policy
9. Monitor and evaluate progress

or vulnerable to the effects of public policies), public health, religion, social services, transportation, and utilities and energy. This broad representation taps the local wisdom and builds comprehensive citizen commitment to initiatives and processes. Clarified in this community structure are citizen roles, community goals, and potential resources.

Leadership development follows the constitution of the structure or committee as step 4. Particular strategies include consultations, conferences, workshops, networking, and assistance in the analysis of scholarly information on community health, specific health topics, or data describing local needs and issues. Within this development process, individuals who have managed sectors other than health or those with no prior leadership experience can become spokespersons and organizers for health. It can be transforming for individuals to realize the health implications of their work, when they had previously seen health as only "the work of health professionals."

Step 5 involves a comprehensive community assessment of strengths, resources, and needs. The process includes existing data describing the population characteristics (e.g., census data) and their health (e.g., morbidity and mortality data), as well as collecting new data through surveys and forums on the perspective and priorities of the citizens. Collaboration with health professionals or higher education institutions can assist with the gathering, presentation, and analysis of these data.

In step 6, community-wide planning for health occurs. Problems are identified, priorities set, actions planned, resources secured, and specific steering groups created to move the work forward. Strong leadership is useful during these processes to capture community energy and mobilize it into beneficial activities. Step 7 involves action: the strategies and programs and policies directed toward the identified goals.

After the community actions for health, step 8 involves sharing data-based information with local, state, and national policy makers as advocacy for healthy public policy. This dialogue and collaboration can further the understanding of the broad implications for health imbedded in most policies and potentially builds a larger network of advocates for health. The final step involves monitoring and evaluating in order to continually improve quality of the program. Data on outcomes are fraught with the challenges discussed previously in connection with the social ecological community development approaches, yet they are necessary to document effect and drive future activities.

CHOOSING PROGRAMS FOR HEALTH PROMOTION AFTER NEEDS IDENTIFICATION

When community leaders, such as public health nurse leaders, have identified a public health issue and available resources and have agreed upon goals and objectives, they might want to consider implementing a prevention program. Information about effective prevention programs has been accumulated and organized to assist community leaders in finding a program that could work in their community. The Institute of Medicine classifies evidence-based programs as universal, selected, and indicated, based upon risk status of the population group to be served. Federal and state agencies and foundations are interested in funding proven programs that are likely to achieve desired outcomes. To help community and public health leaders select programs that work, Center for Substance Abuse Prevention (CSAP) and Office of Juvenile Justice and Delinquency Prevention (OJJDP) compile lists of programs and categorize them as promising, effective, or model programs. Information about these programs can be accessed at www.modelprograms.samhsa.gov and www.strengtheningfamilies.org.

Public health nurse leaders can start by investigating existing programs and selecting programs they believe will work in their community. In addition to the content area, public health nurse leaders should consider programs that have evidence of effectiveness when implemented with a population group that resembles their community and with resources available in their community. Cost is often a major concern. An evidence-based prevention program might be too expensive, yet implementing a program that doesn't achieve desired outcomes is not a good investment. Acknowledging the lack of easy, definitive answers, *Getting to Outcomes*, a technical report developed by RAND and sponsored by the Centers for Disease Control and Prevention (CDC), suggests carefully determining the need for adaptation and making adaptations with quality and careful thought (Chinman, Imm, & Wandersman, 2004). Common wisdom for a local planning group includes determining what components of the program need to be adapted and why; understanding

New Castle Healthy Cities/Henry County Healthy Communities

New Castle, Indiana, became a Healthy City in 1988 as part of a statewide Healthy Cities Indiana grant. The grant was funded by the W. K. Kellogg Foundation and involved partnerships with Indiana University School of Nursing, Indiana Public Health Association, and six Indiana cities. The initiative was later known as CityNet Healthy Cities.

IUSON extended an invitation to New Castle's mayor and health officer, explaining the principles of the Healthy Cities Model and the benefits to their community health. Their interest and commitment represented the city's official political endorsement—and thus began their healthy city journey. One author (JRW), who was a New Castle citizen and an IUSON research assistant and doctoral student, networked with the various citizens to constitute a multisectoral Health Cities Committee. The various segments of the community to participate initially and over the years included the public schools, government, banking, health professionals, ministerial association, labor, business, the arts, and underrepresented population groups. The initiative continues today—15 years later. They have redefined their geographical scope to include the entire rural county and have renamed the committee the Healthy Communities of Henry County (HCHC).

Initial activities involved a comprehensive community assessment, with technical support and consultation by IUSON nursing faculty. Census data and morbidity and mortality figures were assembled by IUSON and analyzed by the committee. Youth and adults were surveyed to ascertain a shared local view of a healthy city. A health behaviors survey was developed by the community, in consultation with IUSON, to ascertain malleable factors related to cardiovascular disease and cancer, the two causes of death for which rates exceeded state and national rates.

The survey was delivered door to door, sampled every neighborhood of the city, and yielded a response rate of 50 percent ($N = 500$). The committee's active participation in the initial survey development and implementation provided a significant turning point in their ownership of the Healthy Cities process. Four years after the initial survey, another survey was administered, asking identical questions for comparison and evaluation purposes.

Several summary points can be drawn from the initial assessment phase. All committee activities have been based on existing data or data generated through participatory action research. The citizen engagement in the assessment strengthened their development and outcomes. Also, the role played by public health nurses in data retrieval and analysis was significant. This technical consultation was a public health nursing contribution to the partnership and did not diminish their community empowerment.

The main structural change sought was to "make the healthy choices the easy choices." The committee focused on increasing health awareness, promoting healthy policies, and creating accessible health programs. Some examples of each include the following: creating and taping of "Healthy Moments" educational messages aired by local radio as public service announcements; writing newspaper articles discussing data that described local health; sponsoring health walks each spring in connection with health presentations and celebrations; promoting recycling days and development of recycling opportunities for the community; sponsoring activities to reduce youth access to tobacco; developing a "Smoke-Free Class of 2000" educational session for educators and administrators of the seventh grade; equipping community members

(continued)

the program's core components and striving to protect the underlying theory; and making careful estimates of resources needed and building in sufficient funding to cover the costs of tracking fidelity to the program and adaptations that will be needed.

Preventing child abuse is an example of a serious public health issue that is complex, long-standing, and seemingly intractable. Attempting to address the entire issue at once can be overwhelming and lead to inertia. Moreover, action might need to be taken before root

causes such as poverty and ignorance are eliminated. It is important to start somewhere and understand how a community-based intervention can potentially contribute to resolving a particular issue and how resolving that issue will benefit the broader community. The question is: Where to begin?

For example, most communities provide broad support for ensuring all children enter school ready to learn and recognize the link between early childhood experiences and school performance. The fact that abuse

⊕ PRACTICE APPLICATION

New Castle Healthy Cities/Henry County Healthy Communities (cont'd)

to develop programs promoting healthy behavior choices; testifying before the city council in favor of a smoke-free ordinance in city builds; and organizing a summer recreation volleyball opportunity for youth. In 1993, they incorporated as a not-for-profit organization so that they could secure funds through local foundations, businesses, and individuals. More recently, HCHC has emphasized physical fitness opportunities and environmental health.

The smoke-free ordinance mentioned previously deserves further explanation, for it is the strongest example of policy advocacy and change. The mayor supported the smoke-free ordinance because it reduced insurance premiums and city costs. HCHC representatives testified during city council hearings on the local data and health implications of secondhand smoke. Through this HCHC testimony and influence, the voices of the citizens were heard, health was explicitly on the political agenda, and health was promoted through public policy change.

A recent focus group of participants involved with HCHC through the years addressed how the healthy city process has influenced the nature of the community and their collective understanding of what they are capable of accomplishing. Highlighted was the unifying effect of volunteers building a playground—including the processes of fundraising, planning, passing city ordinances, and actually building the playground equipment. Socioeconomic barriers were broken down and potential interpersonal gaps were closed as inmates worked next to lawyers, and children worked

next to grandparents. The playground continues today as a visible reminder of collective and empowering action to promote health. The HCHC reports that the healthy cities process helped build structures, pass some policies, and provide some resources to make health behaviors affordable and available to all. The process has given the county a progressive energetic feel and contributed to a collective empowerment regarding problem solving.

Sustainability success is another lesson to learn from the HCHC practice application. Factors identified by the community in a focus group conducted by a nurse researcher include the importance of visionary leadership, strong board members, outstanding volunteers, and periodic grant/funding success. The Healthy Cities Model provided them with a framework for continual engagement in an ongoing process of community health promotion and collective attention to hometown quality of life and well-being.

Through the Healthy Cities process, community capacity building occurred, giving citizens the mechanism, confidence, and inspiration to focus on community health and to address health challenges. The Healthy Cities process empowered and provided the process for ongoing health promotion initiatives. For example, New Castle and Henry County, like many other counties, identified the need to support at-risk families and to prevent child abuse with interventions that promote healthy family structures and interactions.

---

and neglect adversely affects a child's ability to learn is an important reason to prevent child maltreatment before it has a chance to occur. Home visiting programs have been effective in preventing abuse by reaching out to at-risk families and reducing or eliminating risk factors such as isolation, stress, interpersonal violence, lack of knowledge of child development, harsh discipline, depression, and other mental health problems (Johnson, 2001; MacLeod & Nelson, 2000; Olds et al., 1997). The Task Force on Community Preventive Services recommends early childhood home visitation to prevent child abuse and neglect based upon a systematic review and strong evidence of effectiveness (Bilukha et al., 2005). For this reason, inclusion of

home visiting programs is recommended as part of a comprehensive approach to achieving school readiness for all children (Gomby, 2003).

Home visiting as an effective strategy to improve the health and well-being of children and families should come as no surprise to public health nurses. After all, this has been the charge of public health nursing for over 100 years. Lillian Wald, credited with founding the movement to establish public health nursing in the United States, and nurses of Henry Street Settlement House were making home visits to families living in the tenements of New York City in 1893. However, today's families are living in a very different world. Home visiting is a recommended approach to preventing child

⊕ RESEARCH APPLICATION

Multi-level Determinants of Retention in a Home-Visiting Child Abuse Prevention Program

Study Purpose

To identify determinants of retention by examining attributes of mothers, home visitors, and communities and to make recommendations for increasing retention rates, thereby increasing effectiveness of home visiting. Home visiting of sufficient duration and intensity is endorsed as a promising strategy to support families, enhance child development, improve parenting behaviors, and prevent child maltreatment. Most home-visiting programs show modest results. Home-visiting programs rely on families voluntarily participating in weekly or biweekly visits for about 3 years. Greater participation (more home visits and longer duration) is associated with greater benefits. However, many programs experience low rates of retention in the program, with about half the families leaving within 12 months. Retention rates vary across communities within the same program.

Methods

Oregon Healthy Start (OHS) is modeled after Healthy Families America and serves families in 14 counties. Maternal characteristics (age, ethnicity, education, marital status, birth outcome) and duration of home visits were abstracted from electronic records of 1,093 families, who had the opportunity to receive home visits for at least a 12-month period of time. Survey data from 71 home visitors, matched to the families by identification numbers, was analyzed for home visitor attributes (age, ethnicity, education, home visiting experience, hours of supervision per month, perspective scale, empathic concern scale). Community violence index was derived from summing rates of homicide, assaults, forcible rapes, and domestic violence arrests. Separate bivariate analyses identified which variables were associated with program retention beyond one year.

Attributes with p values less than .10 were retained for hierarchical general linear modeling (HGLM).

Findings

Forty-five percent of mothers left the program prior to one year. In the final HGLM analysis, community violence index, hours of supervision, mother's age, and mother's ethnicity (Hispanic) were significant predictors. Each 1-unit increase in community violence reduced the likelihood of retention for one year by 13 percent. Every hour of supervision increased the odds of staying one year by 89 percent. Forty-eight percent of the Hispanic mothers stayed in the program for one year. Retention increased by 4 percent for each year of the mother's age.

Implications

Healthy Families America home-visiting programs need to adapt in order to retain those families who live in more violent communities. Adaptations also need to be considered to meet the scheduling needs of younger mothers. For example, "home visits" might need to occur in places other than the home. Some visits with teen mothers could occur at school. Identifying safe locations could facilitate evening visits to families who work during the day and live in more violent communities. More direct supervision of home visitors is a promising, practical way to increase retention of families.

Reference

McGuigan, W. M., Katzev, A. R., & Pratt, C. C. (2003). Multi-level determinants of retention in a home-visiting child abuse prevention program. *Child Abuse & Neglect, 27,* 363–380.

---

maltreatment, but not all home-visiting programs are equally effective (Bilukha et al., 2005; Chaffin, 2004; 2005; Duggan et al., 2004; Gomby, Culross, & Behrman, 1999). For example, Nurse-Family Partnership (NFP), a model program with a strong track record of demonstrated effectiveness in preventing child abuse, is not as effective when intimate partner violence

is present (Eckenrode et al., 2000). Moreover, the NFP program has restrictive eligibility criteria for the population to be served, and home visitors must meet certain qualifications. Eligibility is limited to first-time mothers, usually young, unmarried, and low income, who enroll in NFP ideally before the 16th week of pregnancy, and home visitors must be registered nurses (Olds et al.,

1997; Olds, Eckenrode, & Kitzman, 2005). Yet, public health nurse leaders realize many at-risk families fail to meet NFP eligibility criteria and communities struggle with a persistent nursing shortage. Fortunately, other effective home-visiting programs exist (Bugental et al., 2002; Mitchell-Herzfeld et al., 2005).

Public health nurse leaders need to select a program that will work in their community. If community leaders have engaged in the Healthy Cities Model, they will have assessed community strengths, have a good sense of existing and available resources, and understand which values the community wants to optimize. The underlying premise of the program model should match the community's perception of the identified need, problem, or issue they wish to address. The community and the program model should share a common understanding of the relationships among underlying factors that are thought to contribute to the problem at hand.

One Success Story: Healthy Families America

Healthy Families America (HFA) is a home-visiting program that was developed by a pediatrician and public health nurse in Hawaii where it had demonstrated success in preventing child abuse among at-risk families. A national not-for-profit organization, Prevent Child Abuse (PCA) America (formerly National Committee to Prevent Child Abuse), concluded the Hawaii program of home visitation (called Healthy Start in Hawaii) was promising and would be appropriate and feasible in most communities (Daro & Harding, 1999). With generous donations from Ronald McDonald House Charities and Freddie Mac Corporation, PCA America proceeded to implement a strategic plan to promote HFA by providing training and technical assistance to help programs get started in local communities and leadership development to help state leaders maintain, sustain, and expand HFA programs.

About the same time, state and local child abuse prevention advocates in Indiana decided to implement a child abuse prevention program that had evidence of effectiveness. After investigating the HFA home visiting program, they recruited one of the authors (JM) to join the state leadership team. As a public health nurse and faculty member, she had developed successful community-based home-visiting programs to prevent infant mortality in rural and urban Indiana counties and was experienced in providing training and technical assis-

tance for multidisciplinary teams of nurses, social workers, and community health workers. She brought two important public health nursing perspectives to the strategic planning and decision-making process. First, public health nurses know that effective programs will not have community-wide impact unless they are taken to scale and sustained over time. Positive outcomes with families will not translate into favorable impacts on community-wide statistics until the program reaches significant numbers of at-risk families, and this takes time. As a result, the state leadership team envisioned Healthy Families Indiana (HF Indiana) as a statewide program from the beginning, and selected a program model that could be expanded over time and sustained in the future. Second, public health nurses know that programs need to be adapted to meet the needs of diverse communities rather than strictly replicated in accordance with the desires of a sponsor or sponsoring organization. Stability and sustainability of community-based programs rely on community support. Community buy-in is fostered when new programs are tailored to the community and blended with existing services that are designed for the same or similar populations. State and local leaders recognized that the HFA model balanced flexibility to meet community needs with fidelity to the program.

Consequently, local leaders expressed keen interest in bringing HFA to their community. In almost every county, local planning bodies already had conducted needs assessments, and prevention of child abuse was one of the top priorities in their plans of action. Plans of action were unique to each county, but HFA was a good fit and the timing was perfect.

Nearly 10 years ago, Lizbeth Schorr commented that Healthy Families Indiana is "living proof that effective replication requires as much wisdom and skill as effective program design" (Schorr, 1997, p. 40). So, what has been accomplished?

HF Indiana grew from six program sites in 1994 to 56 program sites in 2000. HF Indiana was the first HFA home-visiting program that Substance Abuse and Mental Health Services Administration and OJJDP evaluated and included in lists of promising, effective, and model programs for selected families with children under age 5. Annually, about 900 HF Indiana home visitors serve over 18,000 families in all 92 counties. Since 1994, the HF Indiana Training and Technical Assistance Project (HFIT&TAP) at Indiana University School of Nursing has provided training and technical assistance for all HF Indiana staff from each site. Each year, over 1,200 attend about 30 training events. HFIT&TAP continues to evolve to meet emerging needs. In 2005–2006, HFIT&TAP converted some of the classroom training into a 12-course, e-learning curriculum, Building Blocks for Healthier Families. Now newly hired staff can receive required training at their own office instead of traveling to a central location. Although training provided by HFIT&TAP is specifically designed to educate home visitors from multiple disciplines, the content reflects public health nursing principles and can be used to augment public health nursing courses.

The major goal of preventing child abuse by strengthening the relationship between mothers and babies and young children is being met. According to the Indiana Department of Child Services, long-term follow-up shows less than 2 percent of HF Indiana families, who receive at least 12 home visits, have substantiated abuse or neglect, even after home visits are discontinued (personal communication, Phyllis Kikendall, 2006). Significant improvement in parent-child interaction is attributed to the number of home visits, controlling for maternal risk factors and demographic characteristics (Harding et al., In Press). With public health nursing leadership, HF Indiana sites currently are involved in research projects funded by Agency for Healthcare Research and Quality, National Institutes of Health, Agency for Children and Families, and local foundations.

Effective Leadership Roles for Public Health Nurses

Public health nurses have leadership opportunities at multiple levels. To enhance their effectiveness at the local level, public health nurses would be wise to carefully consider recommendations made by the Annie E. Casey Foundation (Hepburn, 2005). The foundation suggests communities gather information about home-visiting program models, identify criteria to select a home-visiting program model, choose a model that can be tailored to fit the community, consider how new models can be coordinated and linked with other existing home-visiting models, and ensure home-visiting is one component of a comprehensive system of supports for families with young children. Public health nurses should strive to improve the health of their community by participating in the decision-making process with other community leaders and organizations. For example, public health nurses are ideally prepared to investigate and evaluate information from online resources that are designed to improve decision making about home visiting and/or school readiness (Chinman, Imm, & Wandersman, 2004; Gomby, 2003; Hepburn, 2005; National Governor's Association Task Force on School Readiness, 2005).

Public health nurses also can exert leadership at national and state levels. Since 1994, one author (JM) has been director of the HFIT&TAP. During a 2-year period of rapid growth, she also was the interim director of HFA at PCA America (Martin, 1999). Her experiences in those national and state leadership positions affirm what Schorr (1997) learned about bringing programs to scale and sustaining them. Schorr (1997) discovered six elements that facilitated making programs "more a matter of deliberate public policy" (p. 60).

1. Combine the essence of a successful intervention with adaptations of components to fit the particular community or population.
2. Have the continuous sponsorship of an organization that can offer expertise, support, legitimization, and clout.
3. Recognize the importance of systems and institutional support.
4. Recognize the importance of people.
5. Use outcomes orientation to measure success.
6. Tackle directly and strategically the obstacles to large-scale change.

Adapt the Essence of a Successful Intervention to Fit a Particular Community

The essence of the HFA home visiting model is distilled into 12 critical elements that are reflected in program standards (Daro & Harding, 1999). Consistent with adapting the essence of a successful intervention, most standards permit or require adaptation to the local community. For example, local HFA programs define the target population and educational requirements for staff, as well as select developmental screening tools and curricula they will use on home visits. HFA programs serve families in over 400 communities across the country. Therefore, local decision making is essential in order to adapt the program model to diverse communities and allow the model to mature over time.

Have the Continuous Sponsorship from an Organization That Offers Expertise, Support, Legitimization, and Clout

PCA America, the sponsoring organization for HFA, supports state leaders and local programs. Expert advice and guidance is available to community leaders who are interested in starting a HFA program. Initially this was provided by the national office. Now it also is being provided by HFA Regional Resource Centers, a concept that is part of a strategic initiative to support statewide systems. PCA America develops and disseminates multiple documents including guides for program planning, advocacy, and accessing funding. The public Web site has a wealth of up-to-date information at www.healthyfamiliesamerica.org. Through PCA America, HFA is at the table when major reviews of home visiting and deliberations occur at the federal level and among voluntary organizations. Strategic partnerships with organizations such as American Academy of Pediatrics, American Nurses Association, National Association of Children's Hospitals and Related Institutions, National Association of Counties, Early Head Start/Head Start, and ZERO TO THREE has resulted in efforts to promote home visiting and advocate for federal funding.

Recognize the Importance of Systems and Institutional Support

Seventy percent of all HF program sites are located in 11 states with multisite systems of 10 or more sites. Supportive infrastructure at the state level fosters expansion of sites. State infrastructure needs to be flexible to meet the needs of new and established sites. HFIT&TAP at Indiana University School of Nursing supports all HF Indiana sites, through a state contract that includes training, quality assurance site visits, technical assistance, and data management and evaluation. Coordination of these state-level support services has been an efficient way to ensure consistency across sites. Since 1994, HFIT&TAP has expanded and adapted to meet growing and changing needs, particularly in the areas of training and data management. Infrastructure flexibility is achieved by keeping permanent staff to a minimum and contracting for services, as needed. HFIT&TAP has been able to meet the needs of diverse program sites and meet program standards, as evidenced by PCA America credentialing all HF Indiana program sites and the state system three different times.

Recognize the Importance of People

The best designed system cannot survive without strong leadership. One inspired leader is not enough. HF Indiana started with a handful of committed advocates and recruited additional people with demonstrated leadership skills. Over time, members of the initial state leadership team assumed different responsibilities, moved to other states, or retired. HF Indiana continues to be a strong, vibrant initiative because the development of new leaders, including public health nurses, is encouraged and fostered. As an example, the HF Indiana Evaluation Workgroup is chaired by a public health nurse, who is program manager for the HF Indiana program site at Indiana University School of Nursing.

Similar to other states, 90 percent of the annual budget for HF Indiana is public dollars, primarily federal dollars administered by the state. Therefore, it is important to maintain support from the governor and top-level state administrators. State policy makers deserve credit for making important funding decisions, and home visitors need to feel their work is valued. Celebrating success is important. When HF Indiana was credentialed by PCA America, over 500 home visitors from local HF Indiana program sites attended a celebration in the Statehouse Rotunda. They were honored to hear their work praised in speeches by the First Lady, the newly appointed director of the state agency, and the PCA America Executive Director. Elected and appointed officials were presented with national awards of excellence for which they received favorable media coverage. Positive public recognition is one of the contributing factors for staff retention and for continued support of HF Indiana across four different administrations, Republican and Democrat alike.

Use Outcomes to Measure Success

Success is not measured by the numbers of HFA program sites or the numbers of families served, but measuring the results of child abuse prevention efforts has particular challenges. First, child maltreatment is hard to measure. Child Protective Service (CPS) standards for substantiating child abuse and neglect vary from state to state and from county to county (USDHHS, 2006). Substantiated maltreatment is the main measure of interest to policy makers, but it is not a good measure. The risk of repeated maltreatment is equally great whether CPS reports are unsubstantiated or substantiated (Drake et al., 2003), but some states expunge

⊕ RESEARCH APPLICATION

Assessing Community Change at Multiple Levels: The Genesis of an Evaluation Framework for California Healthy Cities Project

Study Purpose

To present the research involved in developing the evaluation framework of the California Healthy Cities project and describe the various public health concepts involved. Changes brought about by community-based citizen participation occur at multiple levels. The complexity of the change process, the variety of health issues addressed, and the range of unique community characteristics make evaluation a daunting task.

Methods

Changes resulting from Healthy Cities projects were identified by citizens involved in local projects. From this full list of change possibilities, major categories were developed, and a draft evaluation framework was proposed. This framework was shared with representatives of the cities to solicit their reactions and prioritize the concepts. City representatives were active participants in the validation and refinement of the evaluation framework.

Findings

The three theoretical orientations that informed the framework were social ecology, community capacity/com-

petence, and urban planning. Changes occurred at five levels: individual, civic participation, organizational, inter-organizational, and community. Examples of changes are new policies, services, programs, and/or changes in the physical environment. Data from city representatives provide linkages between concepts and community change.

Implications

Evaluation research in community development and community health promotion is critical to document results, test approaches, develop valid measures, and refine concepts. Refining evaluation precision provides data to improve practice and illuminate the process of community change.

Reference

Kegler, M. C., Twiss, J. M., & Look, V. (2000). Assessing community change at multiple levels: The genesis of an evaluation framework for the California Healthy Cities project. *Health Education & Behavior, 27*(6), 760–779.

---

unsubstantiated CPS reports immediately upon determination or shortly thereafter (National Clearinghouse on Child Abuse and Neglect Information, 2003). Home visitors are mandated to report suspected maltreatment so presence of a home visitor simultaneously can increase CPS reports, even substantiated reports, and decrease risk of maltreatment.

Second, HFA and other home-visiting programs usually are funded as service projects, not research projects. Most local and state funding agencies are not comfortable with randomly assigning at-risk families to a control group that does not receive any home visits. When random assignment is possible, differences among groups are minimized because families in the control group either receive fewer services by design, or families might participate in similar community-based

family strengthening programs such as Early Head Start or Parents as Teachers on their own.

Third, randomized clinical trials are challenging to conduct with at-risk populations. Highest risk subjects can be difficult to engage, and attrition is high. Available outcome tools are not powerful enough to detect small changes over time or comprehensive enough to measure the broad range of factors addressed by home visiting programs (Wollesen & Peifer, 2005). Even when research demonstrates efficacy in well-designed, resource-rich programs, the same results cannot be guaranteed in the real world Still, it is more likely when evidence-based practice is implemented consistently (Chinman, Imm, & Wandersman, 2004). For this reason, HFA created a credentialing process to ensure all HFA programs adhere to agreed upon evidence-based standards.

Tackle Obstacles to Large-Scale Change

At the national level, proponents of the major home visiting programs are working collaboratively to shift federal resources from treatment to prevention. This required reframing child abuse as a public health issue instead of as a social welfare or criminal justice issue (Martin, Green, & Gielen, 2008). A key strategy is to craft a consistent message and promote the concept of home visiting, instead of splintering off and promoting a preferred home visiting program. This requires setting realistic expectations by balancing the promise of success with mixed results from rigorous evaluations (Sherwood, 2005).

In Indiana, creating a sustainable funding stream for HF Indiana was of paramount importance. Without resources, HF Indiana would remain a small demonstration site, unable to reach a significant number of families and unable to make a difference in populations. On the surface, the challenge was money. However, the greater challenge was to develop a broad understanding about the importance of preventing child maltreatment—from the agency perspective. Agencies that primarily were concerned with health, social welfare, education, mental health, or criminal justice also needed to be concerned about child abuse. Once agency leaders understood the connection between their primary mission and child abuse, they realized efforts to meet their stated objectives would be futile, without preventing child abuse. Consequently, they recognized the need to shift some of their funding toward supporting efforts to prevent child abuse, regardless of which agency would receive the money and take the lead.

At the local level, HF Indiana fosters collaboration over competition. From the beginning, each county could submit only one proposal for funding. As a result, multiple agencies collaborated to submit a single proposal, instead of submitting competing proposals. Proposals were stronger because agencies worked together and contributed the best each one had to offer. As HF Indiana expanded, community leaders in counties without HF Indiana program sites decided to join existing programs in adjacent counties and become a "branch office." The long-standing tradition of programs staying within geopolitical boundaries was erased, resulting in HF Indiana program sites serving multiple counties.

What is a common theme at each level—national, state, and local? Efforts are collaborative instead of competitive, and results are promising, but not perfect. This is a work in progress. When community leaders, agencies, and programs decide to relinquish some resources and control, they discover the results are better than what they could have achieved in isolation.

LINKING HEALTHY CITIES AND HEALTHY FAMILIES

Each community develops characteristics and patterns of accomplishing work that influence the health status and quality of life of residents. Communities with urgent health needs are often those challenged with

---

⊕ POLICY HIGHLIGHT

Policy Scope and Influence

National policies with grand scope and substantial budgets capture the imagination when pondering policy as a tool for health promotion and social change. However, local policies, city ordinances, and institutional procedures that govern daily lives have great influence on health. The Healthy Cities Model purports that policies closest to the daily lives of individuals and families can promote health, alter the public debate, and get health on the formal agenda of decision makers. The following examples were discussed in more detail earlier in the chapter:

⊕ A city ordinance banned indoor smoking in public buildings based in part on HCHC data and testimony.

⊕ The development and implementation of a comprehensive land use policy in this rural area encouraged biking and hiking rather than requiring cars for transportation; a HCHC board member sits on this board and reports a change in mindset regarding "making the healthy choices the easy choices."

⊕ A proposal to build a skate park on city property, though defeated by the city council, packed the council chambers with teenage boys who were engaged in the process and subsequent mayoral election; citizen participation is a required first step for policy advocacy and community health in the Healthy Cities Model.

meager political, human, and financial resources to initiate and sustain programs that promote health. Public health nurses work in partnership with communities to navigate the path from their current situation to one of greater health, mindful that journeys involving community development, capacity building, and citizen engagement yield greater and more enduring benefits. Public health nurse leaders play a variety of roles in assisting the community to understand the possibilities and potential programs, as well as developing the local leaders and support for the actions.

Public health nurse leaders who mobilize communities to promote health need an array of communication, political, and analytical skills. Rather than a "cookie-cutter" approach where right and wrong actions are obvious, the process involves matching unique community tendencies to various theoretical approaches. Public health nurses, who are knowledgeable about different approaches, are able to adapt and customize strategies. Interpersonal and mass communication skills, matched with political insights and sensitivity, equip the nurse to lead change efforts.

This chapter describes two community development models that public health nurse leaders can use to promote public health—Healthy Cities and Healthy Families. Using these models and their steps can not only engender a shared definition of health and a sense of community but also build consensus around a particular health issue and priority. The steps of the model are iterative and can provide a way to provide ongoing assessment, gather data, and encourage community action. The community that has built capacity for collective health promotion work through a community development model can more readily identify and choose a program to address the prioritized health issue. In this chapter, the Healthy Families program, which was designed to prevent child maltreatment by strengthening families, was used as an example.

This blending of models and programs demonstrates to public health nurses the requisite creativity in assisting and empowering communities to actively participate in their own health promotion. Public health nurses serve the vital roles of consultant, content expert, facilitator, and advocate for health by creatively adapting what they know to the challenges of the community. Creating communities in which health promotion initiatives can take root, flourish, and even expand is transformative work that requires an engaged community and a creative and inspired public health workforce.

CRITICAL THINKING ACTIVITIES

1. Identifying the health issue of highest priority to the community is an important process. What strategies would you use to begin the process and to validate the outcome? Who would be the key players?

2. Community health promotion is a collaborative process. What are some appropriate roles for health professionals? For citizens? For government officials?

3. When would the Healthy Cities model be the most effective strategy for community development and health promotion?

4. When would you know the actions for community health promotion were achieving the results desired by citizens and health professionals? What if the results desired by citizens varied from those desired by health professionals?

5. Recall the six elements identified by Schorr (1997) to fully implement and sustain community initiatives and reflect on the Healthy Cities practice application of HCHC. Explore how each of the elements was or was not addressed by the HCHC, and as a public health nursing leader make suggestions for ways to improve the process and success.

6. Why is it difficult to demonstrate effectiveness in a voluntary child abuse prevention program? How can evaluation measure the impact of such a program or set of services?

7. What are the rates of child maltreatment in your state? What proportion of CPS referrals is investigated? Of those investigated, what proportion is substantiated? When does your state expunge unsubstantiated CPS reports? How does your state compare with other states? How would you find out? What area do you think needs improving and what would you recommend?

KEY TERMS

child maltreatment

community development for
health promotion

effective program

evidence-based program

Healthy Cities

healthy public policies

model program

multisectoral

participatory development

social ecological approach

KEY CONCEPTS

⊕ Community development approaches originate
from a variety of theoretical orientations.

⊕ The Healthy Cities model is a social ecological
approach to community health promotion and
problem solving.

⊕ The Healthy Cities approach builds capacity
through a shared vision of health, common community values, and diverse citizen participation.

⊕ Improvement in community statistics will not be
seen until effective interventions reach significant
numbers of at-risk families.

⊕ Community leaders should make well-informed
decisions based upon sound selection criteria.

⊕ Program models need to be adapted to meet the
needs of families in diverse communities.

⊕ Evaluations of home-visiting programs show
mixed results. Pre- and postevaluations demonstrate positive changes, but findings from randomized trials are less impressive.

⊕ Public health nurses can be effective leaders at
the local, state, and national level.

REFERENCES

Bilukha, O., Hahn, R. A., Crosby, A., Fullilove, M. T., Liber-
man, A., Moscicki, E., Snyder, S., Tuma, F., Corso, P.,
Schofield, A., & Briss, P. A. (2005). The effectiveness of
early childhood home visitation in preventing violence:
A systematic review. *American Journal of Preventive
Medicine, 28*(2 Suppl. 1), 11–39.

Bugental, D. B., Ellerson, P. C., Lin, E. K., Rainey, B., Koko-
tovic, A., & O'Hara, N. (2002). A cognitive approach
to child abuse prevention. *Journal of Family Psychology,
16*(3), 243–258.

Chaffin, M. (2004). Is it time to rethink healthy start/healthy
families? *Child Abuse & Neglect, 28*(6), 589–595.

Chaffin, M. (2005). "Is it time to rethink healthy start/healthy
families?" Response to Letters. *Child Abuse & Neglect,
29*(3), 241–249.

Chinman, M., Imm, P., & Wandersman, A (2004). *Getting to
outcomes 2004: Promoting accountability through methods
and tools for planning, implementation, and evaluation.*
Santa Monica: RAND Corporation Technical Report.
Available online at http://www.rand.org/publications/TR/
TR10/.

Daro, D., & Harding, K. (1999). Healthy families America:
Using research to enhance practice. *The Future of Children,
9*(1), 152–176. Available online at www.futureofchildren.org

Drake, B., Jonson-Reid, M., Way, I., & & Chung, S. (2003).
Substantiation and recidivism. *Child Maltreatment, 8*(4),
248–260.

Duggan, A., McFarlane, E., Fuddy, L., Burrell, L., Higman,
S. M., Windham, A., & Sia, C. (2004). Randomized trial
of a statewide home visiting program: Impact in preventing child abuse and neglect. *Child Abuse & Neglect, 28*(6),
597–622.

Duhl, L. J. (1996). An ecohistory of health: The role of
"healthy cities." *American Journal of Health Promotion,
10*(4), 258–261.

Duhl, L. J. (2000). *The social entrepreneurship of change.* Put-
nam Valley, NY: Cogent Publishing.

Eckenrode, J., Ganzel, B., Henderson, C. R., Smith, E., Olds,
D., Powers, J., Cole, R., & Kitzman, H. (2000). Preventing child abuse and neglect with a program of nurse
home visitation: The limiting effects of domestic violence.
Journal of the American Medical Association, 284(11),
1385–1391.

Flynn, B.C. (1996). Healthy cities: Toward worldwide health
promotion. *Annual Review of Public Health, 7,* 299–309.

Gomby, D. (2003). *Building school readiness through home
visitation.* Sacramento: First 5 California Children and

Families Commission. Full text available at www.ccfc
.ca.gov.

Gomby, D., Culross, P., & Behrman, R.. (1999). Home visiting: Recent program evaluations—Analysis and recommendations. *Future of Children, 9*(1), 4–223.

Green, L. W., Richard, L., & Potvin, L. (1996). Ecological foundations of health promotion. *American Journal of Health Promotion. 10*(4), 270–281.

Hancock, T. (1997). Healthy cities and communities: Past, present and future. *National Civic Review, 86*(1), 11–22.

Hancock, T., & Duhl, L. (1988). *Promoting health in the urban context.* WHO Health Cities Paper 1. Copenhagen: World Health Organization.

Harding, K., Galano, J., Huntington, L., Martin, J., & Schellenbach, C. (2008). Healthy families America effectiveness: A synthesis of support. *Journal of Prevention and Intervention in the Community.*

Hepburn, K. (2005). *Families as primary partners in their child's development and school readiness.* Baltimore: The Annie E. Casey Foundation. Full text available at www
.aecf.org.

Johnson, K., (2001). *No place like home: State home visiting policies and programs.* New York: The Commonwealth Fund. Full text available at www.cmwf.org.

Kegler, M. C., Twiss, J. M., & Look, V. (2000). Assessing community change at multiple levels: The genesis of an evaluation framework for the California healthy cities project. *Health Education & Behavior, 27*(6), 760–779.

Kikendall, P. (2006). Healthy Families Indiana State Coordinator, Department of Child Services, personal communication.

Lee, P. (2000). Healthy Communities: A young movement that can revolutionize public health. *Public Health Reports, 115* (2), 114–115.

MacLeod, J., & Nelson, G. (2000). Programs for the promotion of family wellness and the prevention of child maltreatment: A meta-analytic review. *Child Abuse & Neglect, 24*(9), 1127–1149.

Martin, J. (1999). Healthy families America. *The Future of Children, 9*(1), 177–178.

Martin, J., Green, L., & Gielen, A. (2008). Potential lessons from public health and health promotion for the prevention of child abuse. *Journal of Prevention and Intervention in the Community.*

McGuigan, W. M., Katzev, A. R., & Pratt, C. C. (2003). Multi-level determinants of retention in a home-visiting child abuse prevention program. *Child Abuse & Neglect, 27*, 363–380.

Mitchell-Herzfeld, S., Izzo, C., Greene, R., Lee, E., & Lowenfels, A. (2005). *Evaluation of healthy families New York: First year program impacts.* Rensselaer, NY: New York

State Office of Children and Family Services, Bureau of Evaluation and Research. Available online at http://www
.ocfs.state.ny.us/main/prevention/assets/HFNY_FirstYear-ProgramImpacts.pdf

National Clearinghouse on Child Abuse and Neglect Information. (2003). *Child Abuse and Neglect State Statute Series Statutes-at-a-Glance, Central Registry/Reporting Records Expungement.* Available online at http://nccanch.acf.hhs
.gov.

National Governor's Association Task Force on School Readiness. (2005*). Building the foundation for bright futures.* Washington, DC: National Governor's Association. Full text available at www.nga.org

Norris, T., & Pittman, M. (2000). The healthy communities movement and the Coalition for Healthier Cities and Communities. *Public Health Reports, 115*(2), 118–124.

Olds, D., Eckenrode, J., Henderson, C. R., Jr., Kitzman, H., Powers, J., Cole, R., Sidora, K., Morris, P., Pettitt, L., & Luckey, D. (1997). Long-term effects of home visitation on maternal life course and child abuse and neglect. Fifteen-year follow-up of a randomized trial. *Journal of the American Medical Association, 278*(8), 637–643.

Olds, D., Eckenrode, J., & Kitzman, H. (2005). Clarifying the impact of the Nurse-Family Partnership on child maltreatment: Response to Chaffin (2004) [letter]. *Child Abuse & Neglect* (29) 3, 229–233.

PAHO. (2002). *Healthy municipalities and communities: Mayors' guide for promoting quality of life.* Washington, DC: Pan American Health Organization.

PAHO (2005). Pan American Health Organization home page. Available www.paho.org.

Schorr, L. B., (1997). *Common purpose: Strengthening families and neighborhoods to rebuild America.* New York: Doubleday.

Sherwood, K. E. (Spring, 2005). Evaluating home visitation: A case study of evaluation at the David and Lucile Packard Foundation. *New Directions for Evaluation, 2005* (105), 59–81.

Stokols, D. (1996). Translating social ecological theory into guidelines for community health promotion. *American Journal of Health Promotion. 10*(4), 282–298.

U.S. Department of Health and Human Services (USDHHS*). *(2006). *Administration on Children Youth, & Families. Child Maltreatment 2004.* Washington, DC: U.S. Government Printing Office. Full report is available online at http://www.acf.hhs.gov/programs/cb/stats_research/index.htm#can.

Wollesen, L., & Peifer, K. (2005). *Life Skills Progression (LSP): An outcome and intervention planning instrument for use with families at risk.* Baltimore: Paul H. Brookes Publishing Co.

World Health Organization Collaborating Center in Healthy Cities. (2005). *Community Health Promotion Model.* Indianapolis: Indiana University School of Nursing.

BIBLIOGRAPHY

Flynn, B.C. (1997). Partnership is healthy cities and communities: A social commitment for advanced practice nurses. *Advanced Practice Nurses Quarterly, 2*(4), 1–5.

Goldstein, G., & Kickbusch, I. (1996). A health city is a better city. *World Health, 90*(1), 4–10.

Hancock, T. (2000). Healthy communities must also be sustainable communities. *Public Health Reports 115*(2, 3), 151–160.

Norris, T., & Pittman M. (2000). The healthy communities movement and the coalition for healthier cities and communities. *Public Health Reports, 115*(2, 3), 118–126.

Pan American Health Organization/WHO (1999*). The healthy municipalities movement: A settings approach and strategy for health promotion in Latin America and the Caribbean.* Washington, DC: author.

Wallerstein, N. (2000). A participatory evaluation model for healthier communities: Developing indicators for New Mexico. *Public Health Reports 115*(2, 3), 1999–210.

RESOURCES

The Alliance for Healthy Cities

Email: alliance/ith@tmd.ac.ip
Web: http://www.alliance-healthycities.com
The Alliance for Healthy Cities is an international network aiming at protecting and enhancing the health of city dwellers. The alliance is a group of cities and other organizations that try to achieve the goal through an approach called Healthy Cities. We believe that international cooperation is an effective and efficient tool to achieve the goal. And we promote the interaction of people who are in the front line of health issues. The Healthy Cities approach was initiated by the World Health Organization. In order to cope with the adverse effects of an urban environment over health, the WHO has been promoting the approach worldwide.

The Future of Children

Email: FOC@princeton.edu
Web: http://www.futureofchildren.org
The Future of Children seeks to promote effective policies and programs for children by providing policy makers, service providers, and the media with timely, objective information based on the best available research. The Future of Children is a publication of The Woodrow Wilson School

of Public and International Affairs at Princeton University and The Brookings Institution. This is the Healthy Families Web site.

The International Healthy Cities Foundation

555 12th Street, 10th Floor
Oakland, California 94607
510-642-1715
FAX: 510-643-6981
Email: hcities@uclink4.berkeley.edu
Web: http://www.healthycities.org
The Web site is a place where people interested in addressing urban and community issues along with concerns about health and quality of life issues in their communities can join and share information. The Web site facilitates linkages among people, issues, and resources in order to support the development of Healthy Cities initiatives. The site includes a searchable database of over 1,000 meritorious solutions to urban issues related to health.

OneWorld United States

3201 New Mexico Avenue NW, Suite 395
Washington, D.C. 20016
202-885-2679
FAX: 202-885-1309
Email: us@oneworld.net
Web: http://us.oneworld.net
OneWorld is a global information network developed to support communication media of the people, by the people, and for the people—everywhere. Its goal is to help build a more just global society through its partnership community. OneWorld encourages people to discover their power—power to speak, connect, and make a difference—by providing access to information and enabling connections between hundreds of organizations and tens of thousands of people around the world. The OneWorld network is driven by the people and organizations it supports—people write the news, provide the video clips, and prepare the radio stories. Through this network, individuals have access to information previously unavailable to them—information that can broaden their world view and enable them to make better decisions.

The Pan American Health Organization (PAHO)

525 23rd Street NW
Washington, D.C. 20037
202-974-3000
Web: http://www.paho.org
PAHO is an international public health agency with 100 years of experience in working to improve health and living standards of the countries of the Americas. It serves as the specialized organization for health of the Inter-American

System. It also serves as the Regional Office for the Americas of the World Health Organization and enjoys international recognition as part of the United Nations system. The Web site provides comprehensive information about Healthy Cities and specific examples and information relevant to Latin and North America.

The World Health Organization (WHO)

Avenue Appia 20
1211 Geneva 27 Switzerland
+ 41-22-791-21-11
FAX: + 41-22-79-3111
Telex: 415 416
Telegraph: UNISANTE GENEVA
Email: info@who.int.
Web: http://www.who.int

The World Health Organization is the United Nations specialized agency for health. It was established on April 7, 1948. WHO's objective, as set out in its Constitution, is the attainment by all peoples of the highest possible level of health. Health is defined in WHO's Constitution as a state of complete physical, mental, and social well-being and not merely the absence of disease or infirmity. WHO is governed by 193 member states through the World Health Assembly. The Health Assembly is composed of representatives from WHO's member states. The main tasks of the World Health Assembly are to approve the WHO program and the budget for the following biennium and to decide major policy questions. The WHO Web site provides rich examples and information on Healthy Cities from an international perspective.

The WHO Collaborating Center for Healthy Cities

Web: http://www.iupui.edu

The WHO Collaborating Center for Healthy Cities resides at Indiana University School of Nursing at IUPUI (Indiana University Purdue University at Indianapolis). Citynet presents a 9-step community health promotion model of great utility.

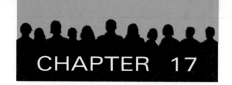

CHAPTER 17

Health Care Management

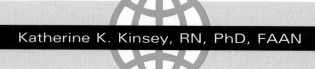

Katherine K. Kinsey, RN, PhD, FAAN

Chapter Outline

🌐 **Management and Public Health Nurses**
　Scope and Standards
　Ounce of Prevention

🌐 **Healthy People 2010**
　Focus Area 23: Public Health Infrastructure

🌐 **Administration and Leadership**
　Organizational Culture
　Community Culture

🌐 **Basics of Internal Management**
　Professional and Personal (Self) Development
　Personnel Management
　Support Services
　Fiscal Management
　Case Management
　Program Management

🌐 **Basics of External Management**
　Public Engagement
　Public Policy
　Globalization

🌐 **Keys to Improvement**

🌐 **Future Orientation**

Learning Objectives

Upon completion of this chapter, the reader will be able to:

1. Define management in the context of public health nursing practice and organizational dynamics.

2. Apply the Scope and Standards of Public Health Nursing Practice in public health settings.

3. Utilize Healthy People 2010 goals and objectives to guide management of public health programs and services.

4. Compare and contrast the terms and functions of managers, organizational leaders, and administrators.

5. Describe professional and personal skills needed to effectively manage personnel, program, and fiscal resources.

6. Identify complexities of community involvement, program improvement, and global issues influencing public health programs.

Public health nurses are uniquely positioned to make lasting differences in the lives of populations they care about and for. In the public health realm, public health nurses provide prevention, early detection, and intervention services in communities, schools, homes, religious organizations, and other institutional settings. Public health nurses, in independent practice or in collaboration with other health, social, and educational professionals, provide direct services to clients and population groups. Frequently, public health nurses are called upon to manage programs, supervise other public health workers, maintain fiscal accountability, contract for services, allocate resources, develop program improvement standards, collaborate with community organizations and the public at large, recognize global threats, and be future oriented.

Managerial positions place public health nurses in the forefront of practice, education and research initiatives to improve the well-being of individuals, families, groups, and communities. Managerial work improves organizational and people skills. The public health nurse manager appreciates the complexity and multiplicity of the health needs of the public and possesses the skills to improve the well-being of one and all. This chapter emphasizes key management elements for public health nurses, promotes opportunities to seek managerial experiences, and serves as a managerial resource guide.

MANAGEMENT AND PUBLIC HEALTH NURSES

Many variables influence the definition of management (noun) and the verb "manage" in the twenty-first century. Abbreviated classic twentieth-century dictionary definitions provided by the unabridged version of *The Random House Dictionary of the English Language* (1969) include: (1) management is the act or manner of handling, direction, or control; (2) manage is to bring about; to succeed in accomplishing; to take charge or care of; to dominate or influence; to handle, direct, govern, or control in action or use. Management in today's public heath arena must be viewed as a term with multiple conditions. The conditions define the use and application of management and managerial approaches. Conditions include the public health nurse's personal interpretation and application of management in everyday life, the organization's expectations about management roles and responsibilities, and external environmental factors. External environmental factors include public policies, legislative decisions, public opinion polls, as well as the introduction of new or recurring public health threats.

Individuals who gravitate to the nursing profession often have basic organizational and managerial skills in their everyday lives. The profession continues to attract a female majority who at a very young age learned how to prioritize and multitask (Braun, 2005). These learned skills serve nursing students well as they progress through demanding and strenuous academic studies. New nursing graduates bring their informal managerial skills to first and subsequent employment experiences.

Schools of nursing offer undergraduate leadership courses; however, managerial courses are typically reserved for advanced study. Yet new and seasoned nurses, particularly public health nurses, are called upon to use their learned managerial skills each and every day. Public health nurses are particularly challenged to perfect their managerial skills given finite resources as well as the unpredictability and suddenness of public health threats, administrative or legislative changes, and changes in public opinion over time.

Public health nurses can be placed in formal management positions because of their recognized skills and expressed interests. Others may be advanced due to longevity, familiarity with the organization and its culture, and personality (good fit with current administration). Regardless of explicit and implicit reasons for offering or accepting management responsibilities in an organization, it is essential for the public health nurse to seek further learning opportunities to improve managerial skills and to understand the organization's mission, vision, and leadership style. The following interpretation of management can serve to guide public health nurses who enter the managerial world:

Management translates the leadership's or organization's vision and mission into productive action and aids in progressing toward public health goals. It is a form of interpretative leadership based on the tenets of public health nursing; communication and collaboration skills; prudent resource allocation; fiscal integrity; and integration of core public health standards, practices, and policies. One constant is being future oriented by understanding the past, managing the present, and anticipating the future. The public health nurse must also appreciate that successes will be built on trust, truth, constancy, confidentiality, listening, and successfully managing change (Robbins, 2003).

Scope and Standards

The Quad Council of Public Health Nursing Organizations includes the American Nurses Association, Council for Community, Primary and Long-Term Care Nursing Practice; the American Public Health Association, Public Health Nursing Section; the Association of Community Health Nursing Educators; and the Association of State and Territorial Directors of Nursing. The Quad Council has put forth the *Public Health Nursing: Scope and Standards of Practice* (2007) published by the American Nurses Association. The publication provides guidance to public health nurses and others in the helping professions to promote and protect the health of populations. It is an effective tool to determine progress toward goals and quality improvement initiatives; to validate the quality of professional services; to promote accountability, advocacy, and social justice for all; and to assist in adapting to new public health challenges. Emphasis is placed on standards of care and professional performance. The standards serve as a framework for critical analyses, as a means for developing accurate reporting measures, and as a tool for identifying areas of need. The document is inclusive of cultural, environmental, geographic factors that may contribute to clinical and programmatic outcomes.

Public health nurse managers will find that the standards guide nursing performance in the field, program management, and evaluation as well as determine areas of improvement and growth. This publication should be a reference tool for every public health nurse and a lasting resource for public health nurse managers. To assist public health nurses in familiarizing themselves with the standards, public health nurse managers could provide a copy of the *Scope and Standards* to staff upon employment and periodically review the standards during clinical conferences.

Ounce of Prevention

An ounce of prevention is worth a pound of cure. Not having a disease or injury in the first place eliminates extraordinary tolls on personal well-being, family life, financial resources, and societal productivity. Benjamin Franklin has been credited for this time-honored wisdom. Others assert that the adage first appeared in H.C. Harburton's 1848 *Book of Wisesaws*. Regardless of its origins, this centuries-old saying holds great relevance in the twenty-first century. The maxim is scientifically valid. For example, data continue to refute the tobacco industry's original assertions that smoking or chewing tobacco does not kill. The marketing and selling of tobacco combined with its purchase and use in one form or another by millions of Americans have contributed to the premature disability and deaths of too many in the United States (Freudenberg, 2005). Furthermore, the costs related to diseases caused by smoking (e.g., hospitalizations, therapies, in-home services) far exceed what private or public insurance covers. This example demonstrates that never smoking (prevention) not only saves lives, it saves money and secures our society's future. Figure 17-1 reinforces the idea that today's pound of cure weighs (in human costs) as much if not more than our forefathers' forecasts.

The reality in today's society is that prevention or cessation of smoking and nicotine addiction is complicated. Public health nurse managers must incorporate both prevention and intervention initiatives at the client level as well as work with policy makers in the fight against tobacco use and nicotine addiction. Published research reinforces the possibilities of developing smoke-free policies within an organization that include smoking cessation workshops and strategies for nonsmokers to avoid secondhand smoke.

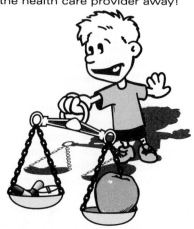

An ounce of prevention is worth a pound of cure

or

An apple a day keeps the health care provider away!

Figure 17-1 Prevention scale.

⊕ RESEARCH APPLICATION

A Longitudinal Assessment of the Impact of Smoke-Free Worksite Policies on Tobacco Use

Study Purpose

To assess the impact of smoke-free work site policies on smoking cessation behaviors.

Methods

Tracked cohort of smokers from the Community Intervention Trial for Smoking Cessation (COMMIT). Data based on 1993 and 2001 telephone surveys to 1967 employed smokers. Data included personal and demographic characteristics, behaviors regarding tobacco use, and work site smoking policies.

Findings

Employees were more likely to reduce cigarette consumption or stop smoking if the work site had more restrictive smoking policies. Respondents who continued to smoke reported that, on average, they reduced daily consumption

by nearly four cigarettes. Workers in environments that prohibited smoking were 2.3 times more likely to have quit smoking than those in environments that did not restrict smoking.

Implications

Policies that enforce 100% smoke-free work sites frame conducive environments for public and individual health. Future studies hold the potential to note a correlation between smoke-free environments and reduced rates of smoking in workers.

Reference

Bauer, J., Hyland, A., Qiang, L., Steger, C., & Cummings, M. (2005). A longitudinal assessment of the impact of smoke-free worksite policies on tobacco use. *American Journal of Public Health, 95*, 1024–1029.

HEALTHY PEOPLE 2010

Science increasingly validates that the economic, family, and community costs of people suffering the aftermaths of accidents, injuries, infectious, and chronic diseases place a tremendous burden on populations as well as the nation. The measured societal and economic burden of disease, disability, and death on American life led to a national planning process for disease prevention and health promotion. In 1979, *Healthy People: The Surgeon's Report on Health Promotion and Disease Prevention* was published. In 1990, Healthy People 2000 was released. Healthy People 2010 represents the third time that 10-year health objectives for the nation have been developed by the U.S. Department of Health and Human Services.

Healthy People 2010 vision is "Healthy People in Healthy Communities." Its overarching goals are to increase both the quality of life and years of healthy life and to eliminate health disparities. Healthy People 2010 (HP 2010) establishes benchmarks for individuals and communities to strive for and represent a social mandate for health care (Carey, 2004). HP 2010 provides a utilitarian framework for public health nurses

involved in case management (individual clients), program management (population focus), or organizational management (human resources, support services, fiscal oversight, etc). For the first time, actions and successes to improve health are guided by a set of leading health indicators reflecting current public health threats. (See Box 17-1).

Healthy People 2010 has 467 objectives in 28 focus areas that incorporate leading health indicators and health improvement initiatives. One essential initiative

BOX 17-1: HP 2010: Leading Health Indicators

Physical activity	Overweight and obesity
Tobacco use	Substance abuse
Responsible sexual behavior	Mental health
Injury and violence	Environmental quality
Immunization	Access to health care

is to improve public health capacity and infrastructure (USDHHS, 2000a). Nurses in public health managerial positions must include focus area 23 (public health infrastructure) as a working goal in their organization.

Focus Area 23: Public Health Infrastructure

The **public health infrastructure** goal is to ensure that federal, tribal, state, and local health agencies have the infrastructure to provide essential public health services effectively. At the local level, health agencies can include an array of providers such as managed care organizations, schools, faith-based groups, and nurse-managed health centers. Sixteen objectives focus on data and information systems, status indicators and priority data needs, workforce, public health organizations, and resources. The focus area incorporates the Essential Public Health Services (see Box 17-2) released by the Public Health Function Steering Committee in the mid 1990s. (www.health.gov/phfunctionsw/public .htm, January 1, 2000).

Public health nurses are directly or indirectly involved in all these services. Public health nurse managers could conduct an annual orientation and review the organization's essential services and outcomes to improve quality, build capacity, and promote prevention initiatives. For example, Objective 17 of Focus Area 23 is to increase the proportion of federal, tribal, state, and local public health agencies that conduct or collaborate on population-based prevention research. Public health nurses responsible for program services or administrative oversight are uniquely positioned to engage diverse and specific population groups in prevention research and to share the findings. These findings will highlight the work of public health nurses and contribute to generalizable knowledge and best practices.

ADMINISTRATION AND LEADERSHIP

Public health nurse managers need to understand the definitions of administration and leadership. These definitions help the public health nurse manager to appreciate an organization's culture (Bhatia, 2003). Organizational cultures contribute to productivity, community credibility, and reputation and guide the public health nurse's relationships and conduct with others in decision-making positions. Organizational understanding

---

BOX 17-2: Essential Public Health Services

1. Monitor heath status to identify community health problems.

2. Diagnose and investigate health problems and health hazards in the community.

3. Inform, educate, and empower people about health issues.

4. Mobilize community partnerships to identify and solve health problems.

5. Develop policies and plans that support individual and community health efforts.

6. Enforce laws and regulations that protect health and ensure safety.

7. Link people to needed personal health services and ensure the provision of health care when otherwise unavailable.

8. Ensure a competent public health and personal health care workforce.

9. Evaluate effectiveness, accessibility, and quality of personal and population-based health services.

10. Research for new insights and innovative solutions to health problems.

---

will be further influenced by the public health nurse's past experiences, education, and collegial interactions and the organizations' construct for future work (Feldman, 2004). The nursing, business, educational, and social service literature offers many interpretations of administration and leadership. In today's dynamic health care environment, there are no single, static definitions. The astute public health nurse manager will use a variety of administration and leadership definitions to deal with vibrant, living, adaptive organizations.

One challenge for public health nurse managers is to understand that people use the terms "management," "administration." and "leadership" interchangeably (Porche, 2004). For the purposes of this chapter, the term **administration** represents the designated work and associated position (job) description with assigned roles and responsibilities within a particular organization. Typically, the work is delineated at the executive level. Organizational charts enable public health nurse managers to understand work and reporting responsibilities. In the Western world, the typical organization continues to be hierarchal where reporting flows up and down; and the status quo is preferred (Senge, 1990).

Defining leadership is challenging. In every organization there are formal leaders as well as informal leaders who do not hold designated key positions. Western society has influenced the concept of formal leadership and leaders. In the United States, leaders and heroes are still viewed as those who faced great challenges to be leaders. Senge, in his seminal work *The Fifth Discipline* (2000), argues that the Western style of leadership assumes that people lack personal vision and are powerless to deal with the forces of change; therefore, only a few great leaders emerge. Organizations that incorporate this perspective define leadership as setting the tone, making key decisions, and manipulating others to reach common goals. This perspective may have been functional in the twentieth century, but it holds little adaptability to the demands and changes occurring in the twenty-first century.

Organizations recognizing the need for proactive change strive to create new learning and system-oriented environments. These organizations want their leaders to be designers, stewards, and teachers (Senge, 2000). Their leaders breathe new life into (inspire) the organization and quietly work to design learning opportunities that support personal mastery and produce real results. Leadership in this environment fosters learning, helps people understand systemic forces that shape change, and builds on the collective will and power to make lasting contributions to society. Public health nurses who work in learning organizations find that there is a collective appreciation of the vision and mission; everyone is valued for his or her work, and the organization recognizes the contributions of formal and informal leaders.

Informal leaders are natural leaders who inspire confidence in others (Senge, 2000). Their ideas, communication skills, and abilities to listen and process, combined with their depth of commitment to lead others, support the organizational culture. Informal leaders are learners and teachers. Astute public health nurses who join a public heath organization quickly recognize the informal leaders who set the tone for the organization, program outcomes, and productive working relationships (Clark, 2004).

Another definition of leadership by Novick and Mays (2001) offers a practical guideline for the public health nurse and clarifies what is expected by the organization. They describe leadership as "the behavior that goes beyond the required performance expectations within an organization or community to provide direction and motivation of the behavior of others" (p. 772). "Going beyond" may be difficult to evaluate; however, assessment of performance in community engagement and employing intervention strategies to prevent or reduce disease or injury is measurable. Many would agree that public health nurses typically go beyond and are emerging formal and informal leaders in many organizations.

Organizational Culture

The organizational culture in which the public health nurse works is important to study and understand because (1) the public health nurse represents the organization in the community; (2) the history and growth of the organization has been shaped by the target community and its needs; (3) the responsiveness of the organization to new and escalating health needs or disease threats will, in part, be influenced by its experience within a particular community. For example, nurse-managed health centers have been established across the nation in underserved neighborhoods in need of quality primary health care services. The identified needs of the community provided the impetus to establish centers in places such as public housing sites, schools, recreation centers, and faith centers. The community has learned about the nurse-managed health centers and the work of nurses in primary and public health. The demand of nurse-managed health centers continues to grow in part because of the responsiveness of this care model to community characteristics and threats. Often community and population threats have been identified by public health nurses employed by nursing centers. Public health nurses work in community settings other than the primary care site. The public health nurses represent the nursing center model wherever they are and whomever they work with and for. Their professionalism and skill base reflects their understanding of the administrative and leadership resources within the organization. The community culture (way of life) and experiences are also critical to understand. The community shapes the organization just as the organization influences the health and well-being of the community.

Community Culture

The culture of a community is influenced by many factors. Factors include geographical location, climate, population base, settlement history (recent émigrés or generations that stay in place), growth potential, politics, economic and living conditions, and ideologies. Richard Hofrichter's edited book *Health and Social Justice: Politics, Ideology, and Inequity in the Distribution of Disease* (2003) analyzes the terrain of health inequities. Public health organizations have been created to address conditions that generated ill health and unequal attention to population groups, particularly the poor and minorities. Public health nurses in management positions must become familiar with the organization's target community or catchment area. Familiarity includes geographic characteristics, demographic profiles of current residents, history of the community, and health, economic, and social indices. Becoming acquainted with the community requires open and respectful dialogue with community leaders and members as well as professionals involved in providing service. Contact with school nurses, principals, hospital staff, visiting nurses, and church pastors will provide additional insight into community resources (assets) as well as the threats to community well-being. What happens in the community can deeply influence the health management decisions of a public health nurse as well as the organization. Public health nurses also follow the local news, including television coverage and publications (newspapers, etc.) that highlight community life and political positions. A politically savvy public health nurse will be able to speak with ease about policies, legislation, and regulations that influence community life and equality of health for all. Furthermore, a public health nurse who studies organizational dynamics and community stresses will be in the forefront of prevention efforts aimed at individual behaviors (Doner & Siegel, 2001).

A public health nurse manager in the forefront of prevention efforts will also be aware of local and regional differences in public health threats. Figure 17-2 typifies three health threats in the twenty-first century. The threats are influenced by geographic location and community culture. Each threat can be addressed through community-based education and behavioral choices to (1) not possess firearms, (2) to take safe driving courses and wear seatbelts, and (3) to learn how to supervise and handle farm equipment safely.

Public health organizations based in rural, suburban, or urban communities prioritize community risk differently and develop public health initiatives appropriate to the population. The local organization's public health nurses are in the position of identifying new or recurrent conditions that might escalate to epidemic or near-epidemic status in particular population groups.

BASICS OF INTERNAL MANAGEMENT

This section examines personal (self) insights and experiences needed to manage others (personnel) involved in public health services. Management basics covered include sound fiscal management, resource allocation, client case management and population-focused program management. Personal, personnel, fiscal, resource, case, and program management are

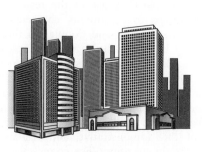

Urban
Impoverished inner city = Aggression, violence, and firearm homicides

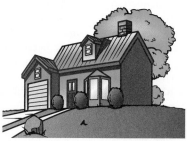

Suburban
Sprawling towns with no public transit = Increase in deaths by automobiles

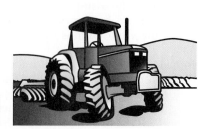

Rural
Agriculture livelihood = Farming injuries and deaths

Figure 17-2 Health threats: Geography and environment.

⊕ PRACTICE APPLICATION

Localized Health Threat

Insects carry disease and pestilence. Certain insects cause human suffering if for no other reason than scratching! Head lice (pediculosis) thrive on humans and spread from person to person in crowded places. Schools, day care, places where many people congregate have repeated outbreaks of head lice. This problem is perceived by many as just a nuisance. That perception changes rapidly if a child brings a note home saying there is a lice problem in school. Even in the twenty-first century, head lice are a pervasive problem. Public health nurse managers are in a position to oversee the efforts of public health nurses and school nurses to deal with head lice problems in schools, camps, day care, and other settings. The consequences of being diagnosed with head lice in a group setting are immediate. Children are excluded from school, treated as "unclean" by other students and teachers, and whispered about. Parents find it hard to understand that head lice do not discriminate. Lice like to be people dwellers—regardless of gender, income, ethnicity, age, and cleanliness—and lice like to reproduce. Under the direction of the public health nurse manager, the public health or school nurse diagnoses the condition, counsels the child, consults with the organization's administrative staff, educates the parents/caregivers about treatment, determines school exclusion until complete eradication, supports and educates the teaching staff and school community about the problem, follows the child(ren) upon return

to school, and begins the screening process all over again. Education includes describing the condition, what must be done to eliminate the pests and associated costs, and adherence to school protocols as well as prevention measures. These measures include no sharing of personal items such as combs, brushes, and hats (prevention) as well as daily head (hair) checks (screening) to diagnose or reassure. This problem may have been identified in only one person; however, the potential rapid spread requires the public health nurse to be proactive. How the public health nurse manager and other professionals share and respond to the problem influences the school, parent, and the community's reactions. People in communities that have known seasonal breakouts may be more informed and calmly attend to the problems. Parents in communities who perceive that their status (economic, housing, social) is being affected are more likely to react with abhorrence and fear. Regardless of community response, the public health nurse manager must prepare public health nurses and school nurses to deal with the problem: answer questions, provide support, and be available to guide and reassure fearful family members. The vigilance of the public health nurse manager regarding a localized health threat reduces the potential for a widespread infestation, and lessons learned can be applied if other health threats present.

interrelated. Experienced public health managers appreciate that the overlap of two or more basics such as funding, resource allocation, and staffing patterns for personnel present interesting opportunities as well as clinical challenges. Public health nurse managers must be mindful that managerial performance internal to the organization must reflect the organization's overall commitment to its target community's needs and interests (Fryer, 2004).

Professional and Personal (Self) Development

Public health nurses in the field as well as those in managerial positions know about "bad hair days." This phrase captures what public health nurses and public health managers can feel during the course of one work day. For example, community engagement is challenging. Programs are scheduled, but few attend. Bad weather complicates the provision of services in homes and community settings. Clients can "be no shows" despite the public health nurse's best efforts to make appointments convenient to the client's schedule. Traveling from point to point is routine for public health nurses. Getting lost, road detours, or wrong directions can frustrate the public health nurse and influence management of time and effort (productivity). Furthermore, in the work environment, people's personalities (quirky behaviors) might influence the public health nurse manager's perception of self as well as the effectiveness of management strategies. In addition, today's multitask and technologically focused environment contribute to the complexity of managerial responsibilities. Another managerial layer is life "outside" of work. How staff manages "outside" life can impact work productivity, work satisfaction, and employee retention (Stewart, 2005).

Public health nurse managers and their staff do have varied resources available to reduce bad hair day experiences at work or in the home. Classic readings are resources. Readings include Blanchard and Johnson's *The One Minute Manager* (2003), Blanchard and Gottry's *The On-Time, On-Target Manager* (2004), as well as Zoglio's *Recharge in Minutes* (2003). Many managers in service industries utilize these and other readings to motivate, inspire, and further develop the clinical and administrative skills of staff. Zoglio (2003) provides quick-lift activities that boost one's sense of self and help balance or manage the ups and downs of everyday life. Revitalization tips start with Chapter One ("I can't think straight") and lead to Chapter Ten ("Just my luck"); they help the reader shift attention from dwelling on what is wrong to giving thanks for life's simple joys. Public health nurse managers can utilize Zoglio's and other authors' insight to reinforce personal and professional development in their staff.

The One Minute Manager (Blanchard & Johnson, 2003) offers simplistic and wise approaches to help people feel good about themselves, be productive, and celebrate life and work. The "secrets" of one-minute goals, one-minute praisings, and one-minute reprimands provide real results. The emphasis on caring and honest communication about what is right and what needs improvement leads to healthier and more productive work environments, and happier workers. Another book, *The On-Time, On-Target Manager* (Blanchard & Gottry, 2004), uses the story of "Bob the Manager" to address the habit of procrastination and how to avoid the stressful, crisis prone, last-minute behaviors that too often end in indecisiveness and poor performance. The allegory proposes practical strategies to prioritize and triage, to delegate, to be committed, and to finish work on time with a sense of accomplishment. The authors highlight "gotta wanna." Gotta wanna people represent the commitment to "the journey as well as the end result. They are committed to the vision. To the truth. To integrity. To the best interest of others" (p. 113).

Other resources for public health nurse managers include mentors and/or confidants whose work and life experiences offer insight and support. Mentors can be those who work in the same or similar service settings with similar managerial responsibilities. Mentors can also be those with dissimilar backgrounds and work environments who share common managerial interests. In the public health arena, mentors or confidants may be discovered serendipitously, and the relationship can be considered akin to "kindred spirits." Public health nurse managers need colleagues who are listeners and problem solvers, who ask difficult questions, and who can recognize the "elephant" in the room (Hammond & Mayfield, 2004).

One technique that helps public health nurse managers understand the challenges of managing one's life (work and home) is journaling. Documenting experiences and feelings about events, situations, and crises allows for immediate ventilation in a nonthreatening manner. Journaling is freeing. Journaling allows for expressive writing and introspection, and rereading the journal allows for reflection and growth. Public health nurse managers can encourage staff to journal and, if interested, share lessons learned and intervention techniques with colleagues, in supervisory conferences and scholarly meetings.

Personnel Management

Public health nurse managers and public health nurses work with and for people. **Personnel** are the human resources who are the organization's and society's capital. Public health nurses in managerial positions appreciate the unique talents and contributions that each staff member makes to client services and the community-focused programs that support the work of administration. However, the process of managing and retaining staff is challenging. Satisfaction with one's work and the work environment combined with the knowledge that advancement opportunities exist are keys to staff retention. Today's public health nurse managers are accountable for staff development and retention as well as productivity (Maguire, Spencer, & Sabatier, 2004).

Nursing Leadership Forum Training programs for public health nurse managers are available to improve managerial skills, competencies, and confidence in managing personnel in today's stressful and unpredictable public health environment. The Nurse Manager Academy offered by The Institute for Johns Hopkins Nursing is a learner-centered educational program. The interactive and collaborative approach builds on adult education theory and teaches reflection-connection-projection techniques. The academy imparts transferable skills in almost every setting, including public health organizations.

Public health nurse managers involved in the management of public health services possess the skills to appreciate the reciprocity and productivity of respectful communication, learning from others and from one's self (Young, Peden-McAlpine, & Kovac, 2001). Public health nurse managers must be prepared to manage self as well as others. Preparation requires ongoing learning through formal and informal methods. Coauthors Heller and Hindle (1998) describe the diverse skills that a manager must employ in a single working day and offer practical advice and illustrations regarding management predicaments and solutions. Their manual serves as a reference source and emphasizes getting the best from people begins through open and honest dialogue and recognizing achievements. Public health nurse managers who employ and use staff intelligently will strengthen the organization's position in the community (Thielen, 2001).

Interviewing and hiring personnel for public health positions will be part of a public health nurse manager's responsibilities. The selection and retention of staff are a responsibility that requires insight. Steps before an employment offer is made include reviewing resumes, conducting face-to-face interviews, contacting references, analyzing the fit of the candidate with the position, and seeking the opinions of others (Eichner, 2005). In the public health field, it is important to have personnel who understand public health principles, express interests in working with diverse populations, value prevention and early intervention, and welcome the challenges presented by the unpredictability of the public health climate in the nation.

Support Services

Public health nurse managers have responsibilities to oversee support services. Support services include personnel such as office managers, receptionists, file clerks, information systems, and outreach workers. Support services also include equipment and technology necessary to implement and evaluate public health services and measure clinical outcomes. Equipment includes stationary and laptop computers, software programs, copiers, faxes, telephone services, pagers, cell telephones, and personal digital assistants (PDAs). The

acceleration of business-related technology means that public health nurses must update skills and arrange for equipment maintenance frequently. Even the space in which personnel work requires management. Safe and work-friendly environments influence staff satisfaction and productivity.

In the public health setting, support services and work environments are influenced by changing fiscal resources and the competing demands of case and/or program management. There is a natural tension managing personnel and support services. Acknowledging this tension with staff is important. Equally important—when resources (support staff, equipment, and space) are finite—is the manager's willingness to involve others in solving problems and creating action plans that address resource allocation, tension producers, and fiscal concerns. Action plans should include comparisons with other organizations involved in public health initiatives as well as internal scrutiny of how resources are managed and related program outcomes.

Fiscal Management

Nurses may enter the public health field with little to no understanding of fiscal management. Too often nurses consider nursing an art and a science but not a business. Nursing, particularly in the public health field, is a business as well as an art and science. Knowing the bottom line and developing business plans for public health programs is an essential skill of public health nurse managers (Kinsey & Buchanan, 2004). Programs cost money, and how programs are funded affects the design, services provided, available resources, and ultimately clinical outcomes. Budgeting processes and accounting practices enable the public health nurse manager to allocate resources effectively and efficiently.

Budgeting refers to the organization's plan to use anticipated funds in relation to expected expenses in various categories. Categories include staff, equipment, operating expenses, travel, consultation, training, and miscellaneous expenditures. Budgeting adheres to the organization's or funding source's funding cycle. The budget details the resources necessary to achieve program outcomes. Budget justifications are provided. For example, a tobacco cessation program may require two full-time staff, one public health nurse, and one health educator. The public health nurse manager would prepare a justification as to why this program needs two staff with different educational preparations.

A periodic review of the budget is required during the budget cycle with accounting procedures in place. Accounting records must be maintained for audit purposes. A general ledger provides information on program performance. It organizes the fiscal information by accounts (e.g., travel, personnel). The general ledger has a year-to-date balance for each account. The public health nurse manager can review the general ledger and know what has been spent or underspent to date. Journal records are also kept. Journal entries record what has been allocated but not yet entered into the general account. For example, an order has been placed for a new copier. The money is committed; however, the copier has not been delivered yet. The date the copier is delivered the expense will be entered in the general ledger. Journal records help the nurse to stay on budget and not overspend in one or more categories.

Public health nurse managers must also understand cash budgets and capital budgets. **Cash budgets** occur when clients or contractors pay for services or goods. **Capital budgets** are in place to acquire and maintain longer term assets such as purchasing or renovating buildings. Zero-base budgeting may be an unfamiliar concept to nurses just entering the public health field. **Zero-base budgeting** requires that there is no budget excess at the end of the fiscal year. Particular grants and contracts are based on zero-based budgets. Each line item is scrutinized and justified. The exact amount of money awarded in a particular contract must be expended—no more, no less. Zero-base budgeting requires weekly if not more frequent scrutiny to determine if expenditures are in line with budget expectations. Figure 17-3 is a reminder about how to manage and calculate dollars at the end of the fiscal cycle.

Expertise with budgets and annual audits enables public health nurse managers to participate in business plan development. Nonprofit public health organizations use business plans to guide their prevention and early intervention work. The business plan considers the development and direction of the organization and how goals will be met. A business plan melds community needs, organizational capacity and mission, and fiscal viability. Business plans are constructed on what is known and documented; however, the unpredictability of public health threats and community changes can immediately and drastically alter a business plan. Public health nurse managers involved in this work understand that a business plan must be flexible and malleable. Otherwise, the organization may not survive in the changing public health environment (Kinsey & Buchanan, 2004).

Zero-based budget = no under or overspending into next fiscal year

$100	$100	$100
- 98	- 100	- 104
$2	$0	-$4
Underspent	Zero Based	Overspent

Figure 17-3 Zero-based budget.

Case Management

Case management of a client's needs and care requirements in public health settings is complex. It is a process by which the provision and coordination of quality health care services are provided to an individual in a cost-effective manner. The services are provided in the home, school, homeless shelter, or other community settings. Case management requires coordination of community resources and linkages with a variety of community-based settings as well as tertiary care settings. The public health nurse manager will use formal and informal lines of communication to optimize a continuum of care. Fragmented services and the lack of affordable, accessible health care for a client who is homebound or in a communal setting will challenge the skills and patience of a public health nurse and the public health nurse manager. Case management also involves the family and wider community. Family members may be essential to optimal case management strategies; likewise, family members can thwart the delivery of service if the needs of the client are misunderstood or tax finite resources.

The term "case management" has been used interchangeably with "program management." For the purposes of this chapter, case management refers to public health services provided to an individual client, whereas program management means a collective group effort to improve a target population's health status. The case management service may be part of a funded program or project; however, the public health nurse and client are involved in interactions that focus on the improvement of the client's well-being. The client's health status will be summarized and reported for program evaluation; however, the case management plan is customized to the individual and accounts for physical, mental, environmental, social, educational, familial, and economic characteristics (Cary, 2004).

The work of a public health nurse with individual clients allows for analysis of health conditions that are common among a cohort of clients. For example, a public health nurse may identify lead poisoning in 10 children whose families live in a six-block radius of the local elementary school. The concern is with each child's health status but now there is an emerging concern that other children, yet unidentified, have been exposed to lead. The collective data inform the public health nurse that a lead poisoning prevention and early intervention program is needed.

Program Management

Program management refers to working with a collective of individuals involved in a service that promotes, protects, and meets the needs of specific populations in the community. Program management involves health planning based on population and community assessments. The assessments enable the formulation and conceptualization of a specific program. Decision trees may be part of the thought processes involved in program design. The value of a program is contrasted with the cost to the taxpayer as well as the costs to the community if the program is not provided. For example, childhood immunizations protect the child and the community at large from infectious diseases. Taxpayers' dollars are needed to support the immunization program, but the cost to the community is less than if children remained unimmunized or underimmunized. In contrast, introducing preventive services for malaria, when only one case has been identified (and that person was infected while touring India), would be a burden to the taxpayers and not of great benefit to the community at large.

Program implementation based on a sound plan requires that public health nurse managers be knowledgeable about available resources and the costs of each activity (Glick, 2004). The manager must account for staff preparedness to implement the program and the knowledge and skill base of all those involved during the implementation and evaluation period. For example, outreach workers are needed for a Childhood Immunization Project for émigré families from Haiti. The outreach workers are unfamiliar with Haitian culture and health beliefs and do not speak French Creole. Their expertise to date has been to engage at-risk families who moved from Puerto Rico to the community and need prenatal care. The outreach workers are fluent in Spanish and are of Puerto Rican heritage. The outreach workers will need an extensive orientation period to conduct culturally sensitive outreach activities to engage Haitian families. The reality is that it might be more cost effective to seek outreach workers more familiar with the Haitian culture and mores.

Program management includes program evaluation. Simply put, evaluation measures the beginning, middle, and end of a planned service. Professionals can claim that a program worked (was effective), but the basis for such a claim is unknown. Did people just like the services or the staff who provided the services and nothing really changed. Did measurable changes occur but the costs incurred were beyond expectation and the program could not be replicated? Not only is the progress of the program targeting a population group and a health need reviewed (formative evaluation), but the conclusion of a program also requires a review of the outcomes and impact on the community (summative evaluation).

Public health nurse managers familiar with advanced planning and evaluation methods including Program Evaluation Review Technique (PERT), Critical Path Method (CPM), and others will factor in the concepts of time and events to allocate resources. Seasoned public health nurse managers will factor in uncertainty in community circumstances. Community circumstances can alter program planning and implementation. Often, natural disasters or near epidemics influence the setting of the services, the quality of services provided, and the outcomes. Public health nurse managers and public health nurses in the field must understand that there can never be 100 percent control of the target population and the program planned. Realistic planning and pragmatic assessment of outcomes and accurate reporting of data are needed. Results of programs that exceed or do not reach target goals are as important to report and document as those that attain target goals and have recognized and lasting community value. Public health nurse managers need to be grounded in reality to be effective in their positions, but also maintain an organizational vision and stay connected with supportive resources in and outside the agency. One excellent resource with newsletters and Webcasts is BetterManagement.com. There are many other Internet resources including the Centers for Disease Control and Prevention that promote organizational strengthening. The choices for public health nurse managers are abundant and should be utilized for personal and professional development.

BASICS OF EXTERNAL MANAGEMENT

Public health managers and leaders understand that building and nurturing relationships with the public advances the public health agenda of the organization, supports Healthy People 2010 goals and objectives, and enables open discourse about family and community assets and needs. Collectively, these form what this chapter refers to as external management. Public health nurse managers open to network opportunities with like-minded professionals as well as those who hold different views can initiate the process of engagement. In addition, public health nurse managers can designate staff with interpersonal and public speaking skills to represent the organization at community and public health forums. In the twenty-first century, any local public health entity is also a part of the regional, national, and international (global) public health workforce and agenda. It is appropriate for public health nurse managers to explore global public health issues and to bring to the table issues that the organization and staff need to be prepared to address. In addition, public policy will be introduced or changed based on local, national and global events. The globalization of the world means that local public health entities can be threatened by Avian flu outbreaks occurring in Hong Kong.

Public Engagement

Striving for positive public engagement is based on simplistic truths (Robbins, 2003) and practices (Senge, 1990). Being present, being consistent, being honest, and being open will engage the public in dialogue and provide for self-interests being set aside to achieve common goals. How functional a public group is over time and the public's ability to attain goals will be based on the individual practices and collective will of the public. For example, a grassroots community group called a public meeting to talk about the number of children in their neighborhoods diagnosed with elevated blood lead levels. The public health nurse manager and other professionals volunteered to conduct a community assessment to determine the need for a lead poisoning prevention educational campaign and in-home screen-

ings for at risk infants and toddlers. The commitment by the public health nurse manager and others indicated to the grassroots group a shared vision to improve the health of children. The grassroots group trusted that the community assessment would be conducted in a professional manner and the information shared with the grassroots group. The public health nurse manager who is honest, forthright, listens, works productively with others, delivers work on time, shares a vision, enjoys diverse groups and opinions, and goes beyond expectations possesses talents that promote public engagement and good citizenship. This public health nurse manager welcomes the challenge of the unknown and recognizes uncertainty as a growth experience.

Public Policy

Public health nurse managers have opportunities to work on internal as well as external policies and legislative decisions that protect and improve the health of the public. Policies are decisions put into action by individuals or groups who study an issue, introduce, and approve a course of action. A public policy is a statement that guides local, regional, and/or national action plans and interventions and is approved by a legislative or sanctioned body. Policies are developed to improve or change conditions of personal and societal well-being. With scientific discoveries, policies have been changed, dropped, and new ones introduced. For example, public policy in many communities or states now eliminates smoking in all public places. These policies were not in place in the 1990s.

Public health nurse managers must be diligent as well as anticipatory about public health threats to the well-being of target populations and society at large. Public policy over time often becomes institutionalized, and the public has limited appreciation as to why the policy occurred. Public health nurse managers must study policies that influence behaviors, analyze the circumstances that created the policies, observe community changes and trend, and, over time, research what are enforceable and acceptable action plans related to the public's health.

Globalization

Public health nurse managers must be mindful that the local scene is now a microcosm of global conditions. What happens in Asia or Africa is just a plane trip away from any locale in the United States. What happens in the next town 12,000 miles away must be considered potential threats to the health and well-being of populations in the public health service arena. The mental imprints of the terrorist attacks on September 11, 2001, and subsequent postal poisonings are lasting reminders that those in the public health field must be prepared to deal with a variety of threats. Likewise the December 2004 tsunami that killed more than 170,000 people in South East Asia reminds all that natural catastrophes can be just as devastating as man-made disasters if not more so. Public health nurse managers keep abreast of local, national, and global threats through Internet resources including online publications and alerts, current professional publications, and the popular press (Hitt, Ireland, & Hoskisson, 2005). Staying current and proactive and instituting "preparedness plans" are essential strategies for health departments. Staff will need in-services and trainings to deal with potential community threats. Infectious disease experts predict that avian flu, Lassa fever, Ebola hemorrhagic fever, and ever-changing strains of influenza have the potential to kill hundreds of thousands if not contained at the local level. Immediate reporting and interventions by officials at the local level must occur. Complacency and fear of economic consequences regarding a particular disease threat may put the world in grave peril. Every public health nurse manager must be part detective and reporter as disease patterns or unusual clusters of health problems emerge.

The idea of globalization is expressed through community demographics. In the twenty-first century, the United States is home to people from all countries and cultures. Public health nurses must be sensitive and aware of diverse cultural interpretations to health and well-being, and the different approaches taken to stay well and free from disease and illness. Adaptive and respectful health care services and public health programs are needed for all groups who represent today's global world.

KEYS TO IMPROVEMENT

How do public health nurse managers improve the quality of services, hire and retain staff, promote staff development, create and sustain learning environments, stay in touch with local and global issues, maintain a sense of balance, enjoy the work, and inspire others to go beyond? Keys to improvement can assist the public health nurse manager in improving services and maintaining productive staff. One key to improvement is for the public health nurse manager to remain open to new experiences and relationships, avoid assumptions, ask questions, encourage differences in opinions, celebrate different approaches to accomplish the goal, and remain principled and honest despite external constraints and/or politics (Wademan, 2005). Wademan interviewed successful executives regarding the best personal advice each received that was applied in their places of employment. The counsel the executives considered to be the best personal advice received included: (1) people are who matters; (2) people are able to change their own rules; (3) take the time to look at things differently; (4) filter outside advice (naysayer); (5) respect your intuition; (6) success can be thwarted by shortcuts; (7) strive beyond easy work; (8) treat every person equally; (9) know the facts and be truthful about the facts; (10) use real data, and demonstrate good judgment.

Keys to improvement are based on good strategies. One strategy is to design, implement, and evaluate practices and polices that use scientific evidence or to generate new evidence on effectiveness, affordability, and application across population groups and even nations (Brownson et al., 2003). Another strategy is to employ and upgrade technology frequently and to be alert to new systems and methods to gather and analyze data. Improvement in one or more interrelated public health services will be based on a public health nurse manager's interpersonal skills; dedication to improvement through communication, technology, and program development; and appreciation of the entirety not just the pieces. One of the essential keys to improvement is the ability to appreciate the sum of the pieces because, in public health practice, the whole is more than the sum of all the parts. Another key is to remain focused (Thomas, 2003). Successful programs left unattended can quickly wither and weaken. Unsuccessful programs require analyses before discarding. The greatest lessons learned and remembered combine successes and failures.

FUTURE ORIENTATION

Public health nurses manage programs, personnel, and resources in the present based on lessons learned and best practices based on research, program replication, and innovation. Future think (orientation) is the framework by which managers anticipate, assess, design, innovate, implement, measure, report, and start all over again. Public health nurse managers focus on the future, work in the present, and deeply value the past. Public health history reveals that science is still very young, and ongoing study modifies past assumptions about health, public needs, and medical interventions. Certain contagious diseases, including leprosy (Hansen's disease), were considered deadly and incurable. Today's findings contradict past scientific assertions. Public health nurse managers must maintain a degree of pragmatic skepticism about published scientific reports since more investigation may either refute or further validate the findings.

The public health nurse manager oriented toward the future possesses a global perspective yet is grounded in local matters. The public health nurse manager committed to the health of the public who shares this commitment and passion with colleagues, staff, administrators and the community will be the leader in the twenty-first century. Visionary and bold public health nurse managers responsible for program management possess the knowledge, dedication, and wherewithal to demonstrate that prevention and early intervention are keys to improving the health of the public.

CRITICAL THINKING ACTIVITIES

1. Why should public health nurses consider managerial positions in community-based organizations?

2. How do you personally define leadership?

3. Name three or more conflicts that could arise between a community-based organization and its target community?

4. What are the essential skills necessary to manage self, personnel, program, and fiscal responsibilities in a public health agency?

5. What support would you need as a public health nurse manager?

6. What managerial strategies can be taken to reduce the threat of global problems occurring in your local community?

KEY TERMS

administration	keys to improvement	program management
budgeting	leadership	public engagement
capital budgets	management	public health infrastructure
case management	organizational culture	public policy
cash budgets	personal (self) insights and experiences	support services
fiscal management		zero-base budgeting
future think	personnel	

KEY CONCEPTS

- Public health nurses are uniquely positioned to make lasting differences in the lives of people they care about and for.

- Managerial positions place public health nurses in the forefront of practice, education, and research initiatives.

- Management is translating the leadership's or organization's vision and mission into productive action and progressing toward public health goals.

- The Scope and Standards of Public Health Nursing and Healthy People 2010 are key references and guides.

- Learning environments help people understand forces that shape change and build on the collective will and power to make lasting contributions to society.

- Community culture shapes public health practice, management styles, and programs.

- Personal, personnel, fiscal, resource, case, and program management are internal management responsibilities.

- External management responsibilities include public engagement, a global perspective, and public policy.

- Keys to improvement are based on valuing self and others and building on lessons learned.

- Public health nurse managers nurture a future orientation that emphasizes prevention.

REFERENCES

American Nurses Association (ANA). *Public Health Nursing: Scope and Standards of Practice* (2007). Washington, DC: American Nurses Association.

Bauer, J., Hyland, A., Qiang, L., Teger, C., & Cummings, M. (2005). A longitudinal assessment of the impact of smoke-free worksite policies on tobacco use. *American Journal of Public Health, 95*(6), 1024–1029.

Bhatia, R. (2003). Swimming upstream in a swift current: Public health institutions and inequality. In R. Hofrichter (Ed.), *Health and social justice* (pp. 557–578). San Francisco: Wiley & Sons.

Blanchard, K., & Gottry, S. (2004). *The on-time, on-target manager: How a last minute manager conquered procrastination.* New York: HarperCollins.

Blanchard, K., & Johnson, S. (2003). *The one minute manager* (3rd ed.). New York: HarperCollins.

Braun Levin, S. (2005). *Inventing the rest of our lives: Women in second adulthood.* New York: Viking.

Brownson, R. C., Baker, E. A., Leet, T. L., & Gillespie, K. N. (2003). *Evidence-based public health.* New York: Oxford.

Cary, A. H. (2004). Case management. In M. Stanhope & J. Lancaster (Eds.), *Community and public health nursing* (6th ed., pp. 413–424). St. Louis: Mosby.

Clark, M. J. (2004). Learning the organization: A model for health system analysis for new nurse administrators. *Nursing Leadership Forum, 9*(1), 28–63.

Doner, L. & Siegel, M. (2001). Public health marketing. In L. F. Novick & G. P. Mays (Eds.), *Public health administration* (pp. 474–509). Gaithersburg, MD: Aspen.

Eichner, J. S. (2005). Labor-management relations. In M. D. Harris (Ed.), *Handbook of home health care administration,* (4th ed., pp. 448–458). Boston: Jones and Bartlett.

Feldman, H. (2004). If I only had a crystal ball: The importance of vision. *Nursing Leadership Forum, 8*(4), 2.

Freudenberg, N. (2005). Public health advocacy to change corporate practices: Implications for health education practice and research. *Health Education & Behavior, 32*(3), 298–319.

Fryer, B. (2004). The micromanager. *Harvard Business Review, 82*(9), 31–40.

Glick, D.F. (2004). Program management. In M. Stanhope & J. Lancaster (Eds.), *Community and public health nursing* (6th ed., pp. 490–515). St. Louis: Mosby.

Hammond, S. A., & Mayfield, A. B. (2004). *Naming elephants: How to surface undiscussables for greater organizational success.* Bend, OR: Thin Book Publishing.

Heller, R., & Hindle, T. (1998). *Essential manager's manual.* New York: DK Publishing.

Hofrichter, R. (2003). *Health and social justice: Politics, ideology, and inequity in the distribution of disease.* San Francisco: Jossey-Bass.

Hitt, M. A., Ireland, R. D., & Hoskisson, R. E. (2005). *Strategic management: Competitiveness and globalization* (6th ed.). Mason, OH: South-Western.

Kinsey, K. K., & Buchanan, M. (2004). The nursing center: A model for community-oriented nursing practice. In M. Stanhope & J. Lancaster (Eds.), *Community and public health nursing* (6th ed., pp. 412–445). St. Louis: Mosby.

Maguire, M. P., Spencer, K. L., & Sabatier, K. H. (2004). The nurse manager academy: An innovative approach to managerial competency development. *Nursing Leadership Forum, 8,* 133–137.

Novick, L. F. & Mays, G. P. (Eds.) (2001). *Public health administration.* Gaithersburg, MD: Aspen.

Porche, D. (2004). *Public and community health nursing practice. A population-based approach.* Thousand Oaks, CA: Sage Publications.

Quad Council of Public Health Nursing Organizations. (1999). *Scope and standards of public health nursing practice.* Washington, DC: American Nurses Association.

Robbins, S. P. (2003). *The truth about managing people.* Upper Saddle River, NJ: Prentice Hall.

Senge, P. M. (1990). *The fifth discipline.* New York: Doubleday.

Stewart, T. A. (2005). Managing yourself. *Harvard Business Review, 83*(1) 100-109.

The Random House Dictionary (1969). New York: Random House.

Thielen, L. (2001). Human resources management. In L. F. Novick & G. P. Mays (Eds.), *Public health administration* (pp. 397–412). Gaithersburg, MD: Aspen.

Thomas, S. A. (2003). Quality management. In J. E. Hitchcock, P. E. Schubert, & S. A. Thomas (Eds.), *Community health nursing: Caring in action* (2nd ed., pp. 413–424). Clifton Park, NY: Thomson Delmar Learning.

U.S. Department of Health and Human Services (USDHHS). (2000a). *Healthy People 2010: Conference edition.*

Washington, DC: Author. Available at http://www.health
.gov/healthypeople.

Wademan, D. (2005). The best advice I ever got. *Harvard
Business Journal, 83*(1), 35–44.

Young, C. E., Peden-McAlpine, C., & Kovac, R. (2001). Organization understanding: Understanding the practice of
expert nurse executives. In H. Feldman (Ed.), *Strategies for
nursing leadership* (pp. 239–263). New York: Springer.

Zoglio, S. (2003). *Recharge in minutes.* Doylestown, PA:
Tower Hill Press.

BIBLIOGRAPHY

Albom, M. (2003). *The five people you meet in heaven.* New
York: Hyperion.

Gibran, K. (1923). *The prophet.* New York: Alfred A. Knopf.

Gladwell, M. (2002). *The tipping point.* Boston: Little, Brown
and Company.

Gladwell, M. (2005). *Blink.* Boston: Little, Brown and
Company.

Miller, W. R., & Rollnick, S. (2002). *Motivational interviewing: Preparing people for change* (2nd ed.). New York: The
Guilford Press.

U.S. Department of Health and Human Services (USDHHS).
(2000b). "Public Health in America Statement." Available
at HYPERLINK "http://www.health.gov/phfunctions/
public.htm" www.health.gov/phfunctions/public.htm.

RESOURCES

American Organization of Nurse Executives (AONE)

Liberty Place
325 Seventh Street NW
Washington, D.C. 20004
202-626-2240
FAX: 202-638-5499
Web: http://www.aone.org

Founded in 1967, AONE, a subsidiary of the American Hospital Association, is a national organization of over 5,000
nurses who design, facilitate, and manage care. Its mission
is to represent nurse leaders who improve health care.
AONE members are leaders in collaboration and catalysts
for innovation. AONE's vision is "Shaping the future of
healthcare through innovative nursing leadership." The
Web site provides information on policy, politics, legislation, and advocacy for nurse executives.

Center on Budget and Policy Priorities

820 1st Street NE, Suite 510
Washington, D.C. 20002
202-408-1080
FAX: 202-408-1056
Email: center@cbpp.org
Web: http://www.cbpp.org

The Center on Budget and Policy Priorities is one of the
nation's premier policy organizations working at the federal and state levels on fiscal policy and public programs
that affect low- and moderate-income families and individuals. The Center conducts research and analysis to inform
public debates over proposed budget and tax policies and
to help ensure that the needs of low-income families and
individuals are considered in these debates. The Center
also develops policy options to alleviate poverty, particularly among working families and examines the short- and
long-term impacts that proposed policies would have on
the health of the economy and on the soundness of federal
and state budgets. Among the issues explored are whether
federal and state governments are fiscally sound and have
sufficient revenue to address critical priorities, both for
low-income populations and for the nation as a whole.

Congressional Budget Office (CBO)

Ford House Office Building, 4th Floor
Second and D Streets SW
Washington, D.C. 20515-6925
202-226-2602
Web: http://www.cbo.gov

CBO was founded on July 12, 1974, with the enactment of
the Congressional Budget and Impoundment Control Act
(P.L. 93-344). The agency began operating on February
24, 1975. CBO issues yearly federal cost estimates and
impact of unfounded mandates on state and local governments, studies, reports, briefs, Monthly Budget Reviews,
letters, and background papers to Congress. CBO also testifies before the Congress as needed on a variety of issues.
Finally, CBO provides up-to-date data on its Web site,
including current budget and economic projections and
information on the status of discretionary appropriations.

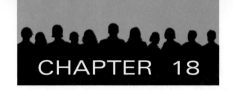

CHAPTER 18

Ethics and Human Rights

Carol Easley Allen, RN, PhD

Cheryl E. Easley, RN, PhD

Chapter Outline

- History of Ethics in Public Health, Nursing, and Public Health Nursing
- Human Rights
- The Intersection of Public Health and Human Rights
- Ethics
  Bioethics
  Principle-Based Ethical Theories
  Ethical Principles
  Moral Rules
  Ethical Theories without Principles
- Cross-Cultural Ethical Perspectives
- Nursing and Other Ethical Codes and Principles
  American Nurses Association Code for Nurses
  International Council of Nurses Code of Ethics for Nurses
  Scope and Standards of Public Health Nursing Practice
  Public Health Leadership Society: Public Health Code of Ethics
- Public Health as Social Justice: Poverty and Health
- Ethical Decision Making in Public Health Nursing
  A Public Health Ethical Decision Making Model
- Selected Issues in Public Health Nursing Ethics
  Global HIV/AIDS
  Genetics and Genomics

Learning Objectives

Upon completion of this chapter, the reader will be able to:

1. Analyze the relationships among public health, public health nursing, ethics, and human rights.
2. Compare principle-based ethical theories and ethical theories without principles.
3. Evaluate the major human rights documents that are relevant to public health and public health nursing ethics.
4. Analyze the major nursing ethics documents.
5. Use the case study method to analyze public health nursing situations.
6. Apply a public health ethical decision-making model to selected issues in public health ethics.

"The mandate to assure and protect the health of the public is an inherently moral one. It carries with it an obligation to care for the well being of others and it implies the possession of an element of power in order to carry out the mandate. The need to exercise power to ensure health and at the same time to avoid the potential abuses of power are at the crux of public health ethics" (Public Health Leadership Society, 2002, p. 5).

This chapter focuses on the intersection of several important concepts: public health, public health nursing, ethics, and human rights. Each of these concepts represents a particular perspective, or worldview, that may or may not be compatible with the other perspectives in every respect. Understanding each perspective and the relationships among the perspectives requires critical thinking: looking at issues from a variety of perspectives, tolerating ambiguity when easy answers are not apparent, and using case study analysis to examine all the nuances of a situation.

"*Public health* is what we, as a society, do collectively to assure the conditions for people to be healthy" (IOM, 1988, p. 1). Even though the Institute of Medicine (IOM) definition stresses society's responsibility to promote the health of the population, an important question remains about the scope of public health. Is public health responsibility confined to the prevention of the immediate causes of injury and disease, such as infectious disease control, or should public health play a role in the alleviation of the larger social and economic problems that play an important role in health and disease, such as poverty, violence, and adequate housing? (Gostin, 2002, p. xix). This issue becomes important as consideration is given to the intersection of public health and ethical concerns.

Ethics has many definitions. It has been viewed as "a generic term for various ways of understanding and examining the moral life" (Beauchamp & Childress, 2001, p. 1). A primary concern of ethics involves the duties of human beings. The study of ethics includes both social morality and philosophical reflection. Morality has reference to widely shared "traditions of belief about right and wrong human conduct" (Beauchamp & Walters, 2003, p.1). By contrast, values are personal beliefs about the worth of objects, ideas, or concepts.

Bioethics is a subfield of ethics that deals with ethical concerns that arise as a result of advances in health care. The concept of bioethics arose in the aftermath of World War II when the Nuremberg Tribunal reviewed the atrocities of Nazi physicians in the name of scientific experimentation during the 1940s. The judgments of the Nuremberg court led to the Nuremberg Code of 1947 that forms a basis for the protection of human subjects in research. As a result of its beginning, bioethics has developed with an emphasis on individual human rights, such as freedom, choice, and self-determination. The self-interests of the person are seen to be more important than the interests of the family, community, or scientific study (Butts & Rich, 2005; Gostin, 2002).

Immediately it can be seen that the concerns of bioethics and public health are not identical. Bioethics emphasizes the rights and interests of the individual, but these factors are not always decisive in public health, and may, in fact, hinder critical thinking about healthy communities. "The field of public health is concerned primarily with prevention rather than treatment, populations rather than individuals, and collective goods rather than personal rights or interests" (Gostin, 2002, p. xxiii). Public health must consider public goods that can be achieved only by collective action, such as clean water, adequate housing, good roads, public safety, and high-quality public education. Only society as a collective can regulate the risks that are shared. Individuals may have to sacrifice some of their self-interest in order to gain the benefits of a safe and healthy society. Bioethics poses the question: What desire and needs does one have as an autonomous, rights-bearing individual? By contrast, public health asks another kind of question: What kind of community does one want and deserve to live in, and what personal interests is one willing to forego to achieve a good society? (Gostin, 2002, xxiv).

HISTORY OF ETHICS IN PUBLIC HEALTH, NURSING, AND PUBLIC HEALTH NURSING

The philosophical basis for modern public health is generally considered to be nineteenth-century utilitarianism. Public health is characterized by a population focus, the primacy of population over individual interests, and the use of coercive powers of the state to enforce public health interventions, such as immunization, reporting, and quarantine.

The issue of balancing interests of the individual against those of the state has played out in various contexts throughout history. In the early 1900s, the concern was smallpox vaccination. The beginning of the HIV/AIDS epidemic in the 1980s gave rise to the question of reporting the results of HIV tests by name to public health authorities. Later issues have related to giving emergency protective powers to governors and state health departments in the face of the anthrax scares subsequent to the terrorist attacks of September 11, 2001. Similar questions may be posed regarding widespread quarantine to combat SARS (severe acute respiratory syndrome) (Rothstein, 2004).

A dark chapter in the history of nursing ethics describes the participation of German nurses in the so-called euthanasia operations of the Third Reich during which over 200,000 innocent people were killed. Grounded in the social Darwinistic ideas of Herbert Spencer, Francis Galton, and Joseph-Arthur de Gobineau, the killings were preceded by a eugenics movement to forcibly sterilize persons suffering from a variety of mental and physical disorders as well as persons exhibiting antisocial behavior, such as prostitutes, homeless persons, petty criminals, and the long-term unemployed.

"Mercy death" was a euphemistic term used by the Nazis to disguise the murder of disabled children and adults, wounded soldiers, and the elderly who were considered to have "life unworthy of life" (Hoskins, 2005, p. 92). The German public and health care professionals were prepared to accept such actions by media propaganda that emphasized the need to divert the services of health care providers and other scarce resources from the care of such inferior persons to the care of injured soldiers. Unlike the current debate regarding euthanasia, the subjects of these actions were not terminally ill, nor were their deaths painless.

German nurses were for the most part voluntarily involved in the killing of many thousands of children and adults by the administration of drug overdoses, air, or lethal compounds. In time, gas chambers and crematoria were installed in the basements of hospitals. Some asserted later that they were coerced or threatened into compliance (although no reprisals were ever carried out), but many nurses felt that they were morally justified in assisting in the deaths of clients or that they were obligated to follow the orders of health care providers. In some cases, the nurses worked in pairs to provide support or to physically restrain and force medication on clients who had realized what was being done and tried to resist. In addition to being illegal even under Nazi era laws, these actions by German nurses violated many of the tenets of human rights and ethics that are discussed in this chapter, including the human rights to life and dignity, and strictures against domination, lies, and harm by health care professionals (Hoskins, 2005; Shields, 2005).

HUMAN RIGHTS

Human rights refer to the basic rights and freedoms to which all humans are entitled, including life, liberty, freedom of thought and expression, equality before the law, and material well-being. There are significant differences between legal rights and moral rights. Legal rights are determined by political constitutions, legislative acts, case law, and executive orders, without reference to moral systems. Moral systems, on the other hand, exist without reference to legal systems. Moral rights serve as a basis for the evaluation of legal rights. Ethical theories can be used to determine whether particular laws are good or bad. Both laws and social practices may violate rights that are derived from moral principles. For example, the U.S. Constitution, the law of the land, protected the slave trade, a violation of human rights, for 50 years. The public health nurse has a responsibility to understand and protect both the legal and the moral rights of clients

A distinction is often drawn between positive and negative rights. A positive right is a right to well-being, usually to receive goods or services. A positive right implies that another person, or society, must provide something to the person who holds the right. If a person has a positive right to health care, then someone must provide that care. Our society has not recognized a legal claim-right to health care. A person is free to seek health care and to make arrangements to receive it, but health care agencies and providers are not legally obligated to provide it. Many public health nurses, as well as other health care professionals, believe that there is a positive right to health care. These health care providers have been leaders in the crusade for a universal right to health care.

Negative rights are rights of noninterference, to be left alone. In contrast to positive rights, no one has to do anything to honor a negative right. For example, if a person holds the negative right of liberty, all others must do is to refrain from interfering with that person (Beauchamp & Walters, 2003; Munson, 2003).

THE INTERSECTION OF PUBLIC HEALTH AND HUMAN RIGHTS

Human rights are rights that all people possess by virtue of being human. These rights are universal in that they inhere in all human beings equally regardless of other duties they may have or statuses that they occupy. Rights are claims or entitlements to something or against someone that are legally or morally recognized. The U.S. Declaration of Independence appeals to natural law in affirming that "all men . . . are endowed by their Creator with certain inalienable Rights," while in the Constitution's Bill of Rights certain rights are established in positive law such that they can be enforced in the courts (Donnelly, 1998; Easley & Allen, 2005; Easley, Marks, & Morgan, 2001).

The catalyst to the formulation of human rights in international law was the atrocities committed by Nazi Germany in the Holocaust during World War II. The Charter of the United Nations that came into existence after the war declares a determination to "reaffirm faith in fundamental human rights" (UN, 1946). In subsequent years the international community moved ahead to codify human rights in law. In 1948, the UN adopted the Universal Declaration of Human Rights (UDHR) (UN, 1948), the foundational human rights that are echoed in many national constitutions and other related documents. The UDHR along with the 1966 International Covenant on Civil and Political Rights (UN, 1966a) and the International Covenant on Economic, Social and Cultural Rights (ICESCR) (UN, 1966b) and protocols thereto form what is termed The International Bill of Human Rights. Included in these and other documents that deal with specific populations such as women, children, prisoners, and racial minorities are assertions of the inalienable dignity of each person and the equality of his or her rights without discrimination.

Recognition of the right to health is referenced in the United Nations Charter and more fully asserted in the Constitution of the World Health Organization (WHO, 1946), which states: "The enjoyment of the highest attainable standard of health is one of the fundamental rights of every human being without distinction of race, religion political belief, economic or social condition" (WHO, 1946). The ICESCR recognizes "the rights of everyone to the enjoyment of the highest attainable standard of physical and mental health" (UN, 1966b). In 1978, the International Conference on Primary Health Care adopted the Declaration of Alma-Ata, which states that each person has a "right to a standard of living adequate for the health and well-being of himself and his family, including food, clothing, housing and medical care and necessary social services, and the right to security in the event of unemployment, sickness, disability, widowhood, old age or other lack of livelihood in circumstances beyond his control" (WHO, 1978).

The term "the right to health" used in international rights documents does not mean that individual human health itself can be legislated or insured by law; instead, it is a shorthand used to denote the more detailed provisions related to health in international law and to emphasize the social and ethical aspects of health care and health status (Leary, 1994; Toebes, 1999). The full conception of the human right to health continues to evolve in the provisions of international instruments such as the 1986 Ottawa Charter for Health Promotion that describes the fundamental conditions and resources for health as "peace, shelter, education, food, income, a stable ecosystem, sustainable resources, social justice and equity" (WHO, 1986). Governments' obligations to achievement of the right to health include the responsibility not only of not violating rights but also of ensuring conditions that help people to realize the whole range of rights that contribute to health (Gruskin, 2004). The individual practice of the public health nurse and his or her advocacy activities are informed by the extent to which the nurse values the notion of a human right to health.

Both human rights and ethics are basically founded in moral philosophy and share many common ideas, but they employ different perspectives. Ethical discourse focuses on the rationale and determination of right behavior, often as they are set forth in codes of behavior for various professions or processes for ethical decision making. Human rights, on the other hand, focus on the legal obligations of nation states to their citizens, which are codified in national and/or international law. Although ultimately both disciplines are concerned that human beings are treated with respect and dignity, in some cases conflicts may occur, for example, when utilitarian ethics, which demands the greatest good for the greatest number, may indicate that individual rights may be subsumed to the good of the whole (Marks, 2001).

In recent decades, stimulated in large part by the human rights issues raised as public health professionals began to confront the international HIV/AIDS epidemic, increased attention has been given to the intersection of health (and public health) and human rights. A foundational writer in this arena was the late Jonathan Mann, until his death Director of the Francois Xavier Bagnoud Center for Health and Human Rights at the Harvard University School of Public Health. Mann (1994) believed that the interaction of health and human rights would contribute more to the advancement of human well-being than either field could alone and proposed three types of linkages:

1. The impact of health policies, programs, and practices on human rights, especially as seen in the use of state power in public health. In carrying out the core public health functions of assessment, policy development, and assurance of public health services, human rights principles could be violated through discrimination of certain vulnerable groups such as HIV positive persons, discrimination in policy formulation, or through measures such as enforced isolation or mandatory testing. Even though it is recognized that in some cases human rights may be limited to protect the community in such areas as public health, this act is restricted in various ways. First of all, certain human rights, including the right to be free from torture or slavery, are considered inviolable under all circumstances. Rules for the restriction of other rights are such restrictions must be strictly necessary to meet the purposes of a democratic society, as non-intrusive as possible; restrictions should not be imposed arbitrarily. In addition, restrictions must be determined by law and must fulfill legitimate objectives.

2. Health impacts resulting from violations of human rights. Serious or possibly life-threatening consequences on health will always result for severe violations of human rights such as torture, inhumane imprisonment, and other attacks on human beings. Further violation of the right to information, failure to provide for safe workplaces, or violations of human dignity may also cause harm to physical or emotional health.

3. Health and human rights: exploring an inextricable linkage. Examples of this connection include the case of HIV/AIDS in which discrimination, stigmatization, and lack of respect for the dignity of the client has increased the risk of vulnerable

groups being exposed to the HIV virus. Further, Mann asserts the importance of health as a precondition to the capacity to realize and enjoy human rights.

In 2000, the American Public Health Association adopted the Principles on Public Health and Human Rights that were developed under the leadership of the International Human Rights Committee (APHA, 2000). See Box 18-1. Continued collaboration of human rights activists and public health workers can be expected over time to result in advances in areas such as the health and human rights of vulnerable groups, the achievement of environmental and occupational safety and health, the protection of human rights in the face of public health emergencies, and the realization of the economic and social conditions that are necessary to the highest attainable standard of health.

BOX 18-1: American Public Health Association Principles on Public Health and Human Rights

1. All human beings are equal in dignity and rights.

2. All human beings are entitled to the enjoyment of all human rights without discrimination.

3. The realization of the highest standard of health requires respect for all human rights, which are indivisible, interdependent, and interrelated.

4. An essential dimension of human rights is the right to health, including conditions that promote and safeguard health and access to culturally acceptable health care.

5. Human rights must not be sacrificed to achieve public health goals, except in extraordinary circumstances, in accordance with the requirements of internationally recognized human rights standards.

6. The active collaboration of public health and human rights workers is a necessary and invaluable means of advancing their common purposes and values.

SOURCE: American Public Health Association (APHA). (2000). *Principles on public health and human rights*. Washington, DC: Author.

ETHICS

Ethics is the branch of philosophy that addresses the question: What is right? There are various approaches to ethics in the literature: those that are simply descriptive or analytical, which do not imply a moral position, and those that do take a moral position. These latter approaches are termed normative ethics. The ethical approach that is most relevant to public health nursing is practical normative ethics: the attempt to develop action guides for particular moral problems. Sometimes called applied ethics, practical normative ethics is the attempt to apply general norms and theories to particular ethical problems. Theory, argument, and analysis are used to examine moral problems and policies (Beauchamp & Walters, 2003).

Bioethics

Modern bioethics derives from two historical themes: traditional medical ethics, which at times was mainly concerned with the proper daily conduct of health care providers; and moral philosophy. One of the earliest documents that have provisions related to the practice of medicine is the *Code of Hammurabi*, written in Babylon around 1750 B.C. *The Hippocratic Oath*, often held up as the guarantee of ethics for medicine, was as much focused on the interests of the medical profession as it was those of clients. With the rise of Christianity, the Hippocratic Oath was modified to render it acceptable to Christians (Harris, 2001; Kuhse & Singer, 1998).

The moral influence of Christianity is noted in the emphasis on love for one's neighbors and the encouraging of charity that led to the establishment of hospitals. *Medical Ethics,* published in 1803 by English health care provider, Thomas Percival, formed the basis of the early codes of medical ethics in America and Britain. As late as the 1940s and 1950s, it continued to influence the code of the World Medical Association. The foundation of this ethical conception was responsibility to the client and to the profession. With more recent developments such as the increase of consumer consciousness, these types of ethical understandings have come under attack. Joseph Fletcher, an American Episcopalian theologian, wrote what was probably the first modern book on bioethics in 1954. Entitled *Morals and Medicine,* its "situation ethics" approach was controversial in its time and veered away from traditional Christian views (Harris, 2001; Kuhse & Singer, 1998).

The other basis for bioethics, moral philosophy, earlier in its history had turned from the consideration of the real-life issues to more scholastic concerns, including the discussion of metaethics. Major social movements of the 1960s and 1970s, including the campaign for nuclear disarmament, the U.S. civil rights movement, the broad-based peace movement, and the protest against the war in Vietnam, led to a refocusing of moral philosophy. Concern for issues of war and peace, the politics of dissent, public and private responsibility, and what is now called bioethics, grew out of this refocusing (Harris, 2001).

The second impetus for the development of bioethics was the development of new medical technologies that raised questions for which there were no answers. One of these was the machine that allowed the dialysis of clients with serious kidney disease. When first introduced, these devices were expensive, and there were not enough of them for all of the clients who could have benefited from their use. A committee set up in a Seattle hospital in 1962 to select clients for dialysis was nicknamed "the God committee" because of the life-and-death nature of the decisions it made. Questions were raised when it was shown that the committee favored clients of the same social class and ethnicity (Kuhse & Singer, 1998).

Further ethical concerns were related to the first heart transplants, made possible largely through the development of the respirator. This and other life-prolonging technologies called into question when a client should be declared dead and who had the authority to make this decision if the client was incompetent to do so. The landmark case regarding Karen Ann Quinlan in 1976 lent credence to the view that health care providers did not have a legal duty to prolong life in all circumstances.

Ethical issues related to informed consent by research subjects came to public attention when it was found that mentally retarded children at Willowbrook State Hospital in New York had been injected with hepatitis virus from 1965 to 1971. Another incident of the same nature was the U.S. Public Health Service Syphilis Study at Tuskegee, Alabama, lasting from the 1930s to the 1970s where life-saving antibiotics were withheld from a cohort of southern black men to study the "natural history" of the untreated disease (Kuhse & Singer, 1998).

Currently the scope of bioethics extends beyond the realms of health care professions and health care to encompass a variety of areas such as environmental ethics, ethics of sexuality and reproduction, ethics of genetic choice and manipulation, and ethics of research. Bioethics has taken on global perspective as its agenda has become the purview of national and international committees concerned with ethics. International documents such as the *Universal Declaration of Human Rights* are increasingly being used as reference points for ethical decision making (Harris, 2001).

Unlike ethics, which had been largely the province of moral philosophers and religious thinkers, bioethics has from the beginning been a multidisciplinary enterprise, involving not only health care providers, and biomedical scientists, but also thinkers from law, economics, and public policy. There are now over 200 bioethical centers around the world, with many national professional organizations and the International Association of Bioethics. Relevant scholarly journals are published in several countries (Kuhse & Singer, 1998).

Principle-Based Ethical Theories

A number of ethical theories have relevance for public health nursing practice. The public health nurse has probably been introduced to several of them as a part of his or her undergraduate education. A few of the theories will briefly be discussed. The reader is referred to the resource material at the end of the chapter for further study.

Utilitarianism

Utilitarianism as an ethical theory finds its roots in the ancient Greek philosophy of hedonism. Hedonism, from the Greek root *hedone* or "pleasure," is the general term for any philosophy that says that pleasure is equivalent to good and pain is equivalent to evil. Utilitarianism also has roots in consequentialism, a group of philosophies that decide whether actions are right entirely with reference to the consequences of the actions, regardless of any moral features the actions may have, such as truthfulness or fidelity. Consequentialist theories seek to judge actions according to the balance of good or bad outcomes that the actions produce. Utilitarianism is also referred to as a *teleological* ethical theory, from the Greek word *telos*, "end" or "goal," because of its emphasis on an external goal or purpose (Beauchamp & Childress, 2001; Beauchamp, & Walters, 2003; Soccio, 2001).

Jeremy Bentham (1748–1832) introduced the principle of utility, which states, "Actions are right in proportion as they tend to promote happiness, wrong as they tend to produce the reverse of happiness." It can also be stated as: "Act always to promote the greatest happiness for the greatest number." Munson (2003) illustrates the principle of utility with the following example. Suppose a woman lies near death in a large hospital. She shows only minimal brain function on an EEG and requires a respirator to breathe. Suppose also that a young man is admitted to the emergency room with severe kidney damage as a result of an automobile accident. He is in need of an immediate kidney transplant. There is a good tissue match with the woman's kidneys. Would it be right to hasten her death possibly by the removal of a kidney?

The principle of utility would probably justify the removal of the woman's kidney. The woman is almost dead, and the man has a good chance of survival if he has the transplant. The woman's life may be shortened by the removal of the kidney, and the surgery itself might kill her, but on balance, more happiness is likely to result from the transplant. If nothing is done, both people are likely to die.

There are a number of objections to utilitarianism. Only a few will be considered. One difficulty that immediately springs to mind is the inability to predict the future. If one is to judge actions by their consequences, then only future outcomes of particular actions can be predicted. What if the only way to achieve a desired outcome is through immoral actions? Utilitarianism might both condone such actions and, in fact, require them. A related problem lies in determining the distinction between actions that are obligatory based on maximizing the good and those that are above and beyond the call of moral obligation. Then there is the problem of unjust distribution of resources and the potential oppression of minorities based on maximizing the greatest good for the greatest number (Beauchamp & Childress, 2001; Wilkens, 1995). Ethical problems that have relevance for public health nurses include the need to balance the use of public health resources for critically ill individuals with need for large-scale public health programs for prevention and health promotion.

Kantian Theories/Deontology

In contrast to utilitarian theories, deontological theories maintain that the rightness or wrongness of human actions is not exclusively, or in the most extreme instance not at all, a function of the consequences of those actions. The most well-known classical deontological philosopher is the German Immanuel Kant (1724–1804). The basic principle of Kant's theory, which evolved over time, was what he called the "categorical imperative." According to this formulation, a person should only act on the maxim that he or she could wish over time would become a universal law. It also asserts that one should never treat another person only as a means to an end, but always at the same time as an end. Kantian ethics are founded in respect for the inherent dignity of each person, due from the person himself and from others. This respect flows from the nature of humans as rational beings. From the principle of not treating people as means to an end arises the idea of duties to the self and to others. These duties are described as "perfect duties" and "imperfect duties."

Prominent among Kant's perfect duties to others are the duty not to kill an innocent person, the duty not to lie, and the duty to keep promises. Perfect duties to oneself include not committing suicide. Imperfect duties, on the other hand, require the pursuit of certain goals, but never at the expense of perfect duties. Imperfect duties include the moral principle of beneficence, which is the duty to contribute to the welfare of others and the duty to develop one's own talents (Mappes & DeGrazia, 2001). Many public health nurses, as well as nurses in general, state that their practice is guided by deontological or Kantian ethics.

Ethical Principles

Most ethical theories accept basic principles as valid in the formation of a framework from which one can think about moral decision making. "A principle is a fundamental standard of conduct from which many other moral standards and judgments draw support for their defense and standing" (Beauchamp & Walters, 2003, p. 21). Ethical principles are grounded in the values found in the common morality and in statements of professional ethics. Ethical principles do not provide complete answers to the moral problems confronted; more information is often needed. But the principles are a starting point for moral reasoning (Beauchamp & Walters, 2003). Ethical principles include autonomy, nonmaleficence, beneficence, and justice.

Autonomy

Autonomy is derived from the Greek words *autos*, "self," and *nomos*, "rule," "governance," or "law." It was applied originally to the Greek city-states, but has been extended to the self-rule of individuals. Its meanings include "self-governance, liberty rights, privacy, individual choice, freedom of the will, causing one's own behavior, and being one's own person" (Beauchamp & Childress, 2001, p. 58). Autonomy is rooted in the concept of the importance of individual freedom and choice. It implies acting according to an individually chosen plan without interference from others (Beauchamp & Walters, 2003). The principle of autonomy may be stated as follows: Rational individuals should be permitted to be self-determining (Beauchamp & Childress, 2001; Munson, 2003, 2004).

Some feminists argue against the notion of the independent self acting in ways that do not consider the community. Recently, feminists have developed the idea of "relational autonomy" that considers the social embeddedness of individuals and the social intersection of such factors as gender, ethnicity, age, and class (Beauchamp & Childress, 2001).

Respect for the autonomy of others is very important, especially in the health care setting. Deontologists would argue that respect for autonomy flows from a recognition of the unconditional worth of each individual. Lack of respect for autonomy means that the person is being treated as a means and not as an end. Utilitarians would support respect for autonomy with the notion that individuals should be allowed to develop according to their personal convictions as long as they do not interfere with the freedom of others (Beauchamp & Childress, 2001).

The principle of respect for autonomy supports several specific moral rules, including telling the truth, respecting privacy, maintaining confidentiality, providing informed consent, and assisting clients in making important decisions when asked (Beauchamp & Childress, 2001). The first statement in the American Nurses Association *Code for Nurses* addresses the worth and dignity of the individual and the right to exercise self-determination (American Nurses Association, 2001).

Nonmaleficence

"Above all [or first] do no harm" is the most common statement of the principle of nonmaleficence, the obligation not to inflict harm on others. The positive version of this principle can be stated as follows: "We ought to act in ways that do not cause needless harm or injury to others" (Munson, 2003, p. 394). In other words, there is a duty to avoid harming other people. This principle is compatible with various ethical theories, such as deontology and utilitarianism. Harm as a concept has a broad range of meanings. Suffice it to say that harm includes significant bodily harms and other setbacks to significant interests, such as psychological, privacy, or liberty interests (Beauchamp & Childress, 2001; Munson, 2003, 2004).

Health care workers are obligated by this principle to be careful, diligent, and knowledgeable in the performance of their professional responsibilities. They must live up to the standard of "due care" that is often found in statements of professional standards. Due care includes protecting clients from exposure to unnecessary risk. With the explosion of knowledge in health care, it is important that health care professionals do not expose clients to risks that may arise from a lack of current or specialized knowledge on the part of the practitioner (Munson, 2003). The principle of nonmaleficence also imposes social duties. One example in the history of public health was in the nineteenth century when great strides were made to fight against disease that society recognized as the need to prevent harm through water treatment, immunization, and quarantine (Munson, 2003).

Beneficence

All health care professionals have a duty to promote the welfare of their clients and to assist them to further their important and legitimate interests; this is termed **beneficence**. This duty implies the provision of appropriate treatment and the duty to make reasonable sacrifices for the sake of clients. Beneficence may also include the notion of utility: the requirement to balance benefits and drawbacks to produce the best overall results. The moral rules associated with beneficence include such examples as protecting and defending the rights of others, helping persons with disabilities, and rescuing persons in danger (Beauchamp & Childress, 2001; Beauchamp & Walters, 2003; Munson, 2003).

The principle of beneficence, like the principle of nonmaleficence, also imposes social duties. Medicare, Medicaid, and prenatal programs are examples of social responses to the need to promote the good of clients. Indirectly, health care research also facilitates the good of the people as a whole. Health care is only one social good that can be provided to the citizens of a country. In the face of limited resources, a society must choose between a number of competing interests such as education, adequate housing, the arts, and many other important and enriching benefits. The society must determine how many of its resources ought to be allocated to health care. The principle of utility has been suggested as a way to balance competing needs. Utility imposes a social duty to do as much good as possible overall, with the recognition that one cannot meet all needs. For example, a public health nurse may decide to require PKU screening for newborns but not to institute mandatory screening for Tay-Sachs. PKU is distributed in the general population; if it is detected early, an effective treatment can be provided. Tay-Sachs, on the other hand, only affects a special segment of the population; early detection makes no difference in the outcome of this disease. Therefore, money spent on mandatory screening of newborns for Tay-Sachs would not be justified by the results produced. It would be better to spend societal resources for other purposes (Beauchamp & Childress, 2001; Beauchamp & Walters, 2003; Munson, 2003, 2004).

Many ethical codes in helping professions include the prevention of harm, a negative duty, but they also assert the duty to promote the client's welfare through the provision of positive benefits. The International Code of Nursing Ethics (1973), for example, states that "the nurse shares with other citizens the responsibility for initiating and supporting action to meet the health and social needs of the public." The range of duties from the prevention of harm to the provision of positive assistance lies along a continuum without clear demarcations. If the two duties come into conflict, the obligation to prevent harm seems to be more compelling than the obligation to do good, but this may not always be the case (Beauchamp & Walters, 2003).

One of the most contested problems associated with the principle of beneficence is whether the duty to do good is a general moral duty, incumbent on everyone, or merely a moral ideal that is not required (i.e., beyond the scope of duty). It would seem that the duty to promote the good of others is inherent in certain professional roles, such as public health nursing, where the very nature of the nurse-client relationship demands it (Beauchamp & Walters, 2003).

The principles of beneficence and autonomy may collide in the context of **paternalism**. In its most positive light, paternalism can be defined as benevolently restricting the freedom of others (i.e., acting for the best good of others without their consent) (Beauchamp & Childress, 2001). Questions of paternalism may arise in relationship to such public health actions as mandatory childhood immunization and laws requiring the use of seatbelts in automobiles and helmets by cyclists.

Justice

Justice requires that we be treated equitably by others and by institutions. This does not mean that one will always have the advantage. For example, individuals pay their share of taxes, even though they may wish to keep the money, in order to support programs for the public good. The rule of triage is respected in the emergency room, so that if a client in critical condition arrives after another client, priority for treatment is given to the client in critical condition (Munson, 2003).

Although there is no single principle of justice, there is a minimal principle, first articulated by Aristotle, which forms the basis of the many justice principles now in existence. Aristotle's **principle of formal justice**, or formal equality, may be stated as follows: "Equals must be treated equally, and unequals must be treated unequally" or "Similar cases ought to be treated in similar ways." The principle of formal justice provides the minimum or core starting point for all theories of justice. The principle is formal because it is like a sentence with blanks; each individual must fill in the information about what factors or features are to be considered relevant in deciding whether cases are similar. The principle does not specify how to determine equality or similarity. For that information, the various theories of justice must be expolored (Beauchamp & Walters, 2003; Munson, 2003).

Justice has two major aspects: noncomparative and comparative justice. **Noncomparative justice** involves making sure that people receive the rights to which they are entitled. **Comparative justice** addresses the fair distribution of social benefits and burdens. This latter form of justice, often called **distributive justice**, is most relevant to issues of public health.

The various theories of distributive justice provide *substantive, or material, principles of justice* and arguments to show why certain factors should be considered relevant in deciding whether cases are similar. The substantive principles can then be used to determine whether particular laws, practices, or policies can be considered just. Material principles identify relevant properties that persons must possess to qualify for a particular distribution. Differences among these principles help explain present disagreements about the distribution of social benefits and burdens. Material principles of justice include the following:

- To each person an equal share
- To each person according to need
- To each person according to effort
- To each person according to contribution
- To each person according to merit
- To each person according to free-market exchanges (Beauchamp & Childress, 2001; Munson, 2003)

Public health nursing ethics must continue to address the tension inherent in balancing competing needs for scarce public health resources. The public health nurse may be called upon to assist communities and health care agencies to decide among such competing interests. How the public health nurse selects and applies material principles of justice will determine the counsel provided for decision making.

Various theories of justice have been developed. These theories attempt to connect properties of persons with morally justifiable distributions of benefits and burdens. Utilitarian theories emphasize a mixture of criteria in order to maximize public utility. Libertarian theories emphasize rights to social and economic liberty by ensuring fair procedures rather than focusing on outcomes. Communitarian theories stress the principles and practices of justice that evolve through traditions and practices in a particular community. Egalitarian theories emphasize equal access to the goods in life that every rational person values with particular reference to the material principles of need and equality (Beauchamp & Childress, 2001; Munson, 2003).

Moral Rules

The four basic ethical principles already discussed—autonomy, nonmaleficence, beneficence, and justice—are central to ethics in the health professions. In addition, rules, rights, and virtues are also important. There is only a loose distinction between principles and rules; for example, some ethicists classify truth-telling as an ethical principle, while others see it as a moral rule. Both principles and rules may function to guide deci-

⊕ RESEARCH APPLICATION

Ethical Issues in Public Health Nursing

Study Purpose

To explore ethical issues in public health nursing in Canada and to begin to identify strategies to support ethical practice.

Methods

In this qualitative study, exploratory descriptive design was used involving interviews with practicing public health nurses. Participants were asked: "Please describe a frequently recurring ethical problem (or problems) that you have experienced in practice—something that has been a common problem for you." Supplemental questions were used to determine what support nurses received when they experienced ethical problems, and how they sought to resolve these problems. The essentially unstructured interviews were tape-recorded and transcribed for thematic analysis.

Findings

The participants were 22 public health nurses, 11 in rural and 11 in urban public health nursing centers. Participants ranged in age from mid-30s to mid-50s and had experience in public health ranging from less than one year to more than 30 years. The analysis revealed five major themes, each with a number of subthemes. The five major themes and the subthemes were (1) relationships with health care professionals: interprofessional and intraprofessional; (2) systems issues: just resource distribution, policy and law as support or constraint, and systems support for nursing practice; (3) character of relationships: context/nature of

the relationship, empowerment versus dependency, and setting boundaries; (4) respect for persons: autonomy, confidentiality, and honoring context; and (5) putting self at risk: values conflicts and physical danger.

Implications

Every aspect of public health nursing was found to have ethical components, but participants' concerns centered on whether their decisions were the "best" in the circumstances. The reality of ethical decision making in public health nursing appears to be in contrast with the essentially linear decision-making frameworks that are found in the literature: gathering data, examining values, considering influencing variables, and making decisions. Instead, in public health nursing ethical issues are rooted in context and highly relational in character. What public health nurses need to support their practice is not a decision-making framework as such but rather opportunities to discuss issues, engage in values clarification, and support and mentor one another. They also need opportunities to engage in dialogue with administrative leaders to educate them about the concerns the nurses face and to discover the values and beliefs that shape administrative practice. The whole system needs to be taken into account when considering support for ethical practice, with a realization that the "client" is multifaceted and complex.

Reference

Oberle, K., & Tenove, S. (2000). Ethical issues in public health nursing. *Nursing Ethics, 7*(5), 425–438.

sion making and action by the public health nurse. Principles provide broad guidelines; rules specify the principles and make them more available for ethical decision making. Several types of moral rules are relevant for public health: substantive rules, authority rules, and procedural rules (Beauchamp & Walters, 2003).

Substantive rules include truth-telling, confidentiality, privacy, foregoing treatment, assisted suicide, informed consent, and the health care rationing. These rules serve to clarify what is required for ethical action (Beauchamp & Walters, 2003).

Authority rules govern decisional authority (i.e., who may and should perform actions). Rules of surrogate authority direct who should make decisions in the place of incompetent persons. Rules of professional authority determine who, if anyone, is able to override the decisions of clients who have made chosen actions that are damaging or poorly considered (Beauchamp & Walters, 2003).

Procedural rules provide for the establishment of appropriate procedures to follow in particular situations. For example, procedural rules may govern the allocation of scarce health care resources or for reporting grievances to higher authorities (Beauchamp & Walters, 2003).

Ethical Theories without Principles

In the past 15 years, there have been challenges to both of the recently dominant ethical theories: deductivism (or grand ethical theories), such as utilitarianism and Kantianism, and principle-based ethics or principlism in which several principles, rules, or duties, none of which routinely takes precedence may be considered relevant in varying circumstances. Challenges to these two ethical frameworks include many different formulations, four of which will be considered in this discussion: (1) feminist and (2) care ethics, both of which derive from the work of Carol Gilligan; (3) virtue ethics; and (4) casuistry, or case-based reasoning (Mappes & DeGrazia, 2001).

Feminist Ethics

In her 1982 book, *In a Different Voice: Psychological Theory and Women's Development*, Carol Gilligan, a contemporary feminist psychologist, challenged the ethical theory of her erstwhile employer, Lawrence Kohlberg who had limited his research on ethical development to privileged white boys and men. She objected to his conclusion that men's moral views were at a higher level than women's, asserting instead the moral development of women was not inferior but rather different: Men thought in terms of rules and justice, and women were much more focused on caring and relationships (Gilligan, 1982). Gilligan interpreted her research data to show that women understood ethical dilemmas in a much more contextualized, narrative way when making decisions as opposed to men who tended to apply abstract rules without full consideration of the surrounding circumstances of the individual case. "Feminist ethicists accept the arguments offered within the realm of 'feminine' ethics which demand that attention be paid to the interdependent, emotionally varied, unequal relationships that shape human lives" (Sherwin & Parish, 2002).

A major task for feminist ethics involves restructuring the power relationships that characterize health care such that the focus moves from crisis management to fostering health empowerment. This approach involves distributing specialized health care knowledge and information for self-help approaches that allow persons to achieve maximum control of his or her own health (Sherwin & Parish, 2002). The feminist perspective supports the public health nursing emphasis on health promotion and prevention through empowering individuals, families, groups, and communities to take responsibility for their health status.

Care Ethics

The ethics of caring deemphasizes rights, principles, and rules in favor of caring interpersonal relationships and context (Mappes & DeGrazia, 2001). Care ethics has been especially attractive to nurses as they have sought to differentiate themselves from medicine (Allmark, 2002). Manning (1998) describes five central ideas in an ethic of care: (1) moral attention to the situation in all its complexity; (2) sympathetic understanding of what others in the situation would want; (3) relationship awareness or cognizance of the networks of relationships that connect the humans in a situation; (4) accommodation for the needs of all who are involved in a situation; (5) and a response that demonstrates caring in concrete action in response to client need.

The implementation of a caring model of health care can be time consuming and is most effective within a relationship characterized by mutual trust. Allmark (2002) criticizes ethics based on care and caring as vague and lacking in normative and descriptive content. He goes on to point out that there has not been an adequate analysis of care that would form a basis for moral meaning for the concept and that care ethicists have not described the issues underlying moral judgments related to caring.

Virtue Ethics

In contrast to deductivism theories and principle-based ethics, which emphasize the moral evaluation of actions, virtue ethics, in the tradition of Plato and Aristotle, emphasize a virtuous character. Virtues may be understood as character traits that are morally valuable such as truthfulness, compassion, or courage. With a focus on the person performing the action, virtue-based ethics is concerned not so much with how to act but with what kind of person to be and what sort of life to lead (Mappes, 2001; Oakley, 1998).

One criticism of virtue ethics is that it is too vague to serve as a criterion for determining rightness. Further there are numerous virtuous characteristics that may be held in varying combinations and degrees by various virtuous persons. How then can it be known what a virtuous person will do in a given circumstance? Such criticisms as these have led to the position by some ethicists that virtue ethics should form an adjunct to rule or principle-based ethics rather than serving as a substitution for them (Mappes, 2001; Oakley, 1998).

Casuistry

Ideas of *casuistry* or case-based reasoning were introduced into bioethics in the late 1980s by Albert Jonsen and Stephen Toulmin. In their work with the National Commission for the Protection of Human Subjects of Biomedical and Behavioral Research, they noted that members of the commission often agreed with *what* ought to be done in certain cases while disagreeing with *why* it should be done. This led them to assert that rather than relying on high-level principles, ethical reasoning should begin from the bottom up (Fulford, Dickenson, & Murray, 2002). Casuists hold that no single unified theory adequately reflects the diversity of moral ideas, nor does ethical reasoning consist of straightforward deduction. Instead, the value of practical wisdom is asserted in a methodology that relies on the examination of "paradigmatic" cases from which some maxim, or specific principle or rule, can be derived to guide moral action (Mappes & DeGrazia, 2001).

The casuistic approach to ethics works best when there is a community of shared underlying values and may call for the careful elucidation of hidden values and concern for minority views. Some critics have noted that there is little fundamental difference between casuistry and principle-based ethics. It is also felt by some ethicists that case-based reasoning relies too heavily on intuition and is unable to move beyond precedent and tradition to address controversial issues (Fulford, Dickenson, & Murray, 2002; Mappes & DeGrazia, 2001).

CROSS-CULTURAL ETHICAL PERSPECTIVES

In recent years, people in the Western world have obtained easy access to the ethical traditions of non-Western secular and religious ethical traditions. This access has provided exposure to systems of health care ethics that do not depend on Greek philosophy or the Hippocratic tradition in medicine. In addition, ethicists from a variety of cultural positions have begun to publish philosophical research that opens important windows on the many ethical traditions that exist in the world today. It is not possible given the scope of this chapter to address the many cultural perspectives that are available, but public health nurses are encouraged to add an investigation of the applicable ethical tradition in their assessment of families and communities.

Annette Dula (2001), an African American bioethicist, correctly notes that the field is dominated by white, male, middle-class professionals. As a result, the voices of women, the poor, and ethnic minorities are not often heard in debates on ethics and health care policy. Dula argues that the development of bioethics perspectives will be enriched by the inclusion of a broader range of viewpoints. In addition to looking at the ethical positions of major world religions, we will explore the ethical statements of selected ethnic groups. In addition to the groups presented in Boxes 18-2 and 18-3, it is important that the public health nurse be alert to the development of the ethical perspectives of American Indians, Latinos, Alaska Natives, Hawaiian Natives, and Pacific Islanders as they become increasingly available in the literature.

Through sensitive listening to cultural narratives and personal stories, the public health nurse may begin to discover the ways that various ethnic groups ground their ethics in common human experiences. This will lead the nurse to respect other cultural traditions. The ethical formulations of many ethnic groups may be much more compatible with feminine or care ethics than with ethical theories that are founded on set principles such as individual autonomy. Ethics in these contexts must be understood in the light of colonization, historical abuse, social marginalization, and disempowerment. Feminist ethics with its goal of empowerment of the oppressed is particularly relevant in regard to the health of ethnic and indigenous populations (Campbell, 2001).

NURSING AND OTHER ETHICAL CODES AND PRINCIPLES

Nursing has developed ethical codes and principles to guide nursing practice. Some are specific to the United States such as the American Nurses Association Code for Nurses. Others are state specific and define the practice of nursing in that state. There are also codes and principles specific to a specialty area in nursing and are used to delineate the practice of nursing within that specialty (Scope and Standards of Public Health Nursing Practice). The International Council of Nurses

BOX 18-2: Cross-Cultural Religious Perspectives

Jewish Ethics

Jewish ethical positions are derived primarily from the Old Testament, particularly from the Torah, and also from the Talmud, the rabbinical teachings. The oldest Jewish document related to medical ethics is the *Oath of Asaph*. Asaph Judaeus was a Jewish medical teacher who probably lived in the sixth century C.E.; his oath was a summary, not only of the ethical obligations for health care providers, but for all Jews. The oath includes prohibitions against certain types of abortions, the administration of poisons, involvement in witchcraft, sexual misconduct, love of money, causing injury or death by any medical treatment, and idolatry. God is acknowledged as the true source of healing and adherence to the divine covenant is encouraged as the impetus for upright behavior and humility (Asaph Judaeus, 2000).

Jewish tradition places ultimate value on the individual human life. The obligation to preserve life is an all-encompassing end in itself, not merely a condition relative to other values. This regard for human life as the supreme value in the Jewish tradition surpasses the value placed on life in the Christian tradition or in Anglo-Saxon common law. Jewish tradition requires that the many ethical issues that arise from this position (e.g., life-preserving treatment, hazardous therapy, informed consent) be referred to the rabbi who serves as an ethicist and will provide an analysis and interpretation of the situation based on Jewish moral tradition (Bleich, 2000).

Catholic Ethics

Like Judaism, Roman Catholicism bases its ethical position on theological considerations. Natural law theory provides the ethical basis for the Catholic perspective. Catholic prohibitions against artificial contraception and abortion are well known. The code of ethics adopted by the National Conference of Catholic Bishops addresses many issues that are of concern to Catholics regarding health care (e.g., the doctrine of double effect, the distinction between ordinary and extraordinary means of preserving life, and the criterion of proportionality). The doctrine of double effect is used to justify actions that cause a serious harm, such as the death of a person, as a side effect of promoting a good result (McIntyre, 2005). The criterion of proportionality is used in bioethics with refer-

ence to the suitability of various means for preserving life. Proportionality involves "studying the type of treatment to be used, its degree of complexity or risk, its cost and the possibilities of using it, and comparing these elements with the result that can be expected, taking into account the state of the sick person and his or her physical and moral resources" (Congregation for the Doctrine of the Faith, 1980, Part IV). Concern for the sick that reflects Jesus' example has motivated Catholic health care for the sick, suffering, and dying throughout history.

The social responsibility of Catholic health care services is based on five normative principles: (1) a commitment to promote and defend human dignity; (2) the biblical mandate to care for the poor; (3) the need to contribute to the common good through the promotion of the economic, political, and social conditions that ensure the protection of fundamental human rights; (4) responsible stewardship of available health care resources; and (5) respect for moral positions that may be in conflict with the moral positions of the Catholic Church with regard to specific medical procedures (National Conference of Catholic Bishops, 2000).

Protestant Ethics

The Protestant religious tradition includes many denominations and subgroups. This diversity makes it difficult to identify a single bioethical perspective. This problem is complicated by the Protestant commitment to the freedom of the layperson to articulate his or her own moral position. However, there is the possibility to trace key themes in the Protestant approach. Ramsey (2000), a former professor of religion at Princeton University, has identified the following themes: covenant fidelity; faithfulness defined by covenant; the role of all, including laypersons, in decisions; and the uniqueness of the religious perspective.

The concept of fidelity to covenant has to do with righteousness between one human being and another. It involves the moral quality and action associated with justice, fairness, faithfulness, the sanctity of life, and charity, among others. These attitudes are those that should characterize the covenant relationship between the health care practitioner and the client.

(continued)

BOX 18-2: Cross-Cultural Religious Perspectives (cont'd)

Muslim/Islamic Ethics

The Islamic approach to health care ethics differs from the ethical literature of both East and West. Significantly informed by the Quranic texts, it is very religious in tone. Traditional ethical writings focus on the role of the health care provider and stress importance of correct moral and ethical behavior in the private life of the health care provider as the prerequisite for correct professional ethics. The health care provider must believe in God and exhibit gratitude to parents and teachers, humility, kindness, mercy, adherence to the teachings of Islam, and other virtues in both public and private life.

Specific duties include keeping abreast of current knowledge, complying with legal professional requirements, recognizing that life begins at conception and that human life cannot be taken away except by God, avoiding harm, following God's guidelines even if they conflict with the desires of the client, and protecting confidentiality, among others.

SOURCE: Based on information in Rahman et al., 2000.

---

has developed a code of ethics that is for the nursing global community.

American Nurses Association Code for Nurses

The American Nurses Association (ANA) Code for Nurses with Interpretive Statements (American Nurses Association, 2001) serves the following purposes:

- It is a succinct statement of the ethical obligations and duties of every individual who enters the nursing profession.

- It is the profession's nonnegotiable ethical standard.

- It is an expression of nursing's own understanding of its commitment to society.

Several aspects of this code have special relevance to public health nursing practice. The first statement, which asserts the dignity of the individual, implies the right to self-determination. It is recognized, however, that each individual is a member of a community, and that in some cases the person's right to self-determination may come into conflict with the welfare of the community. In harmony with the position taken by the general statements on human rights, the ANA Code requires that the restriction of individual rights is a serious deviation.

International Council of Nurses Code of Ethics for Nurses

The code of the International Council of Nurses (ICN, 2000) was adopted initially in 1953 and has been revised and reaffirmed periodically since then with the most recent instance in 2000. The preamble describes the responsibility and scope of nursing and asserts basic human rights principles. The ICN also provides suggestions for application of the code.

Scope and Standards of Public Health Nursing Practice

The *Scope and Standards of Public Health Nursing Practice* was developed through a joint effort of the organizations that make up the Quad Council of Public Health Nursing Organizations (Quad Council, 1999): the American Nurses Association, Council for Community, Primary, and Long-Term Care Nursing Practice; the American Public Health Association, Public Health Nursing Section; the Association of Community Health Nursing Educators; and the Association of State and Territorial Directors of Nursing. This document replaced previous separate statements of the American Nurses Association and the American Public Health Association, Public Health Nursing Section.

One of the seven tenets that describe the scope of public health nursing practice is relevant to concerns of distributive justice: "Stewardship of and allocation of available resources supports the maximum population health benefit gain" (Quad Council, 1999, p. 4). Public health nurses accept the *ANA Code of Ethics with Interpretive Statements* as an ethical standard. They are admonished to apply the basic human rights of autonomy, self-determination, and pursuance of health promotion to the communities that they work with as clients (Quad Council, 1999). The section on

BOX 18-3: Cross-Cultural Ethnic Perspectives

African American Ethics

Dula (2001) states that the African American ethical perspectives come from two bases: (1) the medical experiences of black people and (2) the legacy of black activist philosophy. She examines several mainstream ethical issues that are particularly relevant to African Americans, such as the birth control movement and other reproductive issues and the Tuskegee experiments. She stresses the value of an African American perspective for the field of bioethics as a whole.

Dula's assessment of the problems that African American experience in the health care delivery system is confirmed by the recent Institute of Medicine report, *Unequal Treatment* (Smedley et al., 2003). African Americans and other ethnic minorities in the United States receive a poorer quality of health care regardless of socioeconomic status. Dula charges bioethicists with a lack of attention to the cultural and societal aspects of health care. "Bioethics cannot be exclusively medical or even ethical. Rather, it must also deal with beliefs, values, cultural traditions, and the economic, political, and social order" (Dula, 2001, p. 82).

Black activist philosophy forms the second basis for an African American bioethics. Black philosophy differs from mainstream philosophy in its emphasis on action and social justice. Bioethics and black activist philosophy overlap in their mutual concerns for distributive justice and fairness, autonomy and paternalism in unequal relationships, and individual and social ills.

The African American perspective on bioethics is also informed by the history of abuses that African Americans, other ethnic minorities, and the poor have experienced in the health care delivery system. Dula cites several examples, notably the disproportionate number of sterilizations among African Americans, Latinas, American Indians, and other poor women during the 1960s and early 1970s. She also recounts the infamous Tuskegee study where over 400 poor and undereducated black men with syphilis were uninformed subjects in a U.S. Public Health Service research program to study the effects of untreated syphilis. The study lasted from 1932 to 1972, despite the discovery of the curative effects of penicillin during this period. This unfortunate chapter in health care investigations provided the impetus for policies to protect the rights of human subjects in research.

Dula concludes that the concerns of large segments of the population, based on their experiences in the health care delivery system, point out the importance of their perspective for the larger field of bioethics. As we confront the ethical and human rights implications of the large number of uninsured people in U.S. society, especially the overrepresentation of the poor and ethnic minorities in this group, it compels public health nurses to examine our responsibility, not only to encourage the expansion of the ethical dialogue but also to advocate for the human rights of disadvantaged groups.

African Ethics

Africa is a vast continent that is home to between 800 and 1,200 diverse cultural and ethnic groups. As a result, it is impossible to describe an explicitly African worldview. The various indigenous perspectives have been colored by Christianity, Islam, and many Western influences so that generalizations about a health-related ethics are difficult. However, traditional patterns of thought that are distinctly African have been identified. Peter Kasenene, a South African theologian, has compared general principles that characterize African ethical thinking with Western ethical principles, and Godfrey Tangwa, an ethicist from Cameroon, has addressed the traditional African perception of a person.

African ethics is based on a worldview rooted in the life-affirming promotion of vitality and fertility of human beings, livestock, and the land. If this state is disrupted by disease, both natural and supernatural means are used to restore a state of well-being. In traditional African societies, moral authority resides in a belief in the ancestors who retain such authority after their deaths. Right action is action in accord with customary norms and standards (Kasenene, 2000).

Kasenene has identified two basic ethical principles that underlie the African perspective. The first, the *vital force principle,* was presented by Placied Tempels, a Belgian missionary to the Congo in 1945, in a book entitled *Bantu Philosophy.* For Tempels, vital force is the meaning of "to be." It is the drive to be stronger and to be protected from misfortune. The opposite of vital force is illness, suffering, fatigue, injustice, oppression, or any

(continued)

BOX 18-3: Cross-Cultural Ethnic Perspectives (cont'd)

other physical or social ill. Vital force descends from God through the ancestors and elders to the individual person who has the duty to promote and protect the vital force of the community (Tempels, 1959).

The second principle, the *communalism principle,* is related to the high value placed on community life. Mbiti, who identified this principle in 1969, discusses the notion that for Africans the individual exists as part of a community: the family, the clan, and the whole ethnic group. "I am, because we are; and since we are, therefore, I am" (Mbiti, 1969, p. 109). The person finds his or her identity within the group; thus, the health of the individual is of significant concern to the community. Each individual is expected to preserve his or her life on behalf of the group.

As could be expected, the emphasis on communalism in traditional African ethical thinking limits the personal autonomy that is stressed in Western ethics. Related concerns such as confidentiality and paternalism become issues as a balance is struck between the rights of the individual and the community's interest in the good of the individual as it relates to the good of the group.

The promotion of good (beneficence) and the prevention of harm (nonmaleficence) are compatible with the principle of vital force. As a result, health care is highly valued; however, since the good of the community is paramount, persons suffering from contagious diseases are traditionally isolated, or may even be helped to die, if they pose a threat to community well-being. The African emphasis on wholeness means that the promotion and restoration of health involves not only physical wholeness but the person's social participation as well.

Justice, which is highly valued, is based on to each according to his or her needs. The communal principle means that justice is primarily a social concern; the good of the community is promoted when the needs of each person are addressed without discrimination, but in recognition of the hierarchical nature of traditional African societies. Each person gives and receives according to his or her social status. In terms of setting priorities for receiving health care, this emphasis on status is giving way to an emphasis on need (Kasenene, 1989.)

Tangwa (2000) describes the traditional African perception of the person as totally different from the Western view. From the African perspective, there is interdependence among humans, supernatural spirits, animals, plants, and inanimate objects and forces, with

the possibility of reincarnation, transmigration, transformation, and transmutation between all these entities. This worldview engenders a respectful attitude toward nature and all living things. Health is seen as the highest value, one that makes all other values possible. Health care in traditional African societies is available to all. Tangwa envisions a combination of the scientific and technological advances of Western health care with the moral values of the traditional African worldview.

Asian Ethics

Asian peoples and cultures differ significantly. The more than 30 Asian nations including China, Japan, India, the Philippines, Cambodia, Nepal, and Thailand, to name a few, can be subdivided into even more languages, cultures, and immigration patterns (ETR Associates, 2004). Ren-Zong Qui, director of the Bioethics Programme at the Chinese Academy of Social Sciences, has examined bioethics in an Asian context. As was noted in the discussion of African ethics, there is no single Asian perspective. But also, as in the case of Africa, some commonalities can be identified.

One of the primary differences between Asian and Western ethical perspectives is the issue of self-interest. In contrast to the Western view that the individual pursuit of self-interest will ultimately favor the interests of the group at large, many Asians view self-interest as self-defeating and in many cases not even moral. The Western approach to bioethics is rooted in the preservation of autonomy and the protection of the rights of the client. Asian bioethics, on the other hand, seeks to achieve a balance between the individualist and communitarian positions, and between rights and duties. In many Asian cultures, the individual is viewed as only relatively independent, and in many cases as interdependent with the community or society. "Society is more than the mere sum of all its members. Thus if an individual did some good or some harm to the community or society, that positive or negative effect would in turn affect all its members—including that same individual" (Qui, 1996, p. 14).

The Western emphasis on rights is not reflected in the traditional Asian perspective. For example, Confucian ethics is more concerned with duties, obligations, and responsibilities than with individual rights. The rights approach has the potential to cause conflicts in the Asian context in the face of such concerns as providing

(continued)

BOX 18-3: Cross-Cultural Ethnic Perspectives (cont'd)

for adequate community resources to insure individual rights, determining who has the obligation to provide rights, and allowing the rights of women in traditionally patriarchal communities (Qui, 1996).

Asians and Westerners differ on many specific issues as well. For instance, in the Chinese view, human life begins at birth, not when the sperm penetrates the ovum, as some Westerners believe. Thus, abortion is not a moral issue in contemporary China. There the moral issue is late abortion, not abortion in and of itself. In many Asian countries, health status information is typically withheld from the client and shared with the family instead or never disclosed at all. This differs significantly from the U.S. practice of full disclosure of information to the client alone. Overpopulation is a serious concern in Asia, but it is usually not an issue in the West (Qui, 1996). The approaches of Asian individuals, families, and communities to bioethical issues are influenced not only by nationality but also by religion. The public health nurse must take into account the ethical perspectives of Confucianism, Buddhism, Hinduism, and Islam as well as the Judeo-Christian traditions to which some Asians adhere.

The Ethics of Indigenous Peoples

The major ideas that shape Western ethics derive from the cultural traditions of Greece, Rome, and Christianity and are based more recently on the work of Anglo-American moralists. These ideas emphasize liberal concepts of individual autonomy and rational egoism and give a lesser place to ideas more compatible with other cultural traditions. When these ideas are projected onto various indigenous populations, they may be seen as perpetuations of colonial practices that have led to the discounting of traditional values. The ethics of the Maori of New Zealand will serve as an example of the ethics of an indigenous people.

In New Zealand, the British colonists developed a founding document, the Treaty of Waitanga, which prom-

ised mutual respect between them and the Maori and the preservation of Maori sovereignty and treasures. Maori ethos embodies the laws of *tapu*, or genealogies, history, traditional knowledge, carving, and nature. *Tapu* teaches the Maori respect for the whole of nature. Postcolonial suppression of Maori culture and language, in addition to progressive urbanization has led to the weakening of traditional values and of a full sense of *taha Maori*, or the Maori perspective.

Along with other indigenous peoples, the Maori regard physical illness as bound up with mental or spiritual ills, so that a Maori client may consider him- or herself to have suffered a weakening of the soul or essential being. Death is seen not only as an end of life but also as a reaffirmation of the identity of the person who has died. Sickness is thought of as a diminishing of the *mana* (divinely given power of the individual) that may be replenished in connection with the life of the extended family or *whanau*. It is not acceptable to treat a Maori person as other than a functioning whole embedded in an extended family with its traditional system of beliefs. Health care ethics that result in individuals being treated without reference to this inclusive reality may be harmful to Maori clients (Campbell, Gillett, & Jones, 2001).

The ethical perspective of the Maori is but one example of the ethics of an indigenous group, albeit an international one. Even though the ethical positions of North American indigenous peoples, such as American Indians and Alaska Natives, are yet to be fully presented in the health care literature, the public health nurse may use the experience of the Maori as a departure point for the investigation of some of the critical ethical issues that may arise in caring for any indigenous group. The nurse should pay attention to the important ethical considerations that surround such concepts as health, the nature of the human being, the relationship between humans and nature, appropriate health care delivery, family relationships, child-rearing and childbearing practices, and death and dying practices, to name a few.

"Ethics" asserts the public health nurse's responsibility to identify situations that present ethical dilemmas or jeopardize human rights and/or freedom and to seek council as needed in dealing with these issues. Public health nurses are to "promote, protect, and preserve autonomy, confidentiality, dignity, and human rights" (Quad Council, 1999, p. 19).

Public Health Leadership Society: Public Health Code of Ethics

The *Principles of the Ethical Practice of Public Health* was developed by many public health professionals associated with the Public Health Leadership Society (2002). The Public Health Code of Ethics Committee comprised representatives from public health practice and education, the Centers for Diseases Control and Prevention, and the American Public Health Association. The code is based on a definition of public health as "what we, as a society, do collectively to assure the conditions for peoples to be healthy," and affirms the World Health Organization's definition of health. See Box 18-4. The values and beliefs that underlie the principles are as follows:

Health

1. Humans have a right to the resources necessary for health.

Community

2. Humans are inherently social and interdependent.

3. The effectiveness of institutions depends heavily on the public's trust.

4. Collaboration is a key element to public health.

5. People and their physical environment are interdependent.

BOX 18-4: Principles of the Ethical Practice of Public Health

1. Public health should address principally the fundamental causes of disease and requirements for health, aiming to prevent adverse health outcomes.

2. Public health should achieve community health in a way that respects the rights of individuals in the community.

3. Public health policies, programs, and priorities should be developed and evaluated through processes that ensure an opportunity for input from community members.

4. Public health should advocate and work for the empowerment of disenfranchised community members, aiming to ensure that the basic resources and conditions necessary for health are accessible to all.

5. Public health should seek the information needed to implement effective policies and programs that protect and promote health.

6. Public health institutions should provide communities with the information they have that is needed for decisions on policies or programs and should obtain the community's consent for their implementation.

7. Public health institutions should act in a timely manner on the information they have within the resources and the mandate given them by the public.

8. Public health programs and policies should incorporate a variety of approaches that anticipate and respect diverse values, beliefs, and cultures in the community.

9. Public health programs and policies should be implemented in a manner that most enhances the physical and social environment.

10. Public health institutions should protect the confidentiality of information that can bring harm to an individual or community if made public. Exceptions must be justified on the basis of the high likelihood of significant harm to the individual or others.

11. Public health institutions should ensure the professional competence of their employees.

12. Public health institutions and their employees should engage in collaborations and affiliations in ways that build the public's trust and the institution's effectiveness.

SOURCE: Public Health Leadership Society, 2002.

6. Each person in a community should have an opportunity to contribute to public discourse.

7. Identifying and promising the fundamental requirements for health in a community are of primary concern to public health.

Bases for Action

8. Knowledge is important and powerful.

9. Science is the basis for much of our public health knowledge.

10. People are responsible to act on the basis of what they know.

11. Action is not based on information alone.

PUBLIC HEALTH AS SOCIAL JUSTICE: POVERTY AND HEALTH

"Doctors usually evaluate patients' vulnerability to serious disease by inquiring about risk factors like cigarette smoking, obesity, hypertension and high cholesterol. But they might be better off asking how much money those patients make, how many years they spent in school and where they stand relative to others in their offices and communities." (Goode, 2001, p. 39)

The relationship of poverty with ill health and death has been known for decades, but a great deal of recent research has provided evidence that social class, as measured not only by income and education but also by relative social standing, is a more powerful predictor of health status than genetics, exposure to carcinogens, or cigarette smoking. This relationship holds true for risks for a wide variety of health problems. The risk varies with the relative wealth or poverty of the individual: the higher the social standing, the lower the risk, and vice versa, even at the higher rungs of the social ladder. In fact, some of the health differences often attributed to ethnicity are really related to socioeconomic status because minorities, such as blacks, are disproportionately represented in the lower income brackets (Goode, 2001; Smedley et al., 2003).

However, for some health conditions, ethnicity seems to be a risk factor regardless of social class (Smedley et al., 2003). Ethical issues related to social justice, the equitable distribution of the benefits and burdens of society, arise when we consider poverty from an international perspective. The public health relationship is highlighted by the realization that decisions related to social justice affect human mortality. Despite a growing global economy, billions of people live lives of severe poverty. In fact, the annual death toll from poverty-related causes worldwide is approximately 18 million, one-third of all human deaths (Pogge, 2005).

People who live below the $2.00 per day World Bank international poverty line constitute 44 percent of the world's population, but they consume only 1.3 percent of the global product. These people would need only 1 percent more of the global product to escape poverty. On the other hand, high-income countries have only 955 million citizens. These people consume about 81 percent of the global product. Their average per capita income is nearly 180 times greater than that of the poor. It is therefore possible to eradicate poverty, and with it the excess morbidity and mortality that it brings (Pogge, 2005). What public health issues does this information raise? Are public health professionals obligated to address the larger social issues that have an impact on human health and well-being?

ETHICAL DECISION MAKING IN PUBLIC HEALTH NURSING

An ethical dilemma exists when there are good reasons for one or more mutually exclusive alternatives. Each alternative has both desirable and undesirable aspects. Ethical dilemmas usually take one of two forms: (1) there is evidence that the act in question is morally right and there is also evidence that the act is morally wrong, but the strength of the evidence on either side is inconclusive; (2) the person believes that he or she is morally obligated to perform two or more mutually exclusive actions, thus he or she cannot do both in the same circumstance (Beauchamp & Childress, 2001; Beauchamp & Walters, 2003).

Ethical dilemmas must be distinguished from clinical dilemmas and issues involving lack of moral courage. Clinical dilemmas occur when the public health professional must decide between two actions or practice interventions that present both advantages and disadvantages. For example, a public health nurse must decide on the best plan to reduce teen pregnancy in the community. She can either present a program through the local school district, the YWCA, or a coalition of churches. Her decision, while important, does not have moral implications. Situations involving lack of moral courage exist when a public health professional knows the morally correct action to take but is afraid or reluctant to act on this knowledge. For instance, a public health nurse knows that he should use his advocacy skills to address a situation of injustice to an ethnic group in the community but hesitates to do so for fear of the political repercussions.

The public health nurse must first determine if the issue that presents is an ethical dilemma or not. A number of ethical decision-making models are presented in the literature that can facilitate the resolution of general health care dilemmas. However, there is another level of ethical decision making that relates to the larger ethical implications of public health interventions, programs, research, and policies. For these types of situations, an ethical decision-making model designed specifically for public health is necessary.

A Public Health Ethical Decision-Making Model

Gostin and Lazzarim (1997) and Kass and Gielen (1998) proposed similar public health ethical decision-making frameworks in the late 1990s. Kass refined her model in 2001. The model she suggests strikes a balance between advancing the public's health and social justice while maximizing individual liberties. This goal is rendered problematic because of the differing historical contexts that saw the rise of public health and bioethics in the United States, as discussed earlier in this chapter.

Public health arose in the context of concern for the health of populations rather than individuals, while bioethics grew to prominence in the face of problems posed by the infringement of individual rights in medical practice and research. As a result, the primary emphasis in bioethics has been the individual rather than the community. Public health thus faces many population-related ethical dilemmas that are not addressed in the existing health care codes of ethics. Public health nurses and other public health professionals often confront issues regarding the appropriate scope of public health programs and interventions and the point at which public health activities infringe on individual rights in ethically troublesome ways (Kass, 1998).

Kass (2001) proposes a framework for the ethical analysis of public health activities that is designed to advance traditional public health goals while maximizing individual liberties and furthering social justice. This six-

step model may be applied to proposed interventions, policy proposals, research initiatives, and programs.

1. *What are the public health goals of the proposed program?* Program goals should be expressed in terms of public health improvement (i.e., the reduction of morbidity or mortality). Even though more specific goals may be formulated, for example, that the participants of a health education program will learn a certain amount of information, the ultimate goal of decreased morbidity and mortality must be in view. The program may also be part of a group of interventions that share in reaching the ultimate public health goal.

2. *How effective is the program in achieving its stated goals?* The program must be based on the belief that it will achieve its stated goals. For example, health education programs may be effective in transmitting information, but the recipients show little or no behavioral change. It is important that the outcomes of public health programs are evaluated to insure that the desired changes have occurred and that these changes have had an effect on the morbidity and mortality of the target group. Again, the proposed program may be part of a group of programs that have the same ultimate goal.

3. *What are the known or potential burdens of the program?* Public health programs may involve a number of burdens or harms, but most cluster into three main categories: risks to privacy and confidentiality, particularly in data collection; risks to liberty and self-determination, especially in public health activities designed to contain the spread of disease; and risks to justice, often seen when public health interventions are targeted only to certain groups with the risk of stigmatization. There may be physical risks as well. For example, mandatory immunization programs may impose health risks to individuals or spraying to prevent mosquito-borne viruses may endanger individuals who are sensitive to the chemicals being sprayed.

4. *Can burdens be minimized? Are there alternative approaches?* Those who propose public health programs are obligated to seek to lessen burdens and harms once they are identified in step 3. Contact tracing in sexually transmitted infections programs is routine; however, this practice may pose a threat to confidentiality and privacy. Yet,

contact tracing is voluntary; there are no penalties for those who refuse to participate. Therefore, public health professionals have an ethical obligation to inform individuals of their right to refuse to disclose the names of their sexual partners or to contact their partners themselves. In addition, if more than one alternative exists to meet a public health goal, public health professionals are required ethically to choose the alternative that poses the fewest risks to moral concerns such as liberty, privacy, or justice, while not compromising the benefits of the program.

5. *Is the program implemented fairly?* This question determines whether or not the demands of distributive justice are satisfied in the fair distribution of the benefits and burdens of the proposed program. This aspect is of vital importance if the program includes restrictive measures. Social harms can result if stereotypes are created or perpetuated such as the notion that certain population groups are more vulnerable to sexually transmitted infections or domestic violence. This problem may be intensified if other population groups use such stereotyping to come to the erroneous belief that they are at little or no risk because they do not fit the risk profile. Another issue is whether public health professionals have an ethical obligation to right existing social injustices, such as poverty or hunger, that have an adverse effect on the public's health.

6. *How can the benefits and burdens of a program be fairly balanced?* After the first five steps of the framework have been addressed, a decision must be made as to whether the expected benefits of the proposed program will justify the identified burdens. Inevitably, there will be disagreements over the potential burdens and benefits inherent in the details of a particular program. For instance, taxpayers may focus on the financial burdens of a clean water program that may benefit future generations, while public health professionals see only its benefits. Procedural justice requires that a fair process of decision making is used to resolve such disagreements. This process must seek a balance between communal interests and the liberty rights of individuals, realizing that some infringements on individual liberty are unavoidable. Democratic processes and open hearings can help to ensure that minority positions are presented and considered. In general, "The greater the burden imposed by a program, the greater must be the expected public health benefit, and the more uneven the benefits and burdens . . . the greater must be the expected benefit" (Kass, 2001, p. 1781).

The use of an ethical framework for the analysis of public health activities demonstrates to the community the integrity of proposed programs. This will increase the community's trust that the work being done is ethically appropriate and that it will further public health improvement and social justice (Kass, 2001). Public health nurses can use the Kass model to evaluate public health programs that they develop or implement.

SELECTED ISSUES IN PUBLIC HEALTH NURSING ETHICS

Key considerations in public health nursing ethics from a human rights perspective can be illustrated by the exploration of many examples in national and international health. Two exemplary issues are discussed here: global HIV/AIDS and genetics and genomics.

Global HIV/AIDS

The HIV/AIDS crisis has been described as the most globalized epidemic in history. Since its inception in 1981, HIV/AIDS has spread to every part of the world, so we can now term it a pandemic. The Joint United Nations Programme on HIV/AIDS (UNAIDS, 2005) estimates that at the end of 2004, 40 million children and adults were living with HIV. Sub-Saharan Africa accounted for two-thirds of these cases, while 1,000,000 cases were in the United States. The rate of infection in Sub-Saharan Africa continues to rise, and new epidemics are developing rapidly in other regions such as Eastern Europe and East Asia (China, India, and Indonesia).

The "feminization" of HIV/AIDS is seen in the increasing number of women who become infected with HIV every year. "Globally, nearly half of all persons infected between the ages of 15 to 49 are women. In Africa, the proportion is reaching 60%" (UNAIDS, 2004, preface). Gender inequality has increased the vulnerability, not only of women, but of entire populations to the spread of HIV infection. Women with HIV or AIDS are more likely to experience dis-

⊕ PRACTICE APPLICATION

Genetic Screening Program

Early in the 1970s many states, with support from the federal government, implemented a major genetic screening program in the African American community to identify children and young adults who had the mutation associated with sickle cell disease. Unfortunately, many of the state programs were flawed by inadequate knowledge of the disease, insufficient sensitivity to ethnocultural issues, and misuse of personal test results data. What followed was that many people who were actually carriers of the mutation were labeled as having sickle cell disease. These people were ostracized by their communities, with the accompanying psychological harm; deprived of employment and educational opportunities, such as participation in school sports activities; and denied health and life insurance (Murray, 2002).

It is said that hindsight is better than foresight. So, imagine serving as a public health nurse in 1972 on a multidisciplinary health care team that is planning a sickle cell screening program for an African American. Given what you know about public health ethics, human rights, and the pitfalls of the past, respond to the following:

1. What are the major ethical and human rights issues inherent in the situation?

2. What plan should the team use to safeguard the ethical and human rights interests of the community during the screening program?

3. How will your team address the ethnocultural implications of the screening program for the African American community?

4. What education about the screening program is necessary and to what groups or individuals should it be provided?

5. Analyze your team's plan using the Kass framework for public health ethical decision making.

crimination and stigmatization (Rodriguez-Garcia & Akhter, 2000; UNAIDS, 2004).

Women are at greater risk of HIV infection than men. Biologically, male-to-female transmission of HIV is twice as likely to occur as female-to-male transmission. The risk to women is compounded by the gender inequality that exists in many societies where men are more powerful in sexual relationships. As a result, for many women, their male partners' sexual behavior is the most important HIV risk factor (UNAIDS, 2004). For example, a married woman in some countries is not able to insist on the use of a condom during sexual intercourse with a husband who may have multiple sex partners or even be infected with HIV.

Women bear a greater burden when families are affected by HIV/AIDS because women are much more likely to be caregivers to family members who develop AIDS or to AIDS orphans. Due to their low social status and lack of economic opportunities in many societies, women often suffer disproportionately when communities are impoverished by HIV/AIDS (UNAIDS, 2004).

The HIV/AIDS pandemic provides an opportunity to examine the intersection of public health, bioethics, and human rights. Bioethical and human rights issues are central to public health strategies for the prevention and control of HIV/AIDS. The violation of human rights, particularly the rights of women and children, plays a direct role in the spread of the virus. In addition, bioethical concerns, for example, international antiretroviral drug testing, are raised in relationship to how the pandemic is being managed in disadvantaged countries.

Awareness of the relationship between public health and human rights in the HIV/AIDS pandemic has deepened over time. Jonathan Mann, a leader in health and human rights, has identified two phases in the strategic linkage between HIV/AIDS and human rights. The first phase involved discrimination, stigmatization, and in some cases, violence to which persons with HIV or AIDS are subjected. They continue to experience exclusion from school, work, travel, marriage, housing, transportation, and access to health care (Mann, 2001; Schleifer, 2004). As a result, many people with HIV or AIDS avoid the health care system, thus decreasing the effectiveness of public health programs designed to prevent and control the spread of the infection. So, for the first time in history, a commitment to preventing discrimination against those infected with and affected by HIV has become a part of the global health strategy for an infectious disease.

The second phase, which extends from the late 1980s to the present, has seen the identification of the connection between the level of respect for the human rights and dignity of individuals and groups and their vulnerability to HIV infection. Mann stated that "the failure to realize human rights and respect human dignity has now been recognized as a major cause—actually as the root cause—of vulnerability to the HIV/AIDS epidemic" (Mann, 1994, p. 11). The realization of this connection has led to the *concept of vulnerability:* persons who are able to make and carry out free and informed decisions are least vulnerable to HIV infection; persons who are ill-informed and who have limited ability to make and carry out freely arrived-at decisions are most vulnerable (Mann, 2001).

Public health nursing practice for those affected by and infected with HIV, both in the United States and abroad, must ensure consideration to their ethical and human rights interests. They must be protected from discrimination and be provided with privacy and confidentiality; equal access to health care and insurance; and basic human resources, such as job security, housing, and educational opportunities.

Genetics and Genomics

Genetics is the study of the functions and effects of single genes and is often associated with diseases such as Down syndrome or Huntington's disease. Genomics is the study, not only of single genes, but also of the entire human genome and the interactions of multiple genes with each other and with the environment (Hernandez, 2005). Genomics has become very important since the mapping of the human genome has pointed to a relationship among genetic factors, environmental exposures, and a variety of chronic diseases. The public health nursing responsibilities for prevention and health promotion created by this relationship are self-evident.

The project to map the human genome is funded by the U.S. Department of Energy (DOE) and the National Institutes of Health (NIH). Since the inception of the project in 1990, these two agencies have devoted a small portion of the budget toward the study of the ethical, legal, and social issues (ELSI) surrounding the availability of genetic information. This effort is

now the world's largest bioethics program, serving as a model for other ELSI programs worldwide. Ethical issues addressed by the ELSI program include fairness in the use of genetic information, privacy and confidentiality, stigmatization, and genetically modified foods, among others (U.S. DOE, 2005). The public health nurse will increasingly be called upon to include genetic and genomic considerations in the care that is provided to clients. It is important that the ethical issues raised by new knowledge and technologies associated with genetics and genomics are addressed in public health nursing interventions.

Public health genetic screening programs have been used for many years to identify persons at risk for genetic diseases. A review of the history of genetic screening highlights the intersection of public health, ethics, and human rights, particularly in the case of ethnic minorities. The public health nurse will sometimes encounter African American clients who are suspicious of screening programs and the health care delivery system in general because of problems their communities encountered with the sickle cell screening program.

In the 1970s, a major effort was implemented to screen African American children and young adults for the mutation that is associated with sickle cell disease. Due to inadequate information, a lack of sensitivity to the ethnocultural issues, and misuse of personal test results, the ethical and human rights interests of many who were tested were compromised. Persons who were carriers of the disease were inaccurately labeled as having sickle cell disease. They were subsequently ostracized; deprived of employment and educational opportunities, such as being allowed to participate in school sports activities; and denied health and life insurance (Murray, 2002). Sensitive to the public health problems that advances in genetics and genomics might pose for some segments of the public, the DOE has sponsored conferences and professional education materials to explore the ethical impact of genetic and genomic information on minority communities (U.S. DOE, 2005).

The term genetic screening refers to "public health programs that survey or test target populations with the aim of detecting individuals at risk of disease for genetic reasons" (Munson, 2003, p. 155). Beginning in the early 1960s with a Massachusetts law that mandated PKU screening for all newborns, the number of public health programs that screen particular populations has increased over the years. Now there are screening programs for over 40 conditions, such as metabolic disorders, hypothyroidism, and chromosome anomalies (Munson, 2003).

Some public health practitioners see a similarity between genetic screening and historical public health measures for the detection and prevention of communicable diseases such as tuberculosis and syphilis. Screening programs allowed the identification and treatment of persons with these diseases and the prevention of spread to others. Genetically based diseases can be compared to communicable diseases in the possibility of spread from an affected person to others. However, rather than spreading horizontally through the population, as in the case of communicable disease, genetic disease is spread vertically through generations. Persons that carry the genes that cause disease can be warned about their risks of having genetically impaired children. The use of genetic screening could give the public health system an opportunity to reach and treat the approximately 3000 babies born each year with diseases where early intervention could be life-saving.

Laws mandating screening programs can be justified by the power of the government to secure the welfare of its citizens. Again, public health measures that are used to control communicable diseases can provide a model to control genetics diseases For example, in the same way that we do not allow parents to decide whether their child is vaccinated against smallpox, we can say that the government also has a duty to identify newborns with PKU so that they can receive the appropriate treatment.

There is an argument, however, against the application of the contagious-disease model to genetic screening programs. Because of the way in which genetic diseases are spread, only a very small segment of the population is at risk, especially when compared to a smallpox epidemic, which could threaten millions of lives. In addition, the lack of follow-up or counseling services for some genetic screening programs leads to questions about the benefits for participants. Being told they are the carriers of a genetic disease may do some people more harm than good.

Thus, public health genetic screening programs raise several ethical questions. Do the benefits of such programs outweigh their liabilities? Are screening programs so valuable that they justify the denial of individual choice that is involved in required participation? What about the rights of parents who do not want to know whether their child has the genes responsible for a particular disease? Is the state justified, in the interest of protecting the child, to require parents to know this information whether they want to or not? (Munson, 2003).

CRITICAL THINKING ACTIVITIES

1. Describe the points at which public health, ethics and bioethics, and human rights agree and the points at which these perspectives disagree.

2. The public health nurse has a choice between offering two public health programs in the community. One program would provide services to a greater number of people who have limited needs; the other program would offer services to a smaller number of people who have great need. Apply two ethical theories to this situation to determine which program the nurse will implement. Did the two theories lead to different decisions?

3. The public health nurse encounters several families that object to having their children immunized. Although the law provides for families in such cases to refuse immunizations without jeopardizing the children's school enrollment, the nurse begins to consider the ethical implications of the requirement for immunization and other public health laws that seem paternalistic. Is there an ethical justification for laws that restrict personal freedom in the name of protecting public health?

4. Angie is a pregnant 17-year-old woman who uses cocaine. The public health nurse cannot convince her to stop even to protect the health of her unborn child. What is the nurse's ethical responsibility in this case? What are the relevant ethical and human rights issues that should be considered?

5. What are the most pressing social ills that have an impact on public health outcomes? If the public health nurse felt an ethical obligation to advocate for the resolution of some of these problems, how would he or she go about it?

KEY TERMS

autonomy	genetics	noncomparative justice
beneficence	genetic screening	nonmaleficence
bioethics	genomics	paternalism
care ethics	hedonism	principle of autonomy
comparative justice or distributive justice	human rights	principle of formal justice
	justice	principle of utility
consequentialism	legal rights	utilitarianism
ethics	morality	values
feminist ethics	moral rights	virtue ethics

KEY CONCEPTS

- There is an integral relationship among the sources of public health nursing ethics: public health, public health nursing, ethics and bioethics, and human rights.

- Ethics, part of a larger branch of philosophy called axiology, addresses the rightness or wrongness of moral action.

- Modern bioethics is a subfield of ethics that addresses ethical concerns that arise as a result of advances in health care.

- Ethical theories, both principle-based and without principles, provide the basis for ethical decision making.

- Human rights refer to the basic rights and freedoms that all humans possess as a result of being human, including life, liberty, freedom of thought and expression, equality before the law, and material well-being.

- The diversity of cultural and ethnic groups implies the need to consider ethical perspectives that differ from the Western perspective of most public health nurses in the United States.

- Nursing and public health have developed a number of codes and sets of principles that outline ethical responsibilities.

- Contemporary health problems, such as global HIV/AIDS, national security threats, such as bioterrorism, and health care advances, such as genetics and genomics, give rise to a number of ethical and human rights issues that the public health nurse must consider when planning health care interventions.

- A broad perspective on public health nursing ethics implies that public health nurses have an ethical obligation to advocate the resolution of social ills that contribute to poor health outcomes such as poverty and the inequitable distribution of health care resource

REFERENCES

Allmark, P. (2002). Can there be an ethics of care? In K. W. M. Fulford, D. L. Dickenson, & T. H. Murray (Eds.), *Healthcare ethics and values: An introductory text with readings and case studies* (63-69). Malden, MA: Blackwell.

American Nurses Association. (2001). *Code for nurses with interpretive statements.* Silver Spring, MD: American Nurses Publishing

American Public Health Association (APHA). (2000). *Principles on public health and human rights.* Washington, DC: Author.

Asaph Judaeus. (2000). The Oath of Asaph. In R. M. Veatch (Ed.), *Cross-cultural perspectives in medical ethics: Readings* (2nd ed., pp. 57–59). Boston: Jones and Bartlett.

Beauchamp, T. L., & Childress, J. F. (Eds.). (2001). *Principles of biomedical ethics* (5th ed.). New York: Oxford.

Beauchamp, T. L., & Walters, L. (Eds.). (2003). *Contemporary issues in bioethics* (6th ed.). Belmont, CA: Wadsworth Thomson Learning.

Bleich, J. D. (2000). An obligation to heal in the Judaic tradition. In R. M. Veatch (Ed.), *Cross-cultural perspectives in medical ethics: Readings* (2nd ed., pp. 62–77). Boston: Jones and Bartlett.

Butts, J., & Rich, K. (2005). *Nursing ethics: Across the curriculum and into practice.* Boston: Jones and Bartlett.

Campbell, A., Gillett, G., & Jones, G. (2001). *Medical ethics* (3rd. ed.). New York: Oxford.

Congregation for the Doctrine of the Faith. (1980). *Congregation for the doctrine of the faith, the declaration* Iura et Bona, Part IV. Rome: The Vatican.

Donnelly, J. (1998). *International human rights* (2nd ed.). Boulder, CO: Westview Press.

Dula, A. (2001). Bioethics: The need for dialogue for African Americans. In W. Teays & L. Purdy (Eds.), *Bioethics, justice, and health care* (pp. 80–89). Belmont, CA: Wadsworth Thomson Learning.

Easley, C. E., & Allen, C. E. (2005). Public health and human rights. *Highlights of the American Public Health Association 132nd Annual Meeting.* Continuing Education Credit Activity. *Medscape.com.*

Easley, C. E., Marks, S. P., & Morgan, R. E. (2001). The challenge and place of international human rights in public health. *AJPH, 91,* 1922–1925.

ETR Associates. (2004). *Eliminating health disparities: Conversations with Asian Americans.* Santa Cruz, CA: ETR Associates.

Fulford, K. W. M., Dickenson D. L. & Murray, T. H. (Eds.). (2002). *Healthcare ethics and values: An introductory text with readings and case studies.* Malden, MA: Blackwell.

Gilligan, C. (1982). *In a different voice: Psychological theory and women's development.* Cambridge, MA: Harvard University Press.

Goode, E. (2001). For good health, it helps to be rich and important. In W. Teays & L. Purdy (Eds.), *Bioethics, justice, and health care* (pp. 39–42). Belmont, CA: Wadsworth Thomson Learning.

Gostin, L. O. (2002). *Public health law and ethics: A reader.* Berkeley: University of California Press.

Gostin, L. O. & Lazzarini, A. (1997). *Human rights and public health in the AIDS pandemic.* New York: Oxford University Press.

Gruskin, S. (2004). Is there a government in the cockpit: A passenger's perspective or global public health: The role of human rights. *Temple Law Review, 77,* 313–333.

Harris, John. (Ed.). (2001). *Bioethics.* New York: Oxford.

Hernandez, L. (Ed.). (2005). *Implications of genomics for public health: Workshop summary. Committee on genomics and the public's health in the 21st century.* U.S. Board on Health Promotion and Disease Prevention. Retrieved April 17, 2005, from http://www.nap.edu/books/0309096073.

Hoskins, S. A. (2005). Nurses and national socialism—A moral dilemma: One historical example of a route to euthanasia. *Nursing Ethics, 12,* 79–91.

Hudson, K. (2006). "End of Life Issues: Pain Management and Enhancing Quality of Life—3 Nursing CEs." Retrieved September 5, 2007 from Dynamic Nursing.com, http://dynamicnursingeducation.com/class.php?class_id=85&pid=20.

International Council of Nurses. (1973). *The ICN Code of Ethics for Nurses.* Retrieved, 2007

Institute of Medicine (IOM). (1988). *The future of public health.* Washington, DC: National Academy Press.

Kasenene, P. (1989). African ethical theory and the four principles. In R. M. Veatch (Ed.), *Cross-cultural perspectives in medical ethics: Readings* (2nd ed., pp. 347–357). Boston: Jones and Bartlett.

Kass, N. E. (2001). An ethics framework for public health. *AJPH, 91,* 1776–1782.

Kass, N. E., & Gielen, A. (1998). The ethics of contact tracing and their implication for women. *Duke Journal of Gender Law & Policy, 5,* 89–102.

Kuhse, H., & Singer, P. (Eds.). (1998). *A companion to bioethics.* Malden, MA: Blackwell.

Leary, V. (1994). The right to health in international human rights law. *Health and human rights: An international journal.* Retrieved May, 16, 2005, from http://www.hsph.harvard.edu/fxbcenter/V1N1leary.htm.

McIntyre, A. (Summer 2005). Doctrine of double effect. In E. N. Zalta (Ed.), *The Stanford encyclopedia of philosophy.* Retrieved May 15, 2006, at http://plato.stanford.edu/archives/sum2005/entries/double-effect.

Mann, J. (1994). *The World Health Organization and global health: Towards a new world order? The Calderone Lecture.* New York: Columbia University School of Public Health.

Mann, J. (2001). Human rights. In R. Smith (Ed.), *The encyclopedia of AIDS: A social, political, cultural, and scientific record of the HIV epidemic.* New York: Penguin Group.

Manning, R. A. (1998). A care approach. In H. Kuhse & P. Singer (Eds.), *A companion to bioethics.* Malden, MA: Blackwell.

Mappes, T. A., & DeGrazia, D. (Eds.). (2001). *Biomedical ethics* (5th ed.). New York: McGraw-Hill.

Marks, S. P. (2001). Jonathan Mann's legacy to the 21st century: The human rights imperative for public health. *Journal of Law, Medicine & Ethics, 29,* 131–138.

Mbiti, J. (1969). *African religions and philosophy.* Oxford: Heinemann.

Munson, R. (2003). *Outcome uncertain: Cases and contexts in bioethics.* Belmont, CA: Wadsworth Thomson Learning.

Munson, R. (2004). *Intervention and reflection: Basic issues in medical ethics* (7th ed.). Belmont, CA: Wadsworth Thomson Learning.

Murray, R. D. (2002). Historical perspective: The sickle cell testing debacle. *Journal for Minority Medical Students,* special supplement, Human Genome Project Black Bag, Spring, BB 15–BB 32. Retrieved May 19, 2005, from http://www.ornl.gov/sci.techresources/Human_Genome/publicat/jmmbbag.pdf.

National Conference of Catholic Bishops. (2000). Ethical and religious directives for Catholic health care services. In R. M. Veatch (Ed.), *Cross-cultural perspectives in medical ethics: Readings* (2nd ed., pp. 77–98). Boston: Jones and Bartlett.

Oakley, J. (1998). A virtue ethics approach. In H. Kuhse & P. Singer (Eds.), *A companion to bioethics* (pp. 86–97). Malden, MA: Blackwell.

Oberle, K., & Tenove, S. (2000). Ethical issues in public health nursing. *Nursing Ethics,* 7, 425–438.

Pogge, T. (2005). Symposium: World poverty and human rights. *Ethics & International Affairs,* 19, 1–7.

Public Health Leadership Society. (2002). *Principles of the ethical practice of public health, version 2.2.* Washington, DC: Public Health Leadership Society.

Quad Council of Public Health Nursing Organizations. (1999). *Scope and Standards of Public Health Nursing Practice.* Washington, DC: American Nurses Publishing.

Qui, R. (1996). Bioethics in an Asian context. *World Health,* 49, 13–15.

Rahman, A., Amine, C., & Elkadi, A. (2000). Islamic code of medical professional ethics. In R. M. Veatch (Ed.), *Cross-cultural perspectives in medical ethics: Readings* (2nd ed., pp. 233–239). Boston: Jones and Bartlett.

Ramsey, P. The patient as person. (2000). In R. M. Veatch (Ed.), *Cross-cultural perspectives in medical ethics: Readings* (2nd ed., pp. 99–104). Boston: Jones and Bartlett.

Rodriquez-Garcia, R., & Akhter, M. N. (2000). Human rights: The foundation of public health practice. *AJPH,* 90, 693–694.

Rothstein, M. A. (2004). Are traditional public health strategies consistent with contemporary American values? Symposium: SARS, Public Health, and Global Governance. *Temple Law Review,* 175–192. Retrieved February 25, 2005, from http://www.temple.edu/illpp/PubsSAR.htm.

Schleifer, R. (2004). *Hated to death: Homophobia, violence and Jamaica's HIV/AIDS epidemic.* New York: Human Rights Watch.

Sherwin, S., & Parish, B. (Eds.). (2002). *Women, medicine, ethics and the law.* Hampshire, Great Britain: Ashgate Publishing.

Shields, L. (2005). Report on: Complicity and compassion: The first international conference on nursing and midwifery in the Third Reich, June 10–11, 2004, Limerick, Republic of Ireland. *Nursing Ethics,* 12, 106, 107.

Smedley, B. D., Stith, A. Y., & Nelson, A. R. (2003). *Unequal treatment: Confronting racial and ethnic disparities in health care.* Washington, DC: National Academies Press.

Soccio, D. (2001). *Archetypes of wisdom: An introduction to philosophy* (4th ed.). Belmont, CA: Wadsworth Thomson Learning.

Tangwa, G. B. (2000). The traditional African perception of a person: Some implications for bioethics. *Hastings Center Report,* 30: 39–43.

Temples, T. (1959). *Bantu philosophy.* Paris: Presence Africaine.

Toebes, B. (1999). Towards an improved understanding of the international human right to health. *Human Rights Quarterly,* 21, 661–679.

United Nations (UN). (1946). *Charter of the United Nations.* Retrieved on February 4, 2005, from http://www.unhchr.ch/udhr.lang/eng.htm.

United Nations (UN). (1948). *Universal Declaration of Human Rights. United Nations.* Retrieved on February 4, 2005, from http://www.un.org/Overview/rights.html.

United Nations (UN). (1966a). *International Covenant on Civil and Political Rights.* Retrieved on February 4, 2005 from http://www.ohchr.org/english/law/ccpr.htm.

United Nations (UN). (1966b). *International Covenant on Economic, Social and Cultural Rights.* Retrieved on February 4, 2005, from http://unhchr.ch/html/menu3/b/a_cescr.htm.

UNAIDS. (2004). *2004 Report on the global AIDS epidemic: 4th global report.* Geneva: Joint United Nations Programme on HIV/AIDS (UNAIDS).

UNAIDS. (2005). *2005 Report on the global AIDS epidemic: 5th global report.* Geneva: Joint United Nations Programme on HIV/AIDS (UNAIDS).

U.S. Department of Energy, Office of Science (U.S. DOE). (2005). *Human genome project information: Ethical, legal, and social issues.* Retrieved on May 19, 2005, from http://www.ornl.gov/sci/techresources/Human_Genome/elsi/elsi.shtml.

Wilkens, S. (1995). *Beyond bumper sticker ethics: An introduction to theories of right and wrong.* Downers Grove, Il: InterVarsity Press.

World Health Organization (WHO). (1946). *Constitution of the World Health Organization.* World Health Organization. Retrieved on May 16, 2005 from http://www.whosea.org/aboutsearo/pdf.

World Health Organization (WHO). (1978). *Declaration of Alma-Ata.* World Health Organization. Retrieved on May 16, 2005, from http://www.euro.who.int/AboutWHO/policy/20010827_1?PrinterFriendly=1&.

World Health Organization (WHO). (1986). *Ottawa Charter for Health Promotion. World Health Organization.* Retrieved on May 16, 2005 from http://www.euro.who .int/AboutWHO/Policy/20010827_2?PrinterFriendly=1&.

BIBLIOGRAPHY

American Nurses Association. (1999). *Scope and standards of public health nursing practice.* Washington, DC: Author.

American Nurses Association. (2004). *Nursing: Scope and standards of practice.* Washington, DC: Author.

Beauchamp, D. E., & Steinbok, B. (Eds.). (1999). *New ethics for the public's health.* New York: Oxford University Press.

Blustein, J., & Fleischman, A. R. (2004). Urban bioethics: Adapting bioethics to the urban context. *Academic Medicine* 79, 1198–1202.

Fry, S. T., & Veatch, R. M. (2006). *Case studies in nursing ethics* (3rd ed.). Boston: Jones and Bartlett.

Fulford, K. W. M., Dickenson, D. L., & Murray, T. H. (Eds.). (2002). *Healthcare ethics and values: An introductory text with readings and case studies.* Malden, MA: Blackwell.

Geiger, H. J. (2003). Protecting civil liberties. In B. S. Levy & V. W. Sidel (Eds.), *Terrorism and public health: A balanced approach to strengthening systems and protecting people* (pp. 322–334). New York: Oxford University Press.

Johnstone, M. (2006). *Bioethics: A nursing perspective* (4th ed.). Sidney, Australia: Churchill Livingstone.

Mann, J. M., Gruskin, S., Grodin, M. A., & Annas G. J. (Eds.). (1999). *Health and human rights: A reader.* New York: Routledge.

Rawls, J. (1999). *A theory of justice* (rev. ed.). Cambridge, MA: Harvard University Press.

Sen, A. (2005). *Ethics, development and disaster.* Digital Library of the Inter-American Initiative on Social Capital, Ethics and Development of the Inter-American Development Bank (IDB). Retrieved on February 20, 2005, from www.ladb.org/ethics.

Simoens, S., Villeneuve, M., & Hurst, J. (2005). *Tackling nurse shortages in OECD countries.* OECE Working Papers. Paris: Organization for Economic Co-operation and Development.

Stillwell, B., Khassoum, D., Zurn, P., Dai Poz, M. R., Adams, O., & Buchan, J. (2003). *Developing evidence-based ethical policies on the migration of health workers: Conceptual and practical challenges.* Human Resources for Health. Retrieved on May 16, 2005, from http://www.human-resources-health.com/content/1/1/8.

Teays, W., & Purdy, L. (Eds.). (2001). *Bioethics, justice, and health care.* Belmont, CA: Wadsworth Thomson Learning.

Veatch, R. M. (Ed.). (2000). *Cross-cultural perspectives in medical ethics* (2nd ed.). Boston: Jones and Bartlett.

Wood-Harper, J. (2005). Informing education policy on MMR: Balancing individual freedoms and collective responsibilities for the promotion of public health. *Nursing Ethics, 12,* 43–58.

RESOURCES

Amnesty International (AI)

5 Penn Plaza, 14th floor
New York, New York 10001
212-807-8400
FAX: 212-463-9193, 212-627-1451
Email: admin-us@aiusa.org
Web: http://www.amnesty.org

AI is a worldwide movement of people who campaign for internationally recognized human rights. AI's vision is of a world in which every person enjoys all of the human rights enshrined in the Universal Declaration of Human Rights and other international human rights standards. In pursuit of this vision, AI's mission is to undertake research and action focused on preventing and ending grave abuses of the rights to physical and mental integrity, freedom of conscience and expression, and freedom from discrimination, within the context of its work to promote all human rights. AI is independent of any government, political ideology, economic interest or religion. It does not support or oppose any government or political system, nor does it support or oppose the views of the victims whose rights it seeks to protect. It is concerned solely with the impartial protection of human rights.

Association of Schools of Public Health (ASPH) Curriculum Resources

1101 15th Street NW, Suite 910
Washington, D.C. 20005
202-296-1099
FAX: 202-296-1252
Email: info@asph.org
Web: http://www.asph.org

The much anticipated *Ethics and Public Health: Model Curriculum* is now available for use by Schools of Public Health and other Health related faculty. The project was a collaborative effort between ASPH, the Health Resources and Services Administration (HRSA), and The Hastings Center. The concept for the model curriculum grew from a rising interest in the ethical, legal, and social aspects of public health policy and practice. With this interest came a demand for the teaching of ethics in health-related schools and for the resource materials to support it. The curriculum is intended as a resource to enhance and encourage thoughtful, well-informed, and critical discussions of ethical issues in the field of public health.

BioMed Central Ltd.

Science Navigation Group
Middlesex House
34-42 Cleveland Street
London W1T 4LB
United Kingdom
+44-0-20-7631-9131
FAX: +44-0-20-7631-9926
Email: info@biomedcentral.com
Web: http://www.biomedcentral.com

BioMed Central is an independent publishing house committed to providing immediate open access to peer-reviewed biomedical research. All original research articles published by BioMed Central are made freely and permanently accessible online immediately upon publication. BioMed Central views open access to research as essential in order to ensure the rapid and efficient communication of research findings. The Web site provides access to these research articles.

Francois-Xavier Bagnoud Center for Health and Human Rights

Harvard School of Public Health
651 Huntington Avenue, 7th floor
Boston, Massachusetts 02115
617-432-0656
FAX: 1-617-432 4310
Email: fxbcenter@igc.org
Web: http://www.hsph.harvard.edu

The center was founded at the Harvard School of Public Health in 1993 through a gift from the Association François-Xavier Bagnoud. The François-Xavier Bagnoud Center for Health and Human Rights is the first academic center to focus exclusively on health and human rights. The center combines the academic strengths of research and teaching with a strong commitment to service and policy development. Center faculty work at international and national levels through collaboration and partnerships with health and human rights practitioners, governmental and nongovernmental organizations, academic institutions, and international agencies to do the following:

- Expand knowledge through scholarship, professional training, and public education
- Develop domestic and international policy focusing on the relationship between health and human rights in a global perspective
- Engage scholars, public health and human rights practitioners, public officials, donors, and activists in the health and human rights movement.

Hastings Center

Web: http://www.ascensionhealth.org

Founded in 1969, The Hastings Center is an independent organization comprised of health care providers and scientists, lawyers, philosophers, corporate executives, and government officials dedicated to advanced research and studies in biomedical ethics. The center publishes *The Hastings Center Report*, a quarterly journal focused on issues in health care ethics. The Web site provides access to the publications.

Human Rights Education Association (HREA)

P.O. Box 382396
Cambridge, Massachusetts 02238
Visiting address:
97 Lowell Road
Concord, Massachusetts 01742
978-341-0200
FAX: 978-341-0201
E-mail: info@hrea.org
Web: http://www.hrea.org

HREA is an international nongovernmental organization that supports human rights learning, the training of activists and professionals. the development of educational materials and programming. and community-building through online technologies. HREA is dedicated to quality education and training to promote understanding, attitudes, and actions to protect human rights and to foster the development of peaceable, free, and just communities. HREA works with individuals, nongovernmental organizations, intergovernmental organizations, and governments interested in implementing human rights education programs. The services provided by HREA are

- Assistance in curriculum and materials development
- Training of professional groups
- Research and evaluation
- Clearinghouse of education and training materials
- Networking human rights advocates and educators

Human Rights Watch

1630 Connecticut Avenue NW, Suite 500
Washington, D.C. 20009
202-612-4321
FAX: 202-612-4333
Email: hrwdc@hrw.org
Web: http://www.hrw.org

Human Rights Watch is a major international human rights organization dedicated to protecting the human rights of people around the world. Its mission is to prevent discrimination, to uphold political freedom, to protect people from inhumane conduct in wartime, and to bring offenders to justice by challenging governments and those who hold power to end abusive practices and respect international human rights law. Human Rights Watch is an independent, nongovernmental organization, supported by contributions from private individuals and foundations worldwide. It accepts no government funds, directly or indirectly.

International Society for Health and Human Rights (ISHHR)

P.O. Box 203
Fairfield NSW 2163
Australia
+61-2-9794-1900
FAX: +61-2-9794-1910
Email: istartts@s054.aone.net.au
Web: http://www.ishhr.org

The aim of this Web site is to bring colleagues a bit closer to each other and represent a forum where information on human rights and useful experiences can be presented and shared. ISHHR has members in almost 50 countries worldwide. The human rights issue is a very important one for health workers, and as health professionals. Sharing with each other on this Web site provides an opportunity for communication between professionals as an active defense of human rights.

Nursing Ethics

Web: http://www.ingentaconnect.com

This is the Web site for accessing online the journal *Nursing Ethics*. Fifty-seven issues of this journal are available online, some free of charge.

Nursing Ethics at Boston College

Web: http://www.bc.edu

This Web site is located at the William F. Connell School of Nursing, Boston University. It provides access to human rights-related book abstracts, lectures, ethics tools, databases, dissertations, library collections, and other human rights links.

Nursing Ethics Network (NEN)

Web: http://jmrileyrn.tripod.com

NEN is a nonprofit organization of professional nurses committed to the advancement of nursing ethics in clinical practice through research, education, and consultation. Members of NEN offer a uniquely focused service to the nursing community that is designed to complement, but not to duplicate, the work of other professional nursing organizations. The Web site provides access to nurses involved in nursing ethics.

People's Movement for Human Rights Education (PDHRE)

The People's Movement for Human Rights Education
Shulamith Koenig, Executive Director
526 West 111th Street
New York, New York 10025
212-749-3156
FAX: 212-666-6325
Email: pdhre@igc.apc.org
Web: http://www.pdhre.org

PMHRE was founded in 1988, as a nonprofit, international service organization that works directly and indirectly with its network of affiliates—primarily women's and social justice organizations—to develop and advance pedagogies for human rights education relevant to people's daily lives in the context of their struggles for social and economic justice and democracy. Its members include experienced educators, human rights experts, United Nations officials, and world renowned advocates and activists who collaborate to conceive, initiate, facilitate, and service projects on education in human rights for social and economic transformation. The organization is dedicated to publishing and disseminating demand-driven human rights training and manuals and teaching materials, and otherwise servicing grassroots and community groups engaged in a creative, contextualized process of human rights learning, reflection, and action.

Physicians for Human Rights (PHR)

2 Arrow Street, Suite 301
Cambridge, Massachusetts 02138
617-301-4200
FAX: 617-301-4250
Web: http://www.phrusa.org

PHR mobilizes health professionals to advance health, dignity, and justice and promotes the right to health for all. Harnessing the specialized skills, rigor, and passion of health care providers, public health specialists, and scientists, PHR investigates human rights abuses and works to stop them.

Public Health Ethics

Office of Continuing Education
North Carolina Institute for Public Health
Campus Box 8165
UNC School of Public Health
Chapel Hill, North Carolina 27599
919-966-4032
FAX 919-966-5692
Email: oce@unc.edu
Web: http://www.sph.unc.edu

The North Carolina Institute for Public Health in Public Health Ethics developed this short online course to explore such questions as: Is there a public health ethic? Is it different from medical ethics? And is it the same as public health laws? The series discusses:

- Why medical ethics doesn't meet the needs of public health
- The values and beliefs inherent to a public health perspective
- Twelve principles for the ethical practice of public health
- How public health's legal powers relate to public health ethics

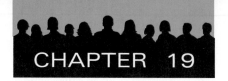

CHAPTER 19

Public Health Nursing Research

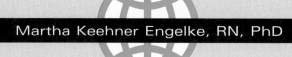

Martha Keehner Engelke, RN, PhD

Chapter Outline

- Research in Public Health Nursing: A Pioneer Who Made a Difference
- The Role of the Public Health Nurse in Research
- Research, Nursing Process, Epidemiology, and Quality Assurance
- Research Priorities in Public Health Nursing
- Types of Research Studies in Public Health Nursing
  Qualitative Research Design
  Quantitative Research Design
- Outcomes Research Related to Public Health Nursing Practice
- Evaluating Research for Evidence-Based Practice

Learning Objectives

Upon completion of this chapter, the reader will be able to:

1. Discuss the role of the public health nurse in using and conducting research

2. Compare and contrast different types of research methods that are used in public health nursing practice

3. Examine specific competencies of the public health nurse specialist and public health nurse generalist in relation to research

4. Describe specific tools that can assist the public health nurse in evaluating outcomes of public health nursing practice

5. Develop a plan that fosters evidence-based public health nursing practice

Throughout history public health nurses have participated in research. In many cases, the research was driven by a need to explain clinical problems that were evident among the clients cared for by the public health nurse. Today, public health nurses collaborate with other health professionals to complete studies that answer critical questions such as "Why do disparities in health outcomes exist for different ethnic groups?" and "Do the interventions of public health nurses make a difference in health outcomes?" The role of public health nurses related to research can range from data collector to principal investigator depending on the educational background and expertise of the nurse. However, all nurses need to have a fundamental understanding of how to evaluate current research and how to use research to provide evidence-based public health nursing. In addition, all nurses should be familiar with specific indicators that are used to evaluate whether public health nursing interventions make a difference for the clients they serve. This knowledge is necessary in an era where budgets are limited and programs are scrutinized on a regular basis to ensure that the best care is delivered in the most efficient and effective manner.

This chapter provides an overview of the role of the public health nurse in relation to research. Specific competencies of the public health nurse generalist and specialist are discussed. Research has elements in common with epidemiology and quality assurance—two other tools used by the public health nurse to document clinical problems and determine appropriate interventions to address these problems. Much progress has been made in developing tools that are sensitive to the interventions and outcomes of public health nursing. However, these tools must be used in well-designed studies if they are to document the outcomes of public health nursing practice.

Finally, the real challenge is ensuring that existing research actually is used in everyday practice. All nurses in public health must value the dissemination and utilization of research. Furthermore, public health nurses need to use research to inform public policy as well as clinical practice. The real pioneers in public health did that. By generating research questions or hypotheses, collecting data in a systematic manner, analyzing the data appropriately, and then disseminating the findings to policy makers and clinicians, our understanding of health and illness has improved significantly. In the best instances, our practice has also changed to reflect this expanded knowledge base. However, in other cases, research has not been integrated into the practice of clinicians, and actual practice is based on tradition or preference rather than concrete evidence.

Research is exciting. It allows the nurse to see fresh new ways of dealing with chronic or difficult problems. Research helps public health nurses to accomplish the fundamental goal of all nursing practice-to make a positive difference in the lives of our clients.

RESEARCH IN PUBLIC HEALTH NURSING: A PIONEER WHO MADE A DIFFERENCE

The history of public health is full of examples of how research has made a difference in practice. This history is elaborated in other sections of this text, particularly chapter 1. Lillian Wald, often referred to as the mother of public health nursing, is an exemplar of important points about research in public health nursing. These are:

- Research questions arise from observations and hunches about clinical problems seen in the nurse's caseload, and public health nurses often have the best understanding of the real world of vulnerable populations.
- To have an impact, nurse researchers must be able to understand the larger societal forces at play and communicate their findings to other clinicians and public policy makers in an effective manner.

Buhler-Wilkerson (1993) suggested that Lillian Wald engaged in three critical experiments that have implications for public health nursing today. These experiments included the invention of public health nursing as a generalist role that included both preventive and sick care, the establishment of a nationwide system of insurance payment for home-based care, and the creation of a national public health nursing service. By collecting data on numbers of visits, clients served, outcomes, and cost, Wald was able to demonstrate the positive impact of her nursing service to clients, insurance companies, and policy holders. Her scope of practice grew, and she established a coalition of agencies that allowed her to provide not only health care but also food, sanitary housing, and ultimately jobs. However, as Buhler-Wilkerson (1993) noted, the long-term impact of Wald's experiments began to wane by the 1920s. This occurred because of complex factors found in society, changes in patterns of disease, and the political reality of the time. In her analysis, Buhler-Wilkerson asked "how might those of us today be guided by Wald's earlier experiments?" She offered several principles from Wald's experiments that are relevant today for public health nursing practice. These are summarized in Box 19-1. As these principles indicate,

Wald's early findings provide guidance for organizing and delivering public health nursing today. Wald's work informs practice and suggests that interventions must consider the social context of the intervention, the economic implications of the intervention, and the ability of the public health nurse to provide comprehensive care to a culturally diverse population. This is the challenge for public health nursing research today and a pioneer in public health nursing who practiced over 100 years ago first discovered these principles.

THE ROLE OF THE PUBLIC HEALTH NURSE IN RESEARCH

The role of the public health nurse related to research will vary based on educational preparation, expertise, and job expectations. In 2000, in response to the Centers for Disease Control and Prevention (CDC) effort to delineate the competencies needed by the public health workforce, the Quad Council of Public Health Nursing Organizations developed a set of national public health nursing competencies. The Quad Council is comprised of the Association of Community Health Educators (ACHNE), the American Nurses Association Congress on Nursing Practice and Economics (ANA), the American Public Health Association—PHN Sections, and the Association of State and Territorial Directors of Nursing (ASTDN). The Quad Council sought to identify competencies for two levels of public health nurses: the staff nurse/generalist and the manager/specialist/consultant. These competencies are found in appendix A.

Although all of the domains are relevant and related to the effective use of research in practice, the area that is most closely aligned to research is the first domain: Analytic Assessment Skills. The specific competencies for this domain are found in Table 19-1. As this table illustrates, all public health nurses (with baccalaureate preparation) should be proficient in defining problems, identifying relevant and appropriate data, and applying ethical principles to the collection, maintenance, use, and dissemination of data for projects developed at the individual and family level. At the population/systems level, the generalist would have knowledge of these areas but would not necessarily be proficient. In contrast, the public health nurse specialist (usually master's prepared) should be proficient in all areas.

In summary, participation in research is a goal for all nurses. At the staff nurse level, the nurse will most likely be involved in identifying researchable prob-

---

BOX 19-1: Guiding Principles for Public Health Nursing Practice from the Early Experiments of Lillian Wald

- Invent a diverse mix of public and private programs that reflect local customs and link with mainstream health care institutions and complement community needs.
- Document cost-effectiveness, benefits valued by society, and client satisfaction as outcomes of care.
- Ensure that you have sufficient control of the structure and process of the practice setting to produce the desired outcomes.
- Examine practices with the reimbursement system that provides payment.
- Articulate the concept of comprehensive community-based nursing care as an innovative solution to the complex needs of vulnerable individuals and families.
- Ensure that practitioners have the training and ability to manage the complexities of community-based care.
- Couple preventive services with health and social needs, rather than offering them in isolation.
- Provide culturally relevant services according to local custom and linguistic preference.

SOURCE: From Buhler-Wilkerson, K. (1993). Bringing care to the people: Lillian Wald's legacy to public health nursing. *American Journal of Public Health, 83*(12): 1778–1786. Reprinted with permission from the American Public Health Association.

TABLE 19-1: Domain 1—Analytic/Assessment Skills of Public Health Nurses

	GENERALIST/STAFF PHN		MANAGER/CNS/CONSULTANT/ PROGRAM SPECIALIST/EXECUTIVE	
	Individuals and Families	Populations/ Systems	Individuals and Families	Populations/ Systems
1 Defines a problem	Proficiency	Knowledge	Proficiency	Proficiency
2 Determines appropriate uses and limitations of both quantitative and qualitative data	Knowledge	Awareness	Proficiency	Proficiency
3 Selects and defines variables relevant to defined public health problems	Knowledge	Knowledge	Proficiency	Proficiency
4 Identifies relevant and appropriate data and information sources	Proficiency	Knowledge	Proficiency	Proficiency
5 Evaluates the integrity and comparability of data and identifies gaps in data sources	Knowledge	Awareness	Proficiency	Proficiency
6 Applies ethical principals to the collection, maintenance, use, and dissemination of data and information	Proficiency	Knowledge	Proficiency	Proficiency
7 Partners with communities to attach meaning to collected quantitative and qualitative data	N/A (see *Note*)	Knowledge	N/A (see *Note*)	Proficiency

(continued)

lems and collaborating with advanced practitioners of research to design studies that can shed light on health problems. All nurses must apply ethical standards to the conduct of research. Assuring that subjects are fully informed about the nature of research as well as any potential benefits and side effects is the responsibility of all nurses. Handling data in a confidential manner that protects the rights of the individual is also a shared responsibility. As nurses gain skill and knowledge in research they will assume a larger role. As will be noted in other areas of this chapter, doctoral-prepared nurses working in conjunction with other disciplines as well as different levels of public health nurses have made important contributions to the science of public health nursing practice.

RESEARCH, NURSING PROCESS, EPIDEMIOLOGY, AND QUALITY ASSURANCE

The nursing process, epidemiology, and quality assurance all have one common denominator with research: They are processes that involve critical thinking and

TABLE 19-1: Domain 1—Analytic/Assessment Skills of Public Health Nurses (cont'd)

	GENERALIST/STAFF PHN		MANAGER/CNS/CONSULTANT/ PROGRAM SPECIALIST/EXECUTIVE	
	Individuals and Families	**Populations/ Systems**	**Individuals and Families**	**Populations/ Systems**
8 Makes relevant inferences from quantitative and qualitative data	Knowledge	Awareness	Proficiency	Proficiency
9 Obtains and interprets information regarding risks and benefits to the community	Knowledge	Knowledge	Proficiency	Proficiency
10 Applies data collection processes, information technology applications, and computer systems storage/retrieval strategies	Knowledge	Awareness	Proficiency	Proficiency
11 Recognizes how the data illuminates ethical, political, scientific, economic, and overall public health issues	Knowledge	Awareness	Proficiency	Proficiency

Note. These competencies, because of their population or system-focused language, do not apply at the individual/family level, but are applicable to the broader context of population-focused public health services and systems.

Adapted from Quad Council of Public Health Nursing Organizations (2004).

problem solving. When using the nursing process, the nurse is challenged to assess, plan, intervene, evaluate, and revise. In general, these steps are very similar to the process that the researcher goes through when defining a problem, choosing a research design, implementing a study and then evaluating the findings. Similarly, the epidemiologist collects data on populations and communities and then looks for patterns in this data. This is often referred to as descriptive epidemiology. When those patterns suggest further research questions, the epidemiologist will frequently design a study using a more rigorous research design. Likewise, quality assurance programs are based on the examination and analysis of data. Quality assurance programs often focus on the improvement of care in a particular agency. Data are collected in specific areas and are used to improve existing programs or to document the need for new programs. In many quality assurance programs, the nurse will "benchmark" the findings. A benchmark is a standard that can be used for comparison. Different agencies can be compared when using a benchmark, and an individual agency can gauge its performance by comparing itself to similar agencies.

So, how does the public health nurse know the difference between these different types of activities? The answer is that it may be difficult to tell. However, one of the hallmarks of research is that the investigator takes the time to delineate the design and the protocol for the research prior to the implementation of the study. In research, the integrity of the intervention must be maintained to ensure that the results are valid and not due to confounding factors. For example, the most rigorous form of research design is the randomized control trial. In this type of design, subjects are randomized to a treatment group and a control group. This type of design provides the best evidence for causality. However, many clinicians are reluctant to implement a study in which half of the subjects do not get an intervention that the clinician has a strong hunch is effective. Researchers in public health clinical sites struggle with the issue of maintaining research integrity within a setting that is primarily designed to provide clinical care. At times, compromises must be made in the design, and in other situations clinicians must approach clinical care in a more systematic manner than is usually found in the agency. This is an ongoing negotiation process during the course of a research study.

Another issue that must be addressed prior to the implementation of a research project is ensuring that the research is conducted according to ethical standards. An Institutional Review Board (IRB) comprised of experienced researchers as well as consumers must review all research. In particular, the IRB reviews research protocols to ensure that all subjects:

- Are informed of the benefits and risks of the research
- Are given an opportunity to accept or decline participation in a manner that does not cause them to be denied usual services
- Have their integrity, dignity, and confidentiality maintained over the course of the study
- Are allowed to stop their participation at any time
- Know who they should contact and what will be done if they have concerns about the study or if they are harmed by the study

In summary, good research requires critical thinking, planning, and attention to detail. The design must be specified, and ethical issues must be addressed prior to the implementation of a research project. As noted in the previous section, the beginning public health nurse must be competent in recognizing the components of an ethical study. Although research requires more rigor than usual quality assurance programs, it should be noted that good research grows out of the practice of the thoughtful nurse who thinks critically or the quality assurance program that is an integral part of an agency's mission.

RESEARCH PRIORITIES IN PUBLIC HEALTH NURSING

One of the questions posed by the public health nurse is: "In what areas do we need research?" The goal of research is to add new knowledge that complements our existing body of knowledge. In many cases, only one or two studies have been done in a particular area, and these studies need to be replicated and confirmed. In other cases, new trends and interventions lead to new areas of inquiry. Two of the major areas of needed research stem from the two broad goals of Healthy People 2010. Research is needed to answer the questions:

- How do we increase the quality and years of healthy life?
- How do we eliminate health disparities?

Within these broad goals, there are several categories for research. In particular, we need to have a better understanding of how the Leading Health Indicators (chapter 5) contribute to health and illness in specific populations. Furthermore, we need to understand how interventions of the public health nurse can have an impact on these goals and these indicators. Key research questions might be:

- Does prenatal home visiting by the public health nurse improve outcomes for African American women at risk for preterm birth?
- Do interventions provided by the hospice nurse have an impact on the quality of life of terminal clients?
- Can school nurses improve healthy life styles among adolescents from rural underserved communities?

The National Institute of Nursing Research (NINR) also provides guidance for research priorities. In 1985, legislation was passed that established the National Center for Nursing Research within the National Institutes of Health (NIH). This was a landmark in that it gave nursing a specific presence within NIH, the federal-level agency most involved with funding for health-related research. This designation came to fruition because of the hard work of nurse researchers who convinced legislators that critical questions related to nursing needed to be answered and nurses were in a unique position to add to our knowledge about health and illness. In 1993, the Center was further upgraded and became an Institute. An Institute is a higher recognition, and this recognition resulted in higher funding levels. Today, the NINR develops priority areas for research, provides money for training nurse researchers, and funds research grants particularly in priority areas. Box 19-2 identifies priority areas for research identified by NINR.

Clearly, these priorities have a high degree of relevance for public health nurses. Management of chronic illness, enhancing health promotion, and end-of-life care are all domains of the public health nurse. In addition, these priorities are very congruent with the major goals of Healthy People 2010: enhancing the quality and years of healthy life and reducing health disparities.

Many nurse researchers have built research programs in areas that are relevant for public health nurses. In 2003, the NINR published a document entitled "Making a Difference: Research Affecting Practice." This document highlights many of the important contributions of nursing research. Table 19-2 highlights some of those nurses who have completed research that has direct implications for public health nursing practice.

TYPES OF RESEARCH STUDIES IN PUBLIC HEALTH NURSING

A wide variety of research study designs are used in public health nursing practice. A thorough discussion of this area is beyond the scope of this chapter. Instead, how different types of design are used to answer different questions and how the public health nurse evaluates existing research for practice will be emphasized. In particular, the reader is challenged to examine the content in this section in relation to other course work related to research.

Research design must be based on the specific research question and the theoretical model that frames

---

BOX 19-2: NINR 2004 Areas of Research Opportunity

Chronic Illnesses or Conditions
Chronic Illness Self-Management and Quality of Life

Behavioral Changes and Interventions
Decreasing Low Birth Weight Infants among Minority Populations
Enhancing Health Promotion among Minority Men

Responding to Compelling Public Health Concerns
End-of-Life: Bridging Life and Death
Nursing Research Training and Centers

---

the question. When a nurse generates a question, that question will have a large bearing on the type of research design that will be needed to answer the question. For example, nurses who are interested in a relatively new phenomenon or a novel intervention might begin with a qualitative approach so that they might better understand the phenomenon. For example, a public health nurse working in a rural area wants to try to develop a culturally appropriate intervention that will increase the prevalence of breastfeeding in a group of Hispanic women. She reviews the literature and studies a variety of programs that have been started in other areas. However, she really would like to know a bit more about the beliefs and experiences related to breastfeeding for the women in her community. Since this type of data does not currently exist, she may use a qualitative approach.

Qualitative Research Design

Qualitative studies are usually approached from one of a variety of philosophical traditions, and the beginning nurse will need some guidance from an experienced qualitative researcher. However, qualitative studies generally are completed in two ways: individual interviews with the members of the target group using

---

⊕ PRACTICE APPLICATION

⊕ Obtain an article by one of the authors in Table 19-2 (or another nurse researcher). Examine the studies in light of your public health nursing clinical experience. How can the findings of this study be used to improve health nursing practice?

TABLE 19-2: Nurse Researchers Who Have Made a Difference in Public Health Nursing Practice

NURSE RESEARCHER	RESEARCH STUDY	FINDINGS
Mary Lou Moore, BSN, PhD	Randomized trial to test the effectiveness of the use of a single personal visit and regular telephone calls to women from 22 to 32 weeks gestation on the incidence of preterm delivery.	Although there was no difference when examining the total sample, in the subgroup of African American women 19 years of age and older, there was a significant difference in both low birth weight rates between intervention and control groups (11.4 percent vs. 17.3 percent) and in preterm births (9.4 percent vs. 12.8 percent).
Carol E. Smith, RN, PhD	Investigated a model of care-giving effectiveness that identified factors that influence outcomes for home-based technologically dependent adults.	Factors that affect outcomes include the relationship between caregiver and client, caregiver preparedness to manage home care, efficient management of resources, and caregiver characteristics such as levels of distress or depression. An intervention to prevent catheter-related infections and reduce hospitalizations in clients receiving total parental nutrition at home resulted in significantly fewer complications in the experimental group when compared to the control group.
N. L. Rothman, RN, EdD	In a community demonstration project, used a holistic approach to engage the adults and children of the targeted community to improve their health and reduce lead levels in children.	At one year, the subjects in the experimental group demonstrated a decrease in lead levels >10 from 57 to 46 percent; in the control group, the difference was 45 percent at baseline and 42 percent at one year. This project highlighted methods to help a community become engaged and take responsibility for a problem.
Loretta Sweet Jemmott, RN, FAAN, PhD	Intervention research on a variety of interventions to reduce high-risk sexual behavior and HIV transmission among African American men and women, African American adolescents, Latino adolescents, and African American and Latino families.	Both one-on-one counseling and small group interventions are appropriate and successful. The interventions can be very short and still be successful. The interventions are designed to be educational, entertaining, culturally sensitive, and gender appropriate.

Note. From National Institute of Nursing Research (2003).

an open or semistructured approach, or focus groups that include members of the target group. Focus groups usually consist of between eight and ten members of the target group, and a leader facilitates the focus group. The skill of the leader is critical in ensuring that all participants feel that their comments are valued and that the information that they provide will be handled confidentially and respectfully.

In the open, semistructured interview, the nurse strives to fully understand the perspective of the client.

Even though there may be a guide for collecting data, it is flexible and might change as the nurse becomes more informed about the topic. In a formal qualitative study, it is important that the nurse has a method for recording the data so that it can be reviewed and analyzed at a later time and by others. This might be accomplished through tape recording or extensive field notes. Qualitative research has been criticized in the past when the researcher did not have a clear framework for assembling and analyzing the data. Whether one is interviewing individuals or conducting focus groups, it is easy for certain comments to "stand out" and overshadow other opinions or statements that are also relevant. Therefore, the qualitative researcher must use a variety of strategies to minimize bias.

The beginning public health nurse is unlikely to have the skills and training to conduct a qualitative study independently. Rather, the nurse will work collaboratively with others. However, public health nurses should be able to evaluate existing qualitative research. Burns and Grove (2003) suggest that there are five standards that should be used to evaluate qualitative studies. These are outlined in Box 19-3.

Quantitative Research Design

Quantitative studies use a variety of research designs. The goal of most quantitative studies is to understand relationships between variables or to establish causality. In addition to concerns related to design, quantitative studies must address issues of measurement and sampling. Burns and Grove (2003) identify several major categories of quantitative research studies. These include descriptive, correlational, quasi-experimental, and experimental.

The descriptive study is focused on describing a phenomenon as it exists. Variables are not manipulated, and no attempt is made to establish causality. Descriptive studies might be further classified as those that examine one sample, more than one sample, or case reports. In a descriptive design, the researcher identifies an area of interest, identifies the variables, develops conceptual and operational definitions of the variables, and describes the variables. Descriptive studies often lay the groundwork for more complex studies.

In the correlational design, the researcher looks for relationships among variables (descriptive correlational design). In some cases, the researcher attempts to predict the value of one variable based on other observed variables (predictive correlational design). One (or several) variables are classified as dependent and other variables are considered to be independent and are used to predict the changes or levels of the dependent variable. Ailinger et al. (2004) used a descriptive correlational design to study tuberculosis knowledge in

---

BOX 19-3: Guidelines for Critiquing Qualitative Studies

1. Descriptive Vividness

Does the researcher describe the data collection processes in a way that the reader can personally experience the event?

2. Methodological Congruence

Does the researcher cite and give references for the philosophical and methodological approach that is used?

Are the following described in a clear and concise manner: subjects, sampling method, data-gathering and data analysis strategies, and processes for informed consent?

3. Analytical Preciseness

Is the decision-making process that the researcher used to transform the concrete data (the words of the subjects) into a more abstract synthesis that imparts meaning to the phenomenon clear and defensible?

4. Theoretical Connectedness

Is the theory developed from this study clearly expressed, logically consistent, reflective of the data, and compatible with other knowledge?

5. Heuristic Relevance

Does the researcher make it possible for the reader to recognize the significance of the study, its applicability to nursing practice, and its influence on future research?

SOURCE: Burns & Grove (2003). *Understanding nursing research*. Philadelphia: Saunders. Adapted with permission.

Latino immigrants receiving latent TB infection (LTBI) therapy. They were interested in whether education, age, or time spent in the United States was correlated with knowledge level. Using a convenience sample of 82 Latino immigrants, they found that most Latino immigrants (80 percent) knew the importance of keeping regular appointments, but many of the subjects did not have a clear understanding of information related to contagiousness. Knowledge was correlated with educational level but not with age or years in the United States. The authors comment that this study suggests specific educational strategies that might be used to meet the needs of this population.

As the researcher moves from describing relationships to testing causality, the design will change to an experimental approach. There are two types of designs in this area: quasi-experimental and experimental. Whenever the researcher moves into the realm of establishing causality through experimentation, three conditions must be met: random assignment, researcher-controlled manipulation of the independent variable, and researcher control of the experimental setting including a control or comparison group. In a quasi-experimental design, one of these conditions, usually the presence of a control group that has been formed through random assignment, is missing. Instead, the experimental group might be compared to a naturally occurring comparison group that is not completely equivalent to the experimental group. In contrast, in the true experimental design, both the experimental and the control group are formed by random assignment. During the experiment, the researcher is able to control the independent variable or the intervention and might manipulate it for different groups. In general, it is often difficult to implement an experimental design in the clinical setting, and true experiments in the clinical setting are often completed within and interdisciplinary team of experienced, highly skilled researchers. Koniak-Griffin et al. (2003) provides one example of the use of a randomized experimental design in her study of predominately Latina and African American adolescent mothers. Mothers were randomized to an experimental group that received preparation for motherhood classes plus intense home visitation by public health nurses from pregnancy through 1 year postbirth. Women randomized to the control group received traditional public health nursing care. The authors found that the intervention resulted in improved outcomes in selected areas of infant and maternal health, and these improvements were sustained for a year following program termination. This type of study is important because the experimental design helps to minimize bias, which gives us more confidence in the findings, and the study focuses on providing evidence about the outcomes of public health nursing practice.

In addition to design, several other factors related to the sample—the instruments and data collection and analysis—must be considered when completing a quantitative study. A thorough discussion of these issues is beyond the scope of this chapter. The beginning public health nurse is rarely in a position to undertake a quantitative study independently. Rather, the nurse would work collaboratively with other members of the team. However, the public health nurse should be able to evaluate existing research for application in practice. Burns and Grove (2003) suggest some guidelines for a beginning research critique that the public health nurse can use. These are found in Box 19-4. Use of these guidelines will help the nurse to evaluate studies and identify the most problematic areas of a research study. The beginner may need some assistance with completing an evaluation of existing research, but with practice, the public health nurse should gain increased skill in understanding research and using good research to guide practice.

OUTCOMES RESEARCH RELATED TO PUBLIC HEALTH NURSING PRACTICE

An important priority for public health nursing research is to document the outcomes of public health nursing practice. As noted earlier, both the history of public health nursing and our present health care delivery system provide evidence for the need to document the effect of our interventions. The problem with this is finding indicators that are sensitive to the work of nursing and finding measurement tools that adequately capture the outcome that the nurse achieves.

Several researchers have focused on developing client outcomes that are sensitive to nursing interventions. What this means is that the outcome can be directly attributed to the actions of the nurse rather than chance, random events, or another confounding factor. The Nursing Outcomes Classification (NOC) scheme was developed by a research team at the University of Iowa. The goal of NOC was to provide a comprehensive classification system of client outcomes that are influenced by nursing. The classification system could then be used

BOX 19-4: Research Critique Guidelines for Quantitative Studies

1. What is the study problem?
2. What is the study purpose?
3. Is the literature review presented?
   a. Are relevant previous studies identified and described?
   b. Are relevant theories and models identified and described?
   c. Are the references current?
   d. Are the studies critiqued by the author?
   e. Is a summary of the current knowledge provided?
4. Is a study framework clearly identified and related to the study being conducted?
5. Are research objectives, questions, or hypotheses used to direct the conduct of the study?
6. Are the major variables or concepts identified and defined (conceptually and operationally)?
7. Is the research design clearly addressed?
   a. Identify the specific design of the study.
   b. Does the study include a treatment or intervention? If so, is the treatment clearly described and consistently implemented?
   c. Are the extraneous variables identified and controlled?

8. Are the following elements of the sample described?
   a. Criteria for inclusion and exclusion from the sample
   b. Method used to obtain the sample
   c. Sample size
   d. Characteristics of the sample
   e. Attrition rate
   f. Procedure for informed consent
9. Are the measurement strategies described with a discussion of reliability and validity?
10. What statistical analyses are included in the research report? Are they appropriate for answering the research question?
11. What is the researcher's interpretation of the findings?
12. What limitations of the study are identified by the researcher?
13. How does the researcher generalize the findings?
14. What implications do the findings have for nursing practice?
15. What suggestions are made for further studies?
16. What are the missing elements of the study?
17. Is the description of the study sufficiently clear to allow replication?

SOURCE: Burns & Grove (2003). *Understanding nursing research*, p. 402–404. Philadelphia: Saunders. Adapted with permission.

to document outcomes and provide a standard language for providing evidence for the value of nursing practice (Head et al., 2004). In contrast to previous outcome classification systems that focused on outcomes that are primarily under the control of the health care provider (such as reducing the blood pressure), NOC was envisioned as a system for capturing the impact of nursing. The NOC taxonomy is a three-level coded organizing structure that currently includes 330 nursing-sensitive outcomes categorized into 29 classes and seven domains (Johnson, Maas, & Moorhead, 2004). Many of the individual outcomes are appropriate for either the acute care or the community setting. For example, the outcome *Knowledge: Behavior* measures the extent of understanding conveyed about the promotion and protection of health. A nurse in the community, a dis-

charge planner in a hospital, or a nurse working in a primary care setting might use this outcome. However, in addition to outcomes related to the individual, there are also two domains that specifically relate to public health nursing outcomes at the community level. The community health domain has two classes:

- Community Well-Being—outcomes that indicate the overall health status and social competence of a population or community
- Community Health Protection—outcomes related to the structure and programs of a community to eliminate or reduce health risks and increase community resistance to health threats.

Another classification system used by public health nurses to document care is the Omaha System developed by the Visiting Nurse Association of Omaha, Nebraska. The Omaha System consists of a Problem Classification Scheme (nursing diagnoses), Problem Rating Scale for outcomes, and an intervention scheme that lists 40 possible problems in four broad domains: environmental, psychosocial, physiological, and health-related behaviors. Barton, Clark, and Baramee (2004) have used the Omaha system in a community-based faculty practice that provides an opportunity for faculty and students to work with immigrant children and families in a Head Start program. The authors found that the Omaha system was an effective way of categorizing their interventions and that there was a statistically significant improvement from admission to discharge in the areas of knowledge, behavior, and status for the clients in the practice.

EVALUATING RESEARCH FOR EVIDENCE-BASED PRACTICE

Although the generation of new knowledge is the main goal of nursing research, clinicians must also be able to integrate existing knowledge from research into practice. As noted earlier, not all public health nurses may have the skills to conduct research independently. However, all public health nurses should be able to use research in their practice. Sometimes it is difficult for beginning nurses to evaluate a study using the criteria described previously. The nurse may not feel confident in completing a critique. Another approach that can be used to evaluate research for practice is to search for evidence in critical reviews that have been completed by reputable experts. There are several of these databases in existence and the growth of the Internet has made these data readily available. Three of the databases that have particular relevance for the public health nurse are listed in Table 19-3. As seen in the examples of reviews that have been completed, these databases provide a wealth of information and are an important tool for public health nurses seeking to integrate the best available evidence into their practice. "The time has come for practitioners from all health care professions to embrace evidence-based practice ... In doing so, clients, healthcare professionals, and healthcare systems will be able to place more confidence in the care that is being delivered and know that the best outcomes for clients and their families are being achieved" (Melnyk & Fineout-Overholt, 2005).

TABLE 19-3: Databases for Systematic Reviews and Clinical Practice Guidelines

TITLE	WEB ADDRESS	PURPOSE	EXAMPLE OF AVAILABLE REVIEWS
The Registered Nurses Association of Ontario (RNAO)	http://www.rnao.org/bestpractices	Provides systematic reviews to guide nursing practice	Assessment and Management of Pain Assessment and Management of Foot Ulcers in Diabetics Establishing Therapeutic Relationships
Cochrane Data Base and Library	http://www.cochrane.org	Provides regularly updated evidence-based health care data bases	Interventions Aimed at Improving Immunization Rates Interventions for Preventing Tobacco-Smoking in Public Places Population-based Interventions for the Prevention of Falls in Older People
Clinical Practice Guidelines	http://www.guideline.gov	Provides a public source for evidence-based clinical practice guidelines	Screening for Obesity in Adults: Recommendations and Rationale Clinical Practice Guidelines for Quality Palliative Care

CRITICAL THINKING ACTIVITIES

1. How would you address the issues outlined by Buhler-Wilkerson if you were involved in a study related to the outcomes of a public health nursing intervention?

2. Examine the Core Competencies for Public Health Nursing found in appendix A. How do they relate to research in public health nursing? For example, how are the skills related to policy development and how is leadership related to public health nursing research?

3. Formulate a question related to public health nursing that might be answered with a qualitative design.

4. Suggest an outcome related to community well-being or community health protection and discuss how public health nursing might have an impact on this outcome.

5. As a new public health nurse in a health department, you suggest a change in practice based on a recent systematic review that you have read. The response to your suggestion is, "We have always done it this way, and the old way works best for us." How would you respond to this?

KEY TERMS

benchmark

correlational design

descriptive epidemiology

descriptive study

experimental study

Institutional Review Board

Nursing Outcomes Classification

Omaha System

qualitative study

quality assurance program

quantitative study

quasi-experimental study

randomized control trial

KEY CONCEPTS

⊕ From the early days of public health nursing, research has been an integral part of practice.

⊕ Public health nurses have different roles, responsibilities, and competencies related to research, and these will expand with increased experience and education.

⊕ The design of a research study is based on many factors including the question to be answered, ethical principles, resources, the current state of knowledge, and the expertise of the research team.

⊕ Measures to evaluate the effectiveness of public health nursing must be sensitive to the interventions and outcomes of public health nursing practice.

⊕ Evidence-based nursing practice is the responsibility of all public health nurses, and the use of best practices is the hallmark of high quality nursing care.

REFERENCES

Ailinger, R., Armstrong, R., Nguyen, N., & Lasus, H. (2004) Latino immigrants knowledge of tuberculosis. *Public Health Nursing, 21*(6): 519–523.

Barton, A., Clark, L., & Baramee, J. (2004). Tracking outcomes in community-based care. *Home Health Care Management and Practice, 16*(3): 171–175.

Buhler-Wilkerson, K. (1993). Bringing care to the people: Lillian Wald's legacy to public health nursing. *American Journal of Public Health, 83*(12): 1778–1786.

Burns, N., & Grove, S. (2003). *Understanding nursing research.* Philadelphia: Saunders.

Johnson, M., Maas, M., & Moorhead, S. (2004). *Iowa Outcomes Project: Nursing outcomes classification* (2nd ed.). St. Louis: Mosby.

Head, B., Aquilino, M., Johnson, M., Reed, D., Maas, M., & Moorhead, S. (2004). Content validity and nursing sensitivity of community-level outcomes from the Nursing Outcomes Classification (NOC). *Journal of Nursing Scholarship, 26*(3), 251–259.

Koniak-Griffin, D., Verzemnieks, I., Anderson, N., Brecht, M., Lesser, J., Kim, S., & Turner-Pluta, C. (2003). Nurse visitation for adolescent mothers. *Nursing Research, 52*(2), 127–136.

Melnyk B., & Fineout-Overholt, E. (2005). *Evidence-based practice in nursing and health care.* Philadelphia: Lippincott Williams & Wilkins.

National Institute of Nursing Research. (2003). *Making a difference, Part II, NINR research results.* Bethesda, MD: National Institutes of Health.

Quad Council of Public Health Nursing Organizations. (2004). Public health nursing competencies. *Public Health Nursing, 21*(5), 443–452.

BIBLIOGRAPHY

Ervin, N. E., & Cowell, J. M. (2004). Integrating research into teaching public health nursing. *Public Health Nursing, 21*(2), 183–190.

Johnson, M., & Maas, M. (Eds.). (1997). *Iowa Outcomes Project. Nursing Outcomes Classification (NOC).* St. Louis: Mosby.

Moss, M. P., & Schell, M. C. (2004). GIS(c): A scientific framework and methodological tool for nursing research. *Advances in Nursing Science, 27*(2), 150–159.

Portillo, C., & Waters, C. (2004). Community partnerships: The cornerstone of community health nursing. *Annual Review of Nursing Research, 22,* 315–329.

RESOURCES

Eastern Nursing Research Society (ENRS)

100 North 20th Street, 4th Floor
Philadelphia, Pennsylvania 19103
215-599-6700
FAX: 215-564-2175
Email: info@enrs-go.org
Web: http://www.enrs-go.org

ENRS has members in the Eastern Region of the United States. Their goals are to advance nursing research in the Northeast region of the United States, facilitate development of nurse researchers, influence development of scientific knowledge base relevant to nursing, and promote research-based nursing practice. Their Web site offers more information about ENRS and links to other nursing organizations.

Midwest Nursing Research Society (MNRS)

10200 West 44th Avenue, Suite 304
Wheat Ridge, Colorado 80033
1-866-908-8617
FAX: 303-422-8894
Email: mnrs@resourcenter.com
Web: http://www.mnrs.org

MNRS, *with membership in the Midwest region of the United States,* advances the scientific basis of nursing practice and promotes development of nurse scientist. Their promoting, disseminating, and utilizing nursing research throughout the Midwest has profoundly influenced the growth in quality and quantity of nursing research for more than 30 years. Their Web site offers more information about MNRS and the many sections of members who share research interests.

National Institute of Nursing Research (NINR)

National Institutes of Health
31 Center Drive, Room 5B10
Bethesda, Maryland 20892-2178
301-496-0207
FAX: 301-480-8845
Web: http://www.ninr.nih.gov

The mission of NINR is to promote and improve the health of individuals, families, communities, and populations. NINR supports and conducts clinical and basic research and research training on health and illness across the lifespan. The research focus encompasses health promotion and disease prevention, quality of life, health disparities, and end-of-life. NINR seeks to extend nursing science by integrating the biological and behavioral sciences, employing new technologies to research questions, improving research methods, and developing the scientists of the future. The Web site includes information about the NINR and research and funding, training investigators, and news and information.

Sigma Theta Tau International (STTI)

550 West North Street
Indianapolis, Indiana 46202
1-888-634-7575; 1-317-634-8171 (international)
Email: stti@stti.iupui.edu
Web: http://www.nursingsociety.org

The mission of STTI is to provide leadership and scholarship
in practice, education, and research to enhance the health
of all people. STTI supports the learning and professional
development of members who strive to improve nursing
care worldwide. Their Web site offers additional information about STTI, membership, and nursing research.

Southern Nursing Research Society (SNRS)

10200 West 44th Avenue, Suite 304
Wheat Ridge, Colorado 80033
1-877-314-SNRS
Email: snrs@resourcenter.com
Web: http://www.snrs.org

SNRS, founded in 1986, is an organization for nursing
researchers in the southern region. There are 14 states
in the SNRS region. The mission is to advance nursing research, promote dissemination and utilization of
research findings, facilitate the career development of
nurses and nursing students as researchers, enhance communication among members, and promote the image of
nursing as a scientific discipline. Their Web site offers
additional information about SNRS, conferences, publications, and research interest groups.

PART 4

PROVISION OF PUBLIC HEALTH NURSING TO VULNERABLE POPULATIONS

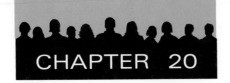

CHAPTER 20

Populations with Infectious and Communicable Disease

Catherine Salveson, RN, MS, PhD

Shelley L. Jones, RN, MS, COHN-S, FAAOHN

Chapter Outline

- Factors that Lead to the Emergence and Reemergence of Infectious and Communicable Disease
- Models of Transmission of Infectious and Communicable Disease
  Natural History of a Disease
  Epidemiological Triangle and the Chain of Transmission
- Levels of Prevention
  Primary Prevention
  Secondary Prevention
  Tertiary Prevention
- Common Infectious and Communicable Diseases
  Food-borne and Water-borne Diseases
  Vector-borne Diseases
  Parasitic Diseases
  Nosocomial Infections
  Respiratory Infections
  Viral Hepatitis
  Sexually Transmitted Infections
- Infectious and Communicable Disease in the Global Community
- The Spectre of Bioterrorism
  Potential Bioterrorism Agents
  What Can Be Done?
- Strategies for Nurses Working with Infectious and Communicable Disease in the Community
  Infectious and Communicable Disease Program Management
  Planning for Pandemic Disease Events
- Infectious and Communicable Disease Resources

Learning Objectives

Upon completion of this chapter, the reader will be able to:

1. Examine factors that lead to the emergence and reemergence of infectious and communicable disease

2. Apply principles from infectious and communicable disease models

3. Use systems for the prevention and control of infectious and communicable disease

4. Differentiate signs, symptoms, and causative agents of common infectious and communicable diseases

5. Describe awareness of infectious and communicable disease in the global community

6. Use public health nursing strategies in the control of infectious and communicable diseases

Human beings share the Earth with an unseen world of microorganisms, many of which are essential partners in the natural world and necessary for human survival. Others are pathogens that are capable of infecting humans and causing disease, disability, and death. The history of the world includes the effects of communicable disease on the rise and fall of great nations and the global migration of entire populations of people (McNeil, 1977). The general public has become increasingly aware of this unseen world, as the public media and entertainment industry have informed them about toxic agents and spreading viruses, from Ebola to antibiotic-resistant bacteria.

The role of public health has always included a commitment to protect the public from infectious or communicable disease, and the control of communicable disease is one of the great successes of public health. In the early 1900s, 40 percent of all deaths in the United States were caused by four communicable diseases—influenza, diphtheria, tuberculosis (TB), and dysentery (Mullen, 1989). By 1997, this had changed dramatically. Pneumonia, influenza, and human immunodeficiency virus (HIV) or acquired immunodeficiency syndrome (AIDS) caused only 4.5 percent of deaths. This change in mortality from communicable disease in the United States is not shared with the rest of the world. The second leading cause of death in the world is still infectious disease, and it is the number one killer of infants and children. The World Health Organization (WHO) expected 58 million deaths worldwide in 2005. Thirty percent of the 58 million deaths that occurred worldwide were caused by microbial agents (WHO, 2005). As we have increasingly become a global community, infectious disease spreads more quickly, and efforts to control it are now shared by public health workers worldwide; consider the worldwide concern about the spread of HIV/AIDS. At the turn of the twenty-first century, public health also faces new challenges worldwide, such as concerns for the mutation of severe acute respiratory syndrome (SARS; also known as Asian avian bird virus), the spread of West Nile virus, antibiotic-resistant tuberculosis, and staphylococcus aureus; and the potential for an N5N1 Asian avian bird influenza worldwide pandemic.

Nurses need to know about communicable disease in all areas of practice, but especially in public health nursing. In this chapter, a background for understanding communicable disease is provided, including the factors that lead to the emergence and reemergence of communicable diseases, models of transmission of communicable diseases, systems for the prevention and control of communicable diseases, common communicable diseases, infectious and communicable diseases in the global community, the threat of bioterrorism, and strategies for the nurse working with infectious and communicable diseases in the community.

FACTORS THAT LEAD TO THE EMERGENCE AND REEMERGENCE OF INFECTIOUS AND COMMUNICABLE DISEASE

Living in a global community includes more than people from diverse cultures speaking different languages. It includes the world of microorganisms that are equally intent on survival. Unfortunately, the survival of many pathogens includes their use of humans for shelter, food, and the perpetuation of their species (Lashley & Durham, 2002). The Institute of Medicine (IOM) report *Emerging Infections: Microbial Threats to Health in the United States* was first published in 1992 and the Forum on Microbial Threats convened in 2003 to follow the initiatives. The report concerned the global nature of emerging infectious diseases, infectious diseases that have newly appeared in a population or that have been known for some time but are rapidly increasing in *incidence* or geographic range. The report emphasized the complacency that currently existed among world health workers. Six important factors in disease emergence and reemergence were identified. These included (1) changes in human demographics and behavior; (2) advances in technology and industry; (3) economic development and changes in land use; (4) commerce; (5) microbial adaptation and change in response to selective pressures; and (6) deterioration in the public health system at the local, state, national, and global levels.

The threat of communicable disease is part of daily living in any community and is increasingly tied to our being a global community (see Figure 20-1). For example, a number of food-borne outbreaks have been linked to imported food, such as *Cyclospora* gastroenteritis in the United States and Canada associated with raspberries imported from Guatemala. Drug resistance is recognized as a national and global problem, as is seen in the continued emergence and intercountry spread of penicillin resistance in *Streptococcus pneumoniae* and the identification of *Staphylococcus aureus* infections caused by strains with partial resistance to vancomycin in Japan, France, and the United States. Human infections caused by an avian strain of influenza in Hong Kong in 1997 provided a reminder of the threat posed by the next influenza epidemic, thought to be associated with the N5N1 virus. The emergence of West Nile virus in New York City in 1999 and its rapid spread through the eastern half of the country emphasized the threats and challenges posed by vector-borne disease. Health care providers need to be aware of emerging diseases in their own and other countries and the critical importance of being connected to a surveillance and response system.

The events of September 11, 2001, began the era of concern regarding threats to our national security. The subsequent unprecedented bioterrorism attacks using germ warfare involving *Bacillus anthracis* sent through the U.S. postal system further dramatized the critical importance of a preparedness and response capacity at the local, state, and national levels. Health care professionals first recognized the illness caused by anthrax, reinforcing the importance of heightened vigilance and familiarity with clinical manifestations of diseases that may result from bioterrorism (Lashley & Durham, 2002). Specific guidelines regarding bioterrorism are included later in this chapter.

Social conditions such as poverty and lack of access to health care create the conditions for an increased incidence of communicable diseases in disadvantaged populations. Despite the continuing challenges, there have been significant successes in disease control. It is believed smallpox had been eradicated from the world; however, frozen viral samples continue to be held for research purposes (WHO 2006). Now, concern exists that smallpox outbreaks may return due to the actions of bioterrorists. Eradication is the elimination of the causative agent. Usually, a disease cannot be totally eradicated; however, a disease can be eliminated from a specific geographic area. Elimination is to have the disease under control. The World Health Organization is working throughout the world to eliminate the polio virus, with the hope of one day eradicating it completely. Historical examples reveal what can happen when an unfamiliar infection attacks a population for the first time. These include the Black Death of the fourteenth century, when one-third of the total population of Europe died, and the cholera epidemics in China and India in the nineteenth century when over 13 percent of the population died (McNeil, 1977). The rise of HIV, the causative agent of AIDS, is another example.

The slow response to the emergence of HIV in the United States in 1981 resulted in the epidemic expanding. By 1993, 1.5 million Americans were infected. The cost grew to over $12 billion annually in research, drug development, education, and treatment efforts. The virus also continued to spread globally. Other countries

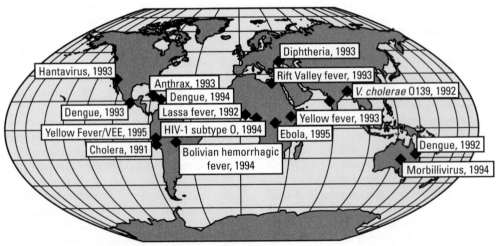

Figure 20-1 Global microbial threats in the 1990s.

⊕ PRACTICE APPLICATION

The Emergence of HIV

In 1981, health care providers began seeing a strange new disease predominantly among gay men in the large metropolitan areas of New York City and San Francisco. They soon discovered that the disease appeared to be contagious and spread through sexual contact. Further investigation revealed that it was also spread through contact with infected blood, and the Centers for Disease Control and Prevention (CDC) issued a report in 1982 warning it might be in the blood supply. Cases had been documented in five people with hemophilia who had received transfusions. The American Association of Blood Banks was reluctant to admit that the nation's blood supply could be contaminated for fear that people would stop donating blood. Anyone who lived a gay lifestyle was urged not to donate blood; however, no official testing began until 1984 when the Hepatitis B antibody test was used to screen people for possible HIV infection. By that time, many people had become infected through routine transfusions. The virus was finally identified in May of 1984, and an antibody test was then developed. It did not take long before the extent of the spread of the virus was confirmed. Over 90 percent of people with hemophilia who had received regular blood transfusions were infected, and people using intravenous drugs had an 87 percent infection rate. Soon it was discovered that women who had sexual relationships with infected men became infected, confirming that the HIV was spreading throughout the entire population (Shilts, 1988).

experienced similar periods of denial regarding the presence and spread of the virus, especially in Africa and increasingly in Asia. The fact that the virus spreads through sexual contact and intravenous drug use makes it culturally difficult to discuss prevention and support those who become infected.

In 2006, the World Health Organization reported 38.6 million people throughout the world were living with HIV. This included over 2.2 million children. It is estimated that in 2006 there were about 14,000 new HIV infections in the world every day. More than 95 percent are in developing countries, and almost 50 percent are women (UNAIDS, 2006). The treatment for those infected has improved in developed countries such as the United States because of the use of antiviral medications: however, these are expensive, difficult to take, and unavailable to most people in the world who have HIV disease. The medication and treatment issues remain a major challenge to those trying to control the spread of the epidemic and help those infected and affected. The WHO General Assembly 2006 High Level Meeting on AIDS brought world leaders together to renew the Declaration of Commitment and target 2015 as the goal for halting and reversing the epidemic (WHO, 2006).

MODELS OF TRANSMISSION OF INFECTIOUS AND COMMUNICABLE DISEASE

Disease is understood as a dynamic process with multiple levels of causation, from disease-producing agents or stimuli in the environment to behavioral factors. The ultimate objective of public health is the prevention of disease to prolong and enhance quality of life. This involves many things as is seen in the constitution of WHO where health is defined as "a state of complete physical, mental and social well being and not just the absence of disease" (WHO, 2006). Models of the transmission of communicable disease have been created to show how disease is initiated and progresses, with a goal of intervening for the purpose of prevention and management.

Natural History of a Disease

Before a disease affects humans, every disease or health condition has precipitating or predisposing causes that are operational in human occupational and living environments. This includes things such as stagnant water,

ase-carrying mosquitoes, or restau-
ndercooked contaminated meat. The
een heredity, social, environmental,
tors can create the circumstances and
stimulus ... disease long before humans are affected.
This interaction of disease-producing factors is called
the period of prepathogenesis. (See Figure 20-2.) Once
humans interact with disease-provoking stimuli, the
period of pathogenesis begins. Combining the process
that happens in the environment with the disease process in humans provides the natural history of a disease
that can lead to recovery, disability or death.

Epidemiological Triangle and the Chain of Transmission

A basic model used in public health to describe infectious disease is called the agent-host-environment epidemiological triangle (see Figure 20-3). Many factors exist
as agents, hosts, or environments in the spread of communicable disease. Changing any one of these factors
can affect how disease is spread. The twenty-first century has seen a significant interruption in the balance

between the environment, the people who live in it,
and the agents that produce disease. This has happened
unknowingly in many circumstances until the damage
has been done, and then the environment for disease
to spread is revealed. For example, the widespread and
intermittent use of antibiotics has created an environment for some organisms to become antibiotic-resistant. The tuberculosis bacillus has become resistant to
the standard treatment of the drugs Rifampin and Iso-
niaid (INH) in part because people have not completed
a full course of treatment and the bacillus adapted to
the medications. The environment can also change,
such as the weather change in the American southwest
that created the conditions for the return of the Hanta-
virus on the Navajo Reservation in 1993.

A particular communicable disease develops in a
given place at a specific time because a specific set of
conditions or events exists. These include the physical
environment, behavioral factors, emotional and psychological influences, biophysical circumstances, and
the influence of the health system. Figure 20-3 shows
the chain of transmission of a communicable disease.
It is called a "chain" because the links that connect one

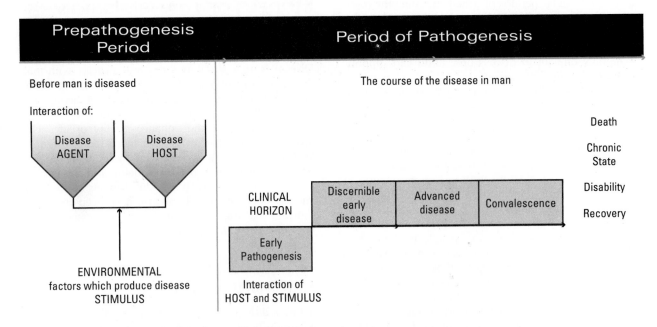

Figure 20-2 Natural history of any disease process in man.

From H. R. Leavell & E. G. Clark (1958). *Preventive Medicine for the Doctor in His Community.* New York: Springer. Copyright 1958. Reprinted with permission of The McGraw-Hill companies.

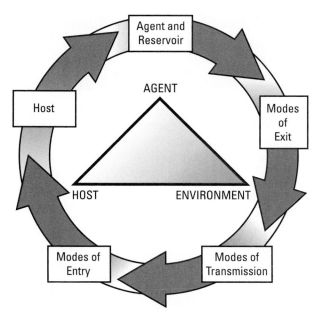

Figure 20-3 Epidemiological triangle and the chain of transmission.

element to another can potentially be broken to stop the spread of a communicable disease. The links in the chain of transmission include the agent and reservoir (all sources of the agent), the modes of exit from the reservoir, the modes of transmission, the modes of entry to the host, and the host (which is part of the reservoir). The model shows the relationship of the links to each other, as well as the relationship of the links to the Epidemiological Triangle. It is easier to see more of the complexities of communicable and infectious disease transmission by studying the chain of transmission.

Agent and Reservoir

There are four main categories of biological agents that cause communicable disease. These are (1) fungi, (2) parasites, (3) bacteria, and (4) viruses. The reservoir of any agent is the sum of all sources of that agent, including human and animal hosts and locations in the environment where the agents may temporarily live. Biological agents are often described based on the etiology and severity of the disease, using epidemiological terms such as infectivity, pathogenicity, toxicity, and antigenicity. Infectivity is the agent's ability to replicate itself in the host in order to grow and spread.

Pathogenicity is the ability of the agent to cause specific signs and symptoms of disease. Virulence refers to the agent's ability to cause severe disease (usually measured by the case fatality ratio of the disease outbreaks). Antigenicity is the agent's ability to stimulate the host's immune system, producing disease-specific antibodies for immunity and future protection of the host. Public health controls of the agent involve treatments that kill the agents to end agent infectivity.

Modes of Exit

The modes of exit from the reservoir are usually described in terms of how agents leave their hosts. Mechanisms of exit are directly related to the body systems of the human or animal host, including the respiratory, gastrointestinal, urinary, and reproductive systems. Exit by the respiratory tract represents almost continuous shedding of the agent through respired air, coughing, sneezing, and touch with contaminated hands and secretions. Agents can be periodically shed from the gastrointestinal tract through defecation and diarrhea. Urinary tract shedding of agents occurs during normal intermittent urination. Agent shedding via the reproductive tract requires direct person-to-person contact and is an intermittent shedding of the agent. In the past, public health efforts to control communicable and infectious diseases at the level of the exit modes involved isolation and quarantine. Current efforts to control modes of transmission focus on frequent hand-washing and avoidance of direct contact with infected body systems.

For specific agents, the mode of entry to a new host is usually the same as the mode of exit from the reservoir for that agent. Disease spread via the gastrointestinal system use modes of entry such as ingestion of contaminated food or water and contaminated hands (fecal-oral route). Influenza and the common cold require close person-to-person contact for sharing of respiratory secretions and airborne droplets.

Modes of Transmission

The environment for transmission includes the social, cultural, biologic, and physical influences on a human host and is called the mode of transmission. It is through the environment that an infectious agent moves out of the reservoir to another host. Many efforts are made to reduce the environmental impact on the spread of disease. This includes things such as large-scale spraying for mosquitoes and ticks, reducing bacterial contamination by requiring all food handlers to be trained in sanitation control in food preparation, and providing clean water and sanitation systems. There are many ways that an infectious agent is spread from an infected person or host to uninfected people. The mode of transmission is often the key to breaking the chain of infection. The three modes of transmission are direct person-to-person, common vehicle, and vectors (see Table 20-1).

Person-to Person Transmission

Person-to-person transmission happens between a parent and child through sperm, placenta, breast milk, or contact with the mother's blood in the birth canal. Sexually transmitted diseases such as syphilis and HIV may be given to infants during birth. Person-to-person spread involves the direct contact of an infected host with an uninfected person. Many agents can be easily spread through the air and through the intimate contacts of sexual partners, family members, other household contacts, and school or child care contacts. Sexually transmitted infections (STIs) are direct person-to-person infections that are challenging to track because people are reluctant to share the names of their sexual contacts, and many diseases do not have significant signs and symptoms early in the disease, such as HIV.

Common Vehicle Transmission

Common vehicle transmission occurs when the infectious agent is able to live outside the host long enough to be transferred through the environment. Common vehicles include water, food, milk, soil, inanimate objects (such as cups, towels, silverware, and toys), and blood or blood products. Public health efforts to control diseases spread by common vehicle transmission cover a wide range of sanitation policies and practices. The public is protected by regular water testing to maintain safe drinking water supplies. Outbreaks of typhoid fever and cholera are almost unknown in the United States because of strict environmental sanitation programs. Food- and milk-borne diseases are controlled by clean food handling regulations. The American Red Cross carefully tests all donated blood to ensure that no infectious agents are spread through blood and blood products.

Vector Transmission

Vectors are animate transmitters of disease. They may be ill with the specific agent or carry it on body parts.

TABLE 20-1: Diseases and Their Modes of Transmission

INFECTIOUS AND COMMUNICABLE DISEASES	MODE OF TRANSMISSION
Poliomyelitis, tuberculosis, influenza, measles, mumps, rubella, scarlet fever, diphtheria, pertussis, hantavirus, respiratory anthrax, smallpox, plague	Airborne
Lice, scabies, smallpox, impetigo	Direct contact
Plague (bubonic), Lyme disease, rabies, malaria	Animal or insect bite
HIV, herpes simplex virus, syphilis, gonorrhea, chlamydia, hepatitis B, C, & D	Sexual contact
Botulism and other food intoxications, such as *Staphlycoccus aureus*, *Clostridium perferingens*	Ingestion
Hepatitis A & E, salmonellosis, typhoid, shigellosis	Oral-fecal ingestion
Hepatitis A,B,C & D, HIV, syphilis	Inoculation by needle
Hookworm, tetanus	Environmental transmission (soil)

Note. From "Infectious Disease Information," National Center for Infectious Diseases, Center for Disease Control and Prevention. Retrieved August 29, 2006, from http://www.cdc.gov/ncidod/diseases/index.htm.

The usual vectors are animals, insects, and birds. West Nile virus is being tracked carefully as it spreads from the east to west coasts of the United States via infected mosquitoes and birds. There are regular public health environmental controls in place for such vector-borne diseases as plague and rabies. The World Health Organization is tracking for the spread of avian flu (see Table 20-4 at the end of this chapter).

The Host

The severity of a communicable disease also depends on characteristics of the animal or human host. Factors that affect how effectively a host can combat an agent include things they cannot control, and other things that they can affect to protect themselves. People at various ages may be more resistant or more susceptible to disease. Small children who have not yet been fully immunized are more susceptible to communicable diseases. Adults may lose their resistance if they do not maintain regular immunizations for agents such as tetanus.

Types of Host Immunity

An individual's ability to be protected from communicable diseases is influenced by natural or acquired immunity. Natural immunity is genetically determined; it is also seen when a specific species is resistant to specific infectious agents. For example, persons with the flu do not infect their pets. For many years, we did not worry about the Asian bird flu because sick chickens did not infect humans. The agent mutated and is now being carefully monitored because it is considered dangerous to humans. Likewise, international panels of experts are engaged in preparations for a potential N5N1 pandemic if the virus found in birds mutates to become infectious to humans.

Acquired immunity is present after a person comes in contact with an agent and his or her body produces antibodies that provide protection from further infection by the same agent. People who have had the measles are immune from having measles again. People acquire immunity in two ways, passively and actively. Passive immunity is provided by mothers through transplacental transfer and through breastfeeding. Maternal antibodies to specific diseases are passed to the infant and protect the child during the vulnerable first months of life. Passive immunity can also be provided through administration of immune globulins or antiserums. These are administered to individuals for short-term protection when exposure to infectious agents is expected and/or the individuals do not have enough time to develop their own antibodies following immunization. Travelers may be given immune globulins prior to going into environments where infectious agents are common. Hepatitis A and rabies are diseases for which preventive immune globulins are commonly used. Active immunity requires that the immune system of a person be activated through having the disease or being immunized against it (see Figure 20-4).

	NATURAL IMMUNITY	ARTIFICIAL IMMUNITY
PASSIVE	• Transplacental transfer	• Gamma globulin

ACTIVE	• Disease or subclinical case
	• Latent immunity
	• Viral diseases
	• Poor antigens
		• Toxoid or vaccine
		  - Injectable
		  - Oral
		  - Nasal
		• Herd immunity

Figure 20-4 Graph of acquired immunity.

Herd immunity is the resistance to the spread of infectious disease in a group because susceptible members are few, making transmission from an infected member unlikely. Herd immunity is the basis of the public health mandates for the immunization of children. When a large percentage of a population (75 to 85 percent) is immunized and resistant to a disease, the agent is less likely to spread, and there are few disease outbreaks. Vaccines help assure that if an agent comes into an environment, the hosts it comes in contact with will have developed antibodies to fight the agent. Hepatitis B is an example of a disease known to be spreading. Public health authorities implemented laws requiring hepatitis B vaccine for the purpose of increasing the herd immunity of the American people. This is being done by routinely immunizing infants and requiring immunization before children enter public schools. Immunization of adolescents is required in many states and is especially targeted to high-risk populations such as children of first generation immigrants from countries with high-prevalence rates of hepatitis B. Health care workers are also required to be immunized.

LEVELS OF PREVENTION

During the 1950's H. R. Leavell and E. G. Clark (1958) wrote a book entitled *Preventive Medicine for the Doctor in His Community*. A model from this book has become a public health classic. The levels of application of preventive measures in the natural history of disease have been a conceptual guide for public health practice and the control of communicable and infectious conditions over the past 60 years (see Figure 20-5). The top third of the model describes theoretical phases of the natural history of any disease. Leavell and Clark describe the activities and responsibilities of the medical practitioner for prevention at each phase of the natural history of a disease. Three levels of prevention are described as a conceptual guide for community practice.

Primary Prevention

Primary prevention is the first defense against communicable disease. "General Health Promotion" includes a variety of lifestyle behaviors and health education to keep people healthy. "Specific Protection" activities are related to preventing a specific disease. The variety of activities includes immunizations to build immunity and chemoprophylaxis to prevent the onset of disease in exposed individuals.

Preventing Disease with Vaccines: Immunization

The most effective way to stop a communicable disease is to prevent outbreaks, and public health promotes the use of vaccines to create immunity. Edward Jenner developed the concept of immunization with his discovery of the first smallpox vaccine in 1796. The discovery that injection of a small particle of a pathogen did not create disease, but could create an immune response that was protective, led to the development of the cholera, rabies, typhoid, and plague vaccines in the late 1800s (National Immunization Program, 2005).

There have been many challenges in convincing people to immunize themselves and their children because very rarely an immunization causes a significant negative reaction creating fear, especially among parents. Taking this small risk into consideration, the mandatory childhood immunizations required for entry into most public schools can only be waived by specific parental request. Effective public health immunization programs include providing access to immunizations, education the public regarding the value of immunizations, and tracking immunizations among families that move frequently. There is growing concern among public health authorities that the lack of immunization registries to track new immigrants and children does not provide the data needed to actively implement successful immunization programs (National Immunization Program, 2005).

Health care providers include immunizations as a part of routine primary care for both children and adults. Older adults receive significant benefit from timely immunizations, especially those living in long-term care or other congregate living facilities. The annual flu vaccine is highly recommended and prioritized for adults older than 65 years, anyone with an immune limitation, and those with many chronic conditions. The Healthy People 2010 national health objectives include increasing immunization rates for a variety of communicable diseases. The Healthy People 2010 Web site provides a comprehensive discussion of these objectives (USDHHS, 2005).

Vaccination is the standard of pediatric practice and is most often given to children between the ages of 19 and 35 months including immunizations for varicella and poliomyelitis; measles, mumps, and rubella; and diphtheria, tetanus, and pertussis. These are administered routinely during well child care in both public and private clinics. Adult vaccine coverage for common diseases such as hepatitis A and B, tetanus, pneumonia, and influenza is not as widespread as childhood vaccination. Adults require boosters for tetanus and diphtheria and unimmunized women of childbearing age increase the risk of congenital rubella syndrome or neonatal tetanus in their infants. Adults and adolescents may also be at risk for varicella if not immunized (National Immunization Program, 2005).

Common sexually transmitted diseases that do not have vaccines available include hepatitis C, D, or E and HIV infection. Research is actively under way in many countries in search of an HIV vaccine to slow the spread of the epidemic. It is more complicated than the development of other vaccines because the HIV mutates constantly and is not controlled completely by the human immune system. Research continues with hopes that a vaccine may also be useful in slowing the progression of the disease in those already infected.

Public health nurses (PHNs) play a critical role promoting immunizations. They are involved with school- and community-based initiatives to plan and implement campaigns to provide education and make immunizations easily available. They are also involved in data-tracking and enforcement programs that ensure those entering schools, from elementary through postsecondary education, are adequately immunized. See Figures 20-6, 20-7, 20-8, and 20-9 for recommended immunization schedules for children, adolescents and adults.

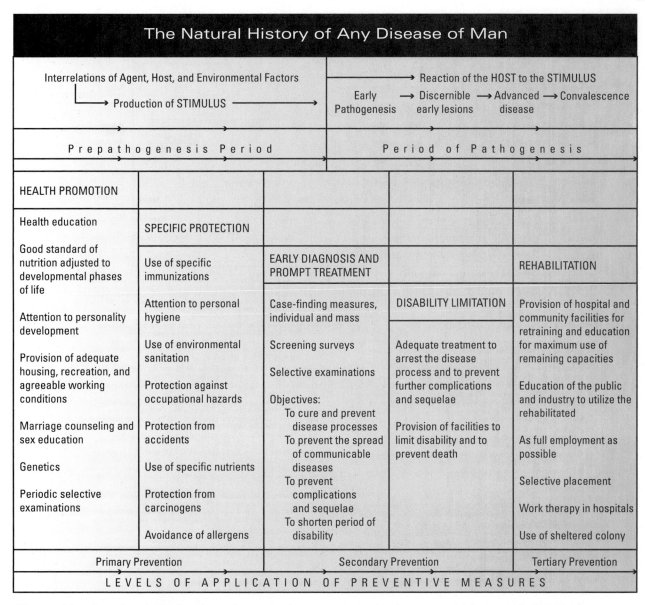

The Natural History of Any Disease of Man

Interrelations of Agent, Host, and Environmental Factors →→ Production of STIMULUS →		Reaction of the HOST to the STIMULUS →→ Early Pathogenesis → Discernible early lesions → Advanced disease → Convalescence		
Prepathogenesis Period		Period of Pathogenesis		
HEALTH PROMOTION Health education Good standard of nutrition adjusted to developmental phases of life Attention to personality development Provision of adequate housing, recreation, and agreeable working conditions Marriage counseling and sex education Genetics Periodic selective examinations	**SPECIFIC PROTECTION** Use of specific immunizations Attention to personal hygiene Use of environmental sanitation Protection against occupational hazards Protection from accidents Use of specific nutrients Protection from carcinogens Avoidance of allergens	**EARLY DIAGNOSIS AND PROMPT TREATMENT** Case-finding measures, individual and mass Screening surveys Selective examinations Objectives: To cure and prevent disease processes To prevent the spread of communicable diseases To prevent complications and sequelae To shorten period of disability	**DISABILITY LIMITATION** Adequate treatment to arrest the disease process and to prevent further complications and sequelae Provision of facilities to limit disability and to prevent death	**REHABILITATION** Provision of hospital and community facilities for retraining and education for maximum use of remaining capacities Education of the public and industry to utilize the rehabilitated As full employment as possible Selective placement Work therapy in hospitals Use of sheltered colony
Primary Prevention		Secondary Prevention		Tertiary Prevention
LEVELS OF APPLICATION OF PREVENTIVE MEASURES				

Figure 20-5 Levels of application of preventive measures in the natural history of disease in man.
From H. R. Leavell & E. G. Clark (1958). *Preventive Medicine for the Doctor in His Community.* New York: Springer. Copyright 1958. Reprinted with permission of The McGraw-Hill companies.

Contact Notification and Chemoprophylaxis

When someone is diagnosed with a communicable disease, they are asked to provide a public health worker with the names of people who are their contacts. This confidential list is used to identify and notify persons who may be infected in order to provide testing. If contacts are found to be infected, treatment is offered to prevent the onset of disease and the exposure of others. Contact notification can be done by either a health care

DEPARTMENT OF HEALTH AND HUMAN SERVICES • CENTERS FOR DISEASE CONTROL AND PREVENTION

Recommended Immunization Schedule for Persons Aged 0–6 Years—UNITED STATES • 2007

Vaccine ▼ Age ▶	Birth	1 month	2 months	4 months	6 months	12 months	15 months	18 months	19–23 months	2–3 years	4–6 years
Hepatitis B[1]	HepB	HepB		see footnote 1		HepB			HepB Series		
Rotavirus[2]			Rota	Rota	Rota						
Diphtheria, Tetanus, Pertussis[3]			DTaP	DTaP	DTaP		DTaP				DTaP
Haemophilus influenzae type b[4]			Hib	Hib	*Hib[4]*	Hib		Hib			
Pneumococcal[5]			PCV	PCV	PCV	PCV			PCV / PPV		
Inactivated Poliovirus			IPV	IPV		IPV					IPV
Influenza[6]						Influenza (Yearly)					
Measles, Mumps, Rubella[7]						MMR					MMR
Varicella[8]						Varicella					Varicella
Hepatitis A[9]						HepA (2 doses)			HepA Series		
Meningococcal[10]									MPSV4		

Range of recommended ages

Catch-up immunization

Certain high-risk groups

This schedule indicates the recommended ages for routine administration of currently licensed childhood vaccines, as of December 1, 2006, for children aged 0–6 years. Additional information is available at http://www.cdc.gov/nip/recs/child-schedule.htm. Any dose not administered at the recommended age should be administered at any subsequent visit, when indicated and feasible. Additional vaccines may be licensed and recommended during the year. Licensed combination vaccines may be used whenever any components of the combination are indicated and other components of the vaccine are not contraindicated and if approved by the Food and Drug Administration for that dose of the series. Providers should consult the respective Advisory Committee on Immunization Practices statement for detailed recommendations. Clinically significant adverse events that follow immunization should be reported to the Vaccine Adverse Event Reporting System (VAERS). Guidance about how to obtain and complete a VAERS form is available at **http://www.vaers, hhs.gov** or by telephone, **800-822-7967**.

1. Hepatitis B vaccine (HepB). *(Minimum age: birth)*
  At birth:
- Administer monovalent HepB to all newborns before hospital discharge.
- If mother is hepatitis surface antigen (HBsAg)-positive, administer HepB and 0.5 mL of hepatitis B immune globulin (HBIG) within 12 hours of birth.
- If mother's HBsAg status is unknown, administer HepB within 12 hours of birth. Determine the HBsAg status as soon as possible and if HBsAg-positive, administer HBIG (no later than age 1 week).
- If mother is HBsAg-negative, the birth dose can only be delayed with physician's order and mother's negative HBsAg laboratory report documented in the infant's medical record.

  After the birth dose:
- The HepB series should be completed with either monovalent HepB or a combination vaccine containing HepB. The second dose should be administered at age 1–2 months. The final dose should be administered at age ≥24 weeks. Infants born to HBsAg-positive mothers should be tested for HBsAg and antibody to HBsAg after completion of ≥3 doses of a licensed HepB series, at age 9–18 months (generally at the next well-child visit).

  4-month dose:
- It is permissible to administer 4 doses of HepB when combination vaccines are administered after the birth dose. If monovalent HepB is used for doses after the birth dose, a dose at age 4 months is not needed.

2. Rotavirus vaccine (Rota). *(Minimum age: 6 weeks)*
- Administer the first dose at age 6–12 weeks. Do not start the series later than age 12 weeks.
- Administer the final dose in the series by age 32 weeks. Do not administer a dose later than age 32 weeks.
- Data on safety and efficacy outside of these age ranges are insufficient.

3. Diphtheria and tetanus toxoids and acellular pertussis vaccine (DTaP). *(Minimum age: 6 weeks)*
- The fourth dose of DTaP may be administered as early as age 12 months, provided 6 months have elapsed since the third dose.
- Administer the final dose in the series at age 4–6 years.

4. *Haemophilus influenzae* type b conjugate vaccine (Hib). *(Minimum age: 6 weeks)*
- If PRP-OMP (PedvaxHIB® or ComVax® [Merck]) is administered at ages 2 and 4 months, a dose at age 6 months is not required.
- TriHiBit® (DTaP/Hib) combination products should not be used for primary immunization but can be used as boosters following any Hib vaccine in children aged ≥12 months.

5. Pneumococcal vaccine. *(Minimum age: 6 weeks for pneumococcal conjugate vaccine [PCV]; 2 years for pneumococcal polysaccharide vaccine [PPV])*
- Administer PCV at ages 24–59 months in certain high-risk groups. Administer PPV to children aged ≥2 years in certain high-risk groups. See *MMWR* 2000;49(No. RR-9):1–35.

6. Influenza vaccine. *(Minimum age: 6 months for trivalent inactivated influenza vaccine [TIV]; 5 years for live, attenuated influenza vaccine [LAIV])*
- All children aged 6–59 months and close contacts of all children aged 0–59 months are recommended to receive influenza vaccine.
- Influenza vaccine is recommended annually for children aged ≥59 months with certain risk factors, health-care workers, and other persons (including household members) in close contact with persons in groups at high risk. See *MMWR* 2006;55(No. RR-10):1–41.
- For healthy persons aged 5–49 years, LAIV may be used as an alternative to TIV.
- Children receiving TIV should receive 0.25 mL if aged 6–35 months or 0.5 mL if aged ≥3 years.
- Children aged <9 years who are receiving influenza vaccine for the first time should receive 2 doses (separated by ≥4 weeks for TIV and ≥6 weeks for LAIV).

7. Measles, mumps, and rubella vaccine (MMR). *(Minimum age: 12 months)*
- Administer the second dose of MMR at age 4–6 years. MMR may be administered before age 4–6 years, provided ≥4 weeks have elapsed since the first dose and both doses are administered at age ≥12 months.

8. Varicella vaccine. *(Minimum age: 12 months)*
- Administer the second dose of varicella vaccine at age 4–6 years. Varicella vaccine may be administered before age 4–6 years, provided that ≥3 months have elapsed since the first dose and both doses are administered at age ≥12 months. If second dose was administered ≥28 days following the first dose, the second dose does not need to be repeated.

9. Hepatitis A vaccine (HepA). *(Minimum age: 12 months)*
- HepA is recommended for all children aged 1 year (i.e., aged 12–23 months). The 2 doses in the series should be administered at least 6 months apart.
- Children not fully vaccinated by age 2 years can be vaccinated at subsequent visits.
- HepA is recommended for certain other groups of children, including in areas where vaccination programs target older children. See *MMWR* 2006;55(No. RR-7):1–23.

10. Meningococcal polysaccharide vaccine (MPSV4). *(Minimum age: 2 years)*
- Administer MPSV4 to children aged 2–10 years with terminal complement deficiencies or anatomic or functional asplenia and certain other high-risk groups. See *MMWR* 2005;54(No. RR-7):1–21.

The Recommended Immunization Schedules for Persons Aged 0–18 Years are approved by the Advisory Committee on Immunization Practices (http://www.cdc.gov/nip/acip), the American Academy of Pediatrics (http://www.aap.org), and the American Academy of Family Physicians (http://www.aafp.org).

SAFER · HEALTHIER · PEOPLE™

CS103164

Figure 20-6 Recommended immunization schedule for persons aged 0–6 years—United States, 2007.

DEPARTMENT OF HEALTH AND HUMAN SERVICES • CENTERS FOR DISEASE CONTROL AND PREVENTION

Recommended Immunization Schedule for Persons Aged 7–18 Years—UNITED STATES • 2007

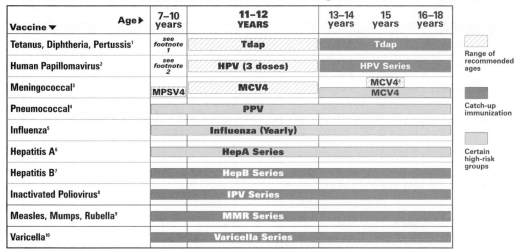

Vaccine ▼ Age ▶	7–10 years	11–12 YEARS	13–14 years	15 years	16–18 years
Tetanus, Diphtheria, Pertussis[1]	see footnote 1	Tdap	Tdap		
Human Papillomavirus[2]	see footnote 2	HPV (3 doses)	HPV Series		
Meningococcal[3]	MPSV4	MCV4	MCV4[3] / MCV4		
Pneumococcal[4]		PPV			
Influenza[5]		Influenza (Yearly)			
Hepatitis A[6]		HepA Series			
Hepatitis B[7]		HepB Series			
Inactivated Poliovirus[8]		IPV Series			
Measles, Mumps, Rubella[9]		MMR Series			
Varicella[10]		Varicella Series			

Range of recommended ages

Catch-up immunization

Certain high-risk groups

This schedule indicates the recommended ages for routine administration of currently licensed childhood vaccines, as of December 1, 2006, for children aged 7–18 years. Additional information is available at http://www.cdc.gov/nip/recs/child-schedule.htm. Any dose not administered at the recommended age should be administered at any subsequent visit, when indicated and feasible. Additional vaccines may be licensed and recommended during the year. Licensed combination vaccines may be used whenever any components of the combination are indicated and other components of the vaccine are not contraindicated and if approved by the Food and Drug Administration for that dose of the series. Providers should consult the respective Advisory Committee on Immunization Practices statement for detailed recommendations. Clinically significant adverse events that follow immunization should be reported to the Vaccine Adverse Event Reporting System (VAERS). Guidance about how to obtain and complete a VAERS form is available at http://www.vaers.hhs.gov or by telephone, 800-822-7967.

1. Tetanus and diphtheria toxoids and acellular pertussis vaccine (Tdap).
(Minimum age: 10 years for BOOSTRIX® and 11 years for ADACEL™)
• Administer at age 11–12 years for those who have completed the recommended childhood DTP/DTaP vaccination series and have not received a tetanus and diphtheria toxoids vaccine (Td) booster dose.
• Adolescents aged 13–18 years who missed the 11–12 year Td/Tdap booster dose should also receive a single dose of Tdap if they have completed the recommended childhood DTP/DTaP vaccination series.

2. Human papillomavirus (HPV). *(Minimum age: 9 years)*
• Administer the first dose of the HPV vaccine series to females at age 11–12 years.
• Administer the second dose 2 months after the first dose and the third dose 6 months after the first dose.
• Administer the HPV vaccine series to females at age 13–18 years if not previously vaccinated.

3. Meningococcal vaccine. *(Minimum age: 11 years for meningococcal conjugate vaccine [MCV4]; 2 years for meningococcal polysaccharide vaccine [MPSV4])*
• Administer MCV4 at age 11–12 years and to previously unvaccinated adolescents at high school entry (at approximately age 15 years).
• Administer MCV4 to previously unvaccinated college freshmen living in dormitories; MPSV4 is an acceptable alternative.
• Vaccination against invasive meningococcal disease is recommended for children and adolescents aged ≥2 years with terminal complement deficiencies or anatomic or functional asplenia and certain other high-risk groups. See *MMWR* 2005;54(No. RR-7):1–21. Use MPSV4 for children aged 2–10 years and MCV4 or MPSV4 for older children.

4. Pneumococcal polysaccharide vaccine (PPV). *(Minimum age: 2 years)*
• Administer for certain high-risk groups. See *MMWR* 1997;46(No. RR-8):1–24, and *MMWR* 2000;49(No. RR-9):1–35.

5. Influenza vaccine. *(Minimum age: 6 months for trivalent inactivated influenza vaccine [TIV]; 5 years for live, attenuated influenza vaccine [LAIV])*
• Influenza vaccine is recommended annually for persons with certain risk factors, health-care workers, and other persons (including household members) in close contact with persons in groups at high risk. See *MMWR* 2006;55 (No. RR-10):1–41.
• For healthy persons aged 5–49 years, LAIV may be used as an alternative to TIV.
• Children aged <9 years who are receiving influenza vaccine for the first time should receive 2 doses (separated by ≥4 weeks for TIV and ≥6 weeks for LAIV).

6. Hepatitis A vaccine (HepA). *(Minimum age: 12 months)*
• The 2 doses in the series should be administered at least 6 months apart.
• HepA is recommended for certain other groups of children, including in areas where vaccination programs target older children. See *MMWR* 2006;55 (No. RR-7):1–23.

7. Hepatitis B vaccine (HepB). *(Minimum age: birth)*
• Administer the 3-dose series to those who were not previously vaccinated.
• A 2-dose series of Recombivax HB® is licensed for children aged 11–15 years.

8. Inactivated poliovirus vaccine (IPV). *(Minimum age: 6 weeks)*
• For children who received an all-IPV or all-oral poliovirus (OPV) series, a fourth dose is not necessary if the third dose was administered at age ≥4 years.
• If both OPV and IPV were administered as part of a series, a total of 4 doses should be administered, regardless of the child's current age.

9. Measles, mumps, and rubella vaccine (MMR). *(Minimum age: 12 months)*
• If not previously vaccinated, administer 2 doses of MMR during any visit, with ≥4 weeks between the doses.

10. Varicella vaccine. *(Minimum age: 12 months)*
• Administer 2 doses of varicella vaccine to persons without evidence of immunity.
• Administer 2 doses of varicella vaccine to persons aged <13 years at least 3 months apart. Do not repeat the second dose, if administered ≥28 days after the first dose.
• Administer 2 doses of varicella vaccine to persons aged ≥13 years at least 4 weeks apart.

The Recommended Immunization Schedules for Persons Aged 0–18 Years are approved by the Advisory Committee on Immunization Practices (http://www.cdc.gov/nip/acip), the American Academy of Pediatrics (http://www.aap.org), and the American Academy of Family Physicians (http://www.aafp.org).

SAFER · HEALTHIER · PEOPLE™

CS100131

Figure 20-7 Recommended immunization schedule for persons aged 7–18—United States, 2007.

Catch-up Immunization Schedule
for Persons Aged 4 Months–18 Years Who Start Late or Who Are More Than 1 Month Behind

UNITED STATES • 2007

The table below provides catch-up schedules and minimum intervals between doses for children whose vaccinations have been delayed. A vaccine series does not need to be restarted, regardless of the time that has elapsed between doses. Use the section appropriate for the child's age.

CATCH-UP SCHEDULE FOR PERSONS AGED 4 MONTHS–6 YEARS

Vaccine	Minimum Age for Dose 1	Minimum Interval Between Doses			
		Dose 1 to Dose 2	Dose 2 to Dose 3	Dose 3 to Dose 4	Dose 4 to Dose 5
Hepatitis B[1]	Birth	4 weeks	8 weeks (and 16 weeks after first dose)		
Rotavirus[2]	6 wks	4 weeks	4 weeks		
Diphtheria, Tetanus, Pertussis[3]	6 wks	4 weeks	4 weeks	6 months	6 months[3]
Haemophilus influenzae type b[4]	6 wks	**4 weeks** if first dose administered at age <12 months **8 weeks (as final dose)** if first dose administered at age 12-14 months **No further doses needed** if first dose administered at age ≥15 months	**4 weeks**[4] if current age <12 months **8 weeks (as final dose)**[4] if current age ≥12 months and second dose administered at age <15 months **No further doses needed** if previous dose administered at age ≥15 months	**8 weeks (as final dose)** This dose only necessary for children aged 12 months–5 years who received 3 doses before age 12 months	
Pneumococcal[5]	6 wks	**4 weeks** if first dose administered at age <12 months and current age <24 months **8 weeks (as final dose)** if first dose administered at age ≥12 months or current age 24–59 months **No further doses needed** for healthy children if first dose administered at age ≥24 months	**4 weeks** if current age <12 months **8 weeks (as final dose)** if current age ≥12 months **No further doses needed** for healthy children if previous dose administered at age ≥24 months	**8 weeks (as final dose)** This dose only necessary for children aged 12 months–5 years who received 3 doses before age 12 months	
Inactivated Poliovirus[6]	6 wks	4 weeks	4 weeks	4 weeks[6]	
Measles, Mumps, Rubella[7]	12 mos	4 weeks			
Varicella[8]	12 mos	3 months			
Hepatitis A[9]	12 mos	6 months			

CATCH-UP SCHEDULE FOR PERSONS AGED 7–18 YEARS

Vaccine	Minimum Age for Dose 1	Dose 1 to Dose 2	Dose 2 to Dose 3	Dose 3 to Dose 4	Dose 4 to Dose 5
Tetanus, Diphtheria/ Tetanus, Diphtheria, Pertussis[10]	7 yrs[10]	4 weeks	**8 weeks** if first dose administered at age <12 months **6 months** if first dose administered at age ≥12 months	**6 months** if first dose administered at age <12 months	
Human Papillomavirus[11]	9 yrs	12 weeks			
Hepatitis A[9]	12 mos	6 months			
Hepatitis B[1]	Birth	4 weeks	8 weeks (and 16 weeks after first dose)		
Inactivated Poliovirus[6]	6 wks	4 weeks	4 weeks	4 weeks[6]	
Measles, Mumps, Rubella[7]	12 mos	4 weeks			
Varicella[8]	12 mos	**4 weeks** if first dose administered at age ≥13 years **3 months** if first dose administered at age <13 years			

1. Hepatitis B vaccine (HepB). *(Minimum age: birth)*
- Administer the 3-dose series to those who were not previously vaccinated.
- A 2-dose series of Recombivax HB® is licensed for children aged 11–15 years.

2. Rotavirus vaccine (Rota). *(Minimum age: 6 weeks)*
- Do not start the series later than age 12 weeks.
- Administer the final dose in the series by age 32 weeks. Do not administer a dose later than age 32 weeks.
- Data on safety and efficacy outside of these age ranges are insufficient.

3. Diphtheria and tetanus toxoids and acellular pertussis vaccine (DTaP). *(Minimum age: 6 weeks)*
- The fifth dose is not necessary if the fourth dose was administered at age ≥4 years.
- DTaP is not indicated for persons aged ≥7 years.

4. *Haemophilus influenzae* type b conjugate vaccine (Hib). *(Minimum age: 6 weeks)*
- Vaccine is not generally recommended for children aged ≥5 years.
- If current age <12 months and the first 2 doses were PRP-OMP (PedvaxHIB® or ComVax® [Merck]), the third (and final) dose should be administered at age 12–15 months and at least 8 weeks after the second dose.
- If first dose was administered at age 7–11 months, administer 2 doses separated by 4 weeks plus a booster at age 12–15 months.

5. Pneumococcal conjugate vaccine (PCV). *(Minimum age: 6 weeks)*
- Vaccine is not generally recommended for children aged ≥5 years.

6. Inactivated poliovirus vaccine (IPV). *(Minimum age: 6 weeks)*
- For children who received an all-IPV or all-oral poliovirus (OPV) series, a fourth dose is not necessary if third dose was administered at age ≥4 years.
- If both OPV and IPV were administered as part of a series, a total of 4 doses should be administered, regardless of the child's current age.

7. Measles, mumps, and rubella vaccine (MMR). *(Minimum age: 12 months)*
- The second dose of MMR is recommended routinely at age 4–6 years but may be administered earlier if desired.
- If not previously vaccinated, administer 2 doses of MMR during any visit with ≥4 weeks between the doses.

8. Varicella vaccine. *(Minimum age: 12 months)*
- The second dose of varicella vaccine is recommended routinely at age 4–6 years but may be administered earlier if desired.
- Do not repeat the second dose in persons aged <13 years if administered ≥28 days after the first dose.

9. Hepatitis A vaccine (HepA). *(Minimum age: 12 months)*
- HepA is recommended for certain groups of children, including in areas where vaccination programs target older children. See *MMWR* 2006;55(No. RR-7):1–23.

10. Tetanus and diphtheria toxoids vaccine (Td) and tetanus and diphtheria toxoids and acellular pertussis vaccine (Tdap). *(Minimum ages: 7 years for Td, 10 years for BOOSTRIX®, and 11 years for ADACEL™)*
- Tdap should be substituted for a single dose of Td in the primary catch-up series or as a booster if age appropriate; use Td for other doses.
- A 5-year interval from the last Td dose is encouraged when Tdap is used as a booster dose. A booster (fourth) dose is needed if any of the previous doses were administered at age <12 months. Refer to ACIP recommendations for further information. See *MMWR* 2006;55(No. RR-3).

11. Human papillomavirus vaccine (HPV). *(Minimum age: 9 years)*
- Administer the HPV vaccine series to females at age 13–18 years if not previously vaccinated.

Information about reporting reactions after immunization is available online at **http://www.vaers.hhs.gov** or by telephone via the 24-hour national toll-free information line 800-822-7967. Suspected cases of vaccine-preventable diseases should be reported to the state or local health department. Additional information, including precautions and contraindications for immunization, is available from the National Center for Immunization and Respiratory Diseases at **http://www.cdc.gov/nip/default.htm** or telephone, **800-CDC-INFO (800-232-4636).**

DEPARTMENT OF HEALTH AND HUMAN SERVICES • CENTERS FOR DISEASE CONTROL AND PREVENTION • SAFER • HEALTHIER • PEOPLE

CS103164

Figure 20-8 Catch-up immunization schedule for persons aged 4 months to 18 years who start late or who are more than 1 month behind—United States, 2007.

Recommended Adult Immunization Schedule
United States, October 2006–September 2007

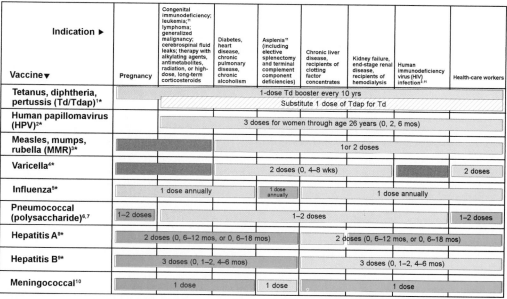

Figure 20-9a Recommended adult immunization schedule—United States, October 2006–September 2007.

Footnotes

1. Tetanus, diphtheria, and acellular pertussis (Td/Tdap) vaccination.
Adults with uncertain histories of a complete primary vaccination series with diphtheria and tetanus toxoid–containing vaccines should begin or complete a primary vaccination series. A primary series for adults is 3 doses; administer the first 2 doses at least 4 weeks apart and the third dose 6–12 months after the second. Administer a booster dose to adults who have completed a primary series and if the last vaccination was received ≥10 years previously. Tdap or tetanus and diphtheria (Td) vaccine may be used; Tdap should replace a single dose of Td for adults aged <65 years who have not previously received a dose of Tdap (either in the primary series, as a booster, or for wound management). Only one of two Tdap products (Adacel® [sanofi pasteur, Swiftwater, Pennsylvania]) is licensed for use in adults. If the person is pregnant and received the last Td vaccination ≥10 years previously, administer Td during the second or third trimester; if the person received the last Td vaccination in <10 years, administer Tdap during the immediate postpartum period. A one-time administration of 1-dose of Tdap with an interval as short as 2 years from a previous Td vaccination is recommended for postpartum women, close contacts of infants aged <12 months, and all health-care workers with direct patient contact. In certain situations, Td can be deferred during pregnancy and Tdap substituted in the immediate postpartum period, or Tdap can be given instead of Td to a pregnant woman after an informed discussion with the woman (see http://www.cdc.gov/nip/publications/acip-list.htm). Consult the ACIP statement for recommendations for administering Td as prophylaxis in wound management (http://www.cdc.gov/mmwr/preview/mmwrhtml/00041645.htm).

2. Human Papillomavirus (HPV) vaccination. HPV vaccination is recommended for all women aged ≤26 years who have not completed the vaccine series. Ideally, vaccine should be administered before potential exposure to HPV through sexual activity; however, women who are sexually active should still be vaccinated. Sexually active women who have not been infected with any of the HPV vaccine types receive the full benefit of the vaccination. Vaccination is less beneficial for women who have already been infected with one or more of the four HPV vaccine types. A complete series consists of 3 doses. The second dose should be administered 2 months after the first dose; the third dose should be administered 6 months after the first dose. Vaccination is not recommended during pregnancy. If a woman is found to be pregnant after initiating the vaccination series, the remainder of the 3-dose regimen should be delayed until after completion of the pregnancy.

3. Measles, Mumps, Rubella (MMR) vaccination. *Measles component:* adults born before 1957 can be considered immune to measles. Adults born during or after 1957 should receive ≥1 dose of MMR unless they have a medical contraindication, documentation of ≥1 dose, history of measles based on health-care provider diagnosis, or laboratory evidence of immunity. A second dose of MMR is recommended for adults who 1) have been recently exposed to measles or in an outbreak setting; 2) were previously vaccinated with killed measles vaccine; 3) have been vaccinated with an unknown type of measles vaccine during 1963–1967; 4) are students in postsecondary educational institutions; 5) work in a health-care facility, or 6) plan to travel internationally. Withhold MMR or other measles-containing vaccines from HIV-infected persons with severe immunosuppression. *Mumps component:* adults born before 1957 can generally be considered immune to mumps. Adults born during or after 1957 should receive 1 dose of MMR unless they have a medical contraindication, history of mumps based on health-care provider diagnosis, or laboratory evidence of immunity. A second dose of MMR is recommended for adults who 1) are in an age group that is affected during a mumps outbreak; 2) are students in postsecondary educational institutions; 3) work in a health-care facility; or 4) plan to travel internationally. For unvaccinated health-care workers born before 1957 who do not have other evidence of mumps immunity, consider giving 1 dose on a routine basis and strongly consider giving a second dose during an outbreak. *Rubella component:* administer 1 dose of MMR vaccine to women whose rubella vaccination history is unreliable or who lack laboratory evidence of immunity. For women of childbearing age, regardless of birth year, routinely determine rubella immunity and counsel women regarding congenital rubella syndrome. Do not vaccinate women who are pregnant or who might become pregnant within 4 weeks of receiving vaccine. Women who do not have evidence of immunity should receive MMR vaccine upon completion or termination of pregnancy and before discharge from the health-care facility.

4. Varicella vaccination. All adults without evidence of immunity to varicella should receive 2 doses of varicella vaccine. Special consideration should be given to those who 1) have close contact with persons at high risk for severe disease (e.g., health-care workers and family contacts of immunocompromised persons) or 2) are at high risk for exposure or transmission (e.g., teachers of young children; child care employees; residents and staff members of institutional settings, including correctional institutions; college students; military personnel; adolescents and adults living in households with children; non-pregnant women of childbearing age; and international travelers). Evidence of immunity to varicella in adults includes any of the following: 1) documentation of 2 doses of varicella vaccine at least 4 weeks apart; 2) U.S.–born before 1980 (although for health-care workers and pregnant women, birth before 1980 should not be considered evidence of immunity); 3) history of varicella based on diagnosis or verification of varicella by a health-care provider (for a patient reporting a history of or presenting with an atypical case, a mild case, or both, health-care providers should seek either an epidemiologic link with a typical varicella case or evidence of laboratory confirmation, if it was performed at the time of acute disease); 4) history of herpes zoster based on health-care provider diagnosis; or 5) laboratory evidence of immunity or laboratory confirmation of disease. Do not vaccinate women who are pregnant or might become pregnant within 4 weeks of receiving the vaccine. Assess pregnant women for evidence of varicella immunity. Women who do not have evidence of immunity should receive dose 1 of varicella vaccine upon completion or termination of pregnancy and before discharge from the health-care facility. Dose 2 should be administered 4–8 weeks after dose 1.

5. Influenza vaccination: *Medical indications:* chronic disorders of the cardiovascular or pulmonary systems, including asthma; chronic metabolic diseases, including diabetes mellitus, renal dysfunction, hemoglobinopathies, or immunosuppression (including immunosuppression caused by medications or HIV); any condition that compromises respiratory function or the handling of respiratory secretions or that can increase the risk of aspiration (e.g., cognitive dysfunction, spinal cord injury, or seizure disorder or other neuromuscular disorder); and pregnancy during the influenza season. No data exist on the risk for severe or complicated influenza disease among persons with asplenia; however, influenza is a risk factor for secondary bacterial infections that can cause severe disease among persons with asplenia. *Occupational indications:* health-care workers and employees of long-term–care and assisted living facilities. *Other indications:* residents of nursing homes and other long-term–care and assisted living facilities; persons likely to transmit influenza to persons at high risk (i.e., in-home household contacts and caregivers of children aged 0–59 months, or persons of all ages with high-risk conditions); and anyone who would like to be vaccinated. Healthy, nonpregnant persons aged 5–49 years without high-risk medical conditions who are not contacts of severely immunocompromised persons in special care units can receive either intranasally administered influenza vaccine (FluMist®) or inactivated vaccine. Other persons should receive the inactivated vaccine.

Figure 20-9b Footnotes.

Footnotes

6. Pneumococcal polysaccharide vaccination. *Medical indications:* chronic disorders of the pulmonary system (excluding asthma); cardiovascular diseases; diabetes mellitus; chronic liver diseases, including liver disease as a result of alcohol abuse (e.g.,cirrhosis); chronic renal failure or nephrotic syndrome; functional or anatomic asplenia (e.g., sickle cell disease or splenectomy [if elective splenectomy is planned, vaccinate at least 2 weeks before surgery]); immunosuppressive conditions (e.g., congenital immunodeficiency, HIV infection [vaccinate as close to diagnosis as possible when CD4 cell counts are highest], leukemia, lymphoma, multiple myeloma, Hodgkin disease, generalized malignancy, organ or bone marrow transplantation); chemotherapy with alkylating agents, antimetabolites, or high-dose, long-term corticosteroids; and cochlear implants. *Other indications:* Alaska Natives and certain American Indian populations and residents of nursing homes or other long-term–care facilities.

7. Revaccination with pneumococcal polysaccharide vaccine. One-time revaccination after 5 years for persons with chronic renal failure or nephrotic syndrome; functional or anatomic asplenia (e.g., sickle cell disease or splenectomy); immunosuppressive conditions (e.g., congenital immuno-deficiency, HIV infection, leukemia, lymphoma, multiple myeloma, Hodgkin disease, generalized malignancy, or organ or bone marrow transplantation); or chemotherapy with alkylating agents, antimetabolites, or high-dose, long-term corticosteroids. For persons aged ≥ 65 years, one-time revaccination if they were vaccinated ≥ 5 years previously and were aged <65 years at the time of primary vaccination.

8. Hepatitis A vaccination. *Medical indications:* persons with chronic liver disease and persons who receive clotting factor concentrates. *Behavioral indications:* men who have sex with men and persons who use illegal drugs. *Occupational indications:* persons working with hepatitis A virus (HAV)–infected primates or with HAV in a research laboratory setting. *Other indications:* persons traveling to or working in countries that have high or intermediate endemicity of hepatitis A (a list of countries is available at http://www.cdc.gov/travel/diseases.htm) and any person who would like to obtain immunity. Current vaccines should be administered in a 2-dose schedule at either 0 and 6–12 months, or 0 and 6–18 months. If the combined hepatitis A and hepatitis B vaccine is used, administer 3 doses at 0, 1, and 6 months .

9. Hepatitis B vaccination. *Medical indications:* Persons with end-stage renal disease, including patients receiving hemodialysis; persons seeking evaluation or treatment for a sexually transmitted disease (STD); persons with HIV infection; persons with chronic liver disease; and persons who receive clotting factor concentrates. *Occupational indications:* health-care workers and public-safety workers who are exposed to blood or other potentially infectious body fluids. *Behavioral indications:* sexually active persons who are not in a long-term, mutually monogamous relationship (i.e., persons with >1 sex partner during the previous 6 months); current or recent injection-drug users; and men who have sex with men. *Other indications:* household contacts and sex partners of persons with chronic hepatitis B virus (HBV) infection; clients and staff members of institutions for persons with developmental disabilities; all clients of STD clinics; international travelers to countries with high or intermediate prevalence of chronic HBV infection (a list of countries is available at http://www.cdc.gov/travel/diseases.htm); and any adult seeking protection from HBV infection. Settings where hepatitis B vaccination is recommended for all adults: STD treatment facilities; HIV testing and treatment facilities; facilities providing drug-abuse treatment and prevention services; health-care settings providing services for injection-drug users or men who have sex with men; correctional facilities; end-stage renal disease programs and facilities for chronic hemodialysis patients; and institutions and nonresidential daycare facilities for persons with developmental disabilities. *Special formulation indications:* for adult patients receiving hemodialysis and other immunocompromised adults, 1 dose of 40 μg/mL (Recombivax HB®) or 2 doses of 20 μg/mL (Engerix-B®).

10. Meningococcal vaccination. *Medical indications:* adults with anatomic or functional asplenia, or terminal complement component deficiencies. *Other indications:* first-year college students living in dormitories; microbiologists who are routinely exposed to isolates of *Neisseria meningitidis;* military recruits; and persons who travel to or live in countries in which meningococcal disease is hyperendemic or epidemic (e.g., the "meningitis belt" of Sub-Saharan Africa during the dry season [December–June]), particularly if contact with local populations will be prolonged. Vaccination is required by the government of Saudi Arabia for all travelers to Mecca during the annual Hajj. Meningococcal conjugate vaccine is preferred for adults with any of the preceeding indications who are aged ≤ 55 years, although meningococcal polysaccharide vaccine (MPSV4) is an acceptable alternative. Revaccination after 5 years might be indicated for adults previously vaccinated with MPSV4 who remain at high risk for infection (e.g., persons residing in areas in which disease is epidemic).

11. Selected conditions for which *Haemophilus influenzae* type b (Hib) vaccination may be used. Hib conjugate vaccines are licensed for children aged 6 weeks–71 months. No efficacy data are available on which to base a recommendation concerning use of Hib vaccine for older children and adults with the chronic conditions associated with an increased risk for Hib disease. However, studies suggest good immunogenicity in patients who have sickle cell disease, leukemia, or HIV infection or have had splenectomies; administering vaccine to these patients is not contraindicated.

This schedule indicates the recommended age groups and medical indications for routine administration of currently licensed vaccines for persons aged ≥ 19 years, as of October 1, 2006. Licensed combination vaccines may be used whenever any components of the combination are indicated and when the vaccine's other components are not contraindicated. For detailed recommendations on all vaccines, including those used primarily for travelers or that are issued during the year, consult the manufacturers' package inserts and the complete statements from the Advisory Committee on Immunization Practices (http://www.cdc.gov/nip/publications/acip-list.htm).

Report all clinically significant postvaccination reactions to the Vaccine Adverse Event Reporting System (VAERS). Reporting forms and instructions on filing a VAERS report are available at http://www.vaers.hhs.gov or by telephone, 800-822-7967.

Information on how to file a Vaccine Injury Compensation Program claim is available at http://www.hrsa.gov/vaccinecompensation or by telephone, 800-338-2382. To file a claim for vaccine injury, contact the U.S. Court of Federal Claims, 717 Madison Place, N.W., Washington, D.C. 20005; telephone, 202-357-6400.

Additional information about the vaccines in this schedule and contraindications for vaccination is also available at http://www.cdc.gov/nip or from the CDC-INFO Contact Center at 800-CDC-INFO (800-232-4636) in English and Spanish, 24 hours a day, 7 days a week.

**Approved by the Advisory Committee on Immunization Practices,
the American College of Obstetricians and Gynecologists, the American Academy of Family Physicians,
and the American College of Physicians**

Figure 20-9c Footnotes.

provider or through client referral. Provider referral occurs when a designated health care provider obtains the names of possible contacts and then notifies them of their need for evaluation and possible treatment. Client referral involves the client notifying his or her contacts personally. Public health nurses are often involved in contact notification. During this process the public health nurse (PHN) may conduct the initial interview in which names and addresses of contacts are provided, make home or worksite visits to inform contacts of their need for testing, and provide education and referral for treatment and follow-up. Contact notification is done to provide access to chemoprophylaxis, the use of antimicrobial drugs to prevent the acquisition of pathogens, for those who may not yet be symptomatic. Prophylaxis may include immediate immunization or booster vaccinations, antitoxins, immune globulins, antibiotics, or antiviral medications. Strict policies and procedures are implemented to ensure that confidentiality is maintained. Common diseases requiring contact notification include gonorrhea, syphilis, diphtheria, tetanus, hepatitis A and B, syphilis, and HIV.

Public health nurses also are often part of the enforcement of chemoprophylaxis to protect the general public or other vulnerable populations. For example, they may be part of directly observed treatment (DOT) to ensure those infected with tuberculosis are not contagious. In DOT, if the nurse cannot personally observe the person taking the TB medication, they are authorized to enlist the assistance of law enforcement to find the infected person and require they take the medication. Some states require all pregnant women to be tested for HIV as part of efforts to provide chemoprophylaxis for the newborn infant. The drug Zidovudine (AZT) is used prenatally, during delivery, and as an elixir for the newborn infant to reduce the transmission of the HIV from mother to child.

Other primary prevention measures include the use of protective clothing to prevent exposure to pathogens or the use of barrier protection, such as condoms for sexually transmitted diseases. Harm reduction strategies such as needle exchange programs for intravenous drug users prevent the spread of hepatitis B, C, and D and HIV. Universal precautions among those in occupations that handle blood, or other body secretions and excretions, provide primary prevention for contagious diseases. For example, improving sanitation and handwashing can reduce the incidence of hepatitis A and E. Public education and planning increases the likelihood of preventing the spread of communicable disease, even among high-risk populations.

Secondary Prevention

When primary prevention fails and infection occurs, secondary prevention provides for early detection through screening, and management of disease progression through diagnosis and treatment. Screening may be part of other community activities or may be targeted to specific populations or locations where high-risk individuals live or work. Public health nurses are often involved in planning and conducting both targeted and public screening events.

Screening

Screening is intended to identify individuals who are not symptomatic and may not yet know they are infected. This would include diseases such as hepatitis A and B, TB, gonorrhea, syphilis, herpes simplex virus (HSV), chlamydia, and HIV. Anonymous testing allows those worried about confidentiality to become informed of their disease status; however, anonymous testing is increasingly being replaced by confidential testing to provide data for disease tracking and contact notification. Same day results are preferred for screening individuals who may not return for follow-up visits.

Screening occurs in many sites throughout the community. Occupational health work site clinics provide confidential access to screening for many people unable or unwilling to access public clinics. Community-based education and outreach programs often include spontaneous screening to those identified to be in need. Donating blood is another way some people access screening because the American Association of Blood Banks requires screening of all donated blood for a variety of communicable diseases, including HIV and Hepatitis C. In the justice system, correctional institutions require TB screening and treatment of all those held for any period of time.

Early Diagnosis

The early diagnosis of a communicable disease is done in two ways. Laboratory tests can be performed to document the presence of the causative organism and/or blood tests can indicate the presence of disease due to specific changes or markers in the blood. The detection of antibodies is a direct way to diagnose diseases such as hepatitis and HIV. For some diseases, such as gonorrhea and chlamydia, the organism must be grown in a culture for identification; the initial diagnosis of other diseases may be based on physical signs and symptoms, followed up by laboratory or blood testing.

Public health nurses collect the blood samples or other specimens for testing at specialized laboratories. They may be involved in informing those involved of the test results and providing education and referral for treatment and follow-up if necessary. They are also included in the collection and processing data for epidemiological investigations.

Treatment

Treatment of a person or population with a communicable disease may be as simple as comfort measures and symptom management or may involve complex interventions and pharmaceutical protocols. As mentioned previously, those living with TB are required by law to manage their disease, and often this is done with the help of community nurses who enforce DOT. The treatment of communicable diseases is guided by national recommendations such as those provided by the CDC for the treatment of sexually transmitted diseases. The diagnosis and initiation of treatment may include confidential notification to appropriate public health authorities for tracking the incidence and prevalence of specific diseases.

When people diagnosed with a communicable disease do not adhere to their treatment regimens, serious complications can happen. Pathogens can become drug-resistant when those taking specific medications fail to complete the full course of treatment. This allows some pathogens to survive and creates an opportunity for others to mutate. *Mycobacterium avium,* gonococcal organisms, and TB are three pathogens that have developed resistance to multiple antibiotics (National Center for Infectious Diseases, 2005). The role of the PHN is to educate and encourage clients to complete their full treatment protocol. Public health nurses may also be involved in advocating for those who experience difficulty accessing diagnosis and treatment.

Tertiary Prevention

Efforts to prevent and detect disease early are not always successful. Tertiary prevention and care is provided for individuals who suffer ongoing long-term physical and emotional challenges from communicable diseases. The focus of tertiary care is the prevention and management of complications of the side effects of treatment, as well as reducing potential harm to others. Public health nurses may have relationships with clients and their families over long periods of time. This may include assisting clients with lifestyle changes, making arrangements for rehabilitative or home-based services, communicating with other health care providers regarding medication dosage changes or simplification of treatment regimens, and planning with family and friends for ongoing support when the progression of disease requires a higher level of care.

Public health nurses are part of interdisciplinary teams when families face the obstacles of long-term management of the consequences of a communicable disease. For example, families with children who have mental retardation or disabilities due to congenital syphilis or rubella face a lifetime of emotional and physical challenges. People living with hepatitis or HIV may need assistance learning how to protect others from infection and how to deal with discrimination. On a policy level, public health nurses advocate for the public support of programs that provide services such as housing, home-care, and financial assistance for clients and families.

COMMON INFECTIOUS AND COMMUNICABLE DISEASES

There are several categories of infectious and communicable diseases; all have implications for the public health nurse.

Food-borne and Water-borne Diseases

Food-borne diseases, including intoxications and infections, are illnesses caused by consuming contaminated food and are often called "food poisoning." These include diseases caused by chemical contaminants such as heavy metals and organic substances; however, the more common food-borne illnesses are due to bacterial toxins in food, and parasitic, viral or bacterial infections. Food intoxication is caused by toxins found in natural sources such as shellfish and mushrooms, in bacterial growth such as botulism, and in chemical contaminants such as mercury poisoning. Food infections come from parasites, viruses, or bacteria found in food. These include pathogens that cause diseases such as trichinosis, salmonellosis, *Escherichia coli* diarrhea, toxoplasmosis, and hepatitis A.

Timing is often a clue to the source of a food-borne illness. Food-borne illness is difficult to identify, especially in single cases. An infectious agent usually causes illness within 12 hours to several days after eating contaminated food. Intoxicants can cause illness within minutes or hours after ingestion. Laboratory analysis of both human and implicated food specimens must be prompt and thorough to identify a causative agent. Food-borne illness may be one of the most common causes of unrecognized and unreported acute illness (Heymann, 2004).

Preventing and controlling any food-borne illness involves avoiding contamination, destroying the contaminant, and preventing further multiplication or spread of the contaminant. Prevention is the responsibility of anyone who handles food and requires attention to the storage, preparation, and cooking of food. The WHO has developed a document for use worldwide called "Five Keys to Safer Food" (see Box 20-1).

Salmonellosis

Salmonellosis is a bacterial illness that is common and usually unreported. It is most serious in infants and small children, but it is dangerous for the elderly and the debilitated. It has onset within 28 hours with symptoms of fever, headache, abdominal pain, diarrhea, and nausea, which make it similar to other gastrointestinal problems. Dehydration may be the greatest risk, and symptoms may persist for several days (Heymann, 2004).

Escherichia coli Diarrhea

Escherichia coli diarrhea came to public attention in 1992 following two outbreaks of illness associated with undercooked hamburgers in a fast-food restaurant. However, *E. coli* may be responsible for over 500 deaths per year. It is a serotype of *E. coli*, which creates a cryotoxin that can cause fatal hemorrhagic colitis. It has been found in roast beef, underpasturized milk and apple cider, alfalfa sprouts, spinach, and municipal water. *Escherichia coli* is diagnosed by onset of severe symptoms including bloody diarrhea and abdominal cramps and may or may not include fever. Children in day care and the elderly in assisted living facilities are at greatest risk for serious disease and complications. Prevention of illness requires thorough cooking of all

---

BOX 20-1: Five Keys to Safer Food

1. Keep clean
2. Separate raw and cooked
3. Cook thoroughly
4. Keep food at safe temperatures
5. Use safe water and raw materials

SOURCE: Heymann (2004). Copyright 2004 by the American Public Health Association.

---

meat and careful washing of fruits and vegetables that may have organic contamination (National Center for Infectious Diseases, 2005).

Vector-borne Diseases

Vectors are carriers of disease and are usually animals, insects, and birds. The vector may be an essential part of the development of the disease and therefore be transmitting the disease biologically, such as mosquitoes that carry malaria. Cockroaches, flies, and ticks are mechanical vectors because they carry the infectious agent on some part of their body. Especially in rural areas where humans live and work closely with agricultural animals, humans may acquire diseases through their contacts with these animals. Anthrax, brucellosis, and mad cow disease are diseases of cattle which may be acquired by humans. Usually, there is no person-to-person transmission, since humans are incidental hosts. Currently, the World Health Organization is monitoring the spread of avian flu. As yet, it is unclear that person-to-person spread is possible. This is a disease of poultry and wild birds that humans can acquire by ingesting the meat of infected birds.

Lyme Disease

In 1975, people in Old Lyme, Connecticut, noticed an increasing incidence of rheumatoid arthritis among their children. In 1982, the cause of this arthritis was found to be Ixodid ticks commonly found on white-tailed deer and white-footed mice. Lyme disease is now the most common vector-borne disease in the United

⊕ RESEARCH APPLICATION

Factors Influencing the Utilization of Lyme Disease-Prevention Behaviors in a High-Risk Population

Study Purpose

To evaluate factors motivating high-risk individuals to implement Lyme disease-prevention behaviors.

Methods

Clients presenting to a Lyme Disease Diagnostic Center in New York State were asked to complete a questionnaire while waiting to be evaluated. The questionnaire included demographic, risk assessment, and Lyme disease-preventive behaviors. Of the 360 respondents who presented at the clinic during the peak Lyme disease season, 219 (61 percent) completed the questionnaire. Bivariate and multivariate analyses were used to examine the association between predictor variables and self-reported behavior to prevent Lyme disease, the outcome variable.

Findings

Ages ranged from 16 to 84, with a mean age being 46 years old. There were an equal number of males and females, 73 percent of the respondents owned pets, 18 percent reported a history of Lyme disease, and 51 per-

cent reported having a family member or friend who had Lyme disease. The mean number of hours spent outdoors per day was 4.6 ($\pm$3.8) hours. Having had Lyme disease or knowing someone with Lyme disease was significantly associated with the use of preventive measures. Older age was significantly associated with the use of personal preventive measures only for persons without prior Lyme disease.

Implications

The study provided information that could be used by public health nurses in developing community prevention programs for Lyme disease. Younger persons without a history of Lyme disease should be targeted for these programs.

Reference

McKenna, D., Faustini, Y., Nowakowski, J., & Wormser, G. P. (2004). Factors influencing the utilization of Lyme disease-prevention behaviors in a high-risk population. *Journal of the American Academy of Nurse Practitioners, 16*(1), 24–30.

States. It is clinically diagnosed by a unique skin lesion called a "bull's eye lesion" because it is a red spot at the site of the bite, followed by spreading rings of inflammation as the infection progresses outward. The lesion develops 3 to 30 days after the tick bite. There may be symptoms of fatigue, headache, fever, stiff neck, muscle aches, enlarged tender lymph nodes, and joint pain. Treatment consists of 10 to 14 days of penicillin or tetracycline. If left untreated, the illness can progress. Stage II involves neurological and cardiac symptoms. Persons who progress to Stage III may have months to years of ongoing attacks of arthritis and arthralgia. A vaccine is in development and will be targeted for use in high-risk areas of the east coast; however, the disease is spreading west throughout the United States (National Center for Infectious Diseases, 2005).

Rocky Mountain Spotted Fever

Dog and wood ticks are the vectors for Rocky Mountain spotted fever. It is most commonly seen in the

south Atlantic and western south-central region of the United States with highest incidence in North Carolina and Oklahoma. Interestingly, it is rarely reported in the Rocky Mountain region. Infection occurs 4 to 6 hours after a tick bite. After an incubation period from 3 to 14 days, the disease is identified by a maculopapular rash on the extremities including the palms of the hands and soles of the feet spreading to the entire body. Blood tests for specific antigens confirm the diagnosis. Antibiotic therapy is required to prevent serious complications with a case fatality rate of 13 to 24 percent without treatment (Heymann, 2004).

Malaria

Malaria is a serious illness affecting up to 300 million people each year and killing 1 million to 2 million people worldwide. Transmission of malaria is through the bite of an infected mosquito. Malaria has been successfully controlled in most temperate-zone countries, but it remains a major cause of illness in many tropical and subtropical areas. For this reason, anyone traveling to areas of the world considered to be endemic for malaria should use mosquito repellent during the day and insecticide-treated mosquito nets while sleeping. Treatment involves antimalarial drugs tailored to the specific type of malaria a person may have and is determined by the area of a country where a person became infected. CDC and WHO provide guides for prevention and treatment of malaria on a country-by-country basis. Travelers can begin prophylaxis several weeks prior to traveling and 4 to 6 weeks upon returning for added protection. Symptoms of cyclical chills and fever should immediately be evaluated for malaria, especially for immigrants and visitors from malaria endemic areas of the world (Heymann, 2004).

Parasitic Diseases

Parasitic diseases are commonly found in tropical climates and in countries with undeveloped disease prevention and control systems. Problems common to developing countries such as lack of sanitation, inadequate access to medications, and insufficient primary care lead to high infection and reinfection rates despite sporadic control efforts by governments and international agencies. Parasitic diseases are classified into four groups of organisms: (1) roundworms (nematodes), (2) tapeworms (cestodes), (3) flukes (trematodes), and (4) single-celled organisms (protozoa). Increased international travel and immigration by people from developing countries increases the potential for the spread of parasitic infections in the United States. Additionally, the HIV epidemic has increased the incidence of parasitic opportunistic infections among immune compromised people, including *Pneumocystst carinii* pneumonia and toxoplasmosis (National Center for Infectious Disease, 2005).

Nurses and health care workers diagnose a parasitic disease by assessing a client's signs and symptoms and questioning about areas of recent travel. Diagnosis includes knowing how and when to collect appropriate laboratory specimens, depending upon which disease is suspected. Health education about compliance with treatment and appropriate measures to prevent the spread of infection to others is important. Drug treatment can effectively control most parasitic infections; however, the cost and availability of drugs to underserved population is often a challenge. Ongoing prevention and control of parasitic diseases includes partnering with clients and communities to improve vector

control, provide support for sanitation and personal hygiene, educate for safer sex practices, and advocate for sanitary disposal of food, water, and waste.

Nosocomial Infections

Nosocomial infections (infections acquired in a hospital setting) may affect anyone who has contact with a hospital. People may be exposed to infectious agents from other clients, hospital staff, or the environment. The treatment of neoplastic and chronic diseases, which involve invasive procedures and often immune-suppressing medications, further enlarges susceptibilities of clients to infectious agents. The CDC maintains the National Nosocomial Infection Surveillance (NNIS) system, which is the source of national data on the epidemiology of nosocomial infections in the United States.

The complex infection surveillance and control programs found in hospitals are managed by infection control specialists who are specifically trained nurses or nurse epidemiologists. They work closely with PHNs when clients with known infectious diseases are admitted or discharged from the hospital, and they often contribute to the data collection and mandatory reporting required by the CDC.

Respiratory Infections

Common respiratory infections include tuberculosis, influenza, and pneumonia.

Tuberculosis

The tubercle bacilli, *Mycobacterium tuberculosis (M. tuberculosis)*, is the causative agent for the leading cause of death from a single infectious agent worldwide. It is estimated that one-third of the world's population, almost 2 billion persons, is infected with *M. tuberculosis* (TB). This includes 8 million new TB cases and approximately 3 million deaths each year. Over 95 percent of TB occurs in developing countries where few health resources exist and concomitant HIV infection is increasing. In the United States, approximately 15 million people are infected. The number of new cases has declined every year since 1992; however, the number of foreign-born people with TB in the United States has increased. Control of TB in foreign-born individuals is most important in the first years of immigration and will remain a public health challenge in the near future. TB has also increased among homeless people, people living with HIV, and people living in correctional institutions and nursing homes (Betts, Chapman, & Penn, 2003).

M. tuberculosis is an airborne pathogen spread by small particle aerosols called droplet nuclei. Droplet nuclei are spread easily by speaking, singing, coughing, or sneezing. Symptoms include fever, cough, chest pains, fatigue, hemoptysis, and weight loss. The incubation period is between 4 and 12 weeks. Active disease usually develops within 6 to 12 months after infection. The complication of extrapulmonary TB occurs in about 5 percent of the cases, whereas 95 per-

cent of those with TB develop latent disease that may not reappear until later in life. Latent infection often reactivates in the elderly, immunocompromised individuals, underweight and malnourished people, substance abusers, and those with diabetes. Concern exists for the increasing incidence of multidrug-resistant TB. During outbreaks of multidrug-resistant TB, mortality rates have been documented at 43 to 89 percent (Heymann, 2004). A national goal for *Healthy People 2010* includes the elimination of TB (less than 1 case per 100,000 population). Meeting this goal will depend on ongoing support for prevention and control, especially among high-risk populations (USDHHS, 2000).

⊕ RESEARCH APPLICATION

Predictors of Influenza Vaccine Acceptance among Healthy Adult Workers

Study Purpose

To assess workers' beliefs that might affect their decision to receive an influenza vaccine.

Methods

This quantitative study used the Health Belief Model to assess workers' perceived susceptibility to and seriousness of influenza, benefits of and barriers to receiving a vaccine, cues that promoted action, knowledge about influenza and vaccine protection, and motivation for protective health behaviors. Workers from a large Midwestern university with an established influenza vaccine program were asked to complete questionnaires before and after the vaccine program ended. The first questionnaire included demographic information and Health Belief Model items. The second questionnaire, given at the end of the vaccine program asked about vaccine acceptance. Data were analyzed using logistic regression to determine variables that predicted acceptance of influenza vaccine.

Findings

Of the 400 workers eligible to participate in the study, 207 completed both questionnaires. The majority (75.5 percent) of the respondents were women, and more than a third (38.6percent) reported they were 50 years and older. Most (75.7 percent) reported they were married, and 74 percent reported being a high school graduate. About half (54.8 percent) reported that they received the vaccine, and of

these, 93 percent reported they got the vaccine from the work site program. Benefits of and barriers to getting the influenza vaccine as well as cues to action predicted vaccine acceptance. In comparison to workers who did not receive an influenza vaccine, workers who did believed they were more susceptible to influenza and that the disease was serious, and they believed there were more benefits and fewer barriers than those who did not receive the vaccine. Neither group was very knowledgeable about influenza or the vaccine.

Implications

Study results indicate that work site education about influenza and the role of the vaccine in preventing influenza is needed. Health education focusing on symptoms, complications, and misconceptions about influenza and the effectiveness of vaccination is needed. In addition, making the program readily available, offering incentives, identifying "champions" who regularly receive a vaccine to promote the program, and developing an influenza vaccination campaign theme are included as strategies to improve vaccine acceptance.

Reference

Blue, C. L., & Valley, J. M. (2002). Predictors of influenza vaccine acceptance among healthy adult workers. *AAOHN Journal, 50,* 226–233.

Multidrug resistant TB (MDR-TB) is a serious concern, one that affects health care workers directly. During the early 1990s, outbreaks were documented in settings such as nursing homes, shelters for the homeless, hospitals, prisons, long-haul flights, and schools. MDR-TB is thought to have been caused as a result of people not completing their full course of treatment with the INH and Rifampin. Specific strains of the TB bacillis have mutated such that they are no longer controlled by these drugs. Worldwide up to 2 percent of TB cases are now due to MDR-TB strains and pose a serious problem. Full compliance with strict infection control procedures is required to prevent the spread of TB both in health care settings and in the community.

Influenza

Influenza is a syndrome caused by infection with influenzia A, B, or C viruses. Epidemics of influenza occur annually in the United States and occasionally worldwide as a pandemic. The annual epidemic lasts 5 to 6 weeks and may affect up to 20 percent of the population with small children most often infected and older adults most often hospitalized (Betts et al., 2003). Each year inactivated flu vaccines are produced to match the expected strain of the virus. If taken sufficiently ahead of time, vaccines can have 70 to 90 percent effectiveness and are especially important in protecting the elderly from influenza-associated pneumonia.

Pneumonia

Any infectious agent that invades a person's lungs may cause pneumonia. Pneumonia results from aspiration of both virulent and nonvirulent organisms that progress to create infection in the lungs. Inhalation of environmental toxic fumes or aspiration of stomach acids can also create inflammatory conditions and the development of secondary bacterial infection in the lungs. Aspiration pneumonia is a high risk for clients with a history of alcoholism or drug abuse.

Pneumonia is normally prevented by the body's natural defenses of the cough reflex, and enhanced protection comes with the use of protective masks or air filtration systems in environments where air-borne contamination is common. Community acquired pneumonia is diagnosed by symptoms of a recent upper respiratory tract infection, chills, fever, and cough associated with chest pain and dyspnea and a chest x-ray. Antibiotics are the treatment of choice and should be started as soon as

a diagnosis is made. Hospitalization and intravenous therapy may be required if there is a delayed response to therapy. Factors that complicate treatment include advanced age, other underlying illness, or immunosuppression for other causes such as HIV infection. Vaccination is important for high-risk groups because of the frequency of occurrence and the potential for antibiotic drug resistance (Betts et al., 2003).

Viral Hepatitis

Inflammation of the liver may be caused by hepatitis. Many things including bacteria, viruses, protozoa, and toxins may cause it. Public health nurses are particularly concerned about the spread of hepatitis A, B, and C. Hepatitis A (HAV) is spread by fecal-oral routes, usually due to inadequate food sanitation or hand-washing after toileting. Infection may spread by contamination to food, water, or milk. HAV is a worldwide concern and most prevalent in regions with sanitation challenges and lack of clean water. An effective HAV vaccine is available and provides protection and is recommended for anyone traveling to the developing world.

Hepatitis B is a blood-borne pathogen and affects over 400 million people worldwide and is responsible for 10 percent of chronic liver disease in the United States (Betts, Chapman, & Penn, 2003). Acute liver failure from HBV only occurs in 1 percent of those infected. Chronic HBV creates fatigue and right upper quadrant discomfort and can be treated with the drugs Interferon and Lamivudine. Community health workers commonly see high rates of HBV among vulnerable populations including the homeless, alcoholics, and IV drug using clients. An effective vaccine is available, and health care workers are often required to be vaccinated.

Hepatitis C (HCV) is a serious public health threat. In the 1980s, it was the most common blood-borne infection in the United States. It was estimated that over 3.9 million people had a positive antibody. About 85 percent of persons infected with HCV develop some degree of chronic liver disease with approximately 15 to 20 percent progressing to end-stage disease causing up to 10,000 deaths each year. The CDC estimates that by 2020 the mortality rate from HCV will triple. HCV is one of the diseases blood banks carefully screen for, and anyone infected with the virus may not donate blood. Treatment includes Interferon and Ribavirin, but these drugs are only indicated in approximately

20 percent of HCV cases (Betts, Chapman, & Penn, 2003; CDC, 2006).

Sexually Transmitted Infections

The public health nurse will care for individuals and groups with sexually transmitted infections, including HIV, venereal warts, herpes, syphilis, and gonorrhea.

HIV

In 1981, an increasing number of gay men in large urban areas on the east and west coasts were becoming ill with a strange disease. In time, they were determined to be infected with the human immunodeficiency virus. HIV has spread throughout the world to become pandemic, affecting over 40 million people in every country in the world (UNAIDS, 2006).

The destruction of a person's immune system makes the person vulnerable to other infections, which are called opportunistic infections because they take the "opportunity" of a person not being able to resist them. The presence of specific opportunistic infections is the basis of the diagnosis of AIDS. A person without HIV would not be vulnerable to these infections. It is known that when these infections are present that HIV is probably also present. An antibody or genetic test can confirm the diagnosis. The severity of the opportunistic infections is influenced by the extent to which HIV has damaged the immune system. The goal of HIV control is to determine as quickly as possible if a person is infected so that immune-preserving medications can be used to prevent HIV from replicating and further damaging the immune system and leaving the person vulnerable to multiple other opportunistic infections.

In the 1990s, new drug treatments called protease inhibitors were discovered. When used in combination with antiretroviral drugs, they are able to prevent HIV from replicating, thereby stopping the progression of the disease. These drugs are expensive and difficult to take due to complex dosing requirements. There is significant humanitarian and political energy being invested in determining how to make these life-saving drugs available to the greatest number of people possible.

Part of the difficulty in controlling the HIV epidemic is the fact that HIV does not produce visible symptoms, often for many years. Therefore infected persons may not know that they are carrying the virus and may continue to practice unsafe sexual or needle-using drug behavior and spread the virus to others. After a person

is infected, it can take up to 90 days for their body to produce antibodies to HIV. Two tests are used to identify these antibodies. The Elisa test is very sensitive and finds potential HIV antibodies, and the Western Blot test is very specific and eliminates any antibody that is not HIV. Used together, these tests provide effective and trustworthy laboratory evaluation. In the late 1990s, genetic tests that detected HIV viral particles were developed. They can be used sooner; however, they are expensive and not as reliable for initial diagnosis. Both the antibody tests and the genetic tests are used by blood banks to test all donated blood.

The primary role of the public health nurse is to promote prevention of the spread of HIV. This is done through public education encouraging everyone to practice safe sex by using condoms for any contact with potentially infected sexual fluids and to not share IV drug needles. Many U.S. communities provide clean needles to those using HIV drugs through "needle exchange programs." It is an effort to prevent the spread of HIV among the drug-using population. When a person suspects they may have become infected, public health nurses encourage them to seek testing. Once diagnosed, people living with HIV need the support of their health care providers to practice safe sex and maintain adherence to the drug protocols required to control the virus. For those whose disease progresses, they may need assistance with case management and accessing medical care. Most importantly, public health nurses are advocates for people living with HIV and educators for others to protect themselves.

Venereal Warts / Condylomata Acuminata

Venereal warts (condylomata acuminata) are caused by the human papillomavirus (HPV). Over 100 types of HPV have been identified. Four to six weeks following infection a woman may develop warts on her genitals and cervix. The infection is self-limiting in women with normal immune function and lasts approximately 8 to 10 months. Treatment is often unsatisfactory and controversial, using cryotherapy and chemical agents to remove the warts. The relapse rate is 75 percent; therefore, once diagnosed with HPV, a woman should continue to be monitored for re-infection (Betts, Chapman, & Penn, 2003).

Women diagnosed with HPV also should be educated about their risk for cervical cancer and the protection available to them. Some "low-risk" types of HPV rarely develop into cancer, but other "high-risk" types, such as HPV-16, HPV-18, HP-31, HP-35, HP-39, and others are associated with cervical cancer and cancer of the vagina and vulva. Although few HPV infections lead to cervical cancer, more than 99 percent of all cervical cancers are related to HPV, and of these, 70 percent are caused by HPV-16 and HPV-18. It is therefore, a critical role of the public health nurse to educate women about HPV and its link to cervical cancer and also to encourage all sexually active women to have regular Pap tests. In June 2006, the U.S. Food and Drug Administration licensed the Gardasil® vaccine for use in girls and women, between the ages of 9 and 26 years. The vaccine protects against four HPV types, which together cause 70 percent of cervical cancers and 90 percent of genital warts. The public health nurse should encourage parents of young girls to get the vaccine before they are sexually active to protect them from HPV. Studies are and will be conducted in the future to determine the benefit from the vaccine for older women, boys, and men.

Herpes Simplex Virus Types 1 and 2

Herpes simplex virus (HSV) types 1 and 2 are usually found in the oral mucosa or genital tract and are clinically diagnosed from localized primary lesions. Initial infection often occurs in childhood or infancy. HSV can be easily transferred from mother to child during birth. The fever and cold blisters normally associated with HSV often occur as reactivation later in life. HSV presents as clear vesicles that erupt and crust over within days. The HSV lesions are highly contagious and infection may spread to other parts of the body and to others. HSV is often found in those with immune suppression from other diseases such as HIV, as well as those who experience high stress in their lifestyle. Genital herpes is caused by HSV-2 and is spread through sexual contact. The incubation period is from 2 to 12 days, but a person is communicable for up to 7 weeks. It is extremely important to practice good hygiene when herpes is present and to use caution regarding the contamination of clothing. Universal precautions should be carefully followed when assisting someone in the care of HSV infection. Acyclovir is the drug of choice and is best used at the earliest possible indication of an outbreak to prevent the formation of vesicles (Heymann, 2004).

Syphilis

Syphilis has long historical roots in all civilizations. After World War II and the discovery of penicillin,

effective treatment became available. Syphilis is characterized by an initial primary lesion, called a chancre, at the point of contact. A characteristic rash appears on the palms of the hands and soles of the feet. The lesion heals, and the rash disappears within weeks; the disease may become asymptomatic for many years while it spreads internally affecting the central nervous system (CNS), the cardiovascular system, and multiple organs. During this time, the person may transmit syphilis to others through sexual contact. Secondary syphilis is often diagnosed as a result of CNS symptoms. For others, first symptoms may include disabling lesions in the aorta of the heart. Syphilis is diagnosed through blood tests such as VDRL (Venereal Disease Research Laboratory) and confirmed using antigen tests. Latency may continue throughout a person's life or may last 5 to 10 years before diagnosis. The disease is most often seen in younger people between the ages of 20 and 29. The number of cases declined in the 1970s and early 1980s, but those figures have been increasing, especially in urban areas and especially in men. Long-acting penicillin in large doses of 2.4 million units IM is the standard of treatment. For those allergic to penicillin, other antibiotic regimens are available; however, they require close surveillance and may take longer (CDC, 2006).

Gonorrhea

Gonorrhea, or gonococcal infection, is a bacterial disease that is prevalent worldwide, especially among young people. Prevalence is highest in lower socioeconomic communities; however, since 1995 an increase in prevalence is being documented in the United States among men who have sex with men. The disease differs in how it first occurs in men and women. In men, 2 to 7 days after exposure, a purulent discharge is present with painful urination. A very small number of cases in men are asymptomatic. In women, the disease presents as a mucopurulent cervicitis, which may be asymptomatic. A woman may first realize she is infected due to bleeding after intercourse. Prepubescent girls are at increased risk of becoming infected in cases of direct genital contact during sexual abuse. A newborn may become infected during the birth process with the infection occurring in their eyes causing conjunctivitis, which can result in blindness. The danger for the health of the community is that a person may transmit the disease for many months if not treated. With treatment by antibiotics, infectivity can be stopped within hours.

A major concern is that the gonococcus has become resistant to some common antimicrobials. When this occurs, efforts must be made to culture the pathogen to develop a treatment that can stop replication and infectivity. It is advised that high-risk people be retested after 1 to 2 months to detect late asymptomatic reactions. Individuals with gonorrhea should be offered confidential testing for HIV and other STIs (i.e., chlamydia testing) because they are at increased risk of infection from other sexually transmitted diseases (Heymann, 2004). Because of the possibility of treatment failure and reoccurrence, it is also important to reexamine and repeat diagnostic testing of individuals who have been treated for an STI (CDC, 2006). The recommended follow-up and test of cure varies with STIs, so the public health nurse should consult treatment guidelines for specific directions.

INFECTIOUS AND COMMUNICABLE DISEASE IN THE GLOBAL COMMUNITY

People are traveling to every region of the globe, moving more freely through once remote regions, and may come in contact with infectious pathogens for which they do not have adequate immunity. It is important for public health nurses to advise anyone traveling to another region of the world to check with a travel clinic for the immunizations recommended for the area they will be visiting. The risk of infection to the traveler may be tied to a specific part of a country or season of the year (such as for malaria), and includes personal health status. Vaccinations taken years earlier, such as tetanus, may need to have a titer test done to determine if sufficient antibodies are still available to provide a first line of defense. Often a vaccination may need to be given to increase specific antibodies prior to traveling. This process can take weeks or months, so it is important for those who are traveling to the developing world to be advised to get their immunization status checked well in advance, and updated if necessary. Traveling to remote regions of the world may require precautions not necessary in more developed areas. It is always important to check whether a person has recently traveled to an exotic place when evaluating for symptoms of disease. Being an informed traveler is important. However, people do not need to be fearful when traveling throughout the world.

⊕ POLICY HIGHLIGHT

HIV and ARVs

The WHO estimates that in 2006 there were over 38 million people living with HIV in the world. In the western world, the number of people dying from HIV fell dramatically during the 1990s due to the effectiveness of antiretroviral (ARV) drugs. These life-saving drugs are available to only one out of eight of the people in the world living with HIV (UNAIDS, 2006). ARVs are being made available to the poorer countries of the world, but not quickly enough. The WHO has a program called 3×5, which was intended to ensure lifetime access to ARV drugs for 3 million people in developing countries by the end of the year 2005 (WHO, 2005). The goal was not reached. The Global Fund against AIDS, Tuberculosis and Malaria hopes that in the near future more money will be provided by the wealthier countries of the world to provide ARVs for all those who need them. To follow the work of those committed to caring for people living with AIDS throughout the world go to http://www.aidscarewatch.org.

The WHO and public health systems of specific countries work together to maintain surveillance of infectious pathogens. Strict travel, immigration, and customs regulations require that both individuals and goods moving around the world be monitored to prevent the spread of disease. This isn't always possible, and occasionally an unexpected pathogen emerges to surprise us. This happened in February 2003 with the SARS epidemic (Heymann, 2004). The causal agent was discovered to be coronavirus. Over 375 people died before the epidemic was controlled. It began in Guangdong Province China and spread to Canada, Singapore, Hong Kong, Taiwan, and Vietnam. The disease followed major airline routes and spread to 20 other sites in Africa, the Americas, Australia, Europe, the Middle East, and the Pacific. The infection spread to hospital workers and their families (Heymann, 2004).

During the SARS outbreak of 2003, the government restricted international travel, schools closed, and business halted while health authorities worked to control the epidemic. Infection control procedures in hospitals and clinics throughout the world were implemented

⊕ PRACTICE APPLICATION

The Occupational Health Nurse and the International Travel Program

In the year 2006, many businesses and industries have joined the global economic community. More than 150 different American companies are known to be multinational corporations. As a result, employees are traveling and living worldwide for their jobs. Occupational health nurses frequently serve as the manager of a company's International Travel Program. The purpose of the travel program is to reduce health risks and ensure the personal health of the traveling worker. The travel program is likely to include the following components:

- ⊕ Travel policies or protocols, including emergency escape plans
- ⊕ Travel agency services and travelers' assistance
- ⊕ Health and safety information related to the destination
- ⊕ Security planning and information
- ⊕ An immunization program
- ⊕ Counseling concerning personal health and medications while traveling
- ⊕ Evaluation of health care services in foreign locations
- ⊕ Education for workers concerning their health resources while they are traveling or living abroad

Because of the complexities of managing and providing so many components of the international travel program, many companies are choosing to outsource selected parts of the program. The occupational health nurse then coordinates with vendors to provide needed international services. One such vendor is an organization called International SOS. This large multinational company provides high-quality medical care and consulting for multinational corporations, insurers, financial institutions and governmental organizations.

The occupational health nurse consults with workers before they travel and when they return. If the employee has acquired an infectious or communicable disease while away, the nurse will consult with the employee to ensure adequate medical care and follow-up, including the surveillance required by local or state public health authorities.

SOURCE: Gochnour, Bruck, & Souza, 2006; International SOS, 2006.

and enlarged as a result of the epidemic. The lessons of SARS inform international activities in preparation for the control the N5N1 virus. WHO maintains ongoing global surveillance for probable and suspect cases of SARS and issues travel recommendations through its *International Health Regulations* (Heymann, 2004).

A specific group of nurses are involved in assisting individuals prepare for international travel and monitoring their health status as they work throughout the world. These occupational health nurses are employed by multinational companies that function throughout the world and increasingly expect their employees to travel.

THE SPECTRE OF BIOTERRORISM

Germ warfare is a term that has been used to describe biological weapons for military purposes. At the start of the new millennium, it is understood that the use of biological agents as weapons extends beyond the military to other international groups. Bioterrorism involves the threat or deliberate use of biological agents to cause illness and/or death in human populations in order to achieve religious, political, or other ideological outcomes. As we entered the twenty-first century, we have had to think about the unthinkable. It is not enough to be concerned about naturally occurring major outbreaks of disease, such as the infectious diseases that have been considered as controlled or eradicated. We are now concerned with biological agents and emerging diseases that can create epidemics by the deliberate actions of humans for specific ends. Terrorists have made effective use of biological agents because they are comparatively easy to acquire, can be modified to easily cause serious disease, and can be very difficult to detect in the environment.

In September 1999, the CDC allocated about $40 million to state and local health departments across the country to expand their ability to detect and respond to biological and chemical agents. The purpose was to provide for an effective response to terrorist acts in the United States. The federal government allocated an additional $133 million for bioterrorism preparedness. In 2006, public health officials at all levels of governmental agencies have been successful in strengthening programmatic efforts to deal with the threats of bioterrorism and provide resources for medical response (Oregon Health Division, January 5, 2000).

Potential Bioterrorism Agents

The CDC has separated biological agents that can be used as bioterrorism agents into three categories. These agents can be naturally occurring. All have been identified as having potential for use in terrorist attacks.

Category A

The Category A organisms or toxins are the highest priority agents in the CDC designation. They pose the highest risk to the public and national security because (1) they can be easily spread or transmitted from person to person; (2) they result in high death rates and have the potential for major public health impact; (3) they might cause public panic and social disruption; and (4) they require special action for public health preparedness. The agents of Category A (Table 20-2) include the following:

- Anthrax (*Bacillus anthracis*)
- Plague (*Yersinia pestis*)
- Smallpox (*Variola major*)
- Botulinum toxin (*Clostridium botulinum*)
- Tularemia (*Francisella tularensis*)
- Hermorrhagic fever (Ebola and Marburg filoviruses; Lassa and Junin arenaviruses)

Category B

Category B bioterrorism agents are designated as the second highest priority agents by CDC. The Category B designation indicates that (1) they are moderately easy to spread; (2) they result in moderate illness rates and low death rates; and (3) they require specific enhancements of CDC's laboratory capacity and enhanced disease surveillance. The agents of Category B include the following:

- Ω Fever (*Coxiella burnetti*)
- Brucellosis (*Brucella* species)
- Glanders (*Burkholderia mallei*)

- Melioidosis—Whitmore Disease (*Burkholderia*)
- Psittacosis (*Chlamydia psittaci*)
- Viral encephalitis (arboviruses and alphaviruses of Venezuela, Eastern, and Western equine encephalitis)
- Ricin toxin (castor beans)
- Typhus fever (*Rickettsea prowazekii*)
- Staphlococcal Enterotoxin B-SEB (*Staphylococcus aureus*)
- Food- and water-borne diseases: cholera (*Vibrio cholerae*), Salmonella species, *Shigella dysenteriae*, *Escherichia coli* O157, *Cryptosporidium parvum*

Category C

Category C agents, the third highest priority category, are emerging pathogens with a potential for engineering for future mass dissemination. They are easily available, are easily produced and spread, and have potential for high morbidity and mortality. They could all be major health threats. The Category C agents include the following.

- Napin virus
- Hantaviruses
- Tick-borne hemorrhagic fever viruses
- Tick-borne encephalitis viruses
- Yellow fever virus
- Multidrug-resistant, *Mycobacterium tuberculosis* (Oregon Health Division, January 2, 2001)

A variety of chemicals can be used as bioterrorism agents. A partial listing of chemical agents is shown in Table 20-3. More information can be located online at http//www.bt.cdc.gov. Contact state or local Poison Control Centers for consultation.

What Can Be Done?

The keys to managing a bioterrorist attack (or naturally occurring large outbreak of disease) is early planning and ongoing infectious disease surveillance. Local health departments, hospitals, laboratories, and health care providers, as well as law enforcement and emergency planners should now have plans in place for local response to disease outbreaks. State and federal health agencies and their resources can be tapped in the event of a bioterrorist attack. The U.S. Department

TABLE 20-2: Bioterrorism Agents—Category A

AGENT	MICROBIOLOGY	RESERVOIR	INCUBATION	TRANSMISSION
Anthrax	Bacillus anthracis, a spore-forming Gram-positive rod	Livestock and wildlife, spores viable in soil for years	Average: 1–7 days Range: 1–60 days	Inhalation and/or ingestion of spores, cutaneous contact with infected animal
Plague	*Yersinia pestis,* a Gram-negative rod	Wild rodents	1–7 days (longer in immunocompromised individuals)	Bites from infected rodents and associated fleas
Smallpox	Variola virus, an orthopoxvirus	Officially, only in designated freezers	7–9 days	Respiratory
Botulism	Neurotoxins produced by the anaerobic Gram-positive rod *Clostridium botulinum*	Spores, ubiquitous in soil	12–36 hours to several days	Inhalation or ingestion of spores
Tularemia	*Francisella tularensis,* a Gram-negative rod	Wild animals (rabbits, beavers, various ticks)	Average: 3–5 days Range: 1–14 days	Tick bites, handling or eating insufficiently cooked meats, drinking contaminated water, inhalation of contaminated soil
Hemorrhagic fever	Ebola and Marburg filoviruses	Unknown Bats?	Average: 5–10 days	Range: 2–19 days Contact with body fluid of infected person

Note. From Oregon Health Division (October 19, 2001). Bioterrorism: Priority agents, *CD Summary, 50,* 52, 1.

of Homeland Security will assume responsibility for the overall management of the event.

We live in a global community, including all countries and continents of the world. An exotic disease can appear anywhere or at any time. Initiating an effective response to bioterrorism events begins at the local level. Alert CHNs, nurse practitioners, and other health care providers should report any unusual events to local or state health authorities. The following should be reported immediately:

⊕ Unusual numbers of undifferentiated febrile illnesses or other medical events believed to be of public health significance

⊕ Anyone with a disease in Category A

⊕ Multiple cases of Category B or C diseases

Depending on the agent or agents used, it may be days or weeks before a bioterrorism incident is known. Early reporting and careful epidemiologic follow-up can minimize the effect to the health of the public.

TABLE 20-3: Major Bioterrorism Chemical Agents

PESTICIDES & OTHER NERVE AGENTS	SYSTEMIC (BLOOD) ASPHYXIANTS	PULMONARY IRRITANTS (CHOKING AGENTS)	VESICANTS (BLISTERING AGENTS)
Sarin	Arsine	Ammonia	Mustard agents:
Tabun	Cyanide agents	Chlorine	Distilled mustard
Soman	Cyanegen chloride	Hydrogen chloride	Mustard gas
VD	Hydrogen cyanide	Phosgene agents	Mustard/lewisite
Organophosphate and methylcarbamate pesticides	Potassium cyanide	Hydrogen fluoride	Nitrogen mustard
	Sodium cyanide		Sesqui mustard
			Sulfur mustard
			Lewisites/chloroarsine agents:
			Lewisite
			Mustard/lewisite
			Phosgene oxime

Note. From the Oregon Department of Human Services (March 25, 2003). Preparing for a chemical terrorist event – A primer. *CD Summary, 52:6,* 1–4.

STRATEGIES FOR NURSES WORKING WITH INFECTIOUS AND COMMUNICABLE DISEASE IN THE COMMUNITY

Many challenges face the community nurse who works directly with infectious and communicable diseases. Nurses are often the first to detect the presence of suspect illness in their clients. The depth and breadth of knowledge required for competent practice in this field is extensive . . . and, that knowledge must be kept current.

Infectious and Communicable Disease Program Management

If the nurse is the epidemiologist in a public health agency, it is the responsibility of the nurse to manage the communicable disease program for that county. Program policies will be guided by federal and state health authorities and their related policies. The surveillance systems for tracking reportable infectious diseases exist at local, state, federal, and international levels of public health agencies. Nurse practitioners, medical providers, and laboratories are required to report confirmed cases. Locally, the nurse epidemiologist conducts case and contact follow-up. Health education is ongoing for health care providers, clients, and other members of the community. A complete immunization administration program is always an ongoing feature of an infectious and communicable disease program.

Communication skills and strategies are at the forefront for relaying information to the public. While individual and small group communication techniques may be the base of a nurse's skills, knowledge of large group and community outreach strategies are now required of all PHNs. Risk communication is a field of communication practice that reaches effectively to the public (U.S. Public Health Service, 1995).

In addition to using risk communication strategies, the public health nurse will want to use the services of a media consultant. Many public health agencies now

⊕ PRACTICE APPLICATION

Case Study of a Bioterrorism Event: It Happened in Oregon

Setting the Scene: Oregon is a beautiful, mostly rural state, especially the high mountain desert on the east side of the snow-capped Cascade Mountains. Land is easy to acquire, and so it was that a little-known religious cult was able to acquire a large tract of land in southeastern Wasco County. The Rajneeshees (followers of the Bhagwan Shree Rajneesh of Poona, India) were intent on building their large religious community, Rajneeshpuram.

The Political Climate: The land was primarily zoned for agricultural purposes. Many tactics were used to try to change the zoning laws, including harassing long-time local residents, importing many people to swell the area's population base to control local elections outcomes, and filing multiple lawsuits against Wasco County and its officials.

First Signs of the Outbreak: In the fall of 1984, people in and around The Dalles, Oregon (county seat of Wasco County), became ill with diarrhea, vomiting, and fever. The victims were sick enough to require hospitalization. The county health department was called to begin the epidemiological investigation.

The Agent: The biological agent causing the outbreak was confirmed by culture as *Salmonella typhimurium*, a common food-borne bacteria. The Oregon State Laboratory determined that this was an unusual strain of *Salmonella*. Consultants were called in from the Centers for Disease Control and Prevention to assist overwhelmed local and state public health resources.

The Extent of the Biocrime: **Biocrime** is the criminal use of biological agents in acts of terrorism. There were several waves of the illness. By the time it was over, 751 people in and around Wasco County had become ill. Of that number, 388 had been confirmed by culture as having *S. typhimurium*. The epidemiological investigation determined that the salad bars in local restaurants were the source of the bacterial contamination. After more than a year of continuing investigation, it was learned that the Rajneeshees had contaminated a number of food and water sources in and around The Dalles, Oregon. They had purchased a culture of *S. typhmurium* from a reputable biological supply company. The next step was to develop ability to grow *S. typhirmurium* in their own laboratory. Prior to the mass contaminations, they had systematically tested their ability to transmit the agent to selected individuals. Finally, they successfully contaminated salad bars in The Dalles with the agent. A criminal investigation was conducted over more than a year. The primary perpetrators were arrested and served time. The Bhahwan Shree Rajneesh was deported and has since died. This incident hardly attracted attention; no one wanted to encourage copycat attacks.

SOURCE: Miller, Engelberg, & Broad (2002); Oregon Health Division (January 2, 2001); Oregon Health Division (January 5, 2000).

hire media specialists to participate as members of the public relations team.

Planning for Pandemic Disease Events

A pandemic is a disease outbreak that occurs over a wide geographic area and affects a high proportion of the population. The outbreak may affect countries worldwide. At this writing, public health agencies around the world are watching for the spread of avian flu (H5N1 in Asia and H7N3 in Canada). The WHO has published the WHO Global Influenza Preparedness Plan. Public health agencies and private business and industry around the world are scrambling to plan for a possible influenza pandemic, whether avian flu or some other variety of influenza. The present WHO global preparedness plan has identified six phases of a pandemic (see Table 20-4). It should be pointed out that currently the avian flu pandemic is at Phase 3 for worldwide planning. Nurses have a number of important roles to play in this planning process.

INFECTIOUS AND COMMUNICABLE DISEASE RESOURCES

Resources abound for the nurse epidemiologist. The field of infectious and communicable disease is very

TABLE 20-4: WHO Phases of Global Influenza: Preparedness Planning

	PHASE DEFINITIONS	OVERARCHING PUBLIC HEALTH GOALS
	Interpandemic Period	
Phase 1	No new influenza virus subtypes have been detected in humans. An influenza virus subtype that has caused human infection may be present in animals. If present in animals, the risk of human infection or disease is considered to be low.	Strengthen influenza pandemic preparedness at the global, regional, national, and subnational levels.
Phase 2	No new influenza virus subtypes have been detected in humans. However, a circulating animal influenza virus subtype poses a substantial risk of human disease.	Minimize the risk of transmission to humans; detect and report such transmission rapidly if it occurs.
	Pandemic Alert Period	
Phase 3	Human infection(s) with a new subtype, but no human-to-human spread, or at most rare instances of spread to a close contact.	Ensure rapid characterization of the new virus subtype and early detection, notification, and response to additional cases.
Phase 4	Small cluster(s) with limited human-to-human transmission but spread is highly localized, suggesting that the virus is not well adapted to humans.	Contain the new virus within limited foci or delay spread to gain time to implement preparedness measures, including vaccine development.
Phase 5	Larger cluster(s) but human-to-human spread still localized, suggesting that the virus is becoming increasingly better adapted to humans, but may not yet be fully transmissible (substantial pandemic risk).	Maximize efforts to contain or delay spread, to possibly avert a pandemic, and to gain time to implement pandemic response measures.
	Pandemic Period	
Phase 6	Pandemic: Increased and sustained transmission in general population.	Minimize the impact of the pandemic.

Note. From WHO (2005). WHO Global Influenza Preparedness Plan.

⊕ PRACTICE APPLICATION

Risk Communication

The nurse who practices in the public arena needs communication skills that can extend beyond individuals and families to the larger community. The skills and techniques of risk communication were developed over the last 20 years of the twentieth century. Risk communication has been defined as "the transmission of information about health and environmental risks, their significance, and the policies for managing them" (Environmental Protection Agency, 1996).

At times, people in communities can be unaware of important health issues or overconcerned about environmental impacts on their health. Peter Sandman developed a public definition of risk: RISK = Hazard + Outrage (1993). Risk communication skills are used by the public health professional to alert the public to health and environmental concerns, while managing potential public outrage. An EPA document lists seven cardinal rules of risk communi-

cation. Using these rules can help to manage communication processes and improve public participation in risk management:

1. Accept and involve the public as a legitimate partner.
2. Plan carefully and evaluate your efforts.
3. Listen to the public's specific concerns.
4. Be honest, frank, and open.
5. Coordinate and collaborate with other credible sources.
6. Meet the needs of the media.
7. Speak clearly and with compassion. (p. 3)

SOURCE: Environmental Protection Agency, 1996; Sandman, 1993; U S Public Health Service, 2006.

dynamic with surveillance and community follow-up at the heart of this work. This chapter concludes with a webliography of online federal resources (USDHHS, 2005). Two key agencies are the WHO and the CDC.

Having a strong knowledge base, the nurse epidemiologist can be an excellent resource for the many health issues that can affect the public.

CRITICAL THINKING ACTIVITIES

1. When you encounter people who ask if you fear becoming infected when caring for someone with a contagious disease, such as HIV or TB, how do you respond? What policies, procedures, and systems are in place to protect you? If you believe you experienced an exposure, what would you do?

2. Imagine you are attending a conference where everyone eats their meals together. After a picnic lunch, several people become very ill and turn to you for help. What would you do? Who would you call? What information would you initially share with the people at the conference? What information would you immediately begin to collect to share with others who may become involved?

3. If you were caring for a family from another part of the world and you suspected that they were spreading an infectious disease, what would you do? Who would you contact? How would you assist them?

4. You are a public health nurse working in the public health department of a major city. You learn of an outbreak of several cases of a reportable infectious disease in a government building. What would make you suspicious about this outbreak? With whom would you discuss your suspicions? What would make you suspicious of a bioattack?

⊕ PRACTICE APPLICATION

Get to Know Your Media Specialist!!

"Through effective media communication, public health officials can engage the public and help them make informed and better decisions" (Hyer & Covello, 2005). Public health professionals know that the media is an important channel for getting information out to the community. Around the world, news is business. It's about change. Whether it is emergency or new information to educate the public, issuing time-sensitive news releases may be the job of the public health nurse or the agency media specialist. A media specialist is a professional health educator or journalist whose job is to assist public health professionals in the preparation of materials to be released to the press. Media contacts include three types of formats, each requiring specific preparation and the assistance of the media specialist.

Every interview is an opportunity to get the public health message before the community. Prepare for interviews; reporters are on a time-line. Start with a "SOCO," the Single Over-riding Communication Objective for the interview. Give no more than three key messages and repeat them three times during the interview. Remember to put the most important message first. Keep answers short and smile.

News releases that are articles, begin with an attention-grabbing headline and a sharp lead paragraph; start with the conclusion. Next, provide background facts to give context. Use active voice and make sentences short and direct. When the news release has been sent, be sure that the agency spokesperson is available and prepared to answer any incoming questions or concerns.

There should be a compelling need for a news conference, as it will provide very high visibility. Such conferences may save time because they allow for responses to all reporters at one time. Preparation is essential. The successful news conference has engaging speakers, real news, and expert visual aids.

The WHO has identified seven steps to effective media communication during public health emergencies. Prepare in advance!

1. Assess media needs, media constraints, and internal media-relation capabilities.
2. Develop goals, plans, and strategies.
3. Train communicators.
4. Prepare messages carefully.
5. Identify media outlets and media activities.
6. Deliver messages.
7. Evaluate messages and performance.

The media specialist employed by your organization is a critical member of the public health staff. Include the media specialist as a member of the program planning teams in any public health agency. This specialist in media communications can write and distribute news releases that are needed for informing community citizens. Get to know your media specialist!

SOURCE: Hyer & Covello, 2005.

KEY TERMS

acquired immunity	common vehicle transmission	herd immunity
active immunity	droplet nuclei	infectivity
antigenicity	elimination	mode of entry
biocrime	emerging infectious disease	mode of exit
biological agents	eradication	mode of transmission
bioterrorism	food-borne disease	natural immunity
chemoprophylaxis	food intoxication	nosocomial infection

KEY TERMS (Cont'd)

passive immunity	reservoir	tertiary prevention
pathogen	risk communication	vector
pathogenicity	secondary prevention	virulence
primary prevention	surveillance system	

KEY CONCEPTS

⊕ Many factors are involved in the emergence and reemergence of communicable disease. These include living in a global community in which individuals travel easily between remote regions of the world, potentially carrying pathogens with them as they move throughout the world. HIV is an example of a pathogen that migrated from Africa throughout the world as people had unprotected sexual contact and shared IV drugs. Changes in the environment also continue to challenge efforts to control communicable disease as nations struggle to ensure clean water, vector control and sanitation to their populations.

⊕ Communicable disease is transmitted in many ways through a chain of infection that includes agents, hosts, and the environment. Pathogens that cause communicable disease have multiple modes of transmission including direct person-to-person, common vehicle routes (such as food, water, blood, serum, or plasma), and vectors (such as animals, insects, and birds).

⊕ People are protected from infectious disease by different types of immunity. This includes the natural immunity that is genetically part of a species. Acquired immunity occurs after a person comes in contact with an infectious agent and builds antibodies that provide ongoing protection. Herd immunity is present when a large percentage of a population is resistant to a disease, often as the result of having been immunized.

⊕ The prevention and control of communicable disease includes primary, secondary, and tertiary activities. Primary prevention is intended to work ahead of an infectious agent to create an environment in which it cannot thrive. This is usually done through healthy behaviors and immunizations to specific pathogens. Secondary prevention involves finding a disease as quickly as possible

through screening, making a diagnosis, and initiating treatment to limit the seriousness of the disease and the infectivity of the pathogen. Tertiary prevention includes supporting adherence to treatment, managing harm reduction activities, and providing rehabilitation and support for acute stages of a disease.

⊕ Common communicable diseases are defined by the mechanism by which they are spread. This includes food and waterborne diseases, vector-borne diseases, parasitic diseases, nosocomial infections, respiratory infections, multi-methods of spread for viral hepatitis, and sexually transmitted diseases.

⊕ International perspectives on communicable disease are necessary as global travel becomes increasingly available to larger numbers of people. Cautions exist for travelers to specific regions of the world, which often require advance immunization and preparation. The World Health Organization and its member nations maintain a complex system of surveillance and reporting of communicable diseases and are increasingly working together to provide the advances of scientific research to all people in the world. Occupational health nurses oversee the international travel programs that protect the health of employees of multinational corporations.

⊕ Current strategies for the nurse working with infectious and communicable diseases are centered in managing surveillance systems for tracking reportable infectious diseases. Using risk communication techniques reaches effectively to the public on critical issues. Using a media specialist augments communications with the community. Effective use of governmental resources enhances planning for pandemic disease events.

REFERENCES

Betts, R. F., Chapman, W. S., & Penn R. L. (2003). *A practical approach to infectious diseases* (5th ed.). Philadelphia: Lippincott Williams & Wilkins.

Blue, C. L., & Valley, J. M. (2002). Predictors of influenza vaccine acceptance among healthy adult workers. *AAOHN Journal, 50,* 226–233.

Centers for Disease Control and Prevention (CDC). (2006). Sexually transmitted diseases treatment guidelines, 2006. *Morbidity and Mortality Weekly Report, 55*(11), 1–94.

Environmental Protection Agency (EPA). (1996). Risk communication and public participation. *EPA's Comparative Risk Projects.* Regional and State Planning Division, 1–2. Retrieved June 11, 2006, from http://www.epa.gov/epahome/programs.htm

Gochnour, M. K., Bruck, A., & Souza, D. (2006). Chapter 16: Examples of occupational health and safety programs. In M. K. Salazar (Ed.) *Core curriculum for occupational and environmental health nursing* (3rd ed.). St. Louis: Saunders/Elsevier, 506–513.

Heymann, D.L. (2004). *Control of communicable diseases manual* (18th ed.). Washington, DC: American Public Health Association.

Hyer, R. N., & Covello, V. T. (2005). *Effective media communication during public health emergencies: A WHO field guide.* Geneva: WHO, ii and 5.

International SOS. (2007). *Worldreach human touch.* Retrieved June 11, 2006, from http://www.internationalsos.com.

Lashley, F. R., & Durham, J. D. (Eds.). (2002). *Emerging infectious diseases: Trends and issues.* New York: Springer.

Leavell, H. R., & Clark, E. G. (1958). Preventive medicine for the doctor in his community. New York: Springer.

Leavell, H. R., & Clark E.G. (1965). *Preventive medicine for the doctor in his community: An epidemiological approach.* New York: McGraw-Hill, 21.

McKenna, D., Faustino, Y., Nowakowski, J., & Wormser, G. P. (2004). Factors influencing the utilization of Lyme disease-prevention behaviors in a high-risk population. *Journal of the American Academy of Nurse Practitioners, 16*(1), 24–30.

McNeil, W .H. (1977). *Plagues and peoples.* New York: Doubleday.

Miller, J., Engelberg, S., & Broad, W. (2002). *Germs: Biological weapons and America's secret war.* New York: A Touchstone Book, 15–33.

Mullan, F. (1989). *Plagues and politics: The story of the United States Public Health Service.* New York: Basic Books Inc.

National Center for Infectious Diseases. (2005). *Antibiotic anitmicrobial resistance. http://www.cdc.gov/ncidod*

National Center for Infectious Diseases, Centers for Disease Control and Prevention. (2007). *Infectious disease information.* Retrieved August 29, 2006, from .

National Immunization Program. (2005). *Vaccines and immunization.* Retrieved August, 2007, from www.cdc.gov

Oregon Health Division. (January 2, 2001). Bioterrorism: Could it happen here? *CD Summary, 50*(1), 1–2.

Oregon Health Division. (October 19, 2001). Bioterrorism: Priority agents. *CD Summary, 50*(22), 1.

Oregon Health Division. (March 25, 2003). Preparing for a chemical terrorist event—A primer. *CD Summary, 52*(6), 1–4.

Oregon Health Division. (January 5, 2000). The spectre of bioterrorism. *CD Summary, 49*(1), 1.

Sandman, P. M. (1993). *Responding to community outrage: Strategies for effective communication.* Fairfax, VA: American Industrial Hygiene Association, 7.

Shilts, R. (1988). *And the band played on.* New York: Viking Penguin.

UNAIDS. (2006). Uniting the world against AIDS. Retrieved August, 2007, from http://www.unaids.org/en/HIV_data/2006GlobalReport/default.asp

U.S. Department of Health and Human Services (USDHHS). (2000). *Healthy People 2010* (Conference edition, in two volumes). Washington, DC: U.S. Government Printing Office.

U.S. Department of Health and Human Services (USDHHS). (2005). *UNAIDS: AIDS epidemic update 2004.* Retrieved November 23, 2004, from http://www.unaids.org.

U.S. Public Health Service (1995). Risk communication: Working with individuals and communities to weigh the odds, *Prevention Report.* Retrieved May 29, 2006, from http://www.osophs.dhhs.gov/pubs/prevrpt/Archives/o5fm1.htm.

World Health Organization (WHO). (1945). *Constitution of the World Health Organization.* Geneva: author, 2. Retrieved September 11, 2006, from http://www.searo.who.int/LinkFiles/About_SEARO_const.pdf.

World Health Organization (WHO). (2006). Important progress seen in tackling AIDS prevention and treatment. . . . *News Release dated May 30, 2006.* Retrieved September 11, 2006, from http://www.who.int/hiv/mediacentre/news60/en /print.html.

World Health Organization (WHO). (2005). Report by the secretariat. *Eleventh General Programme of Work, 2006–2015, # EB 117/16.* Geneva: author, paragraph #34. Retrieved September 11, 2006, from http://www.who.int/gb/ebwha/pdf_files/EB117_16-en.pdf.

World Health Organization (WHO). (2006). Smallpox eradication: Destruction of variola virus stocks. *Report of the Secretariat, EB # 117/33.* Retrieved September 11, 2006, from http://www.who.int/gb/ebwha/pdf_files/EB117/B117_33-en.pdf.

World Health Organization (WHO). (2005). *WHO global influenza preparedness plan.* Geneva: author, 2.

BIBLIOGRAPHY

Ayres, J. R. de C. M., Paiva, V., Franca Jr., I., Gravato, R., Lacerda, R., Della Negra, M., de S. Marques, H. H., Galano, E., Lecussan, P., Segurado, A. C., & Silva, M. H. (2006). Vulnerability, human rights, and comprehensive health care needs of young people living with HIV/AIDS. *American Journal of Public Health.* 96(6). Washington, DC: *American Journal of Public Health,* 96(6), 1001–1006.

Brookesmith, P. (1997). *Biohazard the hot zone and beyond: Mankind's battle against deadly disease.* New York: Barnes & Noble.

Centers for Disease Control and Prevention (CDC). (2006). Sexually transmitted diseases treatment guidelines, 2006. *Morbidity and Mortality Weekly Report,* 55(11), 1–94.

Cleveland Clinic Foundation. (2001). *Handbook of infectious diseases.* Springhouse, PA: Springhouse Corporation.

Diamond, J. (1999). *Guns, germs, and steel: The fates of human societies.* New York: Norton.

Fong, I. W., & Alibek, K. (Eds.). (2005). *Bioterrorism and infectious agents: A new dilemma for the 21st century.* New York: Springer.

Garrett, L., (1994). *The coming plague: Newly emerging diseases in a world out of balance.* New York: Farrar, Straus and Giroux.

Laskley, F. R., & Durham, K. D. (Eds.). (2003). *Emerging infectious diseases: Trends and issues.* New York: Springer.

Leavell, H. R., and Clark, E. G. (1958). *Preventive medicine for the doctor and his community.* New York: McGraw-Hill.

Mayo, A. M., & Cobler, S. (2004). Flu vaccines and patient decision making: What we need to know. *Journal of the American Academy of Nurse Practitioners,* 16, 402–410.

Mayer, K. H., & Pizer, H. F. (2000), *The emergence of AIDS: The impact on immunology, microbiology and public health.* Washington, DC: American Public Health Association.

Mol, C. J., & Koethe, S. M. (2006). QuantiFERON-TB GOLD—An innovation in tuberculosis screening. *AAOHN Journal,* 54, 245–247.

Mosca, N. W., Sweeney, P. M., Hazy, J. M., & Brenner, P. (2005). Assessing bioterrorism and disaster preparedness

training needs for school nurses. *Journal of Public Health Management & Practice* (Supplement), S38–44.

Myers, W. P., Westenhouse, J. L., Flood, J., & Riley, L. W. (2006). An ecological study of tuberculosis transmission in California. *American Journal of Public Health,* 96, 685–690.

Office of the Assistant Secretary for Public Affairs (2005). Appendix B: Websites. *Terrorism and other public health emergencies: A reference guide for media.* Washington, DC: U. S. Department of Health and Human Services, 226–231.

Rein, D. B., Honeycutt, A. A., Rojas-Smith, L., & Hersey, J. C. (2006). Impact of the CDC's section 317 immunization grants program funding on childhood vaccination coverage. *American Journal of Public Health,* 96, 1548–1553.

Serdobova, I., & Kjeny, M-P. (2006). Assembling a global vaccine development pipeline for infectious diseases in the developing world. *American Journal of Public Health,* 96, 1554–1559.

Vélez-McEvoy, M. (2006). Prevention and control of infectious diseases in the workplace—Prevención y control de enfermedades infecciosas en el lugar de trabajo. *AAOHN Journal,* 54, 148–152.

White, C. G., Shinder, F. S., Shinder, A. L., & Dyer, D. L. (2001). Reduction of illness absenteeism in elementary schools using an alcohol-free instant hand sanitizer. *Journal of School Nursing,* 17, 258–265.

World Health Organization. (January 23, 2006). *3X5 Progress Report 2006.* Available: http://www.who.int/gb/e/e-eb117.html.

World Health Organization. (2005). HIV/AIDS: Report by the secretariat. *Universal access to prevention, care and treatment, EB117.6.* Available: http://www.who.int/bg/ebwha/pdf_files/EB117/B117_6-en.pdf.

World Health Organization. (2005). Proceedings of the meeting. *Partners' consultation on WHO 11th General Programme of Work (GPW) "Together towards a healthier future."* Stockholm: author. Available: http://www.who.int/gb/e/e_eb117.html.

World Health Organization. (2005). Report by the secretariat. *Eleventh General Programme of Work, 2006-2015, # EB 117/16.* Geneva; author. Available: http://www.who.int/gb/ebwha/pdf_files/EB117_16-en.pdf.

World Health Organization. (2003). *Country focus: Progress report, Biennium 2002–2003.* Geneva: author. Available: http://www.who.int/countryfocus/resources/country_focus_progress_report-202-2005.pdf.

World Health Organization. (2002). *Health in the millennium development goals.* Available: http://www.who.int/mdg/goals/en/print.html.

RESOURCES

Center for Biologics Evaluation and Research (CBER)

1401 Rockville Pike, Suite 200N
Rockville, MD 20852-1448
1-800-835-4709; 301-827-1800
Email: octma@cber.fda.gov
Web: http://www.fda.gov

CBER protects and enhances the public health through the regulation of biological and related products including blood, vaccines, tissue, allergenics, and biological therapeutics. CBER is committed to a product approval process that maximizes the benefits and minimizes the risks to clients of the biological product. The Web site offers information about new products and topics such as influenza virus vaccine, product recall and withdrawal, and client news and safety information.

Center for Food Safety and Applied Nutrition (CFSAN)

Food and Drug Administration
5600 Fishers Lane
Rockville, Maryland 20857
1-888-463-6332
Web: http://vm.cfsan.fda.gov

The CFSAN, an agency of the Food and Drug Administration (FDA), is responsible for promoting and protecting the public's health by ensuring that the nation's food supply is safe, sanitary, wholesome, and honestly labeled, and that cosmetic products are safe and properly labeled. Although the U.S. food supply is among the world's safest, the increase in the variety of foods and the convenience items available, as well as the complexity of the food industry and the technologies used in food production and packaging, has brought with it public health concerns. Recent news, information about national food safety programs, FDA documents, and special interest areas can be located at this Web site.

Centers for Disease Control and Prevention (CDC)

1600 Clifton Road
Atlanta, Georgia 30333
404-639-3311, 1-800-311-3435
Web: http://www.cdc.gov

The CDC, founded in 1946 to help control malaria, is one of the 13 major operating components of the U.S. Department of Health and Human Services. The CDC has remained at the forefront of public health efforts to prevent and control infectious and chronic diseases, injuries, workplace hazards, disabilities, and environmental health threats. Today, CDC is globally recognized for conducting research and investigations and for its action-oriented approach. The Web site has an abundance of information on infectious and communicable diseases as well as information for prevention. The Division of Global Migration and Quarantine (DGMQ), a department of the CDC, is committed to reducing morbidity and mortality due to infectious diseases among immigrants, refugees, international travelers, and other mobile populations that cross international borders. In addition, the DGMQ promotes border health and prevents the introduction of infectious agents into the United States. The Web site for the DGMQ is http://www.cdc.gov/ncidod/dq/.

Food Safety and Inspection Service (FSIS)

U.S. Department of Health & Human Services
200 Independence Avenue SW
Washington, D.C. 20201
402-344-5000, Hotline 1-800-233-3935
FAX: 402-344-5005
Email: TechCenter@fsis.usda.gov
Web: http://www.fsis.usda.gov

The FSIS is the public health agency in the U.S. Department of Agriculture responsible for ensuring that the nation's commercial supply of meat, poultry, and egg products is safe, wholesome, and correctly labeled and packaged. There are many offices that make up the FSIS. Details about these offices as well as educational materials, regulation and policy, food defense, and emergency response information can be found on the FSIS Web site.

National Institute for Occupational Safety and Health (NIOSH)

Centers for Disease Control and Prevention
1600 Clifton Road
Atlanta, Georgia 30333
1-800-35-NIOSH
Web: http://www.cdc.gov

NIOSH, part of the Centers for Disease Control and Prevention in the U.S. Department of Health and Human Services, is the federal agency responsible for conducting research and making recommendations for the prevention of work-related injury and illness. Their disease and injury program targets prevention of infectious diseases such as influenza, blood-borne infectious diseases, severe acute respiratory syndrome (SARS), tuberculosis, and West Nile virus.

National Vaccine Program Office (NVPO)

U.S. Department of Health & Human Services
200 Independence Avenue SW
Washington, D.C. 20201
202-619-0257, 1-877-696-6775 (toll free)
Web: http://www.hhs.gov

NVPO, part of the U.S. Department of Health & Human Services, has responsibility for coordinating and ensuring collaboration among the many federal agencies involved in vaccine and immunization activities. The National Vaccine Plan and various reports and recommendations relevant to infectious diseases can be found at the NVPO's Web site.

Pan American Health Organization (PAHO)

525 23rd Street NW
Washington, D.C. 20037
202-974-3000
Web: http://www.PAHO.org

(PAHO is an international public health agency with 100 years of experience in working to improve health and living standards of the 35 countries of the Americas. It serves as the specialized organization for health of the Inter-American System. It also serves as the Regional Office for the Americas of the World Health Organization and enjoys international recognition as part of the United Nations system. PAHO's mission is to lead strategic collaborative efforts among member states and other partners to promote equity in health, to combat disease, and to improve the quality of, and lengthen, the lives of the peoples of the Americas.

U.S. Department of Agriculture (USDA)

1400 Independence Avenue SW
Washington, D.C. 20250
Web: http://www.usda.gov

The USDA's mission is to provide leadership on food, agriculture, natural resources, and related issues based on sound public policy, the best available science, and efficient management. They work to control and prevent infectious diseases in animals, thereby protecting people. Their Web site contains many publications on such topics as emerging infectious diseases, requirements for import of animals, food-borne illness, and state agriculture regulations.

U.S. Department of Homeland Security (DHS)

Washington, D.C. 20528
202-282-8000, 202-282-8495
Web: http://www.dhs.gov

DHS's mission is to lead the unified national effort to secure America. It strives to prevent and deter terrorist attacks and protect against and respond to threats and hazards to the nation. It ensures safe and secure borders, welcomes lawful immigrants and visitors, and promotes the free-flow of commerce. Its programs include protecting communities from biological weapons by securing incoming freight, the nation's rail systems, and harmful insider threats. It also planned the national strategy for pandemic influenza which includes (1) detecting human or animal outbreaks that occur anywhere in the world; (2) protecting the American people by stockpiling vaccines and antiviral drugs while improving the capacity to produce new vaccines; and 3) preparing to respond at the federal, state, and local levels in the event an avian or pandemic influenza reaches the United States.

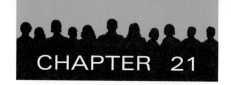

CHAPTER 21

Populations with Chronic Diseases

Susan J. Appel, CCRN, APRN-BC (ACNP & FNP), PhD

Chapter Outline

- Causes of Morbidity and Mortality
- Shift from Acute to Chronic Disease
  - Aging Population
  - Obesity Epidemic
- Increasing Prevalence of Type 2 Diabetes
- Diseases of the Cardiovascular System
  - Coronary Heart Disease
  - Modifiable Risk Factors
- Contextual Risk Factors and Chronic Diseases
- Caregiver Burden
- Disease Trajectory
- Public Health Nursing Consideration for Screening for and Management of Chronic Diseases

Learning Objectives

Upon completion of this chapter, the reader will be able to:

1. Investigate the role of technological developments for the changes in the trends of morbidity and mortality.

2. Analyze the economic and social impacts of chronic diseases on ill individuals, caregivers, and society.

3. Scrutinize the factors that have accelerated the growth of chronic diseases as the top causes of morbidity and mortality.

4. Designate the role of public health nursing in the prevention and management of chronic diseases.

5. Define the concept of caregiver burden when providing care for an individual with a chronic disease.

6. Formulate population-focused nursing interventions for screening, prevention, and management of chronic diseases.

Chronic illness is defined as a pathological process that persists for three or more weeks. The term "chronic" is derived from the Greek word *khronos,* meaning "for the time" (askoxford.com, 2004). This contrasts with acute illness, which describes an illness of a sudden onset and a limited duration. Nearly all individuals affected by chronic disease will inevitably need to spend the remainder of their lives coping with the impact of long-term health-related problems. Etiologies of chronic diseases are multifactorial, having been linked to genetics, environmental factors, and unhealthy lifestyle behaviors. The major contribution of the public health nurse and advanced practice nurse working within society will be to continue to assist aggregate individuals to modify their lifestyle behaviors. Fortunately, many risk factors for chronic diseases, such as tobacco use, sedentary lifestyle, and improper diet, are modifiable. Preventive strategies that enhance healthy lifestyle behaviors will provide opportunities for intervention and potentially will serve to reduce the prevalence of chronic disease.

Healthy People 2010 have delineated objectives aimed at reducing the occurrence and pervasive deleterious sequelae of chronic disease within our society (USDHHS, 2000). The economic impact of chronic illnesses on the United States health care dollar is projected to remain our greatest expenditure. Equally, those faced with a lifelong chronic disease are likely to experience a reduced quality of life. Never before has there been such a need for behavioral scientists, cross-disciplinary collaboration, translational research, and education of the public concerning the link between lifestyle and diseases.

Public health nurses are strategically placed within society and the health care system to provide an important role in the long-term screening, prevention, and management of chronic disease. Substantial bodies of literature exist to descriptively illustrate what it is like to either have a chronic disease or be a caregiver to someone who is chronically ill (see Table 21-1). Qualitative research focused on chronic disease, has given a voice to those affected by ongoing illness. In providing this voice it has opened a window for healthcare providers to witness the actual lived experiences of the chronically ill and their caregivers.

Middle-range or practice nursing theories are being increasingly developed from experiences of the chronically ill to better provide the nurse with a conceptual framework to explore various aspects of chronic disease.

The goal of middle-range theory is to serve as a foundation for grounding of conceptual thought and then identification of where interventions should be focused (Appel, Giger, & Davidhizar, 2005). Ultimately, middle-range nursing theories serve to guide theory-based interventions, in order to reduce complications and thus minimize disability (Appel et al., 2005). An example of a middle-range nursing theory is the Theory of Uncertainty by Mishel (Mishel, 1999). The Theory of Uncertainty has more recently been reconceptualized by Mishel and Clayton (2003), specifically for those individuals living with continual uncertainty (i.e., living with a chronic disease or facing the possibility of recurrence) (Mishel & Clayton, 2003). Insights learned from the personal struggles of the chronically ill and guidance from middle-range theories will potentially hold the key to finding efficacious interventions for the optimal management of chronic disease. However, there seems to be a gap between the information in the research literature and health care practice. Nursing is in a key position to adapt evidenced based knowledge for use in clinical practice. Evidenced based knowledge can be used when testing theories, developing cost-effective interventions, promoting health, preventing illness, assisting individuals to maintain or to recover function, and ultimately to enhance quality of life (Melkus et al., 2002; Sekula, DeSantis, & Gianetti, 2003; Whittemore et al., 2003). The gap between theory, research, and health care practice needs to be bridged in order to prevent, manage, and reduce the deleterious impacts of chronic illness (Goodfellow, 2004; Hutchinson & Johnston, 2004; Ogilvie et al., 2004; Williamson, Webb, & Abelson-Mitchell, 2004). Thus, it is imperative that evidenced-based interventions designed to prevent and manage chronic disease, which have been tested by researchers, be applied within the practice of public health nursing.

CAUSES OF MORBIDITY AND MORTALITY

Over the past five decades, the causes of morbidity (illness rates) and mortality (death rates) have changed. These changes were primarily due to the advent of antibiotic therapy and refinements in public health services. Decreases in rates of infection specifically resulted from the improvements in sanitation, clean drinking water, and dissemination of immunizations (Dore, 2000; Sakula, 2004; Wood & Halfon, 1996). Likewise, dur-

TABLE 21-1: Research Studies: Giving a Voice to Those Affected by Chronic Illness

STUDY	MAJOR THEME(S) OR FINDINGS
Alexander, I. M. (2004). Characteristics of and problems with primary care interactions experienced by an ethnically diverse group of women. *JAANP, 16*(7), 300–310.	Caring Respect Trust One-on-one communication
Bottorff, J. L., Johnson, J. L., Moffat, B., Grewal, J., Ratner, P. A., & Kalaw, C. (2004). Adolescent constructions of nicotine addiction. *Cancer Journal of Nursing Research, 36*(1), 22–39.	Acting addicted "to be cool" Passive role Role of nicotine exposure leading to addiction
Carter-Edwards, L., Skelly, A., Cagle, C. S., & Appel, S. J. (2004). "They care, but don't understand:" Family support of African American women with type 2 diabetes. *The Diabetes Educator, 30*(3), 493–501.	Social support comes from many sources Lack of understanding of needs from social network Health care providers can help by teaching families about the possible needs of their clients with T2D
Dawson, S., Kristjanson, L. J., Toye, C. M., & Flett P. (2004). Living with Huntington's disease: Need for supportive care. *Nursing Health Science, 6*(2), 123–30.	Adjusting to the impact of the illness Surviving the search for essential information Gathering practical support from many sources Bolstering the spirit Choreographing individual care Fearing the future
Goldstein, N. E., Concato, J., Fried, T. R., Kasl, S. V., Johnson-Hurzeler, R., Bradley, & E. H. (2004). Factors associated with caregiver burden among caregivers of terminally ill patients with cancer. *Journal of Paliatitive Care, 20*(1), 38–43.	Intensity of caregiver burden related to: Limited social network Restrictions on own activities Younger age
Kralik, D. (2002). The quest for ordinariness: Transition experienced by midlife women living with chronic illness. *Journal of Advanced Nursing, 39*(2), 146–154.	Transition in chronic illness Extraordinariness Ordinariness Change as an impetus to transition

(continued)

TABLE 21-1: Research Studies: Giving a Voice to Those Affected by Chronic Illness (cont'd)

STUDY	MAJOR THEME(S) OR FINDINGS
MacDermott, A. F. (2002). Living with angina pectoris—A phenomenological study. *European Journal of Cardiovascular Nursing, 1*(4), 265–272.	Limitation and adjustment Resignation Indignation Caution Reluctant compliance Surprise The unknown
Sheppard, V. B., Williams, K. P., & Richardson, J. T. (2004). Women's priorities for lay health home visitors: Implications for eliminating health disparities among underserved women. *Journal of Health Social Policy, 18*(3), 19–35.	Lack of social support Creation of a mother-to-mother relationship
Thorne, S. E., & Paterson, B. L. (2001). Health care professionals support for self-care management in chronic illness: Insights from diabetes research. *Patient Education and Counseling, 42*(1), 81–90.	Social context Trajectory Uniqueness
Trollvik, A., & Severinsson, E. (2004). Parents' experiences of asthma: Process from chaos to coping. *Nursing Health Science, 6*(2), 93–99.	Feelings of uncertainty, helplessness, and guilt Need for support and help from health care professionals Adaptation to everyday life Development of coping strategies Need to "try out" new strategies Importance of a mutual dialogue between health care professionals and parents

ing the last fifty years there have been significant new scientific advancements made in the field of health care providing new therapies for disease management (McCool & Simeone, 2002). These scientific and technological advances have led to more effective management of acute illnesses and to some degree management of chronic diseases. All of these factors have worked together to change the trends in morbidity and mortality from acute infectious diseases to chronic diseases

(see Table 21-2 and Figure 21-1) (Ahmad, Lopez, & Inoue, 2000; Judson, 2004).

SHIFT FROM ACUTE TO CHRONIC DISEASE

Over the years, the prevalence of chronic diseases has steadily increased in both adults and children. It is predicted that the increase in chronic diseases will gain steadily in momentum. Two primary reasons thought to contribute to the continued expansions in the prevalence of chronic over acute diseases are (1) the aging population in North America and (2) the obesity epidemic.

Aging Population

People are living longer than ever before, are surviving with chronic diseases, and are consistently requiring more health care resources throughout their lives. Likewise, it is estimated that in the next thirty years, when all the baby boomers have reached retirement age, there will be two retirees for each person in the workforce (Benko, 2003; Knickman & Snell, 2002; Lee & Miller, 2002). This is likely to place an undue burden on our country's health care resources. By the year 2011, when the majority of baby boomers will have retired, our health care system is heading for one

of its biggest financial challenges (Knickman & Snell, 2002). Although not all chronic diseases are amenable to lifestyle interventions, those that are will be especially important. This will be particularly true if Americans are not able to learn to modify their risk factors, live healthier lives, and make interventions to modify amenable risk factors that have been linked to reducing chronic diseases. Projections are that by 2011, 17 percent of the gross domestic product (GDP) will be spent on health care expenditures (NCHS, 2003). In 2003, health care was about 15 percent of the GDP as the United States was spending $5,635 per every man, woman, and child in this society for health care (NCHS, 2006). Health care costs four times as much for a person older than 65 years of age than it does for a person younger than 45 years of age (Seshamani & Gray, 2004; NCHS, 2003). Therefore, by the year 2011, it is estimated that 17 percent of our GDP will be spent on health care resources (Lee & Miller, 2002; NCHS, 2003). This will represent the biggest increase in demand for health care ever experienced by the

---

TABLE 21-2: The Fifteen Leading Causes of Death in the United States in 2000

1. Heart disease
2. Cancer
3. Stroke
4. Chronic lower respiratory diseases
5. Accidents
6. Diabetes
7. Influenza and pneumonia
8. Alzheimer's disease
9. Kidney disease
10. Septicemia (blood poisoning)
11. Suicide
12. Chronic liver disease and cirrhosis
13. Hypertension (high blood pressure)
14. Homicide
15. Pneumonia resulting from breathing particles or fluid into the lungs

Rank based on number of deaths.

Note. From USNCHS (2003). *U.S. National Center for Health Statistics, National Vital Statistics Report*, vol. 52, no. 3, September 18, 2003. Web: www. cdc.gov/nchs, retrieved: August 7, 2004.

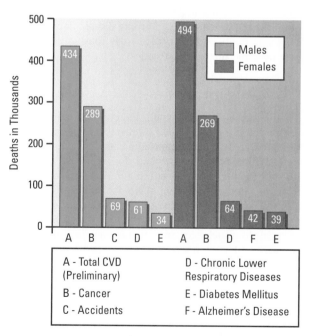

Figure 21-1 Leading causes of death for all males and females.

From CDC/NCHS. Centers for Disease Control and Prevention (CDC) (1999). Behavioral Risk Factor Surveillance System (BRFSS). Retrieved from http://www.cdc.gov/nccdphp/aag/aag_brfss.htm.

⊕ RESEARCH APPLICATION

Evaluating Research

Choose two of the research articles related to different aspects of chronic illness listed in Table 21-1, and compare them for the following:

- ⊕ Do the articles specify different disease trajectories?
- ⊕ If two different disease trajectories are explained, which one would you find harder to live with? What might be the pros and cons of each?
- ⊕ Do either of the articles describe or indicate the presence of caregiver burden? If so, how? Are suggestions made how to minimize this burden?

- ⊕ In the two articles, which chronic disease described do you think has the highest degree of uncertainty?
- ⊕ As a community health nurse visiting families who have a family member with a chronic illness, what community resources would potentially assist those in the two articles you have chosen?

United States (Pati et al., 2004; Tu, 2004). The general population of the United States will be made up of an overwhelming elderly population, who will be supported by a much smaller workforce (Terry, 2002). Therefore, primary and secondary prevention are key to reducing the prevalence of chronic diseases and for battling this financial health care crisis that will be occurring over the next three decades.

Obesity Epidemic

The obesity epidemic has affected children, adolescents, and adults (Holt, 2005; Ramsey & Glenn, 2002). Obesity is defined for adults as having a body mass index (BMI) of over 30 and for children and adolescents, a sex- and age-specific BMI at or above the 95th percentile, based on revised Centers for Disease Control and Prevention (CDC) growth charts (NCHS, 2001; USDHHS,2001). The obesity epidemic is greater in rural, low-socioeconomic regions and has disproportionately affected minorities within the United States (Kumanyika, 2002; Ramsey & Glenn, 2002). This epidemic can be directly linked to the etiology of numerous chronic diseases: hypertension, type 2 diabetes, cardiovascular diseases, osteoarthritis, polycystic ovarian disease, sleep apnea, and some forms of cancer (Zimmet, 2003). The CDC has been able to determine and monitor the presence of the obesity epidemic through the use of survey research. The CDC survey, known as the Behavioral Risk Factor Surveillance System, was carried out by asking adult participants questions via

the telephone (CDC, 1999). One major question each individual was asked: "How much do you weigh and what is your height?" Even with the understanding that most people may underreport their weight, and overreport their height, the results over time showed disquieting trends toward a growing national epidemic of obesity. The epidemic that has occurred in adults is about a 50 to 60 percent increase over the 1990s. However, the epidemic of obesity in children has taken place at an even more rapid pace than that of adults.

⊕ POLICY HIGHLIGHT

Chronic Disease Prevention

Most of the Centers for Disease Control and Prevention (CDC) chronic disease programs are funded through the Labor/Department of Health and Human Services/Education Appropriations Bill "Chronic Disease Prevention and Health Promotion." This money supports the CDC's work in chronic diseases such as diabetes, cancer, heart disease, arthritis, and stroke prevention as well as promoting behaviors such as healthy nutrition, physical activity, oral hygiene, and prevention programs to reduce obesity and tobacco use. The CDC works with state health departments to develop comprehensive, sustainable prevention programs that target the leading causes of death and disability and the risk factors that cause them. All states receive funding for "basic implementation" of the CDC's chronic disease programs.

It is now common to find young children being diagnosed with type 2 diabetes mellitus (ADA, 2000). Type 2 diabetes was once only considered a disease of adulthood. The future of this generation of children, who are already manifesting an elevated cardiac risk profile, will be potentially fraught with higher rates of type 2 diabetes. Likewise, the youth who experience high rates of type 2 diabetes will undoubtedly also be manifesting premature cardiovascular diseases and other associated deleterious sequellae fostering chronic diseases.

Prevalence of Obesity

Results from the National Health and Nutrition Examination Survey (NHANES 1999-2000), estimated that 64.5 percent of the U.S. population would meet the criteria for being overweight (BMI>25) (Flegal et al., 2007). The prevalence of obesity (BMI>30), regardless of gender, was 30.5 percent. Obesity prevalence was highest among adult Mexican Americans and non-Hispanic blacks. Black women had the highest prevalence of both overweight and obesity (Flegal et al., 2007). (See Figure 21-2.)

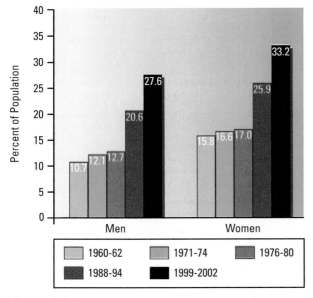

Figure 21-2 Age-adjusted prevalence of obesity in Americans ages 20–74 by sex and survey. (NHES, 1960–1962; NGANES, 1971–1974, 1976–1980, 1988–1994, 1999–2000).

From CDC/NCHS. Centers for Disease Control and Prevention (CDC) (1999). Behavioral Risk Factor Surveillance System (BRFSS). Retrieved from http://www.cdc.gov/nccdphp/aag/aag_brfss.htm.

TABLE 21-3: Body Mass Index Categories for Adults

BMI	CATEGORY
< 18.5	Underweight
18.5–24.9	Normal weight
25–29.9	Overweight
30–34.9	Class I Obesity
35–39.9	Class II Obesity
> 40.0	Class III Extreme Obesity

SOURCE: NHL&BI (1998).

Calculating BMI (http://nhlbisupport.com/bmi/bmicalc .htm):

Formulas for calculating BMI:

$$BMI = \frac{(\text{Weight in pounds})}{(\text{Height in inches}) \times (\text{Height in inches})} \times 703$$

or

$$BMI = \frac{(\text{Weight in kilograms})}{(\text{Height in cm}) \times (\text{Height in cm})} \times 10{,}000$$

Note. NHL&BI (1998). *The evidence: Clinical guidelines on the identification, evaluation, and treatment of overweight and obesity in adults.* National Institutes of Health.

Body mass index is a simple and widely accepted measure used to assess an individual's body habitus. The BMI takes into account weight in relationship to an individual's height, and the formula is weight in kilograms divided by height in meters squared (kg/m2) (NHL&BI, 1998). A determination can be made using BMI if an individual is underweight, normal weight, overweight, or obese (see Table 21-3). A normal range for BMI is 20 to 24.9 m/kg2 (NHL&BI, 1998). In general, it is estimated that 34 percent of the American adult population are overweight (BMI>25–29.9 kg/m²) and 27 percent are obese (BMI>30 kg/m²). That is, one out of every five adults living within the United States fall into either the overweight or obese BMI categories (CDC, 2004; NHL&BI, 1998).

When closely analyzing age-adjusted prevalence of obesity among race/ethnicity groups the differences were mainly seen among women. The age-adjusted prevalence of obesity was 36.0 percent in African American non-Hispanic women, 25.6 percent in Hispanic women, and 20.2 percent in white non-Hispanic women (CDC, 2004; NHL&BI, 1998). It is these same groups of women, with the two highest prevalence rates of obesity, who are now also experiencing the highest prevalence rates of type 2 diabetes and premature morbidity and mortality from diseases of the cardiovascular system.

Obesity as a Risk Factor for Type 2 Diabetes and Cardiovascular Diseases

The obesity epidemic is strongly associated with the onset of chronic disease. Two major chronic diseases that have been directly linked to obesity-related etiologies are hypertension and type 2 diabetes (Tu, 2004). Hypertension and type 2 diabetes have led directly to an increased prevalence in coronary heart disease, myocardial infarctions, congestive heart failure, and stroke (AHA, 2007; Ford, 2004a). The medical health care community considers having diabetes mellitus such a powerful risk factor for fostering the development of chronic diseases such as cardiovascular diseases, that it has been labeled as a "coronary heart disease risk equialevant" (NCEP, 2001). It has been widely supported by research that having pre-diabetes, metabolic syndrome, and/or frank type 2 diabetes mellitus leads to an accelerated development of coronary heart disease (Grundy, 2005; Grundy et al., 2005). In short, individuals with type 2 diabetes are in such a precarious cardiac risk situation that their risk for an acute cardiac event is considered equal to an individual who has already have had a myocardial infarction (NCEP, 2001). Therefore, maximal public health attention needs to be placed on preventing, managing, and minimizing obesity and its related complications.

Screening for pre-diabetes Two major risk factors for diabetes are impaired fasting glucose (IFG) (fasting glucose $\geq$ 100 mg/dL) and impaired glucose tolerance (IGT) (two-hour post oral glucose challenge test, with a glucose 140–199 mg/dL); these criteria have been used to define pre-diabetes (ADA, 2005). The American Diabetes Association (ADA) estimated that there are approximately 22 million individuals in the United States who can be categorized as having pre-diabetes (Ford, 2004b). Therefore, individuals manifesting pre-diabetes are high risk for the development of metabolic syndrome and/or frank type 2 diabetes (CDC, 2005; Grundy et al., 2005). Individuals with pre-diabetes do not always possess the other two components needed to meet the criteria for having metabolic syndrome. However, many of those who possess impaired fasting glucose can also be categorized as having the metabolic syndrome and an increased risk for cardiovascular diseases (Grundy et al., 2005).

Screening for metabolic syndrome The metabolic syndrome is a group of risk factors believed to serve as a precursor for the development of both type 2 diabetes, and ultimately the vascular injury leading to macrovascular cardiovascular diseases (Grundy, 2005; Reaven, Abbasi, & McLaughlin, 2004). Not everyone who develops cardiovascular disease will already have manifested type 2 diabetes, but those who do are already at a much higher risk for cardiac events such as acute myocardial infarction or stroke (Bibbins-Domingo et al., 2004; NCEP, 2001; Stern, Williams, & Hunt, 2005). Individuals with type 2 diabetes are two to four times as likely to develop cardiovascular related diseases (i.e., hypertension, coronary artery disease, myocardial infarctions, peripheral vascular diseases, heart failure, and/or stroke) (AHA, 2007). The core of the metabolic syndrome is central abdominal obesity, around which the other components of the syndrome tend to cluster (Reaven, Abbasi, & McLaughlin, 2004). Early in metabolic syndrome, individuals may have normal fasting glucose levels, but as the syndrome worsens, impaired fasting glucose may develop. In many cases, impaired fasting glucose eventually leads to chronic levels of hyperglycemia and the criteria for type 2 diabetes is met (ADA, 2005). Components of the metabolic syndrome defined by the National Cholesterol Educational Panel (NCEP) Adult Treatment Panel III (ATP III) include central abdominal obesity, hypertension, elevated fasting glucose, elevated triglycerides, and low high-density lipoproteins (HDL) (Harmel & Berra, 2003). According to the NCEP ATP III, for the criteria to diagnose metabolic syndrome to be met, an individual must possess three or more of the five components.

Initial presentation of metabolic syndrome may consist of a normal fasting glucose level (i.e., euglycemic). Euglycemia is commonly present early in the syndrome due to a chronic state of elevated plasma insulin or hyperinsulinemia (Appel, 2005; Reaven, 2002). However, later in the syndrome, when the pancreas is not able to continue the production of sufficient amounts of insulin, hyperglycemia will result (Adami et al., 2001; Anderson et al., 2001). Once the pancreas fails to produce sufficient insulin, glucose homeostasis is disrupted, leading to hyperglycemia and to findings such as impaired fasting glucose, glucose intolerance, and ultimately type 2 diabetes (fasting glucose > 126 mg/dL) (ADA, 2005; Reaven, 1988).

Screening for type 2 diabetes The metabolic syndrome is considered to be a modifiable risk factor for type 2 diabetes, heart diseases, and/or stroke (AHA, 2007). The distinct and well-described pathway known as the metabolic syndrome makes it ideal for early recognition, and management of interventions to disrupt its deleterious progression (Appel, Jones, & Kennedy-Malone, 2004). Without such interventions, the final sequela of the metabolic syndrome such as type 2 diabetes commonly occurs. Type 2 diabetes imposes an increased risk for stroke that is three to four times greater than for nondiabetics (AHA, 2007. Therefore, individuals with either pre-diabetes or metabolic syndrome should be screened regularly for the development of frank type 2 diabetes. Once significant suspicion for risk of type 2 diabetes is recognized, the American Diabetes Association (ADA) recommends screening for diabetes mellitus, by first obtaining a fasting glucose test. However, if the fasting glucose is normal and suspicion still exists as to the individual's ability to metabolize glucose, testing should proceed with use of a two-hour oral glucose tolerance test (OGTT) (ADA, 2005). In general, screening for type 2 diabetes should begin in all adults at age 45 and be repeated every three years. However, the ADA also has made provisions for early screening among individuals who manifest a higher risk for type 2 diabetes. For example, a higher level of suspicion for presence of type 2 diabetes needs to be employed with individuals who are known to have the propensity for insulin resistance. These individuals are commonly members of the minority groups within the United States who are currently experiencing health disparities (i.e., African Americans, Hispanics, Native Americans, or Pacific Islanders) (ADA, 2005). In short, the public health nurse can make a significant impact on risk factors for diabetes mellitus simply by identifying high-risk groups within the community and recommending screening.

Screening for insulin resistance The main underlying pathology of the metabolic syndrome is

insulin resistance, a diminished tissue response to insulin, that can be identified by use of laboratory data, formulas, history, and/or physiological findings (see Table 21-4, for history and noninvasive exam findings indicative of insulin resistance) (Appel, Giger, & Floyd, 2004; Hunter et al., 2000; Matthews et al., 1985; Monzillo & Hamdy, 2003). Obtaining a measure for insulin resistance will assist the public health nurse in the determination, if a client who appears to be at low risk is actually at high risk for type 2 diabetes and/or cardiovascular diseases (Appel, 2005; Appel, Moore, Giger; 2006; Appel, Giger & Floyd, 2004). Early recognition of insulin resistance is especially optimal as this allows for more time for an individual to employ lifestyle adjustments. Hence, prompt detection of insulin resistance preceding the development of further pathology will permit interference with the disease trajectory. The interruption of these pathways consisting of risk factors known to lead to the metabolic syndrome and its sequelae are likely to allow opportunities for both primary and secondary prevention.

Although insulin resistance is not contained within the NCEP's criteria for diagnosing metabolic syndrome, it is contained within the World Health (WHO) and American College of Endocrinology (ACE) criteria (AACE, 2003; Balakau & Charles, 1999). Early recognition of insulin resistance may be of particular importance for managing health disparities among certain at-risk populations such as African Americans, who may develop insulin resistance early in their progression along the pathway leading to pre-diabetes, metabolic syndrome, type 2 diabetes, and ultimately vascular injury associated with cardiovascular disease (Appel, 2005; Hanley et al., 2003). The NCEP did not include a direct marker of insulin resistance but instead decided to rely on the fact that there is generally a positive association between hypertriglyceridemia and hyperinsulinemia. However, the same association does not always hold true among the African American population (Appel, 2006; Liao, Kwon, Shaughnessy et al., 2004). Several large epidemiological studies have found that dyslipidemias differ by race. Most recently the findings of the Insulin Resistance Atherosclerosis Study (IRAS) revealed that African Americans in general had significantly higher HDL cholesterol ($p < 0.001$) and lower triglyceride levels ($p < 0.001$), versus either Caucasians or Hispanics (Haffner et al., 1999). Comparable conclusions regarding racial differences in lipid profiles have been drawn from other large epidemiological studies such as

⊕ RESEARCH APPLICATION

Is There a Need for Screening for Type 2 Diabetes in Seventh Graders?

Study Purpose

To determine if a screening program for type 2 diabetes in a seventh-grade population is warranted as well as to increase health care providers' awareness of the need for this screening.

Methods

Diabetes questionnaires were sent to each participant's parent or guardian. The questionnaire assessed for family history of diabetes, any currently diagnosed participant with diabetes, and physical activity. Other data obtained were age, ethnicity, gender, height, weight, blood pressure, acanthosis nigricans.

Findings

Results indicated that there is a need for screening for type 2 diabetes in a seventh-grade population.

Implications

The role of the nurse practitioner (NP) is to increase health professionals' and the public's awareness of risk factors related to adolescents and type 2 diabetes by client education both in areas of health promotion and disease prevention. NP-directed educational programs could include diabetic education in health classes in cooperation with the school nurse and/or health teacher and community-based diabetic forums addressing this topic.

Reference

Whitaker, J. A., Davis, K. L., & Lauer, C. (2004). Is there a need for screening for type 2 diabetes in seventh graders? *Journal of the American Academy of Nurse Practitioners,* *16*(11), 496–501.

---

the Charleston Heart Study and Atherosclerosis Risk in Communities (ARIC) study (Knapp et al., 1992; Metcalf et al., 1998). Furthermore, Haffner and colleagues (1999), found in the IRAS that the strong association reported between triglyceride levels and insulin resistance (i.e., hyperinsulinemia) does not hold in African Americans, suggesting that, absent a separate insulin resistance marker, the NCEP criteria for metabolic syndrome may underestimate heart disease risk among African American individuals (Appel et al., 2006; Appel et al., 2007; Haffner et al., 1999).

Not as much is known regarding the exact role insulin resistance plays in escalating cardiovascular risk. However, there is ample evidence to indicate a valid link exists between hyperinsulinemia and development of cardiovascular diseases (Alessi et al., 1997). Insulin levels are not commonly measured in primary care settings as are other risk factors. This is because the norms for hyperinsulinemia have not been fully established when an individual has hyperglycemia, but norms are established for euglycemic individuals with hyperinsulinemia (Monzillo & Hamdy, 2003). Evidence indicates that insulin levels $\geq$ 17 uU/ml are indicative of the

presence of insulin resistance and present an increased risk for development of metabolic syndrome, subsequently type 2 diabetes and cardiovascular diseases (McMurray et al., 2000; Monzillo & Hamdy, 2003). There are also many noninvasive history and physical examination findings that are indicative of hyperinsulinemia (see Table 21-4). These are particularly useful for public health nurses to be aware of for potential use during community screening among at-risk minority populations.

Screening for acanthosis nigricans Although insulin levels are not yet commonly measured in primary care, there are other risk markers such as acanthosis nigricans that can easily be screened for in the public health setting (i.e., health fairs, clinics, or schools) (Burke et al., 1999; Cordain, Eades, & Eades, 2003; Kobaissi et al., 2004; Ten & Maclaren, 2004). Use of acanthosis nigricans screening in the schools of the southwestern United States has been successful in finding children at risk for disruptions in their glucose homeostasis (i.e., pre-diabetes, metabolic syndrome, and/or diabetes mellitus).

TABLE 21-4: Noninvasive History and Physical Findings Indicative of Insulin Resistance

GENERAL FINDINGS

Acanthosis nigricans	Verrucous, velvety hyperpigmentation on back of neck, vulva, axillae, groin, knees, elbows, or submammary regions
Cutaneous acrochordons acne	Skin tags
Findings unique to women	
Android appearance	Central obesity, male body habitus (muscularity), clitorimegaly, alopecia (male pattern vertex or crown baldness)
Hirsutism	Inappropriate locations of hair growth: face, chin, chest, perineum
Menstrual dysfunction	Amenorrhea, infertility, increased libido
Gestational diabetes	May have not been diagnosed, but suspicion increases with a history of having given birth to a $\geq$ 9 pound baby

Note: From Goodheart, H.P. (2000). "Hirsutism: Pathogenisis and causes." *Women's Health in Primary Care*, 3(5), 329–337, and Mukhtar, Q.C. (2001). "Prevalence of acanthosis nigricans and its association with hyperinsulinemia in New Mexico adolescents." *Journal of Adolescent Health*, 28(5), 372–376.

Acanthosis nigricans screenings have been extensively used for identifying undiagnosed children and adolescents of Hispanic decent as being insulin resistant and/or having frank type 2 diabetes. Acanthosis nigricans (AN) is characterized by hyperpigmentation of velvety plaques on body folds (e.g., back of the neck, axillae, groin, elbows, or knees) (Mukhtar, 2001). Acanthosis nigricans presents as a smooth and often raised plaque, first noticed at the back of the neck, in a single line (+1); in extreme cases (+4), extending to the frontal plane of the neck and being clearly visible when standing in front of the individual (Burke et al., 1999). Use of acanthosis screening among African American women has shown a positive correlation with several markers of insulin resistance (Appel et al., 2005). Although acanthosis nigricans may commonly be found in all body folds, the back of the neck is commonly used for screening because it is a nonintrusive location for the client and is easily recognizable by the examiner.

Burke and colleagues (1999) demonstrate that the acanthosis nigricans when found is usually first located on the neck, and the neck has the highest sensitivity (93 percent) for insulin resistance. When acanthosis was present in only one location, 99 percent of the time it was found on the neck, compared to any of the other sites. Thus, if acanthosis nigricans was present at all, it was found on the back of the neck (Burke et al., 1999, p. 1658). Burke's 0–4 scale is commonly used to rate the severity of acanthosis nigricans on the neck (Burke et al., 1999).). Acanthosis nigricans has been successfully used as a screening tool to identify those either with insulin resistance or at high risk for development of type 2 diabetes. Further research using the mere presence or absence of acanthosis nigricans during screenings has been especially useful within the Hispanic and African American populations (Bent et al., 1998; Burke et al., 1999). All clients should be assessed for acanthosis nigricans as a risk marker for developing insulin resistance and/or type 2 diabetes (Appel, Ginger, & Floyd, 2004a; Appel, Jones, & Kennedy-Malone, 2004b; Cordain, Eades, & Eades, 2003).

The exact etiology of acanthosis nigricans is not known. However, it is believed that acanthosis nigricans is caused by the hyperinsulinemia stimulating the melanocytes (skin cells) to produce more melanin. Hyperinsulinemia is also believed to cause the binding of insulin to insulin-like growth factor receptors on keratinocytes and fibroblasts, with resultant hyperplasia of the skin (Cruz & Hud, 1992). Recent studies focusing on metabolic risk for cardiovascular diseases have identified that insulin resistance may result from inflammation (Kriketos et al., 2004; Yudkin et al. 2004).

Screening for chronic inflammatory states

Chronic inflammation among low-risk individuals is now being commonly determined by measuring high-sensitivity C-reactive protein (hs-CRP) (Ridker, 2001). Increased hs-CRP levels can be an indication of the presence of hyperinsulinemia associated with systemic inflammation. There is scientific support that hs-CRP is a robust predictor of risk for the occurrence of coronary heart disease. A study by Ridker et al. (2002) found that CRP is a significant predictor of risk for cardiovascular disease beyond that of elevated levels of low-density lipoprotein cholesterol (LDL-C; Ridker et al., 2002). Another study has revealed that having an elevated hs-CRP level may in fact be harmful in its own right and a risk factor for CVD (Ridker et al., 2003). One cause for this alarm is that hs-CRP has been found to elevate plasminogen activator inhibitor-1 (PAI-1), which then fosters a hypercoagulable state (Devaraj, Xu, & Jialal, 2003). Elevated plasma levels of PAI-1 are strongly associated with dysfibrinolysis, a dysfunction of the clotting system, causing an increased propensity for thrombus formation; it is also associated with a worsened prognosis in the presence of a myocardial infarction (Alessi & Juhan-Vague, 2004; Soeki et al., 2002).

Thus risk for development of chronic diseases such as type 2 diabetes and/or cardiovascular diseases may be identified years in advanced of symptomatic pathology (Anderson et al., 2004a; Fagerberg, 2004; Stern et al., 2004). This provides optimal opportunities for public health nurses to plan interventions focused on screening for the related risk markers (see Box 21-1) and risk factors prior to the development of frank pathology (Appel et al., 2002b).

INCREASING PREVALENCE OF TYPE 2 DIABETES

Diabetes has been the subject of much attention both in the lay public's media and in health care literature. This attention has occurred over the past several decades, as increasing prevalence rates for type 2 diabetes have steadily accelerated secondarily to the obesity rates. Recent estimations for the prevalence of type 2 diabetes in the United States reveal that 18.2 million individuals have the disease (NCHS, 2003). It is also believed that over 5 million of these individuals are unaware that they have type 2 diabetes (ADA, 2005; NCHS, 2003). This is a particularly dangerous situation for these uninformed individuals because the complications of type 2 diabetes are insidious in the beginning, but they can quickly lead to both significant micro- and marcovascular injury (Baumelou et al., 2005; Kernan & Inzucci, 2004; Uwaifo & Ratner, 2003).

Diabetes mellitus is the fifth leading cause of death in the general population of the United States. Among African American women, diabetes is the third leading cause of death (AHA, 2007 NCHS, 2003). Consequently, diabetes mellitus is also the major cause of blindness, nontraumatic amputations, and end-stage renal disease among the population of the United States (NCHS, 2003). Diabetes mellitus is undoubtedly a major cause of coronary heart disease-related deaths. Adults with diabetes are two to four times more likely to experience mortality related to coronary heart disease than someone without diabetes (AHA). In fact, 65 percent of diabetes-related deaths are due to heart disease (AHA, 2007 NCHS, 2003). Likewise, approximately 73 percent of adults with diabetes will also have hypertension. Consequently, the risk of stroke is two to four times higher in persons with diabetes (AHA, 2007. Hence, diabetes is a multisystem disease because it affects eye sight (it is the leading cause of blindness);

BOX 21-1

A *risk marker* is a factor that indicates an individual is possibly at risk. However, a risk marker itself doesn't actually cause the physiological risk. Examples are hypertension as a risk factor for stroke and low socioeconomic status (SES) as a risk marker for stroke and other cardiovascular diseases.

the kidney (it leads to end-stage renal failure); and neuropathy (approximately 60 to 70 percent of the persons with diabetes experience some form of neuropathy) (Walker, 2005). Neuropathy is a major predisposing risk factor for amputations (Aszmann, Tassler, & Dellon, 2004; Walker, 2005). The pathological impacts of diabetes are almost too many to discuss within the scope of this chapter. In short, as a member of the health care team, the public health nurse should make every effort to teach health behaviors to avoid the onset of type 2 diabetes and screen individuals within their communities for early signs of risk such as pre-diabetes or the metabolic syndrome. Once frank disease occurs, every effort should be made to implement interventions to minimize its deleterious sequelae.

DISEASES OF THE CARDIOVASCULAR SYSTEM

Coronary heart disease is the number one killer of both men and women in the United States (AHA, 2007). Cardiovascular diseases remain the leading cause of occupational disability among adults. Stroke alone accounts for the disability of more than a million Americans each year (see Figure 21-3) (AHA 2007; NCHS, 2003). Morbidity and mortality from cardiovascular-related diseases places an enormous economic burden on the health system. The economic impact will become even more notable as the numbers of elderly grow larger and the population ages. For 2005, the estimated cost of health care expenditures and lost productivity related to cardiovascular diseases is expected to mount to over $393 billion (AHA, 2007).

Cardiovascular disease, including coronary heart disease, stroke, and heart failure, remains the leading cause of death and disability in the United States despite improvements in prevention, detection, and treatment (AHA, 2007). There is a common misperception that coronary heart disease is a man's illness (AHA, 2007). Yet heart disease places a substantial burden on the morbidity and mortality of women's health (Aikawa et al., 2005; Bello & Mosca, 2004). As illustrated in Figure 21-4, as of 1985 more women began dying from heart disease than men (AHA, 2007). Although women tend to develop the symptoms of heart disease later in life than men, they have a worse prognosis and are more likely to die from an acute cardiac event (AHA, 2007). This delay in manifestation of the symptoms of cardiovascular-related diseases may be explained by the

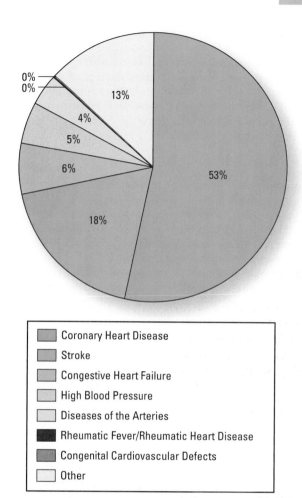

Figure 21-3 Percentage breakdown of deaths from CVD in the United States: 2002 Preliminary.

From CDC/NCHS. Centers for Disease Control and Prevention (CDC) (1999). Behavioral Risk Factor Surveillance System (BRFSS). Retrieved from http://www.cdc.gov/nccdphp/aag/aag_brfss.htm.

physiologic protection of their endogenous hormones. As women near menopause, they begin to lose the protective effects of estrogen (Anderson et al., 2004b). During postmenopausal years, their risk for heart disease accelerates with aging. The death rate from heart disease is approximately three times greater than from breast cancer; this is the case among both white and African American women (AHA, 2007). However, contemporary studies have revealed that many women are still more concerned with dying from breast or reproductive-related cancers than death from heart disease (Hughes & Hayman, 2004). Thus, the American Heart Association has initiated several major campaigns to increase the awareness among women of their risk for heart disease. This is especially appropriate and timely as cardiovascular disease is a killer of people in the prime of life, with more than half of all deaths occurring among women (AHA, 2007).

Coronary Heart Disease

Coronary heart disease is the most significant cause of mortality within the United States, causing 493,382 deaths in 2002, which equates to one out of every five deaths (AHA, 2007). Approximately 83 percent of deaths due to coronary heart disease occur among individuals older than 65 years of age, as this is the leading cause of death among this age group (AHA, 2007). Although women tend to have myocardial infarctions later in life than men, 38 percent of women versus only 25 percent of men die within one year after an acute myocardial infarction (AHA, 2007).

The American Heart Association estimated that in 2002 better than 1 million Americans had either a new or recurrent coronary event, and that about one-third died (AHA, 2007). Similarly, every 26 seconds, an American will suffer an acute coronary event leading to a myocardial infarction, and about every minute someone will die from such an event (AHA, 2007). Each year more than 250,000 people will die of myocardial infarctions (AHA, 2007). Forty-one percent of individuals who experience a myocardial infarction will die within one year (AHA, 2007). Approximately 335,000 deaths that occur each year are located either in the Emergency Department or before the client reaches the hospital (AHA, 2007). This may well be related to the fact that 50 percent of men versus 64 percent of women die from sudden cardiac deaths that occur among individuals without prior symptoms indicative of cardiovascular diseases (AHA, 2007).

Coronary heart disease, also called ischemic heart disease, or acute coronary syndrome refers to atherosclerosis of the arteries that supply the heart muscle. Atherosclerosis is a disorder that can arise from beginning to end of the arterial circulation. It is a general word that refers to the solidifying or hardening of the arteries. Atherosclerosis results from the deposits of substances such as cholesterol, platelets, foam cells, and calcium, and from clotting of the blood (Boyle, 2005). When these substances congregate on the inner

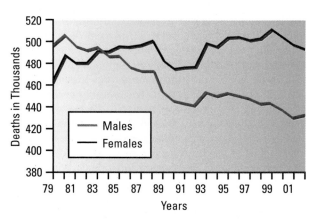

Figure 21-4 CVD mortality trends for males and females in the United States: 1979–2002.
From CDC/NCHS. Centers for Disease Control and Prevention (CDC) (1999). Behavioral Risk Factor Surveillance System (BRFSS). Retrieved from http://www.cdc.gov/nccdphp/aag/aag_brfss.htm.

walls of an artery, it is referred to as plaque. Plaque buildup inside of the arteries may either partially or totally occlude the blood flow. Various pathological events may then occur, such as a formation of thrombus or hemorrhage under the plaque. A hemorrhage under the plaque will cause it to rupture and further occlude the artery (Boyle, 2005). Similarly, a blood clot (or thrombus) may form on the surface of the plaque-enhancing ischemia because the blood flow through the artery is limited. When either one or both of these pathologies occur, acute ischemia results from low flow through the coronary circulation leading to an acute myocardial infarction (Boyle, 2005). Although atherosclerosis develops slowly over time, it is believed to begin early in life (Belay, Belamarich, & Racine, 2004; Lavezzi, Ottaviani, & Matturri, 2005). However, a rapid increase in the amount of plaque and the propensity for thrombus tends to occur as people age and develop central obesity (AHA, 2007). The presence of a hypercoagulable state is associated with the inflammation caused by obesity, which fosters an environment supportive for thrombus formation (Alessi & Juhan-Vague, 2004). In the fifth or sixth decade of life, many individuals become symptomatic due to the presence of atherosclerosis (AHA, 2007). Typically, men begin to manifest the ill effects of atherosclerosis about ten years earlier than their female counterparts (AHA, 2007; Foster & Mallik, 1998; Moser et al., 2005). However, once women are postmenopausal, they frequently manifest signs and symptoms of atherosclerosis.

When a coronary artery becomes occluded by a thrombus and/or ruptured plaque that leads to total occlusion of flow to the artery, then an acute myocardial infarction will likely occur (Boyle, 2005; Falk, 1992; Naghavi et al., 2003). Insufficient blood supply may result from a reduction of blood flow through one or more of the coronary arteries. Cardiac cells are reliant on blood flow through the coronary circulation to supply oxygen, glucose, and various other nutrients for optimal functioning of cardiac tissue. Lacking a sufficient flow of blood, the cardiac cells become irritable or ischemic; this can often be manifested by life-threatening dysrhythmias (i.e., premature ventricular contractions, ventricular tachycardia, and ventricular fibrillation) (Katayama et al., 2005). Ultimately, ischemic cardiac cells become necrotic and die. When an acute cardiac event occurs, urgent emergency management is required to minimize the zone of injury within the heart from extending, injuring, or killing additional cardiac cells and then escalating the risk for sudden cardiac death (Katayama et al., 2005).

Subjective symptoms experienced during an acute cardiac event often vary from one individual to another. However, specific populations such as women, the elderly, and clients with diabetes tend to experience atypical symptoms and patterns of chest pain (McSweeney et al., 2003). Therefore, clients from these populations are in need of special teaching regarding the possible variations of their symptoms that may represent an impending myocardial infarction. The old adage "Time is Tissue" is still appropriate to highlight the priority need for prudent attention in response to the signs of ischemia (Bold & Luedtke, 2001; Wilkinson et al., 2002). Therefore, contributions of the public health nurses are focused on teaching the public how to react with the onset of signs/symptoms of an acute cardiac event. Likewise, a special emphasis is also needed to alert the public to the possible variations the symptoms of an acute cardiac event may manifest among special populations.

Modifiable Risk Factors

Traditionally, risk factors for coronary heart disease or stroke are similar and have been divided between those that are modifiable and those that are nonmodifiable. Risk factors that are considered to be modifiable include (1) tobacco use and passive exposure to smoke from tobacco, (2) obesity, (3) elevated blood cholesterol (dyslipidemia), (4) high blood pressure (hypertension), (5) physical inactivity, and (6) high fat dietary practices (AHA, 2007). Likewise, excessive alcohol use and the presence of high levels of stress have also been shown to lend a propensity toward the development of cardiovascular diseases (Kurihara et al., 2004).

Nonmodifiable risk factors for coronary artery disease include genetics, family history, gender, race, and increasing age. Although it is important for public health nurses to be aware of the nonmodifiable risk factors for cardiovascular disease because these will assist in identification of high-risk groups, public health nurse should focus primarily on the modifiable risk factors, which will be potentially amenable to intervention. Major modifiable risk factors for cardiovascular diseases are reviewed in the following section.

Tobacco Use

Abuses of tobacco products as a group are one of the single largest contributors to premature risk for having a myocardial infarction. Research has shown that smokers are two times more likely to have a myocardial infarction than their nonsmoker counterparts (AHA, 2007). Similarly, smokers are between two and four times more likely to experience sudden death (AHA, 2007; Bernhard et al., 2003). Even passive smoke exposure has also been implicated as a risk for development of coronary heart disease. For those who are able to stop smoking, the ability for the lungs to recover from tobacco use is promising. It is believed that within three years after termination of tobacco use, the risk for sudden cardiac death becomes equal to that of an individual who has never smoked. Dzien and colleagues (2004) found that smokers also had higher fasting glucose levels and were more likely to manifest insulin resistance. Similarly, it was found that smokers not only had reduced HDL cholesterol (HDL-C) levels but also elevated fibrinolytic profiles predisposing them to thrombus formation (i.e., elevated levels of plasma plasminogen activator inhibitor-1) (Appel et al., 2007: Dzien et al., 2004; Minami et al., 2002). Although smokers commonly have levels of BMI that fall into the normal range category, they also have a propensity to manifest central obesity (Sato et al., 1992). Even though it is a common finding that intense smokers may have a BMI that is normal, they tend to have larger waist circumferences than nonsmokers, placing smokers at additional risk for development of metabolic syndrome (den Tonkelaar et al., 1990; Jastrzebska, Goracy, & Naruszewicz, 2003; Seidell et al., 1991). As discussed, smokers have commonly been found to have chronically lower levels of HDL-C, higher fasting levels of glucose, central obesity, and insulin resistance (Maeda, Noguchi, & Fukui, 2003; Sato et al., 1992).

Central Obesity

Ample evidence suggests that increased risk for coronary heart disease can at least be partly accounted for with central obesity at the core surrounded by the cluster of symptoms known as metabolic syndrome (Janssen, Katzmarzyk, & Ross, 2002; Lemieux et al., 2000). As such, central obesity has been found to be a risk factor common to all other metabolic syndrome components as well as an independent risk factor for chronic diseases (Nieves et al., 2003). Prospective studies of adults have shown that central obesity confers an increased risk for cardiovascular diseases (Girman et al., 2004; Goran & Gower, 1998). Recently, Palaniappan and colleagues (2004) analyzed data from the IRAS (Palaniappan et al., 2004). A major finding indicated the best predictor for development of metabolic syndrome was an increased waist circumference (OR: 1.7; CI 1.3-2.0) (Palaniappan et al., 2004). This suggests that central obesity may pave the way for the development of other metabolic syndrome components. Over the last fifty years it has become apparent that deep abdominal visceral adipocyte tissues are metabolically active and excrete many deleterious metabolic substrates (i.e., angiotensin, PAI-1, and numerous cytokines) (Vaughan, 2002; Vaughan, Lazos, & Tong, 1995). Central obesity has been strongly implicated as the preliminary event leading to insulin resistance by triggering of triglycerides to be broken down into free fatty acids (FFA), then flowing directly into the liver via the portal veins and fostering insulin resistance (Alessi, Morange, & Juhan-Vague, 2000; Reaven, 2002; Yoo et al., 2004). Studies have identified the deep visceral adipose tissue (VAT) as one major culprit in the excreting of excess plasma levels of PAI-1 (Kelley et al., 2000). Both hyperinsulinemia and hypertriglyceridemia have been found to stimulate the abdominal adipocytes to release increased PAI-1 fostering a hypercoagulable state leading to increased occurrences of thrombus and thus acute cardiac events.

Dyslipidemia

Elevated levels of blood lipids such as total cholesterol, LDL-C, elevated triglycerides, and/or low levels of HDL-C have been repeatedly demonstrated to significantly increase the risk for coronary heart disease. This is especially true if other risk factors are present. The NCEP considers a LDL-C level below 70 mg/dL as being optimal, especially in an individual who has had a myocardial infarction, diabetes mellitus, or another coronary heart disease equivalent (NCEP, 2001).

Triglyceride levels $\geq$ 150 mg/dL are strongly associated with coronary heart disease (NCEP, 2001). Increasing evidence suggests that centrally obese individuals with hypertriglyceridemia or low HDL-C may have abnormal fibrolytic systems, exemplified by elevated plasma levels of PAI-1 (Cimminiello et al., 1997; Soderberg et al., 1999). It is also known that high levels of HDL-C protect against coronary heart disease and may serve further to activate the fibrolytic system (Saku et al., 1985). Thus, it has been postulated that low levels of HDL-C impair fibrinolysis and can contribute to atherothrombic events associated with dyslipidemias. Likewise, studies that examined the association between central obesity, plasma haemostatic factors, and metabolic parameters have found PAI-1 to be independently associated with central obesity (Abbasi et al., 1999; Cigolini et al., 1996; Lemieux et al., 2000). When allowances were made for BMI and insulin levels, triglycerides were the only other variable positively associated with and in an independent relationship to PAI-1 and central obesity (Cigolini et al., 1996; Rodriguez et al., 2002). These studies suggest that the common dyslipidemias associated with risk for cardiovascular disease may be compounded by abnormal fibrolytic responses. Low HDL-C for men is $\leq$ 40 mg/dL and for women < 50 mg/dL (NCEP, 2001). The NCEP recommends first screening and treating LDL-C and then HDL-C. Ideally HDL-C should be $\geq$ 60 mg/dL and then it is considered as a negative risk factor (NCEP, 2001). Numerous factors have been found to lower HDL-C levels. Several studies have examined the association between smoking and central obesity.

In summary, the NCEP ATP III criteria recommend that healthy adults age 20 and older should have a fasting lipoprotein profile (i.e., total cholesterol, LDL-C, HDL-C, triglycerides) once every five years (NCEP, 2001). Individuals with additional risks for coronary heart disease, such as smoking, central obesity, prediabetes, metabolic syndrome, diabetes, previous myocardial infarction, or stroke, may need more frequent screening. Elevated levels of cholesterol can be controlled through diet modification, increased physical activity, and use of lipid-lowering agents.

Hypertension

Hypertension increases the heart's afterload by triggering it to enlarge and weaken. Therefore, hypertension increases the risk for a number of diseases, including congestive heart failure, end-stage kidney disease, myocardial infarction, and stroke (AHA, 2007). When other risk factors are present, the risk from hypertension increases exponentially. The deleterious effects of hypertension can be controlled to some extent by diet, weight loss, physical activity, salt restriction intake, and antihypertensive medications.

One in four Americans is affected by hypertension, which is a major precursor to life-threatening diseases (AHA, 2005). Figure 21-5 shows age-adjusted trends for high blood pressure in America. Non-Hispanic black

men and women have continued to have the highest prevalence for high blood pressure. For both whites and blacks, the prevalence of high blood pressure decreased between 1988 and 1994, but then increased between 1999 to 2002. Although awareness of hypertension has improved over the past two decades, hypertension continues to contribute significantly to mortality and morbidity among adults and particularly within minority populations. There appears to be physiologic differences among ethnic groups that predispose some to hypertension over other groups. African Americans have been found to be at greatest risk due to a heightened level of cardiac vascular reactivity and the propensity for excessive vasoconstriction (Alpert & Barnard, 2001). It is imperative that the public health nurse not lose sight of the fact that hypertension is also a component of the metabolic syndrome and needs to be viewed as potentially part of a larger group of risk factors acting in synergy to produce vascular injury

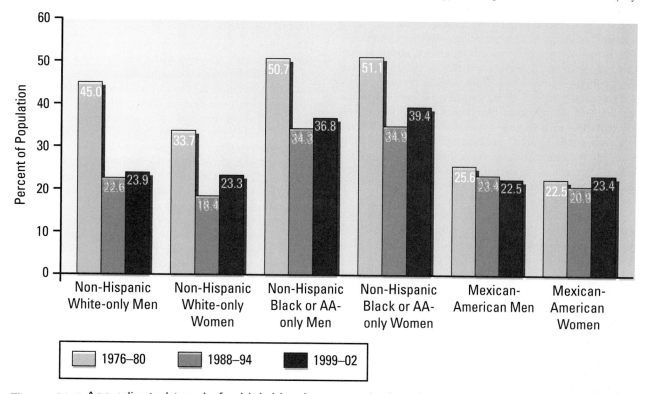

Figure 21-5 Age-adjusted trends for high blood pressure in America age 20–74 by race/ethnicity, sex, and survey (NHANES, 1976–1980, 1988–1994, 1999–2002).

From CDC/NCHS. Centers for Disease Control and Prevention (CDC) (1999). Behavioral Risk Factor Surveillance System (BRFSS). Retrieved from http://www.cdc.gov/nccdphp/aag/aag_brfss.htm. Data based on a single measure of blood pressure.

(Herdegen, 2002; Smith et al., 2005). Therefore, secreening for risk factors such as central obesity, dyslipidemia, and insulin resistance may play an important role in preventing and managing hypertension. Community-based screening and blood pressure management programs have began to offer hope in reaching the higher risk populations of the United States.

Ward and colleagues (2000) in the Community Hypertension Intervention Project (CHIP), a four-year longitudinal study, investigated the environmental and psychosocial factors related to treatment adherence with 1,367 urban-dwelling minority participants (75 percent black and 25 percent Hispanic). Prior to the study, the majority of clients within the clinics did not have appropriately controlled hypertension, and at any one time the clinic would have 45 percent no-show rates for blood pressure management follow-up (Ward et al., 2000). The study examined effects of traditional hypertension care combined with three interventions to improve client compliance (Ward et al., 2000). Participants were randomized to one of three groups: individualized counseling sessions; home visits/discussion groups; or computerized appointment-tracking system, all were managed in either the local hospital-based clinic or a private clinic in the community (Ward et al., 2000). Approximately, 65 percent of the participants remained in blood pressure ranges out of control. The investigators concluded that for the clients with improved control, structural changes at the clinic site, along with the targeted interventions, improved client satisfaction, increased treatment adherence, and improve blood pressure control (Ward et al., 2000).

Examples of community screening efforts for hypertension and promotion of cardiovascular health are abundant within the literature. Nussinovitch and colleagues (2005) conducted blood pressure screenings in high schools and found a prevalence of 76 percent. Boys $\geq$ 17 years of age had significantly higher blood pressures when their body mass index exceeded 17 kg/m^2 (Nussinovitch et al., 2005). The findings of these investigators point to the need for early screening of children and adolescents for hypertension.

Gabbay and colleges conducted a randomized controlled study with two arms, one usual diabetic care ($n = 182$) and the second arm nurse case managed ($n = 150$). Results showed a significant decrease in blood pressure and diabetic-related problems and/or complications among the case managed group (Gabbay et al., 2005). Similarly, close contact seems to provide

improved health outcomes as several studies showed better hypertension control and cardiovascular health outcomes with the use of lay health advisers among minority populations (Kim et al., 2004; Kobetz et al., 2005; Rankin, 2004).

Physical Inactivity

Physical inactivity plays a considerable role in the development of metabolic syndrome, type 2 diabetes, and cardiovascular diseases. Recommendations are that aerobic exercises should be incorporate into the day for at least 20 minutes. Suggested activities include aerobics, jogging, and vigorous walking (AHA, 2007). As a rule of thumb, any exercise that makes you breathe hard and your heart beat rapidly should provide this benefit. Recent research has revealed that even modest levels of low-intensity exercise will provide increased cardiovascular benefit. Examples of these activities include walking for pleasure, gardening, housework, and dancing.

High-Fat Diet

Diets low in fat can help to prevent cardiovascular disease. Research has revealed that diets low in fat and high in both vegetables and fruits play a significant role in preventing atherosclerotic disease (AHA, 2007). Intake of high amounts of dietary fiber that help lower blood cholesterol and the antioxidants contained within these foods serve to assist in lipoprotein oxidation. Conversely, consumption of saturated fat, dietary cholesterol, and red meat has increased the occurrence of heart disease. One of the most ideal dietary interventions for minimizing the development of hypertension and other cardiovascular diseases is the plan called Dietary Approaches to Stop Hypertension (DASH) (i.e., a low-calorie, low-cholesterol diet, with plenty of fruits, vegetables, and fiber) (Ard et al., 2004). DASH is considered an eating style that can be adopted. Like diet, physical activity is the mainstay of treating the ill effects of insulin resistance. When both of these lifestyle alterations are achieved, the metabolic profile has been found to significantly improve.

CONTEXTUAL RISK FACTORS AND CHRONIC DISEASES

Contextual risk factors can be defined as circumstances or variables beyond the control of the individual that may serve to increase morbidity, and/or mor-

⊕ RESEARCH APPLICATION

Midlife Women's Adherence to Home-Based Walking during Maintenance

Study Purpose

To describe midlife women's maintenance of walking following the intervention phase of a 24-week, home-based walking program, and to identify the effects of background characteristics, self-efficacy for overcoming barriers to exercise, and adherence to walking during the intervention phase on retention and adherence to walking.

Methods

Black and white women participants ($N = 90$) aged 40–65 years who completed a 24-week, home-based walking program. Self-efficacy for overcoming barriers to exercise, maximal aerobic fitness, and percentage of body fat were measured at baseline, 24 weeks, and 48 weeks. Adherence was measured with heart-rate monitors and an exercise log.

Findings

Retention was 80 percent during maintenance. On average, the women who reported walking during maintenance adhered to 64 percent of the expected walks during that phase. Examination of the total number of walks and the number and sequence of weeks without a walk revealed dynamic patterns. The multiple regression model explained 40 percent of the variance in adherence during the maintenance phase.

Implications

These results suggest that both self-efficacy for overcoming barriers and adherence during the intervention phase play a role in women's walking adherence. The findings reflect dynamic patterns of adopting and maintaining new behavior.

Reference

Wilbur, J., Vassalo, A., Chandler, P., McDevitt, J., & Miller, A. M (2005). Midlife women's adherence to home-based walking during maintenance. *Nursing Research, 54*(1), 33–40.

tality associated with chronic diseases such as type 2 diabetes, stroke, or coronary heart disease (Appel et al., 2002). Individuals of low socioeconomic status are particularly vulnerable to the impact of their environment and the context in which they live. In general, contextual risk factors may include, but are not limited to, the following: being a single parent, sole head of household, living in a geographically medically underserved region of the United States, lack of a consistent primary care provider, limited information from the health care system, lacking easy access to transportation, and residing in a low-income region of the United States (Appel et al., 2002; Flaskerud & Nyamathi, 2002; Mansfield, Wilson, Kobrinski & Mitchell, 1999).

Research conducted by Mansfield and colleagues (1999) revealed that women living within certain contexts were more at risk for premature morbidity and mortality. Mansfield et al. (1999) found that being a single-parent, female head of household and residing within the southern United States was a major risk fac-

tor for premature mortality. One rationale may be that the southern United States is one of the lowest socioeconomic areas. Likewise, being a single parent may also contribute to limited resources and lower income status. The southern United States also contains some of the largest groups of minorities who tend to possess lower incomes than whites. Traditionally, the South has not provided many resources for its minority groups. The historical aspects of the southern United States may still today play a role in fostering hidden discrimination, limiting resources, and leading to chronic diseases. It is highly likely that residing in a lower-income area facilitates being confronted with contextual factors that increase risks for chronic diseases, by increasing the scarcity of both informational health and financial resources. This scarcity may exacerbate differences in what economists refer to as opportunity cost, defined as "the synergy of time and money required to access available services" (Airhihenbuwa, 2001, p. 268). Opportunity cost provides a further explanation for the apparent disparity in health among minority

⊕ POLICY HIGHLIGHT

Nonmodifiable Risk Factors

The persistent cardiovascular health disparities that exist between African Americans and whites have remained steady over the last several decades. Traditionally, death rates from cardiovascular diseases have remained consistently higher among African Americans than whites, until advanced age. In 2002, coronary heart disease death rates were 220.5 for white males and 250.5 for African American males, 131.2 white females and 169.7 African American females (AHA, 2007: NCHS, 2003). There are numerous hypothesis as to why this disparity persists (i.e., slave health deficit, low SES, etc.) (Appel, Harrell, & Deng, 2002; Appel et al., 2005; Randall, 2002). However, it is worth noting that even the presence of the traditional risk factors for cardiovascular disease combined with the impact of low SES fail to account in full for this deficit. The report from the Institute of Medicine is full of examples where minorities, especially African Americans, have not received optimal medical treatment in spite of insurance status (Betancourt, 2002).

Historically in the United States, the incidence and mortality rates for cardiovascular disease go up as socioeconomic status goes down (Mansfield et al., 1999). The greatest improvements in death rates have occurred for the highest levels of SES (i.e., higher income, education among workers in white-collar jobs) (AHA, 2007; Cohen, Farley, & Mason, 2003; Wong et al., 2002). Although the role of family history is not completely understood, it undoubtedly plays a major part in predicting premature heart disease. Research supports the fact that positive family history for heart disease often identifies an individual at greater risk for development of premature coronary heart disease. This risk is theorized to occur via multiple factors that cluster in families (i.e., genetics; learned lifestyle behaviors leading to physical inactivity, obesity, smoking, high fat diet).

As client advocates, what can public health nurses do to promote policy and procedure adjustments to ensure equitable care across racial, gender, and economic barriers?

populations and thus may explain the presence of chronic diseases among certain populations.

The aforementioned definition of cost is comparable to that used in economics, which take into account what has been "forgone," relinquished or given up, to gain another good or service (Shiell, 1997). This use of cost provides a more accurate foundation for understanding choices made in low-income families (Shiell et al., 2002). If a low-income individual who has limited resources chooses to acquire more of one commodity, he or she can do so only by doing away with, or relinquishing consumption of another good or service (Appel et al., 2005). In short, a health care consumer who earns an income at or below the poverty line is likely to be confronted with greater levels of opportunity costs than a consumer with higher earnings.

In the past when low-income individuals commonly obtained health care from public institutions, they did so by trading their time for their limited money. Commonly, they encounter prolonged waiting times due to overburdening of these public health care services. Even today when services are offered to low-income individuals on a sliding scale or to Medicaid recipients, they are faced with the need to allow additional time to gain access. The idea that "cost" can be incurred in both monetary and nonmonetary ways is an important premise for public health nurses to consider when analyzing health outcomes among vulnerable populations (Appel et al., 2005; Shiell et al., 2002). Obviously, opportunity cost among low-income individuals is much more exaggerated than among the middle class (Appel et al., 2005). Understanding the impact of opportunity cost becomes critical when public health nurses attempt to make a positive impact on health outcomes. This may help avoid the cycle of "blaming the victim" for the outcome of poor health.

An in-depth understanding of the specific opportunity costs encountered by low-income individuals residing in the nurse's community can help to explain how these individuals are making rational choices when using their limited resources. The value of understanding opportunity cost for public health nurses is that this understanding may guide the public health nurse in designing more efficacious health programs that do not create additional barriers for vulnerable populations. Reducing barriers to health care resources by reducing the opportunity cost for low-income and underserved individuals may enhance heart health behaviors.

Vulnerable populations are either unaware of the deleterious outcomes of ignoring health care concerns and/or are overcome with the competing choices they face when trying to survive on a low income (Airhihenbuwa, 2001; Appel et al., 2002; Appel et al., 2005). All of these competing choices are made in the context of the scarcity of resources. Low-income individuals must decide how to distribute the few assets that they do possess. Public health nurses need to understand that some of these individuals will place the needs of their children and other family members above their own needs. Contextual circumstances and competing choices may contribute to lack of utilization of public health programs. Because the traditional risk factors for many chronic diseases do not fully account for the occurrences of health disparities among vulnerable populations, it is quite plausible that multiple factors work in concert to worsen health outcomes among the chronically ill.

CAREGIVER BURDEN

Currently, chronic diseases are pervasive in our society, affecting the neonate to the elderly, and not only impacting chronically ill individuals but also their families and friends who all too often are caregivers. Caregiver burden is an overwhelming feeling of loss of control of one's own life in lieu of taking care of a chronically ill person. Caregiver burden, defined as physical, emotional, and financial stress or burden experienced by a caregiver of a frail person, is a growing phenomenon increasingly reducing the quality of life of those who choose to care for the chronically ill (Gitlin et al., 2003; Lidell, 2002). Not only is caregiving an additional role for spouses and children of the chronically ill, but it also affects grandparents who are increasingly placed in situations of being the primary caregiver of a grandchild with a chronic illness. Being a caregiver to a chronically ill person is commonly an additional role that falls under the supervision of women within the United States.

The public health nurse can do much by assessing and reassessing caregivers for symptoms of extreme burden and assist them with the use of available community resources. Predictors for development of extreme caregiver burden have been identified within the literature as being social isolation, limited family

or social support, little knowledge of either the disease or the ill person's possible responses to the disease, lack of or inability to communicate directly with the ill person, a history of poor coping patterns, strain in the relationship prior to the illness, and guilty feeling of the caregiver (Caap-Ahlgren & Dehlin, 2002; Fried et al., 2005; Goldstein et al., 2004; Nabors, Seacat, & Rosenthal, 2002; Williamson & Shaffer, 2001). Likewise, the public health nurse should assess for protective factors supporting the caregiver such as available family and friends, ability of the caregiver to solve problems, a history of positive coping skills, and knowledge of the disease or condition (Kaufer et al., 2005; Williamson & Shaffer, 2001). Interventions the public health nurse may need to consider in order to minimize caregiver burden should be focused on reducing social isolation by identifying community agencies with resources such as adult day care and temporary sitters. Likewise, the nurse should provide the caregiver with additional information concerning the health status of the ill individual and their expected responses to the illness. The nurse may need to serve as a liaison between the ill individual and the caregiver in order to assist them in the development of realistic expectations for each other.

In general, it is known that the burden of the caregiver increases over time and worsens when there is minimal or no communication between the ill individual and the caregiver (Fried et al., 2005; Nabors, Seacat, & Rosenthal, 2002). Similarly, the greater the psychological maladjustment or the less functional ability of the chronically ill person the more likely the caregiver is to experience excessive burden and the effects of depression (Caap-Ahlgren & Dehlin, 2002; Calhoun, Beckham & Bosworth, 2002). Public health nurses need to be the most concerned with the caregiver who has limited social support, for they are at risk for experiencing the greatest burden (Goldstein et al., 2004).

When chronic diseases are not successfully prevented, they need to be managed, and commonly the chronically ill require care from others. Management of chronic diseases needs to focus on maximizing normal function and reducing the progression of the disease. It is important for public health nurses to understand the specific elements of chronic diseases. There are many examples given in the qualitative literature related to the plight of the chronically ill and the associated impact on the caregiver. Table 21-1 provides a starting point for a fuller exploration of the concept of caregiver burden.

DISEASE TRAJECTORY

Chronic diseases have rapidly become the United States' number one health concern. Thus, public health nurses are assuming a progressively more important role in assisting the communities and families they serve to manage the care of the chronically ill. More families are now providing at-home supervision and care for their ill family members and for increasingly long periods of time. Two common chronic diseases where families provide home care for individuals with downward illness trajectories are multiple sclerosis and Alzheimer's disease. Multiple sclerosis (MS) can be particularly challenging in that there is often the occurrence of remissions and acute exacerbation. Thus, the course of MS is very unpredictable, whereas the illness of Alzheimer's is primarily a downward trajectory.

Therefore, expertise with the progression of specific chronic diseases is needed to enhance the success of public health efforts. The idea of a disease trajectory offers a way for nurses to acquire a fuller appreciation of the dynamic nature of chronic disease. The trajectory, or course, of a chronic disease may vary considerably depending on specific disease processes (Jablonski, 2004). Commonly, chronic disease trajectories are characterized by periods of remission and recurrence (Bostrom & Ahlstrom, 2004). Periods of recurrence may require extended periods of time in an acute care environment, focused acute home care, and ultimately rehabilitation. The more chaotic the disease trajectory, the greater the uncertainty faced by the client and their caregivers. Unpredictability of the disease

---

⊕ PRACTICE APPLICATION

Know Your Own State

⊕ Determine your state's major chronic health problems and where your state ranks compared to the other states in the United States. What percentage of the population in your state is obese, has type 2 diabetes, dies from coronary artery disease or stroke, belongs to a racial minority group, or is older than age 65?

⊕ How does your state rank compared to the list of chronic health problems in the United States listed in Table 21-2?

⊕ Identify the most pressing health issues in your community.

⊕ Make a list of community-based resources found in your city to deal with these chronic health problems.

Note: Many states have a Healthy (name of your state) People 2010 subreport on the Department of Health Web site. Also it is common for local and state Health Departments to publish on the Web reports concerning the health issues in the state and specific counties.

---

trajectory produces increased anxiety, uncertainty, and reduced independence. The results are impaired function of activities for daily living, limitations in self-care, development of emotional dysfunctions, and changes in self-image. In short, the unpredictable nature of a chronic disease profoundly impacts the quality of life achievable by those affected. The greater the knowledge by the public health team of the client's illness and the possible pathway(s) a specific disease trajectory can take, the better prepared the team will be to assist the caregiver to access resources in a timely manner.

PUBLIC HEALTH NURSING CONSIDERATION FOR SCREENING FOR AND MANAGEMENT OF CHRONIC DISEASES

The needs of our nation have shifted over the past fifty years from that of care for acute infectious ill-

---

⊕ POLICY HIGHLIGHT

WHO Goals

The World Health Organization has a vision to reduce death rates from all chronic diseases by 2 percent per year over and above existing trends during the next ten years. This bold goal would result in the prevention of 36 million chronic disease deaths worldwide by 2015, most of these being in low- and middle-income countries. This goal would extend the lives for the benefits of the individual, families, and communities and would also result in economic dividends for countries around the globe.

nesses to chronic diseases. Likewise, the role of the public health nurse has shifted from the care of individuals and their families to that of larger populations. Tackling the predicament of the increasing prevalence of chronic diseases within the United States presents public health nurses with an array of challenges that are both complicated and grueling. Managing this challenge was particularly overwhelming when the focus was once primarily on the health of individuals and their families versus the current shift to improving health outcomes among aggregate populations. The equations for improving the health status of various populations are certainly not without tribulation. Successfully reducing the occurrences of chronic diseases is unlikely without support from social, political, and economic forces. It has long been evident within the United States that financial resources are a fundamental prerequisite for attempting to reach and then maintaining adequate health. It is not inconsequential that the same populations faced with the highest prevalence of chronic diseases are those who have historically been marginalized. Development of an increased appreciation for the contextual aspects faced by the poor and underserved may assist the health care team in better understanding choices made in the face of limited resources, repressed by lack of education, improvised contextual environmental circumstances, and low social position. Public health nurses are in an excellent position to advocate for populations concerning the ongoing discourse about wealth, social position, and health outcomes. The role of public health nurses is to carry out the populace's health care campaign. In performing this role, nurses are positioned to increase public awareness of health disparities within the context of the community's environment. This potentially may lead to the development of needs-oriented new services purposely fashioned for specific communities. Ultimately, this can lead to culturally specific programs where the community has become a stakeholder and has a vested interest in successful outcome.

CRITICAL THINKING ACTIVITIES

1. Explain why chronic illnesses have replaced acute illnesses as the primary causes of morbidity and mortality in the United States.

2. What is the role of evidence-based nursing practice in the prevention or management of chronic illness?

3. Describe the purpose for implementing collaborative and community-based participatory research activities in order to prevent or manage chronic illness.

4. Why is it beneficial for the nurse to consider the trajectory a chronic illness?

5. What type of trajectory would you expect for the following chronic illnesses: (a) diabetes mellitus, (b) stroke, (c) heart disease, and (d) Alzheimer's disease?

KEY TERMS

acute illness	disease trajectory	mortality
chronic illness	insulin resistance	obesity
caregiver burden	metabolic syndrome	pre-diabetes
contextual risk factors	morbidity	

KEY CONCEPTS

- Technological advances have allowed public health nurses to better screen, prevent, and manage acute and chronic disease in the community.

- Chronic disease results in a tremendous negative economic and social impact on individuals, families, communities, and nations.

- The obesity epidemic, tobacco use, inactivity, and aging population has accelerated the growth of chronic diseases such as cardiovascular disease and diabetes.

- The overall physical, emotional, and financial costs of caregiving are collectively referred to as caregiver burden. Public health nurses are uniquely positioned to partner with community organizations to address caregiving responsibilities within families and community resources to prevent the stresses resulting from caring for loved ones.

REFERENCES

Abbasi, F., McLaughlin, T., Lamendola, C., Lipinska, I., Tofler, G., & Reaven, G. M. (1999). Comparison of plasminogen activator inhibitor-1 concentration in insulin-resistant versus insulin-sensitive healthy women. *Arteriosclerosis, Thrombosis, and Vascular Biology, 19*(11), 2818–2821.

Adami, G. F., Ravera, G., Marinari, G. M., Camerini, G., & Scopinaro, N. (2001). Metabolic syndrome in severely obese patients. *Obesity Surgery, 11*(5), 543–545.

Ahmad, O. B., Lopez, A. D., & Inoue, M. (2000). The decline in child mortality: A reappraisal. *Bulletin of the World Health Organization, 78*(10), 1175–1191.

Aikawa, V. N., Bambirra, A. P., Seoane, L. A., Bensenor, I. M., & Lotufo, P. A. (2005). Higher burden of hemorrhagic stroke among women. *Neuroepidemiology, 24*(4), 209–213.

Airhihenbuwa, C. O. (2001). Health promotion and disease prevention strategies for African Americans: A conceptual model. In R. L. Brathwaite & S. E. Taylor (Eds.), *Health Issues in the Black Community* (pp. 267–280). San Francisco: Jossey-Bass Publishers.

Alessi, M. C., & Juhan-Vague, I. (2004). Contribution of PAI-1 in cardiovascular pathology. *Archives des Maladies du Coeur et des Vaisseaux, 9*(6), 673–678.

Alessi, M. C., Morange, P., & Juhan-Vague, I. (2000). Fat cell function and fibrinolysis. *Hormorne and Metabolic Research, 32*(11–12), 504–508.

Alessi, M. C., Peiretti, F., Morange, P., Henry, M., Nalbone, G., & Juhan-Vague, I. (1997). Production of plasminogen activator inhibitor 1 by human adipose tissue: Possible link between visceral fat accumulation and vascular disease. *Diabetes, 46*(5), 860–867.

Alpert, B. S., & Barnard, M. (2001). Prevention of essential hypertension in minority populations. *Progress in Pediatric Cardiology, 12*(2), 189–193.

American College of Endocrinology (ACE). (2003). American College of Endocrinology and American Association of Endocrinologist's joint position statement on the insulin resistance syndrome. *Endocrine Practice, 9*(3), 236–239.

American Diabetes Association (ADA). (2000). Type 2 diabetes in children and adolescents. *Diabetes Care, 23*, 381–389.

American Diabetes Association (ADA). (2005). American Diabetes Association: Position statement: Screening for diabetes. *Diabetes Care, 25*(Supplement), S21–S24

American Heart Association. (2007) *American Heart Association, Heart and Stroke Statistical Update 2007.* Dallas: TX: .

Anderson, G. L., Limacher, M., Assaf, A. R., Bassford, T., Beresford, S. A., Black, H., Bonds, D., Brunner, R., Brzyski, R., Caan, B., Chlebowski, R., Curb, D., Gass, M., Hays, J., Heiss, G., Hendrix, S., Howard, B. V., Hsia, J., Hubbell, A., Jackson, R., Johnson, K. C., Judd, H., Kotchen, J. M., Kuller, L., LaCroix, A. Z., Lane, D., Langer, R. D., Lasser, N., Lewis, C. E., Manson, J., Margolis, K., Ockene, J., O'Sullivan, M. J., Phillips, L., Prentice, R. L., Ritenbaugh, C., Robbins, J., Rossouw, J. E., Sarto, G., Stefanick, M. L., Van Horn, L., Wactawski-Wende, J., Wallace, R., & Wassertheil-Smoller, S. (2004a). Effects of conjugated equine estrogen in postmenopausal women with hysterectomy: the Women's Health Initiative randomized controlled trial. *Journal of the American Medical Association, 291*(14), 1701–1712.

Anderson, J. L., Horne, B. D., Jones, H. U., Reyna, S. P., Carlquist, J. F., Bair, T. L., Pearson, R. R., Lappe, D. L., & Muhlestein, J. B. (2004b). Which features of the metabolic syndrome predict the prevalence and clinical outcomes of angiographic coronary artery disease? *Cardiology, 101*(4), 185–193.

Anderson, P. J., Critchley, J. A., Chan, J. C., Cockram, C. S., Lee, Z. S., Thomas, G. N., & Tomlinson, B. (2001). Factor analysis of the metabolic syndrome: Obesity vs insulin resistance as the central abnormality. *International Journal of Obesity and Related Metabolic Disorders, 25*(12), 1782–1788.

Appel S.J., Phadke P., Hunter G., et al. (2007). Racial differences in PAI-1 levels among healthy African-American and Caucasian women. Paper presented at the American Heart Association 47th Annual Conference on Cardiovascular Disease Epidemiology and Prevention, in association with the Council on Nutrition, Physical Activity, and Metabolism. Buena Vista Palace, Orlando, FL.

Appel S.J. (2006). Metabolic syndrome: Fact or fiction. *Journal of American Academy of Nurse Practitioners.* 18, 255–257.

Appel, S. J., Moore, T. M., & Giger, J.N. (2006). An overview and update on the metabolic syndrome: Implications for identifying cardiometabolic risk among African-American women. *Journal of the National Black Nurses Association, 17*(2), 48–63.

Appel, S.J. (2005). Calculating insulin resistance in the primary care setting: Why should we worry about insulin levels in euglycemic patients? *Journal of the American Academy of Nurse Practitioners, 17,* 331–336.

Appel, S. J., Harrell, J. S., Davenport, M., & Hu, J. (2002a). Association of central obesity with the metabolic syndrome and plasminogen activator inhibitor-1 in youth. *Circulation: Supplement, 106*(19), II-666.

Appel, S. J., Harrell, J. S., & Deng, S. (2002b). Racial and socioeconomic differences in risk factors for cardiovascular disease among Southern rural women. *Nursing Research, 51*(3), 140–147.

Appel, S. J., Giger, J. N., & Floyd, N. A. (2004a). Dysmetabolic syndrome: Reducing cardiovascular risk. *Nurse Practitioner, 29*(10), 18–35; quiz 35-37.

Appel, S., Jones, E., & Kennedy-Malone, L. (2004b). Central obesity and the metabolic syndrome: Implications for primary care providers. *Journal of the American Academy of Nurse Practitioners, 16*(8), 335–342.

Appel, S. J., Giger, J.N., & Davidhizar, R. E. (2005a). Opportunity cost: The impact of contextual risk factors on the cardiovascular health of low-income rural southern African-American women. *Journal of Cardiovascular Nursing, 20*(5), 315–324.

Appel, S. J., Floyd, N. A., Giger, J. N., Weaver, M. T., Luo, H., Hannah, T., & Ovalle, F. (2005b). African American women, metabolic syndrome, and national cholesterol education program criteria: A pilot study. *Nursing Research, 54*(5), 339–346.

Ard, J. D., Coffman, C. J., Lin, P. H., & Svetkey, L. P. (2004). One-year follow-up study of blood pressure and dietary patterns in dietary approaches to stop hypertension (DASH)-sodium participants. *American Journal of Hypertension, 17*(12 Pt 1), 1156–1162.

Askoxford.com (2004). http://www.askoxford.com/asktheexperts/faq/aboutwordorigins/lovenil?view=uk [August 27, 2004].

Aszmann, O., Tassler, P. L., & Dellon, A. L. (2004). Changing the natural history of diabetic neuropathy: Incidence of ulcer/amputation in the contralateral limb of patients with a unilateral nerve decompression procedure. *Annals of Plastic Surgery, 53*(6), 517–522.

Balakau, B., & Charles, M. A. (1999). Comment on the provisional report from the WHO consultation: European Group for the Study of Insulin Resistance (EGIR). *Diabetes Medicine, 16,* 442–443.

Belay, B., Belamarich, P., & Racine, A. D. (2004). Pediatric precursors of adult atherosclerosis. *Pediatrics in Review, 25*(1), 4–16.

Bello, N., & Mosca, L. (2004). Epidemiology of coronary heart disease in women. *Progress in Cardiovascular Diseases, 46*(4), 287–295.

Benko, L. B. (2003). Boomer bust? While hospitals increase capacity to prepare for an onslaught of aging baby boomers, some say medical advances and health awareness mean those extra beds will stay empty. *Modern Healthcare, 33*(30), 24–28.

Bent, K. N., Shuster, G. F., Hurley, J. S., Frye, D., Loflin, P., & Brubaker, C. (1998). Acanthosis nigricans as an early clinical proxy marker of increased risk of type 2 diabetes. *Public Health Nursing, 15*(6), 415–421.

Bernhard, D., Pfister, G., Huck, C. W., Kind, M., Salvenmoser, W., Bonn, G. K., & Wick, G. (2003). Disruption of vascular endothelial homeostasis by tobacco smoke: Impact on atherosclerosis. *The Journal of the Federation of American Societies for Experimental Biology, 17*(15), 2302–2304.

Betancourt, J. R. (2002). IOM highlights health disparities: implications for health plans. *Healthplan, 43*(4), 30–33, 36.

Bibbins-Domingo, K., Lin, F., Vittinghoff, E., Barrett-Connor, E., Hulley, S. B., Grady, D., & Shlipak, M. G. (2004). Predictors of heart failure among women with coronary disease. *Circulation, 110*(11), 1424–1430.

Bold, S. P., & Luedtke, G. (2001). Time is muscle. The Cape Cod Chest Pain Task Force helps shorten AMI discovery-to-treatment times. *Journal of Emergency Medical Services, 26*(4), 52–55.

Bostrom, K., & Ahlstrom, G. (2004). Living with a chronic deteriorating disease: The trajectory with muscular dystrophy over ten years. *Disability and Rehabilitation, 26*(23), 1388–1398.

Boyle, J. J. (2005). Macrophage activation in atherosclerosis: Pathogenesis and pharmacology of plaque rupture. *Current Vascular Pharmacology, 3*(1), 63–68.

Burke, J. P., Hale, D. E., Hazuda, H. P., & Stern, M. P. (1999). A quantitative scale of acanthosis nigricans. *Diabetes Care, 22*(10), 1655–1659.

Caap-Ahlgren, M., & Dehlin, O. (2002). Factors of importance to the caregiver burden experienced by family caregivers of Parkinson's disease patients. *Aging Clinical and Experimental Research, 14*(5), 371–377.

Calhoun, P. S., Beckham, J. C., & Bosworth, H. B. (2002). Caregiver burden and psychological distress in partners of veterans with chronic posttraumatic stress disorder. *Journal of Trauma Stress, 15*(3), 205–212.

Centers for Disease Control and Prevention (CDC). (1999). *Behavioral Risk Factor Surveillance System (BRFSS).* Retrieved November 25, 2002, from http://www.cdc.gov/nccdphp/aag/aag_brfss.htm.

Centers for Disease Control and Prevention (CDC). (2002). *Overweight and obesity: US trends 1985 to 2002.* Retrieved April 3, 2004, from http://www.cdc.gov/nccdphp/dnpa/obesity/trend/maps/index.htm.

Centers for Disease Control and Prevention (CDC). (2005). *National diabetes fact sheet.* Retrieved June 1, 2006, from http://www.cdc.gov/diabetes/pubs/facterrata.htm.

Cigolini, M., Targher, G., Bergamo Andreis, I. A., Tonoli, M., Agostino, G., & De Sandre, G. (1996). Visceral fat accumulation and its relation to plasma hemostatic factors in healthy men. *Arteriosclerosis, Thrombosis and Vascular Biology, 16*(3), 368–374.

Cimminiello, C., Vigorelli, P., Piliego, T., Soncini, M., Toschi, V., Arpaia, G., Perolini, S., & Bonfardeci, C. (1997). Fibrinolytic response in subjects with hypertriglyceridemia and low HDL cholesterol. *Biomedicine and Pharmacotherapy, 51*(4), 164–169.

Cohen, D. A., Farley, T. A., & Mason, K. (2003). Why is poverty unhealthy? Social and physical mediators. *Social Science and Medicine, 57*(9), 1631–1641.

Cordain, L., Eades, M. R., & Eades, M. D. (2003). Hyperinsulinemic diseases of civilization: More than just Syndrome X. *Comparative Biochemistry and Physiology Part A: Molecular and Integrative Physiology, 136*(1), 95–112.

Cruz, P. D., & Hud, J. A. (1992). Excess insulin binding to insulin-like growth factor receptors: Proposed mechanism for acanthosis nigricans. *Journal of Investigative Dermatology, 98,* 682S–85S.

Dellon, A. L. (2004). Diabetic neuropathy: Review of a surgical approach to restore sensation, relieve pain, and prevent ulceration and amputation. *Foot and Ankle International, 25*(10), 749–755.

Den Tonkelaar, I., Seidell, J. C., van Noord, P. A., & Baanders-van Halewijn, E. A. (1990). Waist-to-hip ratio in Dutch women and its relationship with self- reported diabetes mellitus, hypertension and cholecystectomy. *Nederlands Tijdschrift voor Geneeskunde, 134*(39), 1900–1902.

Devaraj, S., Xu, D. Y., & Jialal, I. (2003). C-reactive protein increases plasminogen activator inhibitor-1 expression and activity in human aortic endothelial cells: Implications for the metabolic syndrome and atherothrombosis. *Circulation, 107*(3), 398–404.

Dore, G. J. (2000). Infectious diseases in the 21st century. Are we entering the hot zone? *Australian Family Physician, 29*(7), 627–630.

Dzien, A., Dzien-Bischinger, C., Hoppichler, F., & Lechleitner, M. (2004). The metabolic syndrome as a link between smoking and cardiovascular disease. *Diabetes, Obesity and Metabolism, 6*(2), 127–132.

Fagerberg, B. (2004). The metabolic syndrome—Time to introduce the diagnosis in routine health care? Reflections on a current American report. *Lakartidningen, 101*(48), 3902, 3905–3906, 3909, 3911.

Falk, E. (1992). Why do plaques rupture? *Circulation, 86* (6 Suppl III), 30–42.

Flaskerud, J. H., & Nyamathi, A. M. (2002). New paradigm for health disparities needed. *Nursing Research, 51*(3), 139.

Flegal, K. M., Carroll, M. D., Ogden, C. L., & Johnson, C. L. (2007). Prevalence and trends in obesity among US adults, 1999–2000. *Journal of the American Medical Association, 26*(14), 1723–1727.

Ford, E. S. (2004a). The metabolic syndrome and mortality from cardiovascular disease and all-causes: Findings from the National Health and Nutrition Examination Survey II Mortality Study. *Atherosclerosis, 173*(2), 309–314.

Ford, E. S. (2004b). Prevalence of the metabolic syndrome in US populations. *Endocrinology and Metabolism Clinics of North America, 33*(2), 333–350.

Foster, S., & Mallik, M. (1998). A comparative study of differences in the referral behavior patterns of men and women who have experienced cardiac-related chest pain. *Intensive and Critical Care Nursing, 14*(4), 192–202.

Fried, T. R., Bradley, E. H., O'Leary, J. R., & Byers, A. L. (2005). Unmet desire for caregiver-patient communication and increased caregiver burden. *Journal of the American Geriatrics Society, 53*(1), 59–65.

Gabbay, R. A., Lendel, I., Saleem, T. M., Shaeffer, G., Adelman, A. M., Mauger, D. T., Collins, M., & Polomano, R. C. (2006). Nurse case management improves blood pressure, emotional distress and diabetes complication screening. *Diabetes Research in Clinical Practice, 71*(1), 28-35.

Girman, C. J., Rhodes, T., Mercuri, M., Pyorala, K., Kjekshus, J., Pedersen, T. R., Beere, P. A., Gotto, A. M., & Clearfield, M. (2004). The metabolic syndrome and risk of major coronary events in the Scandinavian Simvastatin

Survival Study (4S) and the Air Force/Texas Coronary Atherosclerosis Prevention Study (AFCAPS/TexCAPS). *The American Journal of Cardiology, 93*(2), 136–141.

Gitlin, L. N., Belle, S. H., Burgio, L. D., Czaja, S. J., Mahoney, D., Gallagher-Thompson, D., Burns, R., Hauck, W. W., Zhang, S., Schulz, R., & Ory, M. G. (2003). Effect of multi-component interventions on caregiver burden and depression: The REACH multi-site initiative at 6-month follow-up. *Psychology and Aging, 18*(3), 361–374.

Goldstein, N. E., Concato, J., Fried, T. R., Kasl, S. V., Johnson-Hurzeler, R., & Bradley, E. H. (2004). Factors associated with caregiver burden among caregivers of terminally ill patients with cancer. *Journal of Palliative Care, 20*(1), 38–43.

Goodfellow, L. M. (2004). Can a journal club bridge the gap between research and practice? *Nurse Educator, 29*(3), 107–10.

Goodheart, H. P. (2000). Hirsutism: Pathogenesis and causes. *Women's Health in Primary Care, 3*(5), 329–337.

Goran, M. I., & Gower, B. A. (1998). Abdominal obesity and cardiovascular risk in children. *Coronary Artery Disease, 9*(8), 483–487.

Grundy, S. M. (2005). Metabolic syndrome scientific statement by the American Heart Association and the National Heart, Lung, and Blood Institute. *Arteriosclerosis, Thrombosis, and Vascular Biology, 25*(11), 2243–2244.

Grundy, S. M., Cleeman, J. I., Daniels, S. R., Donato, K. A., Eckel, R. H., Franklin, B. A., Gordon, D. J., Krauss, R. M., Savage, P. J., Smith, S. C. Jr., Spertus, J. A., & Costa, F. (2005). Diagnosis and management of the metabolic syndrome: Diagnosis and management of the metabolic syndrome: An American Heart Association/National Heart, Lung, and Blood Institute Scientific Statement. *Circulation, 112*(17), e285–290.

Haffner, S. M., D'Agostino, R. Jr., Goff, D., Howard, B., Festa, A., Saad, M. F., & Mykkanen, L. (1999). LDL size in African Americans, Hispanics, and non-Hispanic whites: The insulin resistance atherosclerosis study. *Arteriosclerosis, Thrombosis, and Vascular Biology, 19*(9), 2234–2240.

Hanley, A. J., Wagenknecht, L. E., D'Agostino, R. B. Jr., Zinman, B., & Haffner, S. M. (2003). Identification of subjects with insulin resistance and beta-cell dysfunction using alternative definitions of the metabolic syndrome. *Diabetes, 52*(11), 2740–2747.

Harmel, A. P., & Berra, K. (2003). Impact of the new National Cholesterol Education Program (NCEP) guidelines on patient management. *Journal of the American Academy of Nurse Practitioners, 15*(8), 350–360.

Herdegen, J. J. (2002). Treating "syndrome X" in minority populations: Begin with the treatment of obesity and hypertension. *Ethnicity and Disease, 12*, 429-432.

Holt, R. I. (2005). Obesity—An epidemic of the twenty-first century: An update for psychiatrists. *Journal of Clinical Psychopharmacology, 19*(6 Suppl), 6–15.

Hughes, S., & Hayman, L. L. (2004). Improving cardiovascular health in women: An opportunity for nursing. *Journal of Cardiovascular Nursing, 19*(2), 145–147.

Hunter, G., Giger, J., Weaver, M., Strickland, O., Zuckerman, P., & Taylor, H. (2000). Fat distribution and cardiovascular disease risk in African-American women. *Journal National Black Nurses Association, 11*(2), 7–11.

Hutchinson, A. M., & Johnston, L. (2004). Bridging the divide: A survey of nurses' opinions regarding barriers to, and facilitators of, research utilization in the practice setting. *Journal of Clinical Nursing, 13*(3), 304–315.

Jablonski, A. (2004). The illness trajectory of end-stage renal disease dialysis patients. *Research and Theory for Nursing Practice, 18*(1), 51–72.

Janssen, I., Fortier, A., Hudson, R., & Ross, R. (2002). Effects of an energy-restrictive diet with or without exercise on abdominal fat, intramuscular fat, and metabolic risk factors in obese women. *Diabetes Care, 25*(3), 431–438.

Jastrzebska, M., Goracy, I., & Naruszewicz, M. (2003). Relationships between fibrinogen, plasminogen activator inhibitor-1, and their gene polymorphisms in current smokers with essential hypertension. *Thrombosis Research, 110*(5–6), 339–344.

Judson, L. (2004). Global childhood chronic illness. *Nursing Administration Quarterly, 28*(1), 60–66.

Katayama, T., Nakashima, H., Takagi, C., Honda, Y., Suzuki, S., & Yano, K. (2005). Predictors of mortality in patients with acute myocardial infarction and cardiogenic shock. *Circulation Journal, 69*(1), 83–88.

Kaufer, D. I., Borson, S., Kershaw, P., & Sadik, K. (2005). Reduction of caregiver burden in Alzheimer's disease by treatment with galantamine. *CNS Spectrums, 10*(6), 481–488.

Kelley, D. E., Thaete, F. L., Troost, F., Huwe, T., & Goodpaster, B. H. (2000). Subdivisions of subcutaneous abdominal adipose tissue and insulin resistance. *American Journal Physiology Endocrinology Metabolism, 278*(5), E941–E948.

Kernan, W. N., & Inzucchi, S. E. (2004). Type 2 diabetes mellitus and insulin resistance: Stroke prevention and management. *Current Treatment Options in Neurology, 6*(6), 443–450.

Kim, S., Koniak-Griffin, D., Flaskerud, J. H., & Guarnero, P. A. (2004). The impact of lay health advisors on cardiovascular health promotion: Using a community-based participatory approach. *Journal of Cardiovascular Nursing, 19*(3), 192–199.

Knapp, R. G., Sutherland, S. E., Keil, J. E., Rust, P. F., & Lackland, D. T. (1992). A comparison of the effects of cholesterol on CHD mortality in black and white women: Twenty-eight years of follow-up in the Charleston Heart Study. *Journal of Clinical Epidemiology, 45*(10), 1119–1129.

Knickman, J. R., & Snell, E. K. (2002). The 2030 problem: Caring for aging baby boomers. *Health Services Research, 37*(4), 849–884.

Kobaissi, H. A., Weigensberg, M. J., Ball, G. D., Cruz, M. L., Shaibi, G. Q., & Goran, M. I. (2004). Relation between acanthosis nigricans and insulin sensitivity in overweight Hispanic children at risk for type 2 diabetes. *Diabetes Care, 27*(6), 1412–1416.

Kobetz, E., Vatalaro, K., Moore, A., & Earp, J. A. (2005). Taking the transtheoretical model into the field: A curriculum for lay health advisors. *Health Promotion Practice, 6*(3), 329–337.

Kriketos, A. D., Greenfield, J. R., Peake, P. W., Furler, S. M., Denyer, G. S., Charlesworth, J. A., & Campbell, L. V. (2004). Inflammation, insulin resistance, and adiposity: A study of first-degree relatives of type 2 diabetic subjects. *Diabetes Care, 27*(8), 2033–2040.

Kumanyika, S. (2002). The minority factor in the obesity epidemic. *Ethnicity and Disease, 12*(3), 316–319.

Kurihara, T., Tomiyama, H., Hashimoto, H., Yamamoto, Y., Yano, E., & Yamashina, A. (2004). Excessive alcohol intake increases the risk of arterial stiffening in men with normal blood pressure. *Hypertension Research, 27*(9), 669–673.

Lavezzi, A. M., Ottaviani, G., & Matturri, L. (2005). Biology of the smooth muscle cells in human atherosclerosis. *Acta Pathologica, Microbiologica et Immunologica Scandinavica, 113*(2), 112–121

Lee, R., & Miller, T. (2002). An approach to forecasting health expenditures, with application to the U.S. Medicare system. *Health Services Research, 37*(5), 1365–1386.

Lemieux, I., Pascot, A., Couillard, C., Lamarche, B., Tchernof, A., Almeras, N., Bergeron, J., Gaudet, D., Tremblay, G., Prud'homme, D., Nadeau, A., & Despres, J. P. (2000). Hypertriglyceridemic waist: A marker of the atherogenic metabolic triad (hyperinsulinemia; hyperapolipoprotein B; small, dense LDL) in men? *Circulation, 102*(2), 179–184.

Lidell, E. (2002). Family support—A burden to patient and caregiver. *European Journal of Cardiovascular Nursing, 1*(2), 149–152.

Liao, Y., Kwon, S., Shaughnessy, S., Wallace, P., Hutto, A., Jenkins, A. J., Klein, R. L., & Garvey, W. T. (2004). Critical evaluation of adult treatment panel III: Criteria in identifying insulin resistance with dyslipidemia. *Diabetes Care, 27*(4), 978-83.

Maeda, K., Noguchi, Y., & Fukui, T. (2003). The effects of cessation from cigarette smoking on the lipid and lipoprotein profiles: A meta-analysis. *Preventive Medicine, 37*(4), 283–290.

Mansfield, C. J., Wilson, J. L., Kobrinski, E. J., & Mitchell, J. (1999). Premature mortality in the United States: The roles of geographic area, socioeconomic status, household type, and availability of medical care. *American Journal of Public Health, 89*(6), 893–898.

Matthews, D. R., Hosker, J. P., Rudenski, A. S., Naylor, B. A., Treacher, D. F., & Turner, R. C. (1985). Homeostasis model assessment: Insulin resistance and beta-cell function from fasting plasma glucose and insulin concentrations in man. *Diabetologia, 28*(7), 412–419.

McCool, W. F., & Simeone, S. A. (2002). Birth in the United States: An overview of trends past and present. *Nursing Clinics of North America, 37*(4), 735–746.

McMurray, R. G., Bauman, M. J., Harrell, J. S., Brown, S., & Bangdiwala, S. I. (2000). Effects of improvement in aerobic power on resting insulin and glucose concentrations in children. *European Journal of Applied Physiology, 81*(1–2), 132–139.

McSweeney, J. C., Cody, M., O'Sullivan, P., Elberson, K., Moser, D. K., & Garvin, B. J. (2003). Women's early warning symptoms of acute myocardial infarction. *Circulation, 108*(21), 2619–2623.

Melkus, G. D., Maillet, N., Novak, J., Womack, J., & Hatch-Clein, A. (2002). Primary care cancer and diabetes complications screening of black women with type 2 diabetes. *Journal of the American Academy of Nurse Practioners, 14*(1), 43–48.

Metcalf, P. A., Sharrett, A. R., Folsom, A. R., Duncan, B. B., Patsch, W., Hutchinson, R. G., Szklo, M., Davis, C. E., & Tyroler, H. A. (1998). African American-white differences in lipids, lipoproteins, and apolipoproteins, by educational attainment, among middle-aged adults: The Atherosclerosis Risk in Communities Study. *American Journal of Epidemiology, 148*(8), 750–760.

Minami, J., Todoroki, M., Yoshii, M., Mita, S., Nishikimi, T., Ishimitsu, T., & Matsuoka, H. (2002). Effects of smoking cessation or alcohol restriction on metabolic and fibrinolytic variables in Japanese men. *Clinical Science (London), 103*(2), 117–122.

Mishel, M. H. (1999). Uncertainty in chronic illness. *Annual Review of Nursing Research, 17,* 269–294.

Mishel, M. H., & Clayton, M. F. (2003). Uncertainty in illness theories. In M. J. Smith & P. Liehr (Eds.), *Middle range theory in advanced practice nursing* (pp. 13–39). New York: Springer.

Monzillo, L. U., & Hamdy, O. (2003). Evaluation of insulin sensitivity in clinical practice and in research settings. *Nutrition Reviews, 61*(12), 397–412.

Moser, D. K., McKinley, S., Dracup, K., & Chung, M. L. (2005). Gender differences in reasons patients delay in seeking treatment for acute myocardial infarction symptoms. *Patient Education and Counseling, 56*(1), 45–54.

Mukhtar, Q. C. G. V. R. M. J. W. (2001). Prevalence of acanthosis nigricans and its association with hyperinsulinemia in New Mexico adolescents. *Journal of Adolescent Health, 28*(5), 372–376.

Nabors, N., Seacat, J., & Rosenthal, M. (2002). Predictors of caregiver burden following traumatic brain injury. *Brain Injury, 16*(12), 1039–1050.

Naghavi, M., Libby, P., Falk, E., Casscells, S. W., Litovsky, S., Rumberger, J., Badimon, J. J., Stefanadis, C., Moreno, P., Pasterkamp, G., Fayad, Z., Stone, P. H., Waxman, S., Raggi, P., Madjid, M., Zarrabi, A., Burke, A., Yuan, C., Fitzgerald, P. J., Siscovick, D. S., de Korte, C. L., Aikawa, M., Juhani Airaksinen, K. E., Assmann, G., Becker, C. R., Chesebro, J. H., Farb, A., Galis, Z. S., Jackson, C., Jang, I. K., Koenig, W., Lodder, R. A., March, K., Demirovic, J., Navab, M., Priori, S. G., Rekhter, M. D., Bahr, R., Grundy, S. M., Mehran, R., Colombo, A., Boerwinkle, E., Ballantyne, C., Insull, W. Jr., Schwartz, R. S., Vogel, R., Serruys, P. W., Hansson, G. K., Faxon, D. P., Kaul, S., Drexler, H., Greenland, P., Muller, J. E., Virmani, R., Ridker, P. M., Zipes, D. P., Shah, P. K., & Willerson, J. T. (2003). From vulnerable plaque to vulnerable patient: A call for new definitions and risk assessment strategies: Part I. *Circulation, 108*(14), 1664–1672.

National Center for Health Statistics (NCHS), Centers for Disease Control and Prevention. (2001). *CDC growth charts: United States.* Available from http://www.cdc.gov/growthcharts/.

National Center for Health Statistics (NCHS), Centers for Disease Control and Prevention. (2003). *The burden of chronic disease and the future of public health.* [slide and audio] Retrieved August 25, 2007, from *http://www.cdc.gov/nccdphp/publications/Burden/bcd_41.htm*

National Center for Health Statistics (NCHS). *Health, United States, 2006 with chartbook on trends in the health of Americans.* Retrieved August, 2007, from http://www.cdc.gov/nchs/data/hus/hus06.pdf.

National Cholesterol Education Program (NCEP). (2001). Executive Summary of the Third Report of the National Cholesterol Education Program (NCEP) Expert Panel on Detection, Evaluation, and Treatment of High Blood Cholesterol in Adults (Adult Treatment Panel III). *Journal of the American Medical Association, 285*(19), 2486–2497.

Nieves, D. J., Cnop, M., Retzlaff, B., Walden, C. E., Brunzell, J. D., Knopp, R. H., & Kahn, S. E. (2003). The atherogenic lipoprotein profile associated with obesity and insulin resistance is largely attributable to intra-abdominal fat. *Diabetes, 52*(1), 172–179.

National Heart Lung &Blood Institute (NHL&BI). (1998). *The evidence: Clinical guidelines on the identification, evaluation, and treatment of overweight and obesity in adults.* National Institutes of Health: Bethesda, MD, NIH.

Nussinovitch, N., Elishkevitz, K., Rosenthal, T., & Nussinovitch, M. (2005). Screening for hypertension in high school. *Clinical Pediatrics, 44*(8), 711–714.

Ogilvie, L., Strang, V., Hayes, P., Raiwet, C., Andruski, L., Heinrich, M., Cullen, K., & Morris, H. (2004). Value and vulnerability: Reflections on joint appointments. *Journal of Professional Nursing, 20*(2), 110–117.

Palaniappan, L., Carnethon, M. R., Wang, Y., Hanley, A. J., Fortmann, S. P., Haffner, S. M., & Wagenknecht, L. (2004). Predictors of the incident metabolic syndrome in adults: The Insulin Resistance Atherosclerosis Study. *Diabetes Care, 27*(3), 788–793.

Pati, S., Keren, R., Alessandrini, E. A., & Schwarz, D. F. (2004). Generational differences in U.S. public spending, 1980–2000: Unlike social welfare spending on the elderly, spending on children is highly vulnerable to economic downturns. *Health Affairs, 23*(5), 131–141.

Ramsey, P. W., & Glenn, L. L. (2002). Obesity and health status in rural, urban, and suburban southern women. *Southern Medical Journal, 95*(7), 666–671.

Randall, V. (2002) *Eliminating the slave health deficit: Using reparations to repair black health.* Retrieved March 4, 2005, from http://www.blink.org.uk/pdescription.asp?key=431&grp=46&cat=140.

Rankin SH. (2004). Commentary: Creative support strategies to improve recovery from cardiac events: Peer support, lay health advisors, and eHealth. *Journal of Cardiovascular Nursing, 19,* 172–173.

Reaven, G. M. (1988). Banting lecture 1988. Role of insulin resistance in human disease. *Diabetes, 37*(12), 1595–1607.

Reaven, G. (2002). Metabolic syndrome: Pathophysiology and implications for management of cardiovascular disease. *Circulation, 106*(3), 286–288.

Reaven, G., Abbasi, F., & McLaughlin, T. (2004). Obesity, insulin resistance, and cardiovascular disease. *Recent Progress in Hormone Research, 59,* 207–223.

Ridker, P. M. (2001). Role of inflammatory biomarkers in prediction of coronary heart disease. *The Lancet, 358*(9286), 946–948.

Ridker, P. M., Buring, J. E., Cook, N. R., & Rifai, N. (2003). C-reactive protein, the metabolic syndrome, and risk of incident cardiovascular events. *Circulation, 107*(3), 391–404.

Ridker, P. M., Rifai, N., Rose, L., Buring, J. E., & Cook, N. R. (2002). Comparison of C-reactive protein and low-density lipoprotein cholesterol levels in the prediction of first cardiovascular events. *The New England Journal of Medicine, 347*(20), 1557–1565.

Rodriguez, C., Pablos-Mendez, A., Palmas, W., Lantigua, R., Mayeux, R., & Berglund, L. (2002). Comparison of modifiable determinants of lipids and lipoprotein levels among African-Americans, Hispanics, and Non-Hispanic Caucasians > or = 65 years of age living in New York City. *The American Journal of Cardiology, 89*(2), 178–183.

Saku, K., Ahmad, M., Glas-Greenwalt, P., & Kashyap, M. L. (1985). Activation of fibrinolysis by apolipoproteins of high density lipoproteins in man. *Thrombosis Research, 39*(1), 1–8.

Sakula, A. (2004). Plaques on London houses of medico-historical interest. Sir Alexander Fleming (1881–1955). *Journal of Medical Biography, 12*(1), 11.

Sato, I., Nishida, M., Okita, K., Nishijima, H., Kojima, S., Matsumura, N., & Yasuda, H. (1992). Beneficial effect of stopping smoking on future cardiac events in male smokers with previous myocardial infarction. *Japanese Circulation Journal, 56*(3), 217–22.

Seidell, J. C., Cigolini, M., Deslypere, J. P., Charzewska, J., Ellsinger, B. M., & Cruz, A. (1991). Body fat distribution in relation to physical activity and smoking habits in 38-year-old European men. The European Fat Distribution Study. *American Journal of Epidemiology, 133*(3), 257–265.

Sekula, L. K., DeSantis, J., & Gianetti, V. (2003). Considerations in the management of the patient with comorbid depression and anxiety. *Journal of the American Academy of Nurse Practitioners, 15*(1), 23–33.

Seshamani, M., & Gray, A. (2004). Time to death and health expenditure: An improved model for the impact of demographic change on health care costs. *Age and Ageing, 33*(6), 556–561.

Shiell, A. (1997). Health outcomes are about choices and values: An economic perspective on the health outcomes movement. *Health Policy, 39*(1), 5–15.

Shiell, A., Donaldson, C., Mitton, C., & Currie, G. (2002). Health economic evaluation. *Journal of Epidemiology and Community Health, 56*(2), 85–88.

Soderberg, S., Olsson, T., Eliasson, M., Johnson, O., & Ahren, B. (1999). Plasma leptin levels are associated with abnormal fibrinolysis in men and postmenopausal women. *Journal of Internal Medicine, 245*(5), 533–543.

Soeki, T., Tamura, Y., Shinohara, H., Sakabe, K., Onose, Y., & Fukuda, N. (2002). Plasma concentrations of fibrinolytic factors in the subacute phase of myocardial infarction predict recurrent myocardial infarction or sudden cardiac death. *International Journal of Cardiology, 85*(2–3), 277–283.

Smith, S. C. Jr., Clark, L. T., Cooper, R. S., Daniels, S. R., Kumanyika, S. K., Ofili, E., Quinones, M. A., Sanchez, E. J., Saunders, E., & Tiukinhoy, S. D. (2005). Discovering the full spectrum of cardiovascular disease: Minority Health Summit 2003: Report of the Obesity, Metabolic Syndrome, and Hypertension Writing Group. *Circulation, 111*(10), e134-9.

Stern, M. P., Williams, K., Gonzalez-Villalpando, C., Hunt, K. J., & Haffner, S. M. (2004). Does the metabolic syndrome improve identification of individuals at risk of type 2 diabetes and/or cardiovascular disease? *Diabetes Care, 27*(11), 2676–2681.

Stern, M. P., Williams, K., & Hunt, K. J. (2005). Impact of diabetes/metabolic syndrome in patients with established cardiovascular disease. *Atherosclerosis Supplements, 6*(2), 3–6.

Ten, S., & Maclaren, N. (2004). Insulin resistance syndrome in children. *Journal of Clinical Endocrinology and Metabolism, 89*(6), 2526–2539.

Terry, K. (2002). The baby boom becomes the elder boom. *Business Health, 20*(1), 10–17.

Tu, H. T. (2004). Rising health costs, medical debt and chronic conditions. *Issue brief (Center for Studying Health System Change), 88*, 1–5.

U.S. Department of Health and Human Services (DHHS). (2000). *Healthy People 2010 (Conference Edition, in Two Volumes)*. Washington, DC: Author.

U.S. Department of Health and Human Services. (2001). *The Surgeon General's call to action to prevent and decrease overweight and obesity*. Rockville, MD: U. S. Department of Health and Human Services, Public Health Service, Office of the Surgeon General. Available from U.S. GPO, Washington, DC.

U.S. National Center for Health Statistics (USNCHS). (2003). *National vital statistics report* [Web Page]. Retrieved August 7, 2004, from www.cdc.gov/nchs.

Uwaifo, G. I., & Ratner, R. E. (2003). The roles of insulin resistance, hyperinsulinemia, and thiazolidinediones in cardiovascular disease. *The American Journal of Medicine, 115 Suppl 8A*, 12S–19S.

Vaughan, D. E. (2002). Angiotensin and vascular fibrinolytic balance. *American Journal of Hypertension, 15* (1 Pt 2), 3S–8S.

Vaughan, D. E., Lazos, S. A., & Tong, K. (1995). Angiotensin II regulates the expression of plasminogen activator inhibitor-1 in cultured endothelial cells. A potential link between the renin-angiotensin system and thrombosis. *The Journal of Clinical Investigation, 95*(3), 995–1001.

Walker, R. (2005). Diabetes and peripheral neuropathy: Keeping people on their own two feet. *British Journal of Community Nursing, 10*(1), 33–36.

Ward, H. J., Morisky, D. E., Lees, N. B., & Fong, R. (2000). A clinic and community-based approach to hypertension control for an underserved minority population: Design and methods. *American Journal of Hypertension, 13*(2), 177–183.

Whitaker, J. A., Davis, K. L., & Lauer, C. (2004). Is there a need for screening for type 2 diabetes in seventh graders? *Journal of the American Academy of Nurse Practitioners, 16*(11), 496–501.

Whittemore, R., Bak, P. S., Melkus, G. D., & Grey, M. (2003). Promoting lifestyle change in the prevention and management of type 2 diabetes. *Journal of the American Academy of Nurse Practitioners, 15*(8), 341–349.

Wilbur, J., Vassalo, A., Chandler, P., McDevitt, J., & Miller, A. M (2005). Midlife women's adherence to home-based walking during maintenance. *Nursing Research, 54*(1), 33–40.

Williamson, G. M., & Shaffer, D. R. (2001). Relationship quality and potentially harmful behaviors by spousal caregivers: How we were then, how we are now. The Family Relationships in Late Life Project. *Psychology and Aging, 16*(2), 217–226.

Williamson, G. R., Webb, C., & Abelson-Mitchell, N. (2004). Developing lecturer practitioner roles using action research. *Journal of Advanced Nursing, 47*(2), 153–164.

Wilkinson, J., Foo, K., Sekhri, N., Cooper, J., Suliman, A., Ranjadayalan, K., & Timmis, A. D. (2002). Interaction between arrival time and thrombolytic treatment in determining early outcome of acute myocardial infarction. *Heart, 88*(6), 583–586.

Wong, M. D., Shapiro, M. F., Boscardin, W. J., & Ettner, S. L. (2002). Contribution of major diseases to disparities in mortality. *New England Journal of Medicine, 347*(20), 1585–1592.

Wood, D. L., & Halfon, N. (1996). The impact of the vaccine for children's program on child immunization delivery. A policy analysis. *Archives of Pediatrics and Adolescent Medicine, 150*(6), 577–581.

Yoo, S., Nicklas, T., Baranowski, T., Zakeri, I. F., Yang, S. J., Srinivasan, S. R., & Berenson, G. S. (2004). Comparison of dietary intakes associated with metabolic syndrome risk factors in young adults: The Bogalusa Heart Study. *American Journal of Clinical Nutrition, 80*(4), 841–848.

Yudkin, J. S., Juhan-Vague, I., Hawe, E., Humphries, S. E., di Minno, G., Margaglione, M., Tremoli, E., Kooistra, T.,

Morange, P. E., Lundman, P., Mohamed-Ali, V., & Hamsten, A. (2004). Low-grade inflammation may play a role in the etiology of the metabolic syndrome in patients with coronary heart disease: The HIFMECH study. *Metabolism, 53*(7), 852–857.

Zimmet, P. (2003). The burden of type 2 diabetes: Are we doing enough? *Diabetes Metabolism, 9*(supplement), 6S9–6S18.

BIBLIOGRAPHY

Appel, L. J. (2003). Lifestyle modification as a means to prevent and treat high blood pressure. *Journal of the American Society of Nephrology, 14*(7 Suppl 2), S99–S102

Benko, L.B. (2003). Boomer bust? While hospitals increase capacity to prepare for an onslaught of aging baby boomers, some say medical advances and health awareness mean those extra beds will stay empty. *Modern Healthcare, 33*(30), 24–28.

Bolton, L. B., Giger, J. N., & Georges, A. (2003). Eliminating structural and racial barriers: a plausible solution to eliminating health disparities. *Journal of the National Black Nurses Association, 14*(1), 57–65.

Bostrom, K., & Ahlstrom, G. (2004). Living with a chronic deteriorating disease: The trajectory with muscular dystrophy over ten years. *Disability and Rehabilitation, 26*(23), 1388–1398.

Burnes Bolton, L., Giger, J. N., & Georges, C. A. (2004). Structural and racial barriers to health care. *Annual Review of Nursing Research, 22*, 39–58.

Carnevale, G. J., Anselmi, V., Busichio, K., & Millis, S. R. (2002). Changes in ratings of caregiver burden following a community-based behavior management program for persons with traumatic brain injury. *Journal of Head Trauma Rehabilitation, 17*(2), 83–95.

Chio, A., Gauthier, A., Calvo, A., Ghiglione, P., & Mutani, R. (2005). Caregiver burden and patients' perception of being a burden in ALS. *Neurology, 64*(10), 1780–1782.

Chobanian, A. V., Bakris, G. L., Black, H. R., Cushman, W. C., Green, L. A., Izzo, J. L., Jr., Jones, D. W., Materson, B. J., Oparil, S., Wright, J. T., Jr., & Roccella, E. J. (2003). The Seventh Report of the Joint National Committee on Prevention, Detection, Evaluation, and Treatment of High Blood Pressure: The JNC 7 report. *Journal of the American Medical Association, 289*(19), 2560–2572.

Cox, R.A., & Torres, C.Z. (2004). Acute heart failure in adults. *Puerto Rico Health Science Journal, 23*(4), 265–267.

Davidhizar, R., Giger, J. N., Poole, V., & Dowd, S. B. (2000). Finding meaning in illness. Can nurses help? *Can Nurse, 96*(4), 39.

Farris, R. P., Haney, D. M., & Dunet, D. O. (2004). Expanding the evidence for health promotion: Developing best practices for WISEWOMAN. *Journal of Women's Health, 13*(5), 634–643.

Fisher, L., Chesla, C. A., Bartz, R. J., Gilliss, C., Skaff, M. A., Sabogal, F., Kanter, R. A., & Lutz, C. P. (1998). The family and type 2 diabetes: A framework for intervention. *Diabetes Education, 24*(5), 599–607.

Oster, A., & Bindman, A.B. (2003). Emergency department visits for ambulatory care sensitive conditions: Insights into preventable hospitalizations. *Medical Care, 41*(2), 198–207.

Rudiger, A., Harjola, V. P., Muller, A., Mattila, E., Saila, P., Nieminen, M., & Follath, F. (2005). Acute heart failure: Clinical presentation, one-year mortality and prognostic factors. *European Journal of Heart Failure, 7*(4), 662–670.

Shah, T., Jonnalagadda, S. S., Kicklighter, J. R., Diwan, S., & Hopkins, B. L. (2005). Prevalence of metabolic syndrome risk factors among young adult Asian Indians. *Journal of Immigrant Health, 7*(2), 117–126.

Van Rooyen, J. M., Huisman, H. W., Eloff, F. C., Laubscher, P. J., Malan, L., Steyn, H. S., & Malan, N. T. (2002). Cardiovascular reactivity in Black South-African males of different age groups: The influence of urbanization. *Ethnicity and Disease, 12*(1), 69–75.

Wheeler, E. C., Klemm, P., Hardie, T., Plowfield, L., Birney, M., Polek, C., & Lynch, K. G. (2004). Racial disparities in hospitalized elderly patients with chronic heart failure. *Journal of Transcultural Nursing, 15*(4), 291–297.

RESOURCES

American Association of Diabetes Educators (AADE)

100 W. Monroe, Suite 400
Chicago, Illinois 60603
1-800-338-3633
Email: aade@aadenet.org
Web: http://www.aadenet.org

The AADE is a multidisciplinary professional membership organization of health care professionals dedicated to integrating successful self-management as a key outcome in the care of people with diabetes and related conditions. AADE promotes healthy living through self-management of diabetes and related conditions.

American Diabetes Association (ADA)

1701 North Beauregard Street
Alexandria, Virginia 22311
1-800-342-2383
Email: AskADA@diabetes.org
Web: http://www.diabetes.org

The ADA is the nation's leading nonprofit health organization providing diabetes research, information, and advocacy. It conducts programs in all fifty states and the District of Columbia, reaching hundreds of communities to prevent and cure diabetes and to improve the lives of all people affected by diabetes. Information about diabetes and diabetes prevention, research and scientific findings, services, policy and advocacy for research and for the rights of people with diabetes can be found at the ADA Web site.

Centers for Disease Control and Prevention (CDC)

1600 Clifton Road.
Atlanta, Georgia 30333
404-639-3311, 1-800-311-3435
Web: http://www.cdc.gov

The CDC includes information on chronic diseases and their prevention, publications such as *Preventing Chronic Disease Journal* and *Morbidity and Mortality Weekly Report*, and state and national data. The CDC's U S. National Center for Health Statistics (http://www.cdc.gov/nchs) is the nation's principal health statistics agency and a rich source of information about America's health.

Centers for Medicare and Medicaid Services (CMS)

7500 Security Boulevard
Baltimore, Maryland 21244
1-866-226-1819
Web: http://www.cms.hhs.gov

The mission of CMS is to ensure effective, up-to-date health care coverage and to promote quality care for beneficiaries. The Web site for CMS is a source of information about Medicare and Medicaid services, regulations, and statistics and trend data.

Health Resources and Services Administration (HRSA)

5600 Fishers Lane
Rockville, Maryland 20857
Web: http://www.hrsa.gov

HRSA, an agency of the U.S. Department of Health and Human Services, has offices throughout the United States and territories. HRSA provides national leadership, program resources and services needed to improve access to health care services for people who are uninsured, isolated or medically underserved. HRSA also oversees organ, tissue and bone marrow donation and supports programs that prepare against bioterrorism, compensate individuals harmed by vaccination, and maintains databases that protect against health care malpractice and health care waste, fraud and abuse.

Indian Health Service (IHS)

The Reyes Building
801 Thompson Avenue, Suite 400
Rockville, Maryland 20852-1627
301-443-3024
Web: http://www.ihs.gov

The mission of the IHS is to raise the physical, mental, social, and spiritual health of American Indians and Alaska Natives to the highest level. The IHS Web site is a resource for American Indian and Alaska Native health history, data and trends, health information, and patient education protocols to ensure that comprehensive, culturally acceptable personal and public health services are available and accessible to American Indian and Alaska Native people.

Juvenile Diabetes Research Foundation International (JDRF)

120 Wall Street, 19th Floor
New York, New York 10005
1-800-533-CURE (2873)
FAX: (212) 785-9595
Email: info@jdrf.org
Web: http://www.jdrf.org

The mission of the JDRF is to find a cure for diabetes and its complications through the support of research. JDRF, with chapters from coast to coast and affiliates around the world, gives more money to diabetes research than any other nonprofit, nongovernmental health agency in the world. The Web site is a resource for education, research and ongoing clinical trials, funding opportunities, and publications relevant to juvenile diabetes.

National Council of La Raza (NCLR)

Raul Yzaguirre Building
1126 16th Street, NW
Washington, D.C. 20036
202-785-1670
FAX: 202-776-1792
Email: comments@nclr.org
Web: http://www.nclr.org

NCLR is the largest Latino civil rights and advocacy organization in the United States. NCLR oversees five key areas—assets/investments, civil rights/immigration, education, employment and economic status, and health. It also provides capacity-building assistance to its affiliates who work at the state and local level to advance opportunities for individuals and families.

National Diabetes Education Program (NDEP)

One Diabetes Way
Bethesda, Maryland 20814-9692
301-496-3583

Email: ndep@mail.nih.gov
Web: http://www.ndep.nih.gov

NDEP is a partnership of the National Institutes of Health, the Centers for Disease Control and Prevention, and more than 200 public and private organizations. The Web site is a resource for diabetes information and health education and campaign materials to prevent and manage diabetes.

National Institute of Diabetes and Digestive and Kidney Disease (NIDDK)

Office of Communications & Public Liaison
Building 31. Room 9A06
31 Center Drive, MSC 2560
Bethesda, Maryland 20892-2560
Web: http://www2.niddk.nih.gov

NIDDK conducts and supports research on many of the most serious diseases affecting public health. The institute supports much of the clinical research on the diseases of internal medicine and related subspecialty fields as well as many basic science disciplines. NIDDK is a resource for health information, research funding opportunities, and reports to Congress and strategic plans relevant to diabetes, digestive, and kidney diseases.

Office of Minority Health, U.S. Department of Health and Human Services (OMH)

The Tower Building
1101 Wootton Parkway, Suite 600
Rockville, Maryland 20852
240-453-2882
FAX: 240-453-2883
Email: info@omhrc.gov
Web: http://www.omhrc.gov

The OMH, established in 1986 by the U.S. Department of Health and Human Services, has a mission to improve and protect the health of racial and ethnic minority populations through the development of health policies and programs that will eliminate health disparities. The OMH offers information on funding, services, and campaigns and initiatives to improve and protect the health of racial and ethnic minority populations.

Veterans' Health Administration Diabetes Program

1-800-827-1000
Web: http://www.va.gov

The goal of the Veteran's Health Administration (VHA) is to provide excellence in patient care, veterans' benefits, and customer satisfaction. The VHA is striving for high-quality, prompt, and seamless service to veterans. Their VHA diabetes program Web site contains information about diabetes and its management and also has links to other professional sites with information on diabetes.

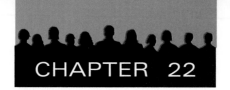

CHAPTER 22

Maternal and Child Populations

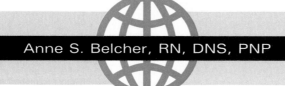

Anne S. Belcher, RN, DNS, PNP

Chapter Outline

- Reduce the Rate of Maternal Deaths
- Reduce the Rate of Fetal and Infant Deaths
- Reduce the Rate of Child Deaths
- Reduce the Rate of Adolescent and Young Adult Deaths
- Reduce the Rate of Pregnancies among Adolescent Females
- Reduce Obesity and Improve Nutrition in Children and Adolescents
  Healthy Eating
  Physical Activity
- Education and Community-Based Programs to Address Maternal and Child Health Issues
- Maternal and Child Health Services and Public Health Nursing

Learning Objectives

Upon completion of this chapter, the reader will be able to:

1. Explore the multidimensional roles of the public health nurse in improving the health and well-being of women, infants, children, and families.

2. Recognize the relationships of the risk factors associated with the current morbidities and mortalities in the maternal child health population.

3. Describe the importance of the Healthy People 2010 Objectives for maternal child health in the practice of the public health nurses.

4. Examine selected community-based approaches and interventions to improve the health of mothers, infants, children, and families.

5. Recognize the challenges associated with reducing obesity and improving nutrition in children and adolescents.

6. Appreciate the importance of the core public health functions in improving the health of the maternal child health population.

Nurses committed to public health are concerned about the health of populations, the impact of their interventions on the defined aggregates, and the evaluation of the outcomes of their work. The core public health functions that are considered essential to nursing practice in the community are assessment, policy development, and assurance. Nurses incorporate assessment by using evidence-based practice (EBP) to form innovative solutions to health problems, extend the EBP to develop healthy public policy, and use EBP to evaluate the effectiveness, quality, and accessibility of population-based services (Quad Council, 2000).

Public health nurses focus on the early detection of risk factors that contribute to undesirable health outcomes for mothers, infants, children, and adolescents. Clinical nurse specialists in public health nursing support maternal-child and adolescent populations by linking them to culturally competent health care services/resources, addressing the critical health disparities in the population groups, and advocating for public policies to meet the Healthy People 2010 Objectives. Chapter 22 highlights the improved health of women, infants, and children; efforts to reduce pregnancies among adolescent females; the growing concern about nutrition and overweight in the maternal child health population; and the importance of education and community-based programs to address the current public health challenges.

REDUCE THE RATE OF MATERNAL DEATHS

Healthy People 2010 Objectives 16-4 and 16-5 are to reduce maternal deaths with a target goal of 3.3 maternal deaths per 100,000 live births and to reduce maternal illness and complications due to pregnancy (USDHHS, 2000). Maternal complications during hospitalized labor and deliveries in 1998 were 31.2 per 100 deliveries. The 2010 target for maternal complications has been set at 24 per 100 deliveries. Three hundred twenty-seven maternal deaths per 100,000 were reported by vital statistics in 1997. Major causes for these maternal deaths were hemorrhage, ectopic pregnancy, pregnancy-induced hypertension, infection, and other complications of pregnancy/childbirth (Berg et al., 1996).

The United States is the only industrialized nation in the world where not all pregnant women receive prenatal care. Selected Healthy People 2010 Objectives for maternal and infant health address risk factors related to inadequate prenatal care. The risk factors associated with maternal mortality include:

- Increasing the number of pregnant women who receive early and adequate prenatal care throughout the pregnancy

- Decreasing the number of maternal complications during hospitalized labor and delivery

- Decreasing the number of women with pregnancy-induced hypertension, embolism, and incidence of infection

- Reducing the number of ectopic pregnancies resulting from tubal scarring, secondary to diagnosed pelvic inflammatory disease

- Increasing abstinence from alcohol, cigarettes, and illicit drug use among pregnant women

In the United States, the percentage of women who receive early prenatal care varies among racial and ethnic groups and geographic area. Access to care depends on the affordability and location of prenatal care services. Approximately three-quarters of all women in the United States receive adequate prenatal care (USDHHS, 2000). Pregnancy outcomes differ within counties located in the same state. Women particularly at risk for poor pregnancy outcomes are those residing in rural areas, those who live near Indian reservations, African American women, and migrant workers (National Rural Health Association, 2001a, 2001b). Public health nurses have a responsibility to encourage women to receive early and adequate prenatal care; maintain a healthy diet throughout the pregnancy; engage in moderate exercise; abstain from the use of tobacco, alcohol, and other illicit substances; avoid potential exposure to infectious diseases; and be safe in caring out the activities of daily living. Prenatal care and education are important components to reducing maternal mortality and complications of pregnancy. The public health nurse will provide screening and education about pregnancy in the clinic, home, or other settings where prenatal care is acquired. The nurse will check for presumptive, probable, and positive signs of pregnancy and assess for factors indicating a high risk pregnancy. Areas for assessment include the biophysical risk assessment for genetic factors, nutritional status, and medical or obstetrical disorders. Psychosocial assessment includes acquiring data related to use of caffeine, tobacco, alcohol, and drugs and assessing attitudes or ambivalence about the pregnancy. The presence of violence and the risks for emotional and physical abuse should also be assessed. Other areas for risk assessment include the client's perceptions on the need for prenatal care supervision, comfort with health care providers and the routine prenatal procedures, possible fears related to parental discovery of the pregnancy, immigration problems, and discovery of certain health habits or lifestyles related to the ethnicity and culture of the mother. Sociodemographic risk assessment includes age, parity, marital status, income, residence, and ethnicity. Environmental risks for consideration include exposure to radiation, chemicals, therapeutic drugs, pollutants, illicit drugs, and mutagenic agents.

Public health nurses working with pregnant women engaging in high-risk behaviors need to stress the importance of eliminating the use of alcohol, tobacco, and drugs in order to achieve a positive pregnancy outcome. Use of these substances is associated with low birth weight, which is a leading cause of infant death or impairment in neurobehavioral outcome (USDHHS, 2000). The nurse should approach these issues of risk assessment and education in a nonjudgmental way, supporting the client and providing educational and community resources for clients to abstain from these habits.

Overall the maternal mortality rate has ranged between 7 and 8 percent per 100,000 live births (occurring in hospitals) since 1982. Maternal mortality rates for hospitalized births among African Americans were 3.6 times the rate of whites in 1997, fluctuating between 18 and 22 deaths per 100,000 live births (CDC, 1998). Shortened hospital stays call for the public health nurse to educate new mothers on the common complications of the postpartum period. Hospital discharge instructions should include information regarding the normal amount and appearance of vaginal discharge for days 1–4 through the second or third week postpartum. Any abnormal bleeding or odor should be reported immediately to the health care provider. Morbidity related to complications of pregnancy includes uterine prolapse, fistulae, incontinence, pain during intercourse, and infertility. Hospitals and local health departments have supported funding for "early discharge programs," which send registered nurses on

⊕ PRACTICE APPLICATION

Benefits of Folic Acid

One of the most important things a woman can do before conception and during early pregnancy to help prevent serious neural tube defects (incomplete development of the brain and spinal cord) is to get enough folic acid every day. Researchers have found that between 50 and 70 percent of neural tube defects can be prevented when women supplement their diet with folic acid, a water-soluble B vitamin. The Centers for Disease Control and Prevention recommends all women of childbearing age eat a diet high in folic acid or take a multivitamin with 0.4 mg of folic acid each day, especially one month prior to conception through the first three months of pregnancy. Despite the recommendations for daily folic acid intake, approximately 3,000 pregnancies are still affected in the United States. Consider the following: Bethany is a public health nurse who has been working with Hispanic women through the county health department. She is interested in developing a culturally appropriate intervention in an effort to promote the use of preconceptual folic acid among the women of childbearing age.

home visits to mothers and infants within 48 hours of an early discharge birth. Maternal and infant assessments and required newborn screening blood work are completed during the visit. Follow-up visits are determined by the results of the assessments.

Nine to 15 percent of women who have recently given birth experience postpartum depression; however, only a small portion of these women are identified as depressed by health care professionals. Postpartum depression should be discussed with the mother, and assessments of coping ability, support networks, financial status, and parent–infant bonding should be conducted by the public health nurse. The Postpartum Depression Checklist (PDC) is an eleven-item checklist designed for use by health personnel to engage the mother in a dialogue about her experiences with early signs of postpartum depression (Beck, 2002). History of addiction, mental health problems, family disruption, conflict, or situational crises are also risk factors for postpartum depression.

REDUCE THE RATE OF FETAL AND INFANT DEATHS

Low birth weight is a significant factor most closely associated with neonatal and infant deaths. Low birth weight has been determined to be the leading cause of death in infants and can be the cause of health problems including respiratory distress, infection, intracranial hemorrhage, blindness, and developmental delay and feeding problems (USDHHS, 2000). Healthy People 2010 Objective 16-10 calls for a reduction in low birth weight and very low birth weight babies. Factors contributing to low birth weight should be considered by the public health nurse. These factors include preterm delivery, inadequate prenatal care, alcohol and tobacco use, drug use, poor nutrition, and exposure to sexually transmitted diseases or (STDs) other viral infection. The average hospital costs associated with a low birth weight delivery are estimated to be three times that of a normal healthy delivery (USDHHS, 2000). Primary interventions for the prevention of low birth weight infants are included as part of early and consistent prenatal care.

In addition to low birth weight, neural tube defects and the presence of fetal alcohol syndrome (FAS) contribute to neonatal and infant morbidity. Evidence indicates that nearly half of all neural tube defects could be prevented with the adequate consumption of folic acid in the first trimester of pregnancy. Public health nurses should encourage women of childbearing age to include 400 micrograms of folic acid in the daily diet. FAS is a preventable cause of cognitive and developmental impairment in infants. Screening for alcohol use prior to and during the prenatal period should be part of the history taking by the public health nurse during the prenatal home visit or clinic appointment.

Injury and illness prevention in the newborn are priorities for the public health nurse working with parents of newborns. Anticipatory guidance is information and education provided to the client in order to take timely action or prevent the onset of a health problem. Anticipatory guidance during home visits should include using rear-facing infant car seats, positioning infant on the back for sleeping, providing a smoke-free environment, avoiding overexposing the infant to the sun, ensuring that the infant is not left alone at any time, and understanding the early signs of illness and the appropriate responses to fever. Environmental assessment suggests that there be working smoke detectors in the home and that the water temperature for an infant be kept below 120°F (USDHHS, 2000).

REDUCE THE RATE OF CHILD DEATHS

The leading causes of death in children between the ages of 1 and 4 are unintentional injuries and motor vehicle accidents. Nurses should be familiar with the Healthy People 2010 Objectives identified for the ages of children they are working with, and targeted health education efforts should emphasize the areas of prevention highlighted in the nation's health objectives for children. Objective 16-2 a, Reduction in deaths of children aged 1–4 from 34.6/100,000 to 18.6/100,000, and Objective 16-2 b, Reduction in deaths of children aged 5–9 from 17.7/100,000 to 12.3/100,000 (USDHHS, 2000).

Motor vehicle injuries are the most common causes of death in both age groups of children. Data for children ages 1–4 indicates that after motor vehicle injuries, drowning, fires, and burns account for the mortality in this age group. Older children ages 5–9 are most likely to die from motor vehicle accidents followed by firearms, including unintentional deaths, homicides, and suicides. Other causes of death in the 1–9 year age group include birth defects, malignant neoplasms, and diseases of the heart (CDC, 2005).

Bright Futures guidelines present a detailed framework for health professionals in partnership with families to promote the developmental health and well-being of children from birth to young adulthood. The following teaching guidelines based on their work can be used as anticipatory guidance for children ages 1–14:

- Use a car safety seat at all times until the child reaches 40 pounds.
- Secure car seats properly in the back seat, preferably in the middle.
- Keep medication, cleaning solutions, and other dangerous substances in childproof containers and out of the reach of children.
- Use safety gates across stairways and guards on windows above the first floor.

- Keep hot water heater temperature below 120°F.
- Cover unused electrical outlets with plastic covers.
- Provide constant supervision for babies using a baby walker and block access to stairways.
- Keep objects and foods that may cause choking away from children (balloons, toys with small parts, coins, hot dogs, peanuts, and hard candies).
- Use fences that completely circle pools and keep gates to pools locked.
- Use smoke detectors in the home. Change batteries once per year, and check the detectors monthly.

- If there is a gun in the home, make sure the gun and the ammunition are locked and separated from each other and out of the reach of children.
- Teach children traffic safety—children under 9 years of age need supervision in crossing streets.
- Teach children when and how to call 911.
- Educate children of all ages and their parents in the proper fit and use of bicycle helmets. (American Academy of Pediatrics, 2002).

Areas of primary prevention for children include immunizations and assessment for iron-deficiency anemia and child abuse. Vaccines are used to produce an

---

⊕ RESEARCH APPLICATION

Rural Parents' Perceptions of Risks Associated with Their Children's Exposure to Radon

Study Purpose

To examine the level of awareness of radon issues, correlates of elective testing behaviors, and the accuracy of risk perception for radon exposures among rural residents receiving public health services.

Methods

Cross-sectional data were collected in the beginning stages of developing the Environmental Risk Reduction through Nursing Intervention and Education (ERRNIE) project to better understand the prevalence and context of radon exposures among rural Montana children. Households with children younger than 6 years of age, referred from the city/county health department, were included in the study. Thirty-one rural households with 71 adults and 60 children participated. All the primary respondents were female, 97 percent Caucasian, and 94 percent between 21 and 40 years of age. Participants completed a radon knowledge and risk perception questionnaire, and homes were tested for radon presence.

Findings

Ten (32 percent) of the houses had a radon level above the Environmental Protection Agency (EPA) action level. Although 65 percent of respondents were accurate in their assessment of risk, 5 (16 percent) who were inaccurate

in their risk assessment had radon exceeding the EPA action level. Adjusting for chance, agreement fell to 21 percent. The general awareness of radon issues was low. About 36 percent disagreed that health effects from radon were serious, and 39 percent disagreed that being around less radon would improve the long-term health of their children. Awareness of radon also was found to be low, with 51.6 percent being neutral or unsure whether radon could cause health problems, 45.2 percent being neutral or unsure about how to find out whether their home was safe or unsafe, and 64 percent being neutral or unsure about taking steps to reduce radon in their home.

Implications

Although the sample size was small, this study provides important information for public health nurses because risk perception has been shown to be a critical factor in radon testing behaviors. Vulnerable rural populations receiving public health services have educational needs about health consequences of radon exposure, risk of exposure, and radon testing.

Reference

Hill, W. G., Butterfield, P., & Larsson, L. S. (2006). Rural parents' perceptions of risks associated with their children's exposure to radon. *Public Health Nursing, 23*(5), 392–399.

immune response in the host. Immunization schedules are complex and change very frequently. Often they are confusing to parents, causing the children to miss doses and placing them at risk for communicable disease. The public health nurse should take the lead with respect to ensuring that the immunizations for infants and children are up to date. The most recent immunization schedule from the Centers for Disease Control can be found in Chapter 20.

REDUCE THE RATE OF ADOLESCENT AND YOUNG ADULT DEATHS

The leading causes of morbidity and mortality among adolescents and young adults are due to unintentional injuries (44 percent), with most of the deaths occurring as a result of motor vehicle accidents. Alcohol was found to be involved in more than half of the fatal accidents in this age group (U.S. Bureau of the Census, 2001). Healthy People 2010 Objective 16-3 is to reduce the number of deaths of adolescents and young adults. Objective 16-3a, Reduction in deaths of adolescents aged 10–14 years from 22.1/100,000 to16.8/100,000, and Objective 16-3b, Reduction in deaths of adolescents aged 15–19 from 70.6/100,000 to 39.8/100,000. Older adolescents are more likely than younger teens to engage in risky behaviors resulting in unintentional injury and death (USDHHS, 2000).

The leading cause of death for adolescents (10–14 years) were motor vehicle crashes, 24.3 percent. Other unintentional injuries contributing to the death rates were falls, drownings, poisonings, homicides, and suicides. The remainder of deaths in the age group was attributed to malignant neoplasms, diseases of the heart, birth defects, and a combination of other medical conditions. Fifty-five percent of the total deaths in the young adolescent age group were due to preventable causes (CDC, 2005). Leading causes of death for adolescents (15–19 years) were motor vehicle crashes, reaching 37.4 percent; falls, drownings, and poisonings, 10.4 percent; homicides, 16.8 percent; suicides, 12.6 percent; and AIDS, 0.2 percent. The remaining 23 percent of the deaths were attributed to malignant neoplasms, diseases of the heart, birth defects, and a combination of other medical conditions. Seventy-seven percent of the deaths attributed to older adolescents

were the result of unnecessary and preventable causes (Hoyert, Kockanck, & Murph, 1999).

Developmentally, adolescents are more likely to dismiss the dangers associated with high-risk behaviors. Adolescents hold firm to the "personal fable" that the negative consequences of their at-risk behaviors will not have personal consequences.

The public health nurse may want to meet with adolescents separately from their parents to identify the health priorities for the adolescents. Adolescence is a time of growing independence where the adolescent begins to "try on" adult roles, yet the adolescent needs the supervision and problem-solving skills of the adults in their lives. According to the family theorist Duvall (1977), healthy families raise adolescents using open communication as the means to balance independence with responsibility. The public health nurse should advocate such crucial parenting skills as setting limits for their children and encouraging responsible behaviors in their children.

Health issues facing adolescents in the twenty-first century include

- ⊕ Establishing dietary and exercise habits

- ⊕ Developing problem-solving and effective coping strategies

- ⊕ Regulating alcohol, drug, and tobacco use

- ⊕ Monitoring early and unprotected sexual activity

⊕ PRACTICE APPLICATION

Dating Violence

Dating violence is becoming a major public health concern. Dating violence occurs when one partner tries to maintain power and control over the other through abuse. It is estimated that one in three teenagers has experienced violence in a dating relationship. Dating violence crosses all racial, economic, and social lines, and most victims are young women. Teen dating violence is influenced by how teenagers look at themselves and others. Young men may believe

they have the right to "control" their female partners in any way necessary, that masculinity is physical aggressiveness, or that they possess their partner. Young women may believe that their boyfriend's jealousy, possessiveness, and even physical abuse is romantic; that abuse is "normal" because their friends are also being abused; or that there is no one to ask for help.

⊕ Driving safely

⊕ Refusing to participate in delinquent and/or violent activities

REDUCE THE RATE OF PREGNANCIES AMONG ADOLESCENT FEMALES

The teen pregnancy rate in the United States is much higher than other comparable countries such as England, Wales, France, Canada, the Netherlands, and Japan (Bachu & O'Connell, 2001). Adolescent pregnancy remains a national issue for the United States. Healthy People 2010 Objective 9-7 is to reduce pregnancies among adolescent females from 68 per 1,000 females aged 15–17 to 43 pregnancies per 1,000 births. Since 1990, pregnancy rates have declined for teens aged 15–17 years (USSDHS, 2000). See Figure 22-1.

Most adolescent childbearing occurs outside of marriage. Seventy-eight percent of births to females younger than 20 years of age in 1997 were out of wedlock as compared to 44 percent out of wedlock births in 1977. Between 1986 and 1991 there was a 24 percent rise in the number of births to teenage mothers. More recently, births to mothers aged 15–19 years of age have declined. The 2002 rate was 41.7 per 1,000 births for Caucasian girls, 73.1 for African American girls, and 92.4 for Hispanic teens (Maternal and Child Health Bureau, 2002).

Adolescent females younger than age 15 experience around 30,000 pregnancies each year. Healthy People

2010 reports widespread consensus that all pregnancies in this age group are high risk, and the target number of pregnancies for girls younger than 15 should be zero (USDHHS, 2000). Statistics report that nearly two-thirds of the pregnancies in the younger age groups end in induced abortion or fetal loss. Teen pregnancies are more likely to result in hypertension, toxemia, anemia, preterm birth, delivery of a low-birth-weight infant, and stillbirth. There has been almost no discernible decline in the annual pregnancy rates for girls 15 years of age or younger (USDHHS, 2000).

Factors that contribute to teen pregnancy include earlier onset of puberty, earlier age at the initiation of

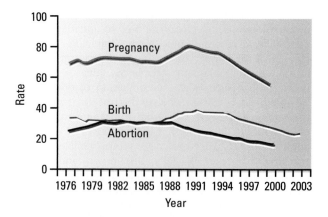

Figure 22-1 Pregnancy, birth, and abortion rates for teenagers.
From National Center for Health Statistics.

intercourse, increased sexual activity, nonuse of contraceptives, and knowledge deficit about sex and conception. Primary prevention is the target goal with respect to teen pregnancy. Comprehensive programs to address teen pregnancy should focus on three goals:

- Delaying or halting participation in sexual activity
- Providing access to contraception and sufficient knowledge and skill to use contraception appropriately.
- Strengthening life goals and encouraging long-term planning.

Sexual activity has increased among teens without a corresponding increase in their knowledge levels about sexual function, risks associated with early sexual behavior, birth control, or procreation. Pregnancy and acquisition of sexually transmitted diseases (STDs) are of low concern to adolescents (Kalmuss et al., 2003). One nonintended consequence of increased sexual activity in teens is the risk of exposure to STDs requiring diagnosis and treatment by the health care delivery system. Each year around four million adolescents contract a STD including chlamydia, gonorrhea, AIDS, syphilis, and hepatitis B (USDHHS, 2000).

Adolescents depend on the health care community to treat and cure STDs they acquire. Education and motivation of teens regarding abstinence and use of contraception to prevent pregnancy and sexually transmitted diseases can be challenging. The public health nurse uses education to assess the individual and target individual risks and behaviors. Primary prevention outcomes of successful education programs for this group include decreasing the spread of STDs, and reduction in the number of unplanned pregnancies. Secondary and tertiary prevention in teen pregnancy focuses on healthier outcomes for the pregnancy including early detection, options counseling, prenatal care, nutritional counseling, childbirth education, parenting education, and safer sex education.

Care coordination is a program that provides a systematic monitoring of the health status of individuals, families and/or groups. Care coordination for pregnant adolescents has been one successful approach to the support services that can be provided to new mothers throughout the pregnancy and following delivery of the newborn. Care coordination has been adopted by the Healthy Families America (HFA) Initiative. HFA is a national initiative to help parents of newborns get

their infants off to a good start. Participation in HFA is voluntary for the participants and is supported with home visiting by public health nurses and community outreach workers. The HFA links families to resources and other services in over 450 communities across the United States (HFA, 2005).

HFA programs have a series of critical elements that represent evidence-based practice related to the implementation of successful home visitation programs. Those care coordination programs promising to adhere to the HFA critical elements are certified as HFA sites. The following are brief descriptions of each element:

Service Initiation

- Initiate services during the prenatal period or at birth.
- Use a standardized assessment tool to systematically identify families who are most in need of services.
- Offer services voluntarily and use positive outreach efforts to build family trust.

Service Content

- Offer services to participating families over the long term (i.e., three to five years), using well-defined criteria for increasing or decreasing frequency of services.
- Ensure that services are culturally competent and materials used reflect the diversity of the population served.
- Ensure that services are comprehensive and focus on supporting the parent as well as supporting parent-child interaction and child development.
- Encourage all families to be linked to a medical provider; families may also be linked to additional health and non-health-related services to meet their needs.
- Limit staff member case loads.

Staff Characteristics

- Service providers are selected based on their ability to establish a trusting relationship with clients.
- All service providers receive basic training in areas such as cultural competency, substance abuse, reporting child abuse, domestic violence, drug-exposed infants, and services in their community.

⊕ Service providers receive thorough training specific to their role to understand the essential components of family assessment and home visitation (HFA, 2005).

Goals of the care coordination programs are to reduce health risks for the mother and infant and to increase the chances that the mother will continue her education after delivery. Olds et al. (1999) reported on the long-term effects (over twenty years) of a Nurse Home Visiting Program. The intervention for the research was short term, from prenatal care to the child's second birthday, yet results indicated a long-term impact on the clients served. Women who participated in the program delayed subsequent pregnancies and were more likely to be actively employed in the workforce, and their children were less likely to have experienced unintentional childhood injuries. Data from the longitudinal follow-up of children born to mothers enrolled in the Nurse Home Visiting Program, indicated that at age 15 children in the study had fewer arrests and convictions, smoked and drank less, and had fewer sexual partners than their peers. Additional long-term studies may determine which strategies are the most successful in achieving the desired outcomes.

⊕ POLICY HIGHLIGHT

California Adolescent Health Collaborative

The California Adolescent Health Collaborative (AHC) is a public-private statewide coalition with the goal of increasing understanding and support for adolescent health and wellness in California. The AHC is a comprehensive, assets-based, multidisciplinary approach to improving the health and well-being of California youth. The program outcome areas include prevention of injury, suicide, teen pregnancy, sexually transmitted illnesses and alcohol, tobacco, and other drug use and promotion of nutrition and physical activity, mental health, oral health, and environmental and occupational health. The AHC is also developing a resource program for providers working with out-of-home youth—those who lack family support and are among the most vulnerable to severe mental health problems (California Adolescent Health Collaborative, 2006).

REDUCE OBESITY AND IMPROVE NUTRITION IN CHILDREN AND ADOLESCENTS

Healthy People 2010 Objective 19-3c is to reduce the proportion of children and adolescents who are overweight and obese. Data collected in 1994 indicated that 11 percent of children ages 6–19 were overweight. The Healthy People 2010 target for this objective is to reduce the percentage of overweight and obese children to 5 percent. The prevalence of overweight among children has more than doubled for preschoolers ages 2–5 and adolescents ages 12–19. Overweight in children 6–11 years has more than tripled since the 1970s. Nearly one-third (31 percent) of children and adolescents ages 6–19 are either at risk or considered at risk for being overweight (Hedley et al., 2004).

Overweight and obesity are major contributors to preventable causes of death. Children and adolescents who are overweight and obese are more likely to be at risk for hypertension, type 2 diabetes, cardiovascular disease, osteoporosis, new onset asthma, and some cancers. Children may develop sleep apnea, mature early, have increased LDL cholesterol, and run the risk of liver and gallbladder diseases (Dietz & Barlow, 2002). Beyond the physical effect of obesity, children and adolescents may also suffer from psychological consequences related to their overweight. The Centers for Disease Control uses the following definitions for measuring childhood overweight:

⊕ *At risk of overweight:* BMI for age >85th percentile to <95th percentile.

⊕ *Overweight:* BMI for age >95th percentile.

Body mass index (BMI) is the ratio of weight to height, a formula in which a person's body weight in kilograms is divided by the square of his or her height in meters. For children ages 2–20 years, BMI is plotted on a growth chart specific for age and gender. Overweight in children and adolescents cannot be measured or discussed in the same terms used with adults. Because of uncertainty about the meaning of weight tables for growing children and a concern about the stigmatizing potential of the term "obesity" some researchers use the CDC terminology "overweight" (Center for Health and Health Care in Schools, 2005).

Genetics is a factor in excess weight, but it does not explain the recent epidemic of overweight children and adolescents. Having overweight parents more than doubles the child's risk of being obese. Genetic characteristics of human populations have not changed in the last two decades, but the prevalence of obesity among children and adults has almost doubled (IOM, 2004). The health care costs associated with childhood and adolescent obesity are substantial. Overweight and obesity are major risk factors for significant diseases including

- *Asthma:* Obese children used more medicine, wheezed more, and made more visits to the emergency room for their asthma than their nonobese peers (Belamarich et al., 2000).

- *Type 2 diabetes:* Impaired glucose tolerance is highly prevalent among children and adolescents with severe obesity regardless of ethnicity. Type 2 diabetes puts these children at risk for blindness, heart and kidney disease, and loss of limbs (Sinha & Fisch, 2002).

- *Cardiovascular risk:* Sixty percent of obese children aged 5–10 years had at least one cardiovascular disease risk factor such as elevated total cholesterol, triglycerides, insulin, or blood pressure (IOM, 2005).

- *Sleep apnea:* Obstructive sleep apnea occurs in 17 percent of obese children and adolescents. These children experience loud snoring, mouth breathing, frequent awakening, daytime sleepiness, and hyperactive behavior, all of which contribute to behavior problems and altered academic performance (Slyper, 1998).

- *Psychosocial consequences:* Overweight children and youth have decreased self-esteem; reported increased rates of loneliness, sadness, and nervousness; and were more likely to smoke and consume alcohol (Strauss, 2000). Overweight adolescents often experience teasing about their weight and are more likely to be socially isolated and outside of the social networks experienced by normal weight adolescents (Eisenberg, Neumark-Sztainer, & Story, 2003).

Two behavioral areas identified to address the obesity problem for children and adolescents in school settings are food consumption and physical activity. The primary goal for obesity prevention and treatment should be healthy eating and increased physical activity.

Healthy Eating

Efforts to increase students' consumption of nutritious foods may be hindered by the availability of junk foods, the impact of advertising on food choices, and private fund-raising efforts that include low-nutrition foods yet support athletic and extracurricular activities. Schools are the primary venue that can be targeted to address food choices available to the K-12 population.

Schools are required to follow the U.S. Department of Agriculture Guidelines for the school lunch program but can promote healthy eating by

- Providing more nutritious food and beverages for foods sold a la carte in the snack bars and limiting sweetened drinks and high-fat, high-sugar snacks in the vending machines

- Expanding the number and variety of healthy food choices available to children and adolescents in schools

- Emphasizing healthful food choices and encouraging moderation in dietary practices rather than overconsumption of food (USDHHS, 2000)

Physical Activity

Physical activity levels in school settings are categorized as organized physical activity and free-time physical activity during nonschool hours. Approximately 38.5 percent of children aged 9–13 participated in organized physical activity and 77.4 percent of children engaged in free-time physical activity during nonschool hours (CDC, 2002). Over half of U.S. students in grades 9–12 were enrolled in physical education classes, and 32.2 percent had a daily physical education class. Of the enrolled students, 83.4 percent reported exercising at least 20 minutes during an average class. About half of all schools reported offering intramural activities or physical activity clubs for students. The CDC survey reported that 84.0 percent of elementary, 77.4 percent of middle/junior high, and 79.5 percent of senior high schools follow national or state physical education standards or guidelines (Burgeson, Wechsler, & Brener, 2001).

Successful interventions for the treatment of obesity in children and adolescents provide gradual increases in activity and targeted reductions in high-fat, high-calorie foods (Barlow & Dietz, 1998). Schools may be the appropriate setting for the promotion of healthy lifestyles in children, but interventions require duplication and repetition in other social settings such as the family. Using the comprehensive school health model developed by CDC the schools can target the whole environment and select strategies that are behaviorally focused.

School-based intervention programs that have been successful include

- Separate, female-only physical education class
- Focus on physical activities selected by the students
- Instruction on the health benefits of physical activity
- Use of the stairs instead of the elevator and walking instead of driving
- Weight control programs that are fun, interactive, and low cost
- Multiple options for physical activity that gradually increase the activity level over time
- Use of program leaders who are currently working to manage their weight or have been overweight in the past (Neumark-Sztainer, Martin, & Story, 2000)

EDUCATION AND COMMUNITY-BASED PROGRAMS TO ADDRESS MATERNAL AND CHILD HEALTH ISSUES

Healthy People Objective 7-2 is to increase the proportion of middle, junior high, and senior high schools that provide school health education to prevent health problems in the following areas: unintentional injury, violence, suicide, tobacco use and addiction, alcohol and other drug use, unintended pregnancy, HIV/AIDS and STD infection, unhealthy dietary patterns, inadequate physical activity, and environmental health (USDHHS, 2000).

Baseline data reported in the School Health Policies and Programs Study (National Center for Chronic Disease Prevention and Health Promotion, 1994) indicated that 26 percent of youth received health education in the identified health behavioral areas. By 2010, the goal is for 70 percent of youth to receive adequate health education in the targeted areas through their state and local school districts (USDHHS, 2000).

The overall goal for educational and community-based programs is to increase the quality, availability, and effectiveness of educational and community-based programs designed to prevent disease and improve health and the quality of life for children and adolescents. Schools are identified as pivotal centers for providing health education to children and adolescents. Healthy People 2010 identified six categories of behaviors that are responsible for more than 70 percent of the illness, disability, and death among adolescents and young adults. Healthy People 2010 suggest that the focus of school health education should address: (a) injury prevention (unintentional and intentional), (b) tobacco use, (c) alcohol and illicit drug use, (d) sexual behaviors that result in unintended pregnancies and sexually transmitted diseases, (e) dietary patterns that cause disease, and (f) inadequate physical activity. Other areas for consideration include environmental health because of its relationship to personal and community health, mental and emotional health, and consumer health (Joint Committee on National Health Education Standards, 1995).

Health literacy has been identified as the overall goal of the National Health Education Standards for youth (USDHHS, 2000). Young people need to be given the tools to find, understand, and use information and services that will lead to improved health. Health education curricula in K–12 schools have been targeted to provide the strategies and instruction time to affect the priority risk behaviors. State and local school health districts are charged with the responsibility to create policies that support effective health education, teacher training, engaging curricula, and continuous quality improvement to ensure that children in grades K–12 have received the education to make sound decisions about health-related behaviors. Teaching strategies should reflect the learning styles of the students and incorporate technology and interaction that supports critical thinking with respect to decisions about behaviors that affect personal health and the health of the community. Family, peers, and the community at large are critical components needed to support long-term health behavior change in adolescents. Health promotion messages should be consistent, culturally appropriate, and designed sequentially to engage the learner from age 5 to age 18 (Kann, Brener, & Allensworth, 2001).

The school health plan for the twenty-first century supports school-based health education, health promotion, physical activity, and health services. The Centers for Disease Control developed the Coordinated School Health Model, which serves as the foundation for the coordinated school health program. The Coordinated School Health Program, which can be seen in Figure 22-2, has eight components identified as being essential for improving health in school settings. These include health education; physical education; health services; counseling, psychological, and social services; healthy school environment; health promotion for staff; and family/community involvement.

School health is viewed beyond heath education classes and health services provided directly to students in school classrooms. The Centers for Disease Control views coordinated school health as the community and components of the model extended to administrators, teachers, and staff as a part of the school community. The school is viewed in the context of the school system and the contributions the school can make to the health of the community at large.

The National Association of School Nurses has called for a comprehensive school health education curriculum that provides programming from kindergarten through twelfth grade that considers the physical, mental, emotional, and social dimensions of health. Health education is designed to motivate students to maintain and improve their health, prevent disease, and reduce

health-related risks (NASN, 2002). Areas of emphasis in the health curriculum include

- Personal health
- Family health
- Community health
- Environmental health
- Sexuality
- Emotional and mental health
- Injury prevention
- Nutrition
- Prevention and control of disease
- Substance use and abuse

MATERNAL AND CHILD HEALTH SERVICES AND PUBLIC HEALTH NURSING

A primary goal for public health nursing is to attain, regain, or maintain the health of mothers, children, and their families in community settings. Specific nursing roles practiced include case finder, care provider, educator, coordinator, case manager, advocate, and change agent. Shrinking resources at the federal, state, and local levels will require resourcefulness on the part of the public health nurse to plan, implement, and evaluate the outcomes for the health services provided.

Evidence-based nursing practice for the public health nurse of the twenty-first century should emphasize:

- Promoting normal growth and development of the individual/family
- Facilitating health promotion and wellness with early screening and developmental assessments
- Enhancing the nutritional and immunologic status of the child/adolescent
- Promoting safe environments for the individual/family
- Improving the health behaviors of the individual/family
- Advocating for healthy public policy for mothers, children, adolescents, and families

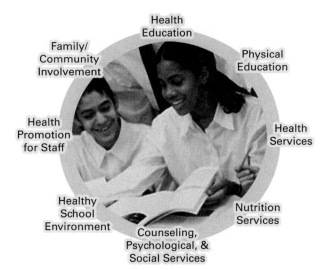

Figure 22-2 Coordinated school health program.

⊕ Monitoring services provided for their accessibility, acceptability, and affordability in meeting the Healthy People 2010 Objectives.

The Healthy People 2010 Objectives offer a systematic approach to improving the health of the maternal, infant, child, and adolescent populations. Objectives by themselves cannot improve the health status of populations, but they do provide a framework for measuring progress toward stated goals over time. Public health nurses committed to improving the health of populations focus on the entire range of factors that determine health rather than personal risk factors for disease. Population-focused practice in maternal child health interfaces with community systems and works to change community norms, attitudes, awareness, practices, behaviors, and policies that affect mothers, infants, children, and adolescents. Use of evidence-based practice at the system level changes organizations, policies, laws, and the structures of systems that impact maternal child health (Minnesota Department of Public Health, 2001).

Interventions at each level of practice contribute to the overall goal of improved population health.

⊕ RESEARCH APPLICATION

Application of the Transtheoretical Model of Behavior Change to the Physical Activity Behavior of WIC Mothers

Study Purpose

To examine the Transtheoretical Model of Behavior Change in relationship to the physical activity behavior of mothers receiving assistance from the Women, Infants, and Children (WIC) program.

Methods

This correlational, descriptive study used purposive sampling to enroll six English-speaking women at each of the five stages of readiness for physical activity ($N = 30$). Variables included physical activity behavior; perceived pros, and decisional balance of physical activity, processes of exercise adoption, self-efficacy for exercise, processes of behavior change, social support for exercise, and stage of physical activity (precontemplation, contemplation, preparation, action, and maintenance).

Findings

Only 38 percent of the women participated in regular physical activity. Stage of behavior change and total physical activity behavior was significantly related. Self-efficacy for physical activity, perceived pros of physical activity, and decisional balance were significant and positively related to stage of physical activity, and perceived cons of physical activity was significant and negatively related to stage of physical activity. Processes of change differed by stage of physical activity.

Implications

Because few WIC mothers engage in physical activity, they represent an at-risk population that could benefit from public health nurses' health promotion interventions that promote physical activity. Public health nurses should assess mothers for stage of physical activity and use behavior change strategies that increase self-efficacy and perceived pros of changing physical activity behavior, decrease perceived cons of changing physical activity behavior, and increase the use of processes of change.

Reference

Fahrenwald, N. L., & Walker, S. N. (2003). Application of the transtheoretical model of behavior change to the physical activity behavior of WIC mothers. *Public Health Nursing, 20,* 307-317.

CRITICAL THINKING ACTIVITIES

1. Examine the health statistics and demographic data related to the health and well-being of either women, infants, children, or families in your geographical area.

   a. What resources are available in your community to support the health of these populations?

   b. What services are available from federal, state, and local resources?

   c. Review the literature with respect to recommended programs and interventions. How do the programs in your geographic area compare to those described in the literature?

   d. Describe the role(s) of the public health nurse in supporting the aggregate you selected.

2. In your role as a public health nurse you have been asked to develop a nutrition and physical activity program for mothers-to-be, a cohort of first grade students, and a group of high school sophomores.

   a. What factors do these programs have in common?

   b. How do the programs for each group differ?

   c. What outcomes would you want to evaluate?

3. As a public health nurse, you have been selected to serve on the assessment team for a coordinated school health program team at the local middle school.

   a. What would be your contribution as a public health nurse to the team?

   a. Describe the focus areas for school health education with this age group?

KEY TERMS

anticipatory guidance	care coordination	evidence-based practice
body mass index	Coordinated School Health Program	

KEY CONCEPTS

- Public health nurses use assessment, assurance, and public policy in their practice to improve the health and well-being of women, infants, children, and families.

- Public health nursing practice occurs with individuals, families, groups, communities, and systems.

- Healthy People 2010 Objectives offer a systematic approach and a framework for public health nursing practice with women, infants, children, and families.

- The Coordinated School Health Program designed by the Centers for Disease Control provides the structure for public health nurses to impact the health and lifestyle choices for students, teachers, school staff and the community.

- Care coordination and the Healthy Families Initiative are evidence-based home visitation programs used to improve pregnancy outcomes for mothers and babies.

- Public health nurses are integral to the development, implementation, and evaluation of programs that impact the major causes of morbidity and mortality of women, infants, children, and families.

REFERENCES

American Academy of Pediatrics. (2002). *Bright futures: Guidelines for health supervision of infants, children and adolescents* (2nd ed.). Available from http://www.brightfutures.org/bf2/pdf/pdf/FrontMatter.pdf.

Bachu, A., & O'Connell, M. (2001). *Fertility of American women: June 2000.* Current Population Reports (P20-543RV). Washington, DC: U.S. Census Bureau.

Barlow, S., & Dietz, W. (1998). Obesity evaluation and treatment: Expert committee recommendations. *Pediatrics, 102*(3), 29–39.

Beck, C. T. (2002). Predictors of postpartum depression: An update. *Nursing Research, 59*(5), 275–285.

Belamarich, P., Luder, E., Kattan, M., Mitchell, H., Islam, S., Lynn, H., & Crain, E. (2000). Do obese inner city children with asthma have more symptoms than non obese children with asthma? *Pediatrics, 106*(6), 1436–1441.

Berg, C. J., Atrash, H. K., Koonin, L. M., & Tucker, M. (1996). Pregnancy related mortality in the United States 1987–1990.*Obstetrics and Gynecology, 88*(2), 161–167.

Burgeson, C., Wechsler, H., & Brener, N. (2001). Physical education activity: Results from the school health policies and program studies 2000. *Journal of School Health, 71*(7), 279–293.

California Adolescent Health Collaborative. (2006). *Investing in adolescent health.* Retrieved November 29, 2006, from http://www.californiateenhealth.org.

Center for Health and Health Care in Schools. (2005). *Childhood overweight: What the research tells us.* Retrieved June 8, 2005, from www.healthinschools.org.

Centers for Disease Control and Prevention (CDC). (1998). Maternal mortality—United States, 1982–1996. *MMWR, 47*(34), 705–707.

Centers for Disease Control and Prevention (CDC). (2002). Physical activity levels among children aged 9–13 years United States 2002. *MMWR 2003, 52*(33), 785–788.

Centers for Disease Control and Prevention (CDC). (2005). Deaths: Leading causes for 2002. *National Vital Statistics Reports, 53*(17), 13.

Dietz, W. H., & Barlow, S. E. (2002). Management of child and adolescent obesity: Summary and recommendations based on reports from pediatricians, pediatric nurse practitioners, and registered dieticians. *Pediatrics, 110,* 236–238.

Duvall, E. M. (1977). *Family development* (5th ed.). Philadelphia: J.B. Lippincott.

Eisenberg, M., Neumark-Sztainer, D., & Story, M. (2003). Associations of weight-based teasing and emotional well being among adolescents. *Archives of Pediatric and Adolescent Medicine, 157,* 733–738.

Fahrenwald, N. L., & Walker, S. N. (2003). Application of the transtheoretical model of behavior change to the physical activity behavior of WIC mothers. *Public Health Nursing, 20,* 307-317.

Fox, H. B., Limb, S. J., McManus, M. A., & Levtov, R. G. (2005). *An analysis of states' capitation methods and pediatric rates, 1997–2003.* Washington, DC: Fox Health Policy Consultants.

Healthy Families America (HFA). (2005). Healthy families America: About us—Critical elements. *Healthy Families America Initiative.* Retrieved June 22, 2005, from http://www.healthyfamiliesamerica.org/about_us/critical_elements.shtml.

Hedley, A., Ogden, C., Johnson, C., Carroll, M. D., Curtin, L.R., & Flegal, K. M., (2004). Prevalence of overweight and obesity among US children, adolescents, and adults, 1999–2002. *Journal of the American Medical Association, 29*(23), 2847–2850.

Hill, W. G., Butterfield, P., & Larsson, L. S. (2006). Rural parents' perceptions of risks associated with their children's exposure to radon. *Public Health Nursing, 23*(5), 392–399.

Hoyert, D. L., Kockanck, K. D., & Murph, S. L. (1999). Deaths: Final data for 1997. *National Vital Statistics Report, 47*(19), 1-15.

Institute of Medicine (IOM), National Academies of Science. (2004). Childhood obesity in the United States: Facts and figures. Retrieved August 27, 2007, from http://www.iom.edu/Object.File/Master/22/606/FINALfactsandfigures2.pdf .

Joint Committee on National Health Education Standards. (1995). *National health education standards: Achieving health literacy.* Atlanta: American Cancer Society.

Kalmuss, D., Davidson, A., Cohall, A., Laraque, D., & Cassell, C. (2003). Preventing sexual risk behaviors and pregnancy among teenagers: Linking research and programs. *Perspectives on Sexual and Reproductive Health, 35*(2), 87–93.

Kann, L., Brener, N. D., & Allensworth, D. D. (2001). Health education: Results from school health policies and programs study 2000. *Journal of School Health, 71*(7), 266–278.

Maternal and Child Health Bureau. (2002). *Child health USA 2002.* Retrieved November 20, 2006, from http://mchb.hrsa.gov/chusa02/main_pages/page_07.htm

Minnesota Department of Public Health Section of Public Health Nursing. (2001). *Public health interventions.* Available at www.health.state.mn.us/divs/chs/phn/.

National Association of School Nurses (NASN). (2002). *Position statement: Coordinated school health education.*

Retrieved May 16, 2005, from www.nasn.org/positions/coordination.htm.

National Center for Chronic Disease Prevention and Health Promotion. (1994). *School Health Policies and Programs Study.* Retrieved August 27, 2007, from http://www.cdc.gov/HealthyYouth/shpps/index.htm

National Rural Health Association, National Agenda for Rural Minority Health. (2001a). *The need for standardized data and information systems issue paper.* Available at www.NRHArural.org.

National Rural Health Association, National Agenda for Rural Minority Health (2001b). *The need for responsive rural health delivery systems issues paper.* Available at www.NRHArural.org.

Neumark-Sztainer, D., Martin, S., & Story, M. (2000). School-based programs for obesity prevention: What do adolescents recommend? *American Journal of Health Promotion, 14*(4), 232–235.

Olds, D. L., Henderson, C. R., Kitzman, H.L., Eckenrode, J.J., Cole, R. E., & Tatelbaum, R. C. (1999). Prenatal and infancy home visitation by nurses: Recent findings. *Future of Children, 9*(1), 44–65.

Quad Council. (2000). *PHN competencies.* Retrieved May 23, 2006, from http://www.astdn.org/publication_quad_council_phn_competencies.htm.

Sinha, R., & Fisch, G. (2002). Prevalence of impaired glucose tolerance among children and adolescents with marked obesity. *New England Journal of Medicine, 346*(11), 802–810.

Slyper, A. H. (1998). Childhood obesity, adipose tissue distribution, and the pediatric practitioner. *Pediatrics, 102*(1), 4–12.

Strauss, R. S., (2000). Childhood obesity and self-esteem. *Pediatrics, 105*(1), 1–5.

U.S. Bureau of the Census. (2001). *Statistical abstracts of the United States 2001. The national data book* (121st ed.). Available online at www.census.gov/statab/www/.

U.S. Department of Health and Human Services (USDHHS). (2000). *Healthy People2010, conference edition: Vol. 2.* Washington, DC: U.S. Government Printing Office.

BIBLIOGRAPHY

Bartlett, T., Lancaster, R., & New, N. (2005). Pediatric obesity: Use a team approach. *Clinical Advisor for Nurse Practitioners 8*(1), 22, 25–28, 31.

Bashe, P., & Greydanus, D. (Ed.). (2003). *Caring for your teenager.* Available from American Academy of Pediatrics, http://www.aap.org/bst/showdetl.cfm?&DID=15&Product_ID=3833&CatID=134.

Bowman, K. G. (2006). Adolescent postpartum care: What daughters want and what their mothers expect to provide. *Pediatric Nursing, 32*(3), 209–215.

Burdette, H. L., & Whitaker, R. C. (2005). A national study of neighborhood safety, outdoor plan, television viewing, and obesity in preschool children. *Pediatrics, 116*(3), 657–662.

Crawford, P. B., Gosliner, W., Strode, P., Samuels, S. E., Burnett, C., Craypo, L., & Yancey, A. K. (2004). Walking the talk: Fit WIC Wellness programs improve self-efficacy in pediatric obesity prevention counseling. *American Journal of Public Health, 94*(9), 1480–1485.

Goldfield, G. S., Mallory, R., Parker, T., Cunningham, T., Legg, C., Lumb, A., Parker, K., Prud'homme, D., Gaboury, I, & Adamo, K. B. (2006). Effects of open-loop feedback on physical activity and television viewing in overweight and obese children: A randomized, controlled trial. *Pediatrics, 118*(1), 157–166.

Haire-Joshu, D., & Nanney, M. S. (2002). Prevention of overweight and obesity in children: Influences on the food environment. *Diabetes Educator, 28*(3), 415–423.

Jago, R., Baranowski, T., Thompson, D., Baranowski, J., & Greaves, K. A. (2005). Sedentary behavior, not TV viewing, predicts physical activity among 3- to 7-year-old children. *Pediatric Exercise Science, 17*(4), 364–376.

Kirk, S., Scott, B. J., & Daniels, S. R. (2005). Pediatric obesity epidemic: Treatment options. *Journal of the American Dietetic Association, 105*(5) Suppl. 1, S44–S51.

Klein, J. D. (2005). Adolescent pregnancy: Current trends and issues: Clinical report. *Pediatrics, 116*(1), 281–286.

Kotch, J. (2005). *Maternal and child health: Programs, problems, and policy in public health* (2nd ed.). Boston: Jones and Bartlett Publishers.

Lloyd, S. L. (2004). Pregnant adolescent reflections of parental communication. *Journal of Community Health Nursing, 21*(4), 239–251.

Logsdon, M. C., & Gennaro, S. (2005). Bioecological model for guiding social support research and interventions with pregnant adolescents. *Issues in Mental Health Nursing, 26*(3), 327–339.

Marcell, A. V., & Bell, D. L. (2006). Making the most of the adolescent male health visit: Part 1: History and anticipatory guidance. *Contemporary Pediatrics, 23*(5), 50–63.

Martyn, K. K., Reifsnider, E., Barry, M. G., Treviño, & Murray, A. (2006). Protective processes of Latina adolescents. *Hispanic Health Care International, 4*(2), 111–124.

Miehl, N. J. (2005). Shaken baby syndrome. *Journal of Forensic Nursing, 1*(3), 111–117.

Ott, M. A., Pfeiffer, E. J., & Fortenberry, J. D. (2006). Perceptions of sexual abstinence among high-risk early and middle adolescents. *Journal of Adolescent Health, 39*(2), 192–198.

Ryan-Wenger, N. A., Sharrer, V. W., & Campbell, K. K. (2005). Changes in children's stressors over the past 30 years. *Pediatric Nursing, 31*(4), 282–288.

Shu, J. (2004). *American Academy of Pediatrics baby and child health.* Available from American Academy of Pediatrics, http://www.aap.org/bst/showdetl. cfm?&DID=15&Product_ID=3980&CatID=134.

RESOURCES

Agency for Healthcare Research and Quality (AHRQ)

John M. Eisenberg Building
540 Gaither Road, Suite 2000
Rockville, Maryland 20850.
Web: http://www.ahrq.gov

AHRQ is the federal agency charged with improving the quality, safety, efficiency, and effectiveness of health care for all Americans. The agency supports health services research that will improve the quality of health care and promote evidence-based decision making. AHRQ invests about 80 percent of its budget in grants and contracts focused on improving health care. The agency conducts and supports research on health care for ethnic and racial minority and other priority populations, as one of its mandates.

Families USA

1201 New York Avenue NW, Suite 1100
Washington, D.C. 20005
202-628-3030
FAX: 202-347-2417
Email: info@familiesusa.org
Web: http://www.familiesusa.org

Families USA is a national nonprofit, nonpartisan organization dedicated to the achievement of high-quality, affordable health care for all Americans. Working at the national, state, and community levels, the organization has earned a national reputation as an effective voice for health care consumers for over 20 years.

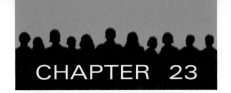

CHAPTER 23

The Elder Population

Eileen K. Rossen, RN, PhD

Ellen Jones, ND, APRN-BC

Chapter Outline

- Theories of Aging
- Culture and Elder Health
- Family as Caregivers
- Health Assessment of Older Adults
  - Environmental Conditions
  - Social Conditions
  - Psychological Conditions
  - Normal Aging Changes to Body Systems
- Health Promotion for Older Adults

Learning Objectives

Upon completion of this chapter, the reader will be able to:

1. Recognize the instrumental role the public health nurse performs in developing and implementing strategies to meet the needs of older adults.

2. Discuss national demographic and health characteristics of older adults.

3. Compare and contrast the usefulness of the major theories of aging.

4. Interpret gender, cohort, and cultural influences on the health of elders using public health nursing concepts.

5. Analyze the family as caregiver.

6. Distinguish normal changes in aging from disease in the following body systems: cardiovascular, pulmonary, gastrointestinal, urinary, musculoskeletal, neurological, integumentary, reproductive, psychosocial, and special senses.

7. Analyze misconceptions in the provision of nursing care of older adults.

8. Formulate health promotion and illness prevention activities for older adults.

ublic health nurses who strive to improve the health of adults aged 65 and older must know the demographic, social, economic, and health characteristics of this large and growing population group to formulate population-based nursing interventions. This chapter will examine the characteristics of the aging population in the United States, explore theories of aging as foundational to understanding the complexity of aging, explore culture and other factors that influence elder health, look at family as caregiver, distinguish normal changes in aging from disease, and discuss appropriate health promotion and illness prevention activities for older adults.

According to the U.S. Census, the population of adults over age 65 is increasing dramatically, numbered 36.3 million in 2004, and is expected to double in size to 71.5 million by 2030 (Administration on Aging, 2005a). Today approximately one in every eight, or 12.4 percent, of the population is 65 years of age or older, and this group is expected to make up 20 percent of the entire population by 2030. The 85+ population is expected to increase from 4.2 million in 2000 to 7.3 million in 2020. In 2004, there were 64,658 (0.18 percent of total population) persons aged 100 or more representing a 73 percent increase from the 1990 figure. In 2004, older women outnumber older men at 21.1 million compared to 15.2 million in 2004 (Administration on Aging, 2005a). Additionally, in 2004, 18.1 percent of persons 65+ were minorities with 8.2 percent being African American; 6.0 percent, Hispanic; 2.9 percent, Asian or Pacific Islander; less than 1 percent, American Indian or Native Alaskan; and 0.6 percent, self-identified as multiracial (Administration of Aging, 2005a).

The social and economic characteristics of older adults in the United States in 2004 revealed that 51 percent of older adults are married, 31 percent are widowed, and 11 percent divorced or separated. Less than 5 percent are never married. A higher percentage of older men (72 percent) than older women (42 percent) are married, whereas 43 percent of older women compared to 14 percent of older men are widowed. Over half of noninstitutionalized older adults (54.7 percent) lived with their spouses, while almost 31 percent (10.7 million) of noninstitutionalized older adults live alone (7.9 million women, 2.8 million men). The majority of older adults lived in metropolitan areas in 2003 (77.4 percent) with over 50 percent living in suburban areas and 27.2 percent living in cities com-

pared to 22.6 percent living in rural areas (Administration on Aging, 2005a). In 2004, the median income of older adults was reported at $21,000 for men and $12,000 for women. Nearly 3.6 million (9.8 percent) older adults reportedly lived below the poverty level in 2004 (Administration on Aging, 2005a). In 2004, older women (12.0 percent) had a higher poverty rate than older men (7.0 percent), and minority elders were more likely to be poor than Caucasians (Administration on Aging, 2005a). Regarding employment, 14.4 percent of Americans aged 65 and older worked in 2004 including 2.8 million men (19 percent) compared to 2.2 million women (11 percent). The educational level of older adults continues to increase with approximately 28 percent having completed high school in 1970 to 70 percent having completed high school in 2004 (Administration on Aging, 2005a; Gist & Hetzel, 2004; USDCESA, 2004).

Health characteristics of older adults living in the United States indicate that approximately 40 percent of noninstitutionalized older adults rated their health as excellent or very good in 2004. Typically, older adults report they have at least one chronic health condition, and many have multiple conditions. In 2002–2003, the most frequently listed conditions were hypertension (51 percent), diagnosed arthritis (48 percent), heart disease (31 percent), cancer (21 percent), diabetes (16 percent), and sinusitis (14 percent) (Administration on Aging, 2005a). Forty-two percent of the population 65 and older reported some type of long-lasting condition or disability (sensory, physical, mental, self-care, or difficulty going outside the home). Over half (57.6 percent) of people 80 years and older had one or more severe disabilities (Administration on Aging, 2005a; Jones, Kennedy-Malone, & Wideman, 2004).

There are a number of professional, governmental, and consumer organizations that work at state and national levels to advocate for education, research, and high standards of health care for older adults. These organizations include the American Nurses Association, American Academy of Nurse Practitioners, Association for Gerontology in Higher Education, Gerontological Society of America, Area Agencies on Aging, National Association of Clinical Nurse Specialists, National Conference of Gerontological Nurse Practitioners, and the National Gerontological Nursing Association. Another resource on aging issues is the White House Conferences on Aging. These conferences are decennial events held to develop recommendations to guide national aging policy for the next 10 years. The American Association of Retired Persons (AARP) is a consumer information, advocacy, and service organization for adults 50 years and older. The Scope and Standards of Gerontological Nursing Practice, disseminated by the American Nurses Association (ANA), defines current practice expectations and competent care standards associated with basic and advanced clinical practice for the specialty of gerontological nursing. According to ANA, the guidelines were developed in consultation with the National Gerontological Nursing Association, National Association of Directors of Nursing Administration in Long Term Care, and National Conference of Gerontological Nurse Practitioners.

THEORIES OF AGING

Theories of aging attempt to organize and explain various factors and dimensions related to the phenomena of aging. Major theories of aging fall into three broad categories: biological, psychological, and sociological. Biological theories are primarily concerned with answering questions related to physiological processes that occur over time and are subdivided into two main categories: programmed and error theories. Psychological theories are broad in scope, are influenced by biology and sociology, and explain behavioral changes and dynamic developmental adaptive processes related to the lives of older adults. Among other concepts, these theories attempt to explain human motivation, self-realization, stages of psychological development, and compensation. Sociological theories focus on social adaptations and related changes in roles and relationships in older adults' life experiences viewed within the context of culture. Refer to Table 23-1.

Older adults are not a homogenous group, and because of the complexity of the aging phenomena, scholars agree that one theory would not be able to explain all aspects of aging. Therefore, public health nurses need to be aware of the various theories and how they may inform their practice with older adults. Biological theories contribute to the public health nurse's understanding of physiological changes with age and thus are better prepared to meet the physical needs of the older population. The psychological theories assist the public health nurse to understand developmental phases and life tasks faced by the aging population. And, the sociological theories enable the public health nurse to see a broad view of older adults, their relationships and roles in society (Meiner, 2005).

CULTURE AND ELDER HEALTH

As the older adult population is dramatically increasing in size, so too is it more diverse. Geographic origin, historical events, cohort position, and gender contribute to these cultural differences. For example, being born in a particular region of the United States contributes to geographical influences of weather patterns, social customs, diet, and so forth. Historical events, such as the Great Depression, also contribute to differences among people as demonstrated by financial savings behaviors. Those who grew up during the Depression spent less and saved more money than those born after the Depression. Because birth circumstances create significant individual differences within any culture, public health nurses, whose role is to integrate community involvement and knowledge about populations with individual and family health and illness experiences, are challenged to understand these differences in order to provide culturally sensitive and competent care.

Culture refers to shared values, beliefs, and behavior by members of a society that serve as guides for interacting within the family, community, and country. Although cultures are unique and none are exactly alike, there are similarities and distinct differences. Culture is universal, found in all parts of the world. Culture is learned and transmitted from one generation to another through socialization and thus provides safety and stability. Variations occur within a culture. Adherence to cultural values, beliefs, and behaviors is variable based on factors such as age, education, social and educational status, language use of the dominant culture, and setting such as urban or rural. Culture is also ethnocentric; that is, each culture places primary value in its own culture and gives their values, beliefs and behaviors a central position.

The meanings of health, illness, and health care practices as well as end-of-life issues are imbedded in values, beliefs, and practices of the culture of the older adult. It is imperative for the public health nurse to be aware of the similarities and differences between his or her culture and the client's culture to provide culturally competent care. Cultural competence and sensitivity indicate an understanding of the issues related to culture, race, gender, social class, and other factors and encompass knowledge, attitudes, and mutual respect (Griffiths et al., 2004).

TABLE 23-1: Theories of Aging

THEORY CATEGORY	THEORY	MAJOR FOCUS
Biological Theories: focus on answering questions concerned with physiologic processes	**Programmed Theories** Genetic Neuronendocrine	These theories claim that aging follows a biological schedule and hypothesize that the body's genetic codes contain cellular commands for regulating reproduction and death.
	Error Theories Wear & Tear Cross-Link Free Radical Somatic DNA Damage	These theories hypothesize that environmental assault on the body causes accumulation of toxic by-products.
Psychological Theories: focus on how a person responds, copes, or adapts to aging.	**Personality Development** Jung's Theory of Individualism	Personality viewed as either extroverted or introverted.
	Erickson's Developmental Theory	Eight stages of development that reflect cultural and societal influences on the development of individual's ego structure.
	Human Motivation Maslow's Hierarchy of Needs	Individuals have an innate internal hierarchy of needs that motivates all human behavior.
Sociological Theories: focus on an individual's changing roles and relationships as he or she ages.	**Disengagement Theory**	Postulates older adults need to withdraw from societal roles and responsibilities as they age.
	Activity Theory	Proposes that older adults need to stay active and engaged in life to age successfully.
	Continuity Theory	Hypothesizes that one should maintain and continue previous life values, habits, and family and social ties of adult life.
	Person-Environment Fit Theory	Examines interrelationships among older adults' competencies and those competencies needed in the individual's environment.

Note. Meiner (2006); Stanley, Blair, & Beare (2005).

FAMILY AS CAREGIVERS

Because the exploding elder population is living longer, there is an increasing need for family caregivers. Family caregivers are women and men of all ages, races, incomes, and educational backgrounds who provide unpaid assistance to a relative or family member who is ill, disabled, or unable to care for self. Although the majority of caregivers are female, a substantial proportion of caregivers are men. It is estimated that 17 percent of households in the United States contain at least one caregiver who provides care to someone 50 years or older, and that 13 percent of caregivers themselves are aged 65 or older (Administration on Aging, 2005b; National Alliance of Caregivers & AARP, 2004). Also, nearly 80 percent of care recipients are 50 years or older (average age is 75), 65 percent being women of whom 42 percent are widowed. Because of women's longevity, older women are usually cared for by adult children, whereas older men are usually cared for by their spouses. In regards to race, white caregivers are more likely than minority caregivers to be age 65 or older. Even though the average duration of caregiving is 4.3 years, older caregivers are more likely to provide care for 10 or more years (National Alliance of Caregivers & AARP, 2004).

Older caregivers (65+) typically are the primary caregiver, live with the care recipient, and report that their health is fair or poor. Age, gender (being female), choice in taking on the role of caregiver, and perceived level of burden are reported factors that appear to predict health declines in caregivers (National Alliance of Caregivers & AARP, 2004). The impact of caregiving includes spending less time with family and friends and giving up vacations, hobbies, and other social activities. Caregivers most impacted by the caregiving role are described as being female, having fair or poor self-rated health, and providing a high level of care (Administration on Aging, 2005b; National Alliance of Caregivers & AARP, 2004). Caregivers report using a variety of coping mechanisms to deal with the demands of caregiving, but prayer is the most commonly used followed by talking with friends and relatives, reading about caregiving, exercising, using the Internet for informa-tion, talking with a professional or spiritual counselor, and last, taking medication.

Caregivers reported that they need more help with or information primarily about finding more time for themselves, keeping the person they care for safe at home, balancing family responsibilities, and managing emotional and physical stress. Caregivers 65 and older are less likely than their younger counterparts to use the Internet or turn to friends for information and are more likely to turn to a health care provider for information (National Alliance of Caregivers & AARP, 2004).

HEALTH ASSESSMENT OF OLDER ADULTS

Many misconceptions surround older adults, especially concerning health and wellness. The truth is that the overwhelming majority of older adults lead independent lives even though they have chronic illnesses and some level of disability. It is also a myth that older adults are totally dependent on others or require constant supervised care. Negative stereotypes of older adults are termed ageism and public health nurses should dispel misconceptions and ageism in their practice. Refer to Box 23-1.

Overall, health and wellness of older adults are influenced by the individual degree of disability and physical illness, the ability to cope with difficulties, individual resilience and adaptability, and the level of familial and societal support for individual difficulties. It is the responsibility of the public health nurse to be able to assess the health status of older adults and to recommend support services where needed such that

⊕ PRACTICE APPLICATION

Client Newly Diagnosed with Type 2 Diabetes

Mr. Chung is a 65-year-old Chinese American who immigrated to the United States when he was 20 years old. He is married and has two adult children who live close by. Mr. Chung's wife was a homemaker who maintains a small home-sewing business. Mr. Chung is a retired textile worker who has a small pension with social security. His only insurance is Medicare. Mr. Chung speaks English, but he is difficult to understand. After seeking medical attention for a wound on his foot that refused to heal, he was diagnosed with type 2 diabetes and elevated cholesterol. As a public health nurse, you have been consulted to evaluate Mr. Chung's wound and help him find therapy for his wound care and diabetes care.

the older adults capitalize on their own abilities and minimize their difficulties. Public health nurses must be able to recognize social, psychological, and environmental issues that are more prevalent among older adults. Likewise, public health nurses need to recognize the physical signs and symptoms of **normal aging** with signs and symptoms that represent disease and injury. For older adults to remain independent, they must be able to access adequate health care. Healthy People 2010 initiatives emphasized the need for older adults to receive health care for illness as well as clinical preventive services that promote activities to improve their quality of life.

Many factors influence successful aging and the degree of health and wellness maintained by older adults (McReynolds & Rossen, 2004; Rossen, Knafl, & Flood, in review; Rowe & Kahn, 1998). When assessing the older adult, public health nurses need to know the various effects environmental, social, psychological, and physical conditions have on the health of older adult populations.

Environmental Conditions

There are many environmental concerns for the older adult; but the most important are adequate food and housing. First, the public health nurse must assess the ability of the older adult to pay for municipal services that include power, temperature control in the home, running water, food, medicines, and medical supplies. The public health nurse must recognize home safety hazards in the home that would make it easy for an older person to fall such as poor lighting, area rugs, and stairs. Safety concerns including fire hazards and lack of smoke detectors should be noted. The kitchen should be assessed for both safety and function. The public health nurse should note any small appliance in the home that is a potential risk for electrocution or fire. Within the living environment, the public health nurse should assess if there is food available and if food can be easily obtained from a local market or delivery service. The overall neighborhood of the older adult should be assessed for safety including the availability of transportation, access to needed services, and nearby neighbors, as well as reported crime and violence rates.

Today, there are many residential housing options for older adults. The most commonly known housing option is institutionalized care provided within nurs-

BOX 23-1: Myths of Aging

Older adults cannot live independently.

Older adults are not happy.

Older adults will have dementia or Alzheimer's.

Older adults are not productive.

Older adults cannot enjoy physical activity.

Older adults are not sexually active.

Older adults refuse change.

ing homes. These facilities offer skilled and unskilled nursing care where residents need round-the-clock care. There are other housing options for older adults that include independent living and assisted living facilities. Independent living allows residents to live in a residential complex that provides extra security and other conveniences such as restaurants, access to health care, and activities that support the older adult lifestyle. Independent living centers require personal purchases similar to home ownership. Assisted living centers offer housing for residents who need minimal assistance. Assisted living centers can be private or subsidized offering housing to older adults with less income. For older adults living at home, services are available such as adult day care that provides a communal place for older adults to go and participate in activities and receive some level of health care services. Home health care services may also be provided to those older adults who wish to remain at home.

Social Conditions

Social support systems are vital to the health and wellness of older adults. Social support has been found to be extremely important in aging successfully and in promoting and maintaining overall long-term health by supporting engagement in life (Rossen, Knafl, & Flood, in review) and by contributing to physical and cognitive functioning. Conversely, social isolation or disengagement is a risk factor of cognitive decline in cognitively intact elders (McReynolds & Rossen, 2004). The public health nurse must ask about and identify those persons who are available to assist the client and provide social support. Family members and children are often the persons older adults rely on, but if they do not live nearby, then the older adult may rely on friends or other members of the community. The public health nurse must also assess other resources of elders such as financial status. It is necessary then for the public health nurse to ask about and identify the economic status of the older adult and their ability to purchase food, housing, and medical services. Older adults that do not have social support systems or funds to pay for services are the most vulnerable.

Psychological Conditions

Multiple factors influence the psychological health of older adults. Older adults who remain relatively healthy with fewer chronic illnesses and disabilities often remain engaged with their family and friends. Older adults who have the opportunity to participate in routine activities, stay involved in meaningful activities, and feel productive in life age successfully and have brighter healthier psychological outlooks than older adults who are limited by multiple debilitating illnesses and physical disabilities that prevent them from remaining active and at home (Rossen, Knafl, & Flood, in press). Older adults who reside in independent or assisted living centers typically remain more engaged than older adults requiring nursing home care.

The majority of older adults experience some degree of vision and hearing loss, which may limit their ability to continue normal activities. Short-term memory loss is common in older adults, which may affect their psychological health. It is the responsibility of the public health nurse to distinguish normal memory loss from more severe dementia or Alzheimer's disease. Personal losses of family members and friends can lead older adults to have feelings of despair and depression.

Sleep disturbances can also contribute to depression since many older adults become discouraged with the inability to sleep through the night, which is a normal occurrence for older adults. Alcohol abuse should not be overlooked among older adults. Severe depression is not a result of normal aging and the prevalence of older adult males committing suicide continues to increase. However, it is normal for older adults to be aware of their own life expectancy and to discuss death and the future with their family and friends (Jones & Beck-Little, 2002).

Despite the realities of growing older with chronic health problems and multiple losses, older adults continue to remain happy (APA, 1998; Rossen & Knafl, 2007; Rossen, Knafl, & Flood, in press). Public health nurses should promote successful aging and overall happiness for the older adult client by encouraging older adults to continue physical activities and social engagements with friends and families. Continued interest in sexuality is an important part of normal aging, and public health nurses should support physical affection. Public health nurses need to emphasize to older adults the necessity to maintain adequate nutrition, exercise, and rest along with health care prevention and maintenance (News ICN on healthy aging, 1999; Jones, York, & Herrick, 2004; McReynolds & Rossen, 2004).

Normal Aging Changes to Body Systems

Physiologic changes are a normal part of aging. The degree to how quickly these changes occur varies among individuals. All of the vital systems are affected with age including cardiovascular, pulmonary, gastrointestinal, urinary, musculoskeletal, neurological,

⊕ PRACTICE APPLICATION

Health Assessment of a New Widow

Mrs. Dobson is a 75-year-old woman who lives alone. Mrs. Dobson has lived alone for 2 years since her husband of 45 years died suddenly from a heart attack. She is a retired school teacher who has always been active in her church and community. She has three children (one daughter, two sons) and five grandchildren who are all successful. However, all her children live over 100 miles from her home. Mrs. Dobson has recently been seen by her primary health care provider where she had a routine preventative exam. Mrs. Dobson did not have any significant physical abnormality; however, as a public health nurse, you have been consulted to evaluate Mrs. Dobson in her home.

integumentary, reproductive, and special senses (Ebersole, Hess, & Luggen, 2004; Ham, Sloan, & Warsaw, 2001; Kennedy-Malone, Fletcher, & Plank, 2004).

⊕ *Cardiovascular System:* Coronary artery disease is the most common cause of death in older adults (AMA, n.d.). Blood pressure rises with age, and the overall cardiac reserve diminishes. Arrhythmias, murmurs, and dilation of the abdominal aorta are also more common in older adults, which may lead to chronic cardiovascular disease. Stroke is the third leading cause of death and the number one cause of disability in older adults. Elevated blood pressure is the number one cause of stroke in older adults (AMA, n.d.).

⊕ *Pulmonary System:* There is a mild decline in pulmonary function including decreased elasticity of alveolar sacs and mucous transport resulting in shortness of breath. However, the majority of pulmonary dysfunction is caused by disease, primarily due to tobacco use, and is not associated with normal age-related changes to the pulmonary system.

⊕ *Gastrointestinal System:* Dental changes are the most universal, especially gum disease and tooth loss. Peristalsis slows through the gastrointestinal system, causing constipation, malabsorption, and esophageal reflux. Often, these conditions are caused by poor diets, drug effects, or underlying disease. The liver and pancreas reduce in

⊕ RESEARCH APPLICATION

Older Men's Health: Motivation, Self-Ratings, and Behaviors

Study Purpose

To explore the relationships among health motivation, self-rated health, and health behaviors in community-dwelling older men.

Methods

A descriptive correlational survey design was used. A convenience sample of 135 mostly white, (78 percent), rural (61 percent), and married (67 percent) community-dwelling men ages 55 to 91 (mean = 70 years) were recruited from various urban and rural settings including senior centers (five urban and two rural), fast food outlets, and community programs. Inclusion criteria included male gender; 55 years of age or older; ability to read, understand, and write English; and absence of obvious cognitive impairments. Participants completed a survey packet that included demographic data (e.g., age, marital status, race, education, income, and presence of others in same household); the Older Men's health program and Screening Inventory (consists of 8 items measuring health of lifestyle, health-promoting activities, health); Health-Promotion Activities of Older Adults Measure (44 items measuring health-promoting behaviors); and the Health Self-Determination Index (17 items measuring health motivation). Descriptive statistics, Pearson's product-moment correlations, and stepwise multiple regression analysis were conducted.

Findings

Older men with more intrinsic motivation rated their health as better and assessed their lifestyles as more healthy than did their counterparts with more extrinsic motivation. Anticipated benefits were significantly related to health-promoting behaviors, health program attendance, and health-screening participation, but the Health Self-Determination Index score did not demonstrate significant relations with any of these three variables.

Implications

These findings suggest that promoting self-motivation may be important to increasing older men's perceptions of health and well-being. Also, the findings indicate that further study of anticipated benefits as a motivator for health-promotion activities and -screening participation is reasonable. Furthermore, this study provides an initial base for developing intervention studies that support the Healthy People 2010 goals of increasing the number of older adults participating in health-promotion activities.

Reference

Loeb, S. J. (2004). Older men's health: Motivation, self-ratings, and behaviors. *Nursing Research 53*(3), 198–206.

size, but without disease their function remains adequate.

- *Urinary System:* Age reduces the peak bladder capacity, and the amount of residual urine increases. The amount of renal blood flow is halved, and the renal tubules are less able to concentrate urine, requiring the kidneys to work through the night when blood flow is increased. Symptoms among women resulting from these changes include nocturia, urgency, and incontinence. Prostatic hypertrophy is common among males resulting in nocturia, decreased urinary stream, and urinary hesitancy. Creatinine clearance declines with age, which causes susceptibility to toxicity from medications that are metabolized within the renal system.

- *Musculoskeletal System:* There are many significant musculoskeletal changes that occur with aging. Muscle mass decreases by 30 percent leading to decreased strength and endurance. Normal aging also can result in slow foot reaction time and decreased vibratory sense in the big toe. The hands may be affected with the fingers loosing strength and the ability to grasp objects. These symptoms are more predominant in older adults suffering from diabetes and arthritis. Osteoporosis is the leading cause of musculoskeletal disability in women. Women older than age 60 should be screened regularly for bone density loss (Neuner et al., 2006). Sarcopenia is the normal loss of muscle mass and affects both men and women. For both men and women injury related to falls is the third leading cause of death and chronic disability leading to older adults' ability to maintain independent living (CDC, 2007a). No matter the cause, weight-bearing physical activity can reduce the susceptibility to changes to the musculoskeletal system, and older adults should be encouraged to maintain an exercise routine consisting of at least 30 minutes of moderate intensity exercise five times a week, weight-bearing exercises three times per week along with daily stretching exercises (CDC, 2007b; Stevens & Olsen, 2000).

- *Neurological System:* Neurological changes can be profound causing numerous changes in function. The most important functional changes cause swaying when going from a sitting to standing position and the inability to stand without swaying with eyes closed. Some medications for cardiovascular disease and elevated blood pressure may enhance these types of side effects. Dehydration may also cause dizziness. Neurological symptoms should be assessed carefully examining medications and nutritional status.

- *Integumentary System:* Perspiration decreases, and then the skin becomes cool and dry. The skin has increased pigmentation, increased cherry angiomas, and wrinkling. Older adults become more susceptible to skin cancers. The hair becomes thinner and gray. Nails thicken and develop ridges.

- *Reproductive System:* For post menopausal women, the ovaries and uterus atrophy. Vaginal secretions become scant, the vaginal mucosa becomes thin and friable resulting in painful intercourse and the need for lubrication, pubic hair decreases, and the breasts become more pendulous. Women may experience complaints with menopausal symptoms such as hot flashes, night sweats, and mood fluctuations. For older men, the prostate enlarges, while the size of the penis and testes decreases, and pubic hair thins. Older adults do experience sexual desire and there are medications available to increase sexual performance. Sexual activity does put older adults at risk for developing sexually transmitted diseases and HIV infections, and older adults should be counseled in prevention (CDC, 2007c).

- *Special Senses:* Visual changes are almost universal among older adults. Beginning around 40 years of age, near vision changes, making it difficult to see objects at close distances. The most common complaint is the need for reading glasses. Light that is able to enter the eye decreases due to reduced pupil size, yellowing to the lens, and opacification of the lens. These changes result in the inability to discriminate blue from green, inability for the eye to adjust from a lighted room to a dark room, and sensitivity to glare. The most common complaint is difficulty in driving at night due to "night blindness." Excessive opacification to the lens is considered a cataract, which may require surgical removal. High-frequency hearing loss, called presbycusis, is common among older adults. Presbycusis causes the inability to discriminate high-pitched sounds, such as hearing *s*, *z*, *sh*, and *ch*. Difficulty hearing sounds of words makes it difficult to interpret speech or to interpret what is being heard in noisy surroundings. Diminished sense of taste and smell may lead to overseasoning foods with salt or sugar. Diminished sensitivity to temperature may lead to overheating food and water temperatures, which increases the risk of burns either when showering or eating. Older adults should be cautioned to test water and food temperature with the wrist or arm and not the fingers and toes to avoid burns.

HEALTH PROMOTION FOR OLDER ADULTS

Health promotion and prevention activities are an integral part of the health care for older adults. Health promotion should include educating older adults about the prevailing views of aging well or aging successfully (Rossen, Knafl, & Flood, in press; Rowe & Kahn, 1998). Older adults should be encouraged to participate in illness prevention to improve quality of life throughout the latter years (Woolf, Jonas, & Lawrence, 1996). Illness prevention recommendations for older adults include health screenings and immunizations, education regarding substance abuse, diet and exercise, sexuality, and preventing injuries (Ebersole, Hess, & Luggen, 2004; Ham, Sloan, & Warsaw, 2001; Kennedy-Malone, Fletcher, & Plank, 2004). Refer to Table 23-2. The table illustrates several tools for measuring physical activity, mental status, depression, alcohol use, nutrition, and social support with older adults.

- *Health Screenings:* Health screenings for older adults include routine measurements for height, weight, BMI, blood pressure, vision, and hearing. Laboratory values should include cholesterol, glucose, hemoglobin and hematocrit, creatinine, and thyroid levels. Diagnostic exams include yearly mammograms for women, prostate exams for men, and a fecal occult blood test. Skin should be examined for any abnormal lesion or wounds that are not healing. Polypharmacy and mental health status should be included in a health screen. Screening for osteoporosis should be included primarily for women, but men with osteoporosis should not be overlooked. Dental exams should be continued throughout older adulthood (USPSTF, 2002).

- *Immunizations:* Unless contraindicated, older adults should receive yearly influenza vaccine, a pneumococcal vaccine every five to ten years, and a tetanus-diphtheria (TD) booster every five to ten years (USPSTF, 2002).

- *Substance Abuse:* Older adults should be assessed for excessive alcohol, drug, and tobacco use. Community resources are available for older adults who wish to seek assistance with smoking or alcohol cessation. Private and community counselors are also available for older adults. Older adults should be encouraged to seek medical attention regardless of the source.

- *Nutrition and Exercise:* Nutritional health should be assessed including amount and types of foods eaten. Regular physical activity should be monitored and encouraged.

- *Sexuality:* Older adults who are sexually active with a new partner need to be educated regarding prevention of sexually transmitted infections and condom use.

- *Injury Prevention:* Older adults are at increased risk for falling with serious injury. Falling accounts for the majority of orthopedic fractures in the older adult population. Prevention of falls includes assessing the individual for their propensity to fall by neurological exams where the ability to go from a standing to sitting position without swaying and the ability to stand still with arms up and eyes closed are assessed. Simply observing the older adult walking with and without assistance indicates whether or not they are able to walk without swaying and stumbling. The *Get Up and Go Test* shown in Box 23-2 is one example of an older adult gait assessment (Mathias, Nayak, & Isaacs, 1986). Accidental falls can always occur if an individual slips or trips on ice, rugs, toys, or other objects on the floor. Older adults should be educated not to walk around outside during icy conditions and reminded that the floor inside their home should be free of items that could cause falling. Older adults should also be encouraged to give up certain activities they did when younger such as climbing ladders. Older adults should continue to wear seat belts. Homes should be equipped with smoke detectors. Older adults feel cold more intensely than younger individuals and often have space heat-

TABLE 23-2: Physical Activity, Psychological, Nutrition, and Social Support Screening Tools for Older Adults

CATEGORY OF MEASUREMENT & INSTRUMENT	TYPE OF INSTRUMENT	NUMBER OF ITEMS	SAMPLE QUESTIONS
Physical Activity			
The Physical Activity Scale for the Elderly[a]	Self Report Measured in participation, days, and duration	32	Over the past 7 days, how often did you participate in sitting activities such as reading, watching TV, or doing handcrafts? (never, seldom, sometimes, often).
Psychological			
Folstein Mini Mental Status[b]	Administered		What is the year? Spell WORLD backwards.
Geriatric Depression Scale (GDS)[c]	Self Report Binary format (yes/no)	11	Do you find life very exciting? Do you feel full of energy?
Michigan Alcoholism Screening Test-Geriatric (MAST-G) Version[d]	Self Report Binary format (yes/no)	24	Does having a few drinks help decrease your shakiness or tremors?
The CAGE[e] Questionnaire (alcoholism)	Administered	4	Have you ever felt you ought to cut down?
Nutrition			
Nutritional Risk Index (NRI)[f]	Self Report Binary format (yes/no)	16	Do you wear dentures? Are you on any kind of special diet? Did you have any trouble swallowing at least 3 days in the past month?
Mini-Nutritional Assessment (MNA)[g]	Anthropometric Measures Self-Report	18	Body mass index (BMI) Does the patient live independently in contrast to a nursing home? Does the patient take more than 3 prescription drugs (per day)?
The DETERMINE Screen[h]	Self Report Binary format (yes/no); plus additional measures (e.g., lab data, height, weight)	10	I eat fewer than 2 meals per day. I eat few fruits or vegetables or milk products. I eat alone most of the time. I am not always physically able to shop, cook, and/or feed myself.

(continued)

TABLE 23-2: Physical Activity, Psychological, Nutrition, and Social Support Screening Tools for Older Adults (cont'd)

CATEGORY OF MEASUREMENT & INSTRUMENT	TYPE OF INSTRUMENT	NUMBER OF ITEMS	SAMPLE QUESTIONS
Social Support			
Iowa Self-Assessment Inventory Social Support Subscale (ISAI)[i]	Self Report 4-point Dichotomous scale	8	There is no one I can turn to in times of stress. There is someone I can talk to about important decisions.
The Multidimensional Scale of Perceived Social Support (MSPSS)[j]	Self-Report Likert Scale	12	There is a special person who is around when I am in need. My family really tries to help me. I can talk about my problems with my family.
Lubben's (1988) Social Network Scale (LSNS)[k]	Self Report	10	How many relatives do you see or hear from at least once a month? When you have an important decision to make, do you have someone you can talk to about it?
Comprehensive			
Iowa Self-Assessment Inventory (ISAI)[l]	Self-Report	56	Identifies resources, status, and abilities in the following seven components: economic resources, emotional balance, physical health status, trusting others, mobility, cognitive status, and social support.

Note. [a]Physical Activity Scale for the Elderly (Hurdle, 2001; Washburn et al., 1993); [b]Folstein Mini-Mental Status (Folstein, Folstein, & McHugh, 1975); [c]GDS (Brink et al., 1982); [d]MAST-G (Blow et al., 1992); [e]CAGE (Ewing, 1989; Hays, Merz, & Nicholas, 1995); [f]NRI (Frisby & Hoeber, 2002); [g]MNA (Wolinsky et al., 1990); [h]DETERMINE (Kane, 2000); [i, j]ISAI (Wakefield, 2001); [j]MSPSS (Wakefield, 2001; Zimet et al., 1988); [k]LSNS (Morris et al., 1990); Mini-Nutritional Assessment (Guigoz, Vellas, & Garry, 1994).

ers in the home to help keep them warm. Space heaters are fire hazards and should be carefully monitored. In case of power outages, older adults should have batteries, flashlights, portable radio, blankets, canned food, and bottled water for emergencies.

Public health nurses have a unique opportunity to improve the quality of life of older adults. Many factors discussed in this chapter influence the health, wellness and successful aging of older adults. Public health nurses interact with community health care professionals and community leaders as well as older adults within their own home, community, and culture. As a result of their influence and direct provision of care, they have the ability to perform individual and community assessments and then to recommend the most appropriate services. Providing health promotion and illness prevention services such as providing access to primary care or opportunities to socialize (with an emphasis on education) and to stay engaged in meaningful activities are all vital to promoting the health and wellness of older adults.

BOX 23-2: Get Up and Go Test

1. Rise from an armless chair without using hands.
2. Stand still momentarily.
3. Walk to a wall ten feet away.
4. Turn around without touching the wall.
5. Walk back to the chair.
6. Turn around.
7. Sit down.

SOURCE: Adapted from Mathias, Nayak, and Isaacs (1986).

CRITICAL THINKING ACTIVITIES

1. Identify an older adult living in the community. Identify and explain the biological, sociological, and psychological theories of aging that best describe the older adult.

2. Visit a community senior center. What are the available health promotion and prevention activities? What activities are missing? How would they contribute to healthy aging?

3. Identify an older adult in your community and visit him or her at home. What safety concerns are present? Is the older adult at risk for falling? Is the older adult at risk for other injuries? How many overall safety concerns did you assess? Based on your assessment, what recommendations would you have to improve safety in the home?

KEY CONCEPTS

⊕ Public health nurses incorporate knowledge of theories of aging and demographic, social, economic, and health and illness characteristics of elders to formulate population-based community interventions that effect the elder population, the family, and the individual.

⊕ Public health nurses integrate knowledge of normal systemic changes in aging and common misconceptions about aging as they work with communities to develop targeted health promotion and disease prevention programs and activities.

⊕ Public health nurses provide health assessments, health education, care management, and primary care to elders and their families.

⊕ Public health nurses collaborate with other health care disciplines and work with professional, governmental, and consumer organizations at the state and national levels to advocate for education, research, and high standards of health care for older adults.

KEY TERMS

ageism

family caregiver

health promotion

illness prevention

normal aging

Scope and Standards of Gerontological Nursing Practice

REFERENCES

Administration on Aging. (2005a). *A profile of older Americans: 2005.* Retrieved from http://www.aogov/PROF/Statistics/profile/2005/2005profile.pdf.

Administration on Aging. (2005b). *Caregiving statistics.* Retrieved August 30, 2007, from http://www.caregiver.org/caregiver/jsp/content_node.jsp?nodeid=439.

American Heart Association (AMA). (n.d.). *Older Americans and cardiovascular disease statistics.* Retrieved June 9, 2006, from http://www.americanheart.org/downloadable/heart/1136584495498OlderAm06.pdf.

American Psychological Association (APA). (1998). *What practitioners should know about working with older adults.* Washington, DC: Office of Public Communications.

Blow, F. C., Brower, K. J., Schulenberg, J. E., Demo-Dananberg, L. M., Young, J. P., & Beresford, T. P. (1992). The Michigan Alcoholism Screening Test—Geriatric Version (MAST-G): A new elderly-specific screening instrument. *Alcoholism: Clinical and Experimental Research 16,* 372.

Brink, T., Yesavage, J., Lum, O., Heersema, P., Adey, M., & Rose, T. (1982). Screening tests for geriatric depression. *Clinical and Experimental Rheutomology, 5,* 147–150.

Centers for Disease Control (CDC). (2007a). *Healthy aging.* Retrieved August 27, 2007, from http://www.cdc.gov/aging/info.htm.

Centers for Disease Control (CDC). (2007b). *Are there special recommendations for older adults?* Retrieved August 27, 2007, from http://www.cdc.gov/nccdphp/dnpa/physical/recommendations/older_adults.htm.

Centers for Disease Control (CDC). (2007c). *Sexually transmitted diseases.* Retrieved August 27, 2007, from http://www.cdc.gov/std/.

Ebersole, P., Hess, P., & Luggen, S. (2004). *Toward healthy aging: Human needs and nursing response* (6th ed.). St. Louis: Mosby.

Ewing, J., (1989). Detecting alcoholism, the CAGE questionnaire. *Journal American Medical Association, 252,* 510.

Folstein, M., Folstein, S., & McHugh, P. (1975). Mini-mental state. A practical method for grading the cognitive state of patients for the clinician. *Journal of Psychiatric Research, 12,* 189–198.

Frisby, W., & Hoeber, L. (2002). Factors affecting the uptake of community recreation as health peromotion for women on low incomes. *Canadian Journal of Public Health, 93*(2):129-133.

Gist, Y. J., & Hetzel, L. I. (2004). *We the people: Aging in the United States.* Census 2000 Special Reports. Available from http://www.census.gov/prod/2004pubs/consr-19.pdf.

Griffiths, R., Johnson, M., Piper, M., & Langdon, R. (2004). A nursing intervention for the quality use of medicines by elderly community clients. *International Journal of Nursing Practice, 10*(4), 166–176.

Guigoz, Y., Vellas, B., & Garry, P. (1994). Mini-nutritional assessment: A practical assessment tool for grading the nutritional state of elderly patients. *Facts and Research in Gerontology, 2,* 15–59.

Ham, R., Sloane, P. D., & Warsaw, G. (Eds.). (2001). *Primary care geriatrics: A case-based approach* (4th ed.). St. Louis: Mosby.

Hays, R. D., Merz, J. F., & Nicholas, R. (1995). Response burden, reliability, and validity of the CAGE, Short MAST, and AUDIT alcohol screening measures. *Behavior Research Methods Instruments Computers, 27*(2), 277–280.

Hurdle, D. E. (2001). Social support: A critical factor in women's health and health promotion. *Health Social Work. 26*(2), 72–79.

Jones, E. D., & Beck-Little, R. (2002). The use of reminiscence therapy for the treatment of depression in rural-dwelling older adults. *Issues in Mental Health Nursing, 23*(3), 279–290.

Jones, E. D., York, R., & Herrick, C. (2004). Intergenerational group demonstrates benefits for youth and older adult members. *Issues in Mental Health and Aging, 25*(8), 753–767.

Jones, E., Kennedy-Malone, L., & Wideman, L. (2004). Early detection of type 2 diabetes among older African-Americans. *Geriatric Nursing, (25)*1, 24–28.

Kane, R. L. (2000). Physiological well-being and health. In R. L. Kane & R. Kane (Eds.), *Assessing older persons* (pp. 49–64). New York: Oxford University Press.

Kennedy-Malone, L., Fletcher, K. R., & Plank, L. M. (2004). *Management guidelines for nurse practitioners working with older adults* (2nd ed.). Philadelphia: Davis.

Loeb, S. J. (2004). Older men's health: Motivation, self-ratings, and behaviors. *Nursing Research 53*(3), 198–206.

Lubben, J. E. (1988). Assessing social networks among elderly populations. *Family & Community Health, 11,* 45–52.

Mathias, S., Nayak, U. S. L., & Isaacs, B. (1986). Balance in elderly patients: The "get-up and go" test. *Archives Physician Medical Rehabilitation, 67*(6), 387.

McReynolds, J. L., & Rossen, E. K. (2004). Importance of physical activity, nutrition, and social support for optimal aging. *Clinical Nurse Specialist, 18*(4), 200–206.

Meiner, S. W. (2005). Theories of aging. In S. E. Meiner & G. Lueckenotte (Eds.), *Gerontologic nursing* (3rd ed., pp. 19–32). St. Louis: Mosby Elsevier

Morris, W., Buckwalter, K., Cleary, T., Gilmer, J., Hatz, D., & Studer, M. (1990). Refinement of the Iowa Self-Assessment Inventory. *The Gerontologist, 30*(2), 243–248

National Alliance for Caregiving & AARP. (2004). *Caregiving in the U.S.* Retrieved May 10, 2005, from http://www.caregiving.org/04finalreport.pdf.

Neuner, J., Binkley, N., Sparapani, R., Purushottam, M., Laud, W., & Nattinger, (2006). Bone density testing in older women and its association with patient age. *Journal of the American Geriatrics Society, 54*(3).

News ICN on healthy aging. (1999). News ICN on healthy aging: A public health and nursing challenge. *Journal of Advanced Nursing 30*(2) 280–281.

Rossen, E. K., & Knafl, K. (2007). The impact of relocation on older women's physical, emotional, and social functioning. *Western Journal of Nursing Research, 29*(2), 183-199 .

Rossen, E. K., Knafl, K., & Flood, M. (in press). "Older women's perceptions of successful aging." *Journal of Activities, Adaptation and Aging.*

Rowe, J. W., & Kahn, R. L. (1998). *Successful aging.* New York: Pantheon Books.

Stanley, M., Blair, K. & Beare, P. G. (2005). *Gerontological nursing,* Philadelphia: F. Davis.

Stevens, J., & Olson, S. (2000). Reducing falls and resulting hip fractures among older women. *Morbidity and Mortality Weekly Report, 49*(RR-2), 3–12.

U.S. Department of Commerce Economics and Statistics Administration (USDCESA). (2004). *We the People: Aging in the United States Census 2000 Special Reports.* Available from http://www.census.gov/prod/2004pubs/censr-19.pdf.

U.S. Preventive Services Task Force (USPSTF). (2002). *US Task Force guide to clinical preventive services* (3rd ed.). McLean, VA: International Medical Publishing.

Wakefield, B. (2001). Altered nutrition: Less than body requirements. In M. L. Maas, K. C. Buckwalter, M. D. Hardy, T. Tripp-Reimer, M. G. Titler, & J. P. Specht (Eds.), *Nursing care of older adults* (pp. 145–157). St. Louis: Mosby.

Washburn, R. , Smith, K. W., Jette, M., & Janney, C. (1993). The physical activity scale for the elderly (PASE): Development and evaluation. *Journal of Clinical Epidemiology. 46*(2), 153–162.

Wolinsky, F., Coe, R., McIntosh, A., Kubena, K., Prendergast, J., Chavez, M., Miller, D., Romeis, J., & Landmann, W. (1990). Progress in the development of a nutritional risk index. *Journal of Nutrition, 120,* 1349–1553.

Woolf, S. H., Jonas, S., & Lawrence, R. S. (Eds.). (1996). *Health promotion and disease prevention in clinical practice.* Philadelphia: Lippincott Williams and Wilkins.

Zimet, G. D., Dahlem, N. W., Zimet, S. G., & Farley, G. K. (1988). The multidimensional scale of perceived social support. *Journal of Personality Assessment, 52*(1), 30–41.

BIBLIOGRAPHY

American Nurses Association (ANA). (2001). *Scope and standards of gerontological nursing* (2nd ed.). Washington, DC: Author.

Muravchick, S. (2003). Physiological changes of aging. *ASA refresher courses in anesthesiology. 31*(1):139–149, 2003.

RESOURCES

National Resource Center for Safe Aging

San Diego State University
6505 Alvarado Road, Suite 211
San Diego, California 92120
619-594-0986
FAX: 619-594-0351
Email: safeaging@sdsu.edu
Web: http://www.safeaging.org

The mission of The National Resource Center for Safe Aging is to gather and share the best information and resources on senior safety, including fall prevention, pedestrian and motor vehicle safety, and prevention of elder abuse. Resources include databases on general, regional, and aging data, as well as best practices and training. These resources are available for public health professionals, older adults, and family members.

The Hartford Institute for Geriatric Nursing

New York University College of Nursing
The John Hartford Foundation Institute for Geriatric Nursing
246 Greene Street
New York, New York 10003
212-998-9018
FAX: 212-995-4561
Email: info@nlihc.org
Web: http://www.hartfordign.org

The mission of the Hartford Institute for Geriatric Nursing is to help nurses provide, teach, learn, and administer best nursing practice to older clients through education, practice, and research.

Hartford Geriatric Nursing Initiative (HGNI)

American Academy of Nursing
Coordinating Center
888 17th Street NW, Suite 800
Washington, D.C. 20006
Email: BAGNC@aannet.org
Web: http://www.geriatricnursing.org; http://www
.hartfordign.org

HGNI was launched in 1995 and confronts the challenges associated with an aging client patient population through an array of programs. With a $60 million investment from the John Hartford Foundation, HGNI is preparing professional nurses to play leadership roles in improving the health of older adults. Programs are aimed at nursing practice, education, research, leadership, and public policy. The program aims are to increase the supply of geriatric nurses and the quality of care they provide by enhancing geriatric nursing training programs that produce the leaders of tomorrow. This Web site was developed by the independent evaluator of the Hartford Geriatric Nursing Initiative, The Measurement Group. This Web site highlights the programs of the Initiative and provides links to other Web sites supported by the Initiative. The Web site also presents emerging evaluation results that show the outcomes and impact of these programs.

The National Council on Aging (NCOA)

NCOA Headquarters
1901 L Street, NW, 4th floor
Washington, D.C. 20036
202-479-1200
FAX: 202-479-0735; TDD: 202-479-6674
Email: info@ncoorg

Founded in 1950, NCOA is dedicated to improving the health and independence of older persons and increasing their continuing contributions to communities, society, and future generations. NCOA is a 501(c)3 organization. At the heart of NCOA is a national network of more than 14,000 organizations and leaders that work together to achieve its mission. NCOA's 3,800 members include senior centers, area agencies on aging, adult day service centers, faith-based service organizations, senior housing facilities, employment services, consumer groups, and leaders from academia, business, and labor. The programs help older people to remain healthy, find jobs, discover new ways to continue to contribute to society after retirement, and take advantage of government and private benefits programs that can improve the quality of their lives. NCOA is also a national voice for both older Americans and community organizations, leading advocacy efforts on important national issues affecting seniors.

The Senior Benefits Checkup developed by NCOA
Web: http://www.benefitscheckup.org

Developed and maintained by the National Council on Aging (NCOA), Benefits Checkup is the nation's most comprehensive Web-based service to screen for benefits programs for seniors with limited income and resources. Benefits Checkup includes more than 1,350 public and private benefits programs from all 50 states and the District of Columbia. Many older people need help paying for prescription drugs, health care, utilities, and other basic needs. Ironically, millions of older Americans—especially those with limited incomes—are eligible for but not receiving benefits from existing federal, state, and local programs. Ranging from heating and energy assistance to prescription savings programs to income supplements, there are many public programs available to seniors in need if they only knew about them and how to apply for them.

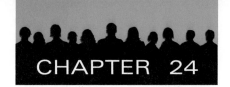

CHAPTER 24

Rural and Migrant Populations

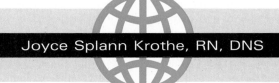

Joyce Splann Krothe, RN, DNS

Chapter Outline

⊕ Rural Defined
⊕ Historical Context
  Federal Initiatives in Rural Health
⊕ Demographics and Health Status Indicators
⊕ Cultural Characteristics of Rural Populations
⊕ Migrant Rural Farmworkers
  Migrant Farmworker Health Issues
  Undocumented Migrant Farmworkers
⊕ Public Health Nursing Practice in Rural
  Communities
  Healthy People 2010 and Primary Health Care Concepts
  Theory Development for Rural Public Health Nursing
  Opportunities for Service Learning and Collaborative Practice
⊕ Health Policy in Rural Settings
⊕ Research in Rural Settings

Learning Objectives

Upon completion of this chapter, the reader will be able to:

1. Develop an understanding of the history of public health nursing practice in rural settings.

2. Describe economic, social, and cultural factors that impact the health status of rural populations.

3. Analyze the role of public health nursing in addressing the unique health care needs of rural populations and addressing the challenges.

4. Apply Healthy People 2010 Health Status Objectives to rural settings.

5. Evaluate appropriate research relevant to rural and migrant health.

6. Assess the role of public health nursing in affecting health policy decisions for rural populations.

People living in rural areas have less access to health care than those in urban areas because of persistent poverty, fewer health services and practitioners, and transportation needed to travel longer distances to access acute and primary preventive services. Public health nurses have historically provided care to people living in rural settings to promote health and prevent illness and injury. This chapter focuses on public health nursing with rural populations. The chapter provides common definitions of the term "rural" and offers a historical context of public health nursing in rural communities; describes characteristics and demographics of rural populations and the unique opportunities and distinct challenges of public health nursing in the setting; and suggests implications related to health policy and research in rural communities.

RURAL DEFINED

There is a lack of consensus in the literature about a universally accepted definition of rural, or an operational definition that clearly distinguishes rural from urban (Anderson & McFarlane, 2000; Baer, Johnson-Webb, & Gesler, 1997; Clark, 2002). Definitions usually address only a single dimension, the distribution of people across space, and ignore the heterogeneity of persons who live in these settings, and the fact that rural and urban are not opposing lifestyles (Rural Information Center Health Service, 2006). The lack of a standardized, clear definition of rural results in a less coordinated approach to define and address the unique health care needs of rural populations (Bushy, 2007).

One way to define rural is by population factors that separate rural from urban. Metropolitan and nonmetropolitan areas are distinctions made by the U.S. Office of Management and Budget. A metropolitan area is defined as one with a population of 50,000 persons or larger. A nonmetropolitan area is defined as one with a population of fewer than 50,000 persons. The Census Bureau classifies counties as metropolitan or nonmetropolitan, as determined by the presence or lack thereof, of a central city or twin city of 50,000 or more population (Office of Management and Budget, 2006).

Another way to define rural is by geographic factors such as geographic location and population density, or in terms of distance from (20 miles), or the time (30 minutes), needed to commute to an urban area. Rural communities have fewer than 2,500 residents or

fewer than 99 persons per square mile. According to the 2000 census, 21 percent of the U.S. population is considered rural. Of this percentage only 5 percent are farm families; the other 95 percent are nonfarm families who reside in rural and frontier settings (U. S .Census Bureau, 2000). "From a health care perspective, the definition of rural involves a combination of the number of people residing in a place, some aspect of geographical distance and space, and recognition of the distance of the place from other nearby health and human services" (American Nurses Association, 1996, p. 6).

The demographic makeup of rural area can be described as mostly younger than age 18 (28 percent) and older than 65 years (30 percent). In the oldest age group (those older than 75), the rural elderly are predominately women with low socioeconomic status (U.S. Census Bureau, 2000). In addition, more rural residents are married and have completed fewer years of formal education than urban residents. Various ethnic groups are also represented in rural settings including African American, Indian, Appalachian, Eskimos, and seasonal and farm workers (U.S. Census Bureau, 2000). Rural minority communities are among the poorest in the United States. The result of a project funded from the Health Resources and Services Administration's Federal Office of Rural Health Policy produced *Rural Healthy People, A Companion Document to Healthy People 2010* (Gamm & Hutchison, 2004). This document identifies health priorities and access to care issues unique to at-risk populations including migrant workers, African Americans, Native Americans, and children and the elderly.

Health Professional Shortage Areas (HPSAs) and Medically Underserved Areas (MUAs), established under the U.S. Public Health Services Act, are federal designations of a geographic area, often a county or a collection of census tracts, that meet the criteria of needing additional primary health care services and providers, a characteristic often associated with rural settings and characteristic of the rural community described in the case study (Indiana State Department of Health, 2003). Other factors that affect the designation include availability of primary care resources in contiguous areas and presence of unusual need, such as high infant mortality or high poverty rates. Federal opportunities available to HPSAs include National Health Service Corps Scholarship and Loan Repayment Programs, Medicare incentive payments, and health education programs through the Rural Health Clinic Services Act

(U.S. Census Bureau, 2000). Figure 24-1 shows primary health care shortage areas for designated populations in the United States. There are increased shortage areas for low-income persons, particularly seasonal and migrant farmworker populations.

HISTORICAL CONTEXT

Rural nursing in the United States has a rich heritage in public health, in particular, maternal child health. The first rural nursing service was established in 1896 in Westchester County, New York, by Mary Morris Wood (Clark, 2002). Box 24-1 briefly summarizes the history of public health nursing in rural settings.

Lillian Wald, a pioneer of public health nursing in urban neighborhoods, influenced the concept and growth of rural public health nursing. In 1912, she convinced the American Red Cross to direct peacetime efforts to develop public health services in rural America. In 1912, the American Red Cross established the Rural Nursing Service, later renamed the Town and Country Nursing Service, to extend public health services to remote rural areas in New York (Clark, 2002). The Town and Country Nursing Service continued until 1947 when it was disbanded due to the rise of official nursing agencies in local and state health departments.

Another early rural nursing concept was the Frontier Nursing Service (FNS), established by Mary Breckenridge

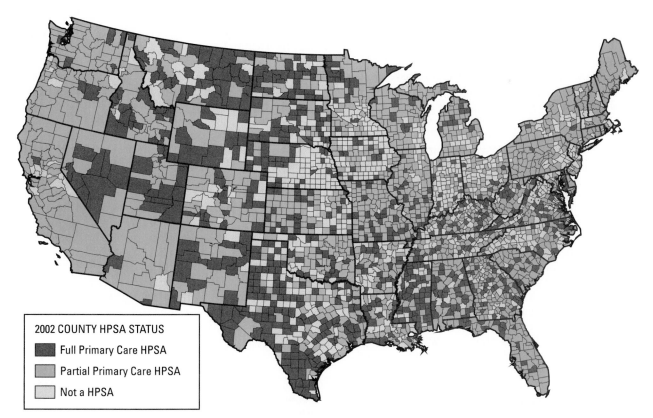

2002 COUNTY HPSA STATUS
- Full Primary Care HPSA
- Partial Primary Care HPSA
- Not a HPSA

Figure 24-1 Health professional shortage areas—primary health designated populations
From U.S. Department of Health and Human Services, Health Resources and Services Administration (2007).

BOX 24-1: History of Public Health Nursing in Rural Settings

1896—First rural nursing service established in Westchester County, New York

1912—Rural Nursing Service established by the American Red Cross

1925—Frontier Nursing Service (FNS) established in rural Kentucky

1939—Frontier School of Midwifery started by the FNS

1999—FNS started community-based family nurse practitioner (FNP) programs

---

in 1925 in rural Leslie County, Kentucky. The purpose of the FNS was to bring primary health care to some of the poorest and most inaccessible counties. It was based on systems of care used in the Highlands and islands of Scotland (Bushy, 2004). Breckenridge's pioneering efforts influenced the development of public health programs geared toward improving the health of inaccessible Appalachian populations. She was instrumental in establishing six outpost nursing centers in rural Kentucky between 1927 and 1930 and introducing the first midwives in the United States.

FNS nurses visited families on horseback. Baseline data on infant and maternal mortality was collected, and evaluation demonstrated the effectiveness of the FNS in reducing pregnancy complications, the number of stillbirths, and infant and maternal mortality and in improving the general health of rural residents. Typical living conditions for residents of rural counties in Kentucky during this period included lack of running water, electricity, or heat. The FNS has continued to grow and still provides public health services to the rural residents of Kentucky.

The Frontier School of Midwifery was started by the FNS in 1939 and has been in continuous operation since that time. In the late 1960s, the FNS recognized the need to provide a more comprehensive education for nurses to provide primary care to families. In 1970, they developed the first certificate program to prepare family nurse practitioners, and the name of the school was changed to the Frontier School of Midwifery and

Family Nursing. In 1999, the community-based family nurse practitioner program was established utilizing distance education options. In 2001, the school began offering a MSN with specialties in midwifery and family nurse practitioner, as well as a certificate in women's health (Frontier Education Center, 2003).

The National Commission on Nurse-Midwifery Education recommended in 1993 that universities expand their nurse-midwifery education programs to increase the number of certified nurse midwives. In response to this recommendation, the Frances Payne Bolton School of Nursing, Case Western Reserve University, and the Community-Based Nurse-Midwifery Education Program collaborated to provide baccalaureate education for nurses with associate degrees to become eligible for a distance learning program of advance training in midwifery (Novotny et al., 1996).

Federal Initiatives in Rural Health

The National Health Service Corps (NHSC), a part of the Health Resources and Services Administration (HRSA), was established in 1972 to provide health manpower for rural areas. Since 1972 they have placed over 20,000 providers in rural and frontier areas. The NHSC provides team-based systems of quality health care, especially for health issues that have the highest racial, ethnic, and socioeconomic disparities.

The National Center for Farmworker Health (NCFH) was established in 1974 in Buda, Texas, and is dedicated to improving the health status of farmworker families by providing human, technical, and information services and products to a network of more than 500 migrant health center service sites in the United States as well as other organizations and individuals serving the farmworker population (National Center for Farmworker Health, 2005).

The Rural Health Clinic Services Act of 1977 was enacted to improve primary health care for medically underserved persons. It allows for reimbursement from Medicare and Medicaid and third-party sources of payment for the services of a nurse practitioner, physician assistant, or nurse midwife in an attempt to improve access to care in underserved areas. Individual states govern the scope of practice and providers. The act stipulates that services are provided in a rural health clinic (RHC).

In 1987, the National Advisory Committee on Rural Health and Human Services was established. It consists of a 21-member citizen panel that advises the Secretary of the U.S. Department of Health and Human Services (USDHHS) on rural health and human services issues.

The Office of Rural Health Policy (ORHP) was authorized by Congress in 1987 to promote better health care in rural America. The ORHP works with local, state, and federal governments as well as the private sector to seek solutions to rural health care problems. It is responsible for policy advocacy and health information development. It serves as a voice for rural communities to inform the Secretary of Health and Human Services of policy impact on rural communities and promotes rural health clinics certified under federal law to provide care in underserved areas (Hitchcock, Schubert & Thomas, 1999). It emphasizes community-oriented planning by actively involving local people.

The Rural Information Center Health Service (RICHS) was initiated in 1987 by ORHP to provide toll-free access nationally to rural residents seeking information on requested topics. It posts information on its Web site regarding funding opportunities, conferences, and publications. The National Rural Recruitment and Retention Network supported by OHRP seeks to improve recruitment and retention of health professionals in rural areas. It consists of 45 state-based organizations assisting health professionals to relocate to rural settings. Table 24-1 summarizes federal initiatives in rural health.

DEMOGRAPHICS AND HEALTH STATUS INDICATORS

Economic indicators of rural settings impact health status. In comparison to urban residents, median income and educational levels in rural areas are lower, poverty and unemployment rates are higher, and the percentage of employers who do not provide health insurance is higher (Rural Information Center Health Service, 2006). Workers in rural settings often comprise a category referred to as "the working poor" because they are self-employed in small family-owned farms and small businesses and because the seasonal nature of farm work places them at increased risk of being uninsured and underinsured. Timely access to emergency services and the availability of specialty care are other issues confronting rural populations.

The following factors that impact health status are characteristic of rural populations: a disproportionate number of very young and elderly residents; health

TABLE 24-1: Federal Initiatives in Rural Health

ORGANIZATION	YEAR	PURPOSE
National Health Service Corps	1972	To provide health manpower for rural areas
National Center for Farmworker Health	1974	To provide services to a network of migrant health centers
Rural Health Clinic Services Act	1977	To improve primary health care for medically under-served populations
Office of Rural Health Policy	1987	To promote better health in rural America
Rural Information Center Health Service	1987	To provide national access to rural residents seeking information on requested topics
National Advisory Committee on Rural Health and Human Services	1987	21-member citizen panel to provide recommendations on rural health to the secretary of DHHS

hazards (e.g., injury, pesticide poisoning); potential for abuse, family violence and neglect, coupled with a lack of resources for mental health services; weather-related hazards (e.g., drought, sun, wind, tornadoes); and geographic isolation, which leads to social isolation and increases the potential for physical and psychological problems; lack of public transportation; and lack of access to specialty care (Bushy, 2004; USDHHHS, 2001).

Rural residents have higher rates of chronic illness than their urban counterparts, including cardiovascular disease, hypertension, and diabetes; higher rates of infant and maternal morbidity and mortality; more psychological problems caused by economic stress; and increased tobacco use (Rural Information Center Health Service, 2006).

Injury-related deaths are 40 percent higher in rural populations than in urban populations, often due to accidents involving agricultural machinery. People living in rural settings are less likely to use preventive screening services. In 1996, 20 percent of the rural population was uninsured compared with 16 percent of the urban population (USDHHS, 2001). Increased occupational health risks exist in rural work settings. Rural residents are more likely to die from complications of injuries due to limited access to health services.

POLICY HIGHLIGHT

Rural Nurse-Managed Clinics

An Indiana statewide initiative to require 20 hours of physician on-sight supervision in all rural nurse-managed clinics was announced. Regional forums were scheduled around the state to discuss the proposed policy. The public health nurses that served as clinic directors networked to coordinate a strategy to voice their concerns related to the proposed policy. The public health nurses were effective in coordinating clients to attend all of the regional meetings and in explaining the resource constraints, both fiscal and personnel, that exist in rural areas where the clinics were located. Their coordinated response led to the state revamping the policy and accepting physician availability for consultation, rather than on-sight supervision. This compromise demonstrated the effectiveness of a coordinated effort on the part of the public health nurses, all of whom worked independently in their respective rural clinics in achieving a policy they could implement.

High-risk industries identified by OSHA in rural areas are forestry, mining, fishing, and agriculture. Associated health risks for these industries include accidents, trauma, selected cancers, and respiratory diseases due to chronic exposure to toxins, pesticides, and herbicides (Lyons, 2003; Bushy, 2004). The lack of a comprehensive surveillance system for reporting injuries in the population makes it difficult to know the extent of injuries (McGuire, 2002).

Mental health and stress-related illnesses are common in rural populations including higher levels of depression (Bushy, 2004). Domestic violence and substance abuse may be unreported or underreported due to lack of available mental health professionals, knowledge of community-based resources, and communication patterns. Misconceptions and stereotypes about mental illness persist in this population; therefore, public health nurses have a role to play in facilitating access to mental health services in culturally acceptable ways and in assuring easy access to health care.

CULTURAL CHARACTERISTICS OF RURAL POPULATIONS

Although each rural community is unique, some commonalities influence public health nursing practice in the setting. These include (1) self-reliance, independence, and individualism of rural residents; (2) time and crisis orientation in relation to health; (3) distrust of outsiders; (4) religious influence; and (5) use of alternative healing remedies, both folk and traditional (Hitchcock, Schubert, & Thomas, 2003).

Health is often tied to the ability to work in rural settings. Although health promotion and disease prevention services are well understood by public health nurses, they may be concepts that are not well understood by members of rural communities, as they may appear unrelated to daily work. Due to the utilitarian viewpoint of health associated with the ability to work by rural populations, health promotion activities may not be valued as the benefits are often long range rather than immediate. Box 24-2 summarizes health problems characteristic of rural populations.

MIGRANT RURAL FARMWORKERS

Migrant rural farmworkers are individuals who move from one region to another in search of farm

BOX 24-2: Health Problems Characteristic of Rural Populations

- Occupational health hazards—injury, exposure to carcinogenic pesticides, infectious disease among migrant rural farmworkers
- Potential for abuse, family violence, and neglect
- Weather-related hazards—drought, sun, wind, tornadoes
- Higher rates of chronic illness, including cardiovascular disease, hypertension, and diabetes
- Higher rates of infant and maternal morbidity and mortality
- Psychological problems caused by economic stress and reluctance to seek assistance

primary health care services due to isolation, lack of transportation, economic barriers, language difficulties, and cultural differences. Even if migrant health centers are available, they often do not offer services during nonwork hours, and unless there is a health crisis, it is unrealistic to expect workers to sacrifice income by leaving work to seek preventive care (Napolitano & Jones, 2004). Chronic poverty, frequent mobility, low literacy, language, cultural, and logistic barriers impede migrant workers' access to social services and cost-effective primary health care (McGuire, 2002). Many migrant workers are not aware of benefits available to them, or they experience difficulty in the application process for benefits due to language or cultural barriers. In addition, migrant farmworkers almost never have health insurance, and lack of portability or reciprocity in Medicaid across state lines creates administrative barriers to coverage for migrant rural workers (NCFH, 2005). In addition to lack of insurance for care, migrant workers often lack transportation to clinics or may be afraid to take the time off work, fearing lost wages or even losing their jobs if they take time off to seek medical care.

Migrant Farmworker Health Issues

Overall, migrant workers suffer a low level of health, much like that of persons in third world nations, suffering from poverty-related health problems such as malnutrition and illness associated with inadequate sanitation (Leon, 2000). Tuberculosis (TB) is another health problem threatening migrant families (NCFH, 2007). In the 1990s, the latest data reported on tuberculosis screening tests among migrant farmworkers in North Carolina, Florida, and Virginia revealed 41, 44, and 48 percent positive tests, respectively. Many farmworkers enter this country from Mexico, and the overall TB incidence is higher in Mexico than in the United States (CDC, 2001). Adjusting for underreporting, the World Health Organization estimates the incidence of pulmonary TB in Mexico to be 45 cases per 100,000, and the prevalence of multidrug-resistant TB (MDR-TB) strains increases concerns regarding the cross-border spread of TB. TB among migrant farmworkers presents a difficult public health problem because the crucial long-term treatment and preventive efforts are impeded by the transient nature of farm work, language barriers, and knowledge deficit about the disease. When treatment is interrupted, the TB strain is more likely to develop into MDR-TB.

or agricultural work of a seasonal or other temporary nature. Migrant farmworkers are required to be absent overnight from their permanent places of residence. There are over 3 million migrant and seasonal farmworkers who travel throughout the United States to follow agricultural crops (NCFH, 2007). According to the 1997–1998 findings of the National Agricultural Workers Survey (NAWS), the average age for migrant workers is 31; 80 percent are men, 84 percent speak Spanish; 12 percent speak English; and the median level of education is the sixth grade (USDHHS, 2001). These workers are the heart of the $28 billion fruit and vegetable industry in the United States as 85 percent of the fruits and vegetables available to bring to our tables are hand cultivated and/or harvested (NCFH, 2007). Migrant workers are crucial to the production and delivery of a wide variety of crops in almost every state in the nation.

Without the health and welfare of migrant workers, U.S. families would not enjoy access to the variety of foods at a reasonable price. Yet, migrant farmworkers are among the poorest, most economically disadvantaged workers, and they work some of the most unhealthy and unsafe jobs in the nation. Allender and Spradley (2005) report that fewer than 20 percent of the estimated four million migrant workers and their families who live in rural areas in the United States use

Dental disease has been identified as one of the top five health problems for migrant farmworkers (Lombardi, 2001). Most migrant workers seek dental care in crisis because of barriers to accessing care such as cost, time factors, and perceptions that treatment would not help them. A health assessment of 652 adult agricultural workers in California revealed that 36.1 percent of males and 29.2 percent of females had at least one untreated decayed tooth compared to 28 percent nationally, and an equal number of males and females had broken or missing teeth (Villarejo et al., 2000). Additionally, gingivitis was the third major dental problem, affecting 14.4 percent of the workers, and nearly half of the respondents reported that they had never been to a dentist. Baby bottle tooth decay (BBTD) is a problem among farmworker children. The prevalence of BBTD among farmworker's children is 20 percent, compared to less than 5 percent in the general population (Lombardi, 2001). Most of the workers reported lack of access to dental care and inadequate knowledge of how to maintain oral hygiene as barriers to oral health. In addition, migrant farmworkers typically do not seek preventive care but rather seek care only when they have a dental emergency. Therefore, primary prevention with applications of fluoride, cleanings, and education are usually not received on a regular basis (Lombardi, 2001).

Workplace injury and illness associated with agricultural work places a high risk of early death for the migrant worker population. The National Institute of Occupational Safety and Health (NIOSH, 1995) identified ergonomic conditions/musculoskeletal injuries, traumatic injuries, respiratory problems, dermatitis, infectious diseases, cancer, and eye problems as migrant health concerns. In a cohort study of injuries in 267 migrant farmworker families in South Texas, workers reported working an average of 6.2 days a week at 10.1 hours per day on farm jobs (Cooper et al., 2006). As the most common workplace hazards, they reported working with knives, cutting tools, tractors, and all-terrain vehicles; doing repetitive hand work and repetitive bending and stooping; working with chemicals; and lifting and moving heavy objects repetitively. The actual injuries reported in a 2-year period were diverse and included cuts, contusions, and abrasions; overexertion strains and fractures; heat stroke; and blisters and rashes. Farmworkers have little training in injury prevention, and transportation to and from the fields where they work often occurs in overcrowded and unsafe vehicles.

Undocumented Migrant Farmworkers

Although human migration has existed for hundreds of thousands of years, immigration in the modern sense refers to movement of people from one nation-state to another, where they are not citizens. Seasonal labor migration is often treated as a form of immigration. The Mexican-origin migrant worker population can be divided into (1) legal residents of the United States who migrate to work in agriculture and (2) citizens of Mexico who come to the United States to work in agriculture. A large percentage enter the United States illegally (undocumented labor), but some enter legally on work visas or approved labor contracts (Cuellar, 2002).

Undocumented migrant workers live in fear of being reported and deported, reside in less than favorable housing that is often overcrowded, and frequently endure discrimination, prejudice, and abuse. In addition, they often come alone with limited resources and language skills. It seems that these stressors can result in harmful mental health effects, but research has found the opposite to be true. For example, Vega et al. (1998) found that lifetime prevalence of psychiatric disorders were lower for Mexican immigrants than for U.S.-born Mexican Americans. More research needs to be done in the area of mental health consequences. In other parts of the country, stressors do result in symptoms of depression, anxiety, and panic attacks, and, as a result, many immigrants refrain from seeking essential health care (DeToledo, Palmerola, & Lowe, 2003). At the University of Miami emergency department, illegal immigrants gave the fear of being deported as the reason for the delay in coming to the hospital. The delay many times resulted in worsened, irreversible conditions such as blindness and stroke.

PUBLIC HEALTH NURSING PRACTICE IN RURAL COMMUNITIES

Health care is shifting to community-based settings as managed care spreads throughout the United States. Health care reform and an emphasis on access to primary health care in rural communities create an opportunity for nurses to achieve innovations in health care (Lyons, 2003).

Public health nursing practice in rural settings requires both professional and personal qualities due to the unique characteristics of the settings. Requisite personal skills and characteristics for public health nursing practice include the following: adaptability, independence, self-reliance, resourcefulness, and ability to prioritize. If the nurse is not a community member, sufficient time for trust to develop is necessary. In rural communities, social and professional roles often overlap and may lead to issues of reduced anonymity and problems with maintaining confidentiality. Developing close relationships with clients may help establish trust in the health care relationship, but it can also serve as a challenge to the nurse who desires a separation between personal and professional relationships.

Anderson and McFarlane (2000) caution that in some communities it may take years for residents to develop trust in health providers and for providers to be considered as community insiders. For example, in the clinic case study included in the chapter, being born in the rural county is the only factor that qualifies one as an insider. Health professionals need to understand this, be sensitive to the community definition of insider status, and most importantly, incorporate insiders in the planning and delivery of health care services. To facilitate the process of being perceived as an insider, it is important for the public health nurse to be visible at events that are considered important in the life of the community. For example, in the case study described, members of the Community Advisory Board emphasized the importance of the public health nurse's visibility at the annual county fair, a marker event for the community.

To work effectively in rural settings, the public health nurse must acknowledge the community's sense of time for meaningful change to take place and recognize that accomplishment of goals often takes far longer than desired or planned.

A public health nurse may be the only health care provider in some rural settings, and because clients vary in age and have diverse health conditions, the nurse must function on a continuum of generalist to specialist, thus maintaining a broad knowledge base and assuming a variety of roles and responsibilities. The nurse must recognize the importance of distinct cultural practices and apply clinical judgment in a manner that is culturally acceptable to rural residents and their families; have expertise in assessment of individuals, families, and communities; and have an expanded knowledge of family and group dynamics. Case management skills and client advocacy are

⊕ POLICY HIGHLIGHT

Hearing Loss in Farmers

Hearing loss of farmers seems inconsistent with the perceived idyllic, peaceful rural farm environment that we often think of. However, the National Safety Council (2005) warns of the presence of high-intensity noise that may result in hearing loss among agricultural workers. In fact, noise-induced hearing loss from tractors, grain dryers, combines, chain saws, grain grinding, and animals is a very large part of the personal lives of most farmers. Because of this, farmers are advised to (1) use hearing protection such as earplugs or muffs from the minute noise begins; (2) consider quiet operation when buying any motorized equipment and keep machinery and equipment well lubricated and well maintained; (3) wear hearing protection if they have to yell to someone 3 feet (two arm's lengths) away; and (4) have a hearing test if ringing in the ears is experienced.

inherent in the role of public health nurses in rural settings.

Reduced opportunities for consultation with colleagues and limited access to continuing education and decreased opportunities for career advancement provide challenges in recruiting and retaining nurses in rural settings. Recent advances in technology including telecommunication and the use of interactive audio, video, and data communications ease the relative isolation of nurses working in rural settings (Hitchcock et al., 2003). The Institute of Medicine (2005) in its report on the future of rural health advocates for investment in an information and communications technology infrastructure to address this problem. Box 24-3 summarizes characteristics of public health nursing practice in rural settings.

Healthy People 2010 and Primary Health Care Concepts

Healthy People 2010 focuses on goals of health promotion, health protection, and disease prevention and outlines a comprehensive, nationwide health promotion and disease prevention agenda. Specifically it seeks to increase both life expectancy and quality of life by

⊕ RESEARCH APPLICATION

Listening to the Quiet Voices of Hispanic Migrant Children about Health

Study Purpose

To answer three research questions related to Hispanic migrant school-aged children's perceptions of their health needs, learning needs, and concerns about health and access to health care.

Methods

Fourteen focus groups were used to hear the voices of 73 migrant children who were attending a summer school program for children of migrant farm workers in south Georgia. Nud*IST software was used to create an index system of the transcribed data.

Findings

Children's ages ranged from 8 to 14 years, and 60 percent of the children were boys. Six themes emerged from the qualitative data: healthy behaviors, acculturation issues, environmental influences, health care actions, health behavior outcomes, and learning needs. The children recognized healthy behaviors as including selecting healthy foods, exercising, getting adequate sleep and rest, taking care of their teeth, attending to personal hygiene, avoiding alcohol and cigarettes, and getting along with others. Acculturation issues included friendships, education, safety, conflict, and difficulty with acquisition of resources. Environmental influences on health included

use of support systems, parental involvement, and parental role-modeling. Health maintenance responses and use of alternative health care practices were identified as health care actions, and health behavior outcomes included perceptions of health care, expectations of health care, and health care recommendations. Their ideas about health learning needs were healthy diet, exercise, water intake, and cleanliness.

Implications

Children of migrant workers reported that they used both Western health care and also alternative health care. Their mothers were their primary caregivers, and their mothers used alternative methods of health care when they were ill. Children voiced fears about living in the United States (e.g., concerns about deportation and prejudice) and also longing for their ethnic foods of Mexico. Hispanic culture is important to these children, and public health nurses need to be aware of and respond to the unique needs of children of migrant workers.

Reference

Wilson, A. H., Pittman, K., & Wold, J. L. (2000). Listening to the quiet voices of Hispanic migrant children about health. *Journal of Pediatric Nursing, 15*(3), 137–147.

---

helping individuals gain knowledge and opportunities to make informed decisions in regard to their health (USDHHS, 2001). It encourages communitywide attention to both individual and collective factors that impact health status. The underlying premise of Healthy People 2010 is that the individual is inseparable from the health of the larger community.

Characteristics associated with access, affordability, acceptability, and availability of health care specific to rural settings include travel distance for tertiary care and ancillary and emergency services; diagnostic testing or specialty treatment modalities may be required due to the geographic isolation of residents in rural settings. Issues related to the lack of public transportation and the cost of fuel are relevant concerns for the public health nurse to consider when planning care.

BOX 24-3: Characteristics of Public Health Nursing Practice in Rural Settings

- ⊕ Independence, self-reliance, resourcefulness, and ability to prioritize are required.
- ⊕ Sufficient time for trust to develop in rural settings is essential for therapeutic public health nursing practice.
- ⊕ Social and professional roles often overlap.
- ⊕ Positive community visibility is essential.

Affordability of health care is an issue in rural settings due to a high percentage of residents who are underinsured and uninsured. Providing options for a reduced or sliding fee scale for services reduces financial barriers to seeking needed health care.

Acceptability is a concept that must be considered due to the unique cultural characteristics of many rural settings. It is important to consider the role of lay providers in extending health care to the community. For example, in the case study described in this chapter, the community health workers employed have no formal preparation in health care, but as lifelong residents of the community, they are an essential component in ensuring that services are planned and delivered within the cultural context acceptable to the rural community.

Availability of care in rural settings relates to lack of resources and also to the times services are offered. Public health nursing services need to be planned to fit the realities of daily life, work schedules, and travel time. Evening and weekend options for care may be needed to accommodate clients who cannot access services during regular daytime hours. Availability of ancillary services for diagnosis and treatment should be considered in contiguous areas to provide necessary diagnostic testing and follow-up.

Theory Development for Rural Public Health Nursing

Health practitioners in rural settings contend that their practice differs markedly from practice in urban settings, yet how it differs is not well articulated. There is a need for an integrated, theoretical approach because nursing models and theories that have been developed in urban settings are not always applicable to rural settings.

Long and Weinert (1999) developed a theoretical approach for rural nursing based on their work in Montana and other rural areas using an ethnographic approach. Three conceptual statements characterize their work: (1) rural dwellers define health primarily as the ability to work, be productive, and do usual tasks (little emphasis is placed on the comfort, the cosmetic, or the life-prolonging aspects of health); (2) rural dwellers are self-reliant and resist accepting help or services from those seen as "outsiders" or from agencies seen as national or regional "welfare" programs; and (3) help is usually sought through an informal system of family, friends, and relatives rather than a formal system.

🌐 POLICY HIGHLIGHT

Fostering Leadership in Rural Areas

The Rural Voices Program was developed by the Health Resources and Services Administration (HRSA) Office of Rural Health Policy (ORHP) and the National Rural Health Association (NRHA) in 2002 to provide leadership training to a select group of the office's grantees. The program is a year long and provides a tailored leadership skill development program for potential rural health leaders and new rural health researchers while ensuring a greater diversity of leadership for rural communities. Participants are brought together through regular conference calls and face-to-face meetings to work on a joint project focusing on a key rural health issue. The intent is to help the participants understand the changing nature of the health policy landscape and provide them with the tools needed to play a leadership role in their rural communities and act as a catalyst for change.

Denham (2003) introduced a family health model based on research with rural Appalachian families. She found that family health is greatly influenced by interactions of household members, more so than by access to health care services. Both the involvement of family members in assessment, decision making, and planning and effective communication are key to positive outcomes from public health nursing interventions. The model is applicable to public health nursing in rural communities given the cultural characteristics described earlier in this chapter.

Opportunities for Service Learning and Collaborative Practice

Recruiting and retaining qualified health professionals, including nurses, in rural settings has historically been difficult. Programs are needed to encourage individuals from rural communities to enter health care professions and to return to the settings for employment. Internships in rural settings for nursing students may help to retain nurses in these settings after graduation. Loan forgiveness programs, such as those available through the National Health Service Corps, provide incentives for health care providers to practice in rural settings.

Recruiting nurses, especially bicultural and bilingual nurses, to rural settings is essential. Providing clinical service-learning experiences for nursing and other health professional students in rural settings may facilitate this process. Curricula should contain content specific to the characteristics and culture of rural settings. Service-learning provides a mechanism that differs from traditional clinical experience by engaging students in active learning while also providing a valuable service to the community; students learn to distinguish *working with* the community in a partnership model from simply *working in* a community as a geographic setting.

Collaborative practice models may facilitate the practice of nurse practitioners, advanced practice nurses, and nurse midwives in rural settings. Implementing a community development model is one way to work effectively in rural settings and to implement collaborative practice. A community development model focuses on the achievement of community goals and includes a true partnership with the community in which power and decision making are shared by community members and health providers (Krothe et al., 2000). The model assumes that desired community change occurs through broad participation by community members. In rural settings, the ability of the public health nurse to collaborate with a wide array of health care providers, including nontraditional providers, such as tribal healers, clergy persons, and herbalists, is important.

HEALTH POLICY IN RURAL SETTINGS

The health care inequities that exist in rural settings have policy implications that require public health nurses to be involved in the policy process. For example, the Balanced Budget Act (BBA) of 1997 introduced changes in Medicare reimbursement that have significant implications for rural health and delivery. Public health centers have been affected by a provision in the BBA that allows states to phase out Medicaid cost-based reimbursement and implement a prospective payment system in rural areas. Nurses need to assume leadership positions in building networks for informal consultation and support to influence policy formula-

⊕ RESEARCH APPLICATION

Evidence-Based Practice and Research Utilization Activities among Rural Nurses

Study Purpose

To identify the extent to which nurses utilize evidence-based practice in rural practice settings; to identify barriers to research utilization in rural areas; and to identify gaps that affect translating research into practice.

Methods

One-hundred and six nurses from six rural practice settings in the southwestern United States participated in this descriptive study using open-ended questionnaires focusing on their current utilization of nursing research findings and previous involvement in nursing research.

Findings

Approximately 21 percent of the participants indicated they utilized research in their rural practice. Barriers to research utilization included rural isolation and the lack of nursing research consultants. Approximately 76 percent of the participants indicated they would be interested in utilizing nursing research if given the opportunity and appropriate support.

Implications

Strategies are needed to encourage nurses in rural practice settings to incorporate evidence-based guidelines in their practice and to increase access to experienced nurses with research backgrounds for consultation. Collaborative efforts should be developed between nursing education and rural practice settings via advanced technology and distance education to address the research isolation experienced by nurses who practice in rural settings.

Reference

Olade, R.A. (2004). Evidence-based practice and research utilization activities among rural nurses. *Journal of Nursing Scholarship, 36*(3), 220–225.

⊕ PRACTICE APPLICATION

County Health Support Clinic

This case study describes the growth and development of a nurse-managed clinic, established in 1996 by the author through a community-campus partnership in a rural midwest community. The rural area where the clinic is located is designated as HPSA and a MUA. In addition to providing health care for uninsured rural residents, the clinic serves as a service-learning site for nursing students and other health professional students in rural health.

A community advisory board, comprised of residents with lifelong ties to the community, guides clinic operation and ensures that services are planned and implemented in a culturally acceptable manner. Utilization of a community development model ensures that the community is actively engaged in planning and implementing health services. For example, in the planning stages of the clinic's development, Brown County Health Promotion Clinic was proposed as a name for the clinic by the university partner. The community advisory board rejected "health promotion" in the name, stating that it was not a concept well understood by community members. Noting that the focus of the clinic was to support the community's health, they officially named the clinic the Brown County Health Support Clinic (Figure 24-2).

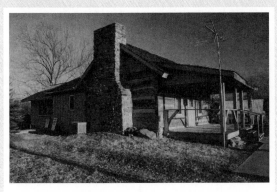

Figure 24-2 The Brown County Health Support Clinic.

Hypertension is a significant problem in the community, which is designated as the "stroke belt" by the state health department; however, community members do not view it as a significant problem. To effectively address the problem, the public health nurse at the clinic worked with area

schools and incorporated nursing students in health promotion activities in conjunction with state-mandated hypertension screening of fourth, seventh, and 11th graders. Students worked with the nurse to design age-appropriate materials related to prevention of hypertension and treatment of the disease for students to share with their families.

A provider agreed to offer needed mental health services at the local mental health office. Despite the need for the services, perceiving that their anonymity could not be assured clients would not go to the mental health office because of its prominent location in the community. Understanding the feelings of the local people, the clinic nurse arranged for mental health services to be offered at the clinic location.

Faculty members are considered to be community outsiders. Acknowledging the community's perception and understanding the consequences of this, community insiders were employed as public health workers and incorporated in all aspects of clinic operations. Lay individuals with lifelong ties to the community serve on the community advisory board, market clinic services, work in the clinic, and represent the clinic at community events and meetings. There was initial resistance to a nurse-managed model of care from members of the medical community, including the local health officer. Public health workers, who are recognized as community insiders, were instrumental in eventually facilitating a collaborative model of health care for rural residents.

Students have been involved since the inception of the project in working with the community to plan and implement culturally acceptable nurse-managed services. They participate in delivering care at the clinic site and in outreach activities and attend community advisory board meetings. Through journals and seminars, which includes community members, students reflect on how the service-learning experience enhanced their understanding of a rural community and the multiple factors that have an impact on health status for residents and consider the role of public health nursing in the health policy arena.

Students confront their misconceptions regarding rural residents who lack health insurance; they had often perceived them to be unwilling to work. They learned, in fact, that they were very hardworking people, often employed in multiple jobs, but lacking access to health care due to the nature of their employment, which was seasonal or in small businesses that did not provide health insurance.

tion at the national level. Examples of activities related to the role of public health nurses in health policy include lobbying for particular bills; developing open communication with local, state, and federal legislators; providing expert testimony; and developing case studies and client profiles to be used in grant writing and other requests for funding.

RESEARCH IN RURAL SETTINGS

Few studies of public health nursing in rural settings exist. Research is needed to demonstrate the evidence-base, efficacy, and cost effectiveness of nurse-managed models of care in rural settings and to study the unique health problems of rural populations. For example, studies related to the long-term health effects of pesticide exposure by rural farmworkers are needed.

Alternative research methodologies, such as ethnographic studies and qualitative methods, should be considered because traditional positivist research paradigms may not be culturally acceptable or appropriate for participants in the research process. For example, in the rural community described in the case study in this chapter, a research instrument to assess clients' knowledge of hypertension that included a written question-naire was not viewed as acceptable. Clients would not complete it and explained that if the researcher wanted to know their thoughts related to hypertension they should engage them in a dialogue regarding it. Subsequent focus group interviews proved to be an effective mechanism to gain knowledge related to hypertension.

Few empirical studies on rural nursing exist. Hartley (2004) described a rural health determinant and urged researchers to describe the environmental and cultural factors that affect health in rural settings. Stressors and rewards of practicing in the settings; health outcomes of nurse-managed services; and empirical data on needs of particular groups of rural residents nationwide are potential areas for nursing research (Bushy, 2004; Rural Policy Research Institute, 1999).

Communicating research results to various audiences such as lay and professional groups, legislators, and policy makers is necessary. Nurses conducting research need to consider appropriate strategies for presenting the results of research findings to multiple audiences. In the preceding Practice Application, rural residents expressed a concern that in the past they had devoted considerable time and resources in research projects only to be left out of the findings and application steps of the process.

CRITICAL THINKING ACTIVITIES

1. Contrast the disparities in health characteristics of rural populations with urban populations.

2. Consider the implications for public health nursing practice in relationship to the unique characteristics and health needs of people who live and work in rural communities.

3. Assess the opportunities and challenges of public health nursing practice in rural settings and propose strategies to address the challenges.

4. Formulate health-related research questions and propose appropriate research methodologies in relation to public health nursing in rural settings.

5. Propose suggestions for public health nurses working in rural settings to become involved in the health policy arena.

6. Suggest further theory development of rural public health nursing.

KEY TERMS

Health Professional Shortage Areas

Medically Underserved Areas

metropolitan

migrant rural farmworker

nonmetropolitan

rural

KEY CONCEPTS

- Public health nursing practice has a long and rich history of practice in rural settings.

- A public health nurse working in a rural setting must be aware of the unique health care needs in order to adequately meet the needs of the populations.

- The public health nurse must be aware of unique challenges in addressing the Healthy People 2010 concepts in rural settings.

- Rural settings present unique challenges and opportunities for public health nursing practice.

- Public health nurses have a responsibility to advocate for health policy that addresses the distinct health care needs of rural populations.

REFERENCES

Allender, J. A., & Spradley, B. W. (2005). *Public health nursing. Promoting and protecting the public's health* (pp. 743–760, 784–808). Philadelphia: Lippincott Williams & Wilkins.

American Nurses' Association. (1996). *Rural/frontier nursing. The challenge to grow.* Washington, DC: Author.

Anderson, E., & McFarlane, J. (2000). *Community as partner: Theory and practice in nursing* (pp. 3–25, 393–401). Philadelphia: Lippincott.

Baer, L. D., Johnson-Webb, K. D., & Gesler, W. M. (1997). What is rural? A focus on urban influence codes. *Journal of Rural Health, 13*(4), 329–333.

Bushy, A. (2004). Community and public health nursing in rural and urban environments. In M. Stanhope & J. Lancaster (Eds.), *Community and public health nursing* (6th ed., pp. 374–395). St. Louis: Mosby.

Bushy, A. (2007). *Rural nursing practice and issues.* American Nurses Association Continuing Education. Retrieved February, 2007, from http://nursingworld.org/mods/mod700/rurlfull.htm.

Centers for Disease Control and Prevention (CDC). (2001). Preventing and controlling tuberculosis along the U.S.–Mexico border. *Morbidity and Mortality Weekly Report, 50*(RR), 1-2). Retrieved February, 2007, from http://www.cdc.gov/mmwr/preview/mmwrhtml/rr5001a1.htm

Clark, M. J. (2002). *Community health nursing: Caring for populations* (4th ed.). Stamford, CT: Prentice Hall.

Cooper, S. P., Burau, K. E., Frankowski, R., Shipp, E. M., Del Junco, D. J., Whitworth, R. E., Sweeney, A. M., Macnaughton, N., Weller, N. F., & Hanis, C. L. (2006). A cohort study of injuries in migrant farm worker families in South Texas. *Annals of Epidemiology, 16*(4), 313–320.

Cuellar, I. (2002). *Mexican-origin migration in the U.S. and mental health consequences.* JSRI Occasional Paper # 40. The Julian Samora Research Institute, Michigan State University, East Lansing, Michigan.

Denham, S. (2003). Family research reveals a new practice model. *Holistic Nursing Practice, 17*(3), 143–151.

DeToledo, J. C., Palmerola, R. A., & Lowe, M. R. (2003). Health care of illegal immigrants post 9-11. *Epilepsy & Behavior, 4,* 764–765.

Frontier Education Center (2003): Retrieved January 25, 2005, from http://www.frontiers.org/html.

Gamm, L. D., & Hutchison, L. L. (Eds.). (2004). *Rural healthy people 2010: A companion document to Healthy People 2010.* College Station, TX: The Texas A&M University System Health Science Center, School of Rural Public Health, Southwest Rural Health Research Center.

Hartley, D. (2004). Rural health disparities, population health, and rural culture. *American Journal of Public Health, 94* (10), 1675–1677.

Hitchcock, J. E., Schubert, P. E., & Thomas, S. A. (Eds.). (2003). *Community health nursing: Caring in action* (2nd ed.). Clifton Park, NY: Thomson Delmar Learning.

Indiana State Department of Health. (2003). *About the Indiana Rural Health Association.* Retrieved February 21, 2005, from http://www.indianaruralhealth.org/.

Institute of Medicine. (2005). *Quality through collaboration. The future of rural health.* Washington, DC: The National Academies Press.

Krothe, J. S., Flynn, B., Ray, D., & Goodwin, S. (2000). Community development through faculty practice in a rural nurse-managed clinic. *Public Health Nursing, 17,* 264–272.

Leon, E. (2000). *The health condition of migrant farmworkers,* JSRI Occasional Paper #71. The Julian Samora Research Institute, Michigan State University, East Lansing, Michigan. Retrieved February, 2007, from http://www.jsri.msu.edu/RandS/research/ops/oc71abs.html.

Lombardi, G. R. (2001). *Migrant health issues: Dental/oral health services.* Migrant Health Monograph Series

Monograph No. 1. National Center for Farmworker Health, Buda, Texas.

Long, K. A., & Weinert, C. (1999). Rural nursing: Developing the theory base. *Scholarly Inquiry for Nursing Practice: An International Journal, 13*(3), 257–269.

Lyons, M.A. (2003). Partnership for healthier rural communities. *Online Journal of Rural Nursing and Health Care, 2*(2). Available: http://www.rno.org/journal/.

McGuire, S. L. (2002). Occupational health nursing. In S. Clemon-Stone, S. L. McGuire, & D. G. Eigsti (Eds.), *Comprehensive public health nursing. Family, aggregate & community practice* (pp. 706–741). St. Louis: Mosby.

Napolitano, M., & Jones, K. D. (2004). Migrant health issues. In M. Stanhope & J. Lancaster (Eds.), *Community and public health nursing* (6th ed., pp. 794–807). St. Louis: Mosby.

National Center for Farmworker Health (NCFH). (2005). Retrieved February 25, 2005 from http://www/ncfh.org/.

National Center for Farmworker Health (NCFH). (2007). *Facts about farmworkers.* Retrieved February, 2007, from www.ncfh.org.

National Institute of Occupational Safety and Health (NIOSH). (1995). *New directions in the surveillance of hired farm worker health and occupational safety.* Cincinnati, OH: U.S. Department of Health and Human Services.

National Safety Council. (2005*). Hearing loss in agriculture workers.* Retrieved July 27, 2006, from http://www.nsc.org/issues/agri/hearingloss.htm.

Novotny, J. M., McHugh, K., Fitzpatrick, J. J., & Severance, D. (1996). A model for collaboration: The Frances Payne Bolton School of Nursing and the Frontier Nursing Service. (Nursing's bigger tent). *Nursing & Health Care: Perspectives on Community, 17*(5), 247-249.

Office of Management and Budget. (2006). *About the Office of Management and Budget.* Retrieved May 29, 2006, from http://www.whitehouse.gov/omb/organization/index.html

Olade, R. A. (2004). Evidence-based practice and research utilization activities among rural nurses. *Journal of Nursing Scholarship, 36*(3), 220–225.

Rural Information Center Health Service. (2006). Retrieved June 12, 2006 from http://www.nal.usda.gov/ric

Rural Policy Research Institute. (1999). *Taking Medicare into the 21st century: Realities of a post BBA world and implications for rural health care.* Columbia: University of Missouri.

U.S. Census Bureau. (2000). *American fact finder.* Retrieved March 3, 2005, from http://factfinder.census.gov.

U.S. Department of Health and Human Services (USDHHS). (2001). *Bureau of Primary Health Care migrant health program.* Retrieved January 11, 2005, from http://www.bphc.hrsa.gov/migrant/

Vega, W. A., Kolody, B., Aguilar-Gaxiola, S., Alderete, E., Catalano, R., & Caraveo-Anduaga, J. (1998). Lifetime prevalence of DSM-III-R psychiatric disorders among urban and rural Mexican Americans in California. *Archives of General Psychiatry, 55,* 771–778.

Villarejo, D., Lighthall, D., Williams, D., Souter, A., Mines, R., Bade, B., Samuels, S., & McCurdy, S. (2000). *Suffering in silence: A report on the health of California's agricultural workers.* Woodland Hills, CA: The California Endowment.

Wilson, A. H., Pittman, K., & Wold, J. L. (2000). Listening to the quiet voices of Hispanic migrant children about health. *Journal of Pediatric Nursing, 15*(3), 137–147.

BIBLIOGRAPHY

Bushy, A. (2005). Rural nursing practice and issues. *Nevada RNformation, 14*(2), 22–29.

Cudney, S., Craig, C., Nichols, E., & Weinert, C. (2004). Barriers to recruiting an adequate sample in rural nursing research. *Online Journal of Rural Nursing & Health Care, 4*(2). Available: http://www.rno.org/journal/.

Lane, A. J., & Martin, M. (2005). Characteristics of rural women who attended a free breast health program. *Online Journal of Rural Nursing & Health Care, 5*(2). Available: http://www.rno.org/journal/.

Morgan, L. L., & Reel, S. J. (2002). Developing cultural competence in rural nursing. *Online Journal of Rural Nursing & Health Care, 3*(1). Available: http://www.rno.org/journal/.

O'Brien, B. L., Anslow, R. M., Begay, W., Pereira, B. A., & Sullivan, M. P. (2002). 21st century rural nursing: Navajo traditional and western medicine. *Nursing Leadership Forum, 9*(2), 67–73.

Rosenthal, K. (2005). What rural nursing stories are you living? *Online Journal of Rural Nursing & Health Care, 5*(1). Available: http://www.rno.org/journal/.

Ward, L. S. (2003). Migrant health policy: History, analysis, and challenge. *Policy, Politics & Nursing Practice, 4*(1), 45–52.

Weinert, C., Lotts, K. C., & Winters, C. A. (2004). The Center for Research on Chronic Health Conditions: A strategy for enhancing rural nursing research. *Nursing Leadership Forum, 9*(2), 67–73.

RESOURCES

Catholic Migrant Farmworker Network (CMFN)

P.O. Box 50026
Boise, Idaho 83705
Email: cmfn@stpaulsboise.org
Web: http://www.cmfn.org

CMFN is a national organization dedicated to pastoral ministry with migrant and seasonal farmworkers. Founded in 1986, the network operates with the support and collaboration of the Office for the Pastoral Care of Migrants and Refugees of the U.S. Catholic Conference. Stories, current issues related to migrant farm work, and links to other information and resources are available at their Web site.

HealthWeb

Web: http://healthweb.org

HealthWeb, supported by the National Library of Medicine, is a collaborative project of the health sciences libraries of the Greater Midwest Region of the National Network of Libraries of Medicine and those of the Committee for Institutional Cooperation. HealthWeb provides organized access to evaluated noncommercial, health-related, Internet-accessible resources. The Web site, http://healthweb .org/rural, provides links to a wide national collection of rural health resources.

National Advisory Committee on Rural Health and Human Services

c/o Office of Rural Health Policy
Health Resources and Services Administration
5600 Fishers Lane, 9A-55
Rockville, Maryland 20857
301-443-0835
FAX: 301-443-2803
Web: http://www.ruralcommittee.hrsa.gov

The National Advisory Committee on Rural Health and Human Services, a 21-member citizens' panel of nationally recognized experts, provides recommendations on rural health and human services issues to the Secretary of the Department of Health and Human Services.

National Center for Farmworker Health (NCFH)

1770 FM 967
Buda, Texas 78610
512-312-2700; 1-800-531-5120
Email: info@ncfh.org
Web: http://www.ncfh.org

NCFH, a private nonprofit corporation established in 1975, has a mission to improve the health status of farmworker families through the appropriate application of human, technical, and information resources. They have a network of more than five hundred migrant health center service sites in the United States as well as other organizations and individuals serving the farmworker population. Their Web site has information about the life of migrant workers, including their housing problems, work conditions, health problems, and their children.

National Rural Health Association (NRHA)

521 E. 63rd Street
Kansas City, Missouri 64110-3329
816-756-3140
FAX: 816-756-3144
Web: http://www.nrharural.org

The NRHA is a national nonprofit organization that provides leadership on rural health issues. Their mission is to improve the health of rural Americans and populations through appropriate and equitable health care services as well as to assist its members in providing leadership on rural issues through advocacy, communications, education, and research. Their Web site is a resource for initiatives, publications, advocacy, and conferences and events—all relevant to rural health.

Rural Information Center (RIC)

National Agricultural Library
10301 Baltimore Avenue, Room 132
Beltsville, Maryland 20705-2351
1-800-633-7701
FAX: 301-504-5181
Web: http://www.nal.usda.gov

The RIC assists local communities by providing information and referral services to local, tribal, state, and federal government officials; community organizations; libraries; businesses; and citizens working to maintain the vitality of America's rural areas. They provide resources and funding programs relevant to rural health, including planning resources, best practices and case studies, information about free or reduced cost medical programs, funding and program assistance, statistics and data resources, and publications relevant to rural health.

U.S. Department of Health and Human Services, Office of Rural Health Policy

Health Resources and Services Administration
5600 Fishers Lane, 9A-55
Rockville, Maryland 20857
301-443-0835
FAX: 301-443-2803
Web: http://www.ruralhealth.hrsa.gov

The Office of Rural Health Policy is a government office located in the Health Resources and Services Administration, promoting better health care service in rural America by informing and advising the U.S. Department of Health and Human Services on matters affecting rural hospitals and health care, coordinating activities within the department that relate to rural health care, and maintaining a national information clearinghouse.

U.S. Department of Labor, National Farm Workers Jobs Program (NFJP)

U.S. Department of Labor
200 Constitution Avenue NW
Washington, D.C. 20210
1-877-US-2JOBS
Web: http://www.doleta.gov

The NFJP assists migrant and other seasonally employed farmworkers and their families to achieve economic self-sufficiency through job training and other services that address their employment-related needs

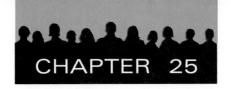

CHAPTER 25

Racial and Ethnic Health Disparities

| Janie Canty-Mitchell, RN, PhD | Barbara Battin Little, RN, DNS |
| Sabrina Robinson, RN, PhD Student | Rasheeta Chandler, RN, PhD Candidate |

Chapter Outline

- **Morbidity and Mortality Trends in Racial/Ethnic Minorities**
  - Diseases of the Heart
  - Cancer
  - Diabetes Mellitus
  - Human Immunodeficiency Virus and Acquired Immune Deficiency Syndrome
  - Perinatal Health Disparities

- **Theoretical Framework of Factors Influencing Racial/Ethnic Minority Disparities**
  - Health Outcomes
  - Population Characteristics
  - Environmental Factors
  - Health Behaviors

- **National Studies, Reports, Initiatives, and Policies to Guide Nursing Interventions**

- **Strategies to Reduce Racial/Ethnic Health Disparities**
  - Assess Population Characteristics
  - Survey Environmental Factors
  - Improve Health Care Access
  - Promote Healthy Behaviors
  - Provide Primary, Secondary, and Tertiary Prevention Strategies

Learning Objectives

Upon completion of this chapter, the reader will be able to:

1. Define key terms: race, ethnicity, minority, and health disparities.

2. Examine specific morbidity and mortality trends in racial/ethnic minorities.

3. Analyze environmental factors, population characteristics, and health behaviors that contribute to racial/ethnic disparities in health outcomes.

4. Critique recommendations from federal agencies and nonprofit organizations for eliminating racial/ethnic health disparities.

5. Evaluate evidenced-based prevention strategies to reduce racial/ethnic minority health disparities.

Eliminating racial and ethnic health disparities is one of the two overarching goals of *Healthy People 2010: Objectives for the Nation* (DHHS, 2000). National, state, and local health providers and policy makers have allocated increased resources to improve health care, health access, treatment, and nursing care to U.S. citizens. These efforts have resulted in an overall improvement in the nation's health, as indicated by declining rates of morbidity and mortality. Despite the success in improving health for all citizens, health disparities persist among racial and ethnic minorities (CDC, 2004a).

Demographic changes in the last decades magnify the importance of addressing racial and ethnic disparities in health and health care. Groups who are currently experiencing poorer health status are predicted to grow in proportion to the total U.S. population (Betancourt, Green, & Ananeh-Firempong, 2003). The 2000 Census data highlighted in Table 25-1 demonstrates that the United States is a racially and ethnically diverse nation (Department of Commerce, 2005). Ethnic and minority populations make up 25 percent of the U.S. population. The Census Bureau projects that in the year 2020 racial and ethnic minorities will increase to 39.2 percent of the population. Higher birth rates and immigration patterns among racial and ethnic minority groups are indicators that the trend of increasing diversity will continue (Department of Commerce, 2005).

Innovative and culturally competent health care, focused public health efforts, and primary prevention programs show the most promise for improving health care and changing lifestyle and behaviors that have resulted in racial and ethnic health disparities. Public health nurses are well suited to (a) synthesize the core public health functions of assessment, health policy, and assurance into clinical practice; (b) plan, implement, and evaluate health promotion programs targeted to racial and ethnic minorities; and (c) collaborate with interdisciplinary teams, community groups, and professional associations to eliminate racial and ethnic health disparities.

Healthy People (HP) 2010 Objectives for the Nation (DHHS, 2000) describes health disparities broadly as "differences [in health status or health care] that occur by gender, race or ethnicity, education or income, disability, geographic location, or sexual orientation (p. 11)." In the Institute of Medicine Report (Smedley, Stith, & Nelson, 2002) health care disparities were described as "differences in quality of healthcare that are not due to access-related factors or clinical needs, preferences, and appropriateness of intervention" (pp. 3–4). The Health Resources and Services Administration (HRSA, 2000), in collaboration with many stakeholders, formulated a definition of health disparities that guided its strategic initiatives to eliminate racial and ethnic health disparities. HRSA defined a health disparity as "a population-specific difference in the presence of disease, health outcomes, or access to health care" (p. 6). The HRSA definition includes both disease and health states, thereby guiding the focus of this chapter.

"Race" and "ethnicity" are terms that have engendered both emotional and intellectual debates. For the

TABLE 25-1: Demographic Profile of the United States: 2000 Census

RACE/ETHNICITY	NUMBER	PERCENT
White	211,460,626	75.1
Black or African American	34,658,190	12.3
Hispanic or Latino (All races)	35,305,818	12.5
Asian	10,242,998	3.6
Native American/Alaskan Native	2,475,956	0.9
Native Hawaiian/Pacific Islander	398,835	0.1
Some other race	15,359,073	5.5
Two or more races	6,826,228	2.4
Total population	281,421,906	100

Note. From Department of Commerce (2005). *U.S. Census 2000.* Retrieved June 1, 2005. from http://www.census.gov/.

TABLE 25-2: U.S. Census Bureau Racial/Ethnic Definitions

RACE/ETHNICITY	DEFINITIONS
Asian	People having origins in any of the original peoples of the Far East, Southeast Asia, or the Indian subcontinent. They include persons who self-identify as "Asian Indian," "Chinese," "Filipino," "Japanese," "Korean," "Vietnamese," "Cambodian," "Hmong," or some other Asian group.
Black or African American	People with origins in any of the black racial groups of Africa. They include people who indicate their race as "Black, African American, or Negro" or provide written entries such as African American, Afro American, Kenyan, Nigerian, or Haitian.
Hispanic or Latino	People who classify themselves in one of the specific Hispanic or Latino categories as: "Mexican, Puerto Rican, Cuban" or those who list themselves as "Other Spanish." Hispanic or Latino origin can be viewed as a heritage, nationality group, lineage, or country of birth of the parents or ancestors before arrival to the United States. People who identify as Spanish, Hispanic, or Latino may be from any race.
Native American and Alaskan Native	People having origins in any of the original peoples of North and South America (including Central America), and who maintain tribal affiliation or community attachment. It includes people who identify themselves as "American Indian," Eskimos, Alaska Indians, or other tribes in the American Indian Detailed Tribal Classification List or in Alaska Native Villages.
Native Hawaiian and Other Pacific Islander	People having origins in any of the original peoples of Hawaii, Guam, Samoa, or other Pacific Islands.
White	People with origins in any of the original peoples of Europe, the Middle East, or North Africa. They include persons who identify as being "white" or report entries such as Irish, German, Italian, Lebanese, Near Easterner, Arab, or Polish.

purposes of this chapter, **race** is a social construct that categorizes an individual or group based on physical and anatomical features, most notably the color of one's skin (Cooper et al., 2002). **Ethnicity** is a cultural construct that categorizes groups of people based on their geographic origins, languages, or cultural similarity in the world. Table 25-1 highlights the number and percentage of the U.S. population by race and ethnicity. Table 25-2 provides the definitions of the various groups as formulated by the U.S. Office of Management and Budget (OMB) for Census 2000 (Department of Commerce, 2005). Census 2000 data assist in calculating morbidity rates, evaluating trends in health status, and monitoring racial and ethnic minority health disparities.

MORBIDITY AND MORTALITY TRENDS IN RACIAL/ETHNIC MINORITIES

Racial and ethnic minorities have a disproportionate burden related to disease, intentional and unintentional injuries, and other health conditions including coronary heart disease, cancer, stroke, diabetes, infant mortality, and HIV/AIDS (DHHS, OMH, 2005). In addition, racial and ethnic minorities have disparate health outcomes associated with asthma, mental illness, homicides, and sexually transmitted diseases (DHHS, OMH, 2005). Several federal agencies conduct surveillance and compile morbidity and mortality reports related to racial and ethnic minority health disparities, as listed in the Resources section of this chapter. Sources of data to monitor health disparities among racial and ethnic minorities include (a) state vital statistics records, (b) hospital discharge data, (c) health utilization data from the Center for Medicare and Medicaid Services (CMS, 2005), and national surveys such as the Behavioral Risk Surveillance Survey and the Youth Health Risk Surveillance Survey (CDC, 2006). For example, the CDC collects data to measure *Healthy People 2010* objectives, including health indicators to monitor the *Healthy People 2010* goal of "eliminating health disparities" (Liao et al., 2004). The National Center for Health Statistics (2006) conducts surveys and compiles epidemiological data on a multitude of health problems, including disparate outcomes related to racial and ethnic minority health disparities.

The Department of Health and Human Services, Office of Minority Health (2005) identified diseases of the heart, all cancers, stroke, and diabetes mellitus as chronic diseases as contributors to the highest numbers of adult deaths in the United States. Rates among minority groups continue to be higher than the white population. There are many identified minority health disparities in health services, health utilization, and health conditions. However, this chapter summarizes only those related to diseases of the heart, cancer, diabetes, HIV/AIDS, and perinatal health disparities. Figure 25-1 illustrates the disparities in age-adjusted mortality rates for coronary artery disease, stroke, and diabetes.

Diseases of the Heart

Diseases of the heart (including coronary heart disease) are the leading cause of death in the United States (AHRQ, 2004; AHA, 2005). Even though age-adjusted mortality rates for heart disease have decreased, African Americans continue to have disparate rates when compared to all other racial/ethnic groups. The Commonwealth Fund Report (McDonough et al., 2004) revealed that gaps in disease, health outcomes, and health utilization related to cardiovascular disease

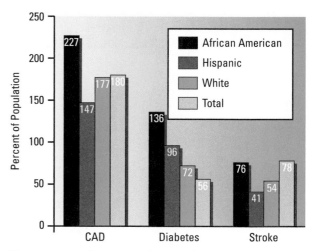

Figure 25-1 Coronary heart disease, stroke, and diabetes mortality rates, 2002.
Note: CAD = Coronary Heart Diseases. CAD and stroke rates are per 100,000 population; diabetes rates are per 1,000 population.
From CDC (2007). *CDC Wonder: Compressed Mortality, 1999-2004 Request.*

depended on the individual's ability to pay, insurance status, and the dynamics of the clinical or institutional settings. However, the majority of studies revealed that racial and ethnic disparities exist in cardiovascular care even after adjusting for confounding variables such as insurance status (McDonough et al., 2004).

Despite overwhelming evidence documenting racial and ethnic differences in cardiovascular care and treatment, Lillie-Blanton and colleagues (2004) reported that national surveys of health providers indicate a lack of awareness of the problem. Fincher et al. (2004) also presented a sociological view of the medical literature on health care provider bias that accounted for racial and ethnic disparities in care of clients with coronary heart disease. These studies provide public health agencies, health providers, policy makers, and voluntary organizations with strategic initiatives to reduce health disparities. These studies reinforce the view that population-focused primary prevention efforts may have the most impact in decreasing racial and ethnic health disparities in cardiovascular morbidity and mortality rates.

Cancer

Researchers have identified health disparities in the incidence of cancer. For example, the incidence rate of cancer is 10 percent higher in African Americans compared to whites. However, the overall cancer mortality rates are 30 percent higher for African Americans compared to whites (McDonough et. al., 2004). Even though Asians and Pacific Islanders on average have indicators that identify them as the healthiest population, women of Vietnamese origin have cervical cancer rates at nearly five times the rate for white women (DHHS, 2000). The Commonwealth Fund Report (McDonough et al., 2004) reported that higher incidences of cancer are due to delayed treatment and inadequate health care for racial and ethnic minorities. Priorities for the nation include interventions and health disparity initiatives to increase cancer screenings, early diagnoses and treatment, and primary prevention efforts for racial and ethnic minorities (AHRQ, 2004; CDC, 2004a, 2004b; DHHS, 2004).

Diabetes Mellitus

Type 2 diabetes mellitus is the sixth leading cause of death in the United States (AHRQ, 2004) and is the leading cause of blindness, end-stage renal disease, and nontraumatic lower extremity amputations (AHRQ, 2004). Mortality rates for diseases of the heart have consistently declined since 2000, but morbidity and mortality rates related to diabetes have increased in all racial and ethnic groups during the same period (CDC, 2004a). Figure 25-2 highlights the increases in diabetes rates between 1998 and 2002 and compares these rates with a *Healthy People 2010* objective related to diabetes. Despite increases in diabetes rates for all groups, African Americans, Hispanics, and Native Americans/ Alaskan Natives have diabetes incidence and mortality rates that are 50 to 100 percent higher than white Americans (AHRQ, 2004; DHHS, 2004; McDonough et al., 2004). Researchers have linked disparate rates of diabetes to factors such as increased body fat and abdominal fat, insulin resistance, and onset of puberty (Abbasi et al., 2002; Burke et al., 2003; Goran, Ball, & Cruz, 2006). Exact mechanisms of how these factors cause diabetes are unknown. Diabetes has reached epidemic proportions in Native Americans and Alaskan Natives, who are 2.6 times more likely to have diagnosed diabetes than white Americans (CDC, 2004a; DHHS, 2005; McDonough et al., 2004). Prevention and management of type 2 diabetes in racial and ethnic minorities is a national concern.

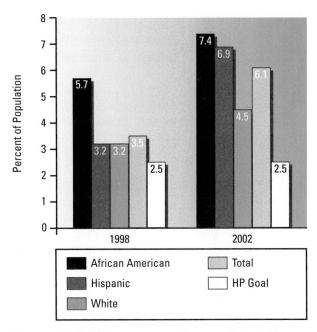

Figure 25-2 Diabetes rates by race/ethnicity compared to Healthy People 2010 objectives, 1998 and 2002.

Human Immunodeficiency Virus and Acquired Immune Deficiency Syndrome

Disproportionate mortality rates are evident among African Americans and Hispanics for 2002. Even though these two racial and ethnic groups make up only 25 percent of the U.S. population, they collectively accounted for 70 percent of newly diagnosed cases. African Americans accounted for 49.6 percent of AIDS cases, even though they account for only 12.3 percent of the U.S. population (CDC, 2006). Table 25-3 summarizes the number and percentage of AIDS cases by race and ethnicity.

Women of African American and Hispanic heritage have disparate rates of AIDS compared to white women, accounting for 83 percent of all new cases in 2003. African American women have higher rates of AIDS than any other racial and ethnic group. The AIDS rate in African American women is 52.2/100,000 compared to rates of 12.4/100,000 in Hispanic women, and 2.0/100,000 in white women (CDC, 2006). Women are more likely than men to become HIV

TABLE 25-3: Number and Percentage of AIDS Cases by Race/Ethnicity

	RACE OR ETHNICITY AIDS CASES (NUMBER) IN 2003	AIDS CASES (%) IN 2003	CUMULATIVE AIDS CASES (NUMBER) THROUGH 2003	CUMULATIVE AIDS CASES (%) THROUGH 2003
Asian/Pacific Islander	497	1.1	7,166	0.8
Black, not Hispanic	21,304	49.6	368,169	40.0
Hispanic	8,757	20.4	172,993	18.8
Native American/ Alaska Native	196	0.5	3,026	0.3
White, not Hispanic	12,222	28.4	376,834	41.0

Note. From Centers for Disease Control and Prevention (CDC). (2006). *Cases of HIV infection and AIDS in the United States, 2000-2004. HIV/AIDS Surveillance Report,* 12(1), 1–35. Available: http://www.cdc.gov/hiv/stats.htm#aidsrace.

infected through heterosexual transmission. In 2003, among 8,733 women who tested positive for HIV at confidential testing sites, heterosexual contact was the source of 80 percent of HIV infections (CDC, 2006). Public health interventions to prevent HIV infection and reduce AIDS related mortality in racial and ethnic minorities must include interdisciplinary and multisector organizations that include public health nurses.

Perinatal Health Disparities

Perinatal health disparities, such as rates of low birth weight and infant mortality, are more prevalent in children born to African American women than to Hispanic or white mothers (CDC, 2002; Martin et al., 2005). Congenital birth defects, conditions related to short gestation and low birth weight, and sudden infant death syndrome (SIDS) are the three leading causes of infant mortality (CDC, 2002). All three causes are higher in infants born to African American women compared to whites or Hispanic women despite the overall improvements in infant mortality rates in the twentieth century.

In 1980, the infant mortality rate was 22.2 per 1,000 live births in African Americans and 10.9 per 1,000 among whites. By the year 2000, these rates had significantly improved for both races, as evidenced in Figure 25-3, to 14 per 1,000 births in African Ameri-

cans and 5.7 per 1,000 live births in whites. Despite these improvements, there are wide gaps or disparities in infant mortality among African Americans and whites, as high as a ratio of 2.5 to 1 infant deaths (CDC, 2002; Martin et al., 2005), as seen in Figure 25-4. A complex set of factors causes infant mortality. Some of these include social and demographic status, risky health behaviors, maternal stress and depression, vaginal infections, and late entry into prenatal care (CDC, 2002, 2004a; Martin et al., 2005). By examining cause-specific differences in rates by race and ethnicity, public health nurses can increase their understanding of infant health disparities, explore interventions to decrease these disparities, and improve the overall health of children.

A major contributor to infant mortality is low-birth weight infants. While infant mortality rates have generally declined over the last 20 years, low-birth weight infant rates per 1,000 live births have increased or remained steady. African Americans have a twofold excess risk of having low-birth weight infants compared to whites (CDC, 2002; Martin et al., 2005). Table 25-4 illustrates the trend in low birth weight among African Americans and whites. In 2004, the rate of low birth weight was 13.7 per 1,000 live births among African Americans and 7.2 per 1,000 live births among whites. If the infant mortality rates among African American women were reduced to the levels of white women,

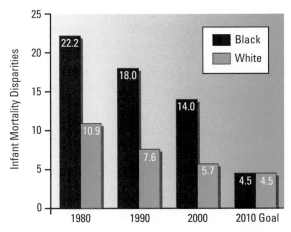

Figure 25-3 Infant mortality disparities between whites and blacks per 1,000 live births.
From CDC (2002). Infant mortality and low birth weight among black and white infants—United States, 1980–2000. *MMWR Morbidity and Mortality Weekly Report, 51*(27), 589–592.

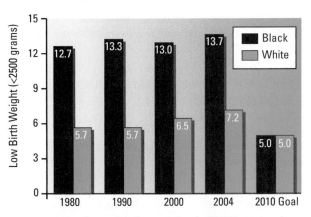

Figure 25-4 Low birth weight (<2500 grams) disparities between whites and blacks per 1,000 live births.
From CDC (2002). Infant mortality and low birth weight among black and white infants—United States, 1980–2000. *MMWR Morbidity and Mortality Weekly Report, 51*(27), and Martin J. A., Hamilton, B. E., Menacker, F., Sutton, P. D., & Mathews, T. J. (2005, November 15). *Preliminary births for 2004: Infant and maternal health.* Hyattsville, MD: NCHS.

U.S. infant mortality rates would be reduced by 44 percent (Matthews, Manacker, & MacDorman, 2003). Clearly, U.S. infant mortality rates are tied to eliminating minority and ethnic health disparities.

The causes of minority health disparities in low birth rates are complex. No one environmental, health-system, or health behavior factor can fully explain causes of disparities in low birth weight. Prior to planning and implementing interventions to address perinatal health disparities, public health nurses must understand and study the population characteristics, environmental factors, and health behaviors that may lead to these distribution and determinants of these disparities. Public health nurses who target interventions

TABLE 25-4: Infant Mortality Rates per 1,000 Live Births by Mother's Race/Ethnicity for 1998 and 2002

MOTHER'S RACE/ETHNICITY	1998	2002
Asian/Pacific Islander	5.5	4.8
Black/African American	13.8	13.8
Hispanic/Latino	5.8	7.0
Native American/Alaskan Native	9.3	8.6
White	6.0	5.8
Total rate	7.2	4.5
Healthy People 2010 Target	4.5	4.5

Note. NCHS (2005). Infant, neonatal, and postneonatal mortality rates, according to detailed race and Hispanic origin of mother: United States selected years 1983–2002. *Health, United States, 2004.* Hyattsville, MD: DHHS.

to minorities with the highest disparities in low-birth weight infants will improve the overall infant mortality for the entire country.

THEORETICAL FRAMEWORK OF FACTORS INFLUENCING RACIAL/ ETHNIC MINORITY DISPARITIES

Policy makers, researchers, epidemiologists, and health providers (including nurses) have identified multiple factors that may contribute to racial and ethnic minority health disparities. Some of these factors include socioeconomic status, cultural beliefs, environment, lifestyle and health behaviors, discrimination and institutional racism, and health care access and utilization (AHRQ, 2004; HRSA, 2000, 2003). Andersen and Davidson (2001) provide a conceptual framework for understanding the factors that may influence health disparities among racial and ethnic minorities. The

authors describe (a) population characteristics, (b) environmental factors, and (c) health behaviors that contribute to health care outcomes. Knowledge of these contributing factors helps to frame public health nursing interventions to eliminate health disparities and assist in achieving *Healthy People 2010 Objectives for the Nation* (DHHS, 2000).

Health Outcomes

Health outcomes included in Andersen and Davidson's model are health access, health utilization, and client satisfaction. Based on national policy reports, health outcomes need to include other factors as well. For the purposes of this chapter, racial and ethnic minority health outcomes include morbidity and mortality rates, incidence of health events (e.g., injuries, teen pregnancies), health access and health utilization (e.g., insurance status, prenatal care, well-child care, emergency room visits), satisfaction with health services,

⊕ PRACTICE APPLICATION

Risks for Low-Birth Weight Infants and Infant Mortality

The infant mortality rate for African Americans in Green County was eight deaths/1,000 live births in 2000 compared to a rate of five deaths/1,000 live births in whites. In 2005, infant mortality among African Americans had increased to 15 deaths/1,000 live births, compared to 5.5/1,000 in whites. Green County had the distinction of having the worse infant mortality rate among African Americans in the United States. Increased and disparate rates of infant mortality between African Americans and white infants produced unwelcome national news for the county.

The State Health Department, in collaboration with the Centers for Disease Control, requested that county health officials develop a plan and strategies to reduce infant mortality among African Americans. The Green County Public Health Department director led the charge to address the infant mortality disparities. Public health nurses, working in collaboration with epidemiologists and community partners, were responsible for assessing population characteristics of all African American infants who died between 2004 through 2005. They were also responsible for conducting interviews with randomly selected mothers whose infants died during this same period. Judy Foster, RN, MSN, director of epidemiological investiga-

tions, assigned team members for selected functions. One team conducted literature reviews to determine the population-based, environmental, and health system factors that contribute to infant mortality. Another team examined the infant birth and death certificates. A third team interviewed women and families whose infants died. A fourth team interviewed health and community partners to determine their perceptions of the predisposing, enabling, and need factors contributing to infant mortality. Results from the epidemiological studies and qualitative interviews will drive health policy changes and health interventions to address the disparate infant outcomes.

Consider the following:

1. What population characteristics would public health nurses assess?

2. What environmental and health system factors contribute to infant mortality?

3. What lifestyle or health behaviors contribute to infant mortality?

4. How does the "weathering effect" contribute to infant mortality?

⊕ RESEARCH APPLICATION

Maternal and Infant Outcomes at One-Year for a Nurse-Health Advocate Home Visiting Program Servicing African Americans and Mexican Americans

Study Purpose

To evaluate the effect of a nurse-health advocate team approach for a home visiting program on the health of mothers and infants.

Methods

A team of registered nurses and trained health advocates conducted home visits to provide health education and case management to mothers and infants.

Findings

Mothers and infants who received home visits compared to families who did not receive home visits had significantly higher rates of immunizations, developmentally

appropriate parenting expectations, and appropriate 12-month infant mental developmental scores.

Implications

Home visiting programs by a nurse-health advocate team can improve maternal and infant outcomes. Effective programs must identify highest risk groups and carefully tailor the culturally appropriate and intensive interventions.

Author

Norr, K. F., Crittenden, K. S., Lehrer, E. L., Reyes, O., Boyd, C. B., Nacion, K. W., et al. (2003). Maternal and infant outcomes at one year for a nurse-health advocate home visiting program serving African Americans and Mexican Americans. *Public Health Nursing, 20*(3), 190–203.

quality of health care, and health-related quality of life (AHRQ, 2004; Andersen & Davidson, 2001; DHHS, 2000). Many of the health outcomes listed here for addressing racial and ethnic minorities are included in *Healthy People 2010 Objectives for the Nation* (DHHS, 2000). Progress toward meeting *Healthy People 2010* objectives (DHHS, 2004) and the elimination of racial and ethnic minority disparities are determined from national surveillance reports, epidemiological studies, funded research, hospital discharge reports, health registries, and national surveys.

Population Characteristics

Andersen and Davidson (2001) describe population characteristics that interact with environmental factors, health system factors, and lifestyle or health behaviors to influence health outcomes. Racial and ethnic health disparities result from complex interactions of these multiple factors. Among population characteristics, Andersen and Davidson postulate that predisposing, enabling, and need factors are specific characteristics that influence health outcomes. Predisposing factors include demographic characteristics such as age, sex,

and race and ethnicity; social structure characteristics such as education, employment, and social support; and health beliefs, such as values and attitudes. Enabling factors are personal and family income, health insurance, health access, and regular source of care and community health personnel and facilities. Need factors are perceived and evaluated need for health services. Perceived needs include the individual, group, or community's perceptions of their health status, health functioning, adherence, and need for services. Evaluated needs include objective measures of the population's health status and treatment provided (Andersen & Davidson, 2001). Population characteristics, such as environmental factors and health behaviors, interact to influence health outcomes in racial and ethnic minorities.

Environmental Factors

In Andersen and Davidson's model, external environmental factors contributing to racial and ethnic health disparities include "economic climate, relative wealth, level of stress and violence, and prevailing norms" of a community (Andersen & Davidson, 2001, p. 14).

Health care system environmental factors are those that may influence access, availability, or acceptance of health care services. Findings from reports such as the Institute of Medicine (Smedley, Stith, & Nelson, 2002), Kaiser Family Foundation (2003), and the Commonwealth Fund (McDonough et al., 2004) indicate that external and health care system environments collectively have contributed greatly to racial and ethnic health care disparities.

The burden of cumulative stressors that accumulate over the life of an individual or group may significantly influence health status and health outcomes (Gee & Payne-Sturges, 2004; Headley et. al., 2004). Headley et al. (2004) term these cumulative stressors the "weathering effect." The authors assert, for example, that chronic morbidity and health disparities in African American women's health status may result from women's "extensive and collective experiences with entrenched social, economic, or political barriers" (Headley et al., 2004, p. 988). Berg, Wilcox, and d'Almada (2001) reinforced this view by noting that long-term deprivation and second-class status, resulting from the effects of racism, cumulative stress, and poverty (or less wealth) may result in cumulative health deterioration, including disparities in perinatal outcomes. The persuasiveness of environmental stress may be an important factor influencing low-birth weight infants and/or infant mortality in women from racial and ethnic backgrounds.

Major influences on external and health system environments are federal, state, and local health policies; available community health resources; organization of services in health care systems; and health care financing (Andersen & Davidson, 2001). Environmental factors influence disparate health outcomes and potentially racial and ethnic health care disparities. Other environmental factors, not included in Andersen and Davidson's conceptual model, that contribute to health outcomes in racial and ethnic minorities include factors such as institutional racism, discriminatory practices in health care settings, and weathering effects (Smedley, Stith, & Nelson, 2002; Papacek et al., 2004).

Health Behaviors

In Andersen and Davidson's conceptual framework, health behaviors include personal health practices and use of health services. Personal health practices are those lifestyle and health risk behaviors that are major contributors to health outcomes. In the *Healthy*

People 2010 document, the leading health indicators include those health behaviors most influenced by lifestyle choices (DHHS, 2000). Personal health practices include tobacco use, substance abuse, physical activity, overweight and obesity, nutritional habits, and responsible sexual behaviors. These are the most amenable to change and most predictive of chronic illnesses within the ten leading causes of death. Reducing racial/ethnic health disparities requires a combination of primary prevention efforts to promote positive health behaviors, environmental and population-focused health initiatives, and quality health and medical care.

Tobacco Use

Cigarette smoking is the leading cause of preventable death and disease in the United States (NCHS, 2006). Smoking is a major risk factor in the leading causes of death such as heart disease, stroke, and cancer (DHHS, OMH, 2005). A current smoker is someone who has smoked 100 cigarettes in their lifetime and reports smoking daily or most days a week (Ahluwalia et al., 2003; CDC, 2002; NCHS, 2006). Smoking is higher among Native Americans with Alaska Natives having the highest rates (DHHS, 2000; GIH, 2003). In one study, the percentage of individuals who smoked ranged from 28.6 to 42.2 percent in African American and Native American communities, respectively (Liao et al., 2004). Smoking among adolescents has increased with 3,000 young people starting each day (DHHS, 2000). In a study by Ellickson et al. (2004), approximately 70 percent of Hispanics and more than 60 percent of African American youths had initiated smoking by the age of 13. *Healthy People 2010 Objectives* state reductions in tobacco use by 12 percent in adults aged 18 years and older and by 19 percent for adolescents in grades 9–12 (DHHS, 2000).

Substance Abuse

Alcohol and illicit drug use are associated with many of the country's most serious diseases including HIV (DHHS, 2000). Binge drinking is having five or more drinks on a single occasion, one or more times in the past 30 days (Ahluwalia et al., 2003; CDC, 2002). Binge drinking is highest among minority males aged 18–24 (Ahluwalia et al., 2003). Buka (2002) states that alcohol and other forms of substance use are associated with diabetes, HIV/AIDS, and liver cirrhosis. Wallace et al. (2002) argue that regardless of the relationship between substance abuse and drug-related consequences, substance use is a great cause of health disparities in minorities. The *Healthy People 2010* objectives, target is to reduce the prevalence of binge drinking and illicit drug use in adults and increase the number of drug- and alcohol-free adolescents aged 12–17 (DHHS, 2000).

Physical Activity

Regular physical activity throughout life is essential in maintaining a healthy body and preventing premature death (DHHS, 2000). Regular physical activity reduces the risk of heart disease, cancer, osteoporosis, and diabetes (NCHS, 2006). In addition, physical activity aids in weight control and loss. Minority populations, particularly African Americans and Hispanics, have the lowest rates of physical activity (Ahluwalia et al., 2003; GIH, 2000). The Racial and Ethnic Approaches to Community Health (REACH) 2010 Risk Factor Survey found the percentage of adults who met physical activity recommendations ranged from 17.3 to 42.9 percent; but when compared with the national average, fewer minority adults met recommendations for moderate or vigorous physical activity (Liao et al., 2004). The *Healthy People 2010* goal is to increase the proportion of adolescents and adults engaging in physical activity by 20 and 15 percent, respectively (DHHS, 2000).

Overweight and Obesity

Overweight and obesity are major risk factors to many preventable causes of death (DHHS, 2000). Overweight and obesity increases the risk of heart disease, hypertension, diabetes, and certain types of cancer (DHHS, 2000; NCHS, 2006). Obesity is more common among members of minority groups. African American and Mexican Americans have a higher prevalence of obesity than their white counterparts. Findings from the National Health and Nutrition Examination Survey (NHANES) indicated that African American and Mexican American children, adolescents, and adults had significantly higher prevalence of overweight and obesity than whites for all ages (Hedley et al., 2004). The *Healthy People 2010* (DHHS, 2000) objective is to reduce the proportion of children and adolescents who are overweight by 6 percent and adults by 8 percent.

Nutritional Habits

Dietary practices that do not allow individuals to get the recommended servings per day predispose certain groups to disease. Minority populations have a higher prevalence of eating unhealthy diets than whites (GIH, 2000). The *National 5-A-Day for Better Health Program* promotes eating five or more servings of fruits and vegetables daily. Results of the REACH 2010 Risk Factor Survey indicated that three-fourths of minorities were not consuming the daily recommendations of fruits and vegetables (Liao et al., 2004). The *Healthy People 2010* objective is to increase the proportion of people two or older who consume at least two servings of fruit, three or more servings of vegetables, and six or more servings of grain or grain products (DHHS, 2000).

Responsible Sexual Behavior

Unprotected sexual behaviors can lead to unintended pregnancies and sexually transmitted diseases including HIV/AIDS (DHHS, 2000). Abstinence is the only method with complete protection. Condoms can be effective if used properly and consistently. Minority groups are more susceptible to having unintended pregnancies and contracting sexually transmitted diseases (STDs) than their white counterparts (DHHS, 2000). Research indicates that women of color are more at risk for HIV due to risky sexual practices such as prostitution, nonuse of condoms, history of STDs, multiple partners, and sex with high-risk partners (Amaro et al., 2001; Sanders-Phillips, 2002). Two *Healthy People 2010* objectives for STDs are to increase the proportion of adolescents who are abstaining from sexual intercourse or using condoms if sexually active and increase the proportion of sexually active individuals who use condoms (DHHS, 2000).

NATIONAL STUDIES, REPORTS, INITIATIVES, AND POLICIES TO GUIDE NURSING INTERVENTIONS

Table 25-5 highlights key policies, reports, and publications that have shaped federal, state, and public health interventions to eliminate racial and ethnic minority health disparities. The landmark IOM Report, *Unequal Treatment: Confronting Racial and Ethnic Disparities in Healthcare* (Smedley, Stith, & Nelson, 2002), documented the extent of racial and ethnic health disparities in the United States, based on a review and synthesis of 175 research publications. The IOM findings indicated that racial and ethnic minorities had lower quality

TABLE 25-5: Landmark Reports, Policies, and Publications Influencing Interventions to Eliminate Racial/Ethnic Health Disparities

PUBLICATIONS	MAJOR EMPHASES
Secretary's Task Force for Black and Minority Health (CDC, 2004a)	Highlighted indicators of racial/ethnic health disparities; recommended creation of an Office of Minority Health in the Department of Health and Human Services (DHHS)
Healthy People 2010 (DHHS, 2000)	Provided national goals, key indicators, and measurable objectives for addressing racial/ethnic health disparities; established base for research, policy, and practice initiatives to address racial/ethnic health disparities
Public Law 106-525: Creation of the National Center on Minority Health and Health Disparities (NCMHD, 2002)	Created the National Center on Minority Health and Health Disparities (NCMHD) in 2000 to serve as a focal point for planning and coordinating minority health and disparities; mandated that NCMHD works with NIH institutes and centers to develop a strategic plan for reducing and eliminating health disparities
Eliminating Health Disparities in the United States (HRSA, 2000)	Addressed strategies to reduce disparities related to diabetes, cardiovascular disease, infant mortality, HIV/AIDS, cancer screening, and immunizations
Unequal Treatment: Confronting Racial and Ethnic Disparities in Health Care (Smedley, Stith, & Nelson, 2002)	Detailed significant variations in the rates of health services and medical procedures by race, even when insurance status, income, age, and severity of conditions are comparable; racial/ethnic minorities are less likely to receive health services or medical procedures and experience a lower quality of health services
Race, Ethnicity, and Health: A Public Health Reader (LaVeist, 2003)	Research publications documenting the environmental, population-focused, health behavior, language, and health system factors influencing minority health; strategies provided to reduce racial/ethnic health disparities
Annual Review of Nursing Research, Eliminating Health Disparities (Villarruel, 2004)	Nursing research to address racial/ethnic health disparities, including race and racism, structural and language barriers, health care access, mental health, immigration, cancer disparities, community partnerships to reduce disparities
A State Policy Agenda to Eliminate Racial and Ethnic Health Disparities (McDonough et al., 2004)	Provided state agencies, policy makers, and health leaders with practical strategies to improve health care coverage, access, and outcomes for racial and ethnic minorities
2004 National Healthcare Disparities Report care (AHRQ, 2004)	Comprehensive national overview of disparities in health among racial, ethnic, and socioeconomic groups in the U.S. population and among priority populations; tracks U.S. progress in eliminating health care disparities
Sullivan Commission on Diversity in the Healthcare Workforce (2004)	Commissioned to address need for diversity in the health care workforce; recommended strategies to increase racial/ethnic minorities in health professions

of health care and worse health outcomes, even when racial/ethnic minorities had similar health care access, insurance status, and income. Racial and ethnic minorities were also less likely to receive health services, pharmacological therapies, and medical procedures than nonminorities.

The IOM report discussed health disparities in the context of broader historic, contemporary, social, and economic inequalities, including the persistence of racial and ethnic discrimination in many sectors of American life. Many sources are contributors to racial and ethnic disparities in health care, including health systems, health care providers, clients, and utilization managers. Research findings supported the bias, stereotyping, prejudice, and clinical uncertainty on the part of health care providers that have contributed greatly to racial and ethnic disparities in health care (Smedley, Stith, & Nelson, 2002).

Public health nurses, working in collaboration and partnership with professional, community, and health service organizations are in key positions to assess racial and ethnic minorities and implement primary, secondary, and tertiary measures to reduce health disparities. Strategic initiatives from the Centers for Disease Control and Prevention (CDC; 1999, 2004a), NCMHD (2002), DHHS (2004), and the DHHS Office of Minority Health (2001, 2005) provide frameworks for national, state, and county-level health interventions.

STRATEGIES TO REDUCE RACIAL/ETHNIC HEALTH DISPARITIES

The DHHS (2004) proposed a public health framework for eliminating health disparities that includes environmental, psychosocial, cultural, as well as health system factors to guide interventions. For example, the CDC targets interventions to reduce disparate health outcomes associated with cardiovascular diseases, cancer, stroke, diabetes, HIV/AIDS, and low birth weight or preterm delivery (DHHS, 2004; Hogan et al., 2001). The IOM Report has also provided recommendations for reducing racial and ethnic health disparities, as highlighted in Table 25-6. The preceding reports, in addition to the Andersen and Davidson's (2001) model, will provide the framework for discussing public health nursing interventions. The Andersen and Davidson model includes key components of the DHHS framework and the IOM recommendations.

Assess Population Characteristics

Andersen and Davidson (2001) address multiple population-related characteristics that influence health outcomes, including predisposing, enabling, and need factors. How and in what context could public health nurses assess these population characteristics in racial and ethnic minority populations? The predisposing, enabling, and need factors can be used to guide public health nurses in assessing characteristics of populations at risk. Predisposing factors that public health nurses could assess include the existing social structure, and educational and employment status of racial and ethnic populations (Abbasi et al., 2002; Goran, Geoff, Ball, & Cruz, 2006). In assessing enabling factors, public health nurses would focus on social support systems, income level or social economic status, and availability of insurance among racial and ethnic populations. Need factors that public health nurses would assess include racial and ethnic populations' perceptions of the need for health services, health education, or health promotion programs, and their beliefs, values, and attitudes about obesity, nutrition, and physical activity. Finally, it is important for public health nurses to assess racial and ethnic populations' level of satisfaction with and acceptance of existing sources of health information, accessing health services, and health education/health promotion programs targeted for them.

Conduct Participatory Action Research and Evaluation

Public health nurses are engaged in both qualitative and quantitative methods to evaluate the effectiveness of initiatives and strategies to improve health outcomes among racial and ethnic minorities. Public health nurses in the role of health advocacy can influence the inclusion of community members in the design, implementation, and evaluation of health disparity interventions or initiatives. **Participatory action research (PAR)** is one method that has been successful with public health nurses. Evaluators who use PAR view targeted populations as collaborators instead of research subjects. PAR has bridged gaps between public health leaders, educators, and the community; created more trust between groups and a greater understanding of community perceptions; decreased evaluator bias and stereotyping; and improved implementation and evaluation of health disparity initiatives (Hughes & Seymour-Rolls, 2000; Jackson et al., 2001). Strategies for involving

TABLE 25-6: Recommendations to Reduce Racial/Ethnic Disparities

General Recommendations

1. Increase awareness of racial/ethnic disparities in health care among key stakeholders.

2. Increase health care providers' awareness of disparities.

Legal, Regulatory, and Policy Interventions

1. Avoid fragmentation of health plans along socioeconomic lines.

2. Strengthen the stability of client-provider relationships in publicly funded health plans.

3. Increase the proportion of underrepresented U.S. racial and ethnic minorities among health professionals.

4. Apply the same managed care protections to publicly funded HMO enrollees that apply to private HMO enrollees.

5. Provide greater resources to the U.S. Department of Health and Human Services Office of Civil Rights to enforce civil laws.

Health System Interventions

1. Promote the consistency and equity of care through evidenced-based guidelines.

2. Structure payment systems to ensure an adequate supply of services to minority clients and limit provider incentives that may promote disparities.

3. Enhance client-provider communications and trust by providing financial incentives for practices that reduce barriers and encourage evidenced-based practice.

4. Support the use of interpretation services where community need exists.

5. Support the use of community health workers.

6. Implement multidisciplinary treatment and preventive care teams.

Education and Empowerment

1. Integrate cross-cultural education into the training of all current and future health professionals.

Data Collection and Monitoring

1. Collect and report data on health care access and utilization by client's race, ethnicity, socioeconomic status, and, where possible, primary language.

2. Include measures of racial and ethnic disparities in performance measurement.

3. Monitor progress toward the elimination of health care disparities.

4. Report racial and ethnic data by federally defined categories, but use subpopulation groups where possible.

Research Needs

1. Conduct further research to identify sources of racial and ethnic disparities and assess promising intervention strategies.

2. Conduct research on ethical issues and other barriers to eliminating disparities.

Note. From Smedley, B. D., Stith, A. Y., & Nelson, A.R. (eds). (2002). *Unequal treatment: confronting racial and ethnicminorities in healthcare, pp. 6-22.* Washington, DC: Institute of Medicine, National Academy Press.

community members include the creation and use of community advisory boards, community focus groups, and public meetings.

Evaluation is a needed component for addressing the effectiveness of health disparity initiatives and interventions at the primary, secondary, or tertiary levels. Evaluation measures include community or population-based satisfaction with health services, perceptions of health care access, perceived effectiveness of community agencies to implement coordinated services, effectiveness of health disparity policies and initiatives, changes in health policy, improvements in health status indictors, lower morbidity and mortality rates, and increased health care access and utilization among racial and ethnic minority populations.

As public health nurses plan, implement, and evaluate health programs for racial and ethnic minority populations, consideration of the multiple influences on health disparities is vital. Collaboration with health professionals and partnerships with racial and ethnic minority communities are increasingly important to the success of public health nursing interventions and research in eliminating health disparities (Portillo & Waters, 2004).

Survey Environmental Factors

Health providers often do not consider environmental interventions in addressing racial and ethnic minority health disparities. Environmental interventions must consider the larger system of society in which racial and ethnic minorities live and work. The limited social and environmental resources available to racial and ethnic minority populations compared to the majority culture influences the compliance with health care provider's recommendations by racial and ethnic populations (Hogan et al., 2001; Lu & Halfon, 2003). Public health nurses can work with the larger community to address sources of urban and community stress for specific minorities and promote efforts to increase community resources, including jobs, adequate housing, adequate child care, a safe and healthy environment, domestic violence shelters, and social services (Lu & Halfon, 2003).

Public health nurses, working in collaboration with health providers and public health agencies, can collaborate with social advocates and community change agents to inform public policy makers on the environmental and social hazards and stressors that affect minority health. Addressing the larger social issues will require working with social services, economic development councils, housing authorities, school readiness coalitions, child care agencies, educational agencies, and environmental health agencies. Increasing interagency and interdisciplinary collaborations to improve integration of services, eliminate environmental hazards, and improve environmental stressors is one of the major strategic objectives to reduce racial and ethnic minority health disparities (Lu & Halfon, 2003). Public health nurses working in partnership with health, social, and community groups can address external environmental hazards through changes or additions in environmental health policies at local, state, and national levels.

Improve Health Care Access

Many racial/ethnic minorities lack access to health care. Delays in seeking health care by racial and ethnic minorities, often caused by limited or no insurance coverage, are one of many factors leading to health disparities (AHRQ, 2004). Even with some insurance coverage, certain health care components (i.e., health screenings) may be inadequately covered by private or public insurance (Lu & Halfon, 2003). In addition, insurance eligibility may be inconsistently applied. For example, in certain states, women eligible for Medicaid during pregnancy are not eligible for family planning services after 60 days postpartum (CMS, 2005). Increasing family planning services to include contraceptive care may help to prevent subsequent pregnancies, provide well-women exams, and screen and treat women for vaginal infections—a primary risk factor for low-birth weight infants.

Insurance coverage for racial and ethnic minorities increases potential access to health screening and early treatment of health problems like diabetes, coronary heart disease, and HIV/AIDS. However, in the absence of public or private health insurance, communities can mobilize to provide health education and health promotion programs, conduct health screenings, and apply for funding to improve access to primary and public health services. Public health nurses can conduct mass screenings and case finding to detect cardiovascular disorders, diabetes, HIV/AIDS, cancer, and mental health problems. Early screening and testing for health disorders are important for making early diagnoses, providing health care treatment, and decreasing health disparities among racial and ethnic minorities (CDC, 2004a; McDonough et al., 2004).

Advocate for Expansion of Mental Health Services

Research indicates that cumulative stressors negatively affect physical and mental health, lifestyle choices and behaviors, and quality of life in children and adults (Headley, 2004; Siantz & Keltner, 2004). Public health nurses as consultants, advocates, health providers, collaborators, and change agents are in positions to assess mental health services within minority communities. They also play key roles in planning, implementing, and evaluating strategies to reduce environmental and psychosocial stressors among racial and ethnic minorities. Improving mental health is a collaborative effort that includes partnerships with public health nurses, health care providers, school nurses, primary care providers, neighborhood groups, and voluntary and faith-based organizations. Community and faith-based organizations, voluntary and social service agencies, public health departments, hospitals, and health professionals are in positions to expand the mental health services and support for racial and ethnic minorities. Public health nurses as advocates can influence health policy decisions to include mental health screenings as a component of all individual, family, and population-based assessments.

Promote Culturally Competent Services

Hernandez and Isaacs (1998) provided four reasons why it is important to provide culturally competent public health services. First, cultural competence brings attention to the important role of culture in the lives of all people. Second, the term connotes that all health providers are in need of becoming culturally competent. Third, cultural competency places an emphasis on people of all racial and ethnic groups becoming culturally competent. Fourth, culturally competent care is a means of improving the effectiveness of physical and mental health outcomes.

Culture refers to integrated patterns of human behavior that include the language, thoughts, communications, actions, customs, beliefs, values, and institutions of racial, ethnic, religious, or social groups (DHHS, OMH, 2001). **Competence** is the capacity to function effectively as an individual and an organization within the context of the cultural beliefs, behaviors, and needs presented by populations and their communities (DHHS, OMH, 2001). **Cultural competence** is a set of congruent behaviors, attitudes, and policies that come together as a system or agency or among professionals and enable that system, agency, or professionals to work effectively in cross-cultural situations (Cross et al., 1989). **Linguistic competence** is the capacity of an organization and its personnel to communicate with persons of limited English proficiency, those who are illiterate or have low literacy skills, and individuals with disabilities.

Public health nurses are in pivotal positions to collaborate and form partnerships with others in the provision of culturally competent care at local, state, and national levels. Strategies could include the promotion and use of bilingual and bicultural staff, cultural brokers, multilingual telecommunication systems, ethnic media in languages other than English, low-literacy and easy-to-read print materials, health literature formatted with pictures and symbols, and health information in alternative formats (Goode & Jones, 2003). The report, *National Standards for Culturally and Linguistically Appropriate Health Services in Health Care* (DHHS, OMH, 2001) provides additional strategies for promoting competence. In addition, the *Compendium of Culturally Competent Initiatives in Healthcare* (Kaiser Family Foundation, 2003) is another resource for use by public health nurses.

Although no one single intervention can reduce health disparities, strong evidence supports the use of culturally and linguistically competent health care providers as a strategy in addressing racial and ethnic minority health disparities (Goode & Harrison, 2000; HRSA, 2000, 2003). Public health nurses are leaders in providing culturally competent care to racial and ethnic minority populations.

Promote Healthy Behaviors

Health risk behaviors are indicators of future health problems. Public health nurses, working within communities, can increase efforts to target lifestyle and health behaviors that lead to coronary heart disease, diabetes, HIV/AIDS, and infant mortality. Health promotion and health education, using participatory action research methods, could be used to develop culturally appropriate and effective health messages to promote healthy behaviors, including lifestyle changes related to food and nutrition, exercise, sexual decision making, and health-seeking behaviors (Portillo & Waters, 2004). Launching health literacy programs may also help to improve utilization of health services and per-

⊕ PRACTICE APPLICATION

Eliminating Disparities

Eliminating health disparities in racial and ethnic minority groups will require multiple strategies that address the population characteristics, environmental factors, and health behaviors. Public health nurses can address these factors on the local, state, and national level through partnerships with community groups. Examples of partnerships may include (a) becoming involved on task forces and advisory boards, (b) assessing population characteristics from focus groups and community organizations, (c) planning and implementing health promotion programs to address health behaviors, (d) advocating for environmental health improvements, and (e) engaging in participatory action research.

sonal health behaviors. For example, the *Folic Acid Campaign, Back to Sleep Campaign*, and teen pregnancy prevention programs helped to improve infant health indicators (CDC, 2002). Public health nurses can plan, implement, and evaluate innovative initiatives to improve nutrition, exercise, and weight control; increase responsible sexual decision making; and improve health-seeking practices in racial and ethnic minorities.

Provide Primary, Secondary, and Tertiary Prevention Strategies

In their multiple roles, public health nurses are engaged in primary, secondary, and tertiary prevention strategies to reduce racial and ethnic minority health disparities. **Primary prevention strategies** aim to reduce the likelihood of susceptibility and incidence of diseases, health conditions, or poor health outcomes in minorities. **Secondary prevention strategies** target early diagnosis and early intervention to prevent premature deaths, disabilities, or injuries. **Tertiary prevention strategies** aim to prevent the further progression or deterioration of a disease, illness, or health problems within minority populations. All of these preventive strategies must also take into account the population characteristics, environmental factors, and health behaviors that act as barriers to minority participation and acceptance of services.

Primary Prevention Strategies

Modifiable risk factors for racial and ethnic minorities include physical inactivity, obesity, poor nutritional habits, and smoking. Bowman and colleagues (2003) documented interventions to reduce modifiable risk behaviors that resulted in decreasing the incidence of Type 2 diabetes. Primary prevention interventions included activities to change modifiable risk factors such as nutrition and weight management; exercise, physical activity, and training; stress management; and smoking cessation. Knowler and colleagues (2002) with the Diabetes Research Group found that lifestyle interventions, including increased physical exercise, weight loss, and reduced fat intake, reduced the risk of diabetes by 58 percent for all race and ethnic populations. Evidenced-based risk-reduction health promotion programs are resources that public health nurses can use to reduce minority health disparities at local, state, and national levels.

⊕ POLICY HIGHLIGHT

Addressing Disparities

In fiscal year 2005, Congress allocated $34.5 million for the CDC's *Racial and Ethnic Approaches to Community Health* (REACH) 2010 program. The REACH 2010 program conducts surveillance and funds projects to eliminate disparities in cardiovascular disease, immunizations, breast and cervical cancer screening and management, diabetes, HIV/AIDS, and infant mortality. The racial and ethnic groups targeted by REACH 2010 are African Americans, American Indians, Alaska Natives, Asian Americans, Hispanics, and Pacific Islanders. Public health nurses working in partnership with community groups can apply for funding or advocate for increased funding to address health disparities in their local communities.

Secondary Prevention Strategies

Screening programs are the best examples of secondary prevention. Based on published research and epidemiological data, secondary prevention measures are most effective in reducing mortality and disparate health outcomes in minority populations. Examples of secondary prevention measures for racial and ethnic minorities include some of the following:

1. Providing culturally appropriate and sensitive population-based assessments
2. Providing yearly physical examinations
3. Performing screening tests (e.g., cholesterol, glucose, HIV, mammogram)
4. Providing case management for acute and chronic illnesses
5. Screening for mental health problems and physical and psychosocial stressors
6. Referring to mental health services for assistance in dealing with family, social, or community stressors
7. Collaborating with health and community groups to market screening programs
8. Educating racial and ethnic minority populations on health risks and behaviors associated with chronic diseases
9. Advocating for health reimbursements to provide mass screening to minority communities

Tertiary Prevention Strategies

Finally, tertiary prevention strategies focus on managing symptoms, providing effective treatment, and preventing further complications such as diabetes-related neuropathies. In the management of type 2 diabetes in racial and ethnic minorities, tertiary prevention strategies include nursing case management, culturally competent family-focused interventions to reduce health risks, stress management, therapeutic communications, and yearly preventive health visits for other health conditions.

CRITICAL THINKING ACTIVITIES

1. Distinguish between the terms race and ethnicity.
2. What national and state surveillance data measure racial and ethnic health disparities?
3. Analyze morbidity and mortality data for your community or state. What racial and ethnic disparities exist in infants and children, adolescents, and adults?
4. What are examples of population characteristics, environmental, and behavioral factors that contribute to racial and ethnic health disparities?
5. Describe at least six historical events, publications, or health policies that influenced interventions to reduce health disparities.
6. What are primary, secondary, and tertiary prevention strategies targeted at individuals, populations, and systems to prevent or reduce racial/ethnic minority health disparities in a community?
7. How could public health nurses collaborate with other community agencies and groups to reduce racial/ethnic health disparities in your community?

KEY TERMS

competence	evaluated needs	health disparities
cultural competence	external environmental factors	health outcomes
culture	health behaviors	linguistic competence
enabling factors	health care disparities	need factors
environmental factors	health care system environmental factors	participatory action research (PAR)
ethnicity		

KEY TERMS (CONT'D)

perceived needs

perinatal health disparities

personal health practices

population characteristics

predisposing factors

primary prevention strategies

race

secondary prevention strategies

tertiary prevention strategies

KEY CONCEPTS

⊕ Health behaviors that influence racial and ethnic minority health disparities include factors such as alcohol and tobacco use, sexual habits, nutrition, exercise, and obesity.

⊕ National studies, commissioned reports and publications, and health policies have influenced efforts to eliminate racial and ethnic minority health disparities.

⊕ Public health nurses work in partnership with other community-based agencies and groups to implement innovative health disparity initiatives, guided by findings and recommendations from national reports and theoretical models.

⊕ Public health nurses provide primary, secondary, and tertiary level interventions to eliminate disparities among minority and ethnic populations.

⊕ Racial and ethnic minorities have a disproportionate burden related to disease and other health conditions, including coronary heart disease, cancer, stroke, diabetes, infant mortality, HIV/AIDS, sexually transmitted diseases, asthma, mental illness, and intentional and unintentional injuries.

⊕ Andersen and Davidson's conceptual model explains relationships among health disparities and population characteristics, environmental factors, and health behaviors that contribute to health outcomes in racial and ethnic minorities.

REFERENCES

Abbasi, F., Brown, W., Lamendola, C., McLaughlin, T., & Reaven, G. M. (2002). Relationship between obesity, insulin resistance, and coronary artery disease risk. *Journal of the American College of Cardiology, 40*(5), 937–943.

Agency for Healthcare Research and Quality (AHRQ). (2004). *2004 National healthcare disparities report: Advancing excellence in health care.* Rockville, MD: Author. Available: www.ahrq.gov.

Ahluwalia, I. B., Mack, K. A., Murphy, W., Mokadad, A. H., & Bales, V. S. (2003). State-specific prevalence of selected chronic diseases-related characteristics—Behavioral Risk Factor Surveillance System. *MMWR Surveillance Summary, 52,* 1–8.

Amaro, H., Raj, A., Vega, R. R., Mangione, T. W., & Norville Perez, L. (2001). Racial/ethnic disparities in the HIV and substance abuse epidemic: Communities responding to the need. *Public Health Reports, 116,* 464–448.

American Heart Association (2005). *Heart disease and stroke statistics: 2005 Update.* Dallas, Texas: American Heart Association. Available: http://www.americanheart.org/.

Andersen, R. M., & Davidson, P. L. (2001). Improving access to health care in America: Individual and contextual indicators. In R. M. Andersen, T. H. Rice, & G. F. Kominski, *Changing the U.S. Health Care System,* 2nd ed. (pp. 3–30). San Francisco: Jossey-Bass.

Anderson, L. M., Scrimshaw, S. C., Fullilove, M. T., Fielding, J. E., Normand, J., & the Task Force on Community Preventive Services. (2003). Culturally competent healthcare systems: A systematic review. *American Journal of Preventive Medicine, 24*(3S), 68–79.

Berg, C. J., Wilcox, L. S., & d'Almada, P. J. (2001). The prevalence of socioeconomic and behavioral characteristics and their impact on very low birth weight in black and white infants in Georgia. *Maternal Child Health Journal, 5*(2), 75–84.

Betancourt, J. R., Green, A. R., & Ananeh-Firempong, O. (2003). Defining cultural competence: A practical framework for addressing racial/ethnic disparities in health and health care. *Public Health Reports, 118,* 293–302.

Bowman, B. A., Gregg, E. W., Williams, D. E., Engelgau, M. M., & Jack, L. (2003). Translating the science of primary, secondary, and tertiary prevention to inform the public health responses to diabetes. *Journal of Public Health Management Practice, 9* (November Supplement), S8–S14.

Buka, S. L. (2002). Disparities in health status and substance use: Ethnicity and socioeconomic factors. *Public Health Reports, 117*(supplement 1), S118–S125.

Burke, J. P., Williams, K., Narayan, K. M. V., Leibson, C., Haffner, S. M.,& Stern, M. P. (2003). A population perspective on diabetes prevention. *Diabetes Care, 26*(7), 1999–2004.

Centers for Disease Control and Prevention (CDC). (1999). *REACH 2010 Risk Factor Survey.* Retrieved June 26, 2006, from http://wonder.cdc.gov/

Centers for Disease Control and Prevention (CDC). (2002). Infant mortality and low birth weight among black and white infants—United States, 1980–2000. *MMWR Morbidity and Mortality Weekly Report, 51*(27), 589–592.

Centers for Disease Control and Prevention (CDC). (2004a). Health disparities experienced by racial/ethnic minority populations. *Morbidity and Mortality Weekly Report, 53*(33), 755-782.

Centers for Disease Control and Prevention (CDC). (2004b). Breast and cervical cancer screening among Korean women-Santa Clara County, California 1994–2002. *Morbidity and Mortality Weekly Report, 53*(33), 765–767.

Centers for Disease Control and Prevention (CDC). (2006). Cases of HIV infection and AIDS in the United States, 2000-2004. *HIV/AIDS Surveillance Report, 12*(1), 1–35. Available: http://www.cdc.gov/hiv/stats.htm#aidsrace.

Centers for Disease Control and Prevention (CDC). (2007). CDC Wonder: Compressed Mortality, 1999-2004 Request. Retrieved September 7, 2007 from http://wonder.cdc.gov/cmf-icd10.html

Centers for Medicare and Medicaid Services (CMS). (2005). *State Medicaid Programs.* Retrieved June 11, 2005, from http://www.cms.hhs.gov/medicaid/statemap.asp.

Cooper, L. A., Hill, M. N., & Powe, N. R. (2002). Designing and evaluating interventions to eliminate racial and ethnic disparities in health care. *Journal of General Internal Medicine 17,* 477–486.

Cross T. L., Barzon, B. J., Dennis, K. W., & Issacs, M. R. (1989). *Towards a culturally competent system of care: A monograph on effective services for minority children who are severely emotionally disturbed.* Washington, DC: CASSP Technical Assistance Center, Georgetown University Child Development Center.

Culhane, J. F., Rauh, V., McCollum, K. F., Hogan, V. K., Agnew, K., & Wadhwa, P. D. (2001). Maternal stress is associated with bacterial vaginosis in human pregnancy. *Maternal and Child Health Journal, 5*(2), 127–134.

Department of Commerce (2005). *U.S. Census 2000.* Retrieved June 1, 2005, from http://www.census.gov/.

Department of Health and Human Services (DHHS). (2000). *Healthy People 2010 objectives for the nation.* Washington, DC: U.S. Government Printing Office. Available: http://www.healthypeople2010.gov.

Department of Health and Human Services (DHHS). (2004, July). *The initiative to eliminate racial and ethnic disparities in health.* Retrieved May 10, 2006, from http://raceandhealth.hhs.gov.

Department of Health and Human Services, Office of Minority Health (DHHS, OMH). (2001). *National standards for culturally and linguistically appropriate services in health care: Final report.* Retrieved June 27, 2006, from http://www.omhrc.gov/clas/.

Department of Health and Human Services, Office of Minority Health (DHHS, OMH). (2005). *Programs and Services.* Retrieved June 11, 2006, from http://www.omhrc.gov/.

Ellickson, P. L., Orlando, M., Tucker, J. S., & Klein, D. J. (2004). From adolescence to young adulthood: Racial/ethnic disparities in smoking. *American Journal of Public Health, 94*(2), 293–299.

Fincher, C., Williams, J. E., MacLean, V., Allison, J. J., Kiefe, C. I., & Canto, J. (2004). Racial disparities in coronary heart disease: A sociological view of the medical literature on physician bias. *Ethnicity and Disease, 14*(3): 360–371.

Gee, G. C. & Payne-Sturges, C. (2004). Environmental health disparities: A framework for integrating psychosocial and environmental concepts. *Environmental Health Perspectives, 112*(17), 1645–1653.

Goode, T. D., & Harrison, S. (2000). *Policy brief 3: Cultural competence in primary health care: Partnerships for a research agenda.* Washington, DC: National Center for Cultural Competence, Georgetown University Center for Child and Human Development. Retrieved June 27, 2006, from http://www.georgetown.edu/research/gucdc/nccc/ncccpolicy3.html.

Goode, T. D., & Jones, W. (2003). *A definition of linguistic competence.* Washington, DC: National Center for Cultural Competence, Georgetown University Center for Child and Human Development. Retrieved June 27, 2006, from www.georgetown.edu/research/gucdc/nccc/framework.html#lc.

Goran, M., Ball, G. D., & Cruz, M. L. (2006). Obesity and Risk of Type 2 Diabetes and Cardiovascular Disease in Children and Adolescents. *Journal of Clinical Endocrinology & Metabolism, 88*(4), 1417–1427.

Grantmakers in Health (GIH). (2000). *Strategies for reducing racial and ethnic disparities in Health.* Retrieved June 27, 2006, from http://www.gih.org/usr_doc/Issue_Brief_5.pdf.

Headley, A. J. (2004). Generations of loss: Contemporary perspectives on black infant mortality. *Journal of the National Medical Association, 96*(7), 987–994.

Hedley, A. A., Ogden, C. L., Carroll, M. D., Curtin, L. R., & Flegal, K. M. (2004). Prevalence of overweight and obesity among U.S. children, adolescents, and adults, 1999–2002. *JAMA, 291*(23), 2847–2850.

Health Resources and Services Administration. (2000). *Eliminating disparities in the United States.* Retrieved June 11, 2005, from: http://www.hrsa.gov.

Health Resources and Services Administration, Bureau of Health Professions (2003, Spring). *Changing Demographics: Implications for Physicians, Nurses, and Other Health Workers.* Retrieved June 11, 2005, from: http://www.hrsa.gov.

Hernandez, M., & Isaacs, M. R. (1998). *Promoting cultural competence in children's mental health services.* Baltimore: Paul H. Brookes Publishing.

Hogan, V. K., Richardson, J. L., Ferre, C. D., Durant, T., & Boisseau, M. (2001). A public health framework for addressing black and white disparities in preterm delivery. *Journal of American Medical Women's Association 56*(4), 177–180, 205.

Hughes, I. & Seymour-Rolls, K. (2000). Participatory Action Research: Getting the Job Done. *Action Research E-Reports, 4.* Available: http://www.fhs.usyd.edu.au/arow/arer/004.htm.

Jackson, F. M., Phillips, M., Hogue, C. J., Curry-Owens, T., et al. (2001). Examining the burdens of gendered racism: Implications for pregnancy outcomes among college-educated African American women. *Maternal Child Health Journal, 5*(2), 95–107.

Kaiser Family Foundation. (2003). *Compendium of cultural competence initiatives in healthcare.* Retrieved June 27, 2006, from http://www.kff.org/content/2003/6067/.

Knowler, W. C., Barrett-Conner, E., Fowler, S. E., Hamman, R. F., Lachin, J. M., Walker, E. A., & Nathan, D. M.; Diabetes Prevention Research Group. (2002). Reduction in type 2 diabetes with lifestyle intervention or metformin. *New England Journal of Medicine, 346*(6), 393–403.

LaVeist, T. A. (Ed.). (2002). *Race, ethnicity, and health: A public health reader.* San Francisco: Jossey-Bass.

Liao, Y., Tucker, P., Okoro, C. A., Giles, W. H., Mokdad, A. H., & Bales Harris, V. (2004). REACH 2010 surveillance for health status in minority communities—United States, 2001–2001. *MMWR Surveillance Summaries, 53*(SS06), 1–36.

Lille-Blanton, M., Maddox, T. M., Rushing, O., & Mensah, G.A. (2004). Disparities in cardiac care: Rising to the challenge of Healthy People 2010. *Journal of the American College of Cardiology, 44*(3): 503–508.

Lu, M. C., & Halfon, N. (2003). Racial and ethnic disparities in birth outcomes: a life-course perspective. *Maternal and Child Health Journal, 7*(1), 13–30.

March of Dimes. (2003). *Low birth weight.* Retrieved June 27, 2006, from http://www.marchofdimes.com/professionals/681_1153.asp

Martin, J. A., Hamilton, B. E., Menacker, F., Sutton, P. D., & Mathews, T. J. (2005, November 15). *Preliminary births for 2004: Infant and maternal health.* Hyattsville, MD: National Center for Health Statistics.

Matthews, T., Manacker, F., & MacDorman, M. (2003). Infant mortality statistics from the 2001 period linked birth/infant death data set. *National Vital Statistics Report, 52*(2) 1-27.

McDonough, J. E., Gibbs, B. K., Scott-Harris, J. L., Kronebusch, K., Navarro, A. M., & Taylor, K. (2004, June). *A state policy agenda to eliminate racial and ethnic health disparities.* Available: http://www.cmwf.org.

National Center on Minority Health and Health Disparities (NCMHD). (2002). *Strategic research plan and budget to reduce and ultimately eliminate health disparities: Fiscal years 2002–2006.* Bethesda, MD: Department of Health and Human Services.

National Center for Health Statistics (NCHS). (2005). Infant, neonatal, and postneonatal mortality rates, according to detailed race and Hispanic origin of mother: United States, selected years 1983–2002. *Health, United States, 2004.* Hyattsville, MD: Department of Health and Human Services.

National Center for Health Statistics (NCHS). (2006). *Health, United States, 2005.* Hyattsville, MD: Department of Health and Human Services.

Norr, K. F., Crittenden, K. S., Lehrer, E. L., Reyes, O., Boyd, C. B., Nacion, K. W., et al. (2003). Maternal and infant outcomes at one year for a nurse-health advocate home visiting program serving African Americans and Mexican Americans. *Public Health Nursing, 20*(3), 190–203.

Papacek, E., Collins, J., Jr., Schulte, N., Goergen, C., & Drolet, A. (2002). Differing postneonatal mortality rates of African-American and white infants in Chicago: An ecologic study. *Maternal and Child Health Journal, 6*, pp. 99–105.

Portillo, C. J., & Waters, C. (2004). Community partnerships: The cornerstone of community health research. *Annual Review of Nursing Research, 22:* 315–329.

Sanders-Phillips, K. (2002). Factors influencing HIV/AIDS in women of color. *Public Health Reports, 117*(Supplement 1), S151–S156.

Siantz, M. L. & Keltner, B. R. (2004). Mental health and disabilities: What we know about racial and ethnic minority children. *Annual Review of Nursing Research, 22*, 265–281.

Smedley, B. D., Stith, A. Y., & Nelson, A. R. (eds.). (2002). *Unequal treatment: confronting racial and ethnic minorities in healthcare.* Washington, DC: Institute of Medicine, National Academy Press.

Sullivan Commission on Diversity in the Healthcare Workforce (2004). Retrieved June 27, 2006, from http://www .sullivancommission.org.

Villarruel, A.M. (2004). Introduction: Eliminating health disparities among racial and ethnic minorities in the United States. *Annual Review of Nursing Research, 22,* 1-6.

Wallace, J. M., Bachman, J. G., O'Malley, P. M., Johnston, L. D., Schulenberg, J. E., & Cooper, S. M. (2002). Tobacco, alcohol, and illicit drug use: Racial and ethnic differences among U.S. high school seniors, 1976–2000. *Public Health Reports, 117*(Supplement 1), S67–S75.

BIBLIOGRAPHY

American Institutes for Research. (2002). *Teaching cultural competence in health care: A review of current concepts, policies and practices.* Report prepared for the Office of Minority Health. Washington, DC: Author.

American Lung Association. (2004). *Trends in asthma morbidity and mortality.* Retrieved February 1, 2005, from http://www.lungusa.org/atf/cf/{7A8D42C2-FCCA-4604-8ADE-7F5D5E762256}/ASTHMA1.pdf.

Burnes, B. L., Giger, J. N., & Georges, C. A. (2004). Structural and racial barriers to health care. *Annual Review of Nursing Research, 22,* 39–58.

Centers for Disease Control and Prevention (CDC). (2002). *2001 BRFSS summary prevalence report.* Retrieved January 25, 2005, from http://www.cdc.gov/brfss/pdf/2001.prvrpt.pdf.

Centers for Disease Control and Prevention (CDC). (2002). *National diabetes surveillance system: Data and trends.* Retrieved January 25, 2005, from http://www.cdc.gov/diabetes/statistics/index.htm

Collins, J., David, R., Symons, R., Handler, A., Wall, S., & Dwyer, L. (2000). Low-income African-American mothers' perception of exposure to racial discrimination and infant birth weight. *Epidemiology, 11*(3), 337–339.

Collins. R., & Winkleby, M. A. (2002). African American women and men at high and low risk for hypertension: A signal detection analysis of NHANES III, 1988–1994. *Preventive Medicine, 35*(4), 303–312.

Eschiti, V. S. (2004). Holistic approach to resolving American Indian/Alaska Native health care disparities. *Journal of Holistic Nursing, 22*(3), 201–208.

Eschiti, V. S. (2005). Cardiovascular disease research in Native Americans. *Journal of Cardiovascular Nursing, 20*(3), 155–161.

Esperat, M. C., Inouye, J., Gonzalez, E. W., Owen, D. C., & Feng, D. (2004). Health disparities among Asian

American and Pacific Islanders. *Annual Review of Nursing Research, 22,* 135–159.

Goode, T. D., & Dunne, C. (2003). *Policy brief 1: Rationale for cultural competence in primary care.* Washington, DC: National Center for Cultural Competence, Georgetown University Center for Child and Human Development. Retrieved October 24, 2003, from http://www.georgetown.edu/research/gucdc/nccc/documents/Policy_Brief_1_2003.pdf.

Grantmakers in Health (GIH). (2003). *Promoting Healthy Behaviors in Erasing the Color Line Report.* Retrieved January 22, 2005, from http://www.gih.org/usr_doc/Erasing_the_Color_Line_Report.pdf.

Hogan, V. K., & Ferre, C. D. (2001). The social context of pregnancy for African American women: Implications for the study and prevention of adverse perinatal outcomes. *Maternal and Child Health Journal, 5*(2), 67–69.

Kaiser Family Foundation. (1999). *Key Facts Race, Ethnicity & Medical Care.* Retrieved October 24, 2003, from http://www.org/content/1999/1523/KEY%20FACTS%20BOOK.pdf.

Kendall, J., & Hatton, D. (2002). Racism as a source of health disparity in families with children with attention deficit hyperactivity disorder. *Advances in Nursing Science, 25*(2): 22–39.

Mattson, S. (2000). Striving for cultural competence: Providing care for the changing face of the U.S. *AWHONN Lifelines, 4*(3), 48–52.

Mayberry, R.M., Mili, F., & Ofili, E. (2002). Racial and ethnic differences in access to medical care. In T.A. LaVeist, Ed., *Race, ethnicity, and health: A public health reader* (pp. 163–197). San Francisco, CA: Jossey-Bass.

McMahon, G. F., Fujioka, K., Singh, B. N., Mendel, C. M., Rowe, E., Rolston, K., Johnson, F., & Mooradian, A. D. (2000). Efficacy and safety of sibutramine in obese white and African American patients with hypertension: A 1-year, double-blind, placebo-controlled, multicenter trial. *Archives of Internal Medicine, 160*(14), 2185–2191.

Murray, L. R. (2003). Sick and tired of being sick and tired: Scientific evidence, methods, and research implications for racial and ethnic disparities in occupational health. *American Journal of Public Health, 93* (2): 221–226.

National Center for Cultural Competence. (2002). *Health Disparities among Ethnic and Racial Groups.* Washington, DC: Georgetown University Center for Child and Human Development. Retrieved October 24, 2003, from http://www.georgetown.edu/research/gucdc/nccc/cultural6.html.

National Institute of Nursing Research (2005). *Strategic plan on reducing health disparities.* Available: http://ninr.nih .gov/ninr/research/diversity/mission.html.

Randall, V. R. (1999). *Other factors affecting health status*. Available: http://academic.udayton.edu/health/08civilrights/01-02-07Environmental.htm.

Siegal, S., Moy, E., & Burstin, H. (2004). Assessing the nation's progress toward elimination of disparities in health care. *Journal of General Internal Medicine, 19*, 195–200.

Stone, J. (2002). Race and healthcare disparities: Overcoming vulnerability. *Theoretical Medicine, 23*, 499–518.

Underwood, S. M., Powe, B., Canales, M., Meade, C. D., & Im, E. O. (2004). Cancer in U.S. ethnic and racial minority populations. *Annual Review of Nursing Research, 22*, 217–263.

Ward, E., Jemal, A., Cokkinides, V., Singh, G. K., Cardinez, C., Ghafoor, A., & Thun, M. (2004). Cancer disparities by race/ethnicity and socioeconomic status. *CA: A Cancer Journal for Clinicians, 54*(2): 78–93.

Wise, P. H. (2003). The anatomy of a disparity in infant mortality. *Annual Review of Public Health, 24*, 341–362.

Yancy, C. W. (2004). The prevention of heart failure in minority communities and discrepancies in health care delivery systems. *Medical Clinics of North America, 88*(5), 1347–1368.

Yeo, S. (2004). Language barriers and access to care. *Annual Review of Nursing Research, 22*, 59–73.

Zambrana, R. E., & Carter-Pokras, O. (2004). Improving health insurance coverage for Latino children: A review of barriers, challenges, and state strategies. *Journal of the National Medical Association, 96*(4), 508–523.

RESOURCES

Agency for Healthcare Research and Quality (AHRQ)

John M. Eisenberg Building
540 Gaither Road, Suite 2000
Rockville, Maryland 20850.
Web: http://www.ahrq.gov

AHRQ is the federal agency charged with improving the quality, safety, efficiency, and effectiveness of health care for all Americans. The agency supports health services research that will improve the quality of health care and promote evidence-based decision-making. AHRQ invests about 80 percent of its budget in grants and contracts focused on improving health care. The agency conducts and supports research on health care for ethnic and racial minority and other priority populations, as one of its mandates.

⊕ Cultural Competency Works Agency for Healthcare Research and Quality
Web: ftp://ftp.hrsa.gov/financeMC/cultural-competence.pdf

This AHRQ document outlines successful practices in delivering culturally competent care including (a) to define culture broadly, (b) to value clients' cultural beliefs, (c) to recognize the complexity in language interpretation, (d) to facilitate learning between providers and communities, (e) to involve the community in defining and addressing service needs, (f) to collaborate with other agencies, (g) to participate in professional staff training, and (h) to institutionalize cultural competence.

⊕ Minority Health Agency for Healthcare Research and Quality
Web: http://www.ahrq.gov

This Web site contains multiple resources for health care researchers, health care providers, and policy makers to address racial and ethnic minority heath disparities, including research documents, requests for proposal, and summaries of funded research.

Centers for Disease Control and Prevention (CDC)

Office of Minority Health (OMH)
1600 Clifton Road
Atlanta, Georgia 30333
404-639-3311
Public Inquiries: (404) 639-3534/ 1-800-311-3435
Web: http://www.cdc.gov

OMH works closely with state, tribal, and local governments, as well as nonprofit organizations to improve health status and eliminate health disparities among Americans of all racial and ethnic groups through policy and practice.

Centers of Disease Control and Prevention (CDC)

Racial and Ethnic Approaches to Community Health (REACH)
4770 Buford Highway NE
Atlanta, Georgia 30341-3717
Web (CDC): http://www.cdc.gov
Web (REACH): http://www.cdc.gov/reach2010/index.htm

CDC is the principal agency in the United States for implementing health promotion strategies to sustain and improve the health of all Americans. The REACH program is a federal initiative that has a goal of eliminating racial and ethnic disparities in health by the year 2010.

Department of Health and Human Services

Minority Women's Health
The National Women's Health Information Center
1-800-994-9662
Web: http://www.4woman.gov

Minority women often have poorer health outcomes than white women. This Web site contains data and related information on the common health risks and concerns of minority women.

Department of Health and Human Services

National Center on Minority Health and Health Disparities (NCMHD)
National Institutes of Health
6707 Democracy Boulevard, Suite 800
Bethesda, Maryland 20892-5465
301-402-1366
FAX: 301-480-4049
Web: http://www.ncmhd.nih.gov
Information Requests: NCMHDinfo@od.nih.gov
NCMHD promotes minority health and leads the National Institute of Health's effort to reduce and ultimately eliminate health disparities. The center supports basic, clinical, social, and behavioral research, promotes research infrastructure and training, fosters emerging programs, and disseminates information to minority and minority serving communities.

Department of Health and Human Services

Office of Minority Health (OMH)
The Tower Building
1101 Wootton Parkway, Suite 600
Rockville, Maryland 20852
1-240-453-2882
FAX: 1-240-453-2883
OMH Resource Center
P.O. Box 37337
Washington, D.C. 20013-7337.
1-800-444-6472.
Web: http://www.omhrc.gov
OMH improves and protects the health of racial and ethnic minority populations through the development of health policies and programs that will eliminate health disparities. It funds grants to address racial and ethnic minority health disparities. Several health disparities initiatives are coordinated by the OMB, including (a) Closing the Gap on Infant Mortality, (b) Minority HIV/AIDS, (c) Community Initiatives to Eliminate Stroke Disparities, and (d) Obesity Abatement in African Americans Campaign.

Health Resources and Services Administration (HRSA)

5600 Fishers Lane
Rockville, Maryland 20857
Web: http://www.hrsa.gov
HRSA is a federal agency whose primary goal is to improve access to health care services for people who are uninsured, isolated, or medically vulnerable. One of the agency's strategic objectives is to eliminate health care disparities. The agency provides funding for initiatives and programs to reduce health care disparities and to increase the pool of racial/ethnic minorities in the health care professions.

The Henry J. Kaiser Family Foundation

Key Facts: Race, Ethnicity and Health Care (#6069)
2400 Sand Hill Road
Menlo Park, California 94025
1-650-854-9400
FAX: 1-650- 854-4800
Web (for foundation): http://www.kff.org
Web (for publication): http://www.kff.org/minorityhealth
The Henry J. Kaiser Family Foundation is an independent, national health philanthropy dedicated to providing information and analysis on health issues to policymakers, the media, and the public. The publication, *Key Facts: Race, Ethnicity, and Medical Care*, is intended to serve as a quick reference source on the health, health insurance coverage, healthcare access and quality among racial/ethnic minority groups in the United States.

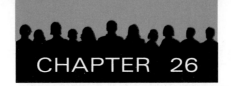

CHAPTER 26

Immigrant and Refugee Populations

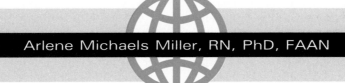

Arlene Michaels Miller, RN, PhD, FAAN

Chapter Outline

⊕ Global Migration Patterns
Trends in Population Movement
Immigration Policies

⊕ Premigration Factors That Affect Health in Immigrants
Socioenvironmental Conditions in Country of Origin
Traumatic Migration Experiences

⊕ Postmigration Factors That Affect Health in Immigrants
Acculturation, Acculturative Stress, and Resilience
Community Context
Workforce and Socioeconomic Issues

⊕ Health Problems with Special Implications for Immigrants and Refugees
Communicable Diseases
Effects of Social Violence, Torture, and Human Trafficking

⊕ Planning and Implementing Care for Immigrants and Refugees

Learning Objectives

Upon completion of this chapter, the reader will be able to:

1. Discuss the impact of recent trends in global migration and immigration policy on the delivery of health care to vulnerable populations.

2. Identify potential long-term effects of premigration factors on health and health care for immigrants and refugees.

3. Discuss the complex interactions among acculturation, community context, socioeconomic status, and postimmigration health.

4. Describe important considerations for assessing health problems to which immigrants and refugees are at particularly high risk.

5. Utilize historical, cultural, and postimmigration factors to plan and implement appropriate health care services and interventions for immigrant and refugee populations.

Global migration has generated an unprecedented amount of ethnic and cultural diversity in many developed countries during the past few decades. In the United States as well as other countries, this phenomenon has created many unique challenges to health services and nursing practice. As public health agencies serve increasingly diverse constituencies, cultural competence has become an essential skill for health care providers. Clients may have premigration experiences that are difficult for providers to comprehend, diseases and health problems that are uncommon in this country, and minimal understanding of this complex and sophisticated health care system. Communication with clients may require specialized language and cultural interpreters (culture brokers) to ensure understanding and establish relationships. Although it is impossible for nurses and other health care providers to master every culture or language, understanding trends in migration, processes of adaptation, risk and resilience patterns, and approaches to developing interventions that are applicable across ethnic and cultural groups comprise an important foundation for public health nursing practice with immigrants and refugees.

GLOBAL MIGRATION PATTERNS

The United Nations High Commissioner for Refugees (UNHCR, 2000) estimates that approximately 150 million people live temporarily or permanently outside their native countries. Although this number represents only about 2.5 percent of the population of the world, recent trends indicate that virtually all developed countries in the world have become destinations of choice for migrants (persons and/or family members moving to another country or region to better their material or social conditions and improve the prospect for themselves or their family).

In addition, the patterns of migration have changed significantly in the past few decades. Immigrants (people who move to a country permamently) to North America during the first half of the twentieth century were most likely to come from European countries. In the years since World War II, several new waves of migration have occurred, during which the predominant source of immigrants (sending countries) shifted.

Trends in Population Movement

Since 1960, emigration from Africa, Asia, and Latin America and the Caribbean has exceeded that from Europe, with most refugees from Southeast Asia arriving after the Vietnam War. Other recent trends include refugees from Eastern Europe following the fall of the Soviet Union in 1991, and immigrants from Middle Eastern and other countries who seek greater social, economic, and political stability. Mexico leads the list of sending countries, and Afghanistan, the Philippines, Pakistan, China, and Colombia are among the others that have high numbers of emigrants—people who leave one country to move permanently to another (Martin & Midgley, 2003).

Countries in Western and Eastern Europe such as Germany and the former Soviet Union, sources of high numbers of emigrants in the past, have now become receiving countries. In some of these receiving countries, population composition is changing more rapidly than existing policies and resources for newcomers. Even in countries with long histories of accepting immigrants and refugees, the effects of accommodating large numbers of people who have unfamiliar cultures requires tremendous effort on the part of health care providers and agencies. In addition, in countries like the United States, many immigrants who are racially similar to dominant groups (i.e., Caucasian) comprise invisible minorities due to their ethnicity and language and may have little understanding of prevailing cultural norms.

The United States and Canada have traditionally had high rates of immigration. The United States is currently accepting more refugees than any other country in the world. The number of immigrants living in the United States tripled during the past 30 years, and immigrants now comprise close to 12 percent of the population. The 32.5 million immigrants who lived in the United States in 2002 accounted for an unprecedented number in U.S. history (Schmidley, 2003), and the Census Bureau estimates that over a million people immigrate annually (Horrigan, 2004). Further, the countries from which refugees emigrate are more diverse than ever. According to the U.S. Office of Refugee Resettlement (2005), 73,851 refugees arrived from over 40 different countries in 2004.

A relatively new phenomenon known as transnationalism reflects fluidity of travel between sending and receiving countries. This is exemplified by (though not limited to) the movement of Mexican-Americans between the United States and Mexico. The United States-Mexico border is recognized as one of the busiest in the world. There are 43 points of entry on the border between the two countries. Every day, more than 800,000 people cross this border, in addition to illegal immigrants who may risk death due to harsh environmental conditions and unscrupulous guides. The United States-Mexico Border Health Commission (USMBHC) was created in 2000 to serve people who reside within 62 miles of this international boundary line. It provides international leadership to optimize health and quality of life along the United States-Mexico border. The health problems that affect the border region have serious repercussions for both nations. Travelers, migrants, and immigrants who cross the border take their health problems with them to other parts of the United States and Mexico. These problems include communicable diseases such as HIV/AIDS and tuberculosis, as well as chronic illnesses such as diabetes, certain cancers, hypertension, and respiratory and gastrointestinal ailments (USMBHC, 2005).

Immigration Policies

All countries have regulations regarding the movement of people from other nations, including passports, visas, and other documents required of travelers as well as immigrants. National policies regarding immigrants tend to divide them into three groups: migrant workers, permanent residents or immigrants, and refugees. Immigration policies may be influenced by special interest groups such as employers and ethnic or humanitarian groups that support immigration, as well as unions and members of the general public who fear loss of jobs, overpopulation, and a drain on national resources. In the United States, policies such as the Refugee Protection Act of 2001 were led by proponents of human rights to assist resettlement of refugees and facilitate permanent resident status and self-sufficiency. More restrictive laws regarding entry of immigrants and refugees were introduced more recently, however, in response to terrorist events such as the September 11, 2001, attack on the World Trade Center in New York City.

The great majority of people who leave their countries of birth are migratory or seasonal workers and their families. A large number are low or unskilled laborers, workers who move, either invited or illegally, to work seasonally in agricultural, mining, and construction jobs (Martin & Midgely, 2003). This international phenomenon is growing as workers are increasingly recruited from poorer countries to those with wealthier economic status. Some are skilled workers whose movement to better developed countries comprises a "brain-

drain" of professionals, many of whom were trained to provide health care in their home countries.

It is estimated that there are 9.3 million undocumented immigrants in the United States, representing approximately one-quarter of the foreign-born population. They have entered or remained in the United States without approval of the Immigration and Naturalization Service. Slightly more than half of the undocumented immigrants are Mexican. Virtually all undocumented men are believed to be in the U.S. labor force, but they and their families are not eligible for health care benefits. Babies born in the United States of undocumented parents become U.S. citizens and are eligible for health services, but their mothers do not receive subsidized prenatal care. Because of their fear of being deported, many undocumented immigrants avoid health care or other public agencies (Passel, Capps, & Fix, 2004; Smith, 2001). Studies suggest that stress regarding legal status contributes to poorer self-reported health (Finch & Vega, 2003).

Although voluntary migration is usually precipitated by a wish for family reunification or improved educational and economic opportunities, the decision to migrate is complex. The initial decision to migrate, when made for economic reasons, is often viewed as a temporary move during which workers will save or send money to family members. Individuals who enter a country as temporary workers or students, however, often end up settling as permanent residents and citizens over time. In the United States, the need for foreign labor to participate in jobs unwanted by citizens will continue to be salient as the population ages and fewer people are capable or interested in taking jobs viewed as less appealing. Migration most commonly occurs from rural to urban locations. Most immigrants are young adult men because families are less likely to make international moves.

Refugees comprise a subset of immigrants who are forced or compelled to leave their countries or communities. Refugees differ from immigrants in that they fear persecution in their home country because of their ethnicity, religion, or political beliefs (Martin & Midgely, 2003). A refugee is defined by the United Nations as a person who, "owing to well-grounded fear of being persecuted for reasons of race, religion, nationality, membership in a particular social group, or political opinion, is outside the country of his nationality and is unable or, owing to such fear, is unwilling to avail himself of the protection of that country" (Bevilacqua, 1983, p. 38).

Approximately 12 million refugees worldwide are presently living outside of their native homeland.

Refugees are eligible for certain services not provided to other immigrants. However, asylum seekers are required to apply for asylum within one year of arriving in the United States. Many refugees are not aware of this policy, and others are not ready to testify within one year because they have experienced traumatic and emotional consequences of abuse in their country of origin (Keller, 2001).

PREMIGRATION FACTORS THAT AFFECT HEALTH IN IMMIGRANTS

Most people prefer to stay in their own countries when they can do so with "safety, dignity, and well-being" (International Labour Office et al., 2001, p. 5). Migration can usually be conceptualized as the result of two categories of factors: push factors and pull factors. Push factors include negative home conditions that impel the decision to migrate, such as loss of job, lack of professional opportunities, overcrowding, famine, war, and disease. Pull factors are positive attributes perceived to exist at the new location, such as better climate, more professional opportunities, better jobs, lower taxes, and more space. People tend to immigrate to countries and communities in which there are already known family members, ethnic neighborhoods, or enclaves of others from their homeland and a need for skilled or unskilled labor. It is important to know about the history and premigration context of individuals and groups as part of the nursing assessment when planning an intervention.

Socioenvironmental Conditions in Country of Origin

Health problems of temporary workers, immigrants, and refugees may occur as a result of socioenvironmental events prior to immigration, including lack of health care services. People from developing countries are at risk for illnesses that result from poverty and malnutrition as well as endemic infectious diseases. Immigrants and refugees may bring health problems that are common in their native country but unusual in the country to which they are migrating. For example, racial and ethnic disparities in later birth outcomes may arise out of prior stressors such as social relationships, housing and nutrition, and discrimination that serve as health risks throughout life (Lu & Halfon, 2003). Further, immigrant and refugee women may have had few opportunities for reproductive health care or cancer screening (Barnes & Harrison, 2004).

Premigration circumstances in countries of origin and reasons for migration may have implications for health care in later life. For example, in addition to coming from a country with the highest rates of cardiovascular disease in the world, 80 percent of all recent Soviet immigrants to the United States are from areas that were most exposed to radiation by the 1986 Chernobyl nuclear power plant disaster and subsequent clean-up efforts. They may have an increased risk for cancer and leukemia, which emphasizes a need for cancer screening in this population.

Traumatic Migration Experiences

Refugees flee their countries of origin for several reasons: they may be victims of natural disasters, warfare, and/or political change. Forced migration refers to compulsory transfer of a group of people, usually by a government. Impelled migration is similar to forced migration but differs in that migrants retain some ability to decide whether to move or not. Refugees are most likely to have been victims of human rights violations. The Universal Declaration of Human Rights is a declaration adopted by the United Nations General Assembly in 1948. Some of these abuses include lack of equal treatment due to race or religion, cruel or unusual punishment such as torture, lack of a fair trial, and denial of freedom of speech (UNHCR, 2005a). They may have experienced social disruption, economic deprivation, and physical violence.

The process of migration, particularly for refugees who lived in temporary camps and shelters, can have a significant long-range impact on health. Families may be separated with loss of the ability to support themselves financially, and children may be sent with strangers to ensure escape to a better country (Fazel & Stein, 2002).

POSTMIGRATION FACTORS THAT AFFECT HEALTH IN IMMIGRANTS

Many complex factors have an impact on mental and physical health after immigration. Understanding the unique social, political, historical, and economic context in which immigrants and refugees live is important for understanding and planning public health nursing services and interventions.

Acculturation, Acculturative Stress, and Resilience

Acculturation is a dynamic process of understanding or adopting specific aspects or characteristics of a new culture. "Acculturation" is a term used broadly to include language, behavior, identity, and values that are maintained or changed when someone comes into contact with another culture. Language acculturation includes, for example, quality of communication skills. Behavioral acculturation is related to adoption of observable aspects of the dominant culture, including lifestyle actions that represent cultural preferences (Berry, 2005). Identity involves the unique integration of two or more ethnicities and implies a sense of belonging as well as commitment to a cultural group that may become part of one's self-concept (Phinney, 2003). Values provide meaning and direction to postmigration life and also affect attitudes toward health and illness.

American culture is continuously being shaped by social processes such as migration. One of the difficulties in assessing acculturation is the lack of consensus regarding the ways to measure this concept, as well as difficulty defining mainstream or dominant "Western" or "American" culture. More research is needed to identify the characteristics of the culture to which new immigrants acculturate since countries like the United States are increasingly characterized by diversity in values, attitudes, beliefs, and behaviors. Although initially viewed by sociologists as a relatively unidimensional process culminating in assimilation to the dominant culture, it is now understood that bicultural or multicultural individuals may be highly acculturated to the mainstream culture while retaining aspects of other cultures (Willgerodt, Miller, & McElmurry, 2002). For some immigrants, acculturation may not be to a mainstream culture but to a new hybrid culture (such as Mexican-American) that has unique characteristics and has developed as a phenomenon of immigration.

Berry's (2005) acculturation framework takes into account both group and individual phenomena. Strategies utilized in the adaptation process can create acculturative stress, which is defined broadly as any stressor that is linked to the acculturation process. According to Berry, individuals decide to what extent they want to maintain their cultural identity and characteristics and to what extent they want to participate in the host society. These decisions result in one of four adaptation or acculturative strategies: assimilation, integration, separation, or marginalization. Assimilation is a strategy in which individuals do not continue to value their native cultural identity and wish to take on only the attributes of the new culture. Separation occurs when individuals avoid those customs of the new culture and value retaining their original culture exclusively. In integration, there is some degree of retention of original culture, while people seek to participate in the new culture as well. Marginalization occurs where there is little possibility or interest in either culture. He believes that integration, an acculturation attitude that is similar to the concept of biculturalism, is most highly related to the best outcomes in terms of health and adjustment.

Some immigrant groups have health profiles that appear to be better than those of the host country shortly after immigration. For example, some foreign-born adults had better ratings on selected health indicators such as self-assessed health than their U.S.-born counterparts (Dey & Lucas, 2006). Similarly, Singh and Siahpush (2002) found that immigrants had lower rates of cardiovascular disease (CVD) than native-born U.S. citizens. One of the most striking and unexpected patterns in terms of health outcomes has been called the Hispanic paradox. Despite socioeconomic and educational disadvantages compared to non-Hispanics, birth outcomes are more favorable among first-generation immigrant Hispanics. This phenomenon has been found particularly among those of Mexican origin. Cultural orientation is a significant predictor of infant birth weight, even after prenatal maternal behaviors such as diet and smoking are considered. Protective factors such as social support networks, healthy dietary practices, and maternal attitudes have been studied and believed to mitigate the adverse effects of poverty and acculturative stress (McGlade, Saha, & Dahlstrom, 2004). The increase in poorer birth outcomes among U.S.-born, compared to Mexican-born, women is attributed in part to negative effects of acculturation.

A decline in health status has been found for some immigrants as the length of time in their new country increases. This has been interpreted to mean that newly acquired conditions are in part responsible (Finch & Vega, 2003; Rubia, Marcos, & Muennig, 2001). When

⊕ RESEARCH APPLICATION

Predictors of Sexual Intercourse and Condom Use Intentions among Spanish-Dominant Latino Youth: A Test of the Planned Behavior Theory

Study Purpose

To identify factors that predict sexual intercourse and condom use for a sample of Latinos who use Spanish as their dominant language.

Methods

Participants were 141 adolescents aged 12–18 (77 girls and 64 boys) who enrolled in a larger intervention study intended to reduce the risk of sexually transmitted HIV in Latino adolescents. Questionnaires included items regarding acculturation level, as well as attitudes, beliefs, and behavior regarding use of condoms and sexual activity.

Findings

The majority of the participants had low scores on the acculturation scale. Attitudes, norms, and beliefs predicted sexual activity and condom use. Compared to U.S. adolescents in the general population, the Latino youth were less likely to report ever engaging in sexual intercourse. Those who were sexually active, however, were less likely to report using a condom during their last sexual experience.

Implications

Interventions need to target adolescents who are more likely to become sexually active as their acculturation levels increase. Also, adolescents who are less acculturated but *do* participate in sexual activity may be at higher risk than their more acculturated peers. The study demonstrates the complex impact of acculturation on health behaviors and the importance of considering acculturation levels for specific behavioral interventions for Latino adolescents.

Author

Villarruel, A. M., Jemmott, J. B., Jemmott, L. S., & Ronis, & D. L. (2004). Predictors of sexual intercourse and condom use intentions among Spanish-dominant Latino youth: A test of the planned behavior theory. *Nursing Research, 53*(3), 172–181.

people abandon previous behaviors that protected their health, behavioral acculturation may be a risk factor for poor health practices, chronic diseases, and mental health problems (Satia et al., 2001). For some ethnic groups, acculturation in the United States has been shown to reduce diet quality and increase selected health problems, including alcohol consumption, obesity, hypertension, and diabetes mellitus (Goel et al., 2004). Cardiovascular disease risk factor prevalence may be high in some immigrant groups on arrival, but it also tends to increase with acculturation and length of time in the United States (Jonnalagadda & Diwan, 2005; Rubia, Marcos, & Muennig, 2001).

Another example that demonstrates a postimmigration decline in health status is the increase in overall cancer rates among immigrants of various countries of origin to become similar to the majority population (Myers & Rodriguez, 2003). It is not clear why these

rates increase, although increased exposure to shared environmental risk factors, as well as changes in dietary habits have been suggested (Arcia et al.., 2001). In addition, immigrants tend to have lower participation in cancer screening activities (Goel et al., 2003).

On the other hand, increased levels of acculturation might improve the health of immigrants from countries with less well-developed health care systems by improving health knowledge. For example, higher acculturation was related to increased leisure physical activity for Mexican-Americans and Asian Indian immigrants (Crespo et al., 2001; Jonnalagadda & Diwan, 2005), and a better CVD risk profile for immigrants from the former Soviet Union (Miller et al., 2004).

Acculturation is a process that unfolds over a relatively extended period of time and generates secondary stressful life events. It may therefore be considered a source of chronic stress (Lazarus & Folkman, 1984).

The impact of acculturative stress contributes to immigrants' increased risk for mental illness and various other psychological health outcomes. Acculturative stressors are those that are directly related to the acculturation process. They include language barriers, financial instability, and social problems such as minority discrimination (Balcazar & Qian, 2000). Depression is potentially one of the most debilitating and common problems for immigrants, particularly among the elderly (Gonzalez, Haan, & Hinton, 2001).

Immigrants and refugees face **xenophobic** (rejection, fear, and stigmatization of foreigners) and **racist** (discrimination of a group of individuals based on racial and ethnic identities, cultures, language, religion, or national origin) reactions in their new countries. Other postimmigration stressors include the loss or absence of strong social support networks. Informal social supports that existed in the country of origin may no longer exist. Ethnic social support contexts are considered to be resources to combat acculturative stress as well as the effects of discrimination. In studies of Korean and Mexican immigrants, social support moderated the impact of perceived discrimination (Finch & Vega, 2003; Noh & Kaspar, 2003). In addition, during the initial postmigration period, the family takes on an important role in what may be a period of social isolation from mainstream society.

Age has consistently been a correlate of psychological symptoms in immigrants, and people who immigrate during or after their midlife years tend to have the most distress. For example, older immigrants from the former Soviet Union tend to have more difficulty adapting to life in the United States than younger immigrants (Miller & Chandler, 2002). Immigration prior to age 12 seems to be most influential in predicting language fluency and adaptation. Women tend to have more difficulty adjusting to life than men following immigration in some ethnic groups, but this seems most related to participation in mainstream culture through employment or educational opportunities. Most studies have found married people and those with families to have fewer psychological symptoms, but families can be a source of stress as well, particularly when there are intergenerational differences in the rates of acculturation (Birman & Trickett, 2001).

Immigration may also provide rich opportunities for challenging and growth-producing experiences, and immigrants demonstrate tremendous resilience in the face of multiple challenges. The concept of **resilience** originated from the field of child development and refers to a capacity to bounce back from adversity. It is seen as a process, not a fixed personality trait, because weaknesses and/or strengths may emerge during transitions throughout life as well as during times of stress. The study of resilience focuses mainly on protective factors that reduce the negative effects of trauma and stress (Southwick, Vythilingam, & Charney, 2005).

Resilience may be an important resource for immigrants to buffer the effects of acculturative stress. Few studies examine resilience for dealing with the challenges related to immigration and acculturation, especially during the early postmigration transition period. Miller and Chandler (2002) found that women who immigrated to the United States from the former Soviet Union who had lower depression scores also report greater resilience. The study of the role of resilience among immigrants has begun relatively recently, and interventions to strengthen resilience in immigrant families are needed (Luthar & Cicchetti, 2000).

Community Context

Community and environmental factors that affect health include the mobility patterns of a particular ethnic group, **ethnic density** (the concentration of people from the same ethnic background living in a community), perceived discrimination, and the availability of social support and networks. The broader community context, including neighborhood social environment, is an important determinant of immigrant health (Schnittker, 2002).

Public health nurses need to recognize residential patterns in order to deliver appropriate health care to groups in ethnically dense locations. Many new immigrants initially settle in neighborhoods with large numbers of people from the same ethnic background. These neighborhoods, called ethnic enclaves, are usually located in urban areas. Such neighborhoods often provide easy access to ethnic amenities, such as special foods and ethnic social networks (Chiswick & Miller, 2005). Ethnic minorities may also rely on **social capital**—the aggregate of individuals' social group networks or geographic space, which includes trust and reciprocity (Carlson and Chamberlain, 2003). Immigrants who lack access to familiar cultural items and social networks may be at higher risk for acculturative stress and isolation than other immigrants. In addition, living in neighborhoods with high ethnic density

⊕ RESEARCH APPLICATION

Predictors of Loneliness in Elderly Korean Women Living in the United States of America

Study Purpose

To examine factors that predict loneliness in elderly Korean-American women.

Methods

Questionnaires were given to 110 Korean immigrant women aged 60 years and older. The questionnaires included items that assessed loneliness, social support, social network size, ethnic attachment to Korean culture, functional status, and sociodemographic characteristics.

Findings

Elderly Korean women had higher loneliness scores than those in other studies. The strongest predictor of loneli-

ness was low satisfaction with social support. Other significant predictors were small social network size, low ethnic attachment, and low functional status.

Implications

Public health nurses need to assess these factors and use them to predict which elderly Korean women are most at risk for loneliness.

Author

Kim, O. (1999). Predictors of loneliness in elderly Korean women living in the United States of America. *J. Advanced Nursing, 29*(5), 1082–1088.

---

may be protective against depression as well as physical health problems (Eschbach et al., 2004; Patel et al., 2003). This may be a result of emotional, financial, and practical support along with the social capital that exists within a community (Frisbie, Cho, & Hummer, 2001).

On the other hand, areas of residential segregation may reflect poverty, group discrimination, and isolation as well as potential for high-risk activities such as gang involvement (Sampson, Morenorr, & Gannon-Rowley, 2002). Excessive reliance on ethnic networks may also postpone or reduce opportunities for acculturation, and contribute to alienation from mainstream culture.

Workforce and Socioeconomic Issues

Although the overall unemployment rates for documented immigrants and native-born adults are similar, the gap between them increases with age. Furthermore, there is a much higher representation of immigrants in lower paying occupations, in part due to language difficulties, lower educational background, and lack of familiarity with the U.S. job market (Mosisa, 2002). Undocumented workers, who are estimated to make up 40 percent of the immigrant workforce, receive even

lower pay and fewer benefits than those with legal status (Capps et al., 2003).

Foreign-born women earn less money than either foreign-born men or native-born women (Capps et al., 2003). For example, home care is dominated by female immigrants and is one of the lowest paying occupations in the United States, along with having a high turnover rate (Stone, 2004). The latter is due not only to poor benefits, but to injury and illness among the workers (Dellve, Lagerstrom, & Hagberg, 2003). Nevertheless, home care workers comprise one of the fastest growing fields of employment, and their number is expected to continue to rise with the proportional increase in the elderly populations in industrialized countries (Hecker, 2004).

Migrant farm workers often live in poverty with their families and have little access to health and social services. The majority of urban migrant workers are men who live away from their families, sending money home for support and returning intermittently. Women may be brought into foreign countries as housekeepers, personal caregivers, and sex workers. These workers are at risk of abuse and exploitation by employers as well as social and cultural alienation, stress, and communicable diseases. They are often resented by or isolated from the native population and have limited health care access because of their legal status. The health and

⊕ POLICY HIGHLIGHTS

Immigration among Nurses

An unresolved immigration policy issue that has global implications for health care is nurse migration from disadvantaged to highly industrialized countries. This is particularly salient for nurses being recruited to the United States from countries such as the Philippines, Africa, and India. Although there has been migration of nurses from these countries for decades, the recently identified shortage in the nursing workforce in the United States led to recommendations that U.S. immigration quotas be expanded or removed for trained nurses from other countries. The loss of trained nurses has significant implications for the health workforce in developing countries, despite the fact that many send money back to support their families. Effects of nurse migration include postimmigration stress and isolation of nurses who are separated from their families. Nurses may have difficulties understanding the U.S. health system, and problems associated with communication and U.S. cultural competence despite English language proficiency. The American Nurses Association and other nursing groups have called instead for strengthening the U.S. infrastructure, including expanding schools of nursing and salaries to accommodate the increased demand for nursing education among U.S. citizens, rather than increasing immigration to solve this problem.

safety of immigrant workers is becoming an important area of study for occupational health professionals.

HEALTH PROBLEMS WITH SPECIAL IMPLICATIONS FOR IMMIGRANTS AND REFUGEES

Immigrants and refugees are at exceptional risk for certain health problems, as well as inadequate immunizations and poor dental health (Fazel & Stein, 2002). Immigrants and refugees are also at risk for stress-related chronic health problems, such as hypertension and digestive problems. Many of the health problems to which they are at risk can be assessed by the ten leading health indicators (LHIs) included in Healthy People 2010. These are physical activity, overweight/obesity, tobacco use, substance abuse, sexual behavior, mental health, injury and violence prevention, environmental quality, immunizations, and access to care. Although data on some of the indicators are limited for foreign-born individuals, the indicators provide a good framework to assess disparities between immigrant and U.S.-born groups (Kandula, Kersey, & Lurie, 2004).

Communicable Diseases

One in three individuals worldwide and 7 million foreign-born persons in the United States are infected with tuberculosis. Most of these cases are acquired in the person's country of origin, and case rates among foreign-born are four to five times higher than among U.S.-born persons. Intestinal parasites (such as hookworm, roundworm, pinworm, and whipworm) are common among some groups of immigrants and refugees but can be asymptomatic. Symptoms vary according to the parasitic infection but can include diarrhea, dyspepsia, constipation, weight loss, and abdominal pain. Migrants usually have carrier rates of hepatitis B similar to individuals in their home country and may be at increased risk for chronic liver disease or hepatocellular carcinoma. In addition, infants born of mothers who are hepatitis B surface antigen positive are likely to be infected (Adams, Gardiner, & Assefi, 2004). As with other infectious diseases, the risk of malaria and HIV/AIDS varies depending on homeland and migration environments.

Effects of Social Violence, Torture, and Human Trafficking

Because of their exposure to war, violence, social discrimination, poverty, and famine, refugees may have high rates of posttraumatic stress disorders and diseases (PTSD), including those contracted in refugee camps as a result of the migration experience (Tulchinsky & Varavikova, 2000). Even immigrants who are not exposed to the trauma of forced migration are susceptible to depression, anxiety, and substance abuse. For example, refugees from the former republic of Yugoslavia (Bosnia-Herzegovina) comprise the largest number of European refugees since World War II due to warfare. In addition to physical illnesses related to war such as hepatitis B, nutritional deficiencies, and injuries, refugees from Bosnia-Herzegovina are at particular risk for posttraumatic stress disorder and other mental health problems.

PTSD is characterized by persistent reexperiencing of traumatic events (recurring nightmares, intrusive thoughts), avoidance of thoughts that remind one of the events, emotional numbing, and increased arousal (hypervigilance, sleep disorders, irritability, difficulty concentrating). PTSD may be expressed through somatic rather than psychiatric symptoms. In addition, traumatic events may lead to adjustment problems, substance abuse, family violence, poor school performance, increased risk taking, and other behavioral problems in vulnerable individuals (Norwood, Ursano, & Fullerton, 2002).

Often, mental health problems in immigrants and refugees are expressed through physical symptoms and are therefore difficult for the health care provider to detect or diagnose. This may be further complicated because mental illness may in fact not be evident until one to two years after immigration. Somatization may be demonstrated by vague symptoms such as headaches, chest pains, palpitations, shortness of breath, fatigue, and sleep disturbances (Barnes, 2001). Expressions of somatization may also be culturally defined and may or may not be presented along with complaints of psychological problems (Mak & Zane, 2004). For example, Pang's (2000) research findings suggest that elderly Korean immigrants may use somatic symptoms to express their distress regarding aging, adjustment, and family issues. It is important for the nurse to assess mental health status even when the primary complaints are comprised of physical health problems.

Interethnic conflict, sexual violence, and disease epidemics may lead to higher mortality for people living in refugee camps than in the countries from which they fled. Other traumatic events include being deprived of food, water, or shelter; being brainwashed; witnessing murder and other violent acts; and being in a combat situation (Adams, Gardiner, & Assefi, 2004). Refugees may also bring a set of hidden problems that result from torture. Between 5 and 35 percent of the world's refugees have experienced torture, and there are an estimated 400,000 to 500,000 survivors of torture now living in the United States. Many are easily overlooked by health professionals without adequate training (Henderson, 2001; McCullough-Zander & Larson, 2004).

The sequelae of torture include physical signs like burn marks, whipping scars, and x-rays that reveal old fractures. Long-term problems related to ritual female genital surgery or female circumcision, and problems related to sexual abuse including rape, may include chronic pelvic inflammatory disease, recurrent urinary tract infection, scar abscesses, and dyspareunia (Adams, Gardiner, & Assefi, 2004).

Human trafficking is the second largest (behind drug trafficking) and fastest growing criminal industry in the world. The United Nations Office on Drugs and Crime (2006; 2007) defines human trafficking as:

> The recruitment, transportation, transfer, harbouring or receipt of persons, by means of the threat or use of force or other forms of coercion . . . for the purpose of exploitation. Exploitation shall include . . . prostitution of others or other forms of sexual exploitation, forced labour or services, slavery or practices similar to slavery, servitude or the removal of organs.

Approximately 800,000 to 900,000 victims are trafficked internationally, and millions more are trafficked within the victims' own countries every year; 17,500 to 18,500 are trafficked into the United States (U.S. Department of Justice, 2005). Trafficking victims often come from vulnerable populations, such as undocumented migrants, runaway youth, and oppressed or marginalized groups.

PLANNING AND IMPLEMENTING CARE FOR IMMIGRANTS AND REFUGEES

Victims of trafficking may have similar medical problems as victims of domestic abuse or rape, including bruises, other signs of battering, sexually transmitted diseases, fear, and depression (USDHHS, 2005). They may be malnourished and/or dehydrated, have poor personal hygiene, and lack any form of identification. Victims who are seen by health care providers for treatment are often kept under surveillance by the trafficker, who acts as translator.

Policies relating to immigrant benefits and health care delivery differ a great deal across receiving countries (Miller & Gross, 2004). In the United States, health services for immigrants and refugees are affected by federal and state policies. Immigrants and refugees might be unaware of governmental policies, which can directly or indirectly affect their health care access or health status.

The Personal Responsibility and Work Opportunities Act of 1996 (Public Law 104-193) shifted responsibility for certain federal programs to the states. This welfare reform law significantly reduced benefits to immigrants, except some designated as having refugee status (Fremsted, 2002). Although some benefits have since been reinstated, the noncitizen immigrant public assistance package is generally much less comprehensive than that of citizens (Ku & Matani, 2001). Immigrants and refugees are not eligible to apply for citizenship until they have resided in the United States for at least five years. Assistance and services for immigrants are, therefore, provided in a highly decentralized context that is extremely difficult to master (IOM, 2001).

The U.S. Public Health Service (USPHS) requires that all immigrants and refugees who want to reside permanently in the United States submit to medical screening in their home country or country of first asylum. This screening mainly detects infectious disease so that they can be treated with drug therapy and detained if necessary. Laboratory work such as tuberculin skin testing, hepatitis B virus serologic testing, and stool ova and parasite examinations or x-rays are performed. Immigrants and refugees from regions with high prevalence of tuberculosis are considered to have positive tuberculin tests if the reaction is greater than 10 mm (Adams, Gardiner, & Assefi, 2004).

The USPHS premigration screening, however, is not comprehensive. Evidence of prior immunization is frequently unavailable, particularly for immigrants from Asian and South American countries (Lifson, Thai, & Hang, 2001). The examination may not identify chronic diseases and has not been helpful for diagnosing mental illness. Continuity of care for problems discovered prior to immigration is difficult due to economic and logistical reasons. Even more problematic is the fact that people who enter the country illegally do not participate in premigration screening, so infectious diseases may not be identified prior to migration. After they arrive in the United States their options for health care are restricted and are usually limited to urgent care treatment in emergency rooms and community clinics.

Immigrants and refugees usually arrive in the United States without basic understanding of its health care system. Their health care needs as well as limited comprehension of the complex U.S. health care system affect accessibility and utilization of services (Aroian, Wu, & Tran, 2005; Ivanov & Buck, 2002). Immigrants and refugees are much less likely to have health insurance than native-born citizens (Ku & Matani, 2001). They may also struggle with nonfinancial barriers such as lack of proficiency in the English language, lack of knowledge about available services, lack of transportation, and limited community resources that would facilitate access to health care services.

Immigrants and refugees who are unfamiliar with, do not trust, or cannot afford Western medicine often prefer to visit indigenous lay healers or use folk remedies to prevent or treat illness. For example, many East and Southeast Asians believe that eating certain foods can bring about a balance or imbalance within the body, which can result in health or illness. Similarly, Vietnamese persons may use forms of dermabrasion

⊕ PRACTICE APPLICATION

Community Wellness Center Programs

Focus groups can be one way to identify components of programs that are culturally appropriate for immigrants. A series of group discussions were held with members of a community wellness center for multicultural older adults in Chicago. Group members included immigrants from Japan, Mexico, and the former Soviet Union. During the discussions, participants talked about their attitudes and beliefs regarding health and health promotion, barriers and benefits of physical activity and other health behaviors, and strategies to motivate other older adults to perform selected activities. Differences were found across the cultural groups that contributed to designing programs that considered culturally specific factors, and findings were also used to evaluate existing programs in the center.

such as coining, cupping, and pinching to treat fevers and influenza. The use of herbal solutions may create side effects, drug interactions, and toxicity, though others may be beneficial and comforting.

Public health nurses are challenged to identify multilevel models and theories that explain how, when, and where interventions can help immigrant populations. Members of each ethnic community need to have access to timely and accurate information that promotes self-care and health awareness. One way to investigate community and environmental factors is to use an existing ecological framework of community health and needs assessment. Through community assessment, nurses can identify areas of immigrant or refugee community needs in order to plan intervention in a focused and goal-oriented manner (Kulig, 2000). A second way to investigate community and environmental factors is to build an interpretive conceptual framework of the community that will enable researchers, practitioners, and policy makers to understand the processes and components needed to promote a healthy community. This includes a comprehensive approach that takes into account the diverse components of the community. For example, socioeconomic status, marital status, and gender can be significant predictors of health and illness.

Public health nurses need to be aware of alternative medicines and health practices that are commonly used among the populations they serve. Western medicine is based on natural science and approaches the human body through analytic approach in order to identify and classify disease. As a result, providers in the United States usually specialize according to anatomy and physiology (e.g., hematology, rheumatology). In contrast, Eastern medicine is based on an overall state of balance between positive (yang) and negative (yin) energy (Kim, 1995). Providers of Eastern medicine treat across structure and functions of the body. For example, the body is seen as a rhythmic microcosm of meridians that represent energy fields of the universe. Certain locations of the body may represent an organ function or movement of blood circulation and each organ also represents a certain set of emotions. A treatment such as acupuncture or massage may target a meridian to improve circulation of energy to a specified part of the body.

Palinkas et al. (2003) suggest that the "journey to wellness" for refugees includes (1) treatment of mental disorders resulting from the refugee experience, (2) treatment of infectious and parasitic diseases acquired in home countries, and (3) prevention of chronic diseases to which immigrants are at risk as a result of living in their new host country. The health history for immigrant clients needs to include the premigration life story, history of infectious diseases, traditional medicine and substance use, sexual history and genital surgery, and trauma history including screening for infectious and sexually transmitted diseases, as well as oral, dental, and visual hearing examinations. Immigrant and refugee women are especially at risk for health problems because they tend to be the caregivers of their families. They often have low rates of breast and cervical cancer screening and higher reports of role burden and stress.

Health promotion for immigrant and refugees requires family- and community-centered comprehensive programs of stress management, behavioral change, and social support networks. Programs need to be tailored to specific cultural attitudes and beliefs (Day & Cohen, 2000; Miller & Iris, 2002). As the population in the United States ages, a larger proportion will be composed of immigrants who are aging in an unfamiliar social milieu. Their families also must deal with the added responsibilities of caring for or finding resources for their elders.

For all ages, a trained medical interpreter is necessary if the nurse is not bilingual or bicultural. They provide meaningful interpretation that goes beyond language translation. An interpreter serves not only as a translator but also as a culture broker who might explain the cultural context of symptoms. Culture brokers also inform health care providers about the way culture affects health and behavior. Issues of privacy, maturity, and family dynamics make family members, especially children, inappropriate for this important task. Organizations such as the American Translators Association and Society of Medical Interpreters promote professionalism and excellence to enhance the provision of health and social services to ethnic communities. Interpretation may be accessed through specialized telephone services in settings where on-site translators are not available.

Public health nurses may need to identify the decision makers in the ethnic community before attempting to implement community-based interventions. Familiarity with religious and cultural practices of the family is also important for designing appropriate individual and family-focused interventions. For example, fatalistic beliefs are a common factor in low rates of cancer screening behaviors and visits to mental health services for some ethnic groups. These beliefs need to be identified in order to establish an effective education and outreach program. Nursing interventions must consider social and cultural factors. Each immigrant group has a unique history and context that may place its individuals at risk for particular health problems but may also be the source of resilience and strength.

CRITICAL THINKING ACTIVITIES

1. In the United States, there are an unprecedented number of immigrants and refugees from countries all over the world. What recent political and social events have changed patterns of global migration? What are the effects of these changing patterns on the delivery of health care in this country?

2. Many premigration factors have long-range effects on health. What information regarding a country of origin would be helpful to know prior to eliciting health information directly from a client? How would you use that information to assess an individual during a health care encounter?

3. Some researchers have suggested that the adaptation strategy of integration or biculturalism is most highly related to positive health and adjustment after immigration. If you do not agree, think of another strategy that is better for the individual or country as a whole.

4. Acculturative stress is believed to contribute to immigrants' increased risk for family problems or mental illness. What are some ways nurses can help decrease this stress? Choose one common stressor related to the process of acculturation and identify ways the nurse might address it in a plan of care.

5. Immigrants and refugees are at higher risk for certain health problems than the general population. How would an assessment of an immigrant or refugee differ from that of a nonimmigrant client, and what would be the most important factors to take into consideration when making such an assessment?

6. Programs are most effective when they are culturally appropriate for a particular ethnic group. Identify a health problem that you would like to address for individuals or families from an immigrant group of your choice. Design a plan to gather information that will help to ensure that your intervention would be culturally appropriate for this group.

KEY TERMS

acculturation	impelled migration	racism
acculturative strategies	integration	receiving country
acculturative stress	marginalization	refugee
assimilation	migrant	resilience
culture broker	migration	sending country
emigrant	migratory or seasonal worker	separation
ethnic density	(also documented migrant worker, itinerant worker)	social capital
forced migration	pull factors	somatization
Hispanic paradox	push factors	transnationalism
immigrant (in general)		xenophobia

KEY CONCEPTS

⊕ Global changes in patterns of migration have resulted in unprecedented numbers of immigrants and refugees who are settling in developed countries around the world. Understanding the factors that contribute to the decision to migrate, and the national policies that affect immigration, provide a foundation for planning and delivering care.

⊕ Premigration factors that affect health in immigrants and refugees include social and environmental characteristics in their home countries such as lack of adequate health care services. The migration experience, such as time spent in refugee camps, war, trauma, torture, and socioeconomic disruption have long-term effects on mental and physical health.

⊕ Acculturation includes language, behavior, identity, and values that may change when a person comes in contact with another culture. For many immigrants, health status declines over time, suggesting that changes due to acculturation or stress increased their vulnerability to disease. Acculturation may also lead to positive health behavior changes and provides an opportunity for challenge and growth.

⊕ Immigrants often experience depression and discrimination, and family can be a source of stress as well as support. Immigrants may be socially isolated if they do not have a social network of people who share their ethnicity, language, or religion.

⊕ Depending on their country of origin, immigrants and refugees may be at particular risk for communicable diseases such as tuberculosis, parasites, hepatitis B, and HIV/AIDS. They may have had inadequate immunizations in their home countries. Cultural expressions of illness may include somatization and symptoms related to non-Western medical beliefs.

⊕ Health programs for immigrants and refugees require family and community centered approaches that are tailored for specific cultural attitudes and beliefs. Nursing interventions need to consider contextual factors that place immigrants at risk as well as individual and cultural characteristics that may be the source of resilience and strength.

REFERENCES

Adams, K. M., Gardiner, L. D., & Assefi, N. (2004). Healthcare challenges from the developing world: Post-immigration refugee medicine. *British Medical Journal, 328,* 1548–1552.

Arcia, E., Skinner, M., Bailey, D., & Correa, V. (2001). Models of acculturation and health behaviors among Latino immigrants to the U.S. *Social Science and Medicine, 53,* 41–53.

Aroian, K. J., Wu, B., & Tran, T. V. (2005). Health care and social service use among Chinese immigrant elders. *Research in Nursing & Health, 28,* 95–105.

Balcazar, H., & Qian, Z. (2000). Immigrant families and sources of stress. In P. C. McKenry & S. J. Price (Eds.), *Families and change: Coping with stressful events and transitions* (pp. 359–377). Thousand Oaks, CA: Sage Publications.

Barnes, D. M. (2001). Mental health screening in a refugee population: A program report. *Journal of Immigrant Health, 3,* 141–149.

Barnes, D. M., & Harrison, C. L. (2004). Refugee women's reproductive health in early resettlement. *Journal of Obstetric, Gynecological, and Neonatal Nursing, 33,* 723–728.

Berry, J. W. (2005). Acculturation: Living successfully in two cultures. *International Journal of Intercultural Relations, 29,* 697–712.

Bevilacqua, A. J. (1983). Who is a refugee? Distinction between economic and political determinants of refugee movements. In J. M. Kitagawa (Ed.), *American refugee policy.* Minneapolis: The Presiding Bishop's Fund for World Relief in collaboration with Winston Press.

Birman, D., & Trickett, E. (2001). Cultural transitions in first-generation immigrants: Acculturation of Soviet Jewish refugee adolescents and parents. *Journal of Cross-Cultural Psychology, 32,* 456–477.

Capps, R., Fix, M., Passel, J. S., Ost, J., & Perez-Lopez, D. (2003). *A profile of the low-wage immigrant workforce.* Retrieved May 29, 2006, from the Urban Institute Immigration Studies Web site: http://www.urban.org/UploadedPDF/310880_lowwage_immig_wkfc.pdf.

Carlson, E. D., & Chamberlain, E. (2003). Social capital, health, and health disparities. *Journal of Nursing Scholarship, 35,* 325–331.

Chiswick, B. R., & Miller, P. W. (2005). Do enclaves matter in immigrant adjustment? *City and Community, 4,* 5–36.

Crespo, C., Smit, E., Carter-Pokras, O., & Andersen, R. (2001). Acculturation and leisure-time physical inactivity in Mexican American adults: Results from NHANES III, 1988–1994. *American Journal of Public Health, 91,* 1254–1257.

Day, K., & Cohen, U. (2000). The role of culture in designing environments for people with dementia: A study of Russian Jewish immigrants. *Environment and Behavior, 32,* 361–399.

Dellve, L., Lagerstrom, M., & Hagberg, M. (2003). Work-system risk factors for permanent work disability among home-care workers: a case-control study. *International Archives of Occupational & Environmental Health, 76,* 216–224.

Dey, A. N., & Lucas, J. W. (2006). Physical and mental health characteristics of U.S.- and foreign-born adults: United States, 1998–2003. *Advance data from vital and health statistics* (no. 369). Hyattsville, MD: National Center for Health Statistics.

Eschbach, K., Ostir G. V., Patel, K. V., Markides, S., & Goodwin, J. S. (2004). Neighborhood context and mortality among older Mexican Americans: Is there a *barrio* advantage? *American Journal of Public Health, 94,* 1807–1812.

Fazel, M., & Stein, S. (2002). The mental health of refugee children. *Archives of Disease in Childhood, 87,* 366–370.

Finch, B. K., & Vega, W. A. (2003). Acculturation stress, social support, and self-rated health among Latinos in California. *Journal of Immigrant Health, 5*(3), 109–117.

Fremsted, S. (2002). *Immigrants and welfare reauthorization.* Washington, DC: Center on Budget and Policy Priorities. Retrieved May 29, 2006, from http://www.cbpp.org.

Frisbie, W. P., Cho, Y., & Hummer, R. A. (2001). Immigration and the health of Asian and Pacific Islander adults in the United States. *American Journal of Epidemiology, 153,* 372–380.

Goel, M. S., McCarthy, E. P., Phillips, R. S., & Wee, C. C. (2004). Obesity among U.S. immigrant subgroups by duration of residence. *JAMA, 292,* 2860–2867.

Goel, M. S., Wee, C. C. McCarthy, E. P., Davis, R. B., Ngo-Metzger, Q., & Phillips, R. S. (2003). Racial and ethnic disparities in cancer screening: The importance of foreign birth as a barrier to care. *Journal of General Internal Medicine, 18,* 1028–1035.

Gonzalez, H. M., Haan, M., & Hinton, L. (2001). Acculturation and the prevalence of depression in older Mexican Americans: Baseline results of the Sacramento Area Latino Study on Aging. *Journal of the American Geriatrics Society, 49,* 948–953.

Hecker, D. E. (2004). Occupational employment projections to 2012. *Monthly Labor Review, 127,* 87–102.

Henderson, S. (2001). New approaches to health care for displaced populations. *JAMA, 285*(9), 1212.

Horrigan, M. W. (2004). Employment projections to 2012: Concepts and context. *Monthly Labor Review, 127,* 3–22.

Institute of Medicine (IOM), Committee on Quality of Health Care in America. (2001). *Crossing the quality chasm: A new health system for the 21st century.* Washington, DC: National Academy Press. Retrieved May 29, 2006, from http://www.iom.edu.

International Labour Office, International Organization for Migration, and Office of the United Nations High Commissioner for Human Rights. (2001). *International migration, racism, discrimination and xenophobia.* Retrieved May 29, 2006, from http://www.ilo.org.

Ivanov L. L., & Buck, K. (2002). Health care utilization patterns of Russian-speaking immigrant women across age groups. *Journal of Immigrant Health, 4,* 17–27.

Jonnalagadda, S. S., & Diwan, S. (2005). Health behaviors, chronic disease prevalence and self-rated health of older Asian Indian immigrants in the U.S. *Journal of Immigrant Health, 7*(2), 75–83.

Kandula, N. R., Kersey, M., & Lurie, N. (2004). Assuring the health of immigrants: What the leading health indicators tell us. *Annual Review of Public Health, 25,* 357–376.

Keller, A. S. (2001). Written testimony in support of the Refugee Protection Act, Allen S. Keller, M.D. *Physicians for Human Rights.* Retrieved May 24, 2006, from http://www.phrusa.org/research/refugees/testimony.html.

Kim, M.T. (1995). Cultural influences on depression in Korean Americans. *Journal of Psychosocial Nursing, 33*(2), 13–18.

Kim, O. (1999). Predictors of loneliness in elderly Korean women living in the United States of America. *J. Advanced Nursing, 29*(5), 1082–1088.

Ku, L., & Matani, S. (2001). Left out: Immigrants' access to health care and insurance. *Health Affairs 20,* 247–256.

Kulig, J. (2000). Community resiliency: The potential for community health nursing theory development. *Public Health Nursing, 17*(5), 374–385.

Lazarus, R. S., & Folkman, S. (1984). *Stress, appraisal, and coping.* New York: Springer.

Lifson, A. R., Thai, D., & Hang, K. (2001). Lack of immunization documentation in Minnesota refugees: Challenges for refugee preventive health care. *Journal of Immigrant Health, 3,* 47–52.

Lu, M. C., & Halfon, N. (2003). Racial and ethnic disparities in birth outcomes: A life-course perspective. *Maternal and Child Health Journal, 7,* 13–30.

Luthar, S., Cicchetti, D., & Becker, B. (2000). The construct of resilience: A critical evaluation and guidelines for future work. *Child Development, 71*(3), 543-562.

Mak, W. W. S., & Zane, N. W. S. (2004). The phenomenon of somatization among community Chinese Americans. *Social Psychiatry and Psychiatric Epidemiology, 39,* 967–974.

Martin, P., & Midgley, E. (2003). Immigration: Shaping and reshaping America. *Population Bulletin 58,* no. 2. Washington, DC: Population Reference Bureau. Retrieved May 29, 2006, from http://www.prb.org/pdg/ImmigShaping America.pdf.

McCullough-Zander, K., & Larson, S. (2004). "The fear is still in me." Caring for survivors of torture: How to identify, assess, and treat those who have endured this extreme trauma. *American Journal of Nursing, 104*(10), 54–64.

McGlade, M. S., Saha, S., & Dahlstrom, M. E. (2004). The Latina paradox: An opportunity for restructuring prenatal care delivery. *American Journal of Public Health, 94,* 2062–2065.

Miller, A. M., & Chandler, P. (2002). Acculturation, resilience, and depression in midlife women from the former Soviet Union. *Nursing Research, 51*(1), 26–32.

Miller, A. M., & Gross, R. (2004). Depression and health of women from the former Soviet Union living in the United States and Israel. *Journal of Immigrant Health, 6*(4), 183–192.

Miller, A. M., & Iris, M. (2002). Health promotion attitudes and strategies in older adults. *Health Education and Behavior, 29,* 249–267.

Miller, A. M., Chandler, P., Wilbur, J., & Sorokin, O. (2004). Acculturation and cardiovascular disease risk factors in midlife immigrant women from the former Soviet Union. *Progress in Cardiovascular Nursing, 19*(2), 47–55.

Mosisa, A. T. (2002). The role of foreign-born workers in the U.S. economy. *Monthly Labor Review, 125,* 3–14.

Myers, H. F., & Rodriguez, N. (2003). Acculturation and physical health in racial and ethnic minorities. In K. M. Chun, P. B. Organista, & G. Marin (Eds.), *Acculturation: Advances in theory, measurement, and applied research* (pp. 163–185). Washington, DC: American Psychological Association.

Noh, S., & Kaspar, V. (2003). Perceived discrimination and depression: Moderating effects of coping, acculturation, and ethnic support. *American Journal of Public Health, 93,* 232–238.

Norwood, A., Ursano, R., & Fullerton, C. (2002). *Disaster psychiatry.* Retrieved May 28, 2006, from http://www.psych.org/psych_pract/principles_and_practice3201.cfm.

Palinkas, L. A., Pickwell, S. M., Brandstein, K., Clark, T. J., Hill, L. L., Moser, R. J., & Osman, A. (2003). *Journal of Immigrant Health, 5,* 19–28.

Pang, K. Y. C. (2000*).* Symptom expression and somatization among elderly Korean immigrants. *Journal of Clinical Geropsychology, 6,* 199–212.

Passel, J. S., Capps, R., & Fix, M. E. (2004). *Undocumented immigrants: Facts and figures.* Retrieved March 24, 2005, from http://www.urban.org/publications/1000587.html.

Patel, K. V., Eschbach, K., Rudkin, L. L., Peek, M. K., & Markides, K. (2003). Neighborhood context and self-rated health in older Mexican Americans. *Annals of Epidemiology, 13,* 620–628.

Phinney, Jean S. (2003). Ethnic identity and acculturation. In K. Chun, P. Balls, & G. Marin, (Eds.), *Acculturation: Advances in Theory, Measurement, and Applied Research* (pp. 63–81). Washington, DC: American Psychological Association.

Rubia, M., Marcos, I., & Muennig, A. (2001). Increased risk of heart disease and stroke among females residing in the U.S. *American Journal of Preventive Medicine, 22,* 30–35.

Sampson, R. J., Morenoff, J.D., & Gannon-Rowley, T. (2002). Assessing "neighborhood effects": Social processes and new directions in research. *Annual Review of Sociology, 28,* 443–478.

Satia, J., Patterson, R., Kristal, A., Hislop, T., Yasui, Y., & Taylor, V. (2001). Development of scales to measure dietary acculturation among Chinese-Americans and Chinese-Canadians. *Journal of the American Dietetic Association, 101,* 548–553.

Schmidley, D. (2003). *The foreign-born population in the United States: March 2002, Current Population Reports (*No. P20-539). Washington, DC: U.S. Census Bureau.

Singh, G., & Siahpush, M. (2002). Ethnic-immigrant differentials in health behaviors, morbidity, and cause-specific mortality in the United States: An analysis of two national data bases. *Human Biology, 74,* 83–109.

Schnittker, J. (2002). Acculturation in context: The self-esteem of Chinese immigrants. *Social Psychology Quarerly, 65,* 56-76.

Smith, L. S. (2001). Health of America's newcomers. *Journal of Community Health Nursing, 18,* 53–68.

Southwick, S. M., Vythilingam, M., & Charney, D. S. (2005). The psychobiology of depression and resilience to stress: Implications for prevention and treatment. *Annual Review of Clinical Psychology, 1,* 255–291.

Stone, R. I. (2004). The direct care worker: The third rail of home care policy. *Annual Review of Public Health, 25,* 521–537.

Tulchinsky, T. H., & Varavikova, E. A. (2000). *The new public health: An introduction for the 21st century.* San Diego: Academic Press.

United Nations High Commissioner for Human Rights. (2005a). *Universal Declaration of Human Rights.* Retrieved May 29, 2006, from http://www.unhchr.ch/udhr/.

United Nations High Commissioner for Refugees (UNHCR). (2000). *The state of the world's refugees: Fifty years of humanitarian action.* Oxford: Oxford University Press.

United Nations Office on Drugs & Crime (UNODC; 2007). *Trafficking in Human Beings.* Retrieved August 21, 2007 from http://www.unodc.org/unodc/en/trafficking_human_beings.html

United Nations Office on Drugs & Crime (UNODC; 2006). *Trafficking in persons: Global patterns.* Retrieved August 21, 2007 from http://www.unodc.org/pdf/traffickinginpersons_report_2006ver2.pdf

U.S. Department of Justice. (2005). *Distinctions between human smuggling and human trafficking.* Retrieved May 29, 2006, from http://www.usdoj.gov/crt/crim/smuggling_trafficking_facts.pdf.

U.S. Department of Health and Human Services (USDHHS), Administration for Children and Families, The Campaign to Rescue and Restore Victims of Human Trafficking. (2005). *Looking beneath the surface: Human trafficking is modern day slavery.* Retrieved May 29, 2006, from http://www.acf.hhs.gov/trafficking/.

United States-Mexico Border Health Commission (USMBHC) (2005). *About the United States–Mexico Border Health Commission.* Retrieved May 28, 2006, from http://www.borderhealth.org/about_us.php.

U.S. Office of Refugee Resettlement (2005). *Refugee Arrivals by Country of Origin and State of Initial Resettlement for FY 2004.* Retrieved May 29, 2006, from http://www.acf.dhhs.gov/programs/orr/data/fy2004RA.htm

Villarruel, A. M., Jemmott, J. B., Jemmott, L. S., & Ronis, & D. L. (2004). Predictors of sexual intercourse and condom use intentions among Spanish-dominant Latino youth: A test of the planned behavior theory. *Nursing Research, 53*(3), 172–181.

Willgerodt, M. A., Miller, A. M., & McElmurry, B. J. (2002). Becoming bicultural: Chinese American women and their development. *Health Care for Women International, 23,* 67–480.

BIBLIOGRAPHY

Cabassa, L. J. (2003). Measuring acculturation: Where we are and where we need to go. *Hispanic Journal of Behavioral Sciences, 25,* 127–146.

Camarota, S. A. (2005). *Immigrants at mid-decade: A snapshot of America's foreign-born population in 2005.* Washington, DC: Center for Immigration Studies.

Carlson, E. D., & Chamberlain, R. M. (2003). Social capital, health, and health disparities. *Journal of Nursing Scholarship, 35,* 325–331.

Kravitz. R., Helms, J., Azari, R., Antonius, D., & Melnikow, J. (2000). Comparing the use of physician time and health care resources among patients speaking English, Spanish, and Russian. *Medical Care, 38,* 728–738.

Lam, B. T. (2005). An integrative model for the study of psychological distress in Vietnamese-American adolescents. *North American Journal of Psychology, 7,* 89–105.

Lee, E. E., & Farran, C. J. (2004). Depression among Korean, Korean American, and Caucasian American family caregivers. *Journal of Transcultural Nursing, 15,* 18–25.

Logan, J. R., Alba, R. D., & Zhang, W. (2002). Immigrant enclaves and ethnic communities in New York and Los Angeles. *American Sociological Review, 67,* 299–322.

Newbold, K. B., & Spindler, J. (2001). Immigrant settlement patterns in Metropolitan Chicago. *Urban Studies, 38,* 1903–1919.

Seng, J. S. (2003). Acknowledging posttraumatic stress effects on health. *Clinical Nurse Specialist, 17,* 34–41.

Trickett, E. J., & Birman, D. (2005). Acculturation, school context, and school outcomes: A differentiated example from refugee adolescents from the former Soviet Union. *Psychology in the Schools, 42,* 27–38.

United Nations High Commission for Refugees (UNHCR). (2005b). *UNHCR: The UN Refugee Agency.* Retrieved May 29, 2006, from http://www.unhcr.org/.

Villarruel, A. M., Jemmott, J. B., Jemmott, L. S., & Ronis, & D. L. (2004). Predictors of sexual intercourse and condom use intentions among Spanish-dominant Latino youth: A test of the planned behavior theory. *Nursing Research, 53*(3), 172–181.

Ward, E., Jemal, A., Cokkinides, V. Singh, G. K., Cardines, C. Ghafoor, A., & Thun, M. (2004). Cancer disparities by race/ethnicity and socioeconomic status. *CA: A Cancer Journal for Clinicians, 54,* 78–93.

Weine, S. M., Raina, D., Zhubi, M., Delesi, M., Huseni, D., Feetham, S., et al. (2003). The TAFES multi-family intervention for Kosovar refugees: A feasibility study. *Journal of Nervous and Mental Disease, 191,* 100–107.

RESOURCES

American Translators Association (ATA)

225 Reinekers Lane, Suite 590
Alexandria, Virginia 22314
(703) 683-6100
FAX: (703) 683-6122
Email: ata@atanet.org
Web: http://www.atanet.org

ATA, founded in 1959, is the largest professional association of translators and interpreters in the United States with over 9,500 members in over 70 countries. ATA's primary goals include fostering and supporting the professional development of translators and interpreters and promoting the translation and interpreting professions. ATA is a professional association founded to advance the translation and interpreting professions and foster the professional development of individual translators and interpreters. Its members include translators, interpreters, teachers, project managers, web and software developers, language company owners, hospitals, universities, and government agencies.

Centers of Disease Control, Division of Global Migration and Quarantine

1600 Clifton Road
Atlanta, Georgia 30333
404-639-4411, 404-639-3534, 1-800-311-3435
Web: http://www.cdc.gov

The Division of Global Migration and Quarantine has statutory responsibility to make and enforce regulations necessary to prevent the introduction, transmission, or spread of communicable diseases from foreign countries into the United States. The Web site describes the policies, criteria, and conduct of required pre-migration physical examinations for immigrants and refugees.

Cross Cultural Health Care Program (CCHP)

270 So. Hanford Street, Suite 208
Seattle, Washington 98134
206-860-0329 or 206-860-0331
FAX: 206-860-0334
Email: administration@xculture.org
Web: http://www.xculture.org

CCHP is an organization that recognizes the diversity and the different ways to health. Its mission is to serve as a bridge between communities and health care institutions to ensure full access to quality health care that is culturally and linguistically appropriate. Includes recommendations about designing culturally competent programs with the collaboration of communities. It is not limited to immigrants and refugees.

EthnoMed

University of Washington
Seattle, Washington
Web: http://www.ethnomed.org

The Web site contains information about cultural beliefs, medical issues, and other related issues pertinent to the health care of recent immigrants to the United States, many of whom are refugees fleeing war-torn parts of the world. It includes culturally specific information about a broad range of immigrant groups.

Refugee Well Being: Partnering for Refugee Health and Well

Web: http://www.refugeewellbeing.samhsa.gov

The Web site provides refugee mental health consultation and technical assistance to federal, state, or local agencies. Site includes access to video and other training media.

The Urban Institute

2100 M Street, NW
Washington, D.C. 20037
202-833-7200
Web: http://www.urban.org

The Urban Institute is a nonpartisan economic and social policy research organization that publishes studies, reports, and books on timely topics worthy of public consideration. It includes, but is not limited to, immigration issues. Its mission is to promote sound social policy and public debate on national priorities. The Urban Institute gathers and analyzes data, conducts policy research, evaluates programs and services, and educates Americans on critical issues and trends.

U.S. Citizenship and Immigration Services (USCIS)

1-800-375-5283
Email: uscis.webmaster@dhs.gov
Web: http://www.uscis.gov

The Web site provides a variety of information on immigration, immigration laws, how to become a citizen of the United States, and other information pertinent to immigration.

U.S. Department of Health and Human Services, Administration for Families and Children, Office of Refugee Resettlement (ORR)

370 L'Enfant Promenade, SW, 6th Floor /East
Washington, D.C. 20447
202-401-9246
FAX: 202-401-5487
Web: http://www.acf.hhs.gov

In the Refugee Act of 1980, Pub. L. No. 96-212, Congress codified and strengthened the United States' historic policy of aiding individuals fleeing persecution in their homelands. The Refugee Act of 1980 provided a formal definition of "refugee," which is virtually identical to the definition in the 1967 United Nations Protocol relating to the Status of Refugees. This definition is found in the Immigration and Nationality Act (INA) at Section 101(a)(42). In addition, the act provided the foundation for today's asylum adjudication process and the development of ORR within the Department of Health and Human Services. ORR's mission is to assist refugees and other special populations, as outlined in ORR regulations, in obtaining economic and social self-sufficiency in their new homes in the United States. To do this, ORR funds and facilitates a variety of programs that offer, among other benefits and services, cash and medical assistance, employment preparation and job placement, skills training, English language training, social adjustment and aid for victims of torture. The mission of ORR is to help refugees, Cuban/Haitian entrants, asylees, and other beneficiaries of our program to establish a new life that is founded on the dignity of economic self-support and encompasses full participation in opportunities that Americans enjoy. The Web site includes a legal definition of refugees and describes eligibility requirements for Refugee Assistance and Services through the Office of Refugee Resettlement

U.S. Department of Health and Human Services, Office of Minority Health (OMH)

P.O. Box 37337
Washington, D.C. 20013-7337
1-800-444-6472
Web: http://www.omhrc.gov

OMH improves and protects the health of racial and ethnic minority populations through the development of health policies and programs that will eliminate health disparities for racial and ethnic minority populations. OMH funds grants to address racial and ethnic minority health disparities. Several health disparities initiatives are coordinated by the Office of Management and Budget, including (a) Closing the Gap on Infant Mortality, (b) Minority HIV/AIDS, (c) Community Initiatives to Eliminate Stroke Disparities, and (d) Obesity Abatement in African Americans Campaign. The Web site describes programs and policies for racial and ethnic minority populations.

U.S. Department of State, Bureau of Population, Refugees, and Migration

U.S. Department of State
2201 C Street NW
Washington, D.C. 20520
202-647-4000
Web: http://www.state.gov

This branch of the U.S. Department of State coordinates U.S. international population policy and promotes its goals through bilateral and multilateral cooperation. The agency oversees admissions of refugees to the United States for permanent resettlement and works closely with the Immigration and Naturalization Service, the Department of Health and Human Services, and various state and private voluntary agencies. This site includes descriptions of refugee programs abroad and in the United States.

U.S. Department of State: How can I recognize trafficking victims?

U.S. Department of State
2201 C Street NW
Washington, D.C. 20520
202-647-4000
Web: http://www.state.gov

The Web site describes resources and screening questions for victims of human trafficking and includes a toll-free number for reporting suspected trafficking cases.

World Health Organization (WHO)

Avenue Appia 20
1211 Geneva 27
Switzerland
+ 41-22-791-21-11
FAX: + 41-22-79-3111
Telex: 415 416
Telegraph: UNISANTE GENEVA
Email: info@who.int.
Web: http://www.who.int

WHO is the United Nations' specialized agency for health. It was established on April 7, 1948. WHO's objective, as set out in its Constitution, is the attainment by all peoples of the highest possible level of health. Health is defined in WHO's Constitution as a state of complete physical, mental, and social well-being and not merely the absence of disease or infirmity. WHO is governed by 193 Member States through the World Health Assembly. The Health Assembly is composed of representatives from WHO's Member States. The main tasks of the World Health Assembly are to approve the WHO program and the budget for the following biennium and to decide major policy questions. The WHO Web site provides rich examples and information on Healthy Cities from an international perspective.

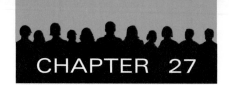

CHAPTER 27

The Homeless Population

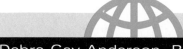

Debra Gay Anderson, RN, BC, PhD

Peggy Riley, RN, MSN

Chapter Outline

⊕ **Health of the Homeless**
   Chronic Versus Acute Health Problems
   Policy Recommendations for Health Care of the Homeless
   Violence
   Mental illness

⊕ **Special Populations**
   Homeless Youth
   Homeless Elderly
   Homeless Families
   Homeless Women
   Homeless Veterans

⊕ **Overall Prevention and Policy Recommendations for the Homeless**
   Ending Chronic Homelessness: Strategies for Action
   Geographic Information System
   Community-Based Homelessness Prevention Program
   National Coalition for the Homeless

Learning Objectives

Upon completion of this chapter, the reader will be able to:

1. Recognize the complexity of homelessness and provide definitions and causes of homelessness.

2. Discuss key factors for the prevention of homelessness in the United States.

3. Describe the health problems facing homeless individuals, families, and communities.

4. Discuss societal factors that contribute to the continuation of homelessness.

5. Interpret the effects of local and national policy and programs on health care and housing for homeless individuals, families, and communities.

6. Discuss issues specific to special populations of homeless: youth, elderly, families, veterans, and the mentally ill.

The definition of homelessness is as complex as homelessness itself. Homelessness, as defined by the Stewart B. McKinney Homeless Assistance Act of 1987, refers to someone who lacks a fixed or permanent, regular, and adequate residence. The act further adds to the definition by stating persons who live in shelters or transitional housing, or those who lack regular sleeping accommodations (persons sleeping in doorways, streets, bus stations, etc.) or those living in their own home or the home of someone else who will be asked to leave within the next month are considered homeless. This definition raises several questions, including: How do you define adequate housing? What is considered an unsuitable place to sleep? Are individuals in jail or detoxification facilities considered homeless? Based on the definition used for homelessness, as well as the accuracy of counting those in shelters, on the street, and doubling up with families and friends, there is quite a disparity in the reported numbers of homeless individuals.

Homelessness in the United States is a social condition that is the result of many factors such as chronic unemployment, domestic violence, poverty, chronic and severe health conditions, mental illness, and substance abuse. There are also a large number of veterans who are homeless. Homelessness is also a result of extreme poverty, war, disease, and severe forces of nature (such as tsunamis in Asia and the hurricanes in the United States).

On any given night in the United States, there are an estimated 500,000 to 760,000 people homeless, one million to two million individuals experience homelessness each year and an estimated 13.5 million people have been homeless at some point in their lifetime due to macro-level (poverty, low-wage jobs, welfare reform, lack of affordable housing, lack of health insurance) and micro-level (domestic violence, mental illness, substance abuse) factors (Anderson & Rayens, 2004; Swigart & Kolb, 2004). Adding to these numbers are runaways or children of families who are homeless. The number of children who are homeless on any given night ranges from 61,500 to 500,000 (Davey & Neff, 2001).

Over the past 20 years the stereotypical face of the homeless has also changed. Many years ago the homeless stereotype was that of an aging male, one who was homeless due to choice or circumstance, namely alcoholism. Today, the homeless population is younger, often employed, and consists of families with children. Approximately 80 percent of homeless families are headed by a female and one-fifth of the homeless women are pregnant (twice the rate of U.S. women in the same reproductive years). Families, with children, account for approximately 41 percent of the homeless population (National Alliance to End Homelessness, 2007).

Although homelessness affects every race and ethnic group, homelessness and the burden of homelessness falls disproportionately on minority communities, affecting the most vulnerable individuals and families within those communities. Vulnerable populations are subgroups of people who are more sensitive to risk factors than others because of their economic, social, physical/environmental, biological, and lifestyle differences. Risk factors of being homeless such as inadequate nutrition, higher rates of chronic disease and disability, inaccessibility and affordability of health care services, and higher rates of injury add to the burden many of these minority communities must face along with already high rates of poverty and health disparities (Barrow et al., 1999).

Being homeless precludes adequate nutrition and appropriate hygiene adding to the complicated health needs of homeless people (Bottomley, Bissonnette, & Snekvik, 2001). Minor medical problems such as sprains or cuts that otherwise would require only rest and proper hygiene to control, often develop into major medical emergencies for persons lacking permanent residence or access to sanitary facilities (Bottomley, 2001).

Key factors for prevention of homelessness are linked with identifying root causes. Poverty has been identified as one of the major contributing factors to homelessness. According to the National Coalition for the Homeless (NCH) (2006a), "in 2004, 12.7% of the U.S. population, or 37 million people, lived in poverty" (p. 1). This puts this population at risk for becoming homeless. This is especially true if medical or financial crisis that creates a dilemma between paying for health care and paying rent occurs.

Other factors identified by the NCH that may lead to increased poverty include

1. Eroding work opportunities (decreasing wages or decreasing value of minimum wage)
2. Decline in public assistance
3. Decline in government supported housing
4. Lack of affordable health care
5. Domestic violence

6. Mental illness

7. Addiction disorders (NCH, 2006a)

Public health nurses must be able to identify risk factors of becoming homeless as well as be aware of specific consequences and risks faced by those that are homeless. One of the core concepts of the public health nurse is advocacy. By understanding some of the issues surrounding homelessness and recognizing the magnitude of the issue of homelessness, public health nurses can become better informed advocates of this vulnerable population.

Therefore, this chapter will focus on homelessness in the United States. We will discuss risk factors of becoming homeless, identify groups at higher risk for homelessness, identify consequences of being homeless, and discuss policy/programs designed to assist the homeless.

HEALTH OF THE HOMELESS

Health problems in homeless people are disproportionately higher than health problems in the general population. Higher rates of drug and alcohol abuse, mental illness, injuries, fractures, dental problems, respiratory tract disease, peripheral vascular disease, hypertension, liver disease, and communicable disease are reported in the homeless population (Swigart & Kolb, 2004). Furthermore, the death rate of homeless adults was almost four times that of the general population with injury, heart disease, liver disease, poisoning, and ill-defined causes accounting for nearly 75 percent of homeless deaths.

The homeless are also at higher risk of overall poor physical health, HIV infection, untreated psychiatric disabilities, and substance abuse. The majority of this increase is due to limited access to health care (Barrow et al., 1999). In a retrospective chart study of a homeless drop-in clinic in the Northeast, Lundy (1999) found the most common reason for a primary care visit to be a physical exam (24 percent). Of the clients at the clinic, 63 percent had a prior hospitalization. The following are reasons for hospitalization: trauma (36 percent), surgery (32 percent), pulmonary problems (8 percent), infectious disease (7 percent), childbirth (5 percent), and detoxification (5 percent). Self-reported substance abuse included tobacco (78 percent), alcohol (65 percent), marijuana (49 percent), cocaine (46 percent), and IV drugs (13 percent). Twenty-nine percent

of those surveyed reported having mental health issues, with 25 percent having depression, 4 percent other psychiatric/mental disorders, 2 percent schizophrenia, and 1 percent bipolar disorder. Mental health symptoms included depression (29 percent), anxiety (19 percent), suicidal ideation (11 percent), and hearing voices (5 percent). Medical problems were reported in 59 percent of the clients, including musculoskeletal problems (15 percent), physical health problems (74 percent), skin problems (25 percent), musculoskeletal pain (22 percent), and cough (21 percent). According to Lundy (1999), traumas were the most common reason for hospitalization of homeless individuals and often the reason for seeking care from a primary care provider. Thirty-nine percent of the homeless tracked had some form of insurance, with the most common being HMO coverage. Seventeen percent reported not having a primary care provider.

Chronic Versus Acute Health Problems

Homeless people are more likely to suffer from every type of chronic health problem, with the exception of obesity, cerebral vascular accidents, and cancer (Bottomley, 2001). Diabetes, tuberculosis (TB), and other such conditions, which require repeated, constant treatment, are difficult to treat or control in persons lacking adequate shelter (Bottomley, 2001). The homeless are at higher risk of TB due to crowded and congregate living arrangements and high-risk behavior practices such as substance abuse or IV drug use (Nyamathi et al., 2005). Compounding these high-risk factors are the high prevalence of chronic disease in the homeless as well as inaccessibility of health care services.

Policy Recommendations for Health Care of the Homeless

Health care for the homeless is complex, and poor health is closely associated with homelessness (NCH, 2006b). The majority of the homeless suffer from multiple health problems, some requiring long-term care and monitoring (i.e. heart disease, diabetes, TB, or HIV). Lack of health insurance remains an issue for the homeless. The homeless are exceptionally vulnerable and at-risk due to barriers such as lack of affordabil-

⊕ PRACTICE APPLICATION

TB Detection Services

Understanding perceptions of homeless persons regarding health promotion and illness prevention efforts is essential to designing programs that are appealing to their needs. Swigart and Kolb (2004) interviewed homeless persons to determine factors influencing their decision to use or reject public health TB detection services. They found that barriers to their utilization of public health TB detection services were their fear of test results, not wanting to be bothered, and fear of being labeled as ill. But, the homeless people also reported encouragement from shelter personnel, the desire to maintain health, a history of lung problems, and the knowledge that living on the street or in crowded quarters as reasons why they utilized public health TB detection services.

Swigart and Kolb (2004) suggested the following guidelines for efforts directed at providing health promotion and disease detection services to homeless people:

- ⊕ Recognize and maximize the positive interest and concern about health in both **sheltered homeless** (those living in shelters or transitional housing) and **street-living homeless** (those living on the streets).
- ⊕ Recognize the period of time in early drug- and alcohol-addiction recovery as an optimal time for emphasis on health promotion and disease detection.
- ⊕ Recognize the important role of shelter personnel and train them to interact in positive ways to enhance compliance to disease detection.
- ⊕ Provide strict confidentiality and privacy during screening activity, particularly for women with potential child-custody problems.

1. How might you organize services provided to a homeless population to serve their needs better?
2. What resources are needed to provide appropriate health promotion and illness prevention services to homeless persons?
3. How can the public health nurse interact with homeless persons to promote health and prevent illness?

ity or inaccessibility to health care. Approximately 55 percent of the homeless population and 73 percent of the homeless obtaining service at Consolidated Health Centers for the homeless are uninsured (compared to 43.6 percent of general population) (NCH, 2006b).

NCH (2006b) has the following recommendations for treating health problems of the homeless:

- ⊕ Provide universal access to affordable health care
- ⊕ Provide accessible public health clinics or centers
- ⊕ Increase funding for health care for the homeless through advocacy to public policy makers
- ⊕ Identify at-risk groups for homelessness
- ⊕ Increase availability of jobs and housing to the homeless through federal, state, and local assistance

Violence

Hate crimes are defined as bias-motivated crimes brought about by prejudice or partiality by the perpetrator against victims belonging to either real or perceived groups (NCH, 2006c). According to NCH, hate crimes against the homeless have increased. Between the years 1999 and 2005, 472 hate crimes were committed against the homeless. A total of 169 deaths were reported along with 303 nonlethal attacks. Types of crime included harassment and physical assault (being set on fire, beaten to death). Crimes were committed in 42 states including Puerto Rico and in 165 cities across the United States. Perpetrator ages ranged from 11 to 75 years and victim ages ranged from 4 months to 74 years of age. Crime was committed against 358 males and 48 females (NCH, 2006c).

Policy Recommendations for Decreasing Hate Crimes

NCH recommends the following to decrease hate crimes:

- ⊕ Increase hate-crime legislation
- ⊕ Ensure hate crimes are publicly acknowledged by the Department of Justice
- ⊕ Create better tracking systems for hate crimes committed against the homeless
- ⊕ Promote police training about hate crimes against the homeless

⊕ Establish Faces of Homelessness Speakers' Bureaus to inform and educate communities about hate crimes and homeless people

Mental Illness

It is estimated that between 20 and 25 percent of the homeless have experienced severe and continuous psychiatric disorders (NCH, 2006d). Schizophrenia, clinical depression, and bipolar disorder were among the most common disorders reported in the homeless population (Folsom et al., 2005). Because 50 percent or more have experienced substance abuse, either as a direct cause of homelessness or related to the stress of being homeless (Koegel et al., 1999), finding a way to improve treatment for the homeless has been a challenge. Treating mental illness in the homeless population presents a challenge due to barriers such as lack of accessibility to health care. Homeless individuals are caught in the daily struggle for survival such as finding shelter for night, finding food, and avoiding violence (Folsom et al, 2005; Koegel et al., 1999, Randolph et al., 2002).

Policy Recommendations for Mental Health Issues

Policy recommendations to assist the homeless mentally ill must be aimed at identifying high-risk groups and increasing accessibility and affordability of services. The National Health Care for the Homeless Council has made the following recommendations:

⊕ Ensure access to and accountability of mainstream addiction and mental health services

⊕ Strengthen existing mental health and addiction services

⊕ End the criminalization of homelessness

⊕ Establish policies and programs that are consistent with emerging evidence-based practice

⊕ Require health plans, including Medicaid, to cover behavioral health services (National Health Care for the Homeless Council, 2004)

SPECIAL POPULATIONS

The individuals comprising the homeless population are not the stereotypes of transient "hobos" or single men sleeping in parks or panhandling on the street. Many factors put people at risk of homelessness: unemployment, low wages, expensive housing, lack of health insurance, and racial discrimination combined with common personal issues such as domestic violence, abuse of alcohol and other drugs, and serious mental and physical illnesses. Therefore, modern homelessness includes youth, the elderly, families, women, and veterans.

Homeless Youth

Homeless youth are defined as those younger than 18 who do not have permanent guardianship by either birth/adopted parents, foster parents, or state institutions (NCH, 2006e). It is estimated that 1.3 million to 2 million youths between the ages of 12 and 17 are homeless (Taylor-Seehafer, 2004).

Causes of youth homelessness fall into three categories: familial problems, economic problems, and residential problems (Hyde, 2005; NCH, 2006e). Familial problems that result in children running away from home or being thrown out include physical (46 percent) or sexual abuse (17 percent), family tension or disputes, and family addictions such as alcohol or substance abuse (Hyde, 2005; NCH, 2006e). NCH (2006e) cites family disruptions as the most frequently named reason for children leaving home to become homeless.

The main economic reason for children becoming homeless is family economic conditions that result in familial homelessness. Reasons for family economic instability can be the result of loss of job or inability to find and sustain work, lack of insurance that results in overwhelming medical bills, lack of affordable housing, or domestic disturbances between parents (Hyde, 2005; NCH, 2006e).

Residential problems or instability also contribute to homeless among youth. Homelessness may be the result of lack of adequate foster care or children living in state institutions becoming too old to live in those institutions yet have no place to go upon discharge (Hyde, 2005; NCH, 2006e).

Another growing body of youth homelessness is the youth's identification with the gay, lesbian, bisexual, and transgender (GLBT) lifestyle. Cochran and colleagues (2002) state that GLBT youth face the challenge of survival on the street as well as the stigma of being a member of a sexual minority group. It is estimated that between 6 and 35 percent of homeless youth may fall into the GLBT category (Cochran et al., 2002). Primary interventions directed toward this population of homeless youth should focus on preventing initial and recurrent episodes of homelessness by providing therapeutic services to assist families in dealing with sexual identity and improving the home environment, therefore reducing the likelihood of the GLBT youth leaving home to become homeless. Secondary interventions are directed toward recognition of particular difficulties GLBT homeless may face and providing services sensitive to issues of sexual orientation (Cochran et al., 2002).

Homeless youth are faced with not only survival but new barriers such as fear of repercussion from authority. Youth may not seek shelter or health care due to fear of being found. Homeless youth have few legitimate opportunities to support themselves financially so many rely on "survival sex" (trading sex for money, drugs, or shelter) or panhandling. Sexual activities increase exposure to sexually transmitted infections (STI), hepatitis B, hepatitis C, and HIV; high rates of substance abuse, depression, and suicide attempts buffer these health risks by helping the teens focus on individual strengths and environmental protective factors (Cochran et al., 2002).

Risk of becoming HIV positive is two to ten times higher in the youth homeless population than that of the same age group of the general population (NCH, 2006e). Rates of major depression have also been found to be higher in this population (three times higher than in general population of same age). With this increased rate comes a higher risk for attempted or actual suicide due to major depression (NCH, 2006e).

Another issue with homeless youth is lack of accessibility to education. Because they have no fixed residence and basic survival needs, homeless youth will not attend school. This lack of education further attenuates chances of long-term poverty, which may lead to increased homelessness (NCH, 2006e).

Policy and Program Recommendations for Homeless Youth

Public health programs aimed at minimizing health risks have been identified as the most effective in dealing with homeless youth. The main emphasis of these programs is on providers with adolescent experience that can focus on the strengths of that population and develop assets for these youth (Taylor-Seehafer, 2004).

Psychosocial support and substance abuse treatment can also minimize health risks. These treatment measures include essential services for the development of caring relationships, case management services, life skills training, support groups, and community mental health referrals (Taylor-Seehafer, 2004). Substance abuse services include easy access and recurrent entry to substance abuse treatment services that are sensitive to the subculture and lifestyle of homeless youths, first-focus on meeting their basic needs (food, clothing, and shelter), and routine screening for childhood abuse; multidisciplinary integrated mental health services focus on reducing the harmful consequences of addictive behavior (Taylor-Seehafer, 2004).

Homeless youth are exposed to a multitude of sexual risks such as rape, sexual victimization, prostitution, commercial sexual exploitation. Many youth engage in survival sex, or the trading of sex to meet their basic needs. Recommendations for reducing risky sexual

⊕ POLICY HIGHLIGHT

No Child Left Behind

The McKinney-Vento Act, originally authorized in 1987 as the Urgent Relief for the Homeless Act, was a landmark federal legislation to address homelessness in America. Congress reauthorized the McKinney-Vento Act as the McKinney-Vento Homeless Education Assistance Improvements Act in the "No Child Left Behind Act" of 2001. The act entitles children who are homeless to a free, appropriate public education and requires schools to address problems that homeless youth face regarding their enrollment, attendance, and success in school. The legislation defines homelessness and recognizes that students in a variety of living situations are homeless. Under the law, schools cannot segregate homeless youth in a separate school program within a school, based on homelessness alone. In addition, schools must immediately enroll homeless students even if they are unable to produce the records normally required by nonhomeless students and they must ensure that homeless children are provided transportation to and from the school. School districts must also designate a local liaison to serve as a primary contact between homeless families, school staff, and other service providers.

behavior include screening and treatment for sexually transmitted diseases, access to contraceptive options, counseling on healthy sexuality and safer sex practices, and counseling to address issues of prior abuse or violence (Taylor-Seehafer, 2004).

In addition to sexual exploitation, homeless youth are also at high risk for exposure to a variety of forms victimization. Their lifestyles and activities of daily living expose them to dangerous people and situations. Recommendations for reducing victimization include providing a drug-free safe place to socialize, group training in conflict resolution and anger management skills, and training in stress reduction and coping skills (Taylor-Seehafer, 2004).

Homeless Elderly

The definition of elder homelessness is an individual older than 50 who lacks a fixed or permanent, regular, and adequate residence (NCH, 2006f; Stewart B. McKinney Act of 1987). Homelessness in the elderly is primarily due to lack of availability of affordable housing coupled with increased poverty due to decreases in wage-earning capability or lack of adequate retirement income (NCH, 2006f).

Elders who are homeless have been found to be more inclined to sleep in the streets as opposed to going to a shelter because they do not trust those at the shelter and are more prone to victimization (theft of personal belongings) or hate crimes (Gibeau, 2001; NCH, 2006c). Health problems are aggravated by age, way of life, and lack of medical treatment. Homeless older adults are more apt to suffer from neurological disorders, such as epilepsy, peripheral neuropathies, and cognitive disorders; gastrointestinal problems; musculoskeletal disorders; and respiratory problems, such as pneumococcal pneumonia, chronic obstructive airway diseases, and TB than the general population (Bottomley, 2001).

Acute illness in the elder homeless is often precipitated by lack of proper nutrition, lack of adequate medical care, lack of support systems, noncompliance with taking medication, substance abuse, or mental illness (Gibeau, 2001). Acute illnesses suddenly become unmanageable chronic disease and disability, further compounding the already compromised older homeless individual.

Poor health is closely linked with homelessness in the older adult population because a serious illness or disability for an older individual already struggling to pay rent can start the slide into homelessness (Bottomley, 2001). Although, for the most part, Medicare covers the elderly population, many older adults have slipped through the system and are no longer eligible. Some have only part A coverage, as many cannot afford the premiums for the voluntary part B coverage, which covers services beyond acute care needs (Bottomley, 2001).

Homelessness results in premature aging as diseases and disorders, such as arthritis, peripheral vascular disease, which are typically seen after the sixth decade of life, may appear in homeless people in their fourth or fifth decade of life. Due to the premature aging, programs for and studies of homeless older adults define elderly homeless as 50 and older, but individuals who are 50 to 65 years of age are too young for Medicare or Social Security (Bruckner, 2001).

Characteristics of Homeless Elderly Men

Homeless elderly nonveteran men are primarily African American, have low levels of education, have significant psychiatric problems, and suffer from chronic diseases such as arthritis, hypertension, diabetes, peripheral vascular disease, alcoholism, and tuberculosis (Bruckner, 2001). The majority were never employed full-time. However, they do have a stable source of income from entitlement programs, but the income is insufficient to meet the needs of housing, food, medical care, and other living expenses (Bruckner, 2001). Homeless elderly men tend to experience a higher rate of social isolation and alienation from families, which oftentimes began earlier in life (Bruckner, 2001). Social isolation is a relative concept with homeless elderly men because they tend to create their own social network for companionship, support, and security (Bruckner, 2001).

Characteristics of Homeless Elderly Women

Homeless elderly women make up a small percentage of the overall homeless population (Bruckner, 2001). Elderly women are vulnerable to becoming homeless after the deaths of their spouses. The homeless elderly women tend to be Caucasian, receive public assistance such as supplemental security income (which is too little to cover living expenses), suffer from psychiatric illnesses (but are less likely to abuse alcohol or other drugs), and have chronic health problems (such as diabetes, arthritis, pneumonia, tuberculosis, and vision and hearing loss) (Bruckner, 2001).

Kisor and Kendal-Wilson (2002) found the stereotypical homeless older woman is a "bag lady." Of the older persons living below the poverty line, 75 percent are women, and most are dependent on social security. Of the older persons living alone and at risk for social isolation, 80 percent are women. Older women are more vulnerable than older men to become homeless. Single older women are more likely to live on a fixed income and are dependent on social security (Kisor & Kendal-Wilson, 2002).

Women may not know about the availability of services and benefits or have trouble applying for them. Because women ages 50 to 62 are ineligible for the major entitlement programs, they are in particular danger of falling through the safety net because there is no income assistance for single adults younger than 62 unless they are severely disabled. Homeless older women tend to mistrust shelters and clinics because they are more prone to maltreatment; consequently, an important encounter for the older homeless woman is adult protective services (Kisor & Kendal-Wilson, 2002). The major reasons for homelessness include inadequate income and mental health difficulties along with disputes with family and friends, relationship violence, and lack of social support (Kiser & Kendal-Wilson, 2002).

Policy and Program Recommendations for the Homeless Elderly

Policy and programs are aimed at improving overall economic, housing, and health circumstances for the aging population. A number of innovative programs exist for the homeless elderly. In some communities, the county social service department coordinates emergency shelter for frail older adults. Accommodations are recruited from church groups and community organization, and the older adult stays until more permanent arrangements are secured. This program has proven to be cost-effective, and the clients served have a high degree of satisfaction (Bruckner, 2001). Another innovative program is a day program where older adults are served exclusively. One such program in Boston provides 100 midday meals a day, along with protection from the weather and street violence, a welcoming place to socialize, access to case management for emergency assistance, housing assistance, access to primary

health care, and access to an alcohol treatment center. A day program in New York offers breakfast, lunch, and snacks, and such services as access to primary health care, access to psychiatric and alcohol rehabilitation services, and housing assistance (Bruckner, 2001).

The three-tiered approach seems to be best. First establish contact and trust to get the individual through the door. Once the individual is inside, address the basic needs of nutrition, primary health care, and a safe environment. Wait until the client is ready and then offer professional help for problems such as mental illness, substance abuse, housing, and access to entitlement programs. Importantly, the programs should be staffed with people who recognize the need for basic human dignity of the clients, who create an environment of safety and trust, and who establish a sense of community (Bruckner, 2001). In addition, the staff, according to homeless older adults, should be able to listen, be caring, and be nonjudgmental (Gibeau, 2001).

Policy recommendations include the following:

- Ensure adequate retirement income such as social security benefits or private retirement.
- Ensure supplemental jobs for the aging who still want to maintain a job
- Ensure adequate and affordable housing
- Provide social support networks such as support groups for the aging
- Provide community programs that have social networking along with resources such as food, shelter, medical care, and financial assistance as needed
- Lobby for improved medical care and benefits such as Medicare and supplemental insurance to provide health care and prescription cost
- Provide resources to grandparents who may be raising grandchildren

Homeless Families

Families with children are one of the fastest growing subpopulations of the homeless in the United States. It is estimated that families account for greater than one-third of the homeless population (NCH, 2006g).

The primary causes for the increase in family homelessness are poverty and lack of affordable

⊕ PRACTICE APPLICATION

Homeless Elderly

Peggy Stuart, a public health nurse working with a city health department, received a referral from a parish nurse at a local church. The parish nurse requested that she assist her in finding medical care and suitable housing for an elderly woman who had come to the church for assistance. The parish nurse reported the woman's family could no longer take care of her because of financial constraints. Although the family moved the elderly woman to an apartment of her own, she left the apartment because her income could not support her, and she was now left to fend for herself on the streets and has been sleeping at various homeless shelters at night.

⊕ What other assessment information do you need?

⊕ Other than housing, what else might the woman need?

⊕ What community resources could be explored? What government resources could be explored?

⊕ What other community workers could be involved in a solution to the woman's needs?

⊕ Provide some logical solutions for the referral.

---

housing (Meadows-Oliver, 2003; NCH, 2006g). Recent studies have found that poverty is increasing especially among single, female-headed households. This may be due to diminishing wages, lack of available jobs, or alterations in federal- and state-funded welfare programs (Meadows-Oliver, 2003). Overall the number of impoverished has risen in the United States. From 2000 to 2004, the number of poor rose by 4.3 million (NCH, 2006g). Because increasing numbers of families and children living below the federal poverty level and because incomes and affordable housing are not keeping up with the trend, more and more families may be forced to become homeless (NCH, 2006g).

Homeless families present a complex set of issues. Children of homeless families tend to be in poorer overall health due to lack of accessibility to health care. These children have higher rates of asthma (due to exposure to elements and environmental pollutants), ear infections, and stomach problems (due to inadequate nutrition and unsanitary living conditions). In addition, children of homeless families tend to have higher rates of behavioral issues and mental health issues (NCH, 2006g).

Education is also compromised in children of homeless families. Barriers such as lack of stable residence, lack of transportation, lack of adequate clothing, lack of nutrition, lack of school supplies, and no permanent school records face homeless families with children (NCH, 2006g).

Homeless families sometimes become separated due to shelter rules, children being placed in foster care or leaving to live with relatives. The stress of day-to-day survival may cause strained relationships between parents causing separation and divorce, further adding to the complexity of being homeless (NCH, 2006g).

Policy and Program Recommendations for Homeless Families

Advocates for homeless families should make strong recommendations to policy makers to end homelessness through job security and affordable family housing. Job and educational training for those without job skills should be a priority. Further, providing affordable, universal health care for families will decrease the likelihood that families will suffer financial ruin from unexpected medical bills (NCH, 2006g).

Homeless Women

It is estimated that 90 percent of homeless families are headed by females. Many of the women become homeless due to relationship violence. Abuse is not a predictor of homelessness, but perhaps the inability to form and maintain relationships is predictive of homelessness. Domestic violence is one of the major contributing factors to homelessness in women. These women are faced with either living in an abusive relationship or becoming homeless (NCH, 2006h).

Anderson and Rayens (2004) investigated the families of origin and the early social support systems of women who had experienced homelessness. They found homeless women scored the lowest regarding social support and reciprocity in relationships, never-homeless women who had experienced an abusive childhood scored the second lowest, and never-homeless women who had not experienced abuse as a child scored the highest and vice versa for scores regarding conflict in relationships. The lack of strength in family of origin and the early support system along with the ensuing difficulty developing and accessing assistance from one's social network may limit a protective relational aspect available to those persons who learned in childhood how to develop relationships. Interventions to reconnect women and their families or to assist women with developing support systems may lessen the physiological, social, and emotional turmoil created by homelessness (Anderson & Rayens, 2004).

Another growing population of homeless women is veterans. In 2000, women veterans made up 5 percent of the total veteran population, and that number is expected to double by 2010 (Gamache, Rosenheck, & Tessler, 2003). Women veterans average 14.1 years of schooling, 46 percent were between the ages of 35 and 49, 54 percent were currently married, 69 percent were non-Hispanic white, 47 percent had annual household incomes than $30,000, and 19 percent lived alone. The risk of homelessness is two to four times greater for women veterans than women nonveterans.

Women veterans possess characteristics that may be risk factors for homelessness. Those risk factors include low income, concomitant posttraumatic stress disorder, and poor physical health per self-assessment. Some potential causes for the high risk of homelessness among veterans are that the veterans in the homeless samples resided in their current cities for shorter lengths of time than had nonveterans, military service may weaken community connections, and the mobility of military service may accompany a reluctance to return home on discharge, resulting in lessened family support when faced with hard times (Gamache, Rosenheck, & Tessler, 2003).

Policy and Program Recommendations for Homeless Women

Policy recommendations are aimed at increasing the safety of victims of domestic violence such as better police protection, more accessible battered shelters, and stricter laws on perpetrators of domestic violence. Specific federal policies, with specific aims of assisting children of homeless women, follow:

- McKinney-Vento Homeless Assistance Act (2001) is a federal law ensuring children the right to attend school regardless of housing circumstances.

- Federal Education Rights and Privacy Act protect the privacy of educational records. Parents must give written permission to allow access to their child's school records. This gives some protection to women who may have emergency protective orders against abusive spouses from locating them or their children.

It has also been recommended that schools assist homeless women by helping them build a strong support system, acting as a resource for referrals for community assistance, providing necessary support and referral to children from abusive homes, and addressing safety needs of women and their children. Above all, it has been recommended that schools become advocates for these victims and their children (McKinney-Vento Homeless Assistance Act, 2001).

Homeless Veterans

According to the Department of Veterans Affairs (DVA, 2007) approximately one-third of all adult homeless are veterans of the armed forces. It is estimated that on any given day there are 200,000 veterans living on the streets or staying in shelters across the country. Specific characteristics of the homeless veteran include being male (33 percent), being a Vietnam veteran (47 percent), serving three or more years in the armed forces (67 percent), being a pre-Vietnam veteran (15 percent), being a post-Vietnam veteran (17 percent), spending some time during military career in a war zone (33 percent), using VA Homeless Services (25 percent), completing high school or GED (85 percent), residing in central cities (79 percent), residing in suburban areas (16 percent), residing in rural areas (5 percent), experiencing drug, alcohol, or mental health issues (76 percent), being age 45 or older (46 percent), needing assistance finding a job (45 percent), and needing assistance finding adequate housing (37 percent) (DVA, 2006).

Homelessness among veterans, as with other homeless populations, is due primarily to lack of affordable

⊕ RESEARCH APPLICATION

Health-Promoting Behaviors of Sheltered Homeless Women

Study Purpose

To describe sociodemographic and personal characteristics, health practices, and health-promoting behaviors in a population of sheltered homeless women from five shelters in the Midwest.

Methods

The descriptive, cross-sectional study sampled 137 women from urban shelters located in the Midwest. In addition to demographic data, health-promoting behaviors were measured with the Health-Promoting Lifestyle Profile II (HPLP II). The HPLP II measures health responsibility, physical activity, nutrition, spiritual growth, interpersonal relations, and stress management. Bivariate descriptive statistics (Pearson's r and Eta correlations) were used to examine relationships among study variables.

Findings

Only 11.7 percent of the women reported accessible health care, citing the emergency room as the usual entry of care. The most frequent barriers to health care were money (63.5 percent) and transportation (32.1 percent). The women's most commonly reported illnesses were asthma (27 percent), chronic bronchitis (25.5 percent), and hyper-

tension (20.4 percent). Most (68.6 percent) of the women used tobacco, with most (47.5 percent) using one or more packs of cigarettes per day. Although 84.7 percent had received medical care and 63.5 percent had a Pap test in the past two years, dental and vision care were reported to be the greatest unmet needs. The lowest scores on the HPLP II were physical activity, nutrition, health responsibility, and stress management.

Implications

Women who are socially and economically deprived can enhance their own health with health promotive behaviors. Access to health care and services are critical to address health disparities in this vulnerable population. Public health nurses can collaborate with food banks, churches, low-income housing, and community centers to develop culturally appropriate holistic care for the physical, psychological, spiritual, and social resources needed by homeless women.

Reference

Wilson, M. (2005). Health-promoting behaviors of sheltered homeless women. *Family and Community Health, 28*(1), 51–63.

---

housing and poverty. Veteran's benefits (decreasing benefits due to federal cutbacks), without supplemental income, is insufficient to meet the needs of housing and food (NCHV, 2006). Other reasons for homelessness in this population are high rates of alcohol and substance abuse due to posttraumatic stress disorder and lack of family and social support systems (NCHV, 2006).

Programs for Homeless Veterans

Available programs specifically address issues surrounding homelessness such as unaffordable housing and poverty. Strong advocacy from nonhomeless veterans as well as concerned groups have encouraged development of specific programs to address the special needs of homeless veterans. Services addressing these specific needs include but are not limited to

- ⊕ VA's Health Care for the Homeless Veterans Program, which provides extensive outreach for physical and psychological examinations, treatment, and referral plus case management
- ⊕ VA's Domiciliary Care for Homeless Veterans, which provides medical care and rehabilitation in a residential setting
- ⊕ Special Outreach and Benefits Assistance, which provides support funding for counselors.
- ⊕ Veterans Benefits Assistance, which serve as a point of contact for referrals to various resources for the homeless
- ⊕ Acquired Property Sales for Homeless Providers Programs, which makes available affordable housing to the homeless from foreclosured VA housing loans

- Readjustment counseling service vet centers, which provide outreach, psychological counseling, support services, and referrals for homeless veterans with mental illness and substance/alcohol abuse
- Drop-in centers, which provide homeless veterans who sleep in the street with a safe, daytime environment where they can take a shower and obtain a meal (DVA, 2006; NCH, 2006i; NCHV, 2006)

Programs are available to assist the homeless veterans, but reaching this population is an issue. Some of the barriers to obtaining these services include distrust of the system, lack of knowledge of all available resources, and inaccessibility of available resources (NCHV, 2006). Identifying and locating this high-risk vulnerable population as well as providing accessible services should be a priority of program coordinators serving this population.

OVERALL PREVENTION AND POLICY RECOMMENDATIONS FOR THE HOMELESS

Recognition of the magnitude of homelessness by advocacy groups and political entities created the federal homelessness task force in 1983. The first homelessness federal task force was created in 1983, called Title V, and provided information to interested parties on obtaining excess federal property. In 1986, responding to growing pressure to address the homelessness issue, Congress passed small portions of the Homeless Persons' Survival Act. In 1987, the Urgent Relief for the Homeless Act was passed by large bipartisan majorities of both congressional houses. The act was renamed the McKinney-Vento Homeless Assistance Act after the death of its chief Republican sponsor, Representative Stewart B. McKinney (Connecticut). On July 22, 1987, President Ronald Regan signed the act into law. Since being passed, it has been amended several times, and according to HUD.gov, provides the best first step to address the needs of a population that is grossly unknown and underrepresented.

According to Green and Kreuter (1999), one of the most effective methods of promoting change is community involvement. Community assessment utilizing models that will promote community uniqueness and individuality is essential. Community strengths as well as identification of community social weakness is best accomplished by a community-based approach; "grounded in the principles of participatory democracy and social justice, community-based programs hold considerable potential for making population changes."

Keeping in mind that each community is diverse is one of the most important concepts. Social problems such as decreased affordable housing or low-wage jobs may not be a problem for every community; therefore, taking a universal approach to policies or programs will not be effective in decreasing homelessness.

Rew and Horner (2003) conducted secondary analysis of qualitative data from three studies. Two distinct types of strengths emerged from the findings: resources and self-improvement. Resources was found to indicate knowledge of environment that enables the homeless to be safer on the streets; to meet the basic survival needs for food, water, shelter, and some medical care; and to develop a community of peers for companionship, guidance, and acceptance. These resources provide internal motivation for self-improvement. Self-improvement skills included enacting healthier behaviors, gaining emotional maturity, and mastering skills for further self-improvement.

Private aid among poor people is the key to keeping millions of homeless people off the streets. Many low-income families, regardless of their own scarcity of resources and inadequate housing, provide the bulk of housing for homeless persons (Kisor & Kendal-Wilson, 2002).

Ending Chronic Homelessness: Strategies for Action

In March 2003, the U.S. Department of Health and Human Services (USDHHS) released "Ending Chronic Homelessness: Strategies for Action," an initiative developed to concentrate on an integrated organization of support systems for people who are chronically homeless. The initiative seeks to enhance access to health and human services, foster state and local responses to homelessness, and prevent new episodes of homelessness. Proposed goals and strategies include increasing accessibility of health and social services for the chronic homeless, empowering state and community partners to improve response to the chronic homeless, working to prevent new episodes of homelessness, and improving the eligibility review process (USDHHS, 2003). A

⊕ POLICY HIGHLIGHT

Not In My Back Yard

"Not In My Back Yard" (NIMBY) is a phenomenon that occurs when residents of a community adopt protectionist attitudes and oppositional tactics to prevent an unwelcome project from developing in their neighborhood. Debates occur when various changes to the neighborhood are proposed including the development of residential or commercial property; introduction of additional infrastructure such as highways, power plants, or wastewater treatment plants; and the construction of culturally unfamiliar functions such as subsidized housing or homeless shelters. An example of NIMBY was a proposal for expansion of a homeless shelter in Des Moine, Iowa (The NIMBY Report, 2006). After being told by city officials that the presence of the homeless shelter was not part of the city's plan for redevelopment of the neighborhood, the Central Iowa Shelter and Services identified a new location for the shelter. After two years, the new neighborhood has protested, "complaining that a disproportionate number of social services had been dumped in their neighborhood and suggested that the shelter would bring sex offenders, predators, and drug addicts to the area." The shelter's board has been reevaluating all of their options, but the future of the shelter is uncertain.

systematic approach to understanding homelessness was utilized in deriving the proposed goals. Committees examined four main areas connected to homelessness. First, a complete epidemiological review was conducted along with a literature review to examine causes and risk factors of long-term and repeated homelessness. Second, an inventory was completed for eight existing USDHHS programs. Third, findings from the first two steps were summarized. Last, forums were held to hear from advocates, communities, resources, and service providers. These steps eventually led to the proposed Strategies for Action (USDHHS, 2003).

Geographic Information System

Wong and Hillier (2001) introduced the use of Geographic Information System (GIS) technology to study patterns of community-based emergency assistance and case management program use to prevent homelessness. GIS, a method of storing, analyzing, and manipulating data that are spatially referenced, has been applied to program development and planning for health care, education, housing, and homelessness with regard to the location of new program sites and the areas that need to be targeted for development. According to Wong and Hillier (2001), the rate of admission to homeless shelters is strongly predicted by demographic and socioeconomic distress factors, which include "concentration of female-headed households with young children, poverty, persons of African-American descent, unemployment, housing abandonment, housing vacancy, housing overcrowding, and high rent-to-income ratio."

Community-Based Homelessness Prevention Program

The goal of the Community-based Homelessness Prevention Program (CHPP) was to help prevent at-risk households from using public shelters by addressing immediate housing needs with emergency cash assistance and by linking at-risk households to community-based social services. The community-based prevention model called for crisis assistance and case management services to be near areas where services were likely to be needed in order to assist with accessibility to and connection with services and agencies. CHPP provided a maximum grant of $1,200 for rent, mortgage, or utility payment; compensation of job search expenses; and six months of case management services. The two-pronged tactic for preventing homelessness with emergency monetary aid and case management services deals with urgent needs and addresses the complex factors that caused the housing crisis reducing the risk of future shelter use (Wong & Hillier, 2001). Based on CHPP and GIS recommendations, six homelessness prevention centers were established in areas of Philadelphia with high use of shelters and a seventh prevention

⊕ PRACTICE APPLICATION

Homeless Clinic

Don, a public health nurse for Kenton County, identified a gap in health care at the Mission for Homeless Persons. Programs at the mission include alcohol recovery services, food service, vocational and educational services, a mental health outreach program, and emergency services for food, clothing, and housing. Case managers at the mission work closely with social workers and mental health professionals in the community, and the mission has a volunteer psychiatrist who provides on-site care. The mission also has a psychiatric nurse specialist who addresses any mental health needs exclusively. Although many social and mental health needs were provided, Don noted that most of the homeless persons have medical health care needs that were being met by case managers with limited assessment skills or experi-

ence and knowledge of medical health care. Don considered engaging the local School of Nursing to provide a Mission clinic for the purpose of assessing and screening for illness, making referrals, and providing health promotion and risk reduction education.

⊕ Who would be key persons to work with at the School of Nursing to begin the foundation of the clinic?

⊕ What resources are needed for such a clinic? What resources may be easily available?

⊕ How would Don work with health care professionals in Kenton County to ensure that referrals would be accepted?

⊕ What clinical projects could the nursing students be involved in?

center located in a downtown area based on public transportation accessibility (Wong & Hillier, 2001).

National Coalition for the Homeless

The NCH is a coalition established to increase public education, policy advocacy, and grassroots organization to end homelessness. Four areas of concentration by the coalition include housing justice, economic justice, health care justice, and civil rights. This organization provides a database of educational information to communities, practitioners, researchers, governmental agencies, general public, and the media. The coalition consists of a 38 member governing board consisting of diverse professional and community backgrounds. Individual members of state and local coalitions strive to increase public awareness of the issue of homelessness. Recommendations are made to Congress and other governmental entities based on evidence-based research to create programs and policies to end homelessness and provide assistance to the homeless across the United States (NCH, 2002a).

NCH has recommended to Congress numerous programs and policies, which include the following:

1. Bringing America Home Act contains components of housing, health, economic justice, civil rights, and education for the homeless.

2. National Housing Trust Fund makes available more affordable housing for the impoverished. This fund includes making new housing available as well as decreasing rent to make housing more affordable for those below the federal poverty level.

3. Reauthorization of HUD McKinney-Vento Homeless Assistance includes Emergency Shelter grants, supportive housing for those experiencing homelessness, Shelter Plus Care to provide rental assistance, and Single Room Occupancy dwelling, which assists those experiencing substance abuse.

4. Housing Opportunities for Persons with AIDS (HOPWA) funds community-based HIV/AIDS housing.

5. Supportive Housing for Persons with Disabilities makes available affordable and accessible housing for the physically or mentally disabled.

6. Health Care for the Homeless (HCH) program provides health care opportunities for the homeless.

7. Education of Homeless Children and Youth (EHCY) allows for mainstreaming of children experiencing homelessness.

8. Creation of Civil Rights Protections for the Homeless ensures that the homeless are given voting privileges and other civil rights liberties (NCH, 2002b).

⊕ RESEARCH APPLICATION

A Different Kind of Clinical Experience: Poverty Up Close and Personal

Study Purpose

To give students a basic understanding of the impact of poverty and health on the poor.

Methods

Fifty-one senior-level nursing students were given a pretest prior to beginning their clinical rotation at a crisis center for the homeless and poor. (Students spent four days a week at this crisis-focused day shelter and multiresource advocacy center during the semester.) Follow-up lectures by instructors were given focusing on four key concepts identified through literature reviews (advocacy, empowerment, hope, and self-esteem). Students were instructed to do no prior research on poverty or homelessness prior to taking the pretest. The pretest included the following questions: (1) People are poor because? (2) You can or cannot recognize a poor person when you see one because? (3) Select and qualify your answer to the following: (a) Poverty is worse for men because? (b) Poverty is worse for women because? (c) Poverty is worse for children because? (d) Poverty is equally bad for all of them because? (4) Poor people could end their poverty if they? (5) For each item below choose does or does not and then describe why: (a) Poverty does or does not affect one's mental well-being because? (b) Poverty does or does not affect one's physical well-being because? (c) Poverty does or does not affect chemical dependencies or substance abuse because? (d) Poverty does or does not contribute to domestic violence because? (e) Poverty does or does not have an impact on parenting skills because? (f) Poverty does or does not affect children's growth, development, or mental health because?

Findings

Pretests confirmed instructor hypotheses of limited understanding by students of the issue of poverty and homelessness. There were significant changes regarding the impact of poverty, making the assumption that the poor could end their poverty, indicating a belief that poverty does have an influence on domestic abuse, increasing awareness of need of increasing public awareness of implications of poverty, and recognizing a need to increase awareness that there are working poor. Thirty-nine percent of the students indicated a strong need for more affordable low-income housing, one-third indicated a need for increasing accessibility of programs aimed at the poor, 29 percent indicated the need for better employment programs for the poor, and 41 percent recognized the need for building trusting relationships with the poor. Overall students indicated both a personal and professional growth with this clinical experience.

Implications

This study demonstrated the need for strong public health education about the affects of poverty and possible resolutions to the issues surrounding poverty that will continue to foster empathy and advocacy for the most vulnerable in the health care system.

Reference

Delashmutt, M. B., & Rankin, E. A. (2005). A different kind of clinical experience: Poverty up close and personal. *Nurse Educator, 30*(4), 143–149.

CRITICAL THINKING ACTIVITIES

1. Discuss the complexity of homelessness and discuss advocacy issues relevant for public health nurses.

2. What are the key factors for the prevention of homelessness in the United States? Knowing those factors, what must the United States do to effect change in homelessness?

3. What are the health problems facing homeless individuals, families, and communities? What are communities doing to address the problems?

4. Read you local newspaper and interpret the effects of local policy and programs on health care and housing for homeless individuals and families in your community.

5. Review the policies related to foster care in your state. What policies contribute to the homelessness of youth and older teens (18 and 19 year olds)?

KEY TERMS

hate crimes

homelessness

sheltered homeless

street-living homeless

vulnerable populations

KEY CONCEPTS

⊕ Homelessness is a complex issue that results from chronic unemployment, domestic violence, poverty, chronic and severe health conditions, mental illness, substance abuse, war, disease, and severe forces of nature.

⊕ Key factors for prevention of homelessness are linked with identifying root causes. Poverty has been identified as one of the major contributing factors to homelessness. Increased poverty results from eroding work opportunities, decline in public assistance, decline in government-supported housing, lack of affordable housing, lack of affordable health care, addiction disorders, domestic violence, and mental illness.

⊕ One of the core concepts of the public health nurse is advocacy. By gaining an understanding of some of the issues surrounding homelessness and the magnitude of the issue of homelessness, public health nurses can become better informed advocates of this vulnerable population.

⊕ Homeless individuals experience significantly more health problems than the general population. Health problems in homeless people are disproportionately higher than health problems in the general population. Higher rates of drug and alcohol abuse, mental illness, injuries, fractures, dental problems, respiratory tract disease, peripheral vascular disease, hypertension, liver disease, and communicable disease are reported in the homeless population (Swigart, 2004). The death rate of homeless adults was almost four times that of the general population with injury, heart disease, liver disease, poisoning, and ill-defined causes accounting for nearly 75 percent of homeless deaths.

⊕ Community health programs aimed at minimizing health risks have been identified as the most effective in dealing with homeless youth, with the main focus on providers with adolescent experience that can focus on the strengths of that population and develop assets for these youth (Taylor-Seehafer, 2004).

⊕ An integrated organization of support systems is necessary to address chronic homelessness and acute homelessness and to prevent new episodes of homelessness. Local, state, and federal agencies, as well as private organizations, must join forces to provide the systematic approach necessary to effect lasting change.

REFERENCES

Anderson, D. G., & Rayens, M. K. (2004). Factors influencing homelessness in women. *Public Health Nursing, 21*(1), 12–23.

Barrow, S. M., Herman, D. B., Cordova, P., & Struening, E. L. (1999). Mortality among homeless shelter residents in New York City. *American Journal of Public Health, 89*(4), 529–534.

Bottomley, J. M. (2001). Health care and homeless older adults. *Topics in Geriatric Rehabilitation, 17*(1), 1–21.

Bottomley, J. M., Bissonnette, A., & Snekvik, V. C. (2001). The lives of homeless older adults: Please, tell them who I am. *Topics in Geriatric Rehabilitation, 16*(4), 50–64.

Bruckner, J. (2001). Walking a mile in their shoes: Sociocultural consideration in elder homelessness. *Topics in Geriatric Rehabilitation, 16*(4), 15–27.

Cochran, B. N., Stewart, A. J., Ginzler, J. A., & Cauce, A. M. (2002). Challenges faced by homeless sexual minorities: Comparison of gay, lesbian, bisexual, and transgender homeless adolescents with their heterosexual counterparts. *American Journal of Public Health, 92*(5), 773–777.

Davey, T. L., & Neff, J. A., (2001). A shelter-based stress-reduction group intervention targeting self-esteem, social competence, and behavior problems among homeless children. *Journal of Social Distress and the Homeless, 10*(3), 279–291.

Delashmutt, M. B., & Rankin, E. A. (2005). A different kind of clinical experience: Poverty up close and personal. *Nurse Educator, 30*(4), 143–149.

Department of Veterans Affairs. (2007). *Overview of homelessness.* Retrieved June 19, 2006, from http://www1.va.gov/homeless/page.cfm?pg=1

Folsom, D. P., Hawthorne, W., Lindamer, L., Gilmer, T., Bailey, A., Golshan, S., Garcia, P., Unützer, J., Hough, R., & Jeste, D. V. (2005). Prevalence and risk factors for homelessness and utilization of mental health services among 10,340 patients with serious mental illness in a large public mental health system. *American Journal of Psychiatry, 162*(2), 370–376.

Gamache, G., Rosenheck, R., & Tessler, R. (2003). Overrepresentation of women veterans among homeless women. *American Journal of Public Health, 93*(7), 1132–1136.

Gibeau, J. L. (2001). Home free: An evolving journey in eradicating elder homelessness. *Topics in Geriatric Rehabilitation, 17*(1), 22–52.

Green, L.W., & Kreuter, M. W. (1999) *Health promotion planning: An educational and ecological approach* (3rd ed., Chapter 8). New York: McGraw-Hill.

Hyde, J. (2005). From home to street: Understanding young people's transitions into homelessness. *Journal of Adolescence, 28*, 171–183.

Kisor, A. J., & Kendal-Wilson, L. (2002). Older homeless women: Reframing the stereotype of the bag lady. *Affilia, 17*(3), 354–370.

Koegel, P., Sullivan, G., Burnam, A., Morton, S. C., & Wenzel, S. (1999). Utilization of mental health substances abuse services among homeless adults in Los Angeles. *Medical Care, 37*(3), 306–317.

Lundy, J. W. (1999). The burden of comorbidity among the homeless at a drop-in clinic. *JAAPA: Journal of the American Academy of Physician Assistants, 4.* Retrieved September 8, 2007, from http://www.jaapa.com/issues/j19990401/j4a032.html

McKinney-Vento Homeless Assistance Act. (2001). Retrieved March 22, 2005, from http://www.hud.gov/offices/cpd/homeless/rulesandregs/laws/index.cfm

Meadows-Oliver, M. (2003). Mothering in public: A meta-synthesis of homeless women with children living in shelters. *Journal for the Specialist in Pediatric Nursing, 8*(4), 130–136.

National Alliance to End Homelessness. (2007). *Homelessness counts.* Washington DC: Author.

National Coalition for the Homeless (NCH). (2002a). *About NCH.* Retrieved June 29, 2005, from http://www.nationalhomeless.org/aboutnch.html.

National Coalition for the Homeless (NCH). (2002b). *Legislation and policy.* Retrieved June 21, 2005, from http://www.nationalhomeless.org/policy/o4agenda.html.

National Coalition for the Homeless (NCH). (2006a). *Why are people homeless?* (NCH fact sheet #1). Retrieved July 25, 2006, from http://www.nationalhomeless.org/publications/facts.html.

National Coalition for the Homeless (NCH). (2006b). *Health care and homelessness* (NCH fact sheet #8). Retrieved July 22, 2006, from http://www.nationalhomeless.org/publications/facts.html.

National Coalition for the Homeless (NCH). (2006c). *Hate crimes and violence against people experiencing homelessness* (NCH fact sheet # 21). Retrieved July 25, 2006, from http://www.nationalhomeless.org/.

National Coalition for the Homeless (NCH). (2006d). *Mental illness and homelessness* (NCH fact sheet #5). Retrieved on June 15, 2005, from http://www.nationalhomeless.org/mentalillness.html.

National Coalition for the Homeless (NCH). (2006e). *Homeless youth* (NCH fact sheet #13). Retrieved on July 25, 2006, from http://www.nationalhomeless.org/homelessyouth.html.

National Coalition for the Homeless (NCH). (2006f). *Homelessness among elderly persons* (NCH fact sheet #15). Retrieved July 25, 2006, from http://www.nationalhomeless.org/publications/facts.html.

National Coalition for the Homeless (NCH). (2006g). *Homeless families with children* (NCH fact sheet #12). Retrieved on July 25, 2006, from http://www.nationalhomeless.org/publications/facts.html

National Coalition for the Homeless (NCH). (2006h). *Domestic violence and homeless* (NCH fact sheet #7). Retrieved July 25, 2006, from http://www.nationalhomeless.org/publications/facts.html.

National Coalition for the Homeless (NCH). (2006i). *Homeless veterans* (NCH fact sheet #14). Retrieved June 19, 2006, from http://www.nationalhomeless.org.

National Coalition for Homeless Veterans (NCHV). (2006). *Facts and media.* Retrieved July 25, 2006, from http://www.nchv.org/background.cfm

National Health Care for the Homeless Council. (2004). *Homelessness and health.* Retrieved July 25, 2006, from http://www.nhchc.org/Advocacy/PolicyPapers/HomelessHealth2006.pdf.

Nyamathi, A., Berg, J., Jones, T., & Leake, B. (2005). Predictors of perceived health status of tuberculosis infected homeless. *Western Journal of Nursing Research, 27*(7), 896–910.

Randolph, F., Blasinsky, M., Morrissey, J. P., Rosenheck, R. A., Cocozza, J., Goldman, H. H., & the ACCESS National Evaluation Team. (2002). Overview of the ACCESS program. *Psychiatric Services, 53*(8), 945–948.

Rew, L., & Horner, S. D. (2003). Personal strengths of homeless adolescents living in a high-risk environment. *Advances in Nursing Science, 26*(2), 90–101.

Swigart, V., & Kolb, R. (2004). Homeless persons' decision to accept or reject public health disease-detection service. *Public Health Nursing, 21*(2), 162–170.

Taylor-Seehafer, M. A. (2004). Positive youth development: Reducing the health risks of homeless youth. *Maternal Child Nursing, 29*(1), 36–40.

The Nimby Report. (2006). Iowa shelter struggles to find suitable location in Des Moines. *The NIMBY Report on the Continuing Struggle for Inclusive Communities* (No. 76). Retrieved September 8, 2007, from http://www.bettercommunities.org/index.cfm?method=nimby.view&nimbyID=88

U.S. Department of Health and Human Services. (2003). *Ending chronic homelessness: Strategies for action. Report from the Secretary's work group on ending chronic homelessness.* Retrieved July 25, 2006, from http://aspe.hhs.gov/hsp/homelessness/strategies03/

Wilson, M. (2005). Health-promoting behaviors of sheltered homeless women. *Family and Community Health, 28*(1), 51–63.

Wong, Y. I., & Hillier, A. E. (2001). Evaluating a community-based homelessness prevention program: A geographic information system approach. *Administration & Social Work, 25*(4), 21–45.

BIBLIOGRAPHY

Kushel, M. B., Hahn, J. A., Evans, J. L., Bangsberg, D. R., & Moss, A. R. (2005). Revolving doors: Imprisonment among the homeless and marginally housed population. *American Journal of Public Health, 95,* 1747–1752.

Kusmer, K. L. (2003). *Down and out, on the road: The homeless in American history.* Oxford: Oxford University Press.

Morris, R., & Strong, L. (2004). The impact of homelessness on the health of families. *The Journal of School Nursing, 20,* 221–227.

O'Sullivan, J., & Lussier-Duynstee, P. (2006). Adolescent homelessness, nursing, and public health policy. *Policy, Politics, & Nursing Practice, 7,* 73–77.

Rosengard, C., Chambers, D. B., Tulsky, J. P., Long, H. L., & Chesney, M. (2001). Value on health: Health concerns and practices of women who are homeless. *Women & Health, 34,* 29–44.

Slesnick, N. (2004). *Our runaway and homeless youth: A guide to understanding.* Westport, CT: Praeger Publishers.

Washington, O. G. M. (2005). Identification and characteristics of older homeless African American women. *Issues in Mental Health Nursing, 26,* 117–136.

Wilde, M. H., Albanese, E. P., Rennells, R., & Bullock, Q. (2004). Development of a student nurses' clinic for homeless men. *Public Health Nursing, 21,* 354–360.

RESOURCES

Health Care for the Homeless (HCH) Programs

202-462-4822, ext. 19
Email: mstoops@nationalhomeless.org
Web: http://www.nationalhomeless.org
HCH provides for primary health care and substance abuse services at locations accessible to people who are homeless; emergency care with referrals to hospitals for inpatient care services and/or other needed services; and outreach services to assist difficult-to-reach homeless persons in accessing care and to provide assistance in establishing eligibility for entitlement programs and housing.

National Alliance to End Homelessness

1518 K Street NW, Suite 206
Washington, D.C. 20005
Email: naeh@naeh.org
Web: http://www.endhomelessness.org

The National Alliance to End Homelessness is a nonprofit organization whose mission is to mobilize the nonprofit, public, and private sectors of society in an alliance to end homelessness.

National Coalition for Homeless Veterans (NCHV)

3331/2 Pennsylvania Avenue SE
Washington, D.C. 20003-1148
1-800-VET-HELP
FAX: 202-546-2063
Email: nchv@nchv.org
NCHV's mission is to end homelessness among veterans by shaping public policy, promoting collaboration, and building the capacity of service providers.

National Coalition for the Homeless (NCH)

2201 P Street NW
Washington, D.C. 20037
202-462-4822
FAX: 202-462-4823
Email: Info@nationalhomeless.org
Web: http://www.nationalhomeless.org
The NCH, founded in 1984, is a national network of people who are currently experiencing or who have experienced homelessness, activists and advocates, community-based and faith-based service providers, and others committed to a single mission. That mission, which is a common bond, is to end homelessness. NCH is committed to creating the systemic and attitudinal changes necessary to prevent and end homelessness. At the same time, it works to meet the immediate needs of people who are currently experiencing homelessness or who are at risk of doing so. NCH takes as its first principle of practice that people who are currently experiencing homelessness or have formerly experienced homelessness must be actively involved in all of its work.

The National Low Income Housing Coalition (NLIHC)

727 15th Street NW, 6th Floor
Washington, D.C. 20005
202 -662-1530
FAX: 202-/93-1973
Email: info@nlihc.org
Web: http://www.nlihc.org
The NLIHC is dedicated solely to ending America's affordable housing crisis. We believe that this is achievable and that the affordable housing crisis is a problem that Americans are capable of solving. Even though the NLIHC is concerned about the housing circumstances of all low-income people, it focuses its advocacy on those with the most serious housing problems, the lowest income households.

National Resource and Training Center on Homelessness and Mental Illness (NRC)

1-800-444-7415
Email: nrtcinfo@cdmgroup.com
Web: http://www.nrchmi.samhsa.gov
The NRC is the only national center specifically focused on the effective organization and delivery of services for people who are homeless and have serious mental illnesses. The Resource Center's activities enable the Center for Mental Health Services to facilitate changes in service systems through field-based knowledge development, synthesis, exchange, and adoption of effective practices.

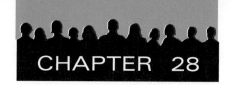

CHAPTER 28

Populations with Substance Abuse

Martha S. Tingen, APRN, BC, PhD

Chapter Outline

- Alcohol Use
- Marijuana Use
- Tobacco Use
- Populations Most at Risk for Alcohol, Marijuana, and Tobacco Abuse
  - School-Aged Populations

Learning Objectives

Upon completion of this chapter, the reader will be able to:

1. Examine the health effects of the primary drugs of substance abuse: alcohol, marijuana, and tobacco.

2. Appraise populations most at risk for alcohol, marijuana, and tobacco abuse.

3. Critique the current state of the science in prevention efforts by a review of current research.

4. Evaluate the pivotal role of public health nursing in addressing alcohol, marijuana, and tobacco use.

In the early 1990s, McGinnis and Foege's (1993) seminal publication on the underlying causes of death in the United States documented that 50 percent of all deaths are from potentially preventable behaviors. The Institute of Medicine (IOM) recently furthered this line of thought and included in their report, *Promoting Health,* that *more than 50 percent* of the ten leading causes of death are based on lifestyle behavior choices (Smedley, Syme, and IOM, 2001).

Healthy People 2010 (USDHHS, 2000b) identifies as a primary goal to "Reduce substance abuse to protect the health, safety, and quality of life for all, especially for children" (p. 26-3). Consistent with this goal is a call for interventions by all health care providers and researchers who focus on providing healthy environments, especially for children, that promote healthy lifestyle behaviors (Smedley, Syme, and IOM, 2001). Because the origins of unhealthy lifestyle behaviors frequently begin in childhood and then manifest the health consequences in adulthood, approaches that target the family and young children are critical and may hold great promise for significant reductions in substance abuse-related mortality and morbidity (CASA, 2004; NCCDPHP, 2004a; Smedley, Syme, and IOM, 2001; USDHHS, 2000a;). These multilevel approaches must include the social and environmental factors that contribute to substance abuse rather than an approach that brings about reductions in specific diseases brought on by the abuse (CASA, 2004; Castrucci et al., 2002; Li, Feigelman, and Stanton, 2000; NCCDPHP, 2004a; Shadel et al., 2000; Smedley et al., 2001; USDHHS, 2000a). Social influence levels include aspects of the individual, family, community, organization {i.e., school/college for children and youth or work environment for adults}, state, and nation (Bandura, 1997; Griffin et al., 2000; Rimal, 2003; Smedley et al., 2001; Wickrama et al., 1999).

Approximately 19.4 million U.S. citizens (9.4 percent of the adult population) meet the clinical criteria for having a substance abuse disorder, being either alcohol or drug use, or both (Grant et al., 2004). Substance abuse classically refers to alcohol, drug, and tobacco misuse. The word "drug" is a term inclusive of many substances such as marijuana, cocaine, inhalants, heroin, steroids, ecstasy, and methamphetamines. This chapter presents information on the primary substances of abuse: alcohol, marijuana, and tobacco.

The numerous health consequences of substance abuse call for involvement by all health care providers.

Public health nurses are in a critical position to impact the health-compromising behaviors of substance abuse. Through their delivery of health care and interactions with clients, public health nurses can foster health-promoting behaviors that are free of substance abuse. This chapter examines the health effects of alcohol, marijuana, and tobacco use, presents information on populations most at risk for abuse of these substances, presents the state-of-the-science in prevention efforts for tobacco use, and evaluates the pivotal role of public health nursing in addressing use of these substances.

ALCOHOL USE

Alcohol use impacts numerous organ systems of the body. The cardiovascular system suffers from long-term abuse of alcohol with an increased risk for hypertension, development of arrhythmias, cardiomyopathies, and potential for stroke (USDHSS, 2000a; NIAAA, 2004). Cirrhosis, one of the ten leading causes of death in the United States, occurs primarily from sustained alcohol abuse (NIAAA, 2004). Additionally, those diagnosed with hepatitis C have even more adverse outcomes when combined with alcohol abuse (USDHSS, 2000b). Cancer of the liver is also associated with alcohol use (ACS, 2003a; NIAAA, 2004). Alcohol intake of more than two drinks per day places individuals at risk for several cancers. There is a clearly established causative effect of alcohol with cancers of the mouth, pharynx, larynx, esophagus, and breast (ACS, 2004b). In individuals who use tobacco in addition to alcohol, the risks of these cancers (mouth, larynx, esophagus) are much greater than the independent effect alone of drinking or smoking (ACS, 2004a).

Fetal alcohol syndrome (FAS) was a term coined more than 30 years ago to describe an array of birth defects occurring in children who were born to mothers who consumed alcohol during pregnancy (NIAAA, 2000). Although there have been numerous publications about alcohol's effects when consumed during the prenatal period, FAS continues to be the number one preventable cause of mental retardation (NIAAA, 2000) and increasing numbers of mothers are drinking during pregnancy (Ebrahim et al., 1999). Children exposed in utero to alcohol often experience growth retardation, facial abnormalities, and brain damage, which manifest as neurological and behavioral problems later in life with resultant academic and employment difficulties (NIAAA, 2000; Thomas et al., 1998).

In addition to damage to bodily systems, 41 percent of all motor vehicle accidents are alcohol related (NIAAA, 2004). Those who consume excessive amounts of alcohol have higher death rates from injuries, violence, suicides, poisoning, fires, drownings, occupational accidents, and high-risk sexual behaviors (CDC, 2004; NIAAA, 2004; USDHHS, 2000a). Alcohol use is also linked to mental health illness and diagnoses. There is a 4.1 and 2.6 times higher risk of mood and anxiety disorders in those with alcohol abuse and dependence, respectively (Grant et al., 2004). There are also significant relationships between disorders of alcohol use and co-occurrence of major depression, dsythymia, panic disorder, mania, hypomania, phobias, and generalized anxiety (Grant et al., 2004). Not only are these co-occurrences having an impact on the alcohol user, but recent evidence also points to the intergenerational transmission of these lifestyle behaviors and health status (Clark et al., 2004). Specifically, children with parents who have a substance abuse disorder are also at risk for transmission of mental health disorders (Clark et al., 2004).

The health consequences of alcohol use have been publicized widely. However, the numerous morbidities and mortalities related to alcohol use have resulted in a steady annual increase since 1992 in economic costs at a rate of 3.8 percent (Harwood, 2000). Nearly $185 billion dollars are spent annually for alcohol-related health and safety costs and productivity losses (Harwood, 2000).

MARIJUANA USE

Approximately 3.1 million Americans, age 12 years and over, use marijuana on a daily or near daily basis (National Household Survey on Drug Use, 2004). Marijuana, the most commonly used illicit drug in the United States, is associated with risky behaviors, especially in youth (NIDA, 2004). These risky behaviors may include driving a vehicle within two hours of use, school absenteeism, theft, assault and battery, property destruction, and high-risk sexual activity (NIDA, 2003; USDHHS, 2000a).

Physiological health effects of marijuana are many and impact the brain, heart, lungs, respiratory system, and immune system (NIDA, 2004). Regarding the brain, short-term adverse effects of marijuana use include difficulties with learning, memory, problem-solving abilities, distorted perceptions, and loss of coordination (NIDA, 2004). Long-term marijuana use results in changes involved in the stress-response system and in the activity of dopamine-containing nerve cells that affect regulation of motivation and reward (NIDA, 2004). The heart is initially affected by marijuana use by an increased rate, and results of one study indicate that the risk of myocardial infarction is more than quadrupled in the first hour after smoking (Mittleman et al., 2001; NIDA, 2004). This risk is believed to occur because marijuana increases blood pressure and heart rate and decreases the oxygen-carrying capacity of the blood (Mittleman et al., 2001).

Marijuana use causes a variety of lung and respiratory outcomes including increased occurrence of respiratory illnesses, cough, mucous production, lung infections, and obstructed airways (NIDA, 2004). Marijuana use doubles to triples the risk of developing cancer of the head and neck (Zhang et al., 1999) and is also associated with cancer of the lung (NIDA, 2004). These cancers are believed to be related to the high carcinogenic hydrocarbons contained in marijuana smoke, which are 50 to 70 percent greater than that contained in tobacco smoke (NIDA, 2004). Delta-9-tetrahydrocannabinol (THC), the main active ingredient in marijuana, is thought to be responsible for impairing the immune system in marijuana users (NIDA, 2004; Zhu et al, 2000). In laboratory studies of mice exposed to THC, those exposed were more likely to develop bacterial infections and tumors than those not exposed (Zhu et al., 2000).

Marijuana use is also associated with a myriad of learning and social behavior problems and mental health disorders (i.e. depression, anxiety, and personality disorders) (NIDA, 2007). Not only does increased use of marijuana compromise the ability to learn and remember information, but it may also result in a slowing of intellectual, job, or social skills (Brook, Cohen & Brook, 1998; Green and Ritter, 2000; NIDA, 2004). Regarding pregnancy outcomes, babies born to mothers who used marijuana are at increased risk of abnormal neurological development (NIDA, 2004). This is often manifested in newborns as increased tremulousness, having a high-pitched cry, or altered response to visual stimuli (NIDA, 2004). Children of mothers who used marijuana during pregnancy have more behavioral problems and exhibit deficits in attentiveness, memory, and decision-making skills in the preschool and early school years (NIDA, 2004). High school students who smoke marijuana have lower grades and graduation rates (Brook, Balka, and Whiteman, 1999; Lynskey & Hall, 2000; NIDA, 2004).

TOBACCO USE

Tobacco use is responsible for approximately 4.9 million premature deaths annually worldwide and continues to be the leading cause of preventable death in the United States (Ezzati and Lopez, 2003; WHO, 1999; 2002). Responsible for 440,000 American deaths per year, nearly 20 percent of all deaths (CDC, 2002; NCCDPHP, 2004b), tobacco use kills more people than AIDS, alcohol, car accidents, fires, illegal drugs, murders, and suicides combined (ACS, 2004b). Forty-six million U.S. adults (22.8 percent of the population) are smokers of which 80 percent initiate the behavior before age 18, and 35 percent become daily smokers by this same age (ACS, 2004b; NCCDPHP, 2004a).

In addition to adult smokers, each day in the United States, 4,000 youth (younger than 18 years of age) try their first cigarette and another 2,000 become regular smokers (ACS, 2004b; NCCDPHP, 2004b). Although there have been minor declines in overall prevalence of tobacco use among youth, rates remain high and continue to increase incrementally with each year of school (ACS, 2004a; CDC, 2002; 2004; USDHHS, 2000a). Nationwide, more than one-third of middle school students have tried cigarettes (ACS, 2004a; 2004b) and by the 10th and 12th grades, 58 and 65 percent of students, respectively, have tried smoking (CDC, 2004). Monitoring the Future, an ongoing study of behaviors, attitudes, and values of U.S. high school students, reports prevalence data that is minimally lower with experimentation by 54 percent of 12th grade students (Johnston et al., 2004).

To reach the Healthy People 2010 goal of reducing youth prevalence of smoking to 16 percent, primary prevention efforts are critical in preventing initiation (USDHHS, 2000a). DiFranza and Wellman (2003) identify that nicotine dependence is the most common life-threatening disorder that affects the pediatric population. Tobacco addiction has its origins in childhood and once initiation occurs, many children quickly lose the ability to halt their behavior due to the addictive nature of nicotine (Sargeant and DiFranza, 2003; DiFranza and Wellman, 2003). Animal studies support that the adolescent brain is especially impacted by the addictive nature of nicotine and with either exposure to nicotine or even one dose of nicotine, structural changes occur in neurons that elicit behavioral changes that endure for the lifespan of the animal (Brown and Kolb, 2001; Leslie et al., 2003; Abreu-Villaca et al., 2003). Similar findings are now evident in humans with nicotine dependence occurring after only several cigarettes (DiFranza et al., 2002a; 2002b) It is established that nicotine is typically the first experimental drug to be used with progression to other substances and other risky behaviors (ACS, 2004b; Botvin et al., 1999; CDC 2004). These animal and human studies emphasize the urgency of primary prevention of tobacco use in youth.

The Surgeon General's report on tobacco use identified that damage from tobacco use affects nearly every organ of the body (NCCDPHP, 2004a). Tobacco use is causally related to the first, second, and third leading causes of death in the United States: coronary heart disease, cancer (lung), and stroke respectively (NCCDPHP, 2004b). Tobacco use is consistently identified as the number one preventable cause of heart disease (AHA, 2002; Eyre et al, 2004; NCCDPHP, 2004a; Rowe, Powell, and Hall, 1999). Smoking is also related to numerous other cardiovascular disorders to include atherosclerosis, congestive heart failure, abdominal aortic aneurysms, myocardial infarctions (MIs), and sudden deaths from MIs (NCCDPHP, 2004a).

Regarding cancer, tobacco use is responsible for 30 percent of all cancers and 87 percent of all lung cancers (ACS, 2003a; 2004a; NCCDPHP, 2004a; Ries et al., 2004). Smokers are 23 times more like to develop lung cancer than nonsmokers (NCCDPHP, 2004b). Smoking is also causally related to mouth, pharynx, larynx, stomach, kidney, bladder, pancreas, and cervical cancers (ACS, 2004a; NCCDPHP, 2004b). Preventing tobacco use onset and exposure and success with cessation are consistently identified as the best strategies for the prevention of lung cancer and many other cancers (ACS, 2003a; 2004a; 2004b; Landis et al., 2000).

Other bodily systems being harmed with tobacco use include the oral cavity, respiratory digestive systems, and eye (ACS, 2004a; NCCDPHP, 2004b). For the oral cavity, in addition to cancers, smokers often develop periodontitis and gum diseases that require extensive dental care. In those who smoke, chronic obstructive pulmonary disease (COPD), emphysema, bronchitis, pneumonia, asthma, airway obstruction, and respiratory infections are common adverse outcomes (NCCDPHP, 2004b). For the digestive system, peptic ulcers are a frequent occurrence. The eyes are greatly impacted by smoking, and smokers have two to three times the risk of developing cataracts than nonsmokers and cataracts are the leading cause of blindness worldwide (NCCDPHP, 2004a). In addition to the harmful effects on the body and the associated human suffering, the economic costs for tobacco use are staggering. For direct medical care of adults with tobacco-attributable illnesses, costs are $75.5 billion annually with an additional cost of $81.9 billion due to lost productivity (CDC, 2002; NCCDPHP, 2004a).

Smoking also has a significant impact on pregnancy and approximately 25 percent or one million of all live births in the United States are from women who smoke (Benowitz et al., 2000). Smoking during pregnancy is associated with a myriad of adverse outcomes to include ectopic pregnancy, premature rupture of membranes, preterm delivery, growth retardation of the baby, increased perinatal mortality, and sudden infant death syndrome (Benowitz et al., 2000; Castles et al., 1999; Melvin, Adams and Miller, 2000; Saraiya et al., 1998). Nicotine affects the developing baby by reducing blood flow through the placenta, resulting in growth retardation and the delivery of a low birth weight (LBW) baby, which is one of the leading causes of infant morbidity and mortality (NCCDPHP, 2004a; USDHHS, 2001). Smoking achieves many of its adverse pregnancy outcomes through several other mechanisms which include (1) nicotine, which acts like a toxin at the cellular level and also as a vasoconstrictor; (2) numerous other components of cigarette smoke (carbon monoxide, nicotine, cyanide, cadmium, lead, methanol, and others) that exert diverse negative effects at the cellular level; (3) alterations in maternal/fetal nutritional state; (4) carbon monoxide, one of the major byproducts of smoking, which binds to hemoglobin causing maternal anemia; and (5) carbon monoxide, which affects the oxygen transport system by decreasing the amount of oxygen transferred from the maternal to fetal blood, resulting in fetal tissue hypoxia (Benowitz et al., 2000).

Tobacco use is different than other substance abuse disorders due to the effects of tobacco smoke exposure on those who are in the environment of the smoker. This is often referred to as **environmental tobacco smoke (ETS)**, passive smoke, or secondhand smoke (SHS) exposure. Tobacco smoke contains approximately 4,000 chemicals, including 200 known poisons, and 43 known carcinogens (ACS, 2002). ETS exposure includes both the inhalation of mainstream smoke exhaled by the smoker and sidestream smoke from a lit cigarette. Studies have shown that there is more tar and nicotine in sidestream smoke than in mainstream smoke (ACS, 2002). Additionally, carbon monoxide, which robs the blood of needed oxygen, is two to 15 times higher in sidestream smoke (ACS, 2002). The World Health Organization (WHO, 1999), estimates that 50 percent of the world's children, or approximately 700 million children, are primarily exposed to ETS in their homes.

Estimates of ETS exposure in the United States are very high with approximately 65 percent of all non-smokers, including children over the age of 4 years, being exposed (USDHHS, 2000b). ETS exposure results in a myriad of health concerns for the pediatric population, many of which are respiratory illnesses, such as asthma, that require numerous hospitalizations and medical treatments. The Healthy People 2010 goal is to reduce this exposure for children who are younger than 6 years of age to no more than 10 percent (USDHHS, 2000b). Results from comparing more than 17,000 children in the United States from smoking versus nonsmoking families revealed that children from smoking families have far greater prevalence of cardiovascular disease (CVD) and cancer morbidity (ACS, 2004a; USDHHS, 2000b). Annually, 45,000 to 60,000 adult CVD deaths and 38,000 cancer deaths result from ETS exposure in nonsmokers (ACS, 2004a; Ries et al., 2004; USDHHS, 2000b). Children who have parents who smoke are at increased risk for tobacco-related diseases due to exposure and the likelihood that many become smokers themselves (Clark and Cornelius, 2004; Distefan et al., 1998; Griffin et al., 2000).

Cotinine, the proximate metabolite of nicotine, is an accurate and objective biochemical marker of smoking status and ETS exposure (Jarvis et al., 2001; 2003). Cotinine measurements can be obtained in several body fluids and mediums to include the hair, saliva, urine, toenails, and plasma (Jarvis et al., 2003) and the sensitivity (96–97 percent) and specificity (99–100 percent) of plasma or salivary analyses for determining smoking status are excellent (Society for Research on Nicotine and Tobacco Subcommittee on Biochemical Verification, 2002). There are ethnic variances in cotinine measurements with blacks having higher cotinine levels than whites (Benowitz et al., 1999). Perez-Stable and colleagues (1998) investigated the underlying mechanisms of higher cotinine levels in blacks than whites and reported that blacks have a mean total clearance of cotinine approximately 20 percent lower. Higher cotinine levels in blacks are attributed to an ethnically associated difference in cotinine metabolism, and this may contribute to the tobacco-related heath disparities, especially the disproportionate rates of cardiovascular disease, various cancers, and overall mortality experienced by blacks as compared to whites (NCCDPHP, 2004a; Ries et al., 2004: USDHHS, 1998).

Currently, 46.2 million U.S. adults use tobacco—25.2 percent of men and 20.7 percent of women (ACS, 2004a; CDC, 2004). It is estimated that 50 percent of those Americans who continue to use tobacco will die prematurely from a smoking-related illness (CDC, 2004; Peto et al., 1994). Seventy percent of all U.S. smokers express that they would like to quit. Of these, 70 percent visit a health care provider each year and 50 percent of these say they have never been advised to quit or provided specific strategies to be successful with quitting (Fiore et al., 2000). These numbers are of grave concern given the numerous resources available to providers to foster quitting in their clients. Originally released in 1996 and updated in 2000, the Public Health Service (PHS) *Treating Tobacco Use and Dependence Clinical Practice Guideline* delineates specific recommendations to be used by health care providers and the health care teams for addressing tobacco use and dependence (Fiore et al., 2000). The guideline identified eight key findings and specific recommendations that should be utilized by health care providers at each client contact. These eight key findings are summarized in Box 28-1.

The *Treating Tobacco Use and Dependence Clinical Practice Guideline* identifies the most important component in addressing tobacco use and dependence as screening or identification of tobacco use (Fiore et al.,

---

BOX 28-1: Summary of the Eight Key Findings of the PHS Guideline

1. Tobacco dependence is a chronic condition that often requires repeated intervention. Effective treatments exist that can produce long-term or even permanent abstinence.

2. Because effective tobacco dependence treatments are available, every client who uses tobacco should be offered at least one of these treatments:
   - Clients *willing* to quit should be provided with identified and effective treatments in the guideline.
   - Clients *unwilling* to quit should be provided with a brief motivational intervention.

3. Clinicians and health care delivery systems (i.e., administrators, insurers, purchasers) should institutionalize consistent identification, documentation, and treatment of every tobacco user who is seen in a health care setting.

4. Brief tobacco dependence treatment is effective and should be offered to every client who uses tobacco.

5. There is a strong dose–response relationship between the intensity of tobacco dependence counseling and its effectiveness. Treatments involving person-to-person contact (i.e., individual or group telephone counseling) are consistently effective, and effectiveness increases with treatment intensity (e.g., minutes of contact).

6. Three types of counseling and behavioral therapies were found to be especially effective and should be used with all clients who are attempting tobacco cessation: problem solving/skills training; intratreatment social support; and extratreatment social support.

7. Except in the presence of contraindications, effective pharmacotherapies for tobacco cessation should be used with all clients attempting to quit. First-line, second-line, and over-the-counter products are identified for use.

8. Tobacco dependence treatments are both clinically effective and cost-effective relative to other medical and disease prevention interventions. Insurers and purchasers should ensure that
   - All insurance plans include as a reimbursed benefit the counseling and pharmacotherapeutic treatments identified as effective in this guideline.
   - Clinicians are reimbursed for providing tobacco dependence treatment.

SOURCE: Adapted from the PHS *Treating Tobacco Use and Dependence* Clinical Practice Guideline (Fiore et al., 2000).

2000). If the client is a tobacco user and expresses willingness to quit, the guideline specifies actions for health care providers to use, referred to as the 5-A's—*Ask, Advise, Assess, Assist,* and *Arrange.* Asking about tobacco use to systematically identify all tobacco users at every client encounter is considered critical. All tobacco users should be strongly *advised* to quit and then *assessed* for their willingness to quit. *Assistance* involves health care providers recommending the combination of appropriate pharmacological and behavioral therapies for cessation. An *arrangement* for follow-up contact should be made for every tobacco user attempting to quit. Specific interventions under each *A* are included in the Clinical Practice Guideline to assist health care providers in helping all tobacco users be successful with cessation efforts.

For tobacco users not willing to make a quit attempt, the guideline recommends the 5-*R*'s model—*Relevance, Risks, Rewards, Roadblocks,* and *Repetition* (Fiore et al., 2000). *Relevance* is a strategy health care providers should use to make tobacco cessation treatments individualized and personalized for each client. *Risks* of smoking should also be personalized, relevant, and include acute, long-term, and environmental risks. *Rewards* of tobacco cessation should be identified by the client as benefits most relevant to them. If the client is not able to identify rewards, the health care provider should point out specific personalized rewards such as improved sense of taste and smell, improved health, saving money, and setting a good example to children. *Roadblocks* should be assessed by asking the client to identify personal barriers to quitting, such as fear of failure, weight gain, or enjoyment of tobacco. *Repetition* involves repeating the 5-*R*'s at each encounter. *Reviewing* the relevance, risks, rewards, and roadblocks with tobacco users at every visit may assist clients to move toward a stage of readiness for beginning cessation treatment.

Efforts by public health nurses and other health care providers should focus on promoting cessation through proven behavioral and pharmacological approaches as recommended in the PHS Guideline (Fiore et al., 2000). Use of this combination approach has been found to yield quit rates that are approximately four times that of no interventions (Fiore et al., 2000). The PHS Guideline (Fiore et al., 2000) and others (Lawrence et al., 2003) also recommend that smoking cessation interventions should be tailored to ethnic/racial groups whenever possible. Since health care provider

🌐 POLICY HIGHLIGHTS

Substance Abuse Prevention

Substance abuse requires multilevel primary and secondary prevention efforts. Several of these efforts involve policy issues and include mass media campaigns; laws and regulations that affect access to substance abuse products; restrictions on advertising (i.e., alcohol and tobacco industries); and increases in the price of alcohol and tobacco products by raising taxes. Grassroots efforts and coalition building have produced many changes through smoke-free ordinances in counties, states, and eating establishments. Public health nurses are called to action to get involved in policy issues, promote change, and thus decrease substance abuse behaviors.

endorsement has been shown to be the strongest factor in prompting health promotion behaviors (Ashby-Hughes and Nickerson, 1999), and the guideline has been demonstrated to be evidenced-based and cost-effective, providers can impact behavioral change in their clients through cessation counseling (Fiore et al., 2000; Godlee, 2003).

POPULATIONS MOST AT RISK FOR ALCOHOL, MARIJUANA, AND TOBACCO ABUSE

Based on established literature, there are strong associations among youth substance use initiation, normative expectations, and behaviors of adults and peers within the social environment (Botvin, 1999; Clark and Cornelius, 2004; Kodl & Mermelstein, 2004; Sargent and DiFranza, 2003). Some authors have identified and coined the process of children adopting their parents' lifestyle behaviors as intergenerational transmission (Rimal, 2003; Wickrama et al., 1999). Substance abuse and the relationship of genetics have also recently been explored (Lerman, Patterson, and Berrettini, 2005; Radel et al., 2005). Information in Tables 28-1 and 28-2 portray the lifetime prevalence and current substance use by ethnicity for high school youth (grades 9 to 12) on alcohol, marijuana, and tobacco (CDC, 2004).

TABLE 28-1: Lifetime Prevalence* of Substance Use by Ethnicity among U.S. High School Students

Ethnicity	ALCOHOL		CIGARETTES		MARIJUANA	
	%	95% CI	%	95% CI	%	95% CI
White	74.4	±3.5	58.1	±3.9	39.8	±3.4
Black	71.4	±3.2	58.4	±4.1	43.3	±4.1
Hispanic	79.5	±3.4	61.9	±3.9	42.7	±3.8

* Ever tried cigarette smoking; ever had one or more drinks of alcohol; ever used marijuana one or more times.

Note. From Centers for Disease Control and Prevention (CDC) (2004). Surveillance summaries: Youth risk behavior surveillance—United States, 2003. May 21, 2004. *Morbidity and Mortality Weekly Report, 53*(SS-2), 1-96.

TABLE 28-2: Current* Substance Use by Ethnicity among U.S. High School Students

Ethnicity	ALCOHOL		CIGARETTES		MARIJUANA	
	%	95% CI	%	95% CI	%	95% CI
White	47.1	±3.0	24.9	±2.4	21.7	±2.3
Black	37.4	±3.3	15.1	±2.8	23.9	**±3.1**
Hispanic	**45.6**	**±2.7**	**18.4**	**±2.3**	**23.8**	**±2.3**

* Smoked cigarettes, drank one or more drinks of alcohol, used marijuana on ≥ 1 of the 30 days before surveyed.

Note. From Centers for Disease Control and Prevention (CDC) (2004). Surveillance summaries: Youth risk behavior surveillance—United States, 2003. May 21, 2004. *Morbidity and Mortality Weekly Report, 53*(SS-2), 1-96.

Although the overall statistics for alcohol, drug, and tobacco use are alarming, there are some populations at increased risk of use. As presented in the tables, white adolescents have the highest percentage of *current use* of alcohol and tobacco (cigarettes), although Hispanic youth also show high usage of both substances (CDC, 2004). Black youth have the highest percentage of *current* marijuana use with white and Hispanic rates being similar. All figures for lifetime prevalence use in all ethnicities are of concern given *at minimum,* nearly 40 percent of all high school students have tried marijuana, 58 percent have tried cigarettes, and 71 percent have tried alcohol (CDC, 2004).

Across adult ethnicities, prevalence rates vary between men and women. In blacks, it is estimated that 26.3 percent of men and 20.8 percent of women smoke (ACS, 2003b). However, smoking prevalence rates are *highest* for American Indian and Alaska Native women at 38.6 percent versus 27.4 percent in men of these cultures (ACS, 2004a). Hispanic women have lower smoking prevalence rates (13.3 percent) than Hispanic men (24 percent) (ACS, 2003a). Additionally, Hispanics who are born in the United States are more likely to become smokers than those who are foreign-born (ACS, 2003a). Asian American women have the lowest smoking rates of all (7.9 percent) with Asian men having higher rates (19.6 percent) (ACS, 2004a). Hispanics have 60 percent higher death rates from liver cancer than all other non-Hispanic ethnicities (Ries et al., 2004). Liver cancer rates are strongly associated with chronic infections of hepatitis B and C viruses; however, alcohol intake is also a strong contributor (ACS, 2004a).

In summary, at *minimum*, 71 percent of all youth are at risk for alcohol experimentation, 40 percent are at risk for marijuana experimentation, and nearly 60 percent are at risk for tobacco experimentation (CDC, 2004). Strategies for primary prevention that target all youth are critical if we are to impact substance abuse and its related health consequences. Numerous approaches are also known, and resources (many of which are culturally sensitive) are readily available to health care providers for assisting clients who are established substance abusers and need secondary prevention efforts (cessation of alcohol, marijuana, and tobacco). Many of these resources are provided at the conclusion of this chapter.

School-Aged Populations

The social environment of the school has been the focus of many primary prevention studies (Botvin et al., 1999; 2003; Epstein, Griffin and Botvin, 2000; Flay, 2000; McGahee and Tingen, 2000; McGahee, Kemp and Tingen, 2000; Peterson et al., 2000; Smith, Tingen and Waller, 2004; Tingen et al., 2006), and one of the most widely published school-based prevention programs is Botvin's LifeSkills Training (LST) Program (Botvin, 1999; 2000; Botvin et al., 1999, 2003; Epstein, Griffin, and Botvin, 2000). The program uses a developmentally appropriate, cognitive behavioral approach and focuses on competency enhancement by teaching and equipping students with life skills to make healthy lifestyle choices regarding avoidance of substance use (Botvin, 1999; 2000). The LST program addresses the three critical domains associated with substance use: resistance skills, personal self-management skills, and general social skills (Botvin, 1999; 2000).

Based on Kandel's (2002) gateway hypothesis of drug use, youth who initiate the behaviors of using cigarettes and alcohol are at greater risk of also experimenting with marijuana and progressing to other illicit drug use. This downward trajectory of drug use beginning in adolescence often continues into early adulthood resulting in delinquent behaviors and compromised physical and mental health. The following research application focuses on the LST prevention approach (Botvin, 1999; 2000).In this study and in prior studies of the LST program, there have been significant reductions between control and intervention groups on self-reported alcohol, marijuana, and smoking frequency and prevalence rates. Results indicate that students who receive the LST program are less likely to initiate risky behaviors because of competence and skill development in the three critical domains of drug use (i.e., resistance skills, personal self-management skills, and general social skills) (Botvin, 1999; 2000).

While findings from the LST interventions are positive, some experts recommend targeting the family for substance use prevention efforts (CASA, 2004; Farkas et al., 1999; 2000; Sargeant and Dalton, 2001; Wakefield et al., 2000). CASA advocates that parent power is the most underutilized tool in preventing substance abuse and that the family is the fundamental social structure in keeping children away from alcohol, tobacco, and other drugs (Califano, 2005). CASA promotes parent involvement and monitoring, a "hands-on" approach that clearly communicates established expectations. This approach results in children with decreased risk for tobacco initiation and also a more positive relationship with their parents than children in "hands-off" environments (Califano, 2005). Studies show that the more often children have dinner with their parents, the less likely they are to initiate smoking, alcohol, and other drugs (Califano, 2005). Household communication regarding health issues plays a critical role in changing health behaviors as well as behavioral determinants (Rimal, 2003). Rivara and colleagues (2004) examined the years of potential life lost (YPLL) that could be reversed from tobacco prevention efforts aimed at youth. They reported smoking prevalence could be decreased by 26 percent and would result in saving 108,466 lives annually and 1.6 million YPLL. Primary prevention of tobacco use with youth is essential to address the public health issues of smoking and other substance abuse behaviors.

Substance abuse impacts nearly every disease entity and affects routine laboratory values and pharmacological interventions of clients treated in public health settings (Andrews and Tingen, 2005). Therefore, in order for public health nurses to provide the highest quality of holistic health care, it is essential that substance abuse be assessed for and treated per established guidelines. All health care providers can and should become educated and effective in assisting their clients with

⊕ RESEARCH APPLICATION

Effectiveness of a Universal Drug Abuse Prevention Approach for Youth at High Risk for Substance Use Initiation

Study Purpose

"To examine the effectiveness of a universal drug abuse prevention approach for youth at high risk of substance use based on their friends' use of alcohol and tobacco and poor grades in school" (Griffin et al., 2003, p.2)

Methods

Randomized, control design with intervention and control groups (N = 758). The sample was 49 percent male and 51 percent female and predominantly minority with 58 percent African-American and 29 percent Hispanic. Sixty one percent were economically disadvantaged and received free lunch at school and 35 percent lived in single-parent households with mothers only. Intervention groups received ten classroom sessions of the LST prevention program in seventh grade followed by nine booster sessions in eighth grade. All sessions were taught by the school classroom teachers who received training on the LST program. Control groups received the standard public school curriculum for substance use.

The specific content of the LST intervention program includes increasing self esteem, saying no to unfair requests, resisting pressure from the media and peers to use drugs, communicating effectively, improving decision-making and problem-solving skills, managing anger and anxiety, and knowing the myths and realities of alcohol, marijuana, and tobacco use. The program addresses all major cognitive, attitudinal, and psychosocial factors that are empirically or theoretically related to alcohol, marijuana, and tobacco use. Information that aims to promote antidrug attitudes, normative expectations, and intentions is also included. Teaching strategies for the LST program include didactic instruction, demonstration, behavioral rehearsal,

feedback, and social reinforcement (National Health Promotion Associates, 2003).

All students were pretested and posttested at one-year follow-up using established self-report measures. To enhance the validity of self-report, carbon monoxide breath samples were collected simultaneously. Four primary outcome measures were assessed: (1) social risk (how many of your friends do you think smoke cigarettes or drink alcohol?); (2) academic risk (what are the typical grades you get in school?); (3) substance use (cigarette, alcohol, marijuana, and inhalant use—frequency and quantity of each); and (4) polydrug use (using tobacco, alcohol, marijuana, and inhalants).

Findings

Students in the intervention groups reported less smoking, drinking, inhalant use, and polydrug use at one-year follow-up than students in the control group. Program effects were statistically significant on all substance use outcomes except marijuana use.

Implications

The universal drug abuse prevention approach appears to be effective for youth at high risk of substance initiation. Follow-up of intervention effects to determine long-term durability in this population is needed.

Author

Griffin, K.W., Botvin, G.J., Nichols, J.R., and Doyle, M.M. (2003). Effectiveness of a universal drug abuse prevention approach for youth at high risk for substance use initiation. *Preventive Medicine, 36,* 1–7.

---

choosing to avoid substance abuse lifestyle behaviors. Nurses in public health are in an opportune position to work with an inclusive approach, targeting not only children and youth, but with adult family members as well in addressing prevention of substance abuse. Only when primary and secondary prevention efforts are consistently implemented using established resources will there be an impact on decreasing substance abuse.

⊕ PRACTICE APPLICATION

A Case Study for Evaluating the Pivotal Role of Public Health Nursing

A client, who is a 20-year-old, white hair stylist presents to the health department today complaining of morning nausea and memory problems. She lives with a male partner and they enjoy evenings of having a few drinks and sometimes smoking pot. She acknowledges they know it is illegal, but it is not hurting anyone and they enjoy it. Both she and her partner also smoke approximately a pack-a-day of cigarettes, but this occurs mostly during the workday. She also shares that in addition to her nausea and memory problems, she has started experiencing anxiety over little things that did not previously bother her. She finds herself anxious about possibly losing her job, how she will then pay her rent, and is also worried her partner may be getting ready to move out. She is unable to identify specific situations or communications that have prompted this anxiety; nevertheless, she is really nervous that these changes may happen. She recently has been inconsistent in taking her birth control pills because she got worried when a friend told her that taking "the pill" and smoking may make her develop blood clots in her legs. Although she has really tried to quit several times, she knows she cannot stop smoking cigarettes because she started when she was 13 and has developed a dependency on them. She is asking for help from the public health nurse for her nausea, anxiety, and memory problems. For public health nurses, the questions in the Critical Thinking Activities section may assist with formulating an individualized plan of care to address the health concerns of this client.

CRITICAL THINKING ACTIVITIES

(Note: The following questions refer to the Practice Application above.)

1. Based on the information the client has shared, what are the five areas of immediate concern for her health?

2. What is the most likely cause of her nausea, her memory problems, and her anxiety?

3. What theoretical aspects might public health nurses consider in providing health care to the client?

4. How would this theoretical information assist public health nurses in identifying health care priorities and planning delivery of care as it applies to substance abuse disorders?

5. What resources are available to public health nurses that may be helpful in providing health care to this client?

6. What resources can public health nurses identify that are available to the client to assist her with these health concerns?

KEY TERMS

cotinine

environmental tobacco smoke (ETS)

fetal alcohol syndrome (FAS)

intergenerational transmission

substance abuse

THC (delta-9-tetrahydrocannabinol)

Treating Tobacco Use and Dependence Clinical Practice Guideline

KEY CONCEPTS

- Substance abuse of alcohol, marijuana, and tobacco has costly health consequences from both a human suffering and economic standpoint.

- Numerous health-related disorders and impairments are preventable through healthy lifestyle behavior choices that include the avoidance of alcohol, marijuana, and tobacco use.

- Alcohol use contributes to 41 percent of motor vehicle accidents, which is the leading cause of death for Americans from birth to age 34.

- There is a high prevalence of co-occurrence of alcohol and mental health disorders.

- Marijuana may quadruple the risk of myocardial infarction within the first hour of smoking.

- Tobacco use harms nearly every organ in the human body.

- The adolescent brain is extremely sensitive to the addictiveness of nicotine.

- Substance use often begins in youth and progresses along a continuum of change with the frequent adding of additional substances and manifestations of health effects in the adult years.

- Broad-based approaches that include multiple social influences are needed for alcohol, marijuana, and tobacco prevention.

- Primary prevention approaches that target all youth are needed to impact alcohol, marijuana, and tobacco use.

- Substance abuse is a chronic disorder, and secondary prevention strategies that are delivered repetitively for alcohol, marijuana, and tobacco use are needed in adult populations.

- Resources for implementing primary and secondary prevention efforts are available.

- Public health nurses are in a pivotal position to implement primary and secondary prevention efforts for alcohol, marijuana, and tobacco use.

REFERENCES

Abreu-Villaca, Y. A., Seidler, F. J., Qiao, D. and Tate, C. A. (2003). *Why do adolescents get addicted to nicotine? Effects on cholinergic systems in a rat model.* (PA1-7). Paper presented at the Society for Research on Nicotine and Tobacco. 9th Annual Meeting, New Orleans.

American Cancer Society (ACS). (2002). *Questions about smoking, tobacco, and health.* Atlanta: Author.

American Cancer Society (ACS). (2003a). *Cancer facts & figures for Hispanics/Latinos 2003–2005.* Atlanta: Author.

American Cancer Society (ACS). (2003b). *Cancer facts & figures for African Americans 2003–2004.* Atlanta: Author.

American Cancer Society (ACS). (2004a). *Cancer facts & figures.* Atlanta: Author.

American Cancer Society (ACS). (2004b). *Cancer prevention & early detection: Facts & figures 2004.* Atlanta: Author.

American Heart Association (AHA). (2002). *Heart facts 2003: African Americans—Cardiovascular diseases still no 1.* Dallas: Author.

Andrews, J. O., and Tingen, M. S. (2005). The effect of smoking, smoking cessation, and passive smoke exposure on common laboratory values in clinical settings: A review of the evidence. *Critical Care Nursing Clinics of North America, 18,* 63–69.

Ashby-Hughes, B., and Nickerson, N. (1999). Provider endorsement: the strongest cue in prompting high-risk adults to receive influenza and pneumococcal immunizations. *Clinical Excellence for Nurse Practitioners, 3*(2), 97–104.

Bandura, A. (1997). *Self-efficacy: The exercise of control.* New York: Freeman.

Benowitz, N. L., Dempsey, D. A., Goldenberg, R. L., Hughes, J. R., Dolan-Mullen, P., Ogburn, P. L., Oncken, C., Orleans, C. T., Slotkin, T. A., Whiteside, H. P., and Yaffe, S. (2000). The use of pharmacotherapies for smoking cessation during pregnancy. *Tobacco Control, 9*(Suppl. III), iii91–iii94.

Benowitz, N. L., Perez-Stable, E. J., Fong, I., Modin, G., Berrera, B., and Jacob, P., III. (1999). Ethnic differences in *N*-glucauronidation of nicotine and cotinine. *Journal of Pharmacology and Experimental Therapeutics, 291,* 1196–1203.

Botvin, G. J. (1999). *Lifeskills training student guide—Level 1* (Elementary School). White Plains, NY: Princeton Health Press.

Botvin, G. J. (2000). *Lifeskills training student guide—Level 1* (Middle School). White Plains, NY: Princeton Health Press.

Botvin, G. J., Griffin, K. W., Diaz, T., Miller, N., and Ifill-Williams, M. (1999). Smoking initiation and escalation in early adolescent girls: One-year follow-up of a school-based prevention intervention for minority youth. *Journal of the American Medical Women's Association, 54,* 139–143.

Botvin, G. J., Griffin, K. W., Paul, E., and Macaulay, A. P. (2003). Preventing tobacco and alcohol use among elementary school students through LifeSkills Training. *Journal of Child and Adolescent Substance Abuse, 12,* 1–17.

Brook, J. S., Balka, E. B., and Whiteman, M. (1999). The risks for late adolescence of early adolescent marijuana use. *American Journal of Public Health, 89*(10), 1549–1554.

Brook, J. S., Cohen, P., and Brook, D. W. (1998). Longitudinal study of co-occurring psychiatric disorders and substance use. *Journal of the American Academy of Child and Adolescent Psychiatry, 37,* 322–330.

Brown, R. W., and Kolb, B. (2001). Nicotine sensitization increases dendritic length and spine density in the nucleus accumbens and cingulated cortex. *Brain Research, 899,* 94–100.

Califano, J. A. Jr. (2005). Parent power: The price young people pay for parental pessimism and nonchalance is high. *America, 193*(13), 13-15.

Castles, A., Adams, E. K., Melvin, C. L., Kelsch, C., and Boulton, M. L. (1999). Effects of smoking during pregnancy. Five meta-analyses. *American Journal of Preventive Medicine, 16*(3), 208–215.

Castrucci, B. C., Gerlach, K. K., Kaufman, N. J., and Orleans, C.T. (2002). The association among adolescents' tobacco use, their beliefs and attitudes, and friends' and parents' opinions of smoking. *Maternal and Child Health Journal, 6*(3), 159–167.

Centers for Disease Control and Prevention (CDC). (2002). Annual smoking-attributable mortality, years of potential life lost, and economic costs—United States, 1995–1999. *Morbidity and Mortality Weekly Report, 51,* 287–320.

Centers for Disease Control and Prevention (CDC). (2004). Surveillance summaries: Youth risk behavior surveillance—United States, 2003. May 21, 2004. *Morbidity and Mortality Weekly Report, 53*(SS-2), 1-96.

Clark D. B., and Cornelius J. (2004). Childhood psychopathology and adult cigarette smoking: A prospective survival analysis in children at high risk for substance use disorders. *Addictive Behaviors, 29,* 837–841.

Clark, D. B., Cornelius, J., Wood, D. S., and Vanyukov, M. (2004). Psychology risk transmission in children of parents with substance use disorders. *The American Journal of Psychiatry, 161,* 685–691.

DiFranza, J. R., and Wellman, R. J. (2003). Preventing cancer by controlling youth tobacco use. *Seminars in Oncology Nursing, 19*(4), 261–267.

DiFranza, J. R., Savageau, J. A., Fletcher, K., Ockene, J. K., Rigotti, N. A., McNeill, A. D., Coleman, M., and Wood, C. (2002a). Measuring the loss of autonomy over nicotine use in adolescents: The DANDY development and assessment of nicotine dependence in youths (DANDY) study. *Archives of Pediatrics & Adolescent Medicine, 156,* 397–403.

DiFranza, J. R., Savageau, J. A., Rigotti, N. A., Fletcher, K., Ockene, J. K., McNeill, A. D., Coleman, M., and Wood, C. (2002b). Development of symptoms of tobacco dependence in youths: 30-month follow-up data from the DANDY study. *Tobacco Control, 11,* 228–235.

Distefan, J. M., Gilpin, E. A., Choi, W. S., and Pierce, J. P. (1998). Parental influences predict adolescent smoking in the United States, 1989–1993. *The Journal of Adolescent Health, 22,* 466–474.

Ebrahim, S. H., Diekman, S. T., Floyd, R. L., and Decoufle, P. (1999). Comparison of binge drinking among pregnant and nonpregnant women, United States, 1991–1995, Part 1. *American Journal of Obstetrics and Gynecology, 180*(1), 1–7.

Epstein, J. A., Griffin, K. W., and Botvin, G. J. (2000). Competence skills help deter smoking among inner city adolescents. *Tobacco Control, 9,* 33–39.

Eyre, H., Kahn, R., Robertson, R. M., Clark, N. G., Doyle, C., Hong, Y., Gansler, T., Glynn, T., Smith, R. A., Taubert, K., Thun, M. J., American Cancer Society, American Diabetes Association, & American Heart Association Collaborative Writing Committee. (2004). Preventing cancer, cardiovascular disease, and diabetes: A common agenda for the American Cancer Society, the American Diabetes Association, and the American Heart Association. *Stroke, 35*(8), 1999–2010.

Ezzati, M., and Lopez, A. (2003). Estimates of global mortality attributable to smoking in 2000. *Lancet, 362,* 847–852.

Farkas, A. J., Distefan, J. M., Choi, W. S., and Pierce, J. P. (1999). Does parental smoking cessation discourage adolescent smoking? *Preventive Medicine, 28,* 213–218.

Farkas, A. J., Gilpin, E. A., White, M. M., and Pierce, J. P. (2000). Association between household and workplace smoking restrictions and adolescent smoking. *The Journal of the American Medical Association, 284,* 717–722.

Fiore, M. C., Bailey, W. C., Cohen, S. J., Dorfman, S. F., Goldstein, M. G., Gritz, E. R., et al. (2000). *Treating tobacco use and dependence. Quick reference guide for clinicians (*Publication No. 1530–6402); *Children and Adolescents, Treating tobacco use and dependence* (AHRQ Publication No. 00-0032). Rockville, MD: U.S. Department of Health and Human Services. Public Health Service. Retrieved on August 18, 2004, from http://www.ahrq.gov/clinic/tobacco/ children.htm.

Flay, B. R. (2000). Approaches to substance use prevention utilizing school curriculum plus social environment change. *Addictive Behaviors, 25*(6), 861–885.

Grant, B. F., Stinson, F. S., Dawson, D. A., Chou, S. P., Dufour, M. C., Compton, W., Pickering, R. P., and Kaplan, K. (2004). Prevalence and co-occurrence of substance use disorders and independent mood and anxiety disorders: Results from the national epidemiologic survey on alcohol and related conditions. *Archives of General Psychiatry, 61,* 807–816.

Green, B. E., and Ritter, C. (2000). Marijuana use and depression. *Journal of Health and Social Behavior, 41*(1), 40–49.

Griffin, K. W., Botvin, G. J., Nichols, T. R., and Doyle, M. M. (2003). Effectiveness of a universal drug abuse prevention approach for youth at risk for substance use initiation. *Preventive Medicine, 36*(1), 1–7.

Griffin, K. W., Botvin, G. J., Scheier, L. M., Diaz, T., and Miller, N. L. (2000). Parenting practices as predictors of substance use, delinquency, and aggression among urban minority youth: Moderating effects of family structure and gender. *Psychology of Addictive Behaviors, 14*(2), 174–184.

Harwood, H. (2000). *Updating estimates of the economic costs of alcohol abuse in the United States: Estimates, update methods, and data report.* Retrieved on January 5, 2005, from http://www.niaaa.nih.gov/publications/economic-2000/index.htm

Jarvis, M. J., Primatesta, P., Boreham, R., Feyerabend, C., and Bryant, A. (2001). Nicotine yield from machine-smoked cigarettes and nicotine intakes in smokers: Evidence from a representative population survey. *Journal of the National Cancer Institute, 93,* 134–138.

Jarvis, M. J., Primatesta, P., Erens, B., Feyerabend, C., and Bryant, A. (2003). Measuring nicotine intake in population surveys: Comparability of saliva cotinine and plasma cotinine estimates. *Nicotine & Tobacco Research, 5,* 349–355.

Johnston, L. D., O'Malley, P. M., Bachman, J. G., and Schulenberg, J. E. (2004). Cigarette smoking among American teens continues to decline, but more slowly than in the past. *University of Michigan News and Information Services.* Ann Arbor, MI. Retrieved on January 6, 2005, from www.monitoringthefuture.org.

Kandel, D. (2002). *Examining the gateway hypothesis: Stages, and pathways of drug involvement.* New York: Cambridge University Press.

Kodl, M. M., and Mermelstein, R. (2004). Beyond modeling: Parenting practices, parental smoking history, and adolescent cigarette smoking. *Addictive Behaviors, 29*(1), 17–32.

Landis, S. H., Steiner, C. B., Bayakly, A. R., McNamara, C., and Powell, K. E. (2000). *Georgia cancer data report.* Publication Number: DPH00.27HW. Georgia Department of Human Resources, Division of Public Health, Cancer Control Section and the American Cancer Society, Southeast Division.

Lawrence, D., Graber, J., Mills, S., Meissner, H., and Warnecke, R. (2003). Smoking cessation interventions in U.S. racial/ethnic minority populations: An assessment of the literature. *Preventive Medicine, 36,* 204–216.

Lerman, C., Patterson, F., and Berrettini, W. (2005). Treating tobacco dependence: State of the science and new directions. *Journal of Clinical Oncology, 23*(2), 311–323.

Leslie, F. M., Lee, A., Oliff, H., and Belluzzi, J. (2003). *Single trial conditioned reinforcement and locomotor sensitization in adolescent rats.* PA1-3. Society for Research on Nicotine and Tobacco, 9th Annual Meeting, New Orleans.

Li, X., Feigelman, S., and Stanton, B. (2000). Perceived parental monitoring and health risk behaviors among urban low-income African-American children and adolescents. *Journal of Adolescent Health, 27,* 43–48.

Lynskey, M., and Hall, W. (2000). The effects of adolescent cannabis use on educational attainment: a review. *Addiction, 95*(11), 1621–1630.

McGahee, T. W., and Tingen, M. S. (2000). The effects of a smoking prevention curriculum on fifth-grade children's attitudes, subjective norms, and refusal skills. *Southern Online Journal of Nursing Research, 1*(2). Retrieved June 21, 2006, from www.snrs.org.

McGahee, T. W., Kemp, V., and Tingen, M. S. (2000). A theoretical model for smoking prevention studies in preteen children. *Pediatric Nursing, 26*(2), 135–141.

McGinnis, J., and Foege, W. (1993). Actual causes of death in the United States. *Journal of the American Medical Association, 270,* 2207–2212.

Melvin, C. L., Adams, E. K., and Miller, V. (2000). Costs of smoking during pregnancy: development of the maternal and child health smoking attributable mortality, morbidity, and economic costs. *Tobacco Control, 9,* 12–15.

Mittleman, M. A., Lewis, R. A., Maclure, M., Sherwood, J. B., and Muller, J. E. (2001). Triggering myocardial infarction by marijuana. *Circulation, 103,* 2805–2809.

National Center on Addiction and Substance Abuse at Columbia University (CASA). (2004). *National survey of American attitudes on substance abuse VI: Teens.* Retrieved October 2, 2004, from http://www.casacolumbia.org/pdshopprov/shop/category.asp?catid=2.

National Center for Chronic Disease Prevention and Health Promotion (NCCDPHP). Tobacco Information and Prevention Source (TIPS). (2004a). *Tobacco use at a glance 2004.* Retrieved October 11, 2004, from http://www.cdc.gov/tobacco/issue.htm.

National Center for Chronic Disease Prevention and Health Promotion (NCCDPHP). (2004b). *The health consequences of smoking: A report of the Surgeon General.*

Retrieved August 18, 2004, from http://www.cdc.gov/tobacco/data_statistics/sgr/sgr_2004/index.htm#lights

National Health Promotion Associates, Inc. (2003). *LifeSkills training products and services* (pp. 1–11). New York: Author.

National Household Survey on Drug Use. (2004). *NIDA InfoFacts—Marijuana.* Retrieved February 2, 2005, from http://www.nida.nih.gov/Infofax/marijuana.html.

National Institute on Alcohol Abuse and Alcoholism (NIAAA). (2000). *Fetal alcohol exposure and the brain—National Institute on Alcohol Abuse and Alcoholism No. 50.* Retrieved February 1, 2005, from http://www.niaaa.nih.gov/publications/aa50.htm.

National Institute on Alcohol Abuse and Alcoholism (NIAAA). (2004). *Surgeon General calls on Americans to face facts about drinking.* Retrieved January 5, 2005, from http://www.niaaa.nih.gov/press/2004/Screenday04.htm.

National Institute on Drug Abuse (NIDA). (2003). *Marijuana: Facts for teens.* (NIH Publication No. 03-4037). Retrieved February 2, 2005, from http://www.nida.nih.gov/MarijBroch/teenpg11-12.html.

National Institute on Drug Abuse (NIDA). (2004). *Marijuana.* Retrieved February 2, 2005, from http://www.nida.nih.gov/Infofax/marijuana.html.

National Institute on Drug Abuse (NIDA). (2007). *Monitoring the Future Survey.* Retrieved September 8, 2007, from http://www.drugabuse.gov/DrugPages/MTF.html

Perez-Stable, E. J., Herrera, B., Jacob, P., and Benowitz, N. L. (1998). Nicotine metabolism and intake in black and white smokers. *Journal of the American Medical Association, 280*(2), 152–156.

Peterson, A. V., Kealey, K. A., Mann, S. L., and Marek, P. M. (2000). Hutchinson Smoking Prevention Project: Long-term randomized trial in school-based tobacco use prevention—Results on smoking. *Journal of the National Cancer Institute, 92*(24), 1979–1991.

Peto, R., Lopez, A., Boreham, J., Thun, M., and Health, C. J. (1994). *Mortality from smoking in developed countries 1950–2000.* New York: Oxford University Press.

Radel, M., Vallejo, R. L., Iwata, N., Arragon, R., Long, J. C., Virkkunen, M., and Goldman, D. (2005). Haplotype-based localization of an alcohol dependence gene to t 5q34 {gamma}aminobutyric acid type A gene cluster. *Archives of General Psychiatry, 62*(1), 47–55.

Ries, L. A. G., Eisner, M. P., Kosary, C. L., Hankey, B. F., Miller, B. A., Clegg, L., Mariotto, A., Feuer, E. J., and Edwards, B. K. (Eds.). (2004). *SEER Cancer Statistics Review, 1975–2001.* Bethesda, MD: National Cancer Institute. Retrieved February 2, 2005, from http://seer.cancer.gov/csr/1975_2001/.

Rimal, R. N. (2003). Intergenerational transmission of health: The role of intrapersonal, interpersonal, and communicative factors. *Health Education and Behavior, 30*(1), 10–28.

Rivara, F. P., Ebel, B. E., Garrison, M. M., Christakis, D. A., Wiehe, S. E., and Levy, D. T. (2004). Prevention of smoking-related deaths in the United States. *American Journal of Preventive Medicine, 27*(2), 118–125.

Rowe, A. K., Powell, K. E., and Hall, V. (1999). *The 1999 Georgia State of the Heart Report.* (Publication number DPH99.3HW). Georgia Department of Human Resources, Division of Public Health, Cardiovascular Health Section, and the American Heart Association, Southeast Affiliate.

Saraiya, M., Berg, C. J., Kendrick, J. S., Strauss, L. T., Atrash, H. K., and Ahn, Y. W. (1998). Cigarette smoking as a risk factor for ectopic pregnancy. *American Journal of Obstetrics and Gynecology, 178*(3), 493–498.

Sargeant, J. D., and Dalton, M. (2001). Does parental disapproval of smoking prevent adolescents from becoming established smokers? *Pediatrics, 108,* 1256–1262.

Sargeant, J. D., and DiFranza, J. R. (2003). Tobacco control for clinicians who treat adolescents. *CA: A Cancer Journal for Clinicians, 53,* 102–123.

Shadel, W. G., Shiffman, S., Niaura, R., Nichter, M., and Abrams, D. B. (2000). Current models of nicotine dependence: What is known and what is needed to advance understanding of tobacco etiology among youth. *Drug and Alcohol Dependence, 59*(Suppl 1), S9–22. Review.

Smedley, B. D., Syme, S. L., and Institute of Medicine (IOM). (2001). *Promoting health: Intervention strategies from social and behavioral research.* Washington, DC: National Academies Press.

Smith, T. M., Tingen, M. S., and Waller, J. (2004). The influence of self-concept and locus of control on rural preadolescent tobacco use. *Southern Online Journal of Nursing Research, 5*(5), 1–23.

Society for Research on Nicotine and Tobacco Subcommittee on Biochemical Verification. (2002). Biochemical verification of tobacco use and cessation. *Nicotine & tobacco research, 4,* 149–159.

Thomas, S. E., Kelly, S. J., Mattson, S. N., and Riley, E. P. (1998). Comparison of social abilities of children with fetal alcohol syndrome to those of children with similar IQ scores and normal controls. *Alcoholism, Clinical and Experimental Research 22*(2), 528–533.

Tingen, M. S., Waller, J. L., Smith, T. M., Baker, R. R., Reyes J., and Treiber, F. A. (2006). Tobacco prevention in children and cessation in family members. *Journal of the American Academy of Nurse Practitioners, 18,* 169–179.

Godlee, R. (Ed.). (2003). *Clinical evidence concise. The international source of the best available evidence for effective care.* London: British Medical Journal.

U.S. Department of Health and Human Services (USDHHS). (1998). *Tobacco use among U.S. racial/ethnic minority groups. A report of the Surgeon General—1998.* Rockville, MD: Office on Smoking and Health, National Center for Chronic Disease Prevention and Health Promotion, Centers for Disease Control and Prevention.

U.S. Department of Health and Human Services (USDHHS). (2000a). *Clinical Practice Guideline: Treating Tobacco Use and Dependence.* AHRQ Publication NO. 00-0032, Rockville, MD: Author.

U.S. Department of Health and Human Services (USDHHS). (2000b). *Healthy People 2010. With understanding and improving health and objectives for improving health* (2 vols.). Washington, DC: U.S. Government Printing Office.

U.S. Department of Health and Human Services (USDHHS). (2001). *Smoking and women's health: A report of the Surgeon General.* Atlanta: Public Health Service, Centers for Disease Control and Prevention, National Center for Chronic Disease Prevention and Health Promotion, Office on Smoking and Health.

Wakefield, M. A., Chaloupka, F. J., Kaufman, N. J., Orleans, C. T., Barker, D. C., and Ruel, E. E. (2000). Effect of restriction on smoking at home, at school, and in public places on teenage smoking: Cross sectional study. *British Medical Journal, 321,* 333–337.

Wickrama, K. A., Conger, R. D., Wallace, L. E., and Elder, G. H., Jr. (1999). The intergenerational transmission of health-risk behaviors: Adolescent lifestyles and gender moderating effects. *Journal of Health and Social Behavior, 40*(3), 258–272.

World Health Organization (WHO). (1999). *Confronting the epidemic: A global agenda for tobacco control research.* Geneva, Switzerland: Research for International Tobacco Control and the World Health Organization.

World Health Organization (WHO). (2002). *The world health report 2002: Reducing risks, extending healthy life.* Geneva: WHO.

Zhang, Z. F., Morgenstern, H., Spitz, M. R., Tashkin, D. P., Yu, G. P., Marshall, J. R., Hsu, T. C., and Schantz, S. P. (1999). Marijuana use and increased risk of squamous cell carcinoma of the head and neck. *Cancer Epidemiology, Biomarkers & Prevention, 8,* 1071–1078.

Zhu, L. X., Sharma, S., Stolina, M., Gardner, B., Roth, M. D., Tashkin, D. P., and Dubinett, S. M. (2000). Delta-9 tetrahydrocannabinol inhibits antitumor immunity by a CB2 receptor-mediated, cytokine-dependent pathway. *J Immunology, 165,* 373–380.

BIBLIOGRAPHY

Agency for Health Care Policy and Research. (2000). *Smoking cessation consumer guide—You can quit smoking.* Rockville, MD: Author.

Agency for Health Care Research and Quality. (2004). *US preventive services task force. Guide to clinical preventive services* (3rd ed., periodic updates). Publication No. 04-IP003. Rockville, MD: Author.

American Cancer Society, Inc. (2006). *When smokers quit—The health benefits over time.* Retrieved September 8, 2007, from http://www.cancer.org/docroot/SPC/content/SPC_1_When_Smokers_Quit.asp?sitearea=PED .

Andrews, J. O., Tingen, M. S., Waller, J. L., and Harper, R. J. (2001). Provider feedback improves adherence with AHCPR smoking cessation guideline. *Preventive Medicine, 33*(5), 101–104.

Cofta-Gunn, L., Wright, K. L., and Wetter, D. W. (2004). Evidence-based treatments for tobacco dependence. *Evidence-Based Preventive Medicine, 1*(1), 7–19.

Hulscher, M. E., Wensing, M., van Der Weijden, T., and Grol, R. (2001). Interventions to implement prevention in primary care (Cochrane Review). *Cochrane Database Syst Rev. 1,* CD000362.

Humair, J. P., and Ward, J. (1998). Smoking-cessation strategies observed in videotaped general practice consultations. *American Journal of Preventive Medicine, 14*(1), 71–72.

Lancaster, T., Silagy, C., and Fowler, G. (2000). Training health professionals in smoking cessation (Cochrane Review). *Cochrane Database Syst Rev. 3,* CD000214.

Sarna, L., Wewers, M.E., Brown, J.K., Lillington, L., and Brecht, M. (2001). Barriers to tobacco cessation in clinical practice: Report from a national survey on oncology nurses. *Nursing Outlook, 49*(4), 166–172.

State of the Science Conference Statement. (2006). *Tobacco Use: Prevention, Cessation, and Control.* Bethesda, MD: National Institutes of Health. Retrieved June 14, 2006, from http://consensus.nih.gov.

University of Wisconsin Medical School. (2003). *Treating tobacco use and dependence: Online continuing medical education course.* Rockville, MD: Agency for Healthcare Research and Quality. Available: http//www.ahrq.gov/clinic/ttudcme.htm.

Zhu, S. H., Anderson, C. M., Tedeschi, G. J., Rosbrook, B., Johnson, C. E., Byrd, M., and Gutierrez-Terrell, E. (2002). Evidence of real-world effectiveness of a telephone quitline for smokers. *New England Journal of Medicine, 347*(14), 1087–1093.

RESOURCES

LifeSkills Training (LST)

National Health Promotion Associates
711 Westchester Avenue
White Plains, New York 10604
914-421-2525 or 1-800-293-4969
FAX: 914-421-2007
Email: lstinfo@nhpamail.com
Web: http://www.lifeskillstraining.com

LST is a substance abuse prevention program for adolescents to reduce the risks of alcohol, tobacco, drug abuse, and violence. This comprehensive program, developed by Dr. Gilbert J. Botvin, targets psychosocial predictors of substance use and other risky behaviors and provides teens with confidence and skills needed to resist pressures that lead to drug use. The LifeSkills Training program is recognized as a Model or Exemplary program by an array of government agencies including the U.S. Department of Education and the Center for Substance Abuse Prevention.

National Institute on Alcohol Abuse and Alcoholism (NIAAA)

5635 Fishers Lane, MSC 9304
Bethesda, Maryland 20892-9304
Email: niaaaweb-r@exchange.nih.gov
Web: http://www.niaaa.gov

The NIAAA provides leadership in the national effort to reduce alcohol-related problems by conducting and supporting research in a wide range of scientific areas including genetics, neuroscience, epidemiology, and the health risks and benefits of alcohol consumption, prevention, and treatment; coordinating and collaborating with other research institutes and federal programs on alcohol-related issues; collaborating with international, national, state, and local institutions, organizations, agencies, and programs engaged in alcohol-related work; and translating and disseminating research findings to health care providers, researchers, policy makers, and the public. The Web site provides numerous pamphlets, resources, and posters for children, adults, and families regarding alcohol use; it also includes "Helping Patients with Alcohol Problems—A Health Practitioner's Guide."

Substance Abuse and Mental Health Services Administration (SAMSHA)

1 Choke Cherry Road
Rockville, Maryland 20857
240-276-2130
FAX: 240-276-2135
Web: http://www.samhsa.gov

SAMSHA, an agency of the U.S. Department of Health and Human Services, was established in 1992 as a services agency to focus attention, programs, and funding on improving the lives of people with or at risk for mental and substance abuse disorders. SAMSHA's mission is to build resilience and facilitate recovery for people with or at risk for mental or substance use disorders. SAMSHA's Substance Abuse Treatment Facility Locator (http://find-treatment.samhsa.gov/) is a searchable directory for locating substance abuse treatment centers.

PART 5

PUBLIC HEALTH NURSING IN THE TWENTY-FIRST CENTURY

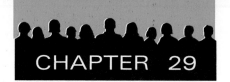

CHAPTER 29

Disaster Preparedness and Public Health Nursing

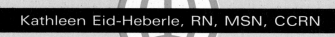

Kathleen Eid-Heberle, RN, MSN, CCRN

Chapter Outline

- **Disasters**
  Natural Disasters
  Man-Made Disasters
  Terrorism

- **Weapons of Mass Destruction**
  Biological Weapons
  Nuclear/ Radiological Weapons
  Chemical Weapons
  Incendiary/ Explosive Weapons

- **Effects of Disasters**
  Effects on Individuals
  Effects on Communities

- **Disease Surveillance**

- **Strategic National Stockpile**

- **Disaster Preparedness**
  Disaster Response and Management
  Public Health Preparedness

Learning Objectives

Upon completion of this chapter, the reader will be able to:

1. Compare the various types of disasters (natural, biological, chemical, nuclear, etc.)

2. Explore the effects of disasters with and without warning on individuals and communities

3. Identify the role and responsibilities of public health nurses responding to disasters

4. Explain the importance of the National Electronic Disease Surveillance System (NEDSS) and the Strategic National Stockpile (SNS)

When disasters strike, nurses must respond effectively and efficiently to mitigate the impact of the incident. Often following a disaster though, such as September 11, 2001 or the hurricanes of 2005, nurses who respond, determined to provide assistance, are not used to their full potential due to a lack of proper training or knowledge concerning disaster response and recovery. It is therefore imperative that nurses, especially public health nurses, acquire a basic understanding of disasters and disaster preparedness, response, and recovery. Public health nurses play a vital role in disaster preparedness; as in most communities, they are an integral part of developing disaster plans, investigating outbreaks, participating in disease surveillance, staffing pharmaceutical dispensaries, helping in shelters, and supporting mass immunization initiatives (Sistrom, 2004). Public health nurses must be *prepared for* disasters and not simply *respond to* them.

DISASTERS

Disasters have been a global concern throughout history. According to the American Red Cross, a disaster is "a threatening or occurring event of such destructive magnitude and force as to dislocate people, separate family members, damage or destroy homes, and injure or kill people. A disaster produces a range and level or immediate suffering and basic human needs that cannot be promptly or adequately addressed by the affected people, and impedes them from initiating and proceeding with their recovery efforts" (ARC, 2003, p. 13). Disasters can occur with little or no warning (e.g, avalanches, tsunamis, fires, and explosions) or with warning (e.g., hurricanes, slow-rinsing floods, winter storms, and droughts). When individuals and communities have time to prepare for a disaster, the effects of the disaster may be mitigated, saving lives and property. Two general classifications of disasters are those that occur naturally and those that are a result of human intervention.

Natural Disasters

Natural disasters are caused by either nature, such as hurricanes, or emerging diseases, such as avian influenza. Disasters related to nature are usually unpreventable and often occur in the same geographical areas because they are related to weather patterns or physical characteristics of a region (FEMA, 2004a).

Disasters attributable to an emerging disease occur when the virus "jumps the species barrier from animals to humans" (p. 100) potentially resulting in a pandemic (USAMRIID, 2004). Once a new disease is introduced into a suitable human population, it spreads rapidly because there is little or no immunity and no available vaccine, bringing with it devastating effects on the medical and public health system (PandemicFlu.gov, 2006). According to USAMRIID (2004), infectious agents such as influenza appear to be occurring more frequently and with greater risk for serious consequences possibly due to "environmental changes, global travel and trade, social upheaval and genetic changes in infectious agents, host or vector populations" (p. 100). Table 29-1 describes some of the larger natural disasters that have occurred throughout history.

Man-Made Disasters

Man-made disasters, or human-generated disasters, can be divided into two categories: accidental or deliberate (Langan, 2005). Major industrial accidents; unplanned releases of nuclear energy; power outages; chemical spills; and fire, or explosions, from hazardous materials such as fuel, chemicals, and nuclear materials are considered accidental disasters. Terrorist bombings or the intentional release of hazardous chemicals are considered deliberate disasters. Differentiating between accidental and deliberate disasters can sometimes be challenging. On August 15, 2003, the biggest power outage in North American history blacked out the northeastern United States and southern Canada affecting approximately 50 million people (DOE, 2003). Initially, this was thought to be the result of a terrorist attack, but it was quickly determined that the cause was technological. Table 29-2 describes selected technological disasters of the twentieth century.

Terrorism

The act of terrorism is designed to injure and kill and instill fear and insecurity in a community. Whether the acts of terrorism involve conventional explosives or weapons of mass destruction (nuclear, biological, chemical, and incendiary/explosive), the result remains the same: they create a climate of fear and panic and draw attention to the terrorists' cause (FEMA, 2004c). Terrorists often target sites that will have the largest impact on communities (ARC, 2002):

TABLE 29-1: Selected Natural Disasters

LOCATION	DATE	DISASTER	EFFECTS
Athens, Greece	430–426 B.C.	Epidemic	The Typhus epidemic devastated Attica, especially Athens.
Pompeii, Italy	79 A.D.	Volcanic eruption	The eruption of Mt. Vesuvius buried the cities of Pompeii and Herculaneum, killing thousands.
Netherlands	1228	Flood	Flooding of the sea caused 100,000 deaths.
Shensi, China	1556	Earthquake	Most deadly earthquake in history, killing 800,000 people.
Ireland	1845–1850	Famine	The famine took as many as one million lives as a result of hunger and disease.
Global	1918	Epidemic	The Spanish influenza killed approximately 25 million people worldwide.
Global	1981–present	Epidemic	The number of deaths worldwide related to AIDS is over 20 million.
Bam, Iran	2003	Earthquake	A 6.7 earthquake struck killing 43,000 people and leveling 70 percent of the buildings.
Southeast Asia earthquake/tsunami	2004	Tsunami	Tsunamis caused by a 9.0 earthquake in the Indian Ocean resulted in over 150,000 deaths in Indonesia, Sri Lanka, India, Thailand, Malaysia, Maldives, Myanmar, and Somalia.
Southeastern United States hurricanes	2006	Hurricane	Hurricanes Katrina, Rita, and Wilma caused extensive destruction in several U.S. states, resulting in approximately 1,300 deaths.

Note. From AVERT (2005), Crossley (2005), NOAA (2006), and Scaruffi (2005).

⊕ Critical Infrastructure Systems—power plants, phone companies, water treatment plants, mass transit systems, and hospitals

⊕ Public Buildings or Assembly Areas—shopping malls, convention centers, entertainment venues, churches, and tourist destinations

⊕ Symbolic or Historic Sites—sites that may have a perceived cultural or social importance, such as the Statue of Liberty

⊕ Controversial Facilities or Businesses—abortion clinics, banks, trade centers, and nuclear facilities

The Code of Federal Regulations (28 C.F.R. Section 0.85) defines **terrorism** as "the unlawful use of force or violence against persons or property to intimidate or coerce a government, the civilian population, or any segment thereof, in furtherance of political or social objective". The Federal Bureau of Investigation (FBI) further identifies terrorism as either domestic or international, depending on the origin, base, and objectives of the terrorist organization.

⊕ **Domestic terrorism** refers to "activities that involve acts dangerous to human life that are a

TABLE 29-2: Selected Technological Disasters

LOCATION	DATE	DISASTER	EFFECTS
Newfoundland, Canada	1912	Transportation accident	The luxury ship, Titanic, struck an iceberg and sank, killing 1,500 people.
Sverdlovsk, U.S.S.R. (now Ekaterinberg, Russia)	1979	Fixed hazardous installation	A filter from a factory producing anthrax was removed for fixing and never replaced, resulting in anthrax spores being emitted into the air, killing at least 68 people.
Bhopal, India	1984	Fixed hazardous installation	At a Union Carbide pesticide plant, 30 tons of methyl isocyanate was released into the air due to poor safety management practices. The accident led to the death of over 2,800 people living in the vicinity and caused respiratory damage and eye damage to over 20,000 others.
Kennedy Space Center, Florida	1986	Transportation accident	A booster failure on the shuttle occurred 73 seconds after lift off, resulting in the breakup of the vehicle and the deaths of all seven crew members.
Chernobyl, Ukraine (formerly U.S.S.R.)	1986	Nuclear power	During a routine test of one of the plant's nuclear reactors, numerous safety procedures were disregarded and a chain reaction led to a core meltdown. Thirty people were killed instantly, and over 135,000 had to be evacuated from within a 20-mile radius of the plant due to extreme levels of radiation.
Prince William Sound, Alaska	1989	Transportation accident	The oil tanker Exxon-Valdez struck the Bligh Reef spilling over 11 million tons of crude oil into the sound, affecting millions of animals, the environment and the fishing industry.
New York, New York	1996	Transportation accident	TWA flight 800 bound for Paris, France, exploded shortly after takeoff from New York, killing all 230 people on board.
Mont Blanc Tunnel, France/ Italy	1999	Transportation accident	A truck passing through the tunnel caught fire, resulting in 35 deaths. Temperature inside the tunnel reached 1,832°F (1,000°C).

Note. From Gulf of Maine Aquarium (2005), NASA (1993), United Nations Environment Program (2002), and EPA (2006).

violation of the criminal laws of the United States or of any state; appear to be intended to intimidate or coerce a civilian population; to influence the policy of a government by mass destruction, assassination, or kidnapping; and occur primarily within the territorial jurisdiction of the United States" [18 U.S.C. § 2331(5)] (FBI, 2004).

⊕ **International terrorism** involves "violent acts or acts dangerous to human life that are a violation of the criminal laws of the United States or any state, or that would be a criminal violation if committed within the jurisdiction of the United States or any state. These acts appear to be intended to intimidate or coerce a civilian population; influence the policy of a government by intimidation or coercion; or affect the conduct of a government by mass destruction, assassination or kidnapping and occur primarily outside the territorial jurisdiction of the United States or transcend national boundaries in terms of the means by which they are accomplished, the persons they appear intended to intimidate or coerce, or the locale in which their perpetrators operate or seek asylum" [18 U.S.C. § 2331(1)] (FBI, 2004).

The FBI also recognizes the emerging threat of cyber-terrorism, which has the potential to damage the United State's national security and interrupt, shut down, or degrade critical national infrastructures, such as energy, transportation, communications, or govern-ment services. According to the Department of Home-land Security (DHS, n.d.), cyber attacks target information technologies (ITs) in three different ways: (1) There is a direct attack against an information system "through the wires" alone (hacking). (2) The attack can be a physical assault against a critical IT element. (3) The attack can be from the inside as a result of compromising a trusted party with access to the system.

Through IT, terrorist have been able to improve communication within their organizations, enable members to quickly coordinate with large number of supporters, allow for continued propaganda, and reach a wide audience for potential financial donors or recruits (Terrorism Files, n.d.).

WEAPONS OF MASS DESTRUCTION

For terrorists to execute incidents with the greatest impact, **weapons of mass destruction** (e.g., biological, nuclear, chemical, and incendiary/explosive weapons) have been used. Chemical agents used in terrorism are likely to cause casualties within an hour or more, whereas biological agents may not be recognized for several days or weeks after their release (Croddy and Ackerman, 2003). Nuclear agents may have an immediate impact if used in connection with explosive agents or may go undetected initially if dispensed in a concealed method. Table 29-3 identifies selected acts of terrorism over the years.

TABLE 29-3: Selected Acts of Terrorism Using Weapons of Mass Destruction

LOCATION	DATE	TERRORIST ACT	EFFECTS
Delphi, Greece	600 B.C.	Biological	The Athenians diverted the river that provided drinking water to Delphi and contaminated it with hellebore roots and excrement. Then they diverted the river back into the city where the inhabitants became violently ill and the Athenians were able to take over the city.
Peloponnesian War	431–404 B.C.	Chemical	The Spartans burned pitch and sulfur, which created toxic fumes eventually enabling them to siege cities.

(continued)

TABLE 29-3: Selected Acts of Terrorism Using Weapons of Mass Destruction (cont'd)

LOCATION	DATE	TERRORIST ACT	EFFECTS
City of Kaffa (now Feodossia, Ukraine)	1346	Biological	The Mongols, who were dying of plague, hurled infected corpses over the city wall into Kaffa. The plague spread within the walls, and the city surrendered to the Mongols.
French and Indian War	1736	Biological	A British commander gave blankets infected with smallpox to a tribe of Ohio Indians. Within a few months the tribe was almost eliminated due to smallpox.
Rajneeshee Religious Cult	1984	Biological	Cult members infected salad bars in 10 restaurants in Dalles, Oregon, to influence county elections. Their goal was to sicken people so they could not vote, and the elections would be won by a cult member running for office. There were 751 reported cases of illnesses attributed to the Salmonella typhimurium contamination.
New York, New York	1993	Explosive	A car bomb was detonated in the garage of the World Trade Center, killing six and injuring 1,000.
Oklahoma City, Oklahoma	1995	Explosive	A car bomb was detonated in front of the Alfred P. Murrah Federal Building, killing 168 people.
Tokyo, Japan	1995	Chemical	The Aum Shinrikyo Cult members released sarin gas on 5 subways killing 12 and injuring 1,500.
United States	2001	Explosive/incendiary	Terrorist attacks with airplanes in New York City, Washington, D.C., and rural Pennsylvania killed over 3,000 people.
United States	2001	Biological	Bacillus anthracis (anthrax) in powder form was mailed to people around the United States, killing 5 and exposing many more.
Madrid, Spain	2004	Explosive	Ten terrorist bombs exploded almost simultaneously during the morning rush hour, killing 190 and injuring more than 1,800.
London, England	2005	Explosives	A series of cocoordinated suicide bombings struck London's public transport system killing 52 and injuring hundreds.

Note. From Fort Worth Public Health Department (2004) and Worldwide Conflicts and Wars (2004).

Public health nurses need to be cognitive of guidelines set forth for prophylaxis and treatment of biological, chemical, and nuclear incidents, including those that address the management of special needs groups such as infants, children, pregnant women, and the elderly. Public health nurses need to be also be prepared to develop and present information concerning medical response to terrorist weapons and other weapons of mass destruction to Emergency Medical Services (EMS), front-line health care providers and the public (APHA, 2001).

Biological Weapons

Briggs and Brinsfield (2003) describe biological terrorism as "the use of microorganisms or toxins derived from living organisms to produce death or disease in humans, animals, or plants" (p. 45). The threat of biological weapons against U.S. military and civilians is a realistic possibility due to the widespread availability of agents, production methods, and dissemination devices (USAMRIID, 2004).

Biological weapons are categorized into three groups; bacterial agents, viral agents, and biological toxins (see Table 29-4), and have three routes of exposure; inhalation, contact and gastrointestinal (USAMRIID, 2004). It may be hours or days before the effects of a biological incident are known, exacerbating the spread of the organism. The detection of a biological outbreak depends on nurses and health care providers who can correctly identify the signs and symptoms of such agents. In turn, it is their responsibility to notify the suspecting diagnosis to the public health officials who will have to initiate an epidemiological investigation to determine the source. If the outbreak is confirmed the public health officials must identify risk factors for the population, implement interventions to control the outbreak, and inform the public (Berkowitz, 2002).

Smallpox

In 1979, the World Health Organization (WHO) officially declared smallpox eradicated (WHO, 2006). Following its eradication, the WHO decided to store the smallpox virus in two laboratories; one at the Centers for Disease Control and Prevention (CDC) in Atlanta and the other at the Institute for Viral Precautions in Moscow, Russia (USAMRIID, 2004). There is now concern in the United States that other countries, hostile to the U.S., have acquired the smallpox virus with the intention of developing offensive programs (USAM-

RIID, 2004). The Centers for Disease Control and Prevention (CDC, 2004a) reports that the deliberate release of smallpox, in order to create an epidemic disease, is now regarded as a possible threat by the U.S., making it vital that public health officials plan and prepare for such an incident.

According to the WHO (2001), smallpox is an acute contagious disease caused by variola virus. Smallpox may initially resemble chickenpox to the health care provider, but there are several key differentiating characteristics (see Table 29-5). Once smallpox has been diagnosed, health care providers must immediately report the findings to the public health department.

In the event of a smallpox outbreak, or any other biological incident, the governor in consultation with public health authorities may declare a state of public health emergency at which time state and local health officials may isolate, quarantine, or vaccinate the public as needed (Center for Law and the Public Health, 2001). The Model State Emergency Health Power Act defines isolation and quarantine as the following (Center for Law and the Public Health, 2001):

- ⊕ **Isolation** is "the physical separation and confinements of an individual or groups of individuals who are *infected* or reasonably believed to be infected with a contagious or possibly contagious disease from non-isolated individuals, to prevent or limit the transmission of the disease to non-isolated individuals" (p. 10).

- ⊕ **Quarantine** is "the physical separation and confinement of and individual or groups of individuals, who are or may have been *exposed* to a contagious or possibly contagious disease and who do not show signs and symptoms of a contagious disease, from non-quarantine individuals, to prevent or limit the transmission of the disease to non-quarantine individuals" (p. 11).

Smallpox Vaccine

The smallpox vaccine is made with a "live" vaccinia virus, a pox-type virus, that enables the body to develop immunity to smallpox. Because the vaccine is a live virus the vaccination site must be cared for carefully so that the vaccine does not spread. The guidelines set forth by the CDC (2004b) for inoculation are as follows:

1. Review client history for contraindications—Some people are at greater risk for complications

TABLE 29-4: Selected Types of Biological Weapons

CATEGORY	DISEASE	CAUSE	MODE OF TRANSMISSION	TRANSMIT PERSON TO PERSON
Bacterial Agents	Anthrax	Anthrax is primarily a zoonotic disease in herbivores. The spores remain dormant until introduced to the right conditions. Humans can contract three forms of anthrax: (a) *inhalation anthrax* when spores from an infected animal or animal product enters the respiratory system or with an intentional aerosol dissemination; (b) *cutaneous anthrax* when spores from an infected animal or animal product enter the body through a cut or abrasion while handling infected materials such as wool, hides, etc.; (c) *gastrointestinal anthrax* from consuming undercooked or raw infected meat.	Inhalation, contact, and gastrointestinal	No
	Pneumonic plague Plague is a zoonotic disease found in rodents and their fleas.	Pneumonic plague can be caused by inhaling the aerosolized bacteria from an infected person or animal.	Inhalation	High
	Tularemia	Tularemia is caused by a bacteria occurring in animals such as rodents and rabbits.	Inhalation, contact, and gastrointestinal	No
Viral Agents	Smallpox	Smallpox is caused by the variola virus and was declared eradicated by the World Health Organization in 1979.	Inhalation and contact	High
	Viral hemorrhagic fever (VHF)	The virus that causes VHF is zoonotic residing in animals such as rodents and arthropods.	Contact	Moderate
Biological toxins	Botulism	Botulism is a muscle-paralyzing disease caused by a nerve toxin. This group of bacteria is commonly found in the soil.	Contact and ingestion	No
	Ricin	Ricin causes cellular death. It is a poison made from the waste left over from processing castor bean.	Inhalation and ingestion	No

(continued)

TABLE 29-4: Selected Types of Biological Weapons (cont'd)

DISEASE	INCUBATION PERIOD	SIGNS AND SYMPTOMS	DURATION OF ILLNESS	TREATMENT
Anthrax	1–7 days	*Inhalation:* Initially similar to a cold or flu progressing to sore throat, mild fever, muscle aches, cough, chest tightness and shortness of breath. *Cutaneous:* small sores that develop into blisters and then into skin ulcers with blackened area in the center. *Gastrointestinal:* nausea, loss of appetite, bloody diarrhea, fever, severe abdominal pain.	*Inhalation:* 3–5 days; *Cutaneous:* 3 weeks; *Gastrointestinal:* 7–10 days	Antibiotics
Pneumonic plague	1–6 days	High fever, headache, weakness progressing to pneumonia, cough, shortness of breath, chest tightness and then dyspnea, cyanosis, and possible death	1–6 days	Antibiotics
Tularemia	2–10 days (average 3–5 days)	Sudden fever, chills, headache, diarrhea, cough, progressive weakness and dsypnea.	Over 2 weeks	Antibiotics
Smallpox	7–17 days (average 12 days)	Fever, malaise, head and body aches followed by a rash then raised bumps forming into pustules which then crust and scab. The scabs fall off in three weeks leaving pitted scars.	3–4 weeks	No treatment; provide supportive medical care.
Viral hemorrhagic fever (VHF)	4–21 days	Vascular system is damaged and the body's ability to regulate itself is impaired. Fever, dizziness, fatigue, bleeding is present from under the skin, in internal organs and from orifices.	Death between 7–16 days	No treatment; provide supportive medical care.
Botulism	1–5 days	Double vision, drooping eyelids, slurred speech, muscle weakness that always descends through the body eventually causing respiratory failure.	Death in 24–72 hours; lasts months if not lethal	Antitoxins
Ricin		*Inhalation:* 4–8 hours *Ingestion:* less than 6 hours *Inhalation:* respiratory difficulties, fever, cough, chest tightness, pulmonary edema resulting in respiratory failure. *Ingestion:* vomiting, diarrhea, dehydration and seizures.	Days	No treatment; provide supportive medical care.

(continued)

TABLE 29-4: Selected Types of Biological Weapons (cont'd)

DISEASE	MORTALITY RATE	STABILITY OF ORGANISM
Anthrax	*Inhalation:* High if untreated; *Cutaneous:* Low: *Gastrointestinal:* Moderate	Very stable; spores remain viable for over 40 years in soil
Pneumonic plague	High unless treated within 12–24 hours.	Stable for several weeks in water, moist soil, and grains
Tularemia	Moderate if untreated.	Months in moist soil
Smallpox	High to moderate	Relatively unstable
Viral hemorrhagic fever (VHF)	High for Zaire strain; moderate with Sudan strain.	Relatively unstable
Botulism	High without respiratory support	Weeks in nonmoving water and food
Ricin	High—death within 36–72 hours from ingestion	Stable

Note. CDC (2004d) and USAMRIID (2004)

⊕ RESEARCH APPLICATION

Planning against Biological Terrorism: Lessons from Outbreak Investigations

Study Purpose

To examine investigations of epidemiological incidents, involving biological agents that could be utilized for bioterrorism, around the world from 1988 to 1999 by the Centers for Disease Control and Prevention's (CDC) Epidemic Intelligence Service (EIS).

Methods

A standardized form was used to assemble data from each EIS investigation. From the reports, information was obtained on "possible bioterrorism, causative agent, location, time from first case to first report of the outbreak, and source of recognition and reporting of the outbreak."

Findings

Of the 1,099 investigated outbreaks, 44 (4.0 percent) were caused by an agent which could be utilized for bioterrorism. The number of days from which an outbreak occurred to the date the identifying agency requested assistance from the CDC was between 0 and 26 days.

Implications

The most critical component for bioterrorism outbreak detection and reporting is the frontline health care professional and the local health departments. Health care professionals must be educated in bioterrorism preparedness in order to shorten the time from detecting an outbreak to reporting it to the public health officials to notification of the CDC. In addition, having a national surveillance system would increase the effectiveness of identifying a bioterrorism incident and reporting it.

Reference

Ashford, D. A. Kaiser, R. M., Bales, M. E., Shutt, K., Patrawalla, A., McShan, A., Tappero, J. W., Perkins, B. A., and Dannenberg, A. L. (2003). Planning against biological terrorism: Lessons from outbreak investigations. *Emerging Infectious Diseases, 9*(5). Retrieved December 30, 2004, from HYPERLINK "http://www.cdc.gov/ncidod/EID/vol9no5/02-0388.htm" http://www.cdc.gov/ncidod/EID/vol9no5/02-0388.htm.

TABLE 29-5: Differentiating Characteristics between Smallpox and Chickenpox

	SMALLPOX	CHICKENPOX
Fever	2–4 days before rash	At time of rash
Rash		
Appearance	Pocks in same stage	Pocks in several stages
Development	Slow	Rapid
Distribution	More pocks on arms and legs	More pocks on body
On palms and soles	Usually present	Usually absent
Death	Usually one in ten die	Very uncommon

Note. From WHO (2001). *WHO slide set on the diagnosis of smallpox.* Retrieved December 30, 2004, from http://www.who.int/emc/diseases/smallpox. Reprinted with permission of WHO.

following vaccination and therefore should not be inoculated unless they have been exposed to the smallpox virus. People who should not receive the vaccine are those who (a) have eczema or atopic dermatitis; (b) have skin conditions such as burns, chickenpox, shingles, impetigo, herpes, severe acne, or psoriasis until the condition has completely healed; (c) have a weakened immune system; (d) are pregnant or plan on becoming pregnant within one month of the vaccination; (e) are breastfeeding; (f) have been diagnosed with a heart condition; (g) are children under 18 and seniors over 65 in nonemergency situations; (h) have a combination of the following conditions, which have been diagnosed by a health care provider: high blood pressure, high cholesterol, and diabetes (CDC, 2004e).

2. Choose the site—The upper arm (deltoid) is the recommended site.

3. Prepare the skin—DO NOT use alcohol to prep the skin as this has shown to inactivate the vaccine virus.

4. Administer the vaccine—The smallpox vaccine is given with a bifurcated (two-pronged) needle that is dipped in the vaccine and pricked to the upper arm numerous times within a few seconds. The pricking is not deep, but will cause soreness and one or two droplets of blood to appear.

5. Absorb excess vaccine—After vaccination, excess vaccine should be absorbed with a sterile gauze and disposed of properly. This will prevent secondary inoculation.

6. Cover the site—Cover the site with a gauze or semipermeable dressing and first aid adhesive tape until a scab forms and drainage ceases.

7. Record the vaccination—The CDC requires that all smallpox administrations be reported.

8. Educate the clients—Clients who have received the smallpox vaccine should be instructed to:

- Not rub or scratch vaccination site.
- Keep site dry and covered.
- Dispose of dressing changes appropriately by putting the contaminated bandages in a sealed plastic bag and throwing them away in the trash.
- Wash all clothing or other materials that come in contact with the vaccination site in hot water.
- Wash hands thoroughly with soap and water after touching anything that has come in contact with the site.
- When the scab falls off discard of it properly by throwing it away in a sealed plastic bag.

⊕ Report any problems by calling the number indicated on the "Post-Vaccination and Follow-Up Information" sheet, calling your health care provider, or visiting the emergency department.

⊕ Return seven days after vaccination to see if the vaccination was successful.

Most people will not experience any adverse reactions to the inoculation other than a low grade fever and a sore arm and redness where the inoculation was administered (CDC, 2004c). In people who do develop a reaction, complications may be minor or life threatening. Minor reactions include secondary inoculation and secondary bacterial infection (cellulitis) of the vaccination site. Major reactions include any involvement with the eyes, entering the bloodstream (lesions will appear everywhere on the skin), and postvaccinal encephalitis (CDC, 2004c).

Nuclear/Radiological Weapons

There are two types of radiological incidents or **Radiological Dispersal Device (RDD)**. The first is the actual detonation of a radiological device, such as a "dirty bomb," which combines a conventional explosive, such as dynamite, with radioactive material (NRC, 2003). According to the U.S. Nuclear Regulatory Commission (NRC, 2003), in most instances, the conventional explosive itself has more immediate lethality than the radioactive material. At the levels created by most probable sources, not enough radiation is present in a dirty bomb to kill people or cause severe illness. Radioactive materials dispensed in the air could contaminate several city blocks (NRC, 2003). "A dirty bomb is in no way similar to a nuclear weapon. The presumed purpose of its use would be therefore not as a Weapon of Mass Destruction but rather as a Weapon of Mass Disruption" (NRC, 2003).

The second type of RDD involves a powerful source of radiation hidden in a public place, such as a trash can, train, or subway, where people passing by may receive a significant dose of radiation without their knowledge (NRC, 2003).

In the event of a nuclear emergency where a power plant is involved, there are two emergency planning zones (EPZ). The first zone covers a 10-mile radius of the plant, where it is possible that people could be harmed by direct radiation exposure. The second zone covers a broader area, usually up to a 50-mile radius from the plant, where radioactive materials could contaminate water supplies, food crops, and livestock (FEMA, n.d.). The release of radioactive material from the plant into the environment is usually characterized by a plume (cloud-like formation) of radioactive gases and particles (FEMA, n.d.).

To mitigate the health effects of a radiological incident, public health officials need to assess the situation to determine whether to evacuate or order in-place sheltering, restrict consumption of locally produced milk and food, distribute potassium iodide tablets, and carry out environmental sampling and illness tracking (Sutton & Gould, 2003). The most effective way to protect the public from radiological exposure is by decreasing the amount of *time* near the source of radiation, increase the *distance* from the radiation source, and increase the *shielding* between the public and the radiation source (CDC, 2003b).

The health effects from a radiological incident may be felt within minutes to days after exposure. Initial symptoms may include nausea, vomiting, and diarrhea which could then progress to acute radiation syndrome (ARS). According to the CDC (2003c), "ARS is an acute illness caused by large amounts of radiation exposure over a brief time (minutes)." The major cause of this syndrome is the depletion of immature parenchymal stem cells. There are three forms of ARS: bone marrow syndrome, which affects the stem cells in the bone marrow; gastrointestinal (GI) syndrome, in which stem cells in the bone marrow and cell lining in the GI tract are dying; and cardiovascular/nervous syndrome, which affects the nervous system (CDC, 2003c).

Chemical Weapons

Hazardous chemicals, which affect people through direct contact, inhalation, or ingestion, can be disseminated by mistake, as in industrial accidents, or intentionally by terrorists (CDC, 2005a). The release may be overt, as with a chemical spill, or covert, as in the deliberate contamination of food, water, or a consumer product (CDC, 2003d). Four categories of agents are:

⊕ Nerve Agents (e.g., sarin and tabun)—Lethal agents that disable enzymes responsible for the transmission of nerve impulses. Victims are exposed to these agents through skin contact or inhalation.

⊕ Vesicant or Blistering Agents (e.g., sulfur mustard, nitrogen mustard, and mustard gas)—Agents that cause blisters on the skin and damage the respiratory tract, mucous membranes, and eyes. Victims are exposed to these agents through skin contact or inhalation.

⊕ Choking Agents (e.g., chlorine, ammonia, and phosgene)—Agents that damage the respiratory tract, causing extensive fluid buildup in the lungs. Victims are exposed to these agents through inhalation.

⊕ Blood Agents (e.g., hydrogen cyanide and arsine)—Agents that interfere with the absorption of oxygen into the bloodstream. Victims are exposed to these agents through inhalation.

Public health professionals, health care providers, and poison control centers must be able to recognize the effects of a chemical incident and implement rapid and appropriate measures for individuals and the community (CDC, 2003d). Following CDC (2003d) guidelines, public health officials would need to (1) provide accurate information to health care providers, clinical laboratories, and poison control centers; (2) monitor the scope of the incident; (3) implement the capacity to receive and investigate any report; (4) implement appropriate protocols, for instance accessing the Laboratory Response Network for Bioterrorism, collecting, transporting, and storing specimens; (5) report to the CDC and local law enforcement if the results of an investigation suggest the intentional release of a chemical agent; and (6) request CDC assistance when necessary.

⊕ PRACTICE APPLICATION

Bioterrorism

Since 9/11 and the subsequent anthrax incidents, much attention has been given to bioterrorism and how to best protect the public. Bioterrorism did not strike the United States for the first time in 2001. In 1984 in The Dalles, Oregon, followers of the Indian guru Bhagwan Shree Rajneesh spiked salad bars at ten restaurants in town with *Salmonella* and sickened about 750 people. The reason for the attack was that the cult members had hoped to incapacitate so many voters that their own candidates for the county elections would win. The plan failed but The Dalles did experience negative economic repercussions.

The Wasco-Sherman Public Health Department received numerous calls about people becoming sick after eating in area restaurants. Within 48 hours of the outbreak, the cause was identified as *Salmonella*, and four days after the first reported case, the Oregon State Public Health Laboratory in Portland identified the agent as an unusual strain of *Salmonella typhimurium*. Approximately eight days after the incident occurred, the Centers for Disease Control and Prevention was contacted for assistance in handling the case. The limited resources that the public health department had made handling such a large case challenging.

Despite thorough investigation by public health officials, no common source for the foods could be identified. The outbreak was initially blamed on the restaurant food handlers, and it was more than a year before the town and country learned the truth behind the illness that plagued The Dalles from cult members turned informants.

As a result of the outbreak, almost 1,000 people had reported symptoms to their health care providers or the hospital of which 751 were confirmed to have *Salmonella* poisoning. The Rajneeshees' attack was the first large-scale use of germ warfare by terrorist in modern U.S. history. Nevertheless, it did not attract much attention, and the public health officials opted not to publish a study of the incident as not to encourage copycats. The case exposed several deficiencies such as accessibility to pathogens from germ banks and lack of communication between law enforcement and public health officials.

Author

DiGiovanni, Jr., C., Reynolds, B., Harwell, R., Stonecipher, E. B., and Burkle, Jr., F. M. (2003). Community reaction to bioterrorism: Prospective study of simulated outbreak. *Emerging Infectious Diseases, 19*(6). Retrieved December 30, 2004, from http://www.cdc.gov/ncidod/EID/vol9no6/02-0769.htm.

Incendiary/Explosive Devices

Most terrorist acts are carried out using small arms, explosives, and incendiaries (Cukier and Chapdelaine, 2003). The hazards from these incendiary weapons are the same as hazards from fires. Smoke inhalation, burns, high temperatures, and dangerous fumes from weapons and other materials being burned can cause serious health problems (ARC, 2002). Incendiary devices can be combined with explosives to amplify the results. After an initial explosion, which creates shockwaves, blast overpressure, and flying debris, there may still be hazards from unstable structures, dangerous debris, or from secondary devices such as hazardous materials. Explosions that occur in confined places such as buildings are associated with greater morbidity and mortality (CDC, 2003a).

Once an explosive or incendiary incident or both has occurred, the threat is usually visible, unlike the effects of biological, chemical, and nuclear incidents in which hours to weeks may pass before an event is detected. According to Cukier and Chapdelaine (2003), this may cause immediate "psychological terror" (p. 165), which may cause chaos and panic. Following an incendiary or explosive incident, the public health department should be in contact with local hospitals to determine their capacity for accepting new clients (CDC, 2003e). This information will need to be communicated to the public; recommending that less seriously injured people go to hospitals outside the affected area.

EFFECTS OF DISASTERS

Disasters not only affect individuals and communities but also can damage a country's economic and productivity abilities (FAO, 2005). According to FEMA (2004b), regardless of the type of disaster—natural, technological, or man-made—"the goal is to mitigate the need for response as opposed to simply increasing the response capabilities." Mitigation can save lives, reduce property damage, protect critical infrastructure, and be cost-effective (FEMA, 2004b).

If individuals or communities have time to prepare for disasters due to warning systems, the effects of the disasters can be reduced. With warning, lives may be saved, property loss may be decreased, responses may be more effective, and human suffering may be reduced. Scientists are continually developing equipment to better predict natural disasters and to disseminate information to the public, such as sheltering and evacuation orders, following a natural or man-made event (FEMA, 2000). Effective warnings should reach every person who is at risk in a timely manner no matter what they are doing or where they are located (FEMA, 2000). To accomplish such a broad distribution, the Working Group on National Disaster Information Systems Subcommittee on Natural Disaster Reduction and the National Science and Technology Council Committee on Environment and Natural Resources recommend that government-owned systems, such as the National Oceanic and Atmospheric Administration (NOAA) Weather Radio and local sirens, must function in collaboration with privately owned systems, such as radio, television, pagers, telephones, Internet, and printed media (FEMA, 2000). This partnership is currently being developed. Certain computers are programmed to respond to warnings by automatically shutting down or appropriately modifying transportation systems, lifelines, and manufacturing processes to further ensure the safety of individuals and communities (FEMA, 2000).

Disasters create great psychological and physical casualties, but those that occur without warning have an even greater effect on people. The lack of warning means that people do not have the opportunity to take safety measures, creating a sense of loss of control, helplessness, vulnerability, and disequilibrium (Briggs and Brinsfield, 2003).

Effects on Individuals

After a disaster, the physiological effects are usually evident by physical pain, injuries, or even death. Short-term emotional effects such as anxiety, fear, and grief may also be apparent. For many victims the mental effects will fade with time but for others the effects may be long term (Ehrenreich, 2001).

Physical Health Effects

Disasters can affect individuals' health in various ways. Individuals may sustain injuries preimpact (evacuating or escaping from the disaster), impact (caused by the disaster), and postimpact (caused by cleaning up after the incident) (ARC, 1999). Physical effects may encompass bone, muscle, and joint injuries; lacerations; rashes; burns; puncture wounds; and possibly death. In addition, individuals may develop stress-related symptoms or exacerbation of preexisting conditions, such as fluctuation in normal vital signs, irritability, gastrointestinal upset, asthma, cardiac problems, headache, and early labor contractions (ARC, 1999).

Mental Health Effects

The emotional effects following a disaster may range from mild anxiety, interpersonal troubles to lasting depression, posttraumatic stress disorder (PTSD), and other emotional disorders (Ehrenreich, 2001). Contributing factors that may increase psychiatric causalities include "terror that strikes a population, lack of information, distortion of threats by news and public media, the direct threat of injury or death, and the horror of exposure to grotesque stimuli" (APA, 2004, p. 13). According to Dr. Dickson Diamond, chief psychiatrist for the FBI and medical consultant to its National Domestic Preparedness Office, people exposed to disasters may not experience signs and symptoms until days or weeks following the event. The more sudden and unexpected the incident, and the more unprepared the society, the greater the long-term psychiatric consequences (APA, 2004). After an incident has occurred, the consequence for the public's health can be extensive as the health care system becomes inundated with "psychogenic casualties"; people who think they may have been exposed to harmful agents or who become alarmed over minor symptoms (Butler, Panzar, and Goldfrank, 2003; Kupersanin, 2000).

After a disaster, demands for medical and mental health services can quickly overwhelm available resources. It is therefore imperative that health officials keep the public informed regarding health concerns related to the disaster. If current and accurate information is not communicated effectively by public health officials, reporters may rely on sources that lack the expertise to get their information. Inaccurate reporting may generate more panic in the community.

Effects on Responders

In addition to providing mental health services to victims and their families, it is essential to provide such services to rescue and relief workers. Rescue workers tend to be dedicated and trained to focus on other's needs, neglecting to take care of their basic needs (APA, 2004). The long hours, breadth of survivors' needs and demands, ambiguous roles, and exposure to human suffering can affect even the most experienced professional. Approximately 20 percent of rescue workers may experience some form of post-traumatic stress disorder

(PTSD) by the end of the first month following a disaster (APA, 2004). To reduce the psychological effects in relief and rescue workers, education concerning general responses to stress, in themselves and their co-workers, should be part of all disaster preparedness trainings (Ehrenreich, 2001). During the disaster response it is imperative that these workers have limited on-duty work hours, rotate from high stress to low stress functions, take adequate breaks, drink plenty of water, eat nutritiously, have periodic debriefings and pair up with another responder so that stress levels may be monitored by one another (SAMHSA, 2003).

Coping with Disasters: A Guidebook to Psychological Disasters (Ehrenreich, 2001) describes four phases that people and communities go through after a disaster.

> Rescue Phase—The first phase may last from a few hours to a couple of days after a disaster. During this phase, the focus is on rescuing and stabilizing the situation. Victims must be provided with shelter, food, medical attention, and clothing.

> Honeymoon Phase—Victims experience this phase within the first weeks after a disaster. During this time, people are relieved at being safe and have unrealistic expectations about recovery.

> Disillusionment Phase—People become more realistic about the long-term effects of the disaster and are disappointed with delayed help. This phase may last from two months to one or two years.

> Reconstruction Phase—In the final phase, people have established a new "pattern of life" (Ehrenreich, 2001, p.21).

The rate at which individuals and communities transition from one phase to another is neither rigid nor distinct. The rate of transition may be influenced by factors such as coping skills, age, ethnicity, recent traumatic life events, financial resources, disability, language barrier, dependency on other people and/or drugs or alcohol, or access to professional help (ARC, 1999; Plum, 2003).

Effects on Communities

A disaster has the potential to overwhelm a community's resources; public service personnel are overworked, public buildings are damaged, resources such as food and medical supplies may become depleted, and there may be an interruption of services. The level at which a community is affected depends on the magnitude of the destruction; the number of people ill, injured, or dead; the number of people seeking medical attention; the extent of the disruption of services (utilities, communication, transportation and sanitation); and the disaster response by authorities (Veenema, 2003a).

Public health nurses must meet the needs of not only individuals and families but also the community. "Restoration of the environment and its resources to pre-disaster conditions is imperative to promote good health and prevent disease" (Veenema, 2003b, p. 171). Public health professionals have a variety of roles when responding to disasters (Levy and Sidel, 2003 and Veenema, 2003b):

- Community Assessment—Assessing the community for the presence, or absence, of clean water, safe food, sanitation, and shelter.

- Diagnosing and Reporting—Diagnosing and reporting illness and injuries, especially those related to biological or chemical incidents, to the appropriate agencies such as the state health department or the CDC.

- Providing Preventative Measure—Educating the public on preventative measures such as appropriate vaccines, prophylactic antimicrobials, and antitoxins and administering such measures when necessary.

- Preventing the Spread of Disease—Responding aggressively to evidence of the transmission of disease in order to prevent an epidemic through the population and educating people on how to prevent the spread of disease.

- Assisting with Outbreak Investigation—Assisting epidemiologists and others in their investigating of the outbreak.

- Discouraging Inappropriate Responses—Discouraging people from taking actions that may be unsafe, such as hoarding antibiotics.

When a disaster does not affect the whole community, public health nurses have the challenge of not only managing the effects of the disaster but also continuing to provide services to their regular clients. In addition, human, financial and other resources may be diverted from local public health programs to meet the needs caused by the disaster (Keck and Erme, 2003). These reallocations of funds and resources can adversely affect individuals and communities.

DISEASE SURVEILLANCE

According to the WHO (2005a), "every country should be able to detect, verify rapidly and respond appropriately to epidemic-prone and emerging disease threats when they arise to minimize their impact on the health and economy of the world's population." The Communicable Diseases Surveillance and Response (CSR) program works to enhance infectious disease surveillance capacity at all levels (international, national, and subnational), including developing early warning mechanisms to detect disease outbreaks (World Health Organization Regional Office for Europe, 2005). CSR is organized throughout the world into nine clusters that work together, exchanging information, coordinating and implementing activities, and planning for the future (WHO, 2005b).

Within the United States, there are currently multiple surveillance systems in place to obtain information from primary-care health care providers, emergency departments, public health labs, community clinics, and local and state health departments. As a result, many of these systems cannot communicate with one another, inhibiting data exchange (CDC, 2005b). To ensure rapid and effective response to an outbreak, secure communication systems must be established, linking all local public health departments to each other, the state, the nation, and the CDC (Conrad and Pearson., 2003). The **Public Health Information Network (PHIN)** currently being developed will integrate capabilities of public health information systems across a wide variety of organizations that participate in public health (CDC, 2005b). This will enable consistent exchange of response, health, and disease-tracking data between public health partners in every community (CDC, 2005b).

The disease surveillance and monitoring component of the PHIN is the **National Electronic Disease Surveillance System (NEDSS)** utilized at the federal, state, and local levels (CDC, n.d.). Information is obtained from hospital admissions, Emergency Department (ED) triage log of chief complaints, ED visit outcome, 911 calls, poison control center calls, unexplained deaths, medical examiner case volume, labs, school/work absenteeism, over-the-counter medication sales, and animal illness or deaths to aid in identifying clusters of unusual infectious diseases that may indicate a biological incident (Broome and Loonsk, 2004). It is most often at the local public health department level that disease surveillance activities occur (Pryor & Veenema, 2003). Local health officials work closely with health care providers and facilities for initial case reporting, follow-up investigation, and provision of feedback (Pryor and Veenema, 2003).

STRATEGIC NATIONAL STOCKPILE

If a public health emergency (terrorist attack, flu outbreak, earthquake, etc.) arises that overwhelms the local health care system, depleting them of medical resources, rapid access to large quantities of pharmaceuticals and medical supplies is vital (CDC, 2005c). Local health authorities may initiate the activation of the CDC's Strategic National Stockpile (SNS) to help meet the needs of a community (CDC, 2005c). The SNS is comprised of large quantities of medicines and medical supplies that can be delivered to any state in the United States (CDC, 2005c). For immediate assistance, within 12 hours, communities can receive supplies via the SNS 12-Hour Push Packages. These are caches of pharmaceuticals, antidotes, and medical supplies designed to provide rapid delivery of a broad spectrum of assets for incidents where the exact cause is unknown (CDC, 2005c). If the incident requires additional pharmaceuticals and/or medical supplies, vendor managed inventory (VMI) supplies can be shipped to arrive within 24 to 36 hours (CDC, 2005c). If the cause of the incident has been identified, VMI can be tailored to provide pharmaceuticals, supplies, and/or products specific to the suspected or confirmed agent(s) (CDC, 2005c).

Accompanying the medical supplies is a team of CDC technical advisers known as the Technical Advisory Response Unit (TARU). The team is comprised of "pharmacists, emergency responders, and logistic experts that will advise local authorities on receiving,

⊕ POLICY HIGHLIGHT

CDC Funding

The American Public Health Association (APHA) has expressed concern to the House Appropriations Subcommittee on Labor, Health and Human Services and Education regarding the public health budget for FY 2007 as it pertains to disaster preparedness. The APHA believes that Congress should support the Centers for Disease Control and Prevention as a whole entity, not just as individual programs within the agency, in order for it to carry out its mission to protect and promote good public health.

The CDC is the command center for protecting the nation's health as it pertains to disaster preparedness, response and recovery for natural disasters (hurricanes), emerging and reemerging infectious diseases (avian influenza), and acts of terrorism (anthrax distribution). As the nation's, and world's, expert resource and response center, the CDC is looked to for accurate information and direction in a crisis or outbreak.

Unfortunately, despite these vital responsibilities, Congress cut overall CDC funding in FY 2006 for the first time in 25 years, and in FY 2007, the President has proposed cutting CDC funding even more, more than 2 percent overall. At a vulnerable time for the nation's health, the APHA believes that these budget cuts would hinder the public's safety, requesting that the proposed cuts not be implemented.

APHA believes that funding for the CDC should be at least $8.5 billion, in addition to funds allocated specifically for preparedness against a potential influenza pandemic. APHA supports the proposed increase in funding for antiterrorism activities, including the increases for the Strategic National Stockpile and the new Botulinum Toxin Research, but cautions that the President's proposed level of funding of the state and local capacity grants continues to reflect a $95 million cut from FY 2005 levels. The APHA requests the restoration of these cuts to ensure that state and local communities can be prepared in the event of an act of terrorism.

distributing, dispensing, replenishing and recovering SNS material" (District of Columbia, n.d.). The Department of Health and Human Services transfers authority of the SNS materials to state and local authorities after it arrives at the designated receiving and storage site (CDC, 2005c). State and local authorities are then responsible for the breakdown and distribution of the SNS supplies, but TARU members will remain on-site in order to assist and advise state and local officials (CDC, 2005c).

DISASTER PREPAREDNESS

According to FEMA, the "disaster life cycle" describes the process through which individuals and communities *prepare* for emergencies and disasters, *respond* to them, help people and communities *recover* from them, mitigate their effects, risk reduction of loss, and prevent disasters reoccurring (see Figure 29-1) (FEMA, 2004e).

FEMA describes the six stages of the disaster cycle as follows (FEMA, 2004d, 2004e):

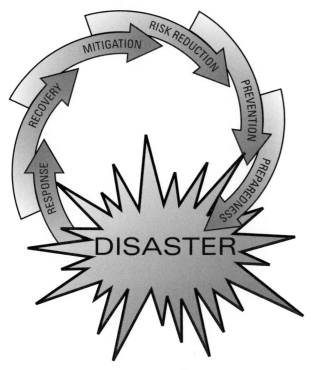

Figure 29-1 Disaster life cycle.
From FEMA (2004e). *About FEMA. What we do.*

- Preparedness Stage—This stage ensures that if a disaster occurs, the emergency management system is prepared to respond safely and effectively as a result of interagency planning, ongoing training and exercises, and public education regarding their own level of preparedness.

- Response Stage—As soon as a disaster is identified, the response stage takes effect. It involves mobilizing and positioning emergency equipment; getting people out of danger; providing food, water, shelter, and medical services; and preventing services and systems from becoming interrupted or damaged.

- Recovery Stage—Rebuilding a community can take months to years depending on the scope of the disaster. Interrupted and damaged infrastructures, buildings, services must be reestablished, and support must be provided for the victims of the disaster.

- Mitigation Stage—By mitigating the effects of disasters, communities become safer, and the loss of property and life is reduced. Two examples of mitigation are retrofitting public buildings to withstand hurricane-strength winds or ground-shaking earthquakes and acquiring damaged homes or businesses in flood-prone areas and returning the property to open space, wetlands, or recreational uses.

- Risk Reduction—As a result of mitigation, the reduction of risk is achieved. As communities require individuals and businesses to comply with guidelines set forth by agencies such as FEMA, the risk of damage and injury is reduced.

- Prevention—Not all emergencies and disasters can be prevented, but for those that can be avoided, every effort should be exercised such as installing fire detectors in homes.

Disaster Response and Management

The National Response Plan (NRP), which supersedes the Federal Response Plan (FRP), is a comprehensive all-hazards plan that was developed to manage domestic incidents through the prevention of, preparedness for, response to, and recovery from terrorism, major natural disasters, and other major emergencies

⊕ PRACTICE APPLICATION

Disaster Preparedness

In response to the events of September 11, 2001, the New York State Nurses Association (NYSNA) was initially unsure of its role and responsibility in the recovery process. Within an hour of the disaster, though, the association organized an Emergency Response Team to assess the situation, determined priorities, arranged transportation, obtained proof of licensure, established communication, and managed volunteers, operations, and public relations. Orr (2002) explains that the organization was "clearly not prepared to respond to a major disaster in which the health care system, and nurses, would be a vital resource to be mobilized."

Following the events of 9/11, the NYSNA used the experience to improve upon its disaster preparedness in several ways: (1) It developed a comprehensive disaster plan from knowledge gained through the experience. This information is available to other nursing organizations so that they may develop a thorough disaster plan. (2) It established guidelines for commu-

nication and information that should be provided to members and the public as well as designated a spokesperson to work with the press. (3) It established and maintained partnerships with governmental and nongovernmental agencies and organizations. (4) It identified the roles and responsibilities of the various disaster relief agencies and organizations. (5) It addressed the disaster educational needs of its members. (6) It planned for support of staff responding to the disaster.

Ready or not, disasters happen, that is why it is imperative that registered nurses, whether working in public health, emergency departments, schools, or clinics, and nursing organizations be educated and trained to respond effectively and efficiently to all types disasters.

Reference

Orr, M. (2002). Ready or not, disasters happen. Online *Journal of Issues in Nursing, 7*(3). Retrieved March 12, 2005, from http://www.nursingworld.org/ojin/topic19/tpc19_2.htm.

(DHS, 2004a). It provides structure and mechanism for the coordination of federal, state, local, and tribal agencies and organizations to respond to emergency situations more quickly, effectively, and efficiently (DHS, 2004a). The plan incorporates best practices from homeland security, emergency management, law enforcement, firefighting, public works, public health, responder and recovery workers, emergency medical services, and the private sector into one plan.

The National Incident Management System (NIMS), provides a consistent nationwide approach for federal, state, local, and tribal governments, private-sector and nongovernmental organizations to work together across jurisdictions to prepare for, prevent, respond to, and recover from domestic incidents regardless of cause, size, or complexity (DHS, 2004b). Homeland Security Presidential Declaration (HSPD) – 5, Management of Domestic Incidents, requires that all federal departments and agencies, and state and local organizations receiving federal funding, adopt the system in their disaster plans (DHS, 2004b).

An element of NIMS is the incident command structure (ICS), which is a management system, or chain of authority, designed to ensure effective communication during a disaster (DHS, 2004b; James, 2005). ICS is the "combination of facilities, equipment, personnel, procedures, and communications operating within a common organizational structure" (DHS, 2004b, p. 130). It is used for all kinds of emergencies and is applicable to small as well as large and complex incidents. ICS is used by various jurisdictions and functional agencies, both public and private, to organize field-level incident management operations (DHS, 2004b).

Public health officials, and other personnel who respond to disasters, must be familiar with the ICS and know their role and responsibilities when it is activated.

Public Health Preparedness

The public health system in the United States is currently undergoing many changes due to new emerging diseases, environmental threats, and bioterrorism. The Council on Linkage Between Academia and Public Health Practice has developed a list of Core Compe-

⊕ RESEARCH APPLICATION

Community Reaction to Bioterrorism: Prospective Study of Simulated Outbreak

Study Purpose

To assess community needs for public information during a bioterrorism-related crisis.

Methods

An 83-minute videotape simulating a series of print and television reports regarding a fictional intentional aerosolized release of Rift Valley fever virus (RVFV) was shown to four groups of people (medical first-responders, medical first-responder spouses or partners, journalists, and others) within the selected community. After viewing the videotape, they were asked to answer questions about their reactions.

Findings

First-responders and their spouses or partners varied in their reactions about reporting for duty during a crisis and receiving vaccinations. Local journalists exhibited considerable personal fear and confusion rendering them

possibly ineffective to communicate information during the incident. All groups demanded, and put more trust in, information from local sources.

Implications

In the event of an actual bioterrorism-related outbreak, local leaders such as private health care providers, government and nongovernment officials, supported by federal health authorities, must take the lead in communicating with local residents.

Reference

DiGiovanni, Jr., C., Reynolds, B., Harwell, Stonecipher, E. B., and Burkle, Jr., F. M. (2003). Community reaction to bioterrorism: Prospective study of simulated outbreak. *Emerging Infectious Diseases, 19*(6). Retrieved December 30, 2004, from http://www.cdc.gov/ncidod/EID/vol9no6/02-0769.htm.

tencies for Public Health Professionals, especially as it pertains to bioterrorism, which represent a "set of skills, knowledge, and attitudes necessary for the broad practice of public health" in this changing environment (Public Health Foundation, n.d.). The eight domains of core competencies and skills according to the Public Health Foundation (n.d.) are: (1) analytic/ assessment skill; (2) policy development/ program planning; (3) communication; (4) cultural competency; (5) community dimensions of practice; (6) basic public health sciences; (7) financial planning and management; and (8) leadership and systems thinking.

Mondy, Cardenas, and Avila (2003) describe the Public Health Nurse Practice Model as a framework for nurses, working with an interdisciplinary public health team, in developing a disaster preparedness plan. The model consists of six steps (Mondy, Cardenas, and Avila, 2003):

1. Assessment—Assess the health status of the population using data, community resources, identi-

fication input from the population, and professional judgment.

2. Diagnosis—Analyze collected assessment data and partner with other disciplines to attach meaning to the data and determine opportunity and needs.

3. Outcome Identification—Participate with other community partners to identify expected outcomes in the population and their health status. Establish outcome objectives in collaboration with the key partners.

4. Planning—Promote and support the development of programs, policies and services that provide interventions that improve the health status of populations. Identify intermediate and process objectives. Implement appropriate interventions.

5. Assurance—Ensure access and availability of programs, policies, resources, and services to the population.

6. Evaluation—Evaluate the health status of the population. The evaluation of the public health programs is a continuous process. When gaps are identified, interventions are modified to resolve the issues.

KEY TERMS

acute radiation syndrome (ARS)

domestic terrorism

incident command structure (ICS)

international terrorism

isolation

National Electronic Disease Surveillance System (NEDSS)

National Incident Management System (NIMS)

National Response Plan (NRP)

natural disasters

Public Health Information Network (PHIN)

quarantine

Radiological Dispersal Device (RDD)

Strategic National Stockpile (SNS)

Technical Advisory Response Unit (TARU)

terrorism

weapons of mass destruction (WMD)

CRITICAL THINKING ACTIVITIES

1. Compare and contrast natural disasters, man-made disasters, and terrorism.

2. An 8-year-old girl is seen by her health care provider for complaints of possible chickenpox. She is diagnosed instead with possible smallpox. What signs and symptoms would differentiate smallpox from chickenpox? What action should the health care provider take? What is the role of the public health nurse in this situation?

3. During a concert taking place in a large indoor facility, people begin to have difficulty breathing and feel as if their throats are burning. What actions would the public health nurse take?

4. An explosion occurs at a major U.S. airport and is determined to be an act of terrorism. What effects would this have physiologically and mentally on individuals and on the community?

5. Through the National Electronic Disease Surveillance System (NEDSS), evidence of intentionally released anthrax is identified causing a public health emergency. What available resources do public heath officials have to supplement the community's medical resources?

6. What is the Public Health Nurse Practice Model and how can it be incorporated into a disaster plan?

KEY CONCEPTS

⊕ Disasters, whether natural or man-made, can have devastating effects on individuals and communities. If a disaster has warning, the impact can be mitigated, but disasters that strike without warning have a greater consequence not only physically but also psychologically on individuals and communities.

⊕ When disasters occur, public health authorities must promptly investigate, diagnose, report, treat, and prevent or mitigate any ill effects in the community. The intentional or unintentional occurrence of certain disasters such as biological, nuclear/ radiological, and chemical can be difficult for public health professionals to differentiate. Through disease surveillance and disaster preparedness, such incidents can be accurately identified and responded to rapidly and efficiently.

⊕ In the ever-changing faces of disasters, it is important that public heath nurses receive proper training and education to contend with a wide spectrum of disasters. It is also essential that partnerships be developed with all agencies and organizations that have roles in disaster preparedness, response, and recovery. Understanding their responsibilities promotes a more effective response following a disaster.

⊕ In the United States, a lot of attention and funding has been provided for disaster preparedness, yet a balance needs to be maintained between funding disaster programs and funding many of the other vital health programs in the community. Diverting resources and staff from other responsibilities to assist with disasters may adversely impact services provided by the public health department.

REFERENCES

American Public Health Association (APHA). (2001). *Emergency medical and public health response to terrorism: Memorandum of understanding.* Retrieved March 2, 2006, from http://www.apha.org/news/press/2001/emsmou.htm.

American Psychiatric Association (APA). (2004). *Disaster psychiatry handbook.* Retrieved January 15, 2006, from http://www.psych.org/disasterpsych/pdfs/apadisasterhandbk.pdf.

American Red Cross (ARC). (1999). *Disaster health services: Overview, instructor's manual.* Publication number 3076–1. Washington, DC: Author.

American Red Cross (ARC). (2002). *Weapons of mass destruction/ terrorism: An overview, instructor's manual.* Publication number 3079–2. Washington, DC: Author.

American Red Cross (ARC). (2003). *Foundations of the disaster services program.* Publication number 3000. Washington, DC: Author.

Ashford, D. A., Kaiser, R. M., Bales, M. E., Shutt, K., Patrawalla, A., McShan, A., Tappero, J. W., Perkins, B. A., and Dannenberg, A. L. (2003). Planning against biological terrorism: Lessons from outbreak investigations. *Emerging Infectious Diseases,* 19(5). Retrieved December 30, 2005, from http://www.cdc.gov/ncidod/EID/vol9no5/02-0388.htm.

AVERT. (January 2005). *World HIV and AIDS statistics.* Retrieved January 10, 2005, from http://www.avert.org/worldstats.htm.

Berkowitz, B. (2002). Public health nursing practice: Aftermath of September 11, 2001. *Online Journal of Issues in Nursing,* 10, 234–245. Retrieved January 10, 2005, from http://www.nursingworld.org/ojin/topic19/tpc19_4.htm

Briggs, S., and Brinsfield, K. (2003). *Advance disaster medical response.* Boston: Harvard Medical International.

Broome, C. and Loonsk, J. (2004). Public health information network—Improving early detection by using a standards-based approach to connecting public health and clinical medicine. *Morbidity and Mortality Weekly Report,* 53(suppl.), 199–202. Retrieved December 30, 2004, from http://www.cdc.gov/ mmwr/preview/ mmwrhtml/ su5301a36. htm.

Butler, A. S., Panzar, A. M., and Goldfrank, L. R. (2003). *Preparing for the psychological consequences of terrorism: A public health strategy.* Retrieved February 20, 2006, from http://darwin.nap.edu/books/0309089530/html/R1.html.

Center for Law and the Public Health. (2001*). Model state emergency health powers ct of 2001.* Retrieved February 20, 2006, from http://www.publichealthlaw.net/MSEHPA/MSEHPA2.pdf.

Centers for Disease Control and Prevention (CDC). (n.d.). *National electronic disease surveillance system (NEDSS). The surveillance and monitoring component of the public health information network.* Retrieved December 28, 2004, from http://www.cdc.gov/ nedss/index.htm.

Centers for Disease Control and Prevention (CDC). (2003a). *Explosions and blast injuries: A primer for clinicians.* Retrieved December 28, 2004, from http://www.bt.cdc.gov/ masstrauma/explosions.asp.

Centers for Disease Control and Prevention (CDC). (2003b). *Radiation facts.* Retrieved December 28, 2004, from http://www.bt.cdc.gov/radiation/facts.asp.

Centers for Disease Control and Prevention (CDC). (2003c). *Acute radiation syndrome.* Retrieved December 28, 2004, from http://www.bt.cdc.gov/radiation/ars.asp.

Centers for Disease Control and Prevention (CDC). (2003d). Recognition of illness associated with exposure to chemical agents—United States, 2003. *Morbidity and Mortality Weekly Report,* 52(39), 938–940. Retrieved December 28, 2004, from http://www.cdc.gov/mmwr/preview/mmwrhtml/mm5239a3.htm.

Centers for Disease Control and Prevention (CDC). (2003e). *Injuries and mass trauma events.* Retrieved December 28, 2004, from http://www.bt.cdc.gov/masstrauma/injuriespro.asp.

Centers for Disease Control and Prevention (CDC). (2004a). *Frequently asked questions about smallpox.* Retrieved December 28, 2004, from http://www.bt.cdc.gov/ agent/smallpox/.disease/faq.asp.

Centers for Disease Control and Prevention (CDC). (2004b). *Smallpox vaccination method.* Retrieved December 28, 2004, from http://www.bt.cdc.gov/agent/smallpox/vaccination/vaccination-method.asp.

Centers for Disease Control and Prevention (CDC). (2004c). *Side effects of smallpox vaccination.* Retrieved December 28, 2004, from http://www.bt.cdc.gov/agent/smallpox/vaccination/reactions-vacc-public.asp.

Centers for Disease Control and Prevention (CDC). (2004d). *Bioterrorism agents/ diseases.* Retrieved December 28, 2004, from http://www.bt.cdc.gov/agent/agentlist.asp.

Centers for Disease Control and Prevention (CDC). (2004e). *People who should NOT get the smallpox vaccine (unless they are exposed to smallpox).* Retrieved December 28, 2004, from http://www.bt.cdc.gov/agent/smallpox/vaccination/contraindications-public.asp.

Centers for Disease Control and Prevention (CDC). (2005a). *Chemical emergencies overview.* Retrieved December 28, 2004, from http://www.bt.cdc.gov/chemical/overview.asp#what.

Centers for Disease Control and Prevention (CDC). (2005b). *Public health information network (PHIN).* Retrieved December 28, 2004, from http://www.cdc.gov/phin/.

Centers for Disease Control and Prevention (CDC). (2005c). *Strategic national stockpile.* Retrieved December 28, 2004 from http://www.bt.cdc.gov/stockpile/.

Conrad, J. L., and Pearson, J. L. (2003). Improving Epidemiology, Surveillance, and Laboratory Capabilities. In Levy, B. S. and Sidel, V. W. (Eds.), *Terrorism and public health. A balanced approach to strengthening systems and protecting people* (270–285). New York: Oxford University Press.

Croddy, E. and Ackerman, G. (2003). Biological and chemical terrorism: A unique threat. In T. G. Veenema (Ed.), *Disaster nursing and emergency preparedness for chemical, biological and radiological terrorism and other hazards* (pp. 300–329). New York: Springer Publishing Company.

Crossley, D. (2005). *Hazards and disasters.* Retrieved December 28, 2004, from http://mnw.eas.slu.edu/hazards.html.

Cukier, W., and Chapdelaine, A. (2003). Small arms, explosives and incendiaries. In B. S. Levy and V. W. Sidel (Eds.), *Terrorism and public health. A balanced approach to strengthening systems and protecting people* (pp. 155–174). New York: Oxford University Press.

DiGiovanni, Jr., C., Reynolds, B., Harwell, R., Stonecipher, E. B., and Burkle, Jr., F. M. (2003). Community reaction to bioterrorism: Prospective study of simulated outbreak. *Emerging Infectious Diseases* 19(6). Retrieved Decem-ber 30, 2005, from http://www.cdc.gov/ncidod/EID/vol9no6/02-0769.htm.

Department of Homeland Security (DHS). (n.d.). *National security emergencies.* Retrieved December 30, 2004, from http://www.dhs.gov/dhspublic/display?theme=14&content=446.

Department of Homeland Security (DHS). (2004a). *National response plan.* Retrieved December 30, 2004, from http://www.dhs.gov/interweb/assetlibrary/NRPbaseplan.pdf.

Department of Homeland Security (DHS). (2004b). *National incident management system.* Retrieved December 30, 2004, from http://www.emergency-management.net/ pdf/NIMS03012004.pdf.

DiGiovanni, Jr., C., Reynolds, B., Harwell, R., Stonecipher, E. B., and Burkle, Jr., F. M. (2003). Community reaction to bioterrorism: Prospective study of simulated outbreak. *Emerging Infectious Diseases* 19(6). Retrieved December 30, 2005, from http://www.cdc.gov/ncidod/EID/vol9no6/02-0769.htm.

District of Columbia. (n.d.). *National repository of life-saving pharmaceuticals and medical supplies.* Retrieved December 30, 2004, from http://bioterrorism.doh.dc.gov/ biot/cwp/view,a,1253,q,553024.asp.

Ehrenreich, J. (October 2001). *Coping with disaster: A guide-book to psychological intervention* (rev. ed.). Retrieved February 20, 2006, from http://www.mhwwb.org/CopingWithDisaster.pdf.

Federal Bureau of Investigation (FBI). (2004). *Terrorism 2000/2001.* Retrieved December 30, 2004, from http://www.fbi.gov/publications/terror/terror2000_2001.htm.

Federal Emergency Management Agency (FEMA). (n.d.). *Technological hazards.* Retrieved December 30, 2004 from http://www.fema.gov/pdf/areyouready/technohazards.pdf.

Federal Emergency Management Agency (FEMA). (2000). *Effective disaster warnings.* Retrieved December 30, 2004, from http://www.fema.gov/pdf/rrr/ndis_rev_oct27.pdf.

Federal Emergency Management Agency (FEMA). (2004a). *Are you ready? An in-depth guide to citizen preparedness.* Retrieved December 30, 2004, from http://www.fema.gov/pdf/areyouready/natural_hazards_1.pdf.

Federal Emergency Management Agency (FEMA). (2004b). *Hazard mitigation: It's not just for natural disasters any more.* Retrieved December 30, 2004, from http://www.fema.gov/fima/antiterrorism/.

Federal Emergency Management Agency (FEMA). (2004c). *General information about terrorism.* Retrieved December 30, 2004, from http://www.fema.gov/hazard/terrorism/info.shtm.

Federal Emergency Management Agency (FEMA). (2004d). *First responder.* Retrieved December 30, 2004, from http://www.fema.gov/fema/first_res.shtm.

Federal Emergency Management Agency (FEMA). (2004e). *About FEMA. What we do.* Retrieved December 30, 2004, from http://www.fema.gov/about/what.shtm.

Food and Agriculture Organization of the United Nations (FAO). (2005). *FAO's emergency activities.* Retrieved December 30, 2004, from http://www.fao.org/FOCUS/E/ disaster/manmad-e.htm.

Fort Worth Public Health Department. (2004). *History of biological terrorism.* Retrieved January 15, 2004, from http://www.fortworthgov.org/health/threats/bio_history1.asp.

Gulf of Maine Aquarium. (2005). *The grave of the Titanic.* Retrieved April 20, 2006, from http://www.gma.org/space1/titanic.html.

James, D. (2005). Organization and implementation of the disaster response. In J. C. Langan & D. C. James (Eds.), *Preparing nurses for disaster management* (pp. 35–54). Upper Saddle River, NJ: Pearson Prentice Hall.

Keck, C. W., and Erme, M. A. (2003). Strengthening the public health system. In B. S. Levy & Sidel (Eds.), *Terrorism and public health. A balanced approach to strengthening systems and protecting people* (pp. 245–269). New York: Oxford University Press.

Kupersanin, E. (July 2000). FBI Psychiatrist urges colleagues to prepare to aid terrorism victims. *Psychiatric News.* Retrieved January 5, 2005, from http://www.psych.org/pnews/00-07-21/fbi.html.

Langan, J. C. (2005). Disasters: A basic overview. In J. C. Langan & D. C. James (Eds.), *Preparing nurses for disaster management* (pp. 1–16). Upper Saddle River, NJ: Pearson Education.

Levy, B. S., and Sidel, V. W. (Eds.). (2003). Challenges that terrorism poses to public health. In B. S. Levy & V. W. Sidel (Eds.), *Terrorism and public health. A balanced approach to strengthening systems and protecting people* (pp. 3–18). New York: Oxford University Press.

Mondy, C., Cardenas, D., and Avila, M. (2003). The role of an advanced practice public health nurse in bioterrorism preparedness. *Public Health Nursing,* 20(6), 422–431. Retrieved December 30, 2004, from http://www.blackwell-synergy.com/openurl?genre=article&sid=nlm:pubmed&issn=0737-1209&date=2003&volume=20&issue=6&spage=422.

National Aeronautics and Space Administration (NASA). (1993). *Challenger.* Retrieved April 20, 2006, from http://science.ksc.nasa.gov/shuttle/resources/orbiters/challenger.html.

National Oceanic and Atmospheric Administration (NOAA). (2006). *Dennis, Katrina, Rita, Stan and Wilma "Retired" from list of storm names international committee selects replacement names for 2011 list.* Retrieved April 10, 2006, from http://www.noaanews.noaa.gov/stories2006/s2607.htm.

Orr, M. (2002). Ready or not, disasters happen. *Online Journal of Issues in Nursing,* 7(3). Retrieved March 12, 2005, from http://www.nursingworld.org/ojin/topic19/tpc19_2.htm.

PandemicFlu.gov. (2006). *General information.* Retrieved April 10, 2006, from http://www.avianflu.gov/general/.

Plum, K.C. (2003). Understanding the psychosocial impact of disasters. In T. G. Veenema (Ed.), *Disaster nursing and emergency preparedness for chemical, biological and radiological terrorism and other hazards* (pp. 62–82). New York: Springer Publishing Company.

Pryor, E. R., and Veenema, T. G. (2003). Surveillance systems for bioterrorism. In T. G. Veenema (Ed.), *Disaster nursing and emergency preparedness for chemical, biological and radiological terrorism and other hazards* (pp. 331–353). New York: Springer Publishing Company.

Public Health Foundation. (n.d.). *Core competencies for public health professionals.* Retrieved January 5, 2005, from http://www.phf.org/ phworkforce.htm#Core%20Competencies.

Scaruffi, P. (2005). *The worst natural disasters ever.* Retrieved December 30, 2004, from http://www.scaruffi.com/politics/disaster.html.

Sistrom, M. (2004). *Bioterrorism preparedness: Procedural heresy and the nature of uncertainty.* Paper presented at the 132nd Annual Meeting of Public Health and the Environment, Washington, DC.

Substance Abuse and Mental Health Services Administration, National Mental Health Information Center (SAMHSA). (2003). *Self-care tips for emergency and disaster response workers.* Retrieved December 30, 2004, from http://www.mentalhealth.samhsa.gov/publications/allpubs/KEN-01-0098/.

Sutton, P. M., and Gould, R. M. (2003). Nuclear, radiological and related weapons. In B. S. Levy & V. W. Sidel (Eds.), *Terrorism and public health. A balanced approach to strengthening systems and protecting people* (pp. 220–242). New York: Oxford University Press.

Terrorism Files. (n.d.). *Weapons & terrorism: Terrorist use of information technology.* Retrieved January 5, 2005, from http://www.terrorismfiles.org/weapons/information_technology.html.

United Nations Environment Program. (2002). *Awareness and preparedness for emergencies on local level.* Retrieved April 20, 2006, from http://www.unepie.org/pc/apell/disasters/lists/technological.html.

U.S. Army Medical Research Institute of Infectious Diseases (USAMRIID). (2004). *USAMRIID's medical management of biological casualties handbook* (5th ed.). Frederick, MD: Author.

U.S. Department of Energy (DOE). (2003). *August 2003 blackout.* Retrieved December 15, 2004, from http://www.electricity.doe.gov/news/blackout.cfm?section=news&level2= blackout#happened.

U.S. Environmental Protection Agency (EPA). (2006). *Exxon Valdez.* Retrieved April 20, 2006, from http://www.epa.gov/oilspill/exxon.htm.

U.S. Nuclear Regulatory Commission (NRC). (2003). *Fact sheet on dirty bombs.* Retrieved December 30, 2004, from http://www.nrc.gov/reading-rm/doc-collections/fact-sheets/dirty-bombs.html.

Veenema, T. G. (Ed.). (2003a). Essentials of disaster planning. *Disaster nursing and emergency preparedness for chemical, biological and radiological terrorism and other hazards* (2–29). New York: Springer Publishing Company.

Veenema, T. G. (Ed.). (2003b). Restoring public health under disaster conditions: Basic sanitation, water and food supply, and shelter. *Disaster nursing and emergency preparedness for chemical, biological and radiological terrorism and other hazards* (pp. 171–189). New York: Springer Publishing Company.

World Health Organization (WHO). (2001). *WHO slide set on the diagnosis of smallpox.* Retrieved December 30, 2004, from http://www.who.int/emc/diseases/smallpox/Africanseries/pages/WHO-Spx-Dx-Africa04-MedRes.htm.

World Health Organization (WHO). (2005a). *Communicable disease surveillance and response.* Retrieved December 30, 2004, from http://www.who.int/csr/en/.

World Health Organization (WHO). (2005b). *Structure and global team.* Retrieved December 30, 2004, from http://www.who.int/csr/about/structure/en/.

World Health Organization (WHO). (2006). *Smallpox.* Retrieved March 20, 2006, from http://www.who.int/csr/disease/smallpox/en/.

World Health Organization Regional Office for Europe. (2005). *Communicable disease surveillance and response.* Retrieved December 30, 2004, from http://www.euro.who.int/surveillance.

Worldwide Conflicts and Wars. (2004). Retrieved December 30, 2004, from http://www.albertarose.org/Disasters/terrorist_acts.html.

BIBLIOGRAPHY

Alibek, A. (1999). *BioHazard.* New York: Random House.

Centers for Disease Control and Prevention (CDC). (2003). *Chemical agents: Facts about personal cleaning and disposal of contaminated clothing.* Available: http://www.bt.cdc.gov/planning/personalcleaningfacts.asp.

Centers for Disease Control and Prevention (CDC). (2006). *Smallpox vaccine administration video.* Available: http://

www.bt.cdc.gov/agent/smallpox/vaccination/administration-video/.

Centers for Disease Control and Prevention (CDC). (2006). *Smallpox: What every clinician should know video.* Available: http://www.bt.cdc.gov/agent/smallpox/training/clinician-know/.

Department of Homeland Security (DHS). (2004). *National response plan. Emergency support function (ESF) annexes.* Available: http://www.dhs.gov/interweb/assetlibrary/NRP_FullText.pdf.

Emergency Management Institute. (2006). *FEMA independent study program.* Available: http://training.fema.gov/EMI-Web/IS/.

National Disaster Medical System. (2006). *Welcome to NDMS.* Available: http://www.oep-ndms.dhhs.gov/index.html.

RESOURCES

American Nurses Association (ANA)

American Nurses Association
8515 Georgia Avenue, Suite 400
Silver Spring, Maryland 20910
1-800-274-4ANA
Web: http://www.nursingworld.org

The ANA was started as the Association of Nursing Alumnae. It later became the American Nurses Association's Congress on Nursing Practice and Economics representing all nurses. The ANA is a professional nursing organization that represents the interest of the 2.9 million registered nurses in the United States and the people for whom they care. The Web site provides various information on ANA activities and access to online nursing journals.

American Public Health Association (APHA)

800 "I" Street NW
Washington, DC 20001-3710
202-777- APHA (2752)
FAX: 202-777-2534
Email: comments@APHA.org
Web: http://www.apha.org

APHA is a nonprofit association of public health professionals from over 50 public health occupations working to improve the public's health and to achieve equity in health status for all. The organization strives to influence policy and set priorities in public health to help prevent disease and promote health. The organization also strives to promote the scientific and professional foundation of public health practice and policy, advocate the conditions for a healthy global society, emphasize prevention, and enhance the ability of members to promote and protect environmental and community health. APHA is an organization that represents more than 50,000 public health professionals worldwide from over 50 occupations of public health.

American Red Cross (ARC)

American Red Cross National Headquarters
2025 E Street NW
Washington, DC 20006
202-303-4498
Web: http://www.redcross.org

Since its founding in 1881 by visionary leader Clara Barton, the American Red Cross has been the nation's premier emergency response organization. As part of a worldwide movement that offers neutral humanitarian care to the victims of war, the American Red Cross distinguished itself by also aiding victims of devastating natural disasters. Over the years, the organization has expanded its services, always with the aim of preventing and relieving suffering. Today, in addition to domestic disaster relief, the American Red Cross offers compassionate services in five other areas: community services that help the needy; support and comfort for military members and their families; the collection, processing, and distribution of lifesaving blood and blood products; educational programs that promote health and safety; and international relief and development programs. The ARC, a humanitarian organization led by volunteers, is guided by its Congressional Charter and the Fundamental Principles of the International Red Cross Movement.

Centers for Disease Control and Prevention (CDC)

1600 Clifton Road
Atlanta, Georgia 30333
404-639-3311; Public Inquiries: 404-639-3534,
    1-800-311-3435
Web: http://www.cdc.gov

CDC is one of the 13 major operating components of the Department of Health and Human Services, the principal agency in the U.S. government for protecting the health and safety of all Americans and for providing essential human services, especially for those people who are least able to help themselves. Since it was founded in 1946, CDC has remained at the forefront of public health efforts to prevent and control infectious and chronic diseases, injuries, workplace hazards, disabilities, and environmental health threats. Today, CDC is globally recognized for conducting research and investigations and for its action oriented approach. CDC applies research and findings to improve people's daily lives and responds to health emergencies—something that distinguishes CDC from its peer agencies.

Department of Homeland Security (DHS)

Washington, D.C. 20528
202-282-8000
Web: http://www.dhs.gov

The National Strategy for Homeland Security and the Homeland Security Act of 2002 served to mobilize and organize our nation to secure the homeland from terrorist attacks. DHS provides resources to federal, state, and local governments and coordinates the transition of multiple agencies and programs into a single, integrated agency focused on protecting the American people and their homeland.

Emergency Nurses Association (ENA)

915 Lee Street
Des Plaines, Illinois 60016-6569
1-800-900-9659
Web: http://www.ena.org

The ENA is a professional member organization that promotes excellence in emergency nursing through leadership, research, education, and advocacy. The Web site is the official Web site for this organization.

Federal Bureau of Investigation (FBI)

J. Edgar Hoover Building
935 Pennsylvania Avenue NW
Washington, D.C. 20535-0001
202-324-3000
Web: http://www.fbi.gov

The FBI investigates violations of federal criminal law; protects the United States from foreign intelligence and terrorist activities; and provides leadership and law enforcement assistance to federal, state, local, and international agencies. The Web site provides information on how to report various crimes.

Federal Emergency Management Agency (FEMA)

500 C Street SW
Washington, D.C. 20472
1-800-621-FEMA (3362)
Web: http://www.fema.gov

FEMA, an entity of the U.S. Department of Homeland Security (DHS) since 2003, leads the effort to prepare the nation for all hazards and effectively manage federal response and recovery efforts following any national incident.

National Institutes of Health (NIH)

9000 Rockville Pike
Bethesda, Maryland 20892
301-496-4000
Web: http://www.nih.gov

NIH is part of the U.S. Department of Health and Human Services. It is the steward of medical and behavioral research for the nation. Its mission is science in pursuit of fundamental knowledge about the nature and behavior of living systems and the application of that knowledge to extend healthy life and reduce the burdens of illness and disability.

Sigma Theta Tau International

550 West North Street
Indianapolis, IN 46202
317-634-8171
FAX 317-634-8188, 1-888-634-7575
Email: memserv@stti.iupui.edu
Web: http://www.nursingsociety.org

In 1922, six nurses founded Sigma Theta Tau at the Indiana University Training School for Nurses, now the Indiana University School of Nursing, in Indianapolis, Indiana. The founders chose the name from the Greek words Storgé, Tharsos, and Timé meaning "love," "courage," and "honor." The honor society became incorporated in 1985 as Sigma Theta Tau International, Inc., a not-for-profit organization with a 501(c)(3) tax status in the United States. The mission of Sigma Theta Tau International is to provide leadership and scholarship in practice, education, and research to enhance the health of all people by supporting the learning and professional development of its members as they strive to improve nursing care worldwide. Sigma Theta Tau is made up of four organizations—the Honor Society of Nursing, Sigma Theta Tau International; Nursing Knowledge International; The International Honor Society of Nursing Building Corporation; and the Sigma Theta Tau International Foundation for Nursing. The vision of all four organizations is to create a global community of nurses who lead using scholarship, knowledge, and technology to improve the health of the world's people.

U.S. Department of Energy (DOE)

100 Independence Avenue SW
Washington, D.C. 20585
1-800-342-5363
FAX: 202-586-4463
Web: http://www.energy.gov

The DOE promotes scientific and technological innovation in advancing the national, economic, and energy security of the United States and ensures environmental cleanup of the national nuclear weapons complex.

U.S. Department of Health and Human Services (DHHS)

200 Independence Avenue SW
Washington, D.C. 20201
202-619-0257, 1-877-696-6775
Web: http://www.dhhs.gov

DHHS is the U.S. government's primary agency involved with protecting the health of all Americans and providing essential human services, especially for people with few resources. The department includes more than 300 programs. The Web site provides health-related publications.

U.S. Department of Homeland Security (DHS)

Office of Grants and Training
810 Seventh Street NW
Washington, D.C. 20531
1-800-368-6498, 8:00 a.m. to 6:00 p.m. EST, Monday–Friday
FAX: 202-786-9920
Web: http://www.ojp.usdoj.gov

The Office of Grants and Training is responsible for providing training, funds for the purchase of equipment, support for the planning and execution of exercises, technical assistance, and other support to assist states and local jurisdictions to prevent, respond to, and recover from acts of terrorism.

U.S. Nuclear Regulatory Commission (USNRC)

Office of Public Affairs (OPA)
Washington, D.C. 20555
1-800-368-5642, 301-415-8200, TDD: 301-415-5575
Web: http://www.nrc.gov

The U.S. Nuclear Regulatory Commission is an independent agency established by the Energy Reorganization Act of 1974 to regulate civilian use of nuclear materials. USNRC is headed by a five-member commission. USNRC's mission is to regulate the nation's civilian use of byproduct, source, and special nuclear materials such as the effects of radiation from nuclear reactors, materials, and waste facilities to ensure adequate protection of public health and safety, to promote the common defense and security, and to protect the environment.

U.S. Army Medical Research Institute of Infectious Diseases (USAMRIID)

Commander
USAMRIID
Attn: MCMR-UIZ-R
1425 Porter Street
Frederick, Maryland 21702-5011
Email: USAMRIIDweb@amedd.army.mil
Web: http://www.usamriid.army.mil

USAMRIID conducts basic and applied research on biological threats resulting in medical solutions to protect military service members. USAMRIID, an organization of the U.S. Army Medical Research and Materiel Command, is the lead medical research laboratory for the U.S. Biological Defense Research Program. The institute plays a key role as the only laboratory in the Department of Defense equipped to safely study highly hazardous infectious agents requiring maximum containment at bio-safety level

(BSL)-4. USAMRID vision is to be the nation's preeminent research laboratory providing cutting-edge medical research for the war fighter against biological threats.

World Health Organization (WHO)

Avenue Appia 20
1211 Geneva 27
Switzerland
+ 41-22-791-21-11
FAX: + 41-22-79-3111
Telex: 415 416
Telegraph: UNISANTE GENEVA
Email: info@who.int.
Web: http://www.who.int

WHO is the United Nations specialized agency for health. It was established on April 7, 1948. WHO's objective, as set out in its constitution, is the attainment by all peoples of the highest possible level of health. Health is defined in WHO's constitution as a state of complete physical, mental and social well-being and not merely the absence of disease or infirmity. WHO is governed by 193 member states through the World Health Assembly, which is composed of representatives from WHO's member states. The main tasks of the World Health Assembly are to approve the WHO program and the budget for the following biennium and to decide major policy questions. The WHO Web site provides rich examples and information on Healthy Cities from an international perspective.

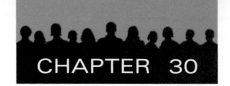

CHAPTER 30

The Future
of Public Health Nursing

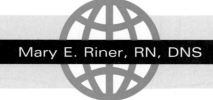

Mary E. Riner, RN, DNS

Chapter Outline

- Health Trends in the Twenty-First Century
  - Health Disparities
  - Lifestyle Issues
  - Immunizations and Medications
  - Access to Health Care
  - Environmental Health
  - Genetics
  - Policy Advocacy
- Futures Thinking
  - Benefits of Futures Thinking
  - Methods of Futures Thinking and Scenario Development
- Public Heath Systems Issues
  - Levels of Leadership
- Quality Improvement
- Public Health Workforce
  - Competency-Based Practice
  - Workforce Trends in Public Health Nursing
- Building Capacity for Community Health Promotion
- Research and Evidence-Based Practice
  - Evidence-Based Practice
  - Best Practices
  - Translational or Dissemination Research
  - Expert Panel Reviews of Evidence

Learning Objectives

Upon completion of this chapter, the reader will be able to:

1. Explore likely health trends and public health nurses' roles in the twenty-first century

2. Examine how futures thinking can benefit public health nursing in the twenty-first century

3. Analyze issues relevant to public health systems for ensuring leadership and quality of services

4. Analyze predicted public health nursing work-force supply, demand, and competencies for practice in the twenty-first century

5. Examine the role of public health nursing in building capacity for community health promotion

6. Examine population-focused research and evidence-based practice issues for public health nurses in the twenty-first century

Preparing now for the future is a challenge for all public health nurses. It is essential for public health nurses to provide leadership to address new and emerging health issues, participate in creating healthy social and physical environments, develop resources necessary to address population health issues, and reduce health disparities in subgroups within communities. Public health nurses who are well informed of health trends will be positioned to interpret their impact on health and better prepared to provide individual and systems level interventions to improve the health of communities. This chapter explores health trends the public health nurse can anticipate in the twenty-first century and discusses futures thinking as a strategy for use in proactively preparing for different possible scenarios. Public health nurse leaders will need to develop a multilevel approach that focuses on the personal, team, and agency levels of actions and outcomes. This multilevel leadership will facilitate addressing workforce issues including supply, education, and competencies. One of the priority areas for public health nurses will be working to build community health promotion capacity. This chapter concludes by examining the contribution of research and evidence-based practice in public health nursing practice in the future.

HEALTH TRENDS IN THE TWENTY-FIRST CENTURY

The focus of public health nursing has always been to reduce the burden of illness, injury, and disease affecting people in the community. Using strategies of education and health promotion, the engineering of environmental controls, and policy enforcement, public health nurses in the twenty-first century will continue to seek to prevent conditions negatively affecting population aggregates at the earliest stage. The core public health functions and interventions will continue to be framed within the context of population health assessment, advocacy and policy development, and assurance that the cost of, accessibility to, and quality of available health services are appropriate to meet the needs of the population. Major public health trends will include health disparities, lifestyle issues, immunizations and medications, access to health care, environmental health, genetics, and policy advocacy.

Health Disparities

Health disparities in access to health care, quality of life, and longevity are realities facing the nation in the twenty-first century. The national health promotion agenda calls for increasing the years of quality life and decreasing disparities in health (USDHHS, 2000). Social status and economic resources have been linked to health outcomes. People having more resources, whether money, knowledge, or social networks will continue to be better positioned to take advantage of new health opportunities relative to those in less-favored positions (Mechanic, 2003). Link and Phelan (1995) refer to social class as a "fundamental cause" (p. 427) of the differences in health status. They observe that risk factors associated with disease and mortality change over time, but that the social class gradient remains. This persistence results from the fact that the advantaged are better positioned to learn about and access new knowledge and technology, whatever these may be, and that typically there will be a lag between the advantaged and the disadvantaged in gaining these benefits. Interventions to reduce health disparities associated with social class in the future will likely result from policy efforts directed at the entire population (Mechanic, 2003). In some cases, policy efforts will need to address specific population groups having unusually high risks, such as persons with AIDS. To the extent that such groups have lacked access to proven interventions, programs to improve access can reduce gaps between population groups.

Health disparities among races will be a major issue to address in moving forward. The U.S. health system spends far more on the "technology" of care (e.g., drugs, devices) than on achieving equity in its accessibility. In a ten-year study of health care spending from 1991 to 2000, researchers contrasted the number of lives saved by medical advances with the number of deaths attributable to excess mortality among African Americans. Medical advances averted approximately 177,000 deaths, but equalizing the mortality rates of whites and African Americans would have averted over 886,000 deaths (Woolf et al., 2004). These findings indicate that achieving equity in making advances in health care equally available to all ethnic groups will reduce disparities on mortality rates.

The distribution of health care providers will continue to make specialty care difficult for some populations, particularly those living in rural communities and the medically indigent living in urban communities, and may continue to exacerbate health disparities. The term **frontier communities** refers to the most sparsely populated and isolated areas of the United States. Frontier and rural communities are more likely to suffer from the national nursing shortage than their urban counterparts because (1) these communities typically lack the economic resources to compete with urban-based employers, (2) nurses are typically not prepared for practice in nonurban settings, and (3) frontier and rural communities depend on nonhospital care settings to a greater extent than their urban counterparts (Frontier Education Center, 2004). Urban-based strategies that emphasize competitive advantage may unwittingly exacerbate frontier and rural shortages. Such communities will increasingly need to adopt "grow your own" approaches such as rural-specific education, in-place education, and funding for education targeted at underserved areas and groups. In addition, the use of technology to provide virtual services and increase the geographic reach of available nurses will be adopted. Use of community health workers will extend health care support and supervision to these communities. Community work that helps people develop more healthy lifestyles is one way public health nurses are likely to influence the future.

Lifestyle Issues

In the next three to five years, illnesses and injuries associated with lifestyle behaviors will require public health nurses to use effective health promotion and disease prevention interventions to engage individuals in choosing risk-reducing behaviors. The three leading causes of death in the United States all have behavioral implications. Risk of stroke is associated with high blood pressure, high cholesterol, diabetes, smoking, physical inactivity, and excessive alcohol intake (American Stroke Association, n.d.). Risks for cancer vary by the type of cancer; however, common lifestyle behavior counseling for public health nurses should focus on reducing excessive sun exposure and the use of tobacco products and on promoting use of early detection tests (American Cancer Society, n.d.). Increased risk of heart disease is associated with smoking, diets high in saturated fat and salt, lack of exercise, being overweight, and noncompliance with medications used in treating heart disease (American Heart Association, n.d.).

Preventive measures and advances with medication and pharmcotherapeutic agents will support lifestyle modifications.

Immunizations and Medications

Educating the public regarding optimal immunization and medication management will be important in the future. Public health nurses are well positioned to address these issues by diligently identifying high-risk groups whose members do not get recommended immunizations or ineffectively manage their medications and by seeking health policy options to overcome resource barriers. Public health nurses can participate in research and use evidence-based practices to

🌐 POLICY HIGHLIGHT

Public Health Nursing Workforce Challenges in Rural Communities

There are more rural than urban public health agencies in states across the country and they face great challenges by nature of their remoteness. They have small staffs and slender budgets yet are expected to provide a wide array of services. Rural public health nurses are less likely to have formal public health training and experience and are more likely to be employed part-time (Rosenblatt, Casey, and Richardson, 2002). Rural public health agencies also have a much smaller team of people with whom to interact and therefore a much narrower range of public health skills represented in the local office. In smaller organizations and rural areas, for example, a registered nurse with no specialized public health education may be both the community's epidemiologist and its health educator (Gebbie, Merrill, and Tilson, 2002). This same registered nurse, possessing primarily on-the-job preparation in outreach and education, also is expected to make important contributions to programs such as HIV prevention, reproductive health, and chronic disease management. Furthermore, the challenges of obtaining continuing education and further training can be immense. For these professionals to be effective and to survive their often-stressful jobs, they must be connected with other professionals at the local, regional, and state levels.

help individuals achieve maximum benefit from their medications.

Preventing antibiotic misuse will be important for preventing development of new antibiotic-resistant diseases and will increase the likelihood that future infections will respond to available drugs. Overuse or misuse of antibiotics means there is a constant demand for creating new drugs, an expensive and time-consuming process that contributes to the overall high cost of drugs.

Another area that will shape public health in the future is the impact of new medications. Due to new uses of antiretroviral drugs, babies born with HIV are becoming rare in the United States. The use of anti-retroviral drugs in HIV positive pregnant women has led to a 67 percent reduction in the risk for perinatal human immunodeficiency virus type 1 (HIV-1) trans-mission (Mofenson, 2002). In 1990, as many as 2,000 babies were born infected with HIV; by 2000, that number was reduced to a just over 200 a year (Mofen-son, 2002).

The cost of prescription drugs will continue to be an economic and political issue in the near future. In addition to rising costs of the drugs, the aging popula-tion will continue to increase in number. Seniors will continue to find it difficult to pay for the multiple medi-cations that allow higher quality of life and will seek ways to lower medication costs. They will engage in efforts to reduce costs including joining prescription dis-count drug programs, using information from the Inter-net for price comparisons, missing prescribed dosages, not filling prescriptions, and obtaining drugs from mar-kets outside the United States. Major issues related to importation of drugs will include quality control, costs of research and development, and increased ability of government organizations to conduct price negotiations (Task Force on Drug Importation, 2004). Advancing technological and medical treatment of conditions must be balanced with issues of access to drugs. Collabora-tion among the diverse groups in the health care field will be needed to find satisfactory solutions.

Access to Health Care

All Americans deserve reliable, affordable, quality health care coverage. Access to health care will continue to be a priority issue in the foreseeable future due to the disparities in health insurance coverage that result in unequal access to health services. Current efforts to

patch together health insurance for specific popula-tions will continue to challenge public health nurses to connect individuals and groups within communities to regular sources of primary health care. Public health nurses will need to understand and advocate for clients in order to help them benefit from new and changing coverage options. Public health nurses will be increas-ingly engaged in community efforts to resolve barriers to health care.

Cover the Uninsured Week town hall meetings began in 2003 as a way to bring together a wide array of people to discuss trends that threaten to increase the number of Americans without health care cover-age, as well as proposals to expand coverage and make health care more affordable while improving its quality. Cover the Uninsured Week has attracted the participa-tion of local, state, and federal elected officials from both parties; faith leaders; business and union leaders; health care providers and nurses; medical and nursing students and educators; as well as Americans without coverage and those struggling to pay for the coverage they have. The discussions are intended to help inform the nation's leaders, including elected officials, about the effect of policy proposals on all Americans, but most especially business owners and individuals who are struggling to pay for benefits, Americans who rely on public programs for health care, and the uninsured. This movement provides resources and suggestions for local groups to use in advocating for insuring all residents.

Environmental Health

Recent gains in understanding the influence of environ-mental factors and conditions on health have occurred in a cooperative atmosphere among researchers, client advocacy groups, and politicians. Through effective integration of basic research, population-based research, and community outreach and education, new initiatives in toxicogenomics, proteomics, and integrations sys-tems biology are being funded (Brown, 2004). Building collaboration among government agencies, profession-als, and interest groups will continue to be vital to the interdisciplinary work needed in creating environmental conditions that support optimal individual and commu-nity life.

Caine (2004) views eliminating health disparities as an environmental justice concern. She calls for three actions: (1) including environmental risk assessment in

⊕ RESEARCH APPLICATION

Reducing Diabetes Health Disparities through Community-Based Participatory Action Research: The Chicago Southeast Diabetes Community Action Coalition

Study Purpose

To address disproportionately high rates of diabetes morbidity and mortality in some of Chicago's medically underserved minority neighborhoods, a group of community residents, medical and social service providers, and a local university founded the Chicago Southeast Diabetes Community Action Coalition. The coalition participated in a Centers for Disease Control and Prevention REACH 2010 Initiative.

Methods

A community-based participatory action research model guided coalition activities from conceptualization through implementation. Capacity-building activities included training on diabetes, coalition building, research methods, and action planning. Other activities sought to increase coalition members' understanding of the social causes and potential solutions for health disparities related to diabetes. Trained coalition members conducted epidemiologic analyses, focus groups, a telephone survey, and a community inventory. All coalition members participated in decisions.

Findings

The participatory process led to increased awareness of the complexities of diabetes in the community and to a state of readiness for social action. Data documented disparities in diabetes.

Implications

The participatory action research approach (a) encouraged key stakeholders outside of the health care sector to participate (e.g., business sector, church groups); (b) permitted an examination of the sociopolitical content affecting the health of the community; (c) provided an opportunity to focus on preventing the onset of diabetes and its complications; and (d) increased understanding of the importance of community research in catalyzing social action aimed at community and systems change.

Reference

Giachello, A. L., Arrom, J. O., Davis, M., Sayad, J. V., Ramirez, D., Nandi, C., and Ramos, C. (2003). Reducing diabetes health disparities through community-based participatory action research: The Chicago southeast diabetes community action coalition. *Public Health Reports, 118*(July–August), 309–323.

client and community health assessments, (2) continuing to bridge the gap between environmental sciences and "traditional" public health, and (3) advocating for science-based policy that links environmental quality to health disparities and furthers environmental justice. These actions can serve as a framework for all public health workers.

Protecting the environment will require a global approach. Though English-speaking countries have access to numerous environmental health publications, that knowledge needs to be available to professionals in sub-Saharan Africa and elsewhere by overcoming language barriers, increasing accessibility to journals, and pursuing other actions. A capacity-building initiative designed to improve the environment and health at a global level currently focuses on increasing access to professional publications in developing countries, such as Mali in sub-Saharan Africa. (Northridge, Sidibe, and Goehl, 2004).

Genetics

Genetics and public health have long been linked and will continue to be linked in the future. From a public policy perspective, genetic diagnostic testing and early interventions have resulted in early identification of disorders such as PKU and the prevention of mental retardation. State legislative bodies across the country are responding to genetic legislative initiatives that will shape the future. These initiatives relate, for example, to embryonic and fetal research; frozen embryos; genetic counselor licensing; genetic privacy; health insurance; human cloning; life, disability, and long-term care insurance; and newborn screening (National Council of State Legislators, n.d.). Policy issues currently of concern to the Association of State and Territorial Health Officers (n.d. a) include cloning of animals or people, bioengineering of food supplies, and DNA detection of sexual and violent offenders. Public health nurses have the opportunity to play a significant role in genetic and other policy advocacy.

Policy Advocacy

In terms of **policy advocacy**, public health nurses have been and will continue to be active in developing health policy in private and public arenas. Nurses will be elected and appointed to local, state, and national office where they can make significant contributions. In addition, nurses will continue to demonstrate the political organizing skills necessary to elect candidates with a pro-health, pro-nursing agenda through involvement in political action committees. A priority goal for public health nurses will be increasing universal access to care.

Academic nursing leaders at Columbia University have proposed a mandatory insurance plan that is "privately administered, community-based, and affordable in cost by a broad group of employers or the public" (Mundinger et al., 2004, paragraph 11). Their proposal calls for nurses to engage in making a business case, as well as a social case, for making essential care affordable to all.

One way to identify future issues for public health nursing action is to look to policy statements issued by influential public health associations. Resolutions recently passed by the American Pubic Health Association, the oldest and largest member organization for promoting public health, are designed as policy statements to guide association advocacy activities. Resolutions are passed at the annual meeting. Some 2004 resolutions relevant to public health nursing include reducing underage alcohol consumption, reducing health disparities in people with disabilities, providing support for community-based participatory research, and promoting public health and education goals through coordinated school health programs (American Public Health Association, 2004).

The National Association of City and County Health Officers (2004) passed two resolutions that could have a significant impact on public health nursing in the future. Voluntary accreditation of local public health agencies is viewed as a long-term strategy to improve quality and accountability of the governmental public health infrastructure. The resolution passed in 2004 calls for the establishment of a voluntary accreditation program. A second resolution passed in 2004 recommends the public health community proceed with caution in adopting national standards for certification within the public health workforce. This resolution is based on the complexity of accommodating the wide variety of academic backgrounds, professional training, and credentials of the workforce; the need for resources to make this feasible; and the lack of evaluation of current state certification programs. The public health community will take action to adopt accreditation and certification programs, similar to those in place in acute and primary care systems. To achieve maximum benefit for the public, this must be well designed and implemented with measurable outcomes.

⊕ POLICY HIGHLIGHT

Using Systems Thinking in Public Policy

Finding and using effective strategies for assisting providers and organizations to adopt tobacco control strategies was a challenge faced by the National Cancer Institute (NCI). The NCI applied a systems thinking model to this challenge in order to increase the impact of tobacco control strategies found to be effective. This policy strategy is known as the Initiative on the Study and Implementation of Systems (ISIS). ISIS was envisioned as a long-term, multiagency initiative to develop and refine transdisciplinary systems thinking for the development, implementation, and coordination of program and policy intervention strategies.

Best et al. (2003) recommend that health promotion programs and policies be designed to integrate multiple disciplinary perspectives in order to achieve better intervention designs. Public health nursing interventions may be more effective if they are based on knowledge from a wide variety of sources.

FUTURES THINKING

Futuring refers to knowing how to think about the future in order to improve it (Cornish, 2004). Futures thinking can help public health nursing to anticipate preferred, possible, and likely future conditions in order to prepare for them. Public health nurses need to have a vision for the future to identify opportunities and risks existing in the environment and to develop thinking patterns that will prepare them for future likely scenarios. Futures thinking is used in health care as well as general business and industry. It is a way of thinking and exploring options that will benefit public health nurses.

Benefits of Futures Thinking

Cornish (2004) describes seven lessons learned by the great explorers in history that can be applied to public health nursing. First, prepare for what you will face in the future. Though we cannot predict the future, public health nurses do need to develop intelligence about what to expect so they will have the ability to have the resources to meet population health needs. Second, anticipate future needs. Public health nurses must play an active part and have a voice and presence in pubic health planning. If public health nurses fail to do this, the consequences may negatively affect the demand for public health nurses and/or their ability to meet population needs. For example, changes in state and local tax revenue will influence the demand for public health nurses. Third, use partial or preliminary information when necessary. Although complete information is most beneficial for decision making, public health nurses must not disdain information just because it may not be adequately detailed. For example, during a biological exposure such as anthrax, public health nurses may need to develop control interventions prior to a confirmation of the specific agent and all exposed persons. In chronic diseases, community interventions must be initiated to address the major causes of morbidity and mortality even as controlled studies of effective behavioral health research continue to be translated for widespread practice. Public health nurses must be able to act while events are still fluid.

The fourth lesson is to expect the unexpected (Cornish, 2004). The unexpected in public health may not necessarily be negative: it may be a great opportunity to propose new solutions such as the one that reduced the prevalence of tuberculosis by using directly observed

treatment (DOT). Public health nurses will need to be ready to deal with the unexpected effectively. This may include becoming experts in social marketing as a way of shifting public discourse about issues like sexually risky behaviors, tobacco use, and infant mortality. The fifth lesson is to think in the long term as well as the short term. Foresight will empower public health nurses to future achievement. A focus on the future will be empowering as public health nurses collaborate with multiple partners to achieve distant goals such as assuring healthy environments in our cities and communities.

The sixth lesson (Cornish, 2004) is to dream productively. Although daily life often involves slogging through routine, occasionally uninspiring tasks that may not be recognized or rewarded, public health nurses must have big and audacious objectives. By having a vision for the future, public health nurses can develop inspiring objectives and strategies for realistically reaching them. The seventh lesson is to learn from predecessors. To mount future campaigns using effective strategies and to avoid pitfalls, public health nurses will need to capitalize on the wisdom of those who have pioneered the field. Lillian Wald had a big audacious goal, arranging for the Metropolitan Life Insurance Company in the 1920s to include home health care as a member benefit. In the future, public health nurses will continue to develop innovative strategies to address health and social burdens faced by communities. One strategy is the development of city health plans for improving health. Rather than continuing the market-driven approach to illness care that characterizes the American health care system, public health nurses can use a Healthy Cities approach. One aspect of the approach is the development of a plan for improving health developed by multiple sectors of the community. This can include increasing the number of miles of hiking/biking trails and reducing the tonnage of solid waste produced by the community.

Methods of Futures Thinking and Scenario Development

Four methods for futuring are described by Cornish (2004): polling, gaming, modeling and simulation, and visioning. Polling involves asking informed people for their views. This is a common strategy that allows a person or organization to gain multiple viewpoints, thereby increasing the pool of potential solutions. Consulting has been a popular way to assist an orga-

⊕ PRACTICE APPLICATION

Public Health Futures Scenario

Institute for the Future developed three scenarios describing possible futures of health and health care in America for the period between 2000 and the year 2010. In the section on public health, they addressed the outlook for public-private partnerships in personal health care. Three scenarios are developed as shown in this section. The three sets of key players whose leadership, management skills, and negotiation capabilities would predict the likelihood of particular scenarios included public health agency directors, private health care providers and organizations, and community-based organizations and leaders.

Scenario One: Public-Private Community Partnerships

In this scenario, the medical services now provided by most government agencies are shifted to the private sector through a variety of public-private partnership. The public health principles—especially those of prevention, shared standards and objectives, and community-based participation—potentiate this partnership. Public health agencies maintain a watchdog role to ensure that vulnerable populations are served, but their focus returns primarily on assessment, policy development, and population-level interventions, such as health systems monitoring or monitoring of food and water sanitation systems.

Scenario Two: Dynamic Competition Rules

Local public health agencies continue to provide medical services, successfully competing with the private sector for both Medicaid and private-pay clients. Competition is both dynamic and effective and is confined to the provision of medical services. In this area,

the advances and achievements in each sector drive improvements in the other's services. For example, the public sector's success in providing wraparound services pushes the private sector to improve its own services in this area. Most of the larger public health functions are provided by the public sector, although the private sector does join in to some extent for the sake of positive public relations.

Scenario Three: Public Health in Tatters

Unable to compete directly with the private sector or to develop successful partnerships, local public health agencies retreat from the provision of medical services, leaving only a skeleton framework of services remaining to fulfill their minimum mandates. The private sector serves all of the insured population, leaving the government health care systems strapped for cash. Without the revenues generated from Medicaid reimbursements and with no additional funding, the public health functions of assessment, policy development, and assurance are in tatters. The "invisible" work of public health, such as water and food safety, becomes very visible as public health systems begin to fail and outbreaks and epidemics spread across the country. In some areas, community leaders begin to assist public health organizations through the private nonprofit sector.

Author

Institute for the Future. (2004). *Health and health care 2010: The forecast, the challenge.* (2nd ed.), p. 182. Princeton, NJ: Jossey-Bass.

nization to work through times of transition. Gaming involves engaging key individuals in working through intellectual exercises designed to portray potential real-life events. This is a strategy used in the military to prepare for alternative scenarios on a battlefield. Gaming has been conducted with high school students to simulate the deliberations of the United Nations. Simulation is the use of a model so as to represent something else. These models can be multidimensional, such as multiple community relationships depicted with Tinkertoy parts or a concept map consisting of various percep-

tions of the word "relationship" that we have in our minds. Computer modeling through Geographic Information Systems (GISs) will become increasingly useful in looking at trends in diseases and other population features relevant to understanding their distribution in populations. The fourth method described by Cornish is visioning. This involves engaging public health nurses in changing their views about the future and then creating a vision of the preferred future. For example, if public health nurses believe that evidence-based practice will be critical to demonstrating the value of services provided to employers and funders (taxpayers), then a future vision must articulate what evidence-based practice will look like when fully implemented.

Many futurists and other consultants have developed programs for visioning the future. A process designed by Bezold, Halperin, and Eng (1993) that parallels the strategic planning process involves five stages of building a vision. The stages include (1) identification of problems, (2) identification of past successes, (3) identification of desires for the future, (4) identification of measurable goals, and (5) identification of resources to achieve those goals. An example of applying the visioning process to the future of public health nursing involves the need for evidence of community-level, nursing-sensitive outcomes that demonstrate the contribution of public health nursing interventions. Efforts are in progress for developing and validating community-level outcomes (Head et al., 2004) and intervention frameworks (Keller et al., 2004). Valid nursing-sensitive outcomes will be developed that demonstrate to employers, funders, and policy makers the unique contributions of public health nurses to the health of populations. A goal for the future is to continue content validity work through funded research by academicians and practitioners.

PUBLIC HEALTH SYSTEMS ISSUES

Approaching public health from a systems planning perspective will allow nurse leaders to take a proactive stance in meeting the multiple, competing demands that must be balanced to improve population health. Using a future orientation to systems planning will allow public health nurse leaders to: think systemically and act strategically; promote change; support the values of the agency and the community; understand the relationship among system inputs, program interventions, and outputs; monitor and evaluate the effects of change; and practice systems thinking at multiple levels of leadership (Rowitz, 2001). Public health nurses will also need to take into consideration events affecting the subsystems in a community as well as events in the supra-system that may affect the community in planning.

Levels of Leadership

Using a multilevel approach to understanding leadership will assist the nurse leader in embracing the full range of skills, knowledge, and behaviors required for providing effective leadership in the future. The first level of leadership includes personal leadership development (Rowitz, 2001). This area will require a commitment to social justice, democracy, and the political process; well-developed communication skills; mentoring skills; decision-making skills; and the ability to balance work and life outside work. The second level, team leadership, will require skills in building and maintaining teams and increasing their effectiveness. The third level, agency leadership, will require the public health nurse leader to develop new models of practice, participate in community health coalitions, interact with privatization initiatives to ensure that population health needs are met; share power through decentralization of responsibilities, embrace communitywide governance of agency and activities, revise values that incorporate changing societal and cultural trends, and embrace new political structures between private, nonprofit, and multiple other government agencies (Rowitz, 2001).

Leadership at the community level will require an understanding of the nature of communities from the multiple perspectives of structure, function, and process. Leadership at this level will involve promoting media advocacy, informing the community of biological threats, linking programs to achieve maximum system benefit (e.g., creating teams that include a public health nurse and environmental specialist), building the community (e.g., conducting town hall meetings on improving access to health care), and building a coalition (e.g., encouraging local communities' efforts to sponsor universal health coverage activities) (Rowitz, 2001). At the professional level, leadership will involve participation in shaping standards of public health nursing practice, contributions to policy discussions regarding funding of advanced practice education, involvement in professional associations through membership in public health nursing organizations, and service in elected and appointed positions of government, philanthropic, and community organizations.

Providing public health nursing leadership in the twenty-first century will involve facing a fluid practice and policy environment in which change is the norm. Public health nursing leaders of the future will need to be prepared to practice on the cutting edge of nursing science and public health science and to advocate for emerging vulnerable populations. Kouzes and Posner (1997) identify five fundamental practices of exemplary leadership that address future challenges for public health nursing leaders. Leaders will need the ability to challenge the process when the status quo no longer serves the public's best interest, inspire a shared vision about the future and enlist others to work toward a common purpose, enable others to act in a spirit of cooperation and mutual trust that strengthens others by sharing power and information, model the way by example and by achieving small wins that build commitment to action, and "encourage the heart" through recognition of contributions and celebration of accomplishments. Leadership requires attention to the quality of services provided in public health agencies.

QUALITY IMPROVEMENT

Performance management is the strategic use of performance standards, measures, progress reports, and ongoing quality improvement efforts to ensure that an agency achieves desired results (Turning Point Program, n.d.). In the case of public health, the ultimate purpose of these efforts is to improve the public's health. Performance management practices can measurably improve public health outputs and outcomes, create efficiencies by working with partners, and help staff and management teams solve problems. By defining results and showing accountability, performance management efforts can help public health agencies communicate what they accomplish to policy makers, employees, and the public.

With increased funding, responsibility, and attention to public health—especially in response to the heightened need for bioterrorism preparedness—there will be greater accountability and expectations for demonstrating performance. Performance management frameworks will increasingly be used for improving public health system performance. The framework for the Turning Point Program (n.d.) includes four key components considered to be classic in quality improvement and tailored to public agencies. Performance standards are objective standards or guidelines that are used to assess an organization's performance (e.g., 80 percent of all clients will rate the health department services as "good" or "excellent"). Performance measures are quantitative measures of capacities, processes, or outcomes relevant to the assessment of a performance indicator (e.g., the number of trained nurse care managers). Reporting of data involves documenting and reporting of progress in meeting standards and targets and sharing of such information through feedback (e.g., quar-

terly audit reports that include steps taken to address areas needing improvement). Quality improvement involves establishing a program or process to manage change and achieve quality improvement in public health policies, programs, or infrastructure based on performance standards, measurements, and reports (e.g., involving community health workers in DOT to decrease the incidence of drug-resistant tuberculosis). While these approaches are not new in health care, they represent under-used accountability processes that public health must engage in to remain viable agencies in the future.

Benefits that performance management can yield for public health nurses using this systems approach include better return on dollars invested in health; greater accountability for funding and increases in the public's trust; reduced duplication of efforts; better understanding of public health accomplishments and priorities among employees, partners, and the public; increased sense of cooperation and teamwork; increased emphasis on quality, rather than quantity; and improved problem solving (Turning Point Program, n.d.). Performance management is integrally linked to the supply and preparation of the public health nursing workforce.

PUBLIC HEALTH WORKFORCE

According to the Institute of Medicine (IOM, 2003, p. 7), the mission of public health is to "fulfill society's interest in assuring conditions in which people can be healthy". The same IOM report identified official government public health agencies' role in fulfilling this mission in terms of the three core public health functions of assessment, policy development, and assurance. It has been 15 years since this report defined these functions for pubic health. Since that time, the public health workforce has continued to be in disarray, underfunded, and uncoordinated in delivery, as well as lacking a competency-based curriculum leading to certification, which is the standard for the majority of other health profession specialties (Gebbie, Merrill, and Tilson, 2002; IOM, 2003; Licktveld et al., 2001; Turnock, 2001).

The seriousness of the current state of affairs has been well stated by Gebbie, Merrill, and Tilson (2002, 3, p. 57): "Without a competent workforce, a public health agency is as useless as a new hospital with no health care workers." Defining the public health workforce and specifying its performance requirements represent equal challenges as the nation anticipates public health needs for the twenty-first century. Persons living in the community are increasingly seeking community-based health promotion programs, protection from deadly toxins and diseases, and prevention of the chronic illnesses that result in higher health care costs, decreased quality of life, and early morbidity. All of these issues speak to the need for public health nurses to base their practice on assessing health status and health needs, developing policies and programs, and ensuring that necessary services are available for the communities they serve.

Competency-Based Practice

The most difficult challenge state and local public health agencies will face in developing the capacity to respond to terrorist events, emerging infectious disease, and other public health threats and emergencies is ensuring that a qualified workforce is available to carry out these functions (Association of State and Territorial Health Officers, n.d a.). Public health nurses will participate in competency-based certification programs that document proficiency in key skills.

The Competencies for Providing Essential Public Health Services were developed by the Council on Linkages Between Academia and Public Health Practice to define those skills, behaviors, knowledge, and attitudes necessary for effective public health practice. There are eight competencies considered critical. For each competency, skill domains are identified including analytic assessment skills, policy development/program planning skills, communication skills, cultural competency skills, community dimension of practice skills, basic public health sciences skills, financial planning and management skills, and leadership and systems thinking skills. The Quad Council of Public Health Nursing Organizations (2004) has leveled these skills for the generalist/ staff public health nurse and the manager/community health nurse/consultant/program specialist/executive. The skill domains and essential competencies can be expected to influence the design and delivery of public health nursing services well into the future.

In 2003, Indiana public health nurses were surveyed to learn about future training needs (Riner, 2003). They were asked to rate the ten essential public health nursing services in terms of additional knowledge, skills, or education they would need to develop in their role as a professional in the next one to three years.

The top three included: mobilize community partnerships to identify and solve health problems; inform, educate, and empower people about health issues; and ensure a competent public health and personal health care workforce.

Emergencies that public health nurses may expect to face in the future may result from natural or manmade disasters. They may occur locally, regionally, nationally, or globally. The magnitude of the emergency will require varying levels of planning and response. Public health nurses will be expected to possess knowledge and skill in assisting communities to plan for, respond to, and recover from emergencies. Regardless of the type or scale of the emergency, public health nurses will need to be prepared to participate. The Core Public Health Worker Competencies for Emergency Preparedness and Response will be used by public health nurses and their agencies as a guide for preparing themselves to effectively participate in the various stages of planning and response (Gebbie, Merrill, and Tilson, 2002). Specifically, these competencies can be used to update/write job descriptions, familiarize new employees with the job and train the existing workforce, and determine current competencies through self-assessment.

Competence in informatics will provide useful guidance for future planning and delivery of services by public health nurses. Public health informatics is defined as the systematic application of information and computer science and technology to public health practice, research, and learning (Yasnoff et al., 2000). Public health informatics competencies are intended to be applicable to currently practicing public health professionals in the United States, though they may be applicable to public health professionals in other countries as well. Three classes of informatics competencies will be useful for public health nurses: those related to (a) the use of information per se for public health practice, (b) the use of information technology to increase one's individual effectiveness as a public health professional, and (c) the management of information technology projects to improve the effectiveness of the public health enterprise (e.g., the state or local health department). For each competency, expertise levels are suggested for three professional workforce segments: front-line staff, senior-level technical staff, and supervisory and management staff (O'Carroll and the Public Health Informatics Competencies Working Group, n.d.).

🌐 RESEARCH APPLICATION

Content Validity and Nursing Sensitivity of Community-Level Outcomes from the Nursing Outcomes Classification (NOC)

Study Purpose

To evaluate the content validity and nursing sensitivity of seven community-level outcomes (Community Competence; Community Health Status; Community Health: Immunity; Community Risk Control; Chronic Disease; Community Risk Control: Communicable Disease; and Community Risk Control: Lead Exposure) from the Nursing Outcomes Classification (NOC).

Methods

A survey research design was used. Questionnaires were mailed to 300 public health nursing experts: 102 nurses responded. Experts evaluated between 11 and 30 indicators for each of the six outcomes for (a) importance of the indicators for measuring the outcome and (b) influence of nursing on the indicators. Content validity and nursing sensitivity of the outcomes were estimated with a modified Fehring technique.

Findings

All outcomes were deemed important: only Community Competence had an outcome content validity score < 0.80. The outcome sensitivity score for Community Health: Immunity was 0.80; other outcome scores ranged from 0.62 to 0.70. Indicator ratios for all 102 indicators met the study criterion for importance, with 87 percent designated as critical and 13 percent as supplemental. Sensitivity ratios reflected judgments that 45 percent of the indicators were sensitive to nursing intervention.

Implications

The study provided evidence of outcome content validity and nursing sensitivity of the study outcomes; further validation research is recommended, followed by testing of the study outcomes in clinical practice. Community-level nursing-sensitive outcomes will potentially enable study of the efficacy and effectiveness of public health interventions focused on improving health of populations and communities.

Reference

Head, B. J., Aquilino, M. L., Johnson, M., Reed, D., Maas, M., and Moorhead, S. (2004). Content validity and nursing sensitivity of community-level outcomes from the nursing outcomes classification (NOC). *Journal of Nursing Scholarship, 36*(3), 251–259.

The informatics competencies will provide a useful tool for education, designing systems, and new learning resources for public health nurses. Proficiency in these competencies will directly assist today's public health nurses to harness the power of modern information technology to the practice of public health.

Three key issues will be pivotal to the expansion of public health informatics in the future (Public Health Informatics Institute, 2004a). Competing priorities must be balanced to allocate resources to integrate informatics into agency need for information management that supports accountability and the delivery of care. Specific informatics training needs that meet complex requirements must replace broad training in basic applications such as word processing and program-specific applications. Adequate staff time and training budgets need to be allocated for learning new systems.

Overcoming the fragmented nature of health information will serve to improve effective health care, especially for children because they are a vulnerable population. Integration of clinical information systems with public health information systems can improve coordination of care for children. Parents, clinicians, insurers, communities, and public health officials will all benefit from timely and accurate information about the children they serve. Integration of public health information systems with clinical information systems can improve coordination of care for children with multiple preventive and therapeutic health care needs. In addition, parents, clinicians, insurers, and public health agencies would all benefit from timely and accurate information about the children they serve (Public Health Informatics, 2004b). Use of competencies to improve and standardize practice is a quality improvement strategy.

Workforce Trends in Public Health Nursing

If current workforce demographic trends are left unchecked, they will have an adverse effect on the capacity of state and local health agencies to carry out their mission. A national survey of state personnel noted that state governments could lose more than 30 percent of their workforce to retirement, private-sector employers, and alternative careers by 2006, and health agencies would be the hardest hit (Carroll and Moss, 2002).

Four major trends were identified in a public health workforce enumeration survey. Results of the survey indicate there will be a rapidly aging public health workforce and shrinking labor pool. Carroll and Moss (2002) found that the ratio of state public health workers to population had dropped from 219 per 100,000 in 1980 to 158 per 100,000 in 2000. This will be further compounded by the high percentage of workers eligible for retirement. The average age of all state public health agency employees is 44 years compared to the average age of American workers of 40. In addition, on average, about 24 percent of each state's pubic health workforce is eligible for retirement compared to 21 percent of all state employees (Carroll and Moss, 2002). The third trend is a chronic shortage of professional public health workers, with vacancy rates in the 11–20 percent range. The fourth trend is high turnover rates, which represents a potentially huge loss of institutional knowledge, leadership, and experience for state health agencies.

The Association of State and Territorial Health Officers also surveyed state public health agencies about workforce trends. Overall public health nurses comprise 11 percent of the total public health workforce and 25 percent of all public health professionals (Carroll and Moss, 2002). Their findings indicate that 30 out of the 38 reporting states indicated that nursing is the occupational class most affected by the workforce shortage, with shortages almost twice that of the next class (30 percent vs. 15 percent for epidemiologists). National projections indicate that by the year 2010 there will be a need for one million additional registered nurses in all health fields (Hecker, 2001). The nursing shortage in the private sector adds to the challenge for the pubic health sector, which must compete for a limited pool of applicants. Part of the public health nurse recruitment challenge will be that young people are increasingly reluctant to enter public health nursing, primarily because of low salaries (Barrett, Greene, and Mariani, 2004). Unfortunately, fiscal conditions in many states do not permit the salary increase necessary to allow state health agencies to effectively compete for limited talent.

State health agencies identified key actions to heading off a workforce crisis. The three most important incentives in attracting and retaining an adequate public health workforce are increased access to advanced education, competitive pay and benefits, and flexible work schedules and telecommuting opportunities (Carroll and Moss, 2002). The International Council of Nurses (ICN) (Buchan and Calman, 2004) developed a policy-based interventions framework to address the global shortage of registered nurses that parallels these national actions. The components of the ICN plan include workforce planning, recruitment and retention, deployment and performance, and utilization and skill mix.

Advanced practice nurses who have master's degrees in public health nursing have the educational background to provide the expertise for effectively managing the nursing health needs of populations and communities. Yet many problems are affecting their status, educational preparation, supply, and demand, including definitions of advance practice nursing that focus on the provision of individual care, biomedicalization of health care systems, lack of federal funding for public health nursing education and practice, changes in public health department infrastructures that focus on the core functions rather than individual services, and shortage of public health nurses (Robertson, 2004). As the field of population-health management continues to evolve and grow in the future, advanced practice public health nurses can be expected to be in increased demand. However, focused advocacy for the role, revision of the work of public health nurses to demonstrate measurable outcomes, and allocation of financial resources will be needed. Advanced practice public health nurses can build capacity within communities for health promotion.

BUILDING CAPACITY FOR COMMUNITY HEALTH PROMOTION

Building capacity for community health promotion will engage public health nurses in work that requires multidisciplinary and community-organizing competence. Capacity building for health promotion refers to enhancing the ability of the health system or organization to develop, implement, and sustain health promotion initiatives and, ultimately, health changes (MacLean et al., 2003). It fosters problem-solving skills that make organizations and communities more competent, not only to address current health issues but also to embark on other health or development issues. Capacity building is a complex and dynamic process involving a multitude of interrelated factors that are influenced by each other. Capacity building requires coherent leadership, a resource center with relevant expertise, a long-term resource commitment, adaptability to changing environments, partners willing to commit time and resources to the project, a willingness to embrace change, and patience (MacLean et al., 2003). Research on community capacity building will provide a scientific basis for advancing this competency.

A significant role of public health nurses in the future will revolve around engaging residents in participating in solving health problems of their communities. Community participation is the process of involving people in the institution of decisions that affect their lives. It involves the mobilization of citizens for the purpose of undertaking activities to improve conditions in the community (DiClemente, Crosby, and Kegles, 2002). Due to the complex nature of chronic diseases, future interventions will be multilayered in order to engage people in the individual, family, and community aspects of their lives and stimulate changes in lifestyle to prevent or reduce illness. Public health nurses will find an increasing amount of their time and energy devoted to developing and working through community partnerships to establish these multilayered interventions.

An important area of effective community partnerships is collaboration. Keller et al. (2004) defines collaboration for public health nursing as "committing two or more persons or organizations to achieve a common goal through enhancing the capacity of one or more of the members to promote and protect health." (p. 456). Coalition building, another skill related to effective community partnership work, "promotes and develops alliance among organizations or constituencies for a common purpose. It builds linkages, solves problems, and/or enhances local leadership to address health concerns" (p. 456). Community organizing "helps community groups to identify common problems or goals, mobilize resources, and develop and implement strategies for reaching the goals they collectively have set." (p. 456). These three skill sets will be basic

tools for public health nurses as they address health concerns of the future within increasingly complex health care systems and community life. Public health nursing work of the future will require engaging multiple partners—health, business, government, education, philanthropy—in improving the health of communities. This multisectoral collaboration is the foundation on which the Healthy Cities program is built.

The Healthy Cities Movement initiated by the World Health Organization in 1986 provides an approach to health promotion that stresses increasing people's control over the determinants of their health, high-level public participation, and intersectoral cooperation (Hancock, 2007). Its aims are increasingly being adopted by community organizations, hospital-based community health departments, and academic centers partnering with communities. The Healthy Cities Movement aims are to create sustainable environments and processes through which governmental and nongovernmental sectors can work in partnership to create healthy public policies, achieve high-level participation in community-driven projects, and ultimately, reduce inequities and disparities among groups (Duhl, 1993; Tsouros, 1995). Community health promotion work will require interventions decisions to be made based on available evidence of expected outcomes.

RESEARCH AND EVIDENCE-BASED PRACTICE

Research relevant to population-level health needs to be conducted by and about public health nurses. Validation of the contribution of public health nursing interventions is needed to address administrative, financial, and policy concerns of this specialty practice in the contemporary health care environment. Seventeen public health nursing interventions with definitions have been proposed by Keller et al. (2004). Researchers and practitioners need to develop strategies for evaluating how nurses implement these roles and the associated impact on population health.

Evidence-Based Practice

Evidence-based practice will be the norm for public health nursing practice in the twenty-first century. Public health nurses will use interventions that have a research basis. Evidence-based practice is a process of using current evidence to guide practice and clinical decision making; it is the Process piece of outcomes management and the application of available research evidence (Titler, 2002). Evidence-based public health is the development, implementation, and evaluation of effective programs and policies in public health through application of principles of scientific reasoning, including systematic uses of data and information systems and appropriate use of program-planning models (Bronson, Gurney, and Land, 1999).

Analytic tools and processes for evaluating evidence will be important in determining when public health action is warranted in the future. According to Bronson, Gurney, and Land (1999), the following methods are all evidence-based public health tools the public health nurse can engage in or use the products of: (1) meta-analysis—synthesis of the findings of multiple independent studies; (2) risk assessment—a systematic approach to characterizing the risks posed to individuals and populations by environmental pollutants and other potentially adverse exposures; (3) economic evaluation—an assessment of the relative appropriateness of expenditures on public health program and polices; (4) public health surveillance—the ongoing, systematic collection, analysis, and interpretation of outcome-specific health data, which are closely integrated with the timely dissemination of these data to those responsible for health policies and interventions; (5) expert panels—professionals who examine scientific studies based on explicit criteria and determine their relevance to health policies and interventions, and (6) consensus conferences—reviews of epidemiologic evidence that occur over a shorter period of time than expert panels.

Best Practices

Health organizations will undertake periodic outcomes management projects to determine the best processes for achieving desired client outcomes, work designed to identify best practices for professionals and organizations. The best practices process will involve systematic information gathering and analysis so that only the most accurate and complete knowledge is incorporated into health care process redesign. Staff will be dedicated to helping to disseminate new knowledge and support colleagues as they integrate this knowledge into daily practices, and competent managers will gather performance data to determine if client care practices have

---

⊕ RESEARCH APPLICATION

Building Capacity for Heart Health Promotion: Results of a 5-year Experience in Nova Scotia, Canada

Study Purpose

To present the outcomes of a capacity-building initiative for heart health promotion.

Methods

Follow-up study combining quantitative and qualitative methods.

Findings

Results included the development of 204 intersectoral partnerships, creation of a health promotion clearinghouse, attendance at 47 workshops by approximately 1,400 participants, diverse research products, implementation of 18 community heart health promotion initiatives, and increased organizational capacity for heart health promotion via varied organizational changes, including policy changes, fund reallocations, and enhanced knowledge and practices.

Implications

Conclusions were that partnership and organizational development were effective mechanisms for building capacity in heart health promotion. This intervention may have implications for large-scale, community-based, chronic-disease prevention projects.

Reference

MacLean, D. R., Farquharson, J., Heath, S., Barkhouse, K., Latter, C., and Joffres, C. (2003). Building capacity for heart health promotion: Results of a 5-year experience in Nova Scotia, Canada. *American Journal of Health Promotion, 17*(3), 202–212.

changed and outcomes improved. In public health the *Best Practices Initiative*, an electronic newsletter, was launched during the summer of 2002 by the Assistant Secretary of Health, Department of Health and Human Services. The purpose is to showcase best practices in public health from across the country to foster an environment of peer learning and collaboration.

Translational or Dissemination Research

Research findings will influence decisions in many areas—individual client care, practice guidelines, commissioning of health care and research, prevention and health promotion, policy development, education, and clinical audit—but only if public health nurses know how to translate knowledge into action (Hains and Donald, 2002). The challenge becomes determining how public health nurses and agencies will involve themselves in the process of translational research. What are the best methods of bringing about public health practice change based on scientific evidence from well-designed studies?

Translational or dissemination research studies have found several key strategies that will prove to be useful in promoting implementation of research findings by public health nurses. They include (1) active rather than passive dissemination approaches, (2) educational outreach and reminders strategies, and (3) multifaceted interventions based on assessment of potential barriers (Grinshaw et al., 2002). Evidence-based practice can also be informed by expert panel reviews.

Communities of practice, or dialogue groups, like journal clubs, that bring together groups of public health nurses for discussing and applying research studies would be a way to move new findings into practice.

These groups could explore how the findings could be adapted to their local communities and their agencies.

Expert Panel Reviews of Evidence

The two primary sources of information that provide expert reviews for public health interventions are the *Guide to Community Preventive Services* and the *Guide to Clinical Preventive Services*. The *Guide to Community Preventive Services* (NCHM, n.d.) summarizes what is known about the effectiveness, economic efficiency, and feasibility of interventions to promote community health and prevent disease. The Task Force on Community Preventive Services makes recommendations for the use of various interventions based on the evidence gathered in the rigorous and systematic scientific reviews of published studies conducted by the review teams of the Community Guide. The findings from the reviews are published in peer-reviewed journals and also made available on an Internet Web site.

The *Guide to Clinical Preventive Services* (AHRQ, 2007) is intended for primary care clinicians: nurses, nurse practitioners, physician assistants, other allied health professionals, and students. It provides recommendations for clinical practice related to screening tests, counseling interventions, immunizations, and chemoprophylactic regimens for the prevention of more than 80 target conditions. The clients for whom these services are recommended include asymptomatic individuals of all age groups and risk categories. Thus, the subject matter is relevant to all of the major primary care specialties: family practice, internal medicine, obstetrics-gynecology, and pediatrics. The recommendations reflect a standardized review of current scientific evidence and include a summary of published clinical research regarding the clinical effectiveness of each preventive service.

CRITICAL THINKING ACTIVITIES

1. Public health policy is developed from the values held by the population and the current scientific knowledge available about a health concern. Give an example of a public health problem you think a nurse, as a policy advocate, should work on. Explain why you chose this problem, and detail how you would begin working on it?

2. Futures thinking is a way to think about the multiple issues that can be expected to influence a situation in the future, such as the role of public health nursing in the twenty-first century. Describe two desired future scenario regarding the role of the public health nurse in using evidence to determine practice guidelines for improving asthma in school-age children.

3. Examine the role of public health nursing in building capacity for community health promotion.

4. Building capacity for community health promotion is a complex process involving community organizing skills that need to be tailored to the dynamics of local communities. How would you as a public health nurse begin to help a community fulfill its desired outcome of establishing a fitness park in an unused lot in their neighborhood?

5. Analyze the public health nursing workforce supply, demand, and education needs for public health agencies in the twenty-first century.

6. It is often difficult to know if the supply of or the demand for public health nurses has resulted in the current shortage in this area of nursing. What issues do you think should be addressed by public health agencies to assist in recruitment and retention of public health nurses?

KEY TERMS

access to health care

capacity building

Cover the Uninsured Week

evidence-based practice

frontier communities

futuring

health disparities

health trends

performance management

performance measures

performance standards

policy advocacy

quality improvement

systems planning perspective

KEY CONCEPTS

⊕ Health trends are important issues for public health nurses to monitor in order to operate proactively within rapidly changing American communities. By understanding trends, the public health nurse can assess the significance of changing health indicators, plan programs and develop resources to respond to emerging health issues or develop new strategies for entrenched problems, and work to ensure that needed services are available.

⊕ Futuring is a process that can help public health nurses think about the future in order to improve it. It encourages systematic thinking about opportunities and risks in the environment and encourages development of likely future scenarios. These scenarios can then be used to develop plans and strategies for achieving the preferred future or preventing an undesired future occurrence.

⊕ The public health workforce of the future will be prepared to lead at the personal, team, agency, and community levels. Public health nurses will embrace national competencies and skills that demonstrate accountability to the public. Agency-level leadership will involve participation in quality improvement initiatives.

⊕ Building community capacity to promote health will require skills in multidisciplinary team building and community organizing. Healthy Cities is an initiative designed to engage community members in promoting health versus health care.

⊕ Evidence-based practice will require skill in translating research into practice, using best practice guidelines, using systematic reviews by expert panels, and participating in conducting research about community-level outcomes sensitive to nursing interventions.

REFERENCES

Agency for Healthcare Research and Quality (AHRQ). (September, 2007). *Guide to Clinical Preventive Services, 2007.* AHRQ Publication No. 07-05100. Rockville, MD. Retrieved October 15, 2007 from .

American Cancer Society (ACS). (n.d.). *Cancer prevention.* Retrieved February 1, 2005, from http://www.cancer.org/docroot/PED/ped_1.asp?sitearea=PED.

American Heart Association (AHA). (n.d.). *Healthy lifestyle.* Retrieved February 1, 2005, from http://www.americanheart.org/presenter.jhtml?identifier=1200009.

American Public Health Association. (2004). Summaries of 2004 policies passed by the APHA Governing Council. *The Nation's Health,* May 29, 2004.

American Stroke Association. (n.d.). *Let's talk about risk factors for stroke.* Retrieved February 1, 2005, from http://www.strokeassociation.org/downloadable/stroke/107523686014550-0065%20ASA%20RiskFactorsStro.pdf.

Association of State and Territorial Health Officers. (n.d. a). *Genomics project.* Retrieved February 1, 2005, from http://www.astho.org/newsletter/newsletters/4/display.php?u=Jmk9NCZwPTc1JnM9NTcx.

Barrett, K., Greene, R., and Mariani, M. (2004). A case of neglect: Why health care is getting worse, even though medicine is getting better. *Governing.* Retrieved February 2, 2005, from www.governing.com/gpp/2004/intro.htm.

Best, A., Moor, G., Holmes, B., Clark, P. I., Bruce, T., Leischow S., Buchholz, K., and Krajnak, J. (2003). Health promotion dissemination and systems thinking: Towards an integrative model. *American Journal of Health Behavior,* 27(Suppl 3): S206–S216.

Bezold, D., Halperin, J. J., and Eng, J. L. (1993). (Eds.) *2020 visions: Health care information standards and technologies.* Based on proceedings of 1992 conference sponsored by the U.S. Pharmacopeial Convention, Rockville, MD: USPC.

Bronson, R. C., Gurney, J. G., and Land, G. H. (1999). Evidence-based decision making in public health. *Journal of Public Health Management Practice, 5*(5), 86–97.

Brown, V. J. (2004). Kenneth Olden, master fencer. *American Journal of Public Health,* 94(11), 1905–1907.

Buchan, J., and Calman, L (2004). *The global shortage of registered nurses: An overview of issues and actions.* Geneva: International Council of Nurses. Retrieved October 15, 2007, from http://www.icn.ch/global/shortage.pdf.

Caine, V. (2004). Eliminating health disparities through environmental justice. *The Nation's Health.* May 3, 2004

Carroll, J. B., and Moss, D. A. (2002). State employee worker shortage: The impending crisis. *Trends Alert.* The Council of State Governments, p. 5.

Cornish, E. (2004). *Futuring: The exploration of the future.* Bethesda, MD: World Future Society.

DiClemente, R. J., Crosby, R. A., and Kegles, M. C. (Eds.). (2002). *Emerging theories in health promotion practice and research: Strategies for improving public health.* San Francisco: Jossey-Bass.

Duhl, L. (1993). Conditions for healthy cities: Diversity, game boards, and social entrepreneurs. *Environment and Urbanization. 5*(2), 112–124.

Frontier Education Center, National Clearinghouse for Frontier Communities. (2004). *Addressing the nursing shortage: Impacts and innovations in frontier America.* (Electronic version.) Retrieved February 7, 2005, from www.frontierus.org.

Gebbie, K., Merrill, J., and Tilson, H. H. (2002). The public health workforce. *Health Affairs. 21*(6), 57–67.

Giachello, A. L., Arrom, J. O., Davis, M., Sayad, J. V., Ramirez, D., Nandi, C., and Ramos, C. (2003). Reducing diabetes health disparities through community-based participatory action research: The Chicago southeast diabetes community action coalition. *Public Health Reports, 118*(July–August), 309–323.

Grimshaw, J., Shirran, L., Thomas, R., Mowatt, G., Fraser C., Bero, L., Grilli, R., Harvey, E., Oxamn, A., and O'Brian, M. A. (2002). Changing provider behavior: An overview of systematic reviews of interventions to promote implementation of research findings fro health care professional. In A. Hains and A. Donald (Eds.), *Getting research findings into practice* (2nd ed.). London: MBJ Publishing Group.

Hains A. and Donald A. (Eds.), *Getting Research Findings into Practice.* 2nd ed London: MBJ Publishing Group.

Hancock, T. (2007). Healthy Cities and Communities. Retrieved October 8, 2007 from http://www.euro.who.int/healthy-cities.

Head, B. J., Aquilino, M. L., Johnson, M., Reed, D., Maas, M., and Moorhead, S. (2004). Content validity and nursing sensitivity of community-level outcomes from the nursing outcomes classification (NOC). *Journal of Nursing Scholarship, 36*(3), 251–259.

Hecker, D. E. (2001). Occupational employment projections to 2010. *Monthly Labor Review, 125*(11) p. 57-84

Institute for the Future. (2004). *Health and health care 2010: The forecast, the Challenge* (2nd ed.), p. 182. Princeton, NJ: Jossey-Bass.

Institute of Medicine. (2003). *The future of the public's health in the 21st century.* Washington, DC: The National Academies Press.

Keller, L. O., Strohschein, S., Schaffer, M. A., and Lia-Hoagberg, B. (2004). Population-based public health interventions: Innovations in practice, teaching, and management, Part II. *Public Health Nursing, 21*(5), 469–487.

Kouzes, J. M., and Posner, B. Z. (1997) *The leadership challenge: How to keep getting extraordinary things done in organizations.* San Francisco: Jossey-Bass.

Licktveld, M. Y., Coiffi, J. P., Baker, Jr., E. L., Bailey, S. B., Gebbie K. Henderson J. V., Jones D. L., Kurz, R. S., Margolis, S., Miner, K., Thielen, L., and Tilson, H. (2001). Partnership for front-line success: A call for a national action agenda on workforce development. *Journal of Public Health Management and Practice,* 7(40): 1–7.

Link, B. G., and Phelan, J. C. (1995). Social conditions as fundamental causes of disease. *Journal of Health and Social Behavior, 36*(extra issue) , pp 80–94.

MacLean, D. R., Farquharson, J., Heath, S., Barkhouse, K., Latter, C., and Joffres, C. (2003). Building capacity for heart health promotion: Results of a 5-year experience in Nova Scotia, Canada. *American Journal of Health Promotion, 17*(3), 202–212, 202-212.

Mechanic, D. (2003). Who shall lead: Is there a future for population health? *Journal of Health Politics, Policy and Law, 28*(2–3), 421-425.

Mofenson, L. M. (November 22, 2002). U.S. Public Health Service task force recommendations of antiretroviral drugs in pregnant HIV-1-Infected for maternal health and interventions to reduce perinatal transmission in the United States. *Morbidity and Mortality Weekly Review.* Retrieved February 1, 2005, from http://www.cdc.gov/mmwr/PDF/RR/RR5118.pdf.

Mundinger, M. O., Thomas, E., Smolowitz, J., and Honig, J. (2004). Essential health care: Affordable for all? *Nursing Economics Journal, 22*(5), 239-244

National Association of City and County Health Officers. (2004). Retrieved June 15, 2006, from http://www.naccho.org/advocacy/NACCHOpositions.cfm.

National Council of State Legislators. (n.d.). *Genetics laws and legislative activity.* Retrieved February 1, 2005, from http://www.ncsl.org/programs/health/genetics/charts.htm.

Northridge, M. E., Sidibe, S., and Goehl, T. J. (2004). Environment and health: Capacity building for the future. *American Journal of Public Health; 94*(11), 1849–1850.

O'Carroll, P. W., and the Public Health Informatics Competencies Working Group. (n.d.) *Informatics competencies for public health professionals: Introduction, background, conceptual approach.* Retrieved January 29, 2005, from http://healthlinks.washington.edu/nwcphp/phi/comps/bg.html.

Public Health Informatics Institute. (2004a). *Research brief: Putting training on track.* Retrieved January 29, 2005, from http://phii.orgFiles/Training.pdf.

Public Health Informatics Institute. (2004b). *Topics in public health informatics: Integrated childhood management systems.* Retrieved January 29, 2004, from http://phii.org/Files/IntegratedCHIS.pdf.

Quad Council of Public Health Nursing Organizations. (2004). Public health nursing competencies. *Public Health Nursing, 21*(5), 443–452.

Riner, M. E. (2003). Public health education and preferred learning styles survey. Indianapolis: Indiana University School of Nursing.

Robertson, J. F. (2004). Does advanced community/public health nursing practice have a future? *Public Health Nursing, 21*(5), 495–500.

Rosenblatt, R., Casey, S., and Richardson, M. (2002). Rural–urban differences in the public health workforce: Local health departments in three rural western states. *American Journal of Public Health, 92*(7), 1102–1105.

Rowitz, L. (2001). *Public health leadership: Putting principles into practice.* Gaithersburg, MD: Aspen Publishers.

Task Force on Community Preventive Services, National Center for Health Marketing (NCHM), Centers for Disease Control and Prevention (n.d.). Guide to Community Preventive Services. Retrieved October 15, 2007 from http://www.thecommunityguide.org/about/default.htm.

Task Force on Drug Importation, U.S. Department of Health and Human Services. (2004). Retrieved February 8, 2005, from http://www.hhs.gov/importtaskforce/.

Titler, M. G. (2002). *Evidence-based practice: Realities and benefits.* A presentation to Clarian Health Systems, Indianapolis, IN (June 17, 2002).

Tsouros, A. (1995). The WHO healthy cities project: State of the art and future plans. *Health Promotion International, 10*(2), 133–141.

Turning Point Program. (n.d.). *From silos to systems: Using performance management to improve the public's health.* Public Health Foundation for the Performance Management National Excellence Collaborative. Retrieved December 10, 2004, from www.turningpointprogram.org.

Turnock, B. J. (2001). Competency-based credentialing of public health administrators in Illinois. *Journal of Public Health Management Practice,* 7(4), 74–82.

U.S. Department of Health and Human Services (USDHHS), Health Resources and Services Administration, Bureau of Health Professionals, National Center for Health Workforce Information and Analysis. (2000). *The Public Health Work Force, Enumeration, 2000,* pp. 25–26, Bethesda: MD.

U.S. Department of Health and Human Services (USDHHS), U.S. Preventive Services Task Force (USPSTF). (n.d.). *Guide to clinical preventive services.* Retrieved December 7, 2003, from http://cpmcnet.columbia.edu/texts/gcps/.

Woolf, S. H., Johnson, R. E., Fryer, G. E., Rust, G., and Satcher, D. (2004). The health impact of resolving racial disparities: An analysis of US mortality data. *American Journal of Public Health, 94*(12), 2078–2081.

Yasnoff, W. A., O'Carroll, P. W., Koo, D., Linkins, R. W., and Kilbourne, E. (2000). Public health informatics: Improving and transforming public health in the information age. *Journal of Public Health Management Practice, 6*(6), 67–75.

BIBLIOGRAPHY

Association of State and Territorial Health Officers. (n.d. b). *State public health employee worker shortage report.* Accessed February 2, 2005, from www.ASTHO.org.

Carty, B. (2000). Nursing informatics: Education for practice. New York: Springer.

Chattopadhyay, S. K., and Carande-Kulis, V. G. (2004). Economics of prevention: The public health research agenda. *Journal of Public Health Management Practice, 10*(5), 467–471.

Centers for Disease Control. (n.d.) *The task force on community preventive services.* Retrieved December 7, 2003, http://www.thecommunityguide.org/overview/default.htm.

Columbia University. (n.d.). *Core public health worker competencies for emergency preparedness and response.* Retrieved January 29, 2004, from http://www.mailman.hs.columbia.edu/CPHP/cdc/COMPETENCIES.pdf.

Council on Linkages Between Academia and Public Health Practice, Public Health Foundation. (2001). *Core competencies for public health professionals.* Retrieved February 5, 2005, from https://www.train.org/DesktopShell.aspx.

Kouzes, J. M., and Posner, B. A. (2005). *The leadership challenge* (3rd ed.). San Francisco: Jossey-Bass.

Minkler, M. (2002). *Community organizing and community building for health.* New Brunswick, NJ: Rutgers University Press.

Office of the Assistant Secretary of Health, U.S. Department of Health and Human Services (2005). *Best practices initiative.* Retrieved February 4, 2005, from http://www.osophs.dhhs.gov/ophs/BestPractice/default.htm.

Provan, K. G., Nakama, L., Veazie, M. A., Teufel-Shone, N. I., and Huddleston, C. (2003). Building community capacity around chronic disease services through a collaborative interorganizational network. *Health Education & Behavior, 30*(6), 646–662.

Smedley, B. D., Stith, A. Y., and Nelson A. R. (Eds.) (2001). *Unequal treatment: Confronting racial and ethic disparities in health care.* Washington, DC: The National Academies Press.

Nussbaum, R. L., McInnes, R. R., Willard, H. F., and Boerkoel, C. F. (2004). *Thompson & Thompson genetics in medicine* (6th ed.). Philadelphia: Saunders.

RESOURCES

Association of State and Territorial Health Officers (ASTHO)

1275 K Street NW, Suite 800
Washington, D.C. 20005-4006
202-371-9090
FAX: 202-371-9797
Web: http://www.astho.org

ASTHO is a national nonprofit organization representing the state and territorial public health agencies of the United States, the U.S. territories, and the District of Columbia. ASTHO's members, the chief health officials of these jurisdictions, are dedicated to formulating and influencing sound public health policy and to assuring excellence in state-based public health practice.

Center for Health Policy Local Public Health Competency for Emergency Response

The Web site contains an article entitled "Core Public Health Worker Competencies for Emergency Preparedness and Response" by the Center for Health Policy, Columbia University School of Nursing. The center is dedicated to research and policy development with a commitment to the improvement of health and health systems.

Committee on Education and Workforce, U.S. House of Representatives

202-225-4527
Web: http://www.house.gov

The Committee and its five subcommittees oversee education and workforce programs that affect and support hundreds of millions of Americans, from school teachers and small business operators to students and retirees. In a changing economy increasingly driven by technology, competition, and knowledge, the Committee on Education and the Workforce works with the Congress to build on vital reforms set in motion by the president.

Council on Linkages Between Academia and Public Health Practice

202-898-5600
FAX: 202-898-5609
Web: http://www.trainingfinder.org

This is the official Web site for the Competencies Feedback Project by the Council on Linkages Between Academia and Public Health Practice, which is comprised of leaders from national organizations representing the public health practice and academic communities. The council grew out of the Public Health Faculty/Agency Forum, which developed recommendations for improving the relevance of public health education to the demands of public health in the practice sector. The need for this improvement, and for public health professionals to place a higher value on practice-specific training and research, were documented by the Institute of Medicine report, The Future of Public Health. This project is supported under a cooperative agreement from the Health Resources and Services Administration. The council's mission is to improve public health practice and education by refining and implementing recommendations of the Public Health Faculty/Agency Forum, establishing links between academia and the agencies of the public health community and creating a process for continuing public health education throughout one's career.

Cover the Uninsured, Robert Wood Johnson Foundation

202-572-2928
Email: info@covertheuninsured.org
Web: http://covertheuninsured.org
Cover the Uninsured is a project of the Robert Wood Johnson Foundation designed to effect broad-based change to bring about health care insurance coverage for all people. This is the official Web site for this organization.

Families USA

1201 New York Avenue NW
Suite 1100
Washington, D.C. 20005
202-628-3030
FAX: 202-347-2417
Email: info@familiesusa.org
Web: http://www.familiesusa.org
Families USA is a national nonprofit, nonpartisan organization dedicated to the achievement of high-quality, affordable health care for all Americans. Working at the national, state, and community levels, the organization has earned a national reputation as an effective voice for health care consumers for over 20 years.

Health Disparities Collaborative

1201 New York Avenue NW
Suite 1100
Washington, D.C. 20005
202-628-3030
FAX: 202-347-2417
Web: http://www.healthdisparities.net
The mission of the Health Disparities Collaborative is to improve access to high-quality, culturally and linguistically competent primary and preventive care for underserved, uninsured, and underinsured Americans.

National Cancer Institute (NCI)

NCI Public Inquiries Office
6116 Executive Boulevard
Room 3036A
Bethesda, Maryland 20892-8322
1-800-422-6237

Web: http://www.cancer.gov
NCI is a component of the National Institutes of Health, one of eight agencies that compose the Public Health Service in the Department of Health and Human Services. The NCI, established under the National Cancer Institute Act of 1937, is the federal government's principal agency for cancer research and training. The National Cancer Act of 1971 broadened the scope and responsibilities of the NCI and created the National Cancer Program. Over the years, legislative amendments have maintained the NCI authorities and responsibilities and added new information dissemination mandates as well as a requirement to assess the incorporation of state-of-the-art cancer treatments into clinical practice. The National Cancer Institute coordinates the National Cancer Program, which conducts and supports research, training, health information dissemination, and other programs with respect to the cause, diagnosis, prevention, and treatment of cancer, rehabilitation from cancer, and the continuing care of cancer clients and the families of cancer clients.

National Center on Minority Health and Health Disparities NCMHD)

National Institutes of Health
6706 Democracy Boulevard, Suite 800
MSC-5465
Bethesda, Maryland 20892-5464
301-402-1366
FAX: 301-480-4049
Email: NCMHDinfo@od.nih.gov
Web: http://ncmhd.nih.gov
The mission of NCMHD is to promote minority health and to lead, coordinate, support, and assess the NIH effort to reduce and ultimately eliminate health disparities. In this effort, NCMHD will conduct and support basic, clinical, social, and behavioral research, promote research infrastructure and training, foster emerging programs, disseminate information, and reach out to minority and other health disparity communities.

Office of Minority Health, Centers for Diseases Control (OMH)

Centers for Disease Control & Prevention
Mailstop E-67
1600 Clifton Road NE
Atlanta, Georgia 30333
404-498-2320
FAX: 404-498-2355
Email: OMH@cdc.gov
Web: http://www.cdc.gov
The mission of OMH is to promote health and quality of life by preventing and controlling the disproportionate burden of disease, injury, and disability among racial and ethnic minority populations. In carrying out its mission, OMH

coordinates White House Executive Orders and Health and Human Services departmental initiatives, supports cooperative agreements for research and professional development, reports on the health status of racial and ethnic minorities in the United States, and initiates strategic partnerships with governmental as well as national and regional organizations.

Racial and Ethnic Approaches to Community Health, Centers for Disease Control

1600 Clifton Road
Atlanta, Georgia 30333
404-639-3311; Public Inquiries: 404-639-3534;
    1-800-311-3435
Web: http://www.cdc.gov
This Web page presents ways to support community coalitions in designing, implementing, and evaluating community-driven strategies to eliminate health disparities.

State of Connecticut Office of Health Care Access

410 Capitol Avenue
MS #13HCA
Hartford, Connecticut 06134-0308
860-418-7001; 1-800-797-9688
FAX: 860-418-7053
Email: Cristine.Vogel@po.state.ct.us
Web: http://www.ct.gov

The mission of the Office of Health Care Access is to ensure that the citizens of Connecticut have access to a quality health care delivery system. The agency will fulfill its mission by advising policy makers of health care issues; informing the public and the industry of statewide and national trends; and designing and directing health care system development.

World Future Society

7910 Woodmont Avenue, Suite 450
Bethesda, Maryland 20814
301-656-8274
E-mail info@wfs.org
Web: http://www.wfs.org
The World Future Society is an association of people interested in how social and technological developments are shaping the future. The society was founded in 1966 and is chartered as a nonprofit educational and scientific organization in Washington, D.C. The society strives to serve as a neutral clearinghouse for ideas about the future. Ideas about the future include forecasts, recommendations, and alternative scenarios. These ideas help people to anticipate what may happen in the next 5, 10, or more years ahead. When people can visualize a better future, then they can begin to create it.

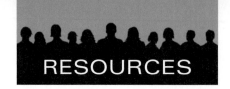
RESOURCES

Adult Literacy Estimates

Web: http://www.casas.org

The Web site provides literacy, education, race/ethnicity, English proficiency, and labor force statistics for any state, county, or city in the United States.

Agency for Healthcare Research and Quality (AHRQ)

John M. Eisenberg Building
540 Gaither Road, Suite 2000
Rockville, Maryland 20850
Web: http://www.ahrq.gov

AHRQ is the federal agency charged with improving the quality, safety, efficiency, and effectiveness of health care for all Americans. The agency supports health services research that will improve the quality of health care and promote evidence-based decision-making. AHRQ invests about 80 percent of its budget in grants and contracts focused on improving health care. The agency conducts and supports research on health care for ethnic and racial minority and other priority populations, as one of its mandates.

Agency for Toxic Substances and Disease Registry (ATSDR)

1825 Century Blvd
Atlanta, Georgia 30345
1-800-343-5436
Web: http://www.atsdr.cdc.gov

ATSDR is a federal public health agency of the U.S. Department of Health and Human Services that uses sound scientific evidence to implement public health interventions, and provides trusted health information to prevent harmful exposures and diseases related to toxic substances.

American Academy of Pediatrics (AAP)

141 Northwest Point Boulevard
Elk Grove Village, Illinois 60007
847-434-4000
FAX: 847-434-8000
Web: http://www.aap.org

The AAP is committed to the attainment of optimal, physical, mental, and social health and well-being for all infants, children, adolescents, and young adults. Their Web site is a resource for health professionals and parents. The site has publications and educational resources on a number of health topics relevant to pediatric and special populations and community health.

American Association of Colleges of Nursing (AACN)

One Dupont Circle NW, Suite 530
Washington, D.C. 20036
202-463-6930
FAX: 202-463-1315
Web: http://www.aacn.nche.edu

AACN is the national voice for America's baccalaureate- and higher-degree nursing education programs. AACN's educational, research, governmental advocacy, data collection, publications, and other programs work to establish quality standards for bachelor's- and graduate-degree nursing education, assist deans and directors to implement those standards, influence the nursing profession to improve health care, and promote public support of baccalaureate and graduate education, research, and practice in nursing—the nation's largest health care profession. The Web site contains government affairs link, bulletins, issue summaries, and briefings of interest to nurses.

American Association of Diabetes Educators (AADE)

100 W. Monroe, Suite 400
Chicago, Illinois 60603
1-800-338-3633
Email: aade@aadenet.org
Web: http://www.aadenet.org

The AADE is a multidisciplinary professional membership organization of health care professionals dedicated to integrating successful self-management as a key outcome in the care of people with diabetes and related conditions. AADE promotes healthy living through self-management of diabetes and related conditions.

American Association of Occupational Health Nurses (AAOHN)

2920 Brandywine Road, Suite 100
Atlanta, Georgia 30341
770-455-7757
FAX: 770-455-7271
Email: aaohn@aaohn.org
Web: http://www.aaohn.org

AAOHN, the largest group of health care professionals serving the workplace, has a mission to ensure occupational and environmental nurses are the authority on health, safety, productivity, and disability management for worker populations. AAOHN is a principal force in furthering the profession of occupational and environmental health nursing by advancing the profession.

American Association of Retired Persons (AARP)

601 E Street NW
Washington, D.C. 20049
202-424-3410
Web: http://www.aarp.org

The AARP, a nonprofit, nonpartisan membership organization for people age 50 and over, is dedicated to enhancing quality of life for all as we age. AARP leads positive social change and deliver value to members through information, advocacy and service.

American Diabetes Association (ADA)

1701 North Beauregard Street
Alexandria, Virginia 22311
1-800-342-2383
Email: AskADA@diabetes.org
Web: http://www.diabetes.org

The ADA is the nation's leading nonprofit health organization providing diabetes research, information, and advocacy. It conducts programs in all fifty states and the District of Columbia, reaching hundreds of communities to prevent and cure diabetes and to improve the lives of all people affected by diabetes. Information about diabetes and diabetes prevention, research and scientific findings, services, policy and advocacy for research and for the rights of people with diabetes can be found at the ADA Web site.

American Health Line

The Advisory Board Company
2445 M Street NW
Washington, D.C. 20037
1-800-717-3245
FAX: 202-266-5700
Web: http://www.americanhealthline.com

American Health Line provides a concise, accurate and nonpartisan synthesis of the days most important and compelling health care news, all delivered via Email by 11:30 A.M. ET. In addition to affording nurses access to the same information that the nation's health care policy makers on Capitol Hill say they can't do their jobs without, a subscription to American Health Line empowers professionals with an array of resources and expertise.

American Heart Association (AHA)

7272 Greenville Avenue
Dallas, Texas 75231
214-373-6300; 1-800-AHA-USA1
Web: http://www.americanheart.org

The AHA is a national voluntary health agency whose mission is to reduce disability and death from cardiovascular diseases and stroke. The AHA is a source for health pro-

motion programs to prevent heart disease and stroke and promote healthy lifestyles. It is also a resource for health care professionals.

American Nurses Association (ANA)

8515 Georgia Avenue, Suite 400
Silver Spring, Maryland 20910
1-800-274-4ANA
Web: http://www.nursingworld.org

The ANA was started as the Association of Nursing Alumnae. It later became the American Nurses Association's Congress on Nursing Practice and Economics representing all nurses. The ANA is a professional nursing organization that represents the interest of the 2.9 million registered nurses in the United States and the people for whom they care. The Web site provides information on ANA activities and access to online nursing journals.

American Organization of Nurse Executives (AONE)

Liberty Place
325 Seventh Street NW
Washington, D.C. 20004
202-626-2240
FAX: 202-638-5499
Web: http://www.aone.org

Founded in 1967, AONE, a subsidiary of the American Hospital Association, is a national organization of over 5,000 nurses who design, facilitate, and manage care. Its mission is to represent nurse leaders who improve health care. AONE members are leaders in collaboration and catalysts for innovation. AONE's vision is "Shaping the future of healthcare through innovative nursing leadership." The Web site provides information on policy, politics, legislation, and advocacy for nurse executives.

American Public Health Association (APHA)

800 "I" Street NW
Washington, DC 20001-3710
202-777- APHA (2752)
FAX: 202-777-2534
Email: comments@APHA.org
Web: http://www.apha.org

APHA is a nonprofit association of public health professionals from over 50 public health occupations working to improve the public's health and to achieve equity in health status for all. The organization strives to influence policy and set priorities in public health to help prevent disease and promote health. The organization also strives to promote the scientific and professional foundation of public health practice and policy, advocate the conditions for a healthy global society, emphasize prevention, and enhance the ability of members to promote and protect environmental and community health. APHA is an organization that represents more than 50,000 public health professionals worldwide from over 50 occupations of public health.

American Public Health Association (APHA), Public Health Nursing (PHN) Section

800 "I" Street NW
Washington, D.C. 20001-3710
202-777-APHA (2752)
FAX: 202-777-2534
Email: comments@APHA.org
Web: http://www.apha.org

This association of public health nurse educators and practitioners operates within the American Public Health Association. The Web site provides information and opportunities for involvement in nationwide PHN issues.

American Red Cross (ARC)

American Red Cross National Headquarters
2025 E Street NW
Washington, DC 20006
202-303-4498
Web: http://www.redcross.org

Since its founding in 1881 by visionary leader Clara Barton, the American Red Cross has been the nation's premier emergency response organization. As part of a worldwide movement that offers neutral humanitarian care to the victims of war, the American Red Cross distinguished itself by also aiding victims of devastating natural disasters. Over the years, the organization has expanded its services, always with the aim of preventing and relieving suffering. Today, in addition to domestic disaster relief, the American Red Cross offers compassionate services in five other areas: community services that help the needy; support and comfort for military members and their families; the collection, processing, and distribution of lifesaving blood and blood products; educational programs that promote health and safety; and international relief and development programs. The ARC, a humanitarian organization led by volunteers, is guided by its Congressional Charter and the Fundamental Principles of the International Red Cross Movement.

American School Health Association (ASHA)

7263 State Route 43
P.O. Box 708
Kent, Ohio 44240
330-678-1601
FAX: 330-768-4526
Email: asha@ashaweb.irg
Web: http://www.ashaweb.org

ASHA is a multidisciplinary association of professionals including administrators, counselors, health educators, school nurses, psychologists, health educators, physical educators, physicians, and social workers. Its mission is to protect and promote the health and well-being of school-age children and youth through coordinated school health programs.

American Translators Association (ATA)

225 Reinekers Lane, Suite 590
Alexandria, Virginia 22314
(703) 683-6100
FAX: (703) 683-6122
Email: ata@atanet.org
Web: http://www.atanet.org

ATA, founded in 1959, is the largest professional association of translators and interpreters in the United States with over 9,500 members in over 70 countries. ATA's primary goals include fostering and supporting the professional development of translators and interpreters and promoting the translation and interpreting professions. ATA is a professional association founded to advance the translation and interpreting professions and foster the professional development of individual translators and interpreters. Its members include translators, interpreters, teachers, project managers, web and software developers, language company owners, hospitals, universities, and government agencies.

America's Health Insurance Plans (AHIP)

601 Pennsylvania Avenue NW
South Building, Suite 500
Washington, D.C. 20004
202-778-3200
FAX: 202-331-7487
Email: ahip@ahip.org
Web: http://www.hiaa.org

AHIP is the national association representing nearly 1,300 member companies providing health insurance coverage to more than 200 million Americans. Member companies offer medical expense insurance, long-term care insurance, disability income insurance, dental insurance, supplemental insurance, stop-loss insurance, and reinsurance to consumers, employers, and public purchasers. AHIP's goal is to provide a unified voice for the health care financing industry, to expand access to high-quality, cost-effective health care to all Americans, and to ensure Americans' financial security through robust insurance markets, product flexibility and innovation, and an abundance of consumer choice.

Amnesty International (AI)

5 Penn Plaza, 14th floor
New York, New York 10001
212-807-8400
FAX: 212-463-9193; 212-627-1451
Email: admin-us@aiusa.org
Web: http://www.amnesty.org

AI is a worldwide movement of people who campaign for internationally recognized human rights. AI's vision is of a world in which every person enjoys all of the human rights enshrined in the Universal Declaration of Human Rights and other international human rights standards. In pursuit of this vision, AI's mission is to undertake research and action focused on preventing and ending grave abuses of the rights to physical and mental integrity, freedom of conscience and expression, and freedom from discrimination, within the context of its work to promote all human rights. AI is independent of any government, political ideology, economic interest or religion. It does not support or oppose any government or political system, nor does it support or oppose the views of the victims whose rights it seeks to protect. It is concerned solely with the impartial protection of human rights.

Association of Community Health Nurse Educators (ACHNE)

10200 W. 44th Avenue, #304
Wheat Ridge, Colorado 80033
303-422-0679
FAX: 303-422-9904
Email: ACHNE@resourcenter.com
Web: http://www.achne.org

ACHNE is an association of educators that teaches community health and public health nursing at universities and colleges. ACHNE provides a meeting ground for thosecommitted to excellence in community and public health nursing education, research, and practice. ACHNE was established in 1978 and is run by elected volunteer leaders who guide the organization in providing networking through the quarterly newsletter and membership directory, and providing educational opportunities through publications and the annual Spring Institute. ACHNE's mission is to promote the public's health by ensuring leadership and excellence in community and public health nursing education, research, and practice. The Web site provides information on workforce issues, PHN/CHN certification, career opportunities, public health nursing graduate education, and links to other Quad Council organizations.

Association of Occupational and Environmental Clinics (AOEC)

1010 Vermont Avenue NW, #513
Washington, D.C. 20005

202-347-4976; 888-347-AOEC (2632)
Email: aoec@aoec.org
Web: http://www.aoec.org

AOEC is a nonprofit organization committed to improving the practice of occupational and environmental health through collaborative research and sharing of information and resources. Since its founding in 1987, the AOEC has grown to a network of more than 60 clinics and more than 250 individuals committed to improving the practice of occupational and environmental medicine through information sharing and collaborative research.

Association of Schools of Public Health (ASPH) Curriculum Resources

1101 15th Street NW, Suite 910
Washington, D.C. 20005
202-296-1099
FAX: 202-296-1252
Email: info@asph.org
Web: http://www.asph.org

The much anticipated Ethics and Public Health: Model Curriculum is now available for use by Schools of Public Health and other Health related faculty. The project was a collaborative effort between ASPH, the Health Resources and Services Administration (HRSA), and The Hastings Center. The concept for the model curriculum grew from a rising interest in the ethical, legal, and social aspects of public health policy and practice. With this interest came a demand for the teaching of ethics in health-related schools and for the resource materials to support it. The curriculum is intended as a resource to enhance and encourage thoughtful, well-informed, and critical discussions of ethical issues in the field of public health.

Association of State and Territorial Directors of Nursing (ASTDN)

1275 K Street NW, Suite 800
Washington, D.C. 20005-4006
202-371-9090
FAX: 202-371-9797
Email: dianakp@health.ok.gov
Web: http://www.astdn.org

The Association of State and Territorial Directors of Nursing began in 1935 as an advisory group of state health department nurses. ASTDN continues today as an active association of public health nursing leaders from across the United States and its territories. ASTDN is an affiliate of the Association of State and Territorial Health Officials (ASTHO). The ASTDN mission is to provide a collegial forum to advance the public health nursing leadership role in protecting and promoting the health of the public. The Web site provides information on publications, population-focused practice, Quad Council competencies,

Partnership Project (CDC and ASTDN), newsletter, and featured state public health nursing profile.

Association of State and Territorial Health Officials (ASTHO)

1275 K Street NW, Suite 800
Washington, D.C. 20005-4006
202-371-9090
FAX: 202-371-9797
Web: http://www.astho.org

The Association of State and Territorial Health Officials (ASTHO) is the national nonprofit organization representing the state and territorial public health agencies of the United States, the U.S. Territories, and the District of Columbia. ASTHO's members, the chief health officials of these jurisdictions, are dedicated to formulating and influencing sound public health policy, and to assuring excellence in state-based public health practice. The Web site provides resources on public health information, workforce issues, law and public health, publications, and many other current issues.

ATSDR's Environmental Health and Nursing Initiative Agency of Toxic Substances and Disease Registry Division of Toxicology and Environmental Medicine

4770 Buford Hwy, NE (Mail Stop F-32)
Atlanta, Georgia 30341-3717
1-800-232-4636
FAX: 770-488-4178
Email: atsdr-nurse@cdc.gov
Web: http://www.atsdr.cdc.gov

This agency promotes and supports nurses' contributions to promoting environmental health for individuals and communities.

B'Tselem (Information Center for Human Rights in the Occupied Territories)

Web: http://www.btselem.org

The Israeli Information Center for Human Rights in the Occupied Territories was established in 1989 by a group of prominent academics, attorneys, journalists, and Knesset members. It endeavors to document and educate the Israeli public and policy makers about human rights violations in the Occupied Territories, combat the phenomenon of denial prevalent among the Israeli public, and help create a human rights culture in Israel. B'Tselem in Hebrew literally means "in the image of" and is also used as a synonym for human dignity. The word is taken from Genesis 1:27 "And God created humans in his image. In the image of God did He create him." It is in this spirit that the first article of the Universal Declaration of Human Rights states that "All human beings are born equal in dignity and rights." As an Israeli human rights organization, B'Tselem acts primarily to change Israeli policy in the Occupied Territories and ensure that its government, which rules the Occupied Territories, protects the human rights of residents there, and complies with its obligations under international law. B'Tselem is independent and is funded by contributions from private individuals in Israel and abroad and from foundations in Israel, Europe, and North America that support human rights activity worldwide.

BioMed Central Ltd.

Science Navigation Group
Middlesex House
34-42 Cleveland Street
London W1T 4LB
United Kingdom
+44-0-20-7631-9131
FAX: +44-0-20-7631-9926
Email: info@biomedcentral.com
Web: http://www.biomedcentral.com

BioMed Central is an independent publishing house committed to providing immediate open access to peer-reviewed biomedical research. All original research articles published by BioMed Central are made freely and permanently accessible online immediately upon publication. BioMed Central views open access to research as essential in order to ensure the rapid and efficient communication of research findings. The Web site provides access to these research articles.

Blue Cross/Blue Shield Association

Web: http://www.bluecares.com

This is the official Web site for the Blue Cross and Blue Shield Association. It features information about Blue Cross/Blue Shield, answers for consumers, and provides consumers with the opportunity to sign up for a Blue Cross/Blue Shield plan on line.

Bureau of National Affairs (BNA)

1231 25th Street NW
Washington, D.C. 20037
1-800-372-1033
FAX: 1-800-253-0332
Email: customercare@bna.com
Web: http://www.bna.com

BNA is a leading publisher of information and analysis products for professionals in law, tax, business, and government. The company's print and electronic products address the full range of legal, legislative, regulatory, and economic developments affecting business. Today, BNA employees in the nation's capital and around the world produce more than 350 news and information services known and valued for their unbiased reporting, including the highly respected Daily Labor Report and Daily Tax Report.

Capitol Hearings

Web: http://www.capitolhearings.org

This Web site is C-SPAN's joint production with Congressional Quarterly to provide a preview story and a daily congressional update of hearings from Capitol Hill that have been presented on C-SPAN.

Catholic Migrant Farmworker Network (CMFN)

P.O. Box 50026
Boise, Idaho 83705
Email: cmfn@stpaulsboise.org
Web: http://www.cmfn.org

CMFN is a national organization dedicated to pastoral ministry with migrant and seasonal farmworkers. Founded in 1986, the network operates with the support and collaboration of the Office for the Pastoral Care of Migrants and Refugees of the U.S. Catholic Conference. Stories, current issues related to migrant farm work, and links to other information and resources are available at their Web site.

Center for Biologics Evaluation and Research (CBER)

1401 Rockville Pike, Suite 200N
Rockville, MD 20852-1448
1-800-835-4709; 301-827-1800
Email: octma@cber.fda.gov
Web: http://www.fda.gov

CBER protects and enhances the public health through the regulation of biological and related products including blood, vaccines, tissue, allergenics, and biological therapeutics. CBER is committed to a product approval process that maximizes the benefits and minimizes the risks to clients of the biological product. The Web site offers information about new products and topics such as influenza virus vaccine, product recall and withdrawal, and client news and safety information.

Center for Food Safety and Applied Nutrition (CFSAN)

Food and Drug Administration
5600 Fishers Lane
Rockville, Maryland 20857
1-888-463-6332
Web: http://vm.cfsan.fda.gov

The CFSAN, an agency of the Food and Drug Administration (FDA), is responsible for promoting and protecting the public's health by ensuring that the nation's food supply is safe, sanitary, wholesome, and honestly labeled, and that cosmetic products are safe and properly labeled. Although the U.S. food supply is among the world's safest, the increase in the variety of foods and the convenience items available, as well as the complexity of the food industry and the technologies used in food production and packaging, has brought with it public health concerns. Recent news, information about national food safety programs, FDA documents, and special interest areas can be located at this Web site.

Center for Health Policy Local Public Health Competency for Emergency Response

Web: http://www.cumc.columbia.edu

The Web site contains an article entitled "Core Public Health Worker Competencies for Emergency Preparedness and Response" by the Center for Health Policy, Columbia University School of Nursing. The center is dedicated to research and policy development with a commitment to the improvement of health and health systems.

Center for Health System Change (HSC)

600 Maryland Avenue SW, #550
Washington, D.C. 20024
202-484-5261
FAX: 202-484-9258
Web: http://www.hschange.org

HSC is a nonpartisan policy research organization located in Washington, D.C. It designs and conducts studies focused on the U.S. health care system to inform the thinking and decisions of policy makers in government and private industry. In addition to this applied use, HSC studies contribute more broadly to the body of health care policy research that enables decision makers to understand change and the national and local market forces driving that change. The mission of HSC is to inform policy makers and private decision makers about how local and national changes in the financing and delivery of health care affect people. HSC strives to provide high-quality, timely, and objective research and analysis that leads to sound policy decisions, with the ultimate goal of improving the health of the American public.

Center for Health, Environment, and Justice (CHEJ)

P.O. Box 6806
Falls Church, Virginia 22040-6806
703-237-2249
Email: chej@chej.org
Web: http://www.chej.org

The CHEJ is a national environmental grassroots organization that assists individuals, families, and communities facing exposures to dangerous environmental chemicals, in the air, water, and soil. CHEJ was involved in establishing some of the first national policies critical to protecting community health like the Superfund Program and Right-to-Know. CHEJ has become the preeminent national leader among grassroots groups reducing the burden of toxic substances on our environment.

Center on Budget and Policy Priorities

820 1st Street NE, #510
Washington, D.C. 20002
202-408-1080
FAX: 202-408-1056
Email: center@cbpp.org
Web: http://www.cbpp.org

The Center on Budget and Policy Priorities is one of the nation's premier policy organizations working at the federal and state levels on fiscal policy and public programs that affect low- and moderate-income families and individuals. The center conducts research and analysis to inform public debates over proposed budget and tax policies and to help ensure that the needs of low-income families and individuals are considered in these debates. The center also develops policy options to alleviate poverty, particularly among working families, and examines the short- and long-term impacts that proposed policies would have on the health of the economy and on the soundness of federal and state budgets. Among the issues explored are whether federal and state governments are fiscally sound and have sufficient revenue to address critical priorities, both for low-income populations and for the nation as a whole.

Centers for Disease Control and Prevention (CDC)

1600 Clifton Road
Atlanta, Georgia 30333
404-639-3311 / Public Inquiries: 404-639-3534 /
1-800-311-3435
Web: http://www.cdc.gov

The CDC is one of the 13 major operating components of the Department of Health and Human Services (HHS), which is the principal agency in the U.S. government for protecting the health and safety of all Americans and for providing essential human services, especially for those people who are least able to help themselves. Since it was founded in 1946, CDC has remained at the forefront of public health efforts to prevent and control infectious and chronic diseases, injuries, workplace hazards, disabilities, and environmental health threats. Today, CDC is globally recognized for conducting research and investigations and for its action-oriented approach. CDC applies research and findings to improve people's daily lives and responds to health emergencies—something that distinguishes CDC from its peer agencies.

Centers for Disease Control and Prevention, Division of Global Migration and Quarantine

1600 Clifton Road
Atlanta, Georgia 30333
404-639-4411, 404-639-3534, 1-800-311-3435
Web: http://www.cdc.gov

The Division of Global Migration and Quarantine has statutory responsibility to make and enforce regulations necessary to prevent the introduction, transmission, or spread of communicable diseases from foreign countries into the United States. The Web site describes the policies, criteria, and conduct of required pre-migration physical examinations for immigrants and refugees.

Centers for Medicare & Medicaid Services (CMS)

7500 Security Boulevard
Baltimore, Maryland 21244
Web: http://new.cms.hhs.gov

CMS is the federal agency responsible for administering Medicare, Medicaid, SCHIP (State Children's Health Insurance), HIPAA (Health Insurance Portability and Accountability Act), CLIA (Clinical Laboratory Improvement Amendments), and several other health programs.

Children's Defense Fund (CDF)

25 E Street NW
Washington, D.C. 20001
202-628-8787; 1-800-233-1200
Email: cdfinfo@childrensdefense.org
Web: http://www.childrensdefense.org

The CDF grew out of the civil rights movement under the leadership of Marian Wright Edelman. It has become the nation's strongest voice for children and families since its founding in 1973. Today, The CDF's Leave No Child Behind® mission is to ensure every child a Healthy Start, a Head Start, a Fair Start, a Safe Start, and a Moral Start in life and successful passage to adulthood with the help of caring families and communities. CDF provides a strong, effective voice for all the children of America who cannot vote, lobby, or speak for themselves.

Children's Environmental Health Network

110 Maryland Avenue NE, Suite 505
Washington, D.C. 20002
202-543-4033
FAX: 202-543-8797
Email: cehn@cehn.org
Web: http://www.cehn.org

The Children's Environmental Health Network is a national organization comprised of multiple disciplines for the purpose of protecting the health of the fetus and the child from environmental health hazards and to promote a healthy environment.

Committee on Education and Workforce, U.S. House of Representatives

202-225-4527

Web: http://www.house.gov

The Committee and its five subcommittees oversee education and workforce programs that affect and support hundreds of millions of Americans, from school teachers and small business operators to students and retirees. In a changing economy increasingly driven by technology, competition, and knowledge, the Committee on Education and the Workforce works with the Congress to build on vital reforms set in motion by the president.

Community Toolbox Work Group on Health Promotion & Community Development

4082 Dole Human Development Center
University of Kansas
1000 Sunnyside Avenue
Lawrence, Kansas 66045-7555
785-864-0533
FAX: 785-864-5281
Email: Toolbox@ku.edu
Web: http://www.ctb.ku.edu

The Community Toolbox is a Web site for a toolkit to support your work in promoting community health and development, providing examples and "how-to" information for assessing community needs and resources. The Toolbox includes practical information about skill building in assessment, strategic planning, leadership, intervention, evaluation, advocacy, marketing; planning, developing, and sustaining a program; problem solving and support; and online forums, resources, and advisers for best practices.

Congressional Budget Office (CBO)

Ford House Office Building, 4th floor
Second and D Streets, SW
Washington, D.C. 20515-6925
202-226-2602
Web: http://www.cbo.gov

CBO was founded on July 12, 1974, with the enactment of the Congressional Budget and Impoundment Control Act (P.L. 93-344). The agency began operating on February 24, 1975. CBO issues yearly federal cost estimates and impact of unfounded mandates on state and local governments, studies, reports, briefs, Monthly Budget Reviews, letters, and background papers to Congress. CBO also tes-

tifies before the Congress as needed on a variety of issues. Finally, CBO provides up-to-date data on its Web site, including current budget and economic projections and information on the status of discretionary appropriations.

Congressional Digest Corporation

4416 East West Highway, Suite 400
Bethesda, Maryland 20814-4568
1-800-637-9915
FAX: 301-634-3189
Email: info@congressionaldigest.com
Web: http://www.congressionaldigest.com

The Web site offers information on political issues from both the pro and con sides as discussed by elected officials.

Congressional E-Mail Directory

Web: http://www.webslingerz.com/jhoffman/congress-email.html

An Email directory for elected officials in Congress.

Congressional Quarterly Legislative Impact, Inc.

1255 22nd Street NW
Washington, D.C. 20037
202-419-8500; 1-800-432-2250
Web: http://www.cq.com

CQ Legislative Impact provides information on pending bills in Congress and current law, so that one can quickly decipher how legislation before Congress would affect existing public law and specific U.S. Code sections.

Constitution Facts

Oak Hill Publishing Company
Box 6473
Naperville, Illinois 60567
1-800-887-6661
FAX 630-904-2737
Web: http://www.constitutionfacts.com

In the early 1990s the first edition of "The U.S. Constitution & Fascinating Facts About It" was published as a resource for law students. Since then, the book has been used by civic organizations, school teachers and police officers, major retailers, and the U.S. armed forces. The Web site was launched in 1996 as a companion to the book to help educate those who want to learn about the Constitution.

Council on Linkages Between Academia and Public Health Practice

202-898-5600
FAX: 202-898-5609
Web: http://www.trainingfinder.org

This is the official Web site for the Competencies Feedback Project by the Council on Linkages Between Academia and Public Health Practice, which is comprised of leaders from national organizations representing the public health practice and academic communities. The council grew out of the Public Health Faculty/Agency Forum, which developed recommendations for improving the relevance of public health education to the demands of public health in the practice sector. The need for this improvement, and for public health professionals to place a higher value on practice-specific training and research, were documented by the Institute of Medicine report, The Future of Public Health. This project is supported under a cooperative agreement from the Health Resources and Services Administration. The council's mission is to improve public health practice and education by refining and implementing recommendations of the Public Health Faculty/Agency Forum, establishing links between academia and the agencies of the public health community and creating a process for continuing public health education throughout one's career.

Cover the Uninsured, Robert Wood Johnson Foundation

202-572-2928
Email: info@covertheuninsured.org
Web: http://covertheuninsured.org
Cover the Uninsured is a project of the Robert Wood Johnson Foundation designed to effect broad-based change to bring about health care insurance coverage for all people. This is the official Web site for this organization.

Cross Cultural Health Care Program (CCHCP)

270 So. Hanford Street, Suite 208
Seattle, Washington 98134
206-860-0329 or 206-860-0331
FAX: 206-860-0334
Email: administration@xculture.org
Web: http://www.xculture.org
CCHCP is an organization that recognizes the diversity and the different ways to health. Its mission is to serve as a bridge between communities and health care institutions to ensure full access to quality health care that is culturally and linguistically appropriate. Includes recommendations about designing culturally competent programs with the collaboration of communities. It is not limited to immigrants and refugees.

Cultural Competency Works Agency for Healthcare Research and Quality

Web: ftp://ftp.hrsa.gov/financeMC/cultural-competence.pdf
This AHRQ document outlines successful practices in delivering culturally competent care including (a) to define culture broadly, (b) to value clients' cultural beliefs, (c) to recognize the complexity in language interpretation, (d) to facilitate learning between providers and communities, (e) to involve the community in defining and addressing service needs, (f) to collaborate with other agencies, (g) to

participate in professional staff training, and (h) to institutionalize cultural competence.

DATA2010

National Center for Health Statistics
Division of Health Promotion Statistics
3311 Toledo Road
Hyattsville, Maryland 20782-2003
301-458-4013 (Health Statistics)
Web: http://wonder.cdc.gov
DATA2010 is an interactive database system developed by the Division of Health Promotion Statistics at the National Center for Health Statistics. It contains the most recent monitoring data for tracking Healthy People 2010 objectives.

Division of Health Promotion Statistics

3311 Toledo Road
Hyattsville, Maryland 20782-2003
301-458-4013 (Health Statistics)
Web: http://wonder.cdc.gov
DATA2010 is an interactive database system developed by the Division of Health Promotion Statistics at the National Center for Health Statistics. It contains the most recent monitoring data for tracking Healthy People 2010 Objectives.

Democratic National Committee

430 S. Capitol Street SE
Washington, D.C. 20003
Web: http://www.democrats.org
This is the official Web site for the Democratic National Committee.

Dietary Guidelines for Americans 2005

Web: http://www.healthierus.gov
The Web site provides new dietary guidelines as well as brochures on how to be healthier, based on the new dietary guidelines, toolkits for health professionals, and press releases. Additional resources are listed at the end of the Web site.

Eastern Nursing Research Society (ENRS)

100 North 20th Street, 4th Floor
Philadelphia, Pennsylvania 19103
215-599-6700
FAX: 215-564-2175
Email: info@enrs-go.org
Web: http://www.enrs-go.org
ENRS has members in the Eastern Region of the United States. Their goals are to advance nursing research in the Northeast region of the United States, facilitate development of nurse researchers, influence development of scientific knowledge base relevant to nursing, and promote

research-based nursing practice. Their Web site offers more information about ENRS and links to other nursing organizations.

Emergency Nurses Association (ENA)

915 Lee Street
Des Plaines, Illinois 60016-6569
1-800-900-9659
Web: http://www.ena.org

The ENA is a professional member organization that promotes excellence in emergency nursing through leadership, research, education, and advocacy. The Web site is the official Web site for this organization.

Employer Health Register

Web: http://www.employerhealth.com

The Employer Health Register is a link to direct employee health specialists with products and services, including health risk appraisals. Published from the Work Loss Data Institute.

EnviRN

Environmental Health Education Center
University of Maryland School of Nursing
655 West Lombard Street, Room 665
Baltimore, Maryland 21201
410-706-1849
Fax: 410-706-0295
Email: enviRN@son.umaryland.edu
Web: http://envirn.umaryland.edu

EnviRN is an interactive and dynamic resource with timely and accurate information on environmental health and nursing for the purpose of preventing environmental disease by improving the knowledge and skills of nurses and health professionals in preventing and intervening with environmental health problems. Based at the University of Maryland's School of Nursing, this resource is a "virtual nursing village" for sharing teaching strategies, practice guidance, information, and research on nursing and environmental health.

Environmental Protection Agency (EPA)

Ariel Rios Building
1200 Pennsylvania Avenue, NW
Washington, D.C. 20460
202-564-4700
Web: http://www.epa.gov

The EPA is a government agency with a mission to protect human health and the environment. The EPA has several federal offices including but not limited to Homeland Security, Children's Health Protection, Civil Rights, Cooperative Environmental Management, Environmental Appeals Board, and Environmental Education. Regional offices are located throughout the United States and are responsible for states' carrying out the mission of the EPA.

The Children's Health Protection site (http://yosemite. epa.gov/ochp/ochpweb.nsf/content/homepage.htm) contains information about children's environmental hazards, health topics, and tips to protect children from environmental hazards. The EPA's aging initiative (http:// www.epa.gov/aging/index.htm) will prioritize and study environmental health hazards to older persons. The Web site provides a wealth of information to protect the environmental health of older persons. IRIS (http://www. epa.gov/iris/index.html), developed by the EPA and its Office of Research and Development, National Center for Environmental Assessment, is a database of human health effects that may result from exposure to various substances found in the environment.

EthnoMed

University of Washington
Seattle, Washington
Web: http://www.ethnomed.org

The Web site contains information about cultural beliefs, medical issues, and other related issues pertinent to the health care of recent immigrants to the United States, many of whom are refugees fleeing war-torn parts of the world. It includes culturally specific information about a broad range of immigrant groups.

Families USA

1201 New York Avenue NW
Suite 1100
Washington, D.C. 20005
202-628-3030
FAX: 202-347-2417
Email: info@familiesusa.org
Web: http://www.familiesusa.org

Families USA is a national nonprofit, nonpartisan organization dedicated to the achievement of high-quality, affordable health care for all Americans. Working at the national, state, and community levels, the organization has earned a national reputation as an effective voice for health care consumers for over 20 years.

Federal Bureau of Investigation (FBI)

J. Edgar Hoover Building
935 Pennsylvania Avenue NW
Washington, D.C. 20535-0001
202-324-3000
Web: http://www.fbi.gov

The FBI investigates violations of federal criminal law; protects the United States from foreign intelligence and terrorist activities; and provides leadership and law enforcement assistance to federal, state, local, and international agencies. The Web site provides information on how to report various crimes.

Federal Emergency Management Agency (FEMA)

500 C Street SW
Washington, D.C. 20472
1-800-621-FEMA (3362)
Web: http://www.fema.gov

FEMA, an entity of the U.S. Department of Homeland Security (DHS) since 2003, leads the effort to prepare the nation for all hazards and effectively manage federal response and recovery efforts following any national incident.

Find Law

Web: http://www.findlaw.com

This is an official site for finding lawyers and legal resources.

FirstGov for Consumers

Email: gateway@ftc.gov
Web: http://www.consumer.gov

FirstGov for Consumers is a link to a broad range of federal departments and information resources for consumers from the U.S. federal government. Information includes food, health and safety, money, transportation, children, and home and community. The site also has an "In the Spotlight" section that highlights new educational and consumer awareness campaigns such as scam alerts and identity theft.

Food and Drug Administration (FDA)

U.S. Food and Drug Administration
5600 Fishers Lane
Rockville, Maryland 20857-0001
1-888-INFO-FDA (1-888-463-6332)
Web: http://www.fda.gov

FDA is a federal agency with the mission of promoting and protecting the public's health by helping consumers receive safe and effective products through market systems in a timely manner, monitoring the safety of products, and helping the public receive accurate, science-based information about products.

Food Safety and Inspection Service (FSIS)

U.S. Department of Health & Human Services
200 Independence Avenue SW
Washington, D.C. 20201
402-344-5000, Hotline 1-800-233-3935
FAX: 402-344-5005
Email: TechCenter@fsis.usda.gov
Web: http://www.fsis.usda.gov

The FSIS is the public health agency in the U.S. Department of Agriculture responsible for ensuring that the nation's commercial supply of meat, poultry, and egg products is safe, wholesome, and correctly labeled and packaged. There are many offices that make up the FSIS. Details about these offices as well as educational materials, regulation and policy, food defense, and emergency response information can be found on the FSIS Web site.

Francois-Xavier Bagnoud Center for Health and Human Rights

Harvard School of Public Health
651 Huntington Avenue, 7th floor
Boston, Massachusetts 02115
617-432-0656
FAX: 1-617-432 4310
Email: fxbcenter@igc.org
Web: http://www.hsph.harvard.edu

The Center for Health and Human Rights was founded at the Harvard School of Public Health in 1993 through a gift from the Association François-Xavier Bagnoud. The François-Xavier Bagnoud Center for Health and Human Rights is the first academic center to focus exclusively on health and human rights. It combines the academic strengths of research and teaching with a strong commitment to service and policy development. Center faculty work at international and national levels through collaboration and partnerships with health and human rights practitioners, governmental and nongovernmental organizations, academic institutions, and international agencies to do the following:

- Expand knowledge through scholarship, professional training, and public education
- Develop domestic and international policy focusing on the relationship between health and human rights in a global perspective
- Engage scholars, public health and human rights practitioners, public officials, donors, and activists in the health and human rights movement.

Free to Grow (FTG)

Mailman School of Public Health
Columbia University
722 West 168th Street, 8th Floor
New York, New York 10032
212-305-8120
FAX: 212-342-1963
Email: info@freetogrow.org
Web: http://www.freetogrow.org

The Free To Grow–Head Start partnership is a national program supported by the Robert Wood Johnson Foundation and the Doris Duke Charitable Foundation to promote substance-free communities. The site offers information on community assessment approaches and links to community assessment strategies. There are 15 Free To Grow sites in the United States collaborating with schools, law enforcement, and mental health programs using community-based efforts to strengthen the environment of young children, families, and communities to prevent substance abuse and child abuse.

General Accounting Office (GAO)

441 G Street NW
Washington, D.C. 20548
202-512-3000
Email: contact@gao.gov
Web: http://www.gao.gov

The U.S. Government Accountability Office (GAO) is an independent, nonpartisan agency that works for Congress. GAO is often called the "congressional watchdog" because it investigates how the federal government spends taxpayer dollars. GAO gathers information to help Congress determine how well executive branch agencies are doing their jobs. GAO's work routinely answers such basic questions as whether government programs are meeting their objectives or providing good service to the public. Ultimately, GAO ensures that government is accountable to the American people. To that end, GAO provides senators and representatives with the best information available—information that is accurate, timely, and balanced—to help them arrive at informed policy decisions.

Guide for Wellness Professionals

Web: http://www.bsu.edu

This Web site provides the reader with history, benefits, limitations, uses, and recommendation for using health risk appraisals. The goal is to help wellness professionals make informed choices from available instruments and vendors.

Hartford Geriatric Nursing Initiative (HGNI)

American Academy of Nursing
Coordinating Center
888 17th Street NW, Suite 800
Washington, D.C. 20006
Email: BAGNC@aannet.org
Web: http://www.geriatricnursing.org; http://www.hartfordign.org

HGNI was launched in 1995 and confronts the challenges associated with an aging client patient population through an array of programs. With a $60 million investment from the John Hartford Foundation, HGNI is preparing professional nurses to play leadership roles in improving the health of older adults. Programs are aimed at nursing practice, education, research, leadership, and public policy. The program aims are to increase the supply of geriatric nurses and the quality of care they provide by enhancing geriatric nursing training programs that produce the leaders of tomorrow. This Web site was developed by the independent evaluator of the Hartford Geriatric Nursing Initiative, The Measurement Group. This Web site highlights the programs of the Initiative and provides links to

other Web sites supported by the Initiative. The Web site also presents emerging evaluation results that show the outcomes and impact of these programs.

Hastings Center

Web: http://www.ascensionhealth.org

Founded in 1969, The Hastings Center is an independent organization comprised of health care providers and scientists, lawyers, philosophers, corporate executives, and government officials dedicated to advanced research and studies in biomedical ethics. The center publishes The Hastings Center Report, a quarterly journal focused on issues in health care ethics. The Web site provides access to the publications.

Health Care Education Association (HCEA)

P.O. Box 388
Florissant, Missouri 63032-0388
1-888-298-3861
FAX: 314-869-5811
Email: Hcea03@cox.net
Web: http://www.hcea-info.org

HCEA is a professional organization of educators whose mission is to support and mentor health care educators to provide a learning community for professionals committed to improving health care and the organizations they serve through education. Full services require membership to the association, but there is information on educational products, programs, and publications that can be accessed without membership.

Health Care for the Homeless (HCH) Programs

202-462-4822, ext. 19
Email: mstoops@nationalhomeless.org
Web: http://www.nationalhomeless.org

HCH provides for primary health care and substance abuse services at locations accessible to people who are homeless; emergency care with referrals to hospitals for inpatient care services and/or other needed services; and outreach services to assist difficult-to-reach homeless persons in accessing care and to provide assistance in establishing eligibility for entitlement programs and housing.

Health Care without Harm (HCWH)

HCWH—U.S. & Canada
Colleen Funkhouser
HCWH Membership Services
1901 North Moore Street, Suite 509
Arlington, Virginia 22209
703-243-0056
FAX: 866-438-5769
Email: cfunkhouser@hcwh.org
Web: http://www.noharm.org

HCWH is an international coalition of hospitals and health care organizations, community groups, health care providers, environmental and religious groups, labor unions, and health-affected constituencies who work collectively to improve health by working to reduce pollution in the health care industry.

Health Disparities Collaborative

1201 New York Avenue NW
Suite 1100
Washington, D.C. 20005
202-628-3030
FAX: 202-347-2417
Web: http://www.healthdisparities.net
The mission of the Health Disparities Collaborative is to improve access to high-quality, culturally and linguistically competent primary and preventive care for underserved, uninsured, and underinsured Americans.

Health Education Assets Library (HEAL)

Email: info@healcentral.org
Web: http://www.healcentral.org
HEAL is a digital library that provides free and accessible digital teaching resources of the highest degree that meet the needs of health sciences educators and learners. Resources go through rigorous peer review to assure high quality materials.

Health Education Resource Exchange (HERE in Washington)

Washington State Department of Health
Office of Health Promotion
P.O. Box 47833
Olympia, Washington 98504-7833
Email: HERE@doh.wa.gov
Web: http://www.doh.wa.gov
The site provides public health education and health promotion projects, materials, and resources in the state of Washington and is designed to help community health professionals share their experience with colleagues around the state. There is a menu including community projects, educational materials, a health educator's toolbox, a link to make connections with other health professionals and organizations, a calendar of conferences and training opportunities, relevant health education literature, and links to other health Web sites.

Health Information

Web: http://www.health.nih.gov
This National Institutes of Health's site provides information on body location/systems, conditions/diseases, health and wellness, health newsletters, health databases, health hotlines, and federal health agencies.

Health Resources and Services Administration (HRSA)

5600 Fishers Lane
Rockville, Maryland 20857
Web: http://www.hrsa.gov
HRSA, an agency of the U.S. Department of Health and Human Services, has offices throughout the United States and territories. HRSA provides national leadership, program resources and services needed to improve access to health care services for people who are uninsured, isolated or medically underserved. To achieve this mission, HRSA provides leadership and financial support to health care providers in every state and U.S. territory. HRSA also oversees organ, tissue and bone marrow donation and supports programs that prepare against bioterrorism, compensate individuals harmed by vaccination, and maintains databases that protect against health care malpractice and health care waste, fraud and abuse.

Healthfinders

National Health Information Center
P.O. Box 1133
Washington, D.C. 20013-1133
Email: healthfinder@nhic.org
Web: http://www.healthfinder.gov
Developed by the DHHS and other federal agencies, Healthfinders is a useful and informative Web site for consumers and health professionals.

Healthier Students Health Risk Appraisals

Web: http://www.csupomona.edu
The Health Risk Appraisals Web site, developed by Jim Grizzell (Student Health Services, California State Polytechnic University, Pomona, CA), provides a slide presentation and other resources from Healthy People 2010 National College Health Objectives. The Web site topics include injury prevention, alcohol abuse, tobacco use, sexual behaviors, dietary behaviors, and physical activity.

Healthier U.S. Government

The U.S. Department of Health and Human Services
200 Independence Avenue SW
Washington, D.C. 20201
202-619-0257; 1-877-696-6775
Web: http://www.healthierus.gov
This Web site is an outline of government Web sites promoting healthy lifestyles. It provides links to physical fitness, disease/illness prevention, nutrition, making healthy choices, and many other government sites.

Healthier Worksite Initiative, Centers for Disease Control and Prevention

1600 Clifton Road
Atlanta, Georgia 30333
404-639-3311
Web: http://www.cdc.gov

The Healthier Worksite Initiative addresses worksite health promotion. The Web site summarizes how to use a health risk appraisal, important considerations for implementation, and ethical considerations. The content source is the Division of Nutrition and Physical Activity, National Center for Chronic Disease Prevention and Health Promotion.

HealthWeb

Web: http://healthweb.org

HealthWeb, supported by the National Library of Medicine, is a collaborative project of the health sciences libraries of the Greater Midwest Region of the National Network of Libraries of Medicine and those of the Committee for Institutional Cooperation. HealthWeb provides organized access to evaluated noncommercial, health-related, Internet-accessible resources. The Web site, http://healthweb.org/rural, provides links to a wide national collection of rural health resources.

Healthy Carolinians, North Carolina Health Assessment

Office of Healthy Carolinians
Division of Public Health
1916 Mail Service Center
Raleigh, North Carolina 27699-1916
919-707-5150
FAX: 919-870-4833
Email: hcinfo@ncmail.net
Web: http://www.healthycarolinians.org

Healthy Carolinians, North Carolina Health Assessment provides links to a community assessment guidebook, assessment information and partnership development, and community health opinion survey.

Healthy People 2010

Web: http://www.healthypeople.gov

Healthy People 2010 provides a framework for prevention for the nation. It is a statement of national health objectives designed to identify the most significant preventable threats to health and to establish national goals to reduce these threats. The Healthy People 2010 home page includes all the national health objectives and publications and data that support them.

Healthy Schools Network, Inc. (HSN)

110 Maryland Avenue NE, Suite 505
Washington, D.C. 20002
202-543-7555
Web: http://www.healthyschools.org

HSN is a nonprofit national organization with a focus on environmental health, dedicated to ensuring that children and school employees have environmentally safe and healthy schools.

Human Rights Education Association (HREA)

P.O. Box 382396
Cambridge, Massachusetts 02238
Visiting address:
97 Lowell Road
Concord, Massachusetts 01742
978-341-0200
FAX: 978-341-0201
E-mail: info@hrea.org
Web: http://www.hrea.org

HREA is an international nongovernmental organization that supports human rights learning, the training of activists and professionals. the development of educational materials and programming. and community-building through online technologies. HREA is dedicated to quality education and training to promote understanding, attitudes, and actions to protect human rights and to foster the development of peaceable, free, and just communities. HREA works with individuals, nongovernmental organizations, intergovernmental organizations, and governments interested in implementing human rights education programs. The services provided by HREA are

- Assistance in Curriculum and Materials Development
- Training of professional groups
- Research and evaluation
- Clearinghouse of education and training materials
- Networking human rights advocates and educators

Human Rights Watch

1630 Connecticut Avenue NW, Suite 500
Washington, D.C. 20009
202-612-4321
FAX: 202-612-4333
Email: hrwdc@hrw.org
Web: http://www.hrw.org

Human Rights Watch is a major international human rights organization dedicated to protecting the human rights of people around the world. Its mission is to prevent discrimination, to uphold political freedom, to protect people from inhumane conduct in wartime, and to bring offenders to justice by challenging governments and those who hold power to end abusive practices and respect international human rights law. Human Rights Watch is an independent, nongovernmental organization, supported by contributions from private individuals and foundations worldwide. It accepts no government funds, directly or indirectly.

Indian Health Service (IHS)

The Reyes Building
801 Thompson Avenue, Suite 400
Rockville, Maryland 20852-1627
301-443-3024
Web: http://www.ihs.gov

The mission of the IHS is to raise the physical, mental, social, and spiritual health of American Indians and Alaska Natives to the highest level. The IHS Web site is a resource for American Indian and Alaska Native health history, data and trends, health information, and patient education protocols to ensure that comprehensive, culturally acceptable personal and public health services are available and accessible to American Indian and Alaska Native people.

Institute of Medicine (IOM)

500 Fifth Street, NW
Washington, D.C. 20001
202-334-2352
FAX: 202-334-1412
Email: iomwww@nas.edu
Web: http://www.iom.edu

IOM, a nonprofit organization, provides scientifically informed advice and information concerning biomedical science, medicine, and health. Its mission is to be an adviser to the nation to improve health. One of its topics is environmental health, and it sponsors a Roundtable on Environmental Health Sciences, Research, and Medicine, established to encourage discussion and dialogue to illuminate environmental issues. An IOM report specific to nursing and the environmental is Nursing, Health, and the Environment, which can be accessed at http://www.nap.edu/books/030905298X/html/index.html.

International Health Economics Association (IHEA)

902-461-4432
Web: http://www.healtheconomics.org

This is the Web site of one of the largest international organization's specifically for health economists. This organization interprets economics quite widely, focusing both on evaluation and on using economic theory to explain individual behaviors and organizational decisions related to health. The Web site is largely aimed at health economics professionals, but it includes several items of interest to those with only an interest in health economics rather than only professionals. In particular, the Web site lists conferences, books, and educational opportunities related to health economics.

International Society for Health and Human Rights (ISHHR)

P.O. Box 203
Fairfield NSW 2163
Australia
+61-2-9794-1900
FAX: +61-2-9794-1910
Email: istartts@s054.aone.net.au
Web: http://www.ishhr.org

The aim of this Web site is to bring colleagues a bit closer to each other and represent a forum where information on human rights and useful experiences can be presented and shared. ISHHR has members in almost 50 countries worldwide. The human rights issue is a very important one for health workers, and as health professionals. Sharing with each other on this Web site provides an opportunity for communication between professionals as an active defense of human rights.

International Society for Pharmacoeconomics and Outcomes Research (USA)

Email: info@ispor.org
Web: http://www.ispor.org

This Web site is the home page of one of the premier organizations supporting professionals whose business is economic evaluation. The word "Pharmacoeconomics" in the title suggests that this organization focuses largely on the evaluation of pharmaceutical products, but this is not the organization's exclusive focus. This Web site lists upcoming conferences, has links to lists of requirements for economic evaluations that have been put forward in different countries, and includes an "educator's tool kit" that lists several books that may be of interest to those learning about pharmacoeconomics and economic evaluation more generally.

Juvenile Diabetes Research Foundation International (JDRF)

120 Wall Street, 19th Floor
New York, New York 10005
1-800-533-CURE (2873)
FAX: (212) 785-9595
Email: info@jdrf.org
Web: http://www.jdrf.org

The mission of the JDRF is to find a cure for diabetes and its complications through the support of research. JDRF, with chapters from coast to coast and affiliates around the world, gives more money to diabetes research than any other nonprofit, nongovernmental health agency in the world. The Web site is a resource for education, research and ongoing clinical trials, funding opportunities, and publications relevant to juvenile diabetes.

Kaiser Family Foundation

2400 Sand Hill Road
Menlo Park, California 94025
650-854-9400
FAX: 650-854-4800
Web: http://www.kff.org

The Henry J. Kaiser Family Foundation is a nonprofit, private operating foundation focusing on the major health care issues facing the nation. The Foundation is an independent voice and source of facts and analysis for policy makers, the media, the health care community, and the general public. KFF develops and runs its own research and communications programs, often in partnership with outside organizations. The Foundation contracts with a wide range of outside individuals and organizations through its programs. The Foundation is not associated with Kaiser Permanente or Kaiser Industries.

KaiserEDU

Web: http://www.kaiserEDU.org

KaiserEDU is an online health policy resource for faculty and students. It is designed to provide students, faculty, and others interested in learning about health policy easy access to the latest data, research, analysis, and developments in health policy. KaiserEDU.org was developed to provide a clearinghouse of introductory materials on major areas of health care policy, particularly for students and faculty in health policy and related disciplines, as well as for anyone interested in learning more about health policy. The site provides a range of resources, including narrated slide lectures and collections of background materials, including research, data, and policy analysis, on the key issues at the forefront of health policy. The site also includes concise summaries of more narrow policy debates along with links to background materials, including policy reports, articles published in the peer-reviewed literature, and key data. Other features include a library of syllabi from health policy courses across the United States, a compilation of fellowships for students and professionals interested in health policy, a summary of the major government agencies involved in health policy, and links to datasets available for further research.

KidsHealth

Web: http://www.kidshealth.org

KidsHealth is a Web site by the Nemours, one of the largest children's health systems. The site is a resource of up-to-date, health care provider-approved information on growth, food and fitness, childhood infections, immunizations, and medical conditions for parents, kids, and teens. There are separate areas for kids, teens, and parents with age-appropriate content and delivery. In-depth features, articles, animations, games, and resources have been developed by experts in the health of children and teens.

LifeSkills Training (LST)

National Health Promotion Associates
711 Westchester Avenue
White Plains, New York 10604
914-421-2525 or 1-800-293-4969
FAX: 914-421-2007
Email: lstinfo@nhpamail.com
Web: http://www.lifeskillstraining.com

LST is a substance abuse prevention program for adolescents to reduce the risks of alcohol, tobacco, drug abuse, and violence. This comprehensive program, developed by Dr. Gilbert J. Botvin, targets psychosocial predictors of substance use and other risky behaviors and provides teens with confidence and skills needed to resist pressures that lead to drug use. The LifeSkills Training program is recognized as a Model or Exemplary program by an array of government agencies including the U.S. Department of Education and the Center for Substance Abuse Prevention.

Mayo Clinic Health Solutions

Mayo Clinic Health Management Resources
Centerplace 4, 200 First Street SW
Rochester, Minnesota 55905
1-800-430-9699
FAX: 507-284-5410
Email: MayoClinicHealthManagementResources@mayo.edu
Web: http://mayoclinichealthmanagementresources.com

This health risk appraisal has a unique emphasis on health education and behavior change. The tool is designed to identify risks within a population, deliver follow-up interventions for those at risk, and track and analyze population health trends over time.

Medicare Payment Advisory Commission (MedPAC)

601 New Jersey Avenue NW, Suite 9000
Washington, D.C. 20001
202-220-3700
Email: webmaster@medpac.gov
Web: http://www.medpac.gov

The Medicare Payment Advisory Commission (MedPAC) is an independent federal body established by the Balanced Budget Act of 1997 (P.L. 105-33) to advise the U.S. Congress on issues affecting the Medicare program. The commission's statutory mandate is quite broad: In addition to advising the Congress on payments to private health plans participating in Medicare and providers in Medicare's traditional fee-for-service program, MedPAC is also tasked with analyzing access to care, quality of care, and other issues affecting Medicare.

Medline Plus

U.S. National Library of Medicine
8600 Rockville Pike
Bethesda, Maryland 20894
Web: http://www.nlm.nih.gov

Medline Plus is a service of the U.S. National Library of
Medicine and the National Institutes of Health, provides
information on health topics, drugs and supplements, and
current health news, and features a medical encyclopedia
and health care directories.

Midwest Nursing Research Society (MNRS)

10200 West 44th Avenue, Suite 304
Wheat Ridge, Colorado 80033
1-866-908-8617
FAX: 303-422-8894
Email: mnrs@resourcenter.com
Web: http://www.mnrs.org

MNRS, with membership in the Midwest region of the United
States, advances the scientific basis of nursing practice and
promotes development of nurse scientist. Their promoting,
disseminating, and utilizing nursing research throughout
the Midwest has profoundly influenced the growth in
quality and quantity of nursing research for more than
30 years. Their Web site offers more information about
MNRS and the many sections of members who share
research interests.

Minority Health Agency for Healthcare Research and Quality

Web: http://www.ahrq.gov

This Web site contains multiple resources for health care
researchers, health care providers, and policy makers
to address racial and ethnic minority heath disparities,
including research documents, requests for proposal, and
summaries of funded research.

National Advisory Committee on Rural Health and Human Services

c/o Office of Rural Health Policy
Health Resources and Services Administration
5600 Fishers Lane, 9A-55
Rockville, Maryland 20857
301-443-0835
FAX: 301-443-2803
Web: http://www.ruralcommittee.hrsa.gov

The National Advisory Committee on Rural Health and
Human Services, a 21-member citizens' panel of nationally
recognized experts, provides recommendations on rural
health and human services issues to the Secretary of the
Department of Health and Human Services.

National Alliance to End Homelessness

1518 K Street NW, Suite 206
Washington, D.C. 20005
Email: naeh@naeh.org
Web: http://www.endhomelessness.org

The National Alliance to End Homelessness is a nonprofit
organization whose mission is to mobilize the nonprofit,
public, and private sectors of society in an alliance to end
homelessness.

National Area Health Education Centers (NAHECs)

109 VIP Drive, Suite 220
Wexford, Pennsylvania 15090
1-888-412-7424
FAX: 724-935-1560
Email: info@nationalahec.org
Web: http://bhpr.hrsa.gov

NAHEC is an academic-community partnership focused on
improving the supply, diversity, distribution and quality
of the health workforce. Health care providers are trained
in rural and underserved sites and are responsive to local
needs.

National Association of Colored Graduate Nurses (NACGN)

8630 Fenton Street, Suite 330
Silver Spring, Maryland 20910-3803
Web: http://www.aaregistry.com

The National Association of Colored Graduate Nurses was
established in 1908 by Martha Franklin to advance public
health training in nursing schools where African Americans were trained.

National Association of Community Health Centers, Inc. (NACHC)

7200 Wisconsin Avenue, Suite 210
Bethesda, Maryland 20814
301-347-0400
FAX: 301-347-0459
Web: http://www.nachc.com

Founded in 1970, NACHC is a nonprofit organization whose
mission is to enhance and expand access to quality,
community-responsive health care for America's medically underserved and uninsured. In serving its mission,
NACHC represents the nation's network of over 1,000
federally qualified health centers (FQHCs), which serve
16 million people through 5,000 sites located in all of the
50 states, Puerto Rico, the District of Columbia, the U.S.
Virgin Islands, and Guam.

National Association of City and County Health Officials (NACCHO)

1100 17th Street, NW, second floor
Washington, D.C. 20036
202-783-5550
Fax: 202-783-1583
Web: http://www.naccho.org

NACCHO is the national voice of local public health agencies across the United States. It supports efforts to protect and promote the public's health through national policies, resources and programs, and effective public health practice and systems.

National Association of Local Boards of Health (NALBOH)

1840 East Gypsy Lane Road
Bowling Green, Ohio 43462
419-353-7714
FAX: 419-352-6278
Email: nalboh@nalboh.org
Web: http://www.nalboh.org

NALBOH vision is to represent the grassroots foundation of public health in America, actively engaging and serving the public by empowering boards of health through education and training. NALBOH's mission is to prepare and strengthen boards of health, empowering them to promote and protect the health of their communities through education, training, and technical assistance. The Web site provides information and links to various health-related organizations that NALBOH works with.

National Association of School Nurses (NASN)

8484 Georgia Avenue, Suite 420
Silver Spring, Maryland 20910
240-821-1130; 1-866-627-6767
FAX: 301-585-1791
Email: nasn@nasn.org
Web: http://www.nasn.org

NASN improves the health and educational success of children and youth by developing and providing leadership to advance school nursing practice. It advances school nursing practice to improve the health of school-aged children and promote their academic success.

National Association of School-Based Health Centers (NASBHC)

202-638-5872, ext 200
Web: http://www.nasbhc.org

NASBHC is a national multidisciplinary group that represents people who support, receive, and provide health care in schools and school-connected programs. The organization provides advocacy, leadership, resources, and technical assistance to build the capacity and sustainability of school-based health care. School health resources are available.

National Black Nurses Association (NBNA)

8630 Fenton Street, Suite 330
Silver Spring, Maryland 20910-3803
FAX: 301-589-3223
Web: http://www.nbna.com

The National Black Nurses Association was organized in 1971 under the leadership of Dr. Lauranne Sams, former dean and professor of nursing, School of Nursing, Tuskegee University, Tuskegee, Alabama. NBNA is a nonprofit organization incorporated on September 2, 1972, in the state of Ohio. The NBNA represents approximately 150,000 African American nurses to "investigate, define and determine what the health care needs of African Americans are and to implement change to make available to African Americans and other minorities health care commensurate with that of the larger society."

National Cancer Institute (NCI)

NCI Public Inquiries Office
6116 Executive Boulevard
Room 3036A
Bethesda, Maryland 20892-8322
1-800-422-6237
Web: http://www.cancer.gov

NCI is a component of the National Institutes of Health, one of eight agencies that compose the Public Health Service in the Department of Health and Human Services. The NCI, established under the National Cancer Institute Act of 1937, is the federal government's principal agency for cancer research and training. The National Cancer Act of 1971 broadened the scope and responsibilities of the NCI and created the National Cancer Program. Over the years, legislative amendments have maintained the NCI authorities and responsibilities and added new information dissemination mandates as well as a requirement to assess the incorporation of state-of-the-art cancer treatments into clinical practice. The National Cancer Institute coordinates the National Cancer Program, which conducts and supports research, training, health information dissemination, and other programs with respect to the cause, diagnosis, prevention, and treatment of cancer, rehabilitation from cancer, and the continuing care of cancer clients and the families of cancer clients.

National Cancer Institute Clear and Simple Program

NCI Public Inquiries Office
6116 Executive Boulevard, Room 3036A
Bethesda, Maryland 20892-8322
1-800-422-6237
Email: cancergovstaff@mail.nih.gov
Web: http://www.cancer.gov

The site provides a basis and introduction for producing health education materials, specifically for those with low literacy levels. The content was developed using the following five: (1) define the target audience, (2) conduct target audience research, (3) develop a concept for the product, (4) develop content and visuals, and (5) pretest and revise draft materials.

National Center for Environmental Health, Centers for Disease Control and Prevention (NCEH)

1600 Clifton Road
Atlanta, Georgia 30333
404-639-3311; 888-232-6348
Email: cdcinfo@cdc.gov
Web: http://www.cdc.gov

The NCEH aims at promoting American's health and quality of life by preventing or controlling illness, disability, or death that results from interactions between people and their environment. NCEH is particularly committed to safeguarding the health of populations that are particularly vulnerable to certain environmental hazards—children, the elderly, and people with disabilities. The NCEH offers data, information, publications, and programs and training opportunities that relate to environmental health.

National Center for Farmworker Health (NCFH)

1770 FM 967
Buda, Texas 78610
512-312-2700; 1-800-531-5120
Email: info@ncfh.org
Web: http://www.ncfh.org

NCFH, a private nonprofit corporation established in 1975, has a mission to improve the health status of farmworker families through the appropriate application of human, technical, and information resources. They have a network of more than five hundred migrant health center service sites in the United States as well as other organizations and individuals serving the farmworker population. Their Web site has information about the life of migrant workers, including their housing problems, work conditions, health problems, and their children.

National Center for Health Statistics (NCHS)

3311 Toledo Road
Hyattsville, Maryland 20782
301-458-4000, toll free data inquiries: 1-866-441-NCHS
Email: nchsquery@cdc.gov
Web: http://www.cdc.gov

The National Center for Health Statistics is a part of the CDC. NCHS provides us with information about the health status of the population and important subgroups. Statistics are used to identify disparities in health status and use of health care by race/ethnicity, socioeconomic status, region, and other important population characteristics. Health statistics from the NCHS are also used to monitor trends in health status and care delivery, identify health problems, and support biomedical and health services research. Statistical information provides information for making policy and program changes and evaluating the impact of policy and programs. Health, United States is an annual report on trends in health statistics. This report can be accessed at http://www.cdc.gov/nchs/hus.htm.

National Center for Policy Analysis (NCPA)

601 Pennsylvania Avenue NW, Suite 900 South Building
Washington, D.C. 20004
202-220-3082
FAX: 202-220-3096
Email: govrel@ncpa.org
Web: http://www.ncpa.org

NCPA is a nonprofit, nonpartisan public policy research organization, established in 1983. The NCPA's goal is to develop and promote private alternatives to government regulation and control, solving problems by relying on the strength of the competitive, entrepreneurial private sector. Topics include reforms in health care, taxes, Social Security, welfare, criminal justice, education, and environmental regulation.

National Center on Minority Health and Health Disparities (NCMHD)

National Institutes of Health
6706 Democracy Boulevard, Suite 800
MSC-5465
Bethesda, Maryland 20892-5464
301-402-1366
FAX: 301-480-4049
Email: NCMHDinfo@od.nih.gov
Web: http://ncmhd.nih.gov

The mission of NCMHD is to promote minority health and to lead, coordinate, support, and assess the NIH effort to reduce and ultimately eliminate health disparities. In this effort, NCMHD will conduct and support basic, clinical, social, and behavioral research, promote research infrastructure and training, foster emerging programs, disseminate information, and reach out to minority and other health disparity communities.

National Cholesterol Education Program, National Heart, Lung, and Blood Institute

Health Information Center
Attention: Web Site
P.O. Box 30105
Bethesda, Maryland 20824-0105
301-592-8573
FAX: 240 629 3246
Email: nhlbiinfo@nhlbi.nih.gov
Web: http://www.nhlbi.nih.gov

The goal of the National Cholesterol Education Program is to reduce the percentage of Americans with high blood cholesterol. Links are provided to program description, roster and meeting notes of the coordinating committee, health-related information for clients as well as health care providers, and clinical practice guidelines for cholesterol management in adults.

National Coalition for Homeless Veterans (NCHV)

3331/2 Pennsylvania Avenue SE
Washington, D.C. 20003-1148
1-800-VET-HELP
FAX: 202-546-2063
Email: nchv@nchv.org

NCHV's mission is to end homelessness among veterans by shaping public policy, promoting collaboration, and building the capacity of service providers.

National Coalition for the Homeless (NCH)

2201 P Street NW
Washington, D.C. 20037
202-462-4822
FAX: 202-462-4823
Email: Info@nationalhomeless.org
Web: http://www.nationalhomeless.org

The NCH, founded in 1984, is a national network of people who are currently experiencing or who have experienced homelessness, activists and advocates, community-based and faith-based service providers, and others committed to a single mission. That mission, which is a common bond, is to end homelessness. NCH is committed to creating the systemic and attitudinal changes necessary to prevent and end homelessness. At the same time, it works to meet the immediate needs of people who are currently experiencing homelessness or who are at risk of doing so. NCH takes as its first principle of practice that people who are currently experiencing homelessness or have formerly experienced homelessness must be actively involved in all of its work.

National Commission for Health Education Credentialing (NCHEC)

1541 Alta Drive, Suite 303
Whitehall, Pennsylvania 18052-5642
1-888-624-3248
FAX: 1-800-813-0727
Web: http://www.nchec.org

NCHEC's mission is to improve the practice of health education and to serve the public and profession of health education by certifying health education specialists, promoting professional development, and strengthening professional preparation and practice. The Web site provides information about responsibilities and competencies for health educators.

National Council of La Raza (NCLR)

Raul Yzaguirre Building
1126 16th Street, NW
Washington, D.C. 20036
202-785-1670
FAX: 202-776-1792
Email: comments@nclr.org
Web: http://www.nclr.org

NCLR is the largest Latino civil rights and advocacy organization in the United States. NCLR oversees five key areas—assets/investments, civil rights/immigration, education, employment and economic status, and health. It also provides capacity-building assistance to its affiliates who work at the state and local level to advance opportunities for individuals and families.

National Diabetes Education Program (NDEP)

One Diabetes Way
Bethesda, Maryland 20814-9692
301-496-3583
Email: ndep@mail.nih.gov
Web: http://www.ndep.nih.gov

NDEP is a partnership of the National Institutes of Health, the Centers for Disease Control and Prevention, and more than 200 public and private organizations. The site provides information on how to prevent or control diabetes, offering resources for health education, awareness campaigns, and partnerships.

National Diabetes Information Clearinghouse

1 Information Way
Bethesda, Maryland 20892-3560
301-654-3333, 1-800-860-8747
FAX: 301-907-8906
Email: ndic@info.niddk.nih.gov
Web: http://www.niddk.nih.gov

The National Diabetes Information Clearinghouse, a service of the National Institute of Diabetes and Digestive and Kidney Diseases, provides educational materials and educational programs on diabetes, digestive diseases, endocrine and metabolic diseases, hematologic diseases, and kidney and urologic diseases.

National Eye Institute's National Eye Health Education Program (NEHEP)

2020 Vision Place
Bethesda, Maryland 20892-3655
301-496-5248
Email: 2020@nei.nih.gov
Web: http://www.nei.nih.gov

NEHEP conducts large-scale public and professional education programs in partnership with national organizations. Their goal is to ensure that vision is a health priority by translating eye and vision research into public and professional education programs. Their Web site provides information about NEHEP's education programs and free educational materials and public service announcements.

National Health Policy Forum (NHPF)

2131 K Street NW, Suite 500
Washington, D.C. 20037
202-872-1390
FAX: 202-862-9837
Email: nhpf@gwu.edu
Web: http://www.nhpf.org

NHPF was created in 1971 by senior-level congressional staff and executive agency decision makers to address their information needs and provide a safe harbor for open and frank conversations. The NHPF seeks to inform the public policy process by helping participants—federal health policy makers in the legislative and executive branches and in congressional support agencies—engage in rigorous, constructive, and respectful dialogue. NHPF is a nonpartisan organization that does not advocate particular policy positions. It provides a forum covering a broad range of health policy topics that allows for honest exchange of ideas and viewpoints.

National High Blood Pressure Education Program (NHBPEP)

NHLBI Health Information Center
P.O. Box 30105
Bethesda, Maryland 20824-0105
301-592-8573
FAX: 301-592-8563
Email: nhlbiinfo@nhlbi.nih.gov
Web: http://www.nhlbi.nih.gov

The NHBPEP is a cooperative effort among professional and voluntary health agencies, state health departments, and many community groups and is coordinated by the National Heart, Lung, and Blood Institute. The goal of the NHBPEP is to reduce death and disability related to high blood pressure through programs of professional, client, and public education. The NHBPEP Web site features links to program description, roster and meeting notes of the coordinating committee, health-related information for clients and health care professionals, and a guide to lowering high blood pressure.

National Institute for Occupational Safety and Health (NIOSH)

Centers for Disease Control and Prevention
1600 Clifton Road
Atlanta, Georgia 30333
1-800-35-NIOSH
Web: http://www.cdc.gov

NIOSH, part of the Centers for Disease Control and Prevention in the U.S. Department of Health and Human Services, is the federal agency responsible for conducting research and making recommendations for the prevention of work-related injury and illness. Their disease and injury program targets prevention of infectious diseases such as influenza, blood-borne infectious diseases, severe acute respiratory syndrome (SARS), tuberculosis, and West Nile virus.

National Institute of Diabetes and Digestive and Kidney Disease (NIDDK)

Office of Communications & Public Liaison
Building 31. Room 9A06
31 Center Drive, MSC 2560
Bethesda, Maryland 20892-2560
Web: http://www2.niddk.nih.gov

NIDDK conducts and supports research on many of the most serious diseases affecting public health. The institute supports much of the clinical research on the diseases of internal medicine and related subspecialty fields as well as many basic science disciplines. NIDDK is a resource for health information, research funding opportunities, and reports to Congress and strategic plans relevant to diabetes, digestive, and kidney diseases.

National Institute of Nursing Research (NINR)

National Institutes of Health
31 Center Drive, Room 5B10
Bethesda, Maryland 20892-2178
301-496-0207
FAX: 301-480-8845
Web: http://www.ninr.nih.gov

The mission of NINR is to promote and improve the health of individuals, families, communities, and populations. NINR supports and conducts clinical and basic research and research training on health and illness across the lifespan. The research focus encompasses health promotion and disease prevention, quality of life, health disparities, and end-of-life. NINR seeks to extend nursing science by integrating the biological and behavioral sciences, employing new technologies to research questions, improving research methods, and developing the scientists of the future. The Web site includes information about the NINR and research and funding, training investigators, and news and information.

National Institute on Alcohol Abuse and Alcoholism (NIAAA)

5635 Fishers Lane, MSC 9304
Bethesda, Maryland 20892-9304
Email: niaaaweb-r@exchange.nih.gov
Web: http://www.niaaa.gov

The NIAAA provides leadership in the national effort to reduce alcohol-related problems by conducting and supporting research in a wide range of scientific areas including genetics, neuroscience, epidemiology, and the health risks and benefits of alcohol consumption, prevention, and treatment; coordinating and collaborating with other research institutes and federal programs on alcohol-related issues; collaborating with international, national, state, and local institutions, organizations, agencies, and programs engaged in alcohol-related work; and translating and disseminating research findings to health care providers, researchers, policy makers, and the public. The Web site provides numerous pamphlets, resources, and posters for children, adults, and families regarding alcohol use; it also includes "Helping Patients with Alcohol Problems—A Health Practitioner's Guide."

National Institutes of Environmental Health Sciences (NIEHS)

P.O. Box 12233
111 T.W. Alexander Drive
Research Triangle Park, North Carolina 27709
919-541-3345
Email: webcenter@niehs.nih.gov
Web: http://www.niehs.nih.gov

The NIEHS has a mission to reduce illness and disability by understanding how the environment influences the development and progression of human disease. The NIEHS focuses on clinical research in environmental health science; basic research to understand basic mechanisms of toxicants in human biology; environmental health research programs to address the cross-cutting problems in human biology and human disease; population-focused research; markers of environmental exposure, early (preclinical) biological response, and genetic susceptibility; and multidisciplinary training for researchers.

National Institutes of Health (NIH)

9000 Rockville Pike
Bethesda, Maryland 20892
301-496-4000
Web: http://www.nih.gov

NIH is part of the U.S. Department of Health and Human Services. It is the steward of medical and behavioral research for the nation. Its mission is science in pursuit of fundamental knowledge about the nature and behavior of living systems and the application of that knowledge to extend healthy life and reduce the burdens of illness and disability.

National Nursing Centers Consortium (NNCC)

260 S Broad Street, 18th floor
Philadelphia, Pennsylvania 19102
215-731-7140
FAX: 215-731-2400
Email:Tine@nncc.us
Web: http://www.nncc.us

NNCC represents nurse-managed health centers serving vulnerable people across the country. It strengthens the capacity of its members to provide quality health care services to vulnerable populations and to eliminate health disparities in underserved communities.

National Republican Congressional Committee (NRCC)

320 First Street S
Washington, D.C. 20003
202-479-7000
Web: http://www.nrcc.org

This is the official Web site for the Republican Party. The NRCC's origins date back to 1866, when the Republican caucuses of the House and Senate formed a "Congressional Committee." Today, the NRCC is organized under Section 527 of the Internal Revenue Code. It supports the election of Republicans to the House through direct financial contributions to candidates and Republican Party organizations; provides technical and research assistance to Republican candidates and Party organizations; encourages voter registration, education, and turnout programs; and engages in other party-building activities.

National Resource and Training Center on Homelessness and Mental Illness (NRC)

1-800-444-7415
Email: nrtcinfo@cdmgroup.com
Web: http://www.nrchmi.samhsa.gov

The NRC is the only national center specifically focused on the effective organization and delivery of services for people who are homeless and have serious mental illnesses. The

Resource Center's activities enable the Center for Mental Health Services to facilitate changes in service systems through field-based knowledge development, synthesis, exchange, and adoption of effective practices.

National Resource Center for Safe Aging

San Diego State University
6505 Alvarado Road, Suite 211
San Diego, California 92120
619-594-0986
FAX: 619-594-0351
Email: safeaging@sdsu.edu
Web: http://www.safeaging.org

The mission of The National Resource Center for Safe Aging is to gather and share the best information and resources on senior safety, including fall prevention, pedestrian and motor vehicle safety, and prevention of elder abuse. Resources include databases on general, regional, and aging data, as well as best practices and training. These resources are available for public health professionals, older adults, and family members.

National Rural Health Association (NRHA)

521 East 63rd Street
Kansas City, Missouri 64110-3329
816-756-3140
FAX: 816-756-3144
Web: http://www.nrharural.org

The NRHA is a national nonprofit membership organization with more than 10,000 members that provides leadership on rural health issues. The association's mission is to improve the health and well-being of rural Americans and to provide leadership on rural health issues through advocacy, communications, education, research, and leadership. The NRHA membership is made up of a diverse collection of individuals and organizations, all of whom share the common bond of an interest in rural health.

National Vaccine Program Office (NVPO)

U.S. Department of Health & Human Services
200 Independence Avenue SW
Washington, D.C. 20201
202-619-0257, 1-877-696-6775
Web: http://www.hhs.gov

NVPO, part of the U.S. Department of Health & Human Services, has responsibility for coordinating and ensuring collaboration among the many federal agencies involved in vaccine and immunization activities. The National Vaccine Plan and various reports and recommendations relevant to infectious diseases can be found at the NVPO's Web site.

Nursing Ethics

Web: http://www.ingentaconnect.com

This is the Web site for accessing online the journal Nursing Ethics. Fifty-seven issues of this journal are available online, some free of charge.

Nursing Ethics at Boston College

Web: http://www.bc.edu

This Web site is located at the William F. Connell School of Nursing, Boston University. It provides access to human rights-related book abstracts, lectures, ethics tools, databases, dissertations, library collections, and other human rights links.

Nursing Ethics Network (NEN)

Web: http://jmrileyrn.tripod.com

NEN is a nonprofit organization of professional nurses committed to the advancement of nursing ethics in clinical practice through research, education, and consultation. Members of NEN offer a uniquely focused service to the nursing community that is designed to complement, but not to duplicate, the work of other professional nursing organizations. The Web site provides access to nurses involved in nursing ethics.

Office of Disease Prevention and Health Promotion

Office of Public Health and Science, Office of the Secretary
1101 Wootton Parkway, Suite LL100
Rockville, Maryland 20852
240-453-8280
FAX: 240-453-8282
Web: http://odphp.osophs.dhhs.gov

The Office of Disease Prevention and Health Promotion, Office of Public Health and Science, Office of the Secretary, U.S. Department of Health and Human Services, works to strengthen the disease prevention and health promotion priorities of the department within the collaborative framework of the HHS agencies.

Office of Minority Health, U.S. Department of Health and Human Services (OMH)

The Tower Building
1101 Wootton Parkway, Suite 600
Rockville, Maryland 20852
240-453-2882
FAX: 240-453-2883
Email: info@omhrc.gov
Web: http://www.omhrc.gov

The OMH, established in 1986 by the U.S. Department of Health and Human Services, has a mission to improve and protect the health of racial and ethnic minority populations through the development of health policies and programs that will eliminate health disparities. The OMH offers information on funding, services, and campaigns and initiatives to improve and protect the health of racial and ethnic minority populations.

Office of Minority Health & Health Disparities (OMHD)

Centers for Disease Control & Prevention
Mailstop E-67
1600 Clifton Road NE
Atlanta, Georgia 30333
404-498-2320
FAX: 404-498-2355
Email: OMH@cdc.gov
Web: http://www.cdc.gov

The mission of OMHD is to promote health and quality of life by preventing and controlling the disproportionate burden of disease, injury, and disability among racial and ethnic minority populations. In carrying out its mission, OMHD coordinates White House Executive Orders and Health and Human Services departmental initiatives, supports cooperative agreements for research and professional development, reports on the health status of racial and ethnic minorities in the United States, and initiates strategic partnerships with governmental as well as national and regional organizations.

Office of the High Commissioner for Human Rights (OHCHR)

Web: http://www.ohchr.org

The OHCHR is a department of the United Nations Secretariat and is mandated to promote and protect the enjoyment and full realization by all people of all rights established in the Charter of the United Nations and in international human rights laws and treaties. The mandate includes preventing human rights violations, securing respect for all human rights, promoting international cooperation to protect human rights, coordinating related activities throughout the United Nations, and strengthening and streamlining the United Nations system in the field of human rights. In addition to its mandated responsibilities, it leads efforts to integrate a human rights approach within all work carried out by United Nations agencies.

OneWorld United States

3201 New Mexico Avenue NW, Suite 395
Washington, D.C. 20016
202-885-2679
FAX: 202-885-1309
Email: us@oneworld.net
Web: http://us.oneworld.net

OneWorld is a global information network developed to support communication media of the people, by the people, and for the people—everywhere. Its goal is to help build a more just global society through its partnership community. OneWorld encourages people to discover their power—power to speak, connect, and make a difference—by providing access to information and enabling connections between hundreds of organizations and tens of thousands of people around the world. The OneWorld network is driven by the people and organizations it supports—people write the news, provide the video clips, and prepare the radio stories. Through this network, individuals have access to information previously unavailable to them—information that can broaden their world view and enable them to make better decisions.

Pan American Health Organization (PAHO)

525 23rd Street NW
Washington, D.C. 20037
202-974-3000
Web: http://www.PAHO.org

(PAHO is an international public health agency with 100 years of experience in working to improve health and living standards of the 35 countries of the Americas. It serves as the specialized organization for health of the Inter-American System. It also serves as the Regional Office for the Americas of the World Health Organization and enjoys international recognition as part of the United Nations system. PAHO's mission is to lead strategic collaborative efforts among member states and other partners to promote equity in health, to combat disease, and to improve the quality of, and lengthen, the lives of the peoples of the Americas.

Partners in Information Access for the Public Health Workforce

Web: http://www.phpartners.org

Partners in Information Access for the Public Health Workforce is a collaboration of resources (U.S. government agencies, public health organizations, and health sciences libraries) for health educators and health promotion specialists. Their website contains resources for health educators and health promotion specialists including links to professional literature, health statistics, grants and funding, education and training, legislation and policy, conferences, and public health professionals and organizations.

People's Charter for Health

Web: http://www.phmovement.org

In the beginning, there were thousands of people across the world working very hard in big and little ways to promote the dream of a world where a healthy life is a reality for all. In the optimistic, joyous, compassionate 1970s, it seemed that this would be possible. And was not the Alma Ata declaration signed by 134 governments in 1978? Did not the declaration promise Health For All by 2000?

When the millennium edged closer and equitable health policy was still not a reality, the optimists did not give up. They knew that the third world had been plunged into debt and that health care was in danger of complete privatization. To remind the world of the commitment made in more hopeful times, the optimists came together in solidarity. People's organizations, civil society organizations, nongovernmental organizations, social activists, health professionals, academics, and researchers came together to make a strong statement against the studied indifference in this crucial area of human life. The First People's Health Assembly was organized in Savar, Bangladesh, in December 2000 to discuss the health for all challenge. In all, 1,453 participants from 75 countries came together to create and endorse a consensus document called the People's Charter for Health. The charter reflects the vision, goals, and principles that unite all the members of the PHM coalition and calls for action. It is the most widely endorsed consensus document on health since the Alma Ata declaration. The Web site provides the entire People's Charter for Health in a pdf file.

People's Movement for Human Rights Education (PMHRE)

The People's Movement for Human Rights Education
Shulamith Koenig, Executive Director
526 West 111th Street
New York, New York 10025
212-749-3156
FAX: 212-666-6325
Email: pdhre@igc.apc.org
Web: http://www.pdhre.org

PMHRE was founded in 1988, as a nonprofit, international service organization that works directly and indirectly with its network of affiliates—primarily women's and social justice organizations—to develop and advance pedagogies for human rights education relevant to people's daily lives in the context of their struggles for social and economic justice and democracy. Its members include experienced educators, human rights experts, United Nations officials, and world renowned advocates and activists who collaborate to conceive, initiate, facilitate, and service projects on education in human rights for social and economic transformation. The organization is dedicated to publishing and disseminating demand-driven human rights training and manuals and teaching materials, and otherwise servicing grassroots and community groups engaged in a creative, contextualized process of human rights learning, reflection, and action.

Pfizer, Inc., Health Communication Initiative

Web: http://www.pfizerhealthliteracy.com

The Pfizer Foundation Health Literacy Community Grants Program funds community-based interventions that improve client outcomes and reduce health disparities. The Partnership for Clear Health Communication offers resources for improving communication with low-literacy persons. The Health Communication Initiative website contains information for public health professionals to ensure that health information is delivered in easy-to-understand, actionable, and culturally relevant terms.

Physicians for Human Rights (PHR)

2 Arrow Street, Suite 301
Cambridge, Massachusetts 02138
617-301-4200
FAX: 617-301-4250
Web: http://www.phrusa.org

PHR mobilizes health professionals to advance health, dignity, and justice and promotes the right to health for all. Harnessing the specialized skills, rigor, and passion of health care providers, public health specialists, and scientists, PHR investigates human rights abuses and works to stop them.

Physicians for Social Responsibility

1875 Connecticut Avenue, NW, Suite 1012
Washington, D.C. 20009
202-667-4260
FAX: 202-667-4201
Email: psrnatl@psr.org
Web: http://www.psr.org

Physicians for Social Responsibility represents medical and public health professions and concerned citizens, working together to protect human life from the gravest threats to human health and survival. Their focus includes toxic chemicals, global warming, air pollution, safe drinking water, nuclear disarmament, and gun violence. The national Physicians for Social Responsibility has several constituencies. One good resource for environmental health material is The Greater Boston Physicians for Social Responsibility. A particularly good publication, In Harm's Way: Toxic Threats to Child Development, can be accessed at http://psr.igc.org/ihwrept/frontmatter.pdf. The publication provides a thorough discussion of the relationship of toxic chemicals and child development.

Protocol Driven Healthcare

Web: http://www.pdhi.com

The Web site provides a comprehensive assessment from self-reported health status information. It is available in both English and Spanish.

Public Health Ethics

Office of Continuing Education
North Carolina Institute for Public Health
Campus Box 8165
UNC School of Public Health
Chapel Hill, North Carolina 27599
919-966-4032
FAX 919-966-5692
Email: oce@unc.edu
Web: http://www.sph.unc.edu

The North Carolina Institute for Public Health in Public Health Ethics developed this short online course to explore such questions as: Is there a public health ethic? Is it different from medical ethics? And is it the same as public health laws? The series discusses:

- Why medical ethics doesn't meet the needs of public health
- The values and beliefs inherent to a public health perspective
- Twelve principles for the ethical practice of public health
- How public health's legal powers relate to public health ethics

Public Health Foundation (PHF)

1300 L Street, N. W., Suite 800
Washington, DC 20005
202-218-4400
FAX: 202-218-4409
Email: info@phf.org
Web: http://www.phf.org

The Public Health Foundation (PHF), a national non-profit organization, devotes its support for research, training and technical assistance to promote health in every community. The PHF works to improve the public health infrastructure and performance by translating complex data for use in practice, promoting evidence-based policies and programs, producing tools and providing technical assistance, disseminating training and educational materials, and developing systems for learning management and organization. Additionally, the PHF helps diverse groups discover common solutions to public health problems and supports public health systems research and national initiatives to improve the nation's public health.

Quackwatch

Web: http://www.quackwatch.com

Quackwatch, a nonprofit corporation, offers a guide to quackery, health fraud, and intelligent decisions. Some of Quackwatch activities include investigating questionable claims, answering inquiries about products and services, distributing reliable publications, improving the quality of health information, and attacking misleading advertising on the Internet.

Rabbis for Human Rights

Hehovharekhavim 9
Jerusalem, Israel 93462
972-2-648-2757
FAX: 972-2-678-3611
Web: http://www.rhr.Israel.net

Rabbis for Human Rights is an international group of rabbis working toward human rights. The Web site provides information on human rights issues and activities of this group.

Racial and Ethnic Approaches to Community Health, Centers for Disease Control

1600 Clifton Road
Atlanta, Georgia 30333
404-639-3311; Public Inquiries: 404-639-3534;
1-800-311-3435
Web: http://www.cdc.gov

This Web page presents ways to support community coalitions in designing, implementing, and evaluating community-driven strategies to eliminate health disparities.

Refugee Well Being: Partnering for Refugee Health and Well Being

Web: http://www.refugeewellbeing.samhsa.gov

The Web site provides refugee mental health consultation and technical assistance to federal, state, or local agencies. Site includes access to video and other training media.

ReliefWeb

ReliefWeb New York
Office for the Coordination of Humanitarian Affairs
United Nations
New York, New York 10017
212-963-1234
Web: http://www.reliefweb.int

ReliefWeb is the global hub for time-critical humanitarian information on Complex Emergencies and Natural Disasters. It is founded within the United Nations Office for the Coordination of Humanitarian Affairs. The Web site provides information on the needs of the humanitarian relief community.

Republican National Committee

310 First Street, SE
Washington, DC
20003
Web: http://www.gop.com

This is the official Web site for the Republican National Committee.

Roll Call Newspaper Online

50F Street NW, Suite 700
Washington, D.C. 20001-1572
202-824-6800
FAX: 202-824-0475
Web: http://www.rollcall.com

This is the online version of the official newspaper of Capitol
Hill. The newspaper provides information, news, and
analysis of Capitol Hill proceedings.

Rural Assistance Center

School of Medicine and Health Sciences, Room 4520
501 North Columbia Road, Stop 9037
Grand Forks, North Dakota 58202-9037
1-800-270-1898
FAX: 1-800-270-1913
Email: info@raconline.org
Web: http://www.raconline.org

Rural Assistance Center was established in 2002 as an information conduit for rural health and human services. The
center helps rural communities and other stakeholders
access available programs, funding, and research that
can help improve and provide quality health and human
services to rural residents. The rural health clinics (RHCs)
program is intended to increase primary care services for
Medicaid and Medicare patients in rural communities.
RHCs can be public, private, or nonprofit. The main
advantage of RHC status is enhanced reimbursement rates
for providing Medicaid and Medicare services in rural
areas. RHCs must be located in rural, underserved areas
and must use midlevel practitioners.

Rural Information Center (RIC)

National Agricultural Library
10301 Baltimore Avenue, Room 132
Beltsville, Maryland 20705-2351
1-800-633-7701
FAX: 301-504-5181
Web: http://www.nal.usda.gov

The RIC assists local communities by providing information
and referral services to local, tribal, state, and federal
government officials; community organizations; libraries;
businesses; and citizens working to maintain the vitality of
America's rural areas. They provide resources and funding programs relevant to rural health, including planning
resources, best practices and case studies, information
about free or reduced cost medical programs, funding and
program assistance, statistics and data resources, and publications relevant to rural health.

Scorecard

c/o Green Media Toolshed
1212 New York Avenue NW, Suite 300
Washington, D.C. 20005
202-464-5350
FAX: 202-776-0110
Email: info@greenmediatoolshed.org
Web: http://www.scorecard.org

Scorecard is a pollution information site. Upon entering a zip
code, pollution information for a particular community
and who is responsible is presented. Information about
geographic areas and companies that have the worst pollution records are also included in this Web site. There is
also information about how to take action as an informed
citizen.

Senate Home Page

For correspondence to U.S. Senators:
Office of Senator (Name)
United States Senate
Washington, D.C. 20510
For correspondence to Senate Committees:
(Name of Committee)
United States Senate
Washington, D.C. 20510
202-224-3121.
Web: http://www.senate.gov

This is the official Web site for the U.S. Senate. It provides
information on how to contact a senator and bills in the
Senate.

Sexuality Information and Education Council of the U.S. School Health Education Clearinghouse (SIECUS)

130 West 42nd Street, Suite 350
New York, New York 10036-7802
212-819-9770
FAX: 212/819-9776
Web: http://www.siecus.org

SIECUS was developed to give professionals easy access to
essential school health information. It provides information from all over the Web in one place on state and local
policies, sexual health promotion programs, national
guidelines, information on curricula, and links to additional information.

Shaping America's Health—Association for Weight Management and Obesity Prevention

1701 North Beauregard Street
Alexandria, Virginia 22311
703-253-4808
Web: http://www.obesityprevention.org

Shaping America's Health is a new organization formed from the American Diabetes Association and the North American Association for the Study of Obesity, aimed at weight loss and weight management. The organization will be involved with educating the public and issuing new clinical guidelines and evidence-based initiatives.

Sigma Theta Tau International

550 West North Street
Indianapolis, IN 46202
317-634-8171
FAX 317-634-8188, 1-888-634-7575
Email: memserv@stti.iupui.edu
Web: http://www.nursingsociety.org

In 1922, six nurses founded Sigma Theta Tau at the Indiana University Training School for Nurses, now the Indiana University School of Nursing, in Indianapolis, Indiana. The founders chose the name from the Greek words Storgé, Tharsos, and Timé meaning "love," "courage," and "honor." The honor society became incorporated in 1985 as Sigma Theta Tau International, Inc., a not-for-profit organization with a 501(c)(3) tax status in the United States. The mission of Sigma Theta Tau International is to provide leadership and scholarship in practice, education, and research to enhance the health of all people by supporting the learning and professional development of its members as they strive to improve nursing care worldwide. Sigma Theta Tau is made up of four organizations—the Honor Society of Nursing, Sigma Theta Tau International; Nursing Knowledge International; The International Honor Society of Nursing Building Corporation; and the Sigma Theta Tau International Foundation for Nursing. The vision of all four organizations is to create a global community of nurses who lead using scholarship, knowledge, and technology to improve the health of the world's people.

Society for Medical Decision Making

100 North 20th Street, 4th floor
Philadelphia, Pennsylvania 19103
215-545-7697
FAX: 215-564-2175
Email: smdm-office@lists.smdm.org
Web: http://www.smdm.org

This is the Web site for a smaller organization focusing on medical decision making broadly. Health economics is only one aspect of medical decision making. The Web site includes education modules that are likely to be of interest to those with limited experience in the area. In particular, there is a list of academic departments with some level of interest in medical decision making. The Web site also includes educational modules, but only members of the organization can access them.

Society for Public Health Education (SOPHE)

750 First Street NE, Suite 910
Washington, D.C. 20002-4242
202-408-9804
FAX: 202-408-9815
Email: info@sophe.org
Web: http://www.sophe.org

SOPHE is an international professional association made up of a diverse membership of health education professionals and students. The society's primary focus on health education promotes healthy behaviors, healthy communities, and healthy environments. The Web site offers additional information about SOPHE as well as meetings and publications of interest to public health professionals.

Southern Nursing Research Society (SNRS)

10200 West 44th Avenue, Suite 304
Wheat Ridge, Colorado 80033
1-877-314-SNRS
Email: snrs@resourcenter.com
Web: http://www.snrs.org

SNRS, founded in 1986, is an organization for nursing researchers in the southern region. There are 14 states in the SNRS region. The mission is to advance nursing research, promote dissemination and utilization of research findings, facilitate the career development of nurses and nursing students as researchers, enhance communication among members, and promote the image of nursing as a scientific discipline. Their Web site offers additional information about SNRS, conferences, publications, and research interest groups.

SpeakOut.com

20720 Beallsville Road
Dickerson, MD 20842
Web: http://www.speakout.com

The Web site provides a forum for political conversations and activity.

State of Connecticut Office of Health Care Access

410 Capitol Avenue
MS #13HCA
Hartford, Connecticut 06134-0308
860-418-7001; 1-800-797-9688
FAX: 860-418-7053
Email: Cristine.Vogel@po.state.ct.us
Web: http://www.ct.gov

The mission of the Office of Health Care Access is to ensure that the citizens of Connecticut have access to a quality health care delivery system. The agency will fulfill its mission by advising policy makers of health care issues;

informing the public and the industry of statewide and national trends; and designing and directing health care system development.

Substance Abuse and Mental Health Services Administration (SAMSHA)

1 Choke Cherry Road
Rockville, Maryland 20857
240-276-2130
FAX: 240-276-2135
Web: http://www.samhsa.gov

SAMSHA, an agency of the U.S. Department of Health and Human Services, was established in 1992 as a services agency to focus attention, programs, and funding on improving the lives of people with or at risk for mental and substance abuse disorders. SAMSHA's mission is to build resilience and facilitate recovery for people with or at risk for mental or substance use disorders. SAMSHA's Substance Abuse Treatment Facility Locator (http://findtreatment.samhsa.gov/) is a searchable directory for locating substance abuse treatment centers.

Surveillance, Epidemiology, and End Results (SEER)

Cancer Statistics Branch
Surveillance Research Program
Division of Cancer Control and Population Sciences
National Cancer Institute
Suite 504, MSC 8316
6116 Executive Boulevard
Bethesda, Maryland 20892-8316
301-496-8510
Web: http://www.seer.cancer.gov

The Surveillance, Epidemiology, and End Results (SEER), a program of the National Cancer Institute, provides information on cancer incidence and survival statistics in the United States. SEER is the only comprehensive source of population-based information that includes stage of cancer at the time of diagnosis and patient survival data. Data come from state registries, so SEER guides states to collect data that are compatible for pooling and improving national cancer estimates. One of SEER's efforts is a Web-based tool for public health workers, State Cancer Profiles, to find cancer statistics for specific states and counties. This effort is a joint project between the National Cancer Institute and the Centers for Disease Control and Prevention and is part of the Cancer Control P.L.A.N.E.T. Web site (http://cancercontrolplanet.cancer.gov) that provides comprehensive cancer resources for public health professionals. SEER is the most complete registry for quality cancer data being reported.

The Alliance for Healthy Cities

Email: alliance/ith@tmd.ac.ip
Web: http://www.alliance-healthycities.com

The Alliance for Healthy Cities is an international network aiming at protecting and enhancing the health of city dwellers. The alliance is a group of cities and other organizations that try to achieve the goal through an approach called Healthy Cities. Healthy Cities believes that international cooperation is an effective and efficient tool to achieve the goal. And the alliance promotes the interaction of people who are in the front line of health issues. The Healthy Cities approach was initiated by the World Health Organization. In order to cope with the adverse effects of an urban environment over health, the WHO has been promoting the approach worldwide.

The Brookings Institution

1775 Massachusetts Avenue NW
Washington, D.C. 20036-2188
202-797-6000
FAX: 202-797-6004
Web: http://www.brook.edu

The Brookings Institution is a private nonprofit organization devoted to independent research and innovative policy solutions. For more than 90 years, Brookings has analyzed current and emerging issues and produced new ideas for the nation and the world. For policy makers and the media, Brookings scholars provide the highest quality research, policy recommendations, and analysis on the full range of public policy issues. Research at the Brookings Institution is conducted to inform the public debate, not advance a political agenda. The scholars at the Brookings Institution are drawn from the United States and abroad— with experience in government and academia—and hold diverse points of view. Brookings's goal is to provide high-quality analysis and recommendations for decision makers in the United States and abroad on the full range of challenges facing an increasingly interdependent world.

The Center for Health and Health Care in Schools (CHHCS)

School of Public Health and Health Services
The George Washington University Medical Center
2121 K Street NW, Suite 250
Washington, D.C. 20037
202-466-3396
FAX: 202-466-3467
Email: CHHCS@GWU.EDU
Web: http://www.healthinschools.org

CHHCS is a nonpartisan policy and program resource center located at The George Washington University School of Public Health and Health Services. CHHCS builds on a 20-year history of testing strategies to strengthen health care delivery systems for children and adolescents. For the past decade, with support from The Robert Wood Johnson Foundation, staff and consultants at the center have worked with institutional leaders, state officials, and clinical providers to maximize outcomes for children through more effective health programming in schools. Members are committed to strengthening health care delivery systems for children and adolescents through effective health programming and health care services in schools.

The Future of Children

Email: FOC@princeton.edu

Web: http://www.futureofchildren.org

The Future of Children seeks to promote effective policies and programs for children by providing policy makers, service providers, and the media with timely, objective information based on the best available research. The Future of Children is a publication of The Woodrow Wilson School of Public and International Affairs at Princeton University and The Brookings Institution. This is the Healthy Families Web site.

The Hartford Institute for Geriatric Nursing

New York University College of Nursing

The John Hartford Foundation Institute for Geriatric Nursing

246 Greene Street

New York, New York 10003

212-998-9018

FAX: 212-995-4561

Email: info@nlihc.org

Web: http://www.hartfordign.org

The mission of the Hartford Institute for Geriatric Nursing is to help nurses provide, teach, learn, and administer best nursing practice to older clients through education, practice, and research.

The Hill

1625 K Street, NW Suite 900

Washington, D.C. 20006

202-628-8500

FAX: 202-628-8503

Web: http://www.hillnews.com

This Web site is an online newspaper for and about the U.S. Congress.

The International Healthy Cities Foundation

555 12th Street, 10th Floor

Oakland, California 94607

510-642-1715

FAX: 510-643-6981

Email: hcities@uclink4.berkeley.edu

Web: http://www.healthycities.org

The Web site is a place where people interested in addressing urban and community issues along with concerns about health and quality of life issues in their communities can join and share information. The Web site facilitates linkages among people, issues, and resources in order to support the development of Healthy Cities initiatives. The site includes a searchable database of over 1,000 meritorious solutions to urban issues related to health.

The Library of Congress

Washington, D.C. 20540

202-707-5000

Web: http://www.lcweb.loc.gov

The Library of Congress is the nation's oldest federal cultural institution and serves as the research arm of Congress. It is also the largest library in the world, with more than 130 million items on approximately 530 miles of bookshelves. Its mission is to make its resources available and useful to the Congress and the American people and to sustain and preserve a universal collection of knowledge and creativity for future generations.

The Library of Congress THOMAS

Web: http://thomas.loc.gov

This Web site was launched in January of 1995. The leadership of the 104th Congress directed the Library of Congress to make federal legislative information freely available to the public. The Web site provides full text of laws and bills in Congress from 1973 to currently.

The National Center for Healthy Housing

10320 Little Pataxent Parkway, Suite 500

Columbia, Maryland 21044

410-992-0712

FAX: 443-539-415010.992.0712 / Fax: 443.539.4150

Web: http://www.centerforhealthyhousing.org

The National Center for Healthy Housing (formerly the National Center for Lead-Safe Housing) was founded as a nonprofit organization in October 1992, to bring the public health, housing, and environmental communities together to combat the nation's epidemic of childhood lead poisoning. It continues its important role in reducing children's risk of lead poisoning and has expanded its mission to help to decrease children's exposure to other hazards in the home including biological, physical, and chemical contaminants in and around the home. The NCHH mission is to develop and promote practical methods to protect children from environmental health hazards in their homes while preserving affordable housing.

The National Council on Aging (NCOA)

NCOA Headquarters
1901 L Street, NW, 4th floor
Washington, D.C. 20036
202-479-1200
FAX: 202-479-0735; TDD: 202-479-6674
Email: info@ncoa.org
Web: http://www.ncoa.org

Founded in 1950, NCOA is dedicated to improving the health and independence of older persons and increasing their continuing contributions to communities, society, and future generations. NCOA is a 501(c)3 organization. At the heart of NCOA is a national network of more than 14,000 organizations and leaders that work together to achieve its mission. NCOA's 3,800 members include senior centers, area agencies on aging, adult day service centers, faith-based service organizations, senior housing facilities, employment services, consumer groups, and leaders from academia, business, and labor. The programs help older people to remain healthy, find jobs, discover new ways to continue to contribute to society after retirement, and take advantage of government and private benefits programs that can improve the quality of their lives. NCOA is also a national voice for both older Americans and community organizations, leading advocacy efforts on important national issues affecting seniors.

The National Low Income Housing Coalition (NLIHC)

727 15th Street NW, 6th Floor
Washington, D.C. 20005
202 -662-1530
FAX: 202-/93-1973
Email: info@nlihc.org
Web: http://www.nlihc.org

The NLIHC is dedicated solely to ending America's affordable housing crisis. The NLIHC believes that this is achievable and that the affordable housing crisis is a problem that Americans are capable of solving. Even though the NLIHC is concerned about the housing circumstances of all low-income people, it focuses its advocacy on those with the most serious housing problems, the lowest income households.

The Peoples' Decade for Human Rights Education (PDHRE)

526 West 111th Street, Suite 4E
New York, New York 10025
212-749-3156
FAX: 212-666-6325
Email: pdhre@igc.org
Web: http://www.pdhre.org

Founded in 1988, the People's Decade of Human Rights Education (PDHRE—International) is a nonprofit, international service organization that works directly and indirectly with its network of affiliates—primarily women's and social justice organizations—to develop and advance pedagogies for human rights education relevant to people's daily lives in the context of their struggles for social and economic justice and democracy. PDHRE's members include experienced educators, human rights experts, United Nations officials, and world renowned advocates and activists who collaborate to conceive, initiate, facilitate, and service projects on education in human rights for social and economic transformation. The organization is dedicated to publishing and disseminating demand-driven human rights training manuals and teaching materials, and otherwise servicing grassroots and community groups engaged in a creative, contextualized process of human rights learning, reflection, and action. PDHRE views human rights as a value system capable of strengthening democratic communities and nations through its emphasis on accountability, reciprocity, and people's equal and informed participation in the decisions that affect their lives.

The Senior Benefits Checkup developed by NCOA

Web: http://www.benefitscheckup.org

Developed and maintained by the National Council on Aging (NCOA), Benefits Checkup is the nation's most comprehensive Web-based service to screen for benefits programs for seniors with limited income and resources. Benefits Checkup includes more than 1,350 public and private benefits programs from all 50 states and the District of Columbia. Many older people need help paying for prescription drugs, health care, utilities, and other basic needs. Ironically, millions of older Americans—especially those with limited incomes—are eligible for but not receiving benefits from existing federal, state, and local programs. Ranging from heating and energy assistance to prescription savings programs to income supplements, there are many public programs available to seniors in need if they only knew about them and how to apply for them.

The Urban Institute

2100 M Street, NW
Washington, D.C. 20037
202-833-7200
Web: http://www.urban.org

The Urban Institute is a nonpartisan economic and social policy research organization that publishes studies, reports, and books on timely topics worthy of public consideration. It includes, but is not limited to, immigration issues. Its mission is to promote sound social policy and public debate on national priorities. The Urban Institute gathers and analyzes data, conducts policy research, evaluates programs and services, and educates Americans on critical issues and trends.

The WHO Collaborating Center for Healthy Cities

Web: http://www.iupui.edu

The WHO Collaborating Center for Healthy Cities resides at Indiana University School of Nursing at IUPUI (Indiana University Purdue University at Indianapolis). Citynet presents a 9-step community health promotion model of great utility.

The World Bank

1818 H Street NW
Washington, D.C. 20433
202-473-1000
FAX: 202-477-6391
Web: http://www.worldbank.org

The World Bank is a vital source of financial and technical assistance to developing countries around the world. The World Bank is a vital source of financial and technical assistance to developing countries around the world. It is not a bank in the common sense. The World Bank is made up of two unique development institutions owned by 184 member countries—the International Bank for Reconstruction and Development (IBRD) and the International Development Association (IDA). Each institution plays a different but supportive role in the mission of global poverty reduction and the improvement of living standards. The IBRD focuses on middle-income and creditworthy poor countries, while IDA focuses on the poorest countries in the world. Together they provide low-interest loans, interest-free credit, and grants to developing countries for education, health, infrastructure, communications and many other purposes.

Toxicology and Environmental Health Information Program at the National Library of Medicine

Specialized Information Services
Two Democracy Plaza, Suite 510
6707 Democracy Boulevard, MSC 5467
Bethesda, Maryland 20892-5467
301-496-1131
FAX: 301-480-3537
Email: tehip@teh.nlm.nih.gov
Web: http://www.sis.nlm.nih.gov

The Toxicology and Environmental Health Information Program has two objectives: (1) to create automated toxicology data banks and (2) to provide toxicology and environmental health information and data services. The National Library of Medicine has a free online toxicology tutorial that can be accessed at http://sis.nlm.nih.gov/
- Tox/ToxTutor.html. There are three tutorials: Basic principles, Toxicokinetics, and Cellular toxicology.

ToxTown

c/o U.S. National Library of Medicine
8600 Rockville Pike
Bethesda, Maryland 20894
1-888-FIND-NLM
Email: tehip@teh.nlm.nih.gov
Web: http://toxtown.nlm.nih.gov

ToxTown is an incredibly useful site for assessing environmental health risks in our everyday lives. The site is from the National Library of Medicine and would be helpful for guiding an environmental nursing assessment. ToxTown provides information about everyday locations where toxic chemicals are found, descriptions of chemicals, Internet links to authoritative chemical information and other resources, and how the environment can impact human health.

Turning Point

Email: turnpt@u.washington.edu
Web: http://www.turningpointprogram.org

Turning Point, started in 1997, was an initiative of The Robert Wood Johnson Foundation and the W. K. Kellogg Foundation. Its mission was to transform and strengthen the public health system in the United States by making it more community-based and collaborative. The initial idea for Turning Point came from the foundations' concerns about the capacity of the public health system to respond to emerging challenges in public health, specifically the system's capacity to work with people from many sectors to improve the health status of all people in a community. Turning Point created a network of 23 public health partners across the country to:
- Define and assess health, prioritize health issues, and take collective action.
- Promote education to decrease the risk of infectious and chronic disease.
- Strengthen environmental health services for clean air and water and safe food.
- Gain access to health care for everyone.
- Improve health status for minority groups.
- U.S. Army Medical Research Institute of Infectious Diseases (USAMRIID)

U.S. Army Medical Research Institute of Infectious Diseases

Commander
USAMRIID
Attn: MCMR-UIZ-R
1425 Porter Street
Frederick, Maryland 21702-5011
Email: USAMRIIDweb@amedd.army.mil
Web: http://www.usamriid.army.mil

USAMRIID conducts basic and applied research on biological threats resulting in medical solutions to protect military service members. USAMRIID, an organization of the U.S. Army Medical Research and Materiel Command, is the lead medical research laboratory for the U.S. Biological Defense Research Program. The institute plays a key role as the only laboratory in the Department of Defense equipped to safely study highly hazardous infectious agents requiring maximum containment at bio-safety level (BSL)-4. USAMRID vision is to be the nation's preeminent research laboratory providing cutting-edge medical research for the war fighter against biological threats.

U.S. Census Bureau

4700 Silver Hill Road
Washington, D.C. 20233-0001
301-763-6440
FAX: 301-457-2654
Email: POL.Policy.Office@census.gov
Web: http://www.census.gov

The Census Bureau serves as the leading source of quality data about the nation's people and economy. The Census Bureau was established in 1790 under the responsibility of Secretary of State Thomas Jefferson. That census, taken by U.S. marshals on horseback, counted 3.9 million inhabitants. Today, in addition to taking a census of the population every 10 years, the Census Bureau conducts censuses of economic activity and state and local governments every 5 years and conducts more than 100 other surveys every year. In addition, the Census Bureau publishes notices informing the public of our collections of information and other activities in the Federal Register and offers international programs and fellowships.

U.S. Citizenship and Immigration Services (USCIS)

1-800-375-5283
Email: uscis.webmaster@dhs.gov
Web: http://www.uscis.gov

The Web site provides a variety of information on immigration, immigration laws, how to become a citizen of the United States, and other information pertinent to immigration.

U.S. Department of Agriculture (USDA)

1400 Independence Avenue SW
Washington, D.C. 20250
Web: http://www.usda.gov

The USDA's mission is to provide leadership on food, agriculture, natural resources, and related issues based on sound public policy, the best available science, and efficient management. They work to control and prevent infectious diseases in animals, thereby protecting people. Their Web site contains many publications on such topics as emerging infectious diseases, requirements for import of animals, food-borne illness, and state agriculture regulations.

U.S. Department of Agriculture, Economic Research Service (ERS)

1400 Independence Avenue SW
Washington, D.C. 20250
202-694-5050
Email: InfoCenter@ers.usda.gov
Web: http://www.ers.usda.gov

The ERS is a resource for a Community Food Security Assessment Toolkit. The toolkit is useful for assessment of household food security and resources, accessibility, availability and affordability, and community production resources. It also has focus group guides and materials to use for assessment.

U.S. Department of Energy (DOE)

100 Independence Avenue SW
Washington, D.C. 20585
1-800-342-5363
FAX: 202-586-4463
Web: http://www.energy.gov

The DOE promotes scientific and technological innovation in advancing the national, economic, and energy security of the United States and ensures environmental cleanup of the national nuclear weapons complex.

U.S. Department of Health and Human Services (DHHS)

200 Independence Avenue, SW
Washington, D.C. 20201
202-619-0257, 1-877-696-6775
Web: www.dhhs.gov

DHHS is the U.S. government's primary agency involved with protecting the health of all Americans and providing essential human services, especially for people with few resources. The Web site provides health related publications.

U.S. Department of Health and Human Services, Administration for Families and Children, Office of Refugee Resettlement (ORR)

370 L'Enfant Promenade, SW, 6th Floor /East
Washington, D.C. 20447
202-401-9246
FAX: 202-401-5487
Web: http://www.acf.hhs.gov

In the Refugee Act of 1980, Pub. L. No. 96-212, Congress codified and strengthened the United States' historic policy of aiding individuals fleeing persecution in their homelands. The Refugee Act of 1980 provided a formal definition of "refugee," which is virtually identical to the definition in the 1967 United Nations Protocol relating to the Status of Refugees. This definition is found in the Immigration and Nationality Act (INA) at Section 101(a)(42).

In addition, the act provided the foundation for today's asylum adjudication process and the development of ORR within the Department of Health and Human Services. ORR's mission is to assist refugees and other special populations, as outlined in ORR regulations, in obtaining economic and social self-sufficiency in their new homes in the United States. To do this, ORR funds and facilitates a variety of programs that offer, among other benefits and services, cash and medical assistance, employment preparation and job placement, skills training, English language training, social adjustment and aid for victims of torture. The mission of ORR is to help refugees, Cuban/Haitian entrants, asylees, and other beneficiaries of our program to establish a new life that is founded on the dignity of economic self-support and encompasses full participation in opportunities that Americans enjoy. The Web site includes a legal definition of refugees and describes eligibility requirements for Refugee Assistance and Services through the Office of Refugee Resettlement.

U.S. Department of Health and Human Services, Office of Minority Health (OMH)

P.O. Box 37337
Washington, D.C. 20013-7337
1-800-444-6472
Web: http://www.omhrc.gov

OMH improves and protects the health of racial and ethnic minority populations through the development of health policies and programs that will eliminate health disparities for racial and ethnic minority populations. OMH funds grants to address racial and ethnic minority health disparities. Several health disparities initiatives are coordinated by the Office of Management and Budget, including (a) Closing the Gap on Infant Mortality, (b) Minority HIV/AIDS, (c) Community Initiatives to Eliminate Stroke Disparities, and (d) Obesity Abatement in African Americans Campaign. The Web site describes programs and policies for racial and ethnic minority populations.

U.S. Department of Health and Human Services, Office of Rural Health Policy

Health Resources and Services Administration
5600 Fishers Lane, 9A-55
Rockville, Maryland 20857
301-443-0835
FAX: 301-443-2803
Web: http://www.ruralhealth.hrsa.gov

The Office of Rural Health Policy is a government office located in the Health Resources and Services Administration, promoting better health care service in rural America by informing and advising the U.S. Department of Health and Human Services on matters affecting rural hospitals and health care, coordinating activities within the department that relate to rural health care, and maintaining a national information clearinghouse.

U.S. Department of Homeland Security (DHS)

Office of Grants and Training
810 Seventh Street NW
Washington, D.C. 20531
1-800-368-6498, 8:00 a.m. to 6:00 p.m. EST, Monday–Friday
FAX: 202-786-9920
Web: http://www.ojp.usdoj.gov

The Office of Grants and Training is responsible for providing training, funds for the purchase of equipment, support for the planning and execution of exercises, technical assistance, and other support to assist states and local jurisdictions to prevent, respond to, and recover from acts of terrorism.

U.S. Department of Labor, National Farm Workers Jobs Program (NFJP)

U.S. Department of Labor
200 Constitution Avenue NW
Washington, D.C. 20210
1-877-US-2JOBS
Web: http://www.doleta.gov

The NFJP assists migrant and other seasonally employed farmworkers and their families to achieve economic self-sufficiency through job training and other services that address their employment-related needs.

U.S. Department of State, Bureau of Population, Refugees, and Migration

U.S. Department of State
2201 C Street NW
Washington, D.C. 20520
202-647-4000
Web: http://www.state.gov

This branch of the U.S. Department of State coordinates U.S. international population policy and promotes its goals through bilateral and multilateral cooperation. The agency oversees admissions of refugees to the United States for permanent resettlement and works closely with the Immigration and Naturalization Service, the Department of Health and Human Services, and various state and private voluntary agencies. This site includes descriptions of refugee programs abroad and in the United States.

U.S. Department of State: How can I recognize trafficking victims?

U.S. Department of State
2201 C Street NW
Washington, D.C. 20520
202-647-4000
Web: http://www.state.gov

The Web site describes resources and screening questions for victims of human trafficking and includes a toll-free number for reporting suspected trafficking cases.

U.S. Government Printing Office (GPO)

732 North Capitol Street NW
Washington, D.C. 20401
202-512-0000
Email: jbradley@gpo.gov
Web: http://www.access.gpo.gov

The U.S. Government Printing Office provides free electronic access to important information products such as federal documents produced by the federal government. The information provided on this site is the official, published version and the information retrieved from GPO Access can be used without restriction, unless specifically noted. This free service is funded by the Federal Depository Library Program and has grown out of Public Law 103-40, known as the Government Printing Office Electronic Information Enhancement Act of 1993.

U.S. House of Representatives Home Page

Washington, D.C. 20515
202-224-3121(202) 225-1904
Web: http://www.house.gov

This is the official Web site of the U.S. House of Representatives.

U.S. Nuclear Regulatory Commission (USNRC)

Office of Public Affairs (OPA)
Washington, D.C. 20555
1-800-368-5642, 301-415-8200, TDD: 301-415-5575
Web: http://www.nrc.gov

The U.S. Nuclear Regulatory Commission is an independent agency established by the Energy Reorganization Act of 1974 to regulate civilian use of nuclear materials. USNRC is headed by a five-member commission. USNRC's mission is to regulate the nation's civilian use of byproduct, source, and special nuclear materials such as the effects of radiation from nuclear reactors, materials, and waste facilities to ensure adequate protection of public health and safety, to promote the common defense and security, and to protect the environment.

United Nations

Web: http://www.un.org

This is the official Web site for the United Nations. The information provided on this Web site includes but is not limited to daily briefings, press releases, documents, publications, and databases.

United Nations Association of the United States of America (UNA–USA)

801 Second Avenue, 2nd floor
New York, New York 10017
212-907-1300
FAX: 212-682-9185
Email: unahq@unausa.org
Web: http://unausa.org

UNA–USA is part of the World Federation of UNAs. It is a center for innovative programs to engage Americans in issues of global concern, from education and HIV/AIDS to peace, security, and international law. Its educational and humanitarian campaigns, including teaching students in urban schools, clearing minefields, and providing school-based support for children living in HIV/AIDS-affected communities in Africa, allow people to make a global impact at the local level. A not-for-profit organization, UNA–USA encourages United States leadership in the United Nations.

United Nations Economic and Social Development

Web: http://www.un.org

One of the UN's central mandates is the promotion of higher standards of living, full employment, and conditions of economic and social progress and development. The UN has unique strengths in promoting development. Its presence is global and its comprehensive mandate spans social, economic and emergency needs. The UN does not represent any particular national or commercial interest. When major policy decisions are taken, all countries, rich and poor, have a voice. This Website provides information on UN's progress in these areas.

United Nations System of Organizations

Web: http://www.unsystem.org

This Web site serves as a portal to Web sites of the United Nations, its funds, programs, and specialized agencies. It also includes links to key projects and initiatives to various joint programs of the UN.

United Nations World Food Program

Via C.G.Viola 68
Parco dei Medici
00148 - Rome - Italy
39-06-65131
FAX: 39-06-6513 2840
Email: wfpinfo@wfp.org
Web: http://www.wfp.org

The UN World Food Program was established to meet one of the Millennium Development Goals, which the United Nations set for the 21st century, halving the proportion of hungry people in the world is top of the list. This Web site provides information concerning progress toward the goal.

URAC

1220 L Street NW, Suite 400
Washington, D.C. 20005
202-216-9010
FAX: 202-216-9006
Web: http://www.urac.org

URAC is an independent, nonprofit organization known as a leader in promoting health care quality through its accreditation and certification programs. URAC offers a wide range of quality benchmarking programs and services that keep pace with the rapid changes in the health care system and provides a symbol of excellence for organizations to validate their commitment to quality and accountability. Through its broad-based governance structure and an inclusive standards development process, URAC ensures that all stakeholders are represented in establishing meaningful quality measures for the entire health care industry. URAC's mission is to promote continuous improvement in the quality and efficiency of health care management through processes of accreditation and education.

Veterans' Health Administration Diabetes Program

1-800-827-1000
Web: http://www.va.gov

The goal of the Veteran's Health Administration (VHA) is to provide excellence in patient care, veterans' benefits, and customer satisfaction. The VHA is striving for high-quality, prompt, and seamless service to veterans. Their VHA diabetes program Web site contains information about diabetes and its management and also has links to other professional sites with information on diabetes.

World Future Society

7910 Woodmont Avenue, Suite 450
Bethesda, Maryland 20814
301-656-8274
E-mail info@wfs.org
Web: http://www.wfs.org

The World Future Society is an association of people interested in how social and technological developments are shaping the future. The society was founded in 1966 and is chartered as a nonprofit educational and scientific organization in Washington, D.C. The society strives to serve as a neutral clearinghouse for ideas about the future. Ideas about the future include forecasts, recommendations, and alternative scenarios. These ideas help people to anticipate what may happen in the next 5, 10, or more years ahead. When people can visualize a better future, then they can begin to create it.

World Health Organization (WHO)

Avenue Appia 20
1211 Geneva 27
Switzerland
+ 41-22-791-21-11
FAX: + 41-22-79-3111
Telex: 415 416
Telegraph: UNISANTE GENEVA
Email: info@who.int.
Web: http://www.who.int

WHO is the United Nations' specialized agency for health. It was established on April 7, 1948. WHO's objective, as set out in its Constitution, is the attainment by all peoples of the highest possible level of health. Health is defined in WHO's Constitution as a state of complete physical, mental, and social well-being and not merely the absence of disease or infirmity. WHO is governed by 193 Member States through the World Health Assembly. The Health Assembly is composed of representatives from WHO's Member States. The main tasks of the World Health Assembly are to approve the WHO program and the budget for the following biennium and to decide major policy questions. The WHO Web site provides rich examples and information on Healthy Cities from an international perspective.

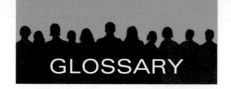

GLOSSARY

access to health care   Opportunity to use health care that is reliable, affordable, appropriate, and of high quality.

acculturation   Dynamic process of understanding or adopting specific aspects or characteristics of a new culture; term used broadly to include language, behavior, identity, and values that are maintained or changed when someone comes into contact with another culture.

acculturative strategies   Adaptation styles defined by Berry (2005) based on relationships between new and native cultures for immigrants or minority groups.

acculturative stress   Any stressor that is linked to the acculturation process.

acquired immunity   Resistance to a disease after a person comes in contact with an agent and the body produces antibodies that protect from further infection by the same agent.

active immunity   Resistance to a disease by the activation of the immune system of a person through having the disease or being immunized against it.

activity-related affect   A subjective positive or negative feeling state about a behavior.

acute illness   Sickness of a sudden onset and a limited duration, usually less than a month.

acute radiation syndrome (ARS)   Acute illness caused by large amounts of radiation exposure over a brief time. There are three forms of ARS: bone marrow syndrome, which affects the stem cells in the bone marrow; gastrointestinal syndrome, in which stem cells in the bone marrow and cell lining in the GI tract are dying; and cardiovascular/nervous syndrome, which affects the nervous system.

administration   Designated work associated with the job description that outlines assigned roles and responsibilities within the organization.

affective skills   Change in interests, attitudes, and values.

ageism   Term used to describe negative stereotyping of older adults.

alien   Any person who is not a citizen or national of the United States.

allocative efficiency   A mix of goods and services wherein no one in society can be better off without making someone else worse off; requires technical efficiency and an allocation of resources across different types of production that leaves no room to reallocate resources without making someone worse off.

American Red Cross   A nonprofit, humanitarian organization founded by nurse Clara Barton in 1881 that provides emergency assistance, disaster relief, and education inside the United States.

androgogy   An adult learning model based on adult autonomy and self-directedness, life experiences, and need for real-life situations.

anticipatory guidance   Information and education provided to the client in order to take timely action or prevent the onset of a health problem.

antigenicity   Agent's ability to stimulate the host's immune system, producing disease specific antibodies for immunity and future protection of the host.

assessment   Core public health function that involves the systematic collection, evaluation, and communication of information on the health of populations.

assimilation   Strategy in which individuals do not continue to value their native cultural identity and wish to take on only the attributes of the new culture.

assurance   Core function through which public health agencies make sure that their communities receive the services necessary to achieve health.

at the margin   Concept of making decisions that focus on spending one more dollar or trying to bring about one more positive health outcome.

autonomy   "Self-governance, liberty rights, privacy, individual choice, freedom of the will, causing one's own behavior, and being one's own person" (Hudson 2006); is rooted in the concept of individual freedom and choice and implies acting according to an individually chosen plan without interference from others.

benchmark   Standard that can be used for comparison.

beneficence   Provision of appropriate treatment and the duty to make reasonable sacrifices for the sake of clients; may also include the notion of utility: the requirement to balance benefits and drawbacks to produce the best overall results.

biocrime   Criminal use of biological agents in acts of terrorism.

bioethics   Subfield of ethics that deals with ethical concerns that arise as a result of advances in health care. Bioethics has developed an emphasis on individual human rights, such as freedom, choice, and self-determination.

biological agents   Fungi, parasites, bacteria, and viruses that cause communicable disease.

bioterrorism   Terrorism using germ warfare or the release of microbial agents with the intent to cause disease.

body mass index   Relationship of body weight and height used by the National Institutes of Health to define overweight and obesity.

brownfields site   Abandoned or underutilized industrial/commercial properties where redevelopment has been impeded by real or perceived environmental contamination.

budgeting   Organization's plan to use anticipated funds in relation to expected expenses in various categories.

capacity building   Enhancing the ability of the health system or organization to develop, implement, and sustain health promotion initiatives and, ultimately, health changes.

capital budgets   Plan to acquire and maintain longer-term assets such as purchasing or renovating buildings.

care coordination   A program that provides a systematic monitoring of the health status of individuals, families, and/or groups.

care ethics   An ethic of care that has five central ideas: (1) moral attention to the situation in all its complexity; (2) sympathetic understanding of what others in the situation would want; (3) relationship awareness or cognizance of the networks of relationships that connect the humans in a situation; (4) accommodation for the needs of all who are involved in a situation; and (5) a response that demonstrates caring in concrete action in response to client need.

caregiver burden   The physical, emotional, and financial stress or burden experienced by a caregiver of an ill person.

case management   Process by which the provision and coordination of quality health care services are provided to an individual in a cost-effective manner.

cash budgets   Plan wherein clients or contractors pay for services or goods.

chemoprophylaxis   Use of antimicrobial drugs to prevent the acquisition of pathogens in an endemic area or to prevent their spread from one person to another.

child maltreatment   An act or failure to act by a parent, caregiver, or other person as defined under state law that results in physical abuse, neglect, medical neglect, sexual abuse, or emotional abuse, or an act or failure to act that presents imminent risk of serious harm to a child.

chronic disease   Any disease with an onset that occurs over time and has a course that lasts over a prolonged period of time, usually three months or more.

cognitive skills   Development of knowledge.

cohort   A group of people followed through time to see if they develop the disease in question; prospective cohort study design follows people before the development of a disease, while retrospective cohort study design begins after the disease is present.

common vehicle transmission   Transmission of an infectious agent through environmental mechanisms such as through water, food, milk, soil, and inanimate objects.

community assessment   Comprehensive process to identify risk factors, health problems, protective factors, assets, needs, strengths, and resources of populations in the community.

community development for health promotion   Environmental change and restructuring, such as eliminating air pollutants or requiring tamper-proof medication bottles; takes into account the interrelationships of diverse personal, institutional, and environmental factors inherent in health and illness, and is a comprehensive perspective.

community health centers (CHCs)   Private, not-for-profit, consumer-directed health care facilities that have the mission of providing high-quality, cost-effective, and comprehensive primary and preventive care to persons who have no health insurance or who are medically underserved.

Community-As-Partner Model   Model used in community assessment with a focus on the community core, subsystems, and perceptions as well as the lines of defense a community possesses.

comparative justice or distributive justice   Fair distribution of social benefits and burdens.

competence   Capacity to function effectively as an individual and an organization within the context of the cultural beliefs, behaviors, and needs presented by populations and their communities.

competency-based practice   Essential skill domains in which public health nurses demonstrate proficiency.

conceptualizing   Articulating thoughts and ideas in an objective format that involves finding solutions to the identified needs.

consequentialism   Group of philosophies that decide whether actions are right entirely with reference to the consequences of the actions, regardless of any moral features the actions may have, such as truthfulness or fidelity. Consequentialist theories seek to judge actions according to the balance of good or bad outcomes that the actions produce.

contextual risk factors   Variables beyond the control of the individual that may serve to increase morbidity and/or mortality associated with chronic diseases.

convenience sample   Individuals included in a study because they are available or happen to be in the right place at the right time.

Coordinated School Health Program   Program of components identified by the Centers for Disease Control as essential for improving health in school settings. The components include health education, physical education, health services, nutrition services, counseling, psychological and social services, healthy school environment, health promotion for staff, and family/community involvement.

copayment   Fixed payment that the insured must pay for each health care provider visit, procedure, treatment, or prescription; payment sharing between the third party payer and the insured; also known as coinsurance.

core competencies   Aptitudes that represent the knowledge, skills and attitudes needed for the practice of public health by a diverse group of professional disciplines (Council on Linkages Between Academic and Public Health Practice): developed through a national consensus process.

Core Functions of Public Health   Activities of assessment, policy development, and assurance that have been identified as critical to the mission of public health.

correlational design   Measures of association used to study relationships among variables.

cost-benefit analysis (CBA)   Comparison of the costs of an intervention with the dollar value of the benefits. Also defined as an economic analysis that measures both costs and outcomes in dollars.

cost-consequence analysis (CCA)   Economic analysis that measures the consequences and costs of each alternative approach.

cost-effectiveness analysis (CEA)   Comparison of the costs of an intervention with the benefits that accrue from that intervention; similar to a cost-benefit analysis except that it is not expected that outcomes will be valued in monetary terms. Also defined as an economic analysis that measures outcomes in the same units across alternatives, typically in dollars per life year.

cost-minimization analysis (CMA)   Economic analysis that assumes each approach has equal effects and compares only the costs between alternative approaches to determine which alternative is least costly.

cost-utility analysis (CUA)   Economic analysis that measures outcomes in quality-adjusted life years and allows comparison across populations and disease states.

cotinine   The proximate metabolite of nicotine; an accurate and objective biochemical marker of smoking status and ETS exposure.

Cover the Uninsured Week   Campaign begun in 2003 as a way to bring together a wide array of people to discuss trends that threaten to increase the number of Americans without health care coverage, as well as proposals to expand coverage and make health care more affordable while improving its quality.

cultural competence   Set of congruent behaviors, attitudes and policies that come together as a system, as an agency, or among professionals and enable that system, agency, or professionals to work effectively in cross-cultural situations.

culture   Integrated patterns of human behavior that include the language, thoughts, communications, actions, customs, beliefs, values, and institutions of racial, ethnic, religious, or social groups.

culture broker   Bilingual/bicultural person whose familiarity with a specific culture permits him or her to provide specialized language and cultural interpretation to ensure understanding and establish relationships between clients and providers.

decibel (dB) Measure of the loudness of a sound; the higher the number of decibels, the louder the sound.

deductibles Amount the insured must pay before the third party payer will pay for health care services.

descriptive epidemiology Study of patterns in population data.

descriptive study Research that describes a phenomenon as it exists.

detailing Assessing the program in terms of the identified solutions and formulating objectives that will meet the program goal.

Diffusion of Innovations Theory Approach used to evaluate the distribution and use of products or health services in the community.

discount rate Difference between the weight on the present and the future; partially a function of market forces and partially determined by stakeholders.

discounting Method of valuation that emphasizes future costs and benefits.

disease trajectory Course of periods of remission and reoccurrence of an illness.

district nursing A geography-based form of trained nursing care for the delivery of services to the "sick poor" in their homes, initiated by William Rathbone and Florence Nightingale in 1861.

domestic terrorism Activities that involve acts dangerous to human life and are a violation of the criminal laws of the United States or of any state; appear to be intended to intimidate or coerce a civilian population; influence the policy of a government by mass destruction, assassination, or kidnapping; and occur primarily within the territorial jurisdiction of the United States.

dose Amount of a substance ingested or absorbed at a given time.

dose–response curve Graphical representation of the relationship between the dose of a substance and the biological response to that substance.

droplet nuclei Small particle aerosols containing pathogenic microorganisms that are exhaled, sneezed, or coughed by an infected person.

ecological model A broad, multideterminant perspective, emphasizing the interconnections among many factors that contribute to health. Also defined as a model of behavior that considers the interaction between people and intrapersonal, sociocultural, policy, and physical-environmental factors.

economic globalization Inextricable linkages through technology, banking systems, geopolitics, foods, clothing, and global systems of trade and investment across state boundaries.

economics Study of how scarce resources are allocated.

Edwin Chadwick (1780–1890) An English civil servant who was one of the major authors of the 1942 "Report into the Sanitary Conditions of the Labouring Population of Great Britain," showing that life expectancy was much lower in English towns than in the countryside and that disease was related to environmental conditions.

effective program Evidence-based program with rigorous evaluation that consistently demonstrates positive outcomes.

e-learning Learning facilitated and enhanced through the use of information and communication technology, including methods such as personal computers, CD-ROMs, video conferencing, Internet, interactive television or satellite broadcast, e-mail, and discussion forums, and may include online interaction between the learner and their teacher or peers.

elimination Having a disease under control in a geographic area.

emerging infectious disease An infectious disease that has newly appeared in a population or that has been known for some time but is rapidly increasing in incidence or geographic range.

emigrant Person leaving a country to move (permanently) to another.

emigration The act of departing or exiting from one State with a view to settling in another.

emotional readiness The internal motivation toward knowledge, beliefs, and skills that will help people solve problems and concerns in their own lives.

enabling factors Elements such as personal and family income, health insurance, health access, and regular source of care, and availability of community health personnel and facilities.

environmental epidemiology Study of the effect of environmental contaminants on human health.

environmental factors Elements that may influence access, availability, or acceptance of health care services.

environmental health   Those aspects of human health, including quality of life, determined by physical, chemical, biological, social, and psychological problems in the environment.

environmental justice   Concept of disproportionate environmental risks that are borne by poor communities and communities of color.

environmental tobacco smoke (ETS)   The tobacco smoke a nonsmoker is exposed to when in proximity to a smoker; includes both the inhalation of mainstream smoke exhaled by the smoker and sidestream smoke from a lit cigarette; also known as passive smoke or secondhand smoke (SHS) exposure.

epidemiological model   Model used in understanding disease and the relationships among three elements—agent, host, and environment.

eradication   Elimination of the causative agent of disease.

essential public health services   The 10 services critical to reaching the vision of healthy people in healthy communities.

ethic   Generic term that refers to understanding and examining the moral life and the duties of human beings; includes both social morality and philosophical reflection.

ethnic density   The concentration of people from the same ethnic background living in a community.

ethnicity   Cultural construct that categorizes groups of people based on their geographic origins, languages, or cultural similarity in the world.

evaluated needs   Objective measures of the population's health status and treatment provided.

evaluating   Assessing those alternatives from the detailing phase related to costs, economic analysis, benefits, and how the program provider, the population, and the community may react to the alternatives.

evidence-based practice   Health care interventions based on rigorous analysis of available scientific evidence. Also defined as the process of using current evidence to guide practice and clinical decision making for the purpose of outcomes management.

evidence-based program   Theory-driven program that has activities related to the theory, and is reasonably well-implemented.

experiential readiness   A person's ability to learn, based on cognitive, affective, and psychomotor abilities.

experimental study   Research that manipulates variables and controls some conditions that could affect the results of the study. Subjects are randomly assigned to either a treatment or a control group.

exposure   The quantitative contact with environmental pollutants and other agents, that the individual or community is experiencing.

external environmental factors   Elements such as economic climate, relative wealth, level of stress and violence, and prevailing norms of a community.

externalities   Method of valuation that emphasizes the way costs and benefits are valued for people who are not the users of preventive services. Also defined as outcomes or side effects of an action or behavior of an individual or firm that affect others without their consent.

family caregiver   Family member who cares for an ill or disabled member of the family.

fate and transport   Processes by which substances are disbursed through the environment, such as leaching and runoff.

federally qualified health centers (FQHCs)   Nonprofit, consumer-directed health care corporations funded with U.S. Public Health Service monies that provide comprehensive primary and preventive health care services; designated as FQHCs because they meet the standards for funding based on rigorous standards for high-quality care and services.

fee-for-service   Charge for services received in which the provider determines the fee or charge and the insured pays through a third party payer (insurance company). The charge is paid in three ways: premiums, deductibles, and copayments.

feminist ethics   Restructuring of the power relationships that characterize health care such that the focus moves from managing crises to fostering health empowerment.

fetal alcohol syndrome (FAS)   An array of birth defects occurring in children who were born to mothers who consumed alcohol during pregnancy.

fiscal management   Supervision and accountability for organizational and/or programmatic funds and allocations.

fixed costs   Set costs or prices for resources.

Florence Nightingale (1820–1910)   An influential English nurse who originated formal training for nurses after organizing a large team that provided direct care to wounded British soldiers during the Crimean War.

focus group   Group of people with similar experiences or interests who meet to discuss their perceptions and perspectives on a topic of interest.

food intoxication   Illness caused by toxins found in natural sources such as shellfish and mushrooms, in bacterial growth such as botulism, and in chemical contaminants such as mercury poisoning.

food-borne disease   Illness caused by consuming food contaminated by toxic substances such as bacteria, parasites, viruses, or chemicals; often called "food poisoning."

forced migration   Compulsory transfer of a group of people, usually by a government.

formal or institutional agenda items   Items that are seriously being considered by decision makers.

formative evaluation   Assessment conducted while the program is still in progress to focus on developing and improving the program.

formulating   Defining the problem based on a needs assessment of the program population.

frontier communities   The most sparsely populated and isolated areas of the United States.

future think   Framework by which a manager anticipates, assesses, designs, innovates, implements, measures, reports, and starts all over again.

futuring   Knowing how to think about the future in order to improve it.

genetic screening   Public health programs that survey or test target populations with the aim of detecting individuals at risk of disease for genetic reasons.

genetics   Study of the functions and effects of single genes.

genomics   Study of both single genes, but also of the entire human genome and the interactions of multiple genes with each other and with the environment.

germ theory   The theory that microorganisms cause infectious diseases.

global   All countries noted on a globe.

global health   Provision of health as a social, economic, and political issue, along with a fundamental human right for all nations and peoples across state boundaries.

Global North   The richer countries in the world such as the United States.

Global South   The poorer countries in the world such as those in sub-Saharan Africa.

globalization   Process of increasing economic, political, and social independence and integration as capital, goods, persons, concepts, images, ideas, and values cross state boundaries.

Great Depression   A massive economic recession that ran from 1929 to approximately 1939 and was felt largely in the United States, bringing with it high unemployment and poverty, bank failures, and dramatically reduced industrial and agricultural production.

hate crimes   Bias-motivated crimes brought about by prejudice or partiality by the perpetrator against victims belonging to either real or perceived groups.

health   A social, economic, and political issue, but above all a fundamental human right for all nations and peoples.

health behaviors   Personal health practices and use of health services.

health care disparities   Differences in quality of health care due to factors other than access-related or clinical needs, preferences, and appropriateness of intervention.

health care system environmental factors   Elements that that may influence access, availability, or acceptance of health care services.

health communication   A strategy to disseminate information necessary to promote and maintain a healthy state and quality of life to individuals, groups, and communities.

health disparities   Differences among subgroups in access to health care and treatment, quality of life, health care outcomes, and longevity of life. Also defined as differences in health status or health care that occurs by gender, race or ethnicity, education or income, disability, geographic location, or sexual orientation.

health education   Planned learning involving some form of communication designed to improve health literacy, including improving knowledge, and developing life skills which are conducive to individual and community health.

Health For All   The goal set by the World Health Organization for countries to achieve by the year 2000.

health literacy   The capacity of individuals to obtain, interpret, and understand basic health information and services and the competence to use such information and services in ways which enhance health.

health outcomes   Included in Andersen and Davidson's model are health access, health utilization, and client satisfaction.

health policies   Directives that pertain to the health and the pursuit of health.

Health Professional Shortage Area (HPSA)   Area designated by the U.S. Health Resources and Services Administration that may have shortages of primary medical, dental, or mental health providers, and may be urban or rural areas, population groups or medical or other public facilities.

health promotion   Activities that are done to promote wellness. Also defined as the process of enabling people to increase control over and to improve their health by reducing differences in current health status and ensuring equal opportunities and resources to enable all people to achieve their fullest health potential.

health risk appraisal tool   Instrument that identifies specific factors in individuals that increase the risk of impairments or disabilities and then recommends behavioral modifications to minimize their impact.

health services pyramid   A visual representation of how the different levels of health care should relate to one another.

health trends   Indicators of health collected over time that show a general direction.

health-promoting behavior   Any behavior that attains a positive health outcome.

Healthy Cities; Healthy Communities   A social ecological approach to development and community health promotion that is a collaborative and local partnership between political leaders and citizens.

healthy public policies   Plans that address the determinants of health and seek a positive impact on health outcomes and quality of life. Also defined as directives whose aim is to create supportive environments that enable people to lead healthy lives; characterized by a focus on health, equity, and accountability for the health impact of the policy.

hedonism   Any philosophy that says that pleasure is equivalent to good and pain is equivalent to evil.

Helvie's energy theory   Theory that views the community as an open system and the population as changing through bound, kinetic, and potential energy.

Henry Street Settlement   A social settlement established in 1893 by Lillian Wald in Manhattan's Lower East Side and initially modeled after Hull House in Chicago.

herd immunity   Resistance to the spread of infectious disease in a group because susceptible members are few, making transmission from an infected member unlikely.

Hispanic paradox   Phenomenon in which most Hispanic immigrant groups, who are characterized by low socioeconomic status, have better than expected health and mortality outcomes when compared to nonimmigrants of similar socioeconomic status.

HMO (health maintenance organization)   Fee-for service health plan where the HMO has a contract with a group of health care providers, both primary care providers and specialists, who have agreed to be responsible for the care provided to enrolled health care consumers. Health care providers under HMOs are paid a fixed fee per client (known as per capita form of reimbursement).

homelessness   Term referring to persons who lack a fixed or permanent, regular, and adequate residence.

Hull House   A social settlement on Chicago's Near West Side that was established in 1889 by Jane Addams and provided social services, activities, and meeting spaces for those in poor urban neighborhoods.

human rights   Basic rights and freedoms to which all humans are entitled, including life, liberty, freedom of thought and expression, equality before the law, and material well-being.

illegal alien or undocumented alien   Alien who enters or stays in a country without the appropriate documentation.

illness prevention   Activities that are done to help prevent or delay illness.

immigrant (in general)   Person entering a country (permanently) from another.

impelled migration   Similar to forced migration but differs in that migrants retain some ability to decide whether to move.

implementing   Putting into action the best plan selected to meet the needs of the target population.

incidence   Proportion of a given population with newly diagnosed diseases during a defined period of time.

incident command structure (ICS)   Model for the command, control, and coordination of a response to an emergency; provides the means to coordinate the efforts of individual agencies.

infectivity   Agent's ability to replicate itself in the host in order to grow and spread.

information/communication systems capacity   A component of the public health infrastructure that includes a current system of guidelines, recommendations, alerts, standards-based information, and communications systems for monitoring disease and communicating within the public health system of public and private health organizations, community organizations, the media, and the public.

Institutional Review Board   Group of experienced researchers and consumers who examine the research according to ethical standards.

insulin resistance   Diminished tissue response to insulin leading to the development of diabetes.

intangibles   Method of valuation that emphasizes non-monetary costs and benefits.

integrated pest management (IPM)   Method of pest control that integrates a variety of chemical and nonchemical techniques to control pests while reducing or minimizing risks to human health and the environment.

integration   Acculturation where there is some degree of retention of original culture, while people seek to participate in the new culture as well.

intergenerational transmission   Term identified and coined by some authors to describe the process of children adopting their parents' lifestyle behaviors.

international terrorism   Violent acts or acts dangerous to human life that appear to be intended to intimidate or coerce a civilian population or to influence the policy of a government. These acts occur primarily outside the territorial jurisdiction of the United States or transcend national boundaries in terms of the means by which they are accomplished, and the persons they appear intended to intimidate or coerce.

interviews   Method of data collection in which the public health nurse asks questions about health, attitudes, beliefs, and health behaviors of community members; performed face-to-face or by telephone.

isolation   Physical separation and confinement of an individual or groups of individuals, who are infected or reasonably believed to be infected with a contagious or possibly contagious disease from nonisolated individuals, to prevent or limit the transmission of the disease to nonisolated individuals.

Jane Addams (1860–1935)   An American social worker and reformer who founded the social settlement Hull House in Chicago and built an international reputation based on her writing, settlement house work, and peace efforts.

John Snow (1813-1858)   A British health care provider who recognized that that cholera was likely transmitted through ingestion and then traced an 1854 London cholera epidemic to the Broad Street pump where contaminated drinking water was being obtained by local residents.

justice   Equitable treatment of individuals.

keys to improvement   Self and organizational approaches that enhance work performance, efficiency, and effectiveness to improve public health initiatives.

Lavinia Dock (1858–1956)   A public health nurse advocate, suffragist, and political activist who worked with Lillian Wald at the Henry Street Settlement House and was a strong supporter of professional nursing training and practice.

leach   Removal of contaminants, such as pesticides or fertilizers, from the soil by water trickling through.

leadership   Behaviors that provide direction and motivation of the behaviors of others by going beyond the organization's or community's expectations.

leading health indicators   Evidence-based major public health concerns in the United States used to measure the health of the nation over the next 10 years.

learner needs   Discrepancy or gaps between knowledge, skills, and abilities or competencies needed for performance and their present level of development.

learner readiness   The time when the learner demonstrates an interest in learning the type or degree of information necessary to maintain optimal health.

learning   A process of change that results in change in knowledge, attitude, skills, and behavior.

learning style   A person's or group's preferred modes and environments for learning and includes cognitive, affective, and psychomotor/physiological dimensions as well as characteristics of instruction and settings for instruction.

legal rights   Rights determined by political constitutions, legislative acts, case law, and executive orders, without reference to moral systems.

liability or tort   "A civil wrong committed against a person or the person's property" and "acts of omissions which unlawfully violate a person's rights by law and for which the appropriate remedy is a common law action for damages by the injured party." (Guido, 2001)

Lillian Wald (1867–1940) A social reformer and political activist who founded the Henry Street Settlement House and became the nurse credited with establishing the profession of public health nursing.

linguistic competence Capacity of an organization and its personnel to communicate with persons of limited English proficiency, those who are illiterate or have low literacy skills, and individuals with disabilities.

lobbying The art of using persuasion to convince a legislator, a government official, the head of an agency, or a state official to comply with a request.

logic models Logical process by which program inputs and activities are intended to create the outcomes or effects.

long-term objectives Broad, long-term statements of expected outcomes.

malpractice Violation of the professional standard of care as defined in state nurse practice acts.

managed care Organized effort by health insurance plans and providers to use financial incentives and organizational arrangements to alter provider and client behavior so that health care services are delivered and utilized in a more efficient and lower cost manner.

managed competition Health insurance provision that builds in competition among insurance companies for buyers such as employers; this competition is considered to be the means for providing lower insurance costs to the consumer.

management Translating the leadership's or organization's vision and mission into productive action and progression toward public health goals.

marginal benefit Value or benefit of a resource.

marginalization Little interest in or possibility maintaining either culture.

McCarthyism A period in American history identified with Wisconsin senator Joseph McCarthy and lasting from approximately 1945 to 1960, in which extreme anticommunist political repression emerged that resulted in hundreds of deportations, cost thousands of Americans their jobs, and brought about two executions.

media Another word for the different environments—air, water, soil.

Medicaid (Title XIX) Insurance program jointly funded by federal and state governments; eligibility is determined by income and resources and is for all ages.

Medically Underserved Areas (MUA) Area designated by the U.S. Health Resources and Services Administration that may have shortages of health care professionals based on an Index of Medical Underservice (IMU) involving four variables—ratio of primary medical care physicians per 1,000 population, infant mortality rate, percentage of the population with incomes below the poverty level, and percentage of the population age 65 or older.

Medicare (Title XVIII) Federal insurance program for individuals 65 years and older and those who are disabled but younger than 65 years.

Medigap Additional health insurance for the elderly and disabled to cover the costs that Medicare does not cover under both Parts A and B.

mental health A state of successful mental functioning, resulting in productive activities, fulfilling relationships, and the ability to adapt to change and cope with adversity.

metabolic syndrome A group of risk factors believed to serve as a precursor for the development of type 2 diabetes and cardiovascular disease.

metropolitan Area having a population of 50,000 or more people.

migrant Persons and/or family members moving to another country or region to better their material or social conditions and improve the prospect for themselves or their family.

migrant health centers Federally funded health centers that provide culturally and linguistically competent health and support services to migrants and seasonal farmworkers and their families.

migrant rural farmworker Individual who moves from one region to another in search of farm or agricultural work of a seasonal or other temporary nature and is required to be absent overnight from his or her permanent place of residence.

migration Process of moving, either across an international border or within a State; encompasses any kind of population people, whatever its length, composition, and causes.

migratory worker or seasonal worker (also documented migrant worker, itinerant worker) "Person who is engaged. . .in a remunerated activity in a State of which he or she is not a national" (Art. 2(1), International Convention on the Protection of the Rights of All Migrant Workers and Members of Their Families, 1990).

Millennium Development Goals (MDGs)
Commitments made by 189 countries "to reduce poverty and hunger, and to tackle ill-health, gender inequality, lack of education, lack of access to clean water and environmental degradation." (WHO, 2004).

mission statement clarification Process of reviewing the mission statement in order to have a clear sense of direction: this will drive the activities and set the expectations of the program development.

mode of entry Description of how agents enter their hosts.

mode of exit Description of how agents leave their hosts.

mode of transmission Environment for transmission including the social, cultural, biologic, and physical influences on a human host.

model program Evidence-based program that meets criteria for effective programs and is ready for dissemination.

moral rights Rights derived from moral principles and serve as a basis for the evaluation of legal rights.

morality Beliefs surrounding right and wrong human conduct.

morbidity Illness or disease rates.

mortality Death rates.

multisectoral Refers to inclusion of various segments of the community to participate in healthy initiatives.

National Electronic Disease Surveillance System (NEDSS) Disease surveillance and monitoring component of the PHIN, utilized at the federal, state and local levels.

National Incident Management System (NIMS) System that provides a consistent nation-wide approach for federal, state, local, and tribal governments and private-sector and nongovernmental organizations to work together across jurisdictions to prepare for, prevent, respond to, and recover from domestic incidents regardless of cause, size, or complexity.

National Response Plan (NRP) Comprehensive all-hazards plan developed to manage domestic incidents through the prevention of, preparedness for, response to, and recovery from terrorism, major natural disasters, and other major emergencies; supersedes the Federal Response Plan (FRP).

natural disasters Acts caused by either nature, such as hurricanes, or emerging diseases, such as avian influenza.

natural immunity Resistance to a specific disease that is genetically determined.

need factors Perceived and evaluated need for health services.

needs assessment Means to identify population-based needs, evaluate a current target population in need of services, identify new target populations that have unmet needs, and provide resources available to meet those needs.

negative valence Being repulsed by or having a negative attitude or belief toward an object, behavior, or outcome of a behavior.

negligence Deviation from the standard of care that an individual would expect in a given situation.

New Deal A comprehensive reform package that included government jobs and social security benefits and was established by U.S. President Franklin D. Roosevelt as a mechanism for reversing the impact of the Great Depression.

Nineteenth Amendment An amendment to the Constitution of the United States that was ratified in 1920 and states that "The right of citizens of the United States to vote shall not be denied or abridged by the United States or by any State on account of sex. Congress shall have power to enforce this article by appropriate legislation."

noise pollution Unwanted, man-made sound that can be harmful to human health. Examples include noise from automobiles, aircraft, construction work, and factories.

noncomparative justice Making sure that people receive the rights to which they are entitled.

nonmaleficence Obligation not to inflict harm on others.

nonmetropolitan Area having population of fewer than 50,000 people.

normal aging Aging changes that occur to the majority of individuals.

nosocomial infection Infection acquired during hospitalization, also called hospital-acquired infection.

nurse-managed health centers Health centers run by nurses to provide comprehensive health services based on community need and the specific needs of vulnerable populations.

nursing assessment   Systematic collection of data about a client's health status, beliefs, and behaviors relevant to developing a health promotion prevention plan.

Nursing Outcomes Classification   Scheme to document client outcomes that are influenced by nursing.

obesity   For adults, having a body mass index of 30 kg/m² or greater; for children and adolescents, a sex- and age-specific BMI at or above the 95th percentile, based on revised Centers for Disease Control and Prevention growth charts.

occupational health nursing   Specialty practice that provides the delivery of health and safety programs and service to workers, groups of workers, populations, and community groups.

Omaha System   Scheme to classify client problems, outcomes, and interventions in environmental, psychosocial, physiological, and health-related behaviors.

opportunity cost   Idea that resources used for one purpose cannot be used for another.

organizational culture   Internal expectations of an organization based on its vision, mission, institutional and community history.

organizational/systems capacity   A public health system infrastructure component that refers to the ability of local, state, and national governmental public health and public health system partners to provide the essential services for the purpose of promoting healthy people in healthy communities.

outcome evaluation   The degree to which the educational objectives were met.

outcome expectancies   Expected outcomes that would occur if the person were to perform the behavior and whether those outcomes had a positive and negative value for the person.

overweight   Being too heavy for one's height. A person is considered overweight if he or she has a body mass index of 25 to 30 kg/m².

participatory action research (PAR)   View in which targeted populations are considered collaborators instead of research subjects. PAR has bridged gaps between public health leaders, educators, and the community; created more trust between groups and a greater understanding of community perceptions; decreased evaluator bias and stereotyping; and improved implementation and evaluation of health disparity initiatives.

participatory development   A style of community health promotion and capacity building that emphasizes citizen involvement, partnerships, and participation.

passive immunity   Resistance to a disease from antibodies provided by mothers through transplacental transfer and breastfeeding or through the administration of immune globulins or antiserums.

paternalism   Benevolently restricting the freedom of others and acting for the best good of others without their consent.

pathogen   Agent or microorganism capable of causing disease.

pathogenicity   Ability of an agent to cause specific signs and symptoms of disease.

pedagogy   Teacher-centered educational model where the teacher decides what, how, and when content will be learned, and whether teaching content has been learned.

Pender's Health Promotion Model   A theoretical perspective that explains factors and relationships influencing the promotion of healthy behaviors and ultimately to the enhancement of health and quality of life.

People's Charter for Health   Document asserting that health is a human right and that health and human rights should prevail over economic and political concerns.

People's Health Assembly (PHA)   A group of individuals across countries that believe health is a fundamental human right that cannot be met without a commitment to equity and social justice. The participants gather to assess the current unjust state of affairs and to map the way forward so that health for all could be achieved.

People's Health Movement (PHM)   International coalition of grassroots organizations dedicated to challenging the prevailing system of health care delivery that is failing to serve most of the poor worldwide.

perceived needs   Individual, group, or community's perceptions of their health status, health functioning, adherence, and need for services.

performance management   Strategic use of performance standards, measures, progress reports, and ongoing quality improvement efforts to ensure that an agency achieves desired results. In the case of public health, the ultimate purpose of these efforts is to improve the public's health.

performance measures   Quantitative measures of capacities, processes, or outcomes relevant to the assessment of a performance indicator.

performance standards   Objective standards or guidelines that are used to assess an organization's performance.

perinatal health disparities Measures of low birth weight and infant mortality rates.

permanent resident alien Alien admitted to the United States as a lawful permanent resident.

persistence Length of time a substance stays in the environment after it has been introduced.

persistent, bioaccumulative, and toxic chemicals (PBTs) Toxic chemicals that are slow to break down (persist), and that accumulate in the bodies of animals and humans, with the highest concentrations found in those animals at the top of the food chain.

personal (self) insights and experiences Life events that influence one's perceptions, assumptions, expectations and relationships.

personal health practices Lifestyle and health risk behaviors that are major contributors to health outcomes.

personnel Human resources who are the organization's and society's capital.

physical activity Any form of exercise or movement produced by skeletal muscles that results in an expenditure of energy. It may include planned activity such as walking, running, playing basketball, or participating in other sports. It may also include other daily activities such as household chores, yard work, and walking the dog. It is recommended that adults get at least 30 minutes and children at least 60 minutes of moderate physical activity most days of the week.

planning Organized, systematic method to conceptualize, detail, implement, and evaluate the effectiveness of a program.

policy advocacy Professional being active in developing health policy in private and public arenas and in being elected and appointed to local, state, and national offices where they can make significant contributions.

policy development A core public health function that involves the development and evaluation of evidence-based public health policies.

politics The art and science of influencing the allocation of scarce resources; it also includes the notion of power.

population characteristics Characteristics such as age, sex, race and ethnicity, education, employment, values and attitudes, income, health insurance, health access, and a regular source of health care that influence health outcomes.

population-based nursing practice Public health nursing interventions with a focus on primary prevention, consideration of broad determinants of health, and the entire population that shares similar health concerns or characteristics.

positive valence Being attracted to or having a positive attitude or belief toward an object, behavior, or outcome of a behavior.

Preferred Provider Organization (PPO) Fee-for service health plan where the consumer chooses health care providers from a select group.

PRECEDE-PROCEED framework Guideline to help program managers identify factors affecting public health and plan targets for intervention, specify objectives, and criteria for evaluation.

pre-diabetes Condition characterized by a fasting blood glucose of > 100 mg/dL or a 2-hour post glucose tolerance blood glucose test of 140–199 mg/dL.

predisposing factors Demographic characteristics such as age, sex, and race and ethnicity; social structure characteristics such as education, employment; and health beliefs, such as values and attitudes.

preference Choice reflecting decision makers' values, wants, or needs.

premium Calculated amount that the insured pays per month for the health insurance plan; The third party payer determines the charge for the premium.

prevalence The proportion of a population that has been diagnosed with a certain disease at a single point in time.

primary care Accessible health services in the community provided by clinicians who practice in the context of the client's family and community to address diverse personal health care needs.

primary health care Model of care defined by the World Health Organization as a combination of primary care and public health care that is made universally accessible to community members and families and is provided at a cost the community and country can afford.

primary prevention Activities directed toward wellness involving specific protection for selected diseases.

primary prevention strategies Efforts to reduce the likelihood of susceptibility and incidence of diseases, health conditions, or poor health outcomes in minorities.

principle of autonomy Idea that rational individuals should be permitted to be self-determining.

principle of formal justice Defined by Aristotle as formal equality that states "Equals must be treated equally, and unequals must be treated unequally" or "Similar cases ought to be treated in similar ways."

principle of utility   Way to balance competing needs; utility imposes a social duty to do as much good as possible overall, with the recognition that one cannot meet all needs.

private insurance   Plans purchased by employers for employees or purchased directly by individuals from insurance carriers.

problem identification   Process of isolating the gap between what is available and what is needed for the stakeholder group.

process evaluation   The documentation and analysis of the way an education program is implemented and conducted at various points during the program.

profit   Net revenue or the amount by which revenue exceeds costs.

program components   Major functions or facets of the program that are to be evaluated.

program development   Strategic alignment of activities undertaken to meet an intended purpose to ensure that an identified problem has the best possible likelihood of success with the adequate resources.

program effects   Intended and unintended results or consequences of the program components.

program evaluation   Use of scientific methods to measure the implementation and outcomes of programs, for decision-making purposes.

program management   A collective of people involved in a service that promotes, protects, and meets the needs of a specific population in the community.

program objectives   Immediate, intermediate, or ultimate/ final aims that the program is meant to achieve.

program outputs   Services provided in the program.

program planning   Organized, systematic method to conceptualize, detail, implement, and evaluate the effectiveness of a program.

prospective payment system   Charges based on prices predetermined by the government rather than the provider, as under the retrospective payment system. For hospital care, the predetermined prices are based on a statistical system known as diagnosis-related groups.

psychomotor skills   Skills requiring physical manipulation.

public engagement   Being present, consistent, and truthful to engage people in dialogue to achieve common goals.

public health   That which "we as a society do collectively to assure the conditions in which people can be healthy" (Institute of Medicine, 1988).

Public Health Information Network (PHIN)   System to integrate the capabilities of public health information systems across a wide variety of organizations that participate in public health, to enable consistent exchange of response, health, and disease tracking data between public health partners in every community.

public health infrastructure   Organization or a group of organizations with established systems of communication, resources and programs that support public health initiatives and possess the ability to be responsive and proactive in time of critical need or threats.

public health nursing   A discipline within nursing that employs knowledge from nursing, social science, and public health science to promote the health of populations.

public health nursing competencies   The intersection of nursing and public health; this set of skills, knowledge, and attitudes is based on the Council of Linkages Core Competencies and serves as a guideline for population-focused public health nursing practice.

public insurance   Plans that are subsidized by the federal and state governments, such as Medicare, Medicaid, and Tri Care.

public policy   Directives formed by governmental bodies at the local, state, and federal levels that affect individual and institutional behaviors; also refers to court rulings dealing with institutions or organizations. Also defined as a statement that guides local, regional, and/or national action plans and interventions and is approved by a legislative or sanctioned body.

pull factors   Positive attributes perceived to exist at the new location, such as better climate, more professional opportunities, better jobs, lower taxes, and more space.

push factors   Negative attributes such as home conditions that impel the decision to migrate, such as loss of job, lack of professional opportunities, overcrowding, famine, war, and disease.

Quad Council of Public Health Nursing Organizations   An alliance of four national nursing organizations that address public health nursing issues: the Association of Community Health Nurse Educators (ACHNE), the American Nurses Association's Congress on Nursing Practice and Economics (ANA), the American Public Health Association—Public Health Nursing

Section (APHA), and the Association of State and Territorial Directors of Nursing (ASTDN).

qualitative study Nonquantitative, multimethod field of inquiry involving methods that describe meanings of phenomena to people.

quality adjusted life year (QALY) Measure that summarizes the quantity and quality of life experienced by clients.

quality assurance program Program that evaluates care of clients to improve existing programs or add new ones.

quality improvement Program or process to manage change and achieve higher standards in public health policies, programs, or infrastructure based on performance standards, measurements, and reports.

quantitative study Research using numbers to describe variables in a study.

quarantine Physical separation and confinement from nonquarantine individuals of an individual or groups of individuals, who are or may have been exposed to a contagious or possibly contagious disease and who do not show signs and symptoms of a contagious disease, to prevent or limit the transmission of the disease to nonquarantine individuals.

quasi-experimental study Research that manipulates variables but cannot control conditions. Subjects are either randomly assigned to a treatment or a control group.

race Social construct that categorizes an individual or group based on physical and anatomical features, most notably the color of one's skin.

racism Discrimination of a group of individuals based on racial and ethnic identities, cultures, language, religion, or national origin.

Radiological Dispersal Device (RDD) There are two types of RDD: detonation of a radiological device, such as a "dirty bomb" (conventional explosive with radioactive material) and radiation hidden in a public place that is not visible.

randomized control trial Study in which research subjects are randomized to either a treatment or a control group to reduce bias of study findings.

rates Measures of frequency of health events that put raw numbers into a frame of reference based on the size of a population.

receiving country Country accepting immigrants from other countries.

refugee Any person who is outside his or her country of nationality and is unable or unwilling to return to that country because of persecution or a well-founded fear of persecution.

relative risk A comparison of two morbidity or mortality rates using a calculation of the ratio of one to the other.

reservation wage Lowest wage at which a person is willing to enter the labor market.

reservoir Sum of all sources where the agents may temporarily live, including human and animal hosts and locations in the environment.

resilience Personal traits that provide the capacity to bounce back from adversity.

retrospective payment system Charges that are based on the actual care and services provided.

risk The probability that an illness or injury will occur within a specified time frame.

risk assessment An evaluation of a substance to identify environmental and/or human health risks resulting from exposure to this chemical. This assessment incorporates the toxicity of the compound with the potential for exposure to determine the risk.

risk communication Field of communication that involves the transmission of information about health and environmental risks, their significance, and the policies for managing them.

Roy's Adaptation Model Community assessment model based on the premise that individuals or populations receive stimuli from the environment. A changing environment may stimulate a person or a population to use coping mechanisms to make an adaptive response.

rural Descriptor for a community with fewer than 2,500 residents or fewer than 99 persons per square mile.

rural health clinics Organizations that provide primary care services to persons with Medicare and Medicaid in rural areas not designated as "urbanized areas" by the U.S. Census Bureau and in locations designated as a Health Professional Shortage Area (HPSA) or a Medically Underserved Area (MUA).

safety net providers Agencies and health care providers who deliver services to people who have trouble accessing affordable, timely, and continuous health care because of financial, cultural, linguistic, or geographic barriers.

sanitary era   A nineteenth-century public health movement that focused on cleanliness and contended that disease is directly caused by dirt and poor hygiene.

school-based health centers   Health centers located on school grounds that provide a variety of preventive, acute, chronic, mental, and behavioral health services to help children and youth achieve optimal health and academic success.

Scope and Standards of Gerontological Nursing Practice   A document published by the American Nurses Association that defines current practice expectations and competent care standards associated with basic and advanced clinical practice for the specialty of gerontological nursing.

screening   The classification of people based on their likelihood of having a disease.

secondary data   Data already collected and archived.

secondary prevention   Level of prevention that focuses on early detection through screening, and rapid management of disease progression through diagnosis and treatment.

secondary prevention strategies   Efforts of early diagnosis and early intervention to prevent premature deaths, disabilities, or injuries.

self-efficacy   A judgment about one's personal capability to organize and carry out a particular action.

sending country   Country that is the source of immigrants.

sensitive   A test that avoids false negatives and finds a large percentage of the true positives.

separation   When individuals avoid those customs of the new culture and value retaining their original culture exclusively.

sheltered homeless   People who are homeless and living in shelters or transitional housing.

Sheppard-Towner Act   A legislative act in place from 1921 to 1930 that increased funding for the federal government's efforts to reduce infant mortality through the provision of maternal and infant health care.

short-term objectives   Specific, clear, and unambiguous descriptions of educational expectations.

social capital   Aggregate of individuals' social group networks or geographic space, which includes trust and reciprocity.

social construction   Target populations viewed by elected officials as advantaged, contenders, dependents, and deviants.

social Darwinism   A social belief that was adapted from Darwin's theories of survival and suggested that the poor were disadvantaged because of their own lack of motivation.

social ecological approach   A perspective that emphasizes the interrelationships of people and their multifaceted environments (e.g., social, institutional, cultural, physical, political, and economic).

social marketing   The application of commercial marketing principles and techniques to promote socially relevant behaviors.

somatization   Vague or generalized somatic symptoms such as headaches, chest pains, palpitations, shortness of breath, fatigue, and sleep disturbances that express emotional distress.

specific   A test that avoids mistaken identifications or false positives and finds a large percentage of the true negatives.

spend down   Practice wherein the elderly dispose of all their liquid assets to an amount determined by the federal government prior to their qualifying for Medicaid.

stakeholder analysis   Study of that group of people who have a vested interest or who may benefit from the program.

Strategic National Stockpile (SNS)   Caches of large quantities of medicines and medical supplies that can be delivered anywhere in the United States to supplement medical resources that are being depleted.

street-living homeless   People who are homeless and living on the streets.

substance abuse   Description for the misuse of alcohol, drugs, and tobacco.

suffrage   The civil right to vote. Women were allowed to vote in the United States after the Nineteenth Amendment was passed in 1920.

summative evaluations   Assessment conducted at the end of a program; it focuses on program outcomes.

Superfund   Federal program administered by the U.S. Environmental Protection Agency that investigates and cleans up the largest and most contaminated sites in the United States.

support services   Personnel such as office managers, receptionists, file clerks, information systems, and outreach workers. Support services also include equipment and technology necessary to implement and evaluate public health services and measure clinical outcomes.

surveillance system Ongoing, systematic tracking of reportable infectious diseases; purpose is to reduce morbidity and mortality and to improve health.

survey Self-report data collected from community residents using questionnaires to obtain information about demographics, knowledge, attitudes, perceptions, opinions, health beliefs, and behaviors.

SWOT Analysis identifying the areas of strengths, weaknesses, opportunities, and threats in program development and planning.

systemic agenda items Policies or issues that are abstract.

systems planning perspective Approach that allows nurse leaders to take a proactive stance in meeting the multiple, competing demands that must be balanced to improve population health.

teaching Act of behavior shaping through a learning process.

teaching-learning process A systematic and strategic problem-solving process that mirrors the nursing process and includes assessing the learner, planning and developing objectives, implementing the plan, and evaluating the teaching-learning encounter.

Technical Advisory Response Unit (TARU) Team of CDC technical advisers, comprised of pharmacists, emergency responders, and logistic experts, who accompany the SNS medical supplies and advise local authorities on receiving, distributing, dispensing, replenishing, and recovering SNS material.

technical efficiency Idea that total costs of producing a quantity of a good or service are being minimized.

technical rate of substitution Ratio representing when the same amount is produced per dollar that is spent on each input.

terrorism Unlawful use of force or violence against persons or property to intimidate or coerce a government, the civilian population, or any segment thereof, in furtherance of political or social objective.

tertiary prevention Level of prevention that focuses on the prevention and management of complications of the side effects of treatment, rehabilitation, as well as reducing potential harm to others.

tertiary prevention strategies Efforts to prevent the further progression or deterioration of a disease, illness, or health problem within minority populations.

THC (delta-9-tetrahydrocannabinol) Main active ingredient in marijuana thought to be responsible for impairing the immune system in marijuana users (NIDA, 2004; Zhu et al., 2000).

third party payer Company or organization, either private or public, that pays or underwrites health care coverage for a business or individual.

toxicity Potential of a substance to have a harmful effect on humans or animals.

toxicology Studies of poisons or chemicals that cause illness.

transnationalism Fluidity of travel of people between sending and receiving countries.

Tri Care Federal health care program for active-duty and retired service personnel, their eligible family members, and survivors.

triadic reciprocal determinism Dynamic and simultaneous interaction of person, environmental factors, and behavior to determine the behavior as well as affect the person and environment in which the behavior occurs.

UN Covenant on Civil and Political Rights Document dealing with persons' negative rights: what governments must not do to their citizens.

UN Covenant on Economic, Social, and Cultural Rights Document dealing with positive rights: what governments must do for their citizens.

uncertainty Idea that multiple outcomes are associated with a probability and the expected outcome (a weighted average based on the probability of each possible outcome) used in decision making.

universal coverage Provision of health insurance by a government for all individuals within a country; also known as a single payer system of health care.

Universal Declaration of Human Rights Declaration with 30 articles that are the basis for all human rights documents. They are the international basis for every person's right to equal dignity, "without distinction of any kind, such as race, color, sex, language, religion, political or other opinion, national or social origin, property, birth or other status." (WHO, 1946).

utilitarianism Ethical theory rooted in the ancient Greek philosophy of hedonism. It basic tenet is to promote the greatest happiness or good for the greatest number.

utility Life satisfaction.

value-expectancy theories　Theories that hold the premise that behavior is a function of the subjective value of an outcome and the subjective expectation that a particular action will achieve that outcome.

values　Personal beliefs about the worth of objects, ideas, or concepts.

variable costs　Costs or prices for resources that vary depending on other factors.

vector　Carrier of disease; usually animals, insects, and birds that transmit disease from a host to a noninfected animal.

virtue ethics　In the tradition of Plato and Aristotle, virtues may be understood as character traits that are morally valuable such as truthfulness, compassion, or courage. Virtue based ethics is concerned not with how to act, but with what kind of person to be and what sort of life to lead.

virulence　Agent's ability to cause severe disease and death.

vulnerable populations　Subgroups of people who are more sensitive to risk factors than others because of their economic, social, physical/environmental, biological, and lifestyle differences.

watershed　Land area that drains water into a stream or other body of water.

weapons of mass destruction (WMD)　Any device, material, or substance used in a manner to cause death or serious injury to persons or significant damage to property.

window of opportunity　Timing for any of the three streams of the policy process (policy stream, problem stream, and political stream) appearing on the political agenda.

windshield survey　Method for collecting data in the community by direct observation.

workforce capacity　A public health system infrastructure dealing with the size and competency of the public health workers in local, state, and national public health agencies, whose function is protecting and promoting the health of the community, and preventing and controlling disease in that community.

working poor or uninsured　Individuals who do not have health insurance, including those working for small companies that do not offer insurance, the self-employed, and part-time and seasonal workers.

World Social Forum (WSF)　Group of economists and grassroots activists who challenged the existing global economic system and declared that a world is possible where people's human rights are respected and nations can develop in peace.

xenophobia　Rejection, fear, and stigmatization of foreigners.

zero-base budgeting　Plan wherein there is no budget excess at the end of the fiscal year.

zoning　Policy and process by which land use is designated as residential, commercial, industrial, parks, or some combination of these.

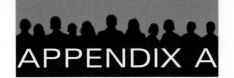

APPENDIX A

Core Competencies for Public Health Nursing Practice

DOMAIN 1 Analytic Assessment Skills

	GENERALIST/STAFF PHN		MANAGER/ CNS/ CONSULTANT/ PROGRAM SPECIALIST/ EXECUTIVE	
	Individuals and Families	Populations/ Systems	Individuals and Families	Populations/ Systems
1. Defines a problem	Proficiency	Knowledge	Proficiency	Proficiency
2. Determines appropriate uses and limitations of both quantitative and qualitative data	Knowledge	Awareness	Proficiency	Proficiency
3. Selects and defines variables relevant to defined public health problems	Knowledge	Knowledge	Proficiency	Proficiency
4. Identifies relevant and appropriate data and information sources	Proficiency	Knowledge	Proficiency	Proficiency
5. Evaluates the integrity and comparability of data and identifies gaps in data sources	Knowledge	Awareness	Proficiency	Proficiency
6. Applies ethical principles to the collection, maintenance, use, and dissemination of data and information	Proficiency	Knowledge	Proficiency	Proficiency
7. Partners with communities to attach meaning to collected quantitative and qualitative data	N/A*	Knowledge	N/A*	Proficiency
8. Makes relevant inferences from quantitative and qualitative data	Knowledge	Awareness	Proficiency	Proficiency
9. Obtains and interprets information regarding risks and benefits to the community	Knowledge	Knowledge	Proficiency	Proficiency
10. Applies data collection processes, information technology applications, and computer systems storage retrieval strategies	Knowledge	Awareness	Proficiency	Proficiency
11. Recognizes how the data illuminates ethical, political, scientific, economic, and overall public health issues	Knowledge	Awareness	Proficiency	Proficiency

* These competencies, because of their population or system-focused language, do not apply at the individual/family level, but are applicable to the broader context of population-focused public health services and systems.

DOMAIN 2 Policy Development / Program Planning Skills

	GENERALIST/ STAFF PHN		MANAGER/ CNS/ CONSULTANT/ PROGRAM SPECIALIST/ EXECUTIVE	
	Individuals and Families	Populations/ Systems	Individuals and Families	Populations/ Systems
1. Collects, summarizes, and interprets information relevant to an issue	Knowledge	Awareness	Proficiency	Proficiency
2. States policy options and writes clear and concise policy statements	Awareness	Awareness	Proficiency	Proficiency
3. Identifies, interprets, and implements public health laws, regulations, and policies related to specific programs	Knowledge	Knowledge	Proficiency	Proficiency
4. Articulates the health, fiscal, administrative, legal, social, and political implications of each policy option	Awareness	Awareness	Proficiency	Proficiency
5. States the feasibility and expected outcomes of each policy option	Awareness	Awareness	Proficiency	Proficiency
6. Utilizes current techniques in decision analysis and health planning	Knowledge	Awareness	Proficiency	Proficiency
7. Decides on the appropriate course of action	Knowledge	Awareness	Proficiency	Proficiency
8. Develops a plan to implement policy, including goals, outcome and process objectives, and implementation steps	Proficiency	Knowledge	Awareness	Proficiency
9. Translates policy into organizational plans, structures, and programs	N/A*	Awareness	N/A*	Proficiency
10. Prepares and implements emergency response plans	Knowledge	Knowledge	Proficiency	Proficiency
11. Develops mechanisms to monitor and evaluate programs for their effectiveness and quality	Knowledge	Knowledge	Proficiency	Proficiency

* These competencies, because of their population or system-focused language, do not apply at the individual/family level, but are applicable to the broader context of population-focused public health services and systems.

DOMAIN 3 Communication Skills

	GENERALIST/ STAFF PHN		MANAGER/ CNS/ CONSULTANT/ PROGRAM SPECIALIST/ EXECUTIVE	
	Individuals and Families	Populations/ Systems	Individuals and Families	Populations/ Systems
1. Communicates effectively both in writing and orally, or in other ways	Proficiency	Knowledge	Proficiency	Proficiency
2. Solicits input from individuals and organizations	Proficiency	Knowledge	Proficiency	Proficiency
3. Advocates for public health programs and resources	Proficiency	Knowledge	Proficiency	Proficiency
4. Leads and participates in groups to address specific issues	Proficiency	Knowledge	Proficiency	Proficiency
5. Uses the media, advanced technologies, and community networks to communicate information	Knowledge	Awareness	Knowledge *	Knowledge*
6. Effectively presents accurate demographic, statistical, programmatic, and scientific information for professional and lay audiences	Knowledge	Knowledge	Proficiency	Proficiency
7. Attitudes: Listens to others in an unbiased manner, respects points of view of others, and promotes the expression of diverse opinions and perspectives	Proficiency	Proficiency	Proficiency	Proficiency

*Reflects ability to determine need for and to utilize experts in these areas.

DOMAIN 4 Cultural Competency Skills

	GENERALIST/ STAFF PHN		MANAGER/ CNS/ CONSULTANT/ PROGRAM SPECIALIST/ EXECUTIVE	
	Individuals and Families	Populations/ Systems	Individuals and Families	Populations/ Systems
1. Utilizes appropriate methods for interacting sensitively, effectively, and professionally with persons from diverse cultural, socioeconomic, educational, racial, ethnic professional backgrounds, and persons of all ages and lifestyle and preferences	Proficiency	Proficiency	Proficiency	Proficiency
2. Identifies the role of cultural, social, and behavioral factors in determining the delivery of public health services	Knowledge	Knowledge	Proficiency	Proficiency
3. Develops and adapts approaches to problems that take into account cultural differences	Proficiency	Knowledge	Proficiency	Proficiency
4. Attitudes: Understands the dynamic forces contributing to cultural diversity	N/A*	Knowledge	N/A*	Proficiency
5. Attitudes: Understands the importance of diverse public health workforce	N/A*	Knowledge	N/A*	Proficiency

* These competencies, because of their population or system-focused language, do not apply at the individual/family level, but are applicable to the broader context of population-focused public health services and systems.

DOMAIN 5 Community Dimensions of Practice Skills

	GENERALIST/ STAFF PHN		MANAGER/ CNS/ CONSULTANT/ PROGRAM SPECIALIST/ EXECUTIVE	
	Individuals and Families	Populations/ Systems	Individuals and Families	Populations/ Systems
1. Establishes and maintains linkages with key stake holders		Knowledge		Proficiency
2. Utilizes leadership, team building, negotiation, and conflict resolution skills to build community partnerships		Knowledge		Proficiency
3. Collaborates with community partners to promote the health of population		Knowledge		Proficiency
4. Identifies how public and private organizations operate within a community		Knowledge		Proficiency
5. Accomplishes effective community engagements		Knowledge		Proficiency
6. Identifies community assets and available resources		Knowledge		Proficiency
7. Develops, implements, and evaluates a community public health assessment		Knowledge		Proficiency
8. Describes the role of government in the delivery of community health services		Knowledge		Proficiency

DOMAIN 6 Basic Public Health Sciences Skills

	GENERALIST/ STAFF PHN		MANAGER/ CNS/ CONSULTANT/ PROGRAM SPECIALIST/ EXECUTIVE	
	Individuals and Families	Populations/ Systems	Individuals and Families	Populations/ Systems
1. Identifies the individual's and organization's responsibilities within the context of the Essential Public Health Services and core functions	Knowledge	Knowledge	Proficiency	Proficiency
2. Defines, assesses, and understands the health status of populations, determinants of health and illness, factors contributing to health promotion and disease prevention, and factors influencing the use of health services	Knowledge	Knowledge	Proficiency	Proficiency
3. Understands the historical development, structure, and interaction of public health and health	Knowledge	Knowledge	Proficiency	Proficiency
4. Identifies and applies basic research methods used in public health	Awareness	Awareness	Knowledge	Knowledge
5. Applies the basic public health sciences including behavioral and social sciences, biostatistics, epidemiology, environmental public health, and prevention of chronic and infectious diseases and injuries	Awareness	Awareness	Knowledge	Knowledge
6. Identifies and retrieves current relevant scientific evidence	Knowledge	Knowledge	Proficiency	Proficiency
7. Identifies the limitations of research and the importance of observations and relationships	Awareness	Awareness	Knowledge	Knowledge
8. Attitudes: Develops a lifelong commitment to rigorous critical thinking	Proficiency	Proficiency	Proficiency	Proficiency

DOMAIN 7 Financial Planning and Management Skills

	GENERALIST/ STAFF PHN		MANAGER/ CNS/ CONSULTANT/ PROGRAM SPECIALIST/ EXECUTIVE	
	Individuals and Families	Populations/ Systems	Individuals and Families	Populations/ Systems
1. Develops and presents a budget		Awareness		Proficiency
2. Manages programs within budget constraints		Knowledge		Proficiency
3. Applies budget processes		Awareness		Proficiency
4. Develops strategies for determining budget priorities		Awareness		Proficiency
5. Monitors program performance		Knowledge		Proficiency
6. Prepares proposals for funding from external sources		Awareness		Proficiency
7. Applies basic human relationship skills to the management of organizations, motivation of personnel, and resolution of conflicts		Knowledge		Proficiency
8. Manages information systems for collection, retrieval, and use of data for decision making		Awareness		Proficiency
9. Negotiates and develops contracts and other documents for the provision of population-based services		Awareness		Proficiency
10. Conducts cost-effectiveness, cost benefit, and cost utility analyses		Awareness		Proficiency

DOMAIN 8 Leadership and Systems Thinking Skills

	GENERALIST/ STAFF PHN		MANAGER/ CNS/ CONSULTANT/ PROGRAM SPECIALIST/ EXECUTIVE	
	Individuals and Families	Populations/ Systems	Individuals and Families	Populations/ Systems
1. Creates a culture of ethical standards within organizations and communities		Knowledge		Proficiency
2. Helps create key values and shared vision and uses these principles to guide action		Knowledge		Proficiency
3. Identifies internal and external issues that may impact delivery of essential public health services (i.e., strategic planning)		Knowledge		Proficiency
4. Facilitates collaboration with internal and external groups to ensure participation of key stakeholders		Knowledge		Proficiency
5. Promotes team and organizational learning		Knowledge		Proficiency
6. Contributes to development, implementation, and monitoring of organizational performance standards		Knowledge		Proficiency
7. Uses the legal and political system to effect change		Knowledge		Proficiency
8. Applies theory of organizational structures to professional practice		Awareness		Proficiency

Note. From Quad Council of Public Health Nursing Organizations. (2004). Public health nursing competencies. *Public Health Nursing, 21*(5), 443–452. Copyright 2004 by Blackwell Publishing.

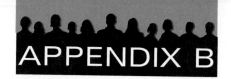

Public Health Nursing: Scope and Standards of Practice

The Standards of Public Health Nursing Practice and the associated measurement criteria are adapted from and reflect the intent of the template language of the Standards of Practice and Standards of Professional Performance presented in *Nursing: Scope and Standards of Practice* (ANA, 2004a).

STANDARDS OF PRACTICE

The six Standards of Practice describe a competent level of public health nursing care as demonstrated by the critical thinking model known as the nursing process. The nursing process includes the components of assessment, diagnosis, outcomes identification, planning, implementation, and evaluation. The nursing process encompasses all significant actions taken by registered nurses and forms the foundation of the nurse's decision-making.

STANDARDS OF PROFESSIONAL PERFORMANCE

Taken together the ten Standards of Professional Performance describe competency in the professional role. The standards address a competency level, including activities related to quality of practice, education, professional practice evaluation, collegiality, collaboration, ethics, research, resource utilization, and leadership. The advocacy standard addresses the unique responsibility of all public health nurses to serve as spokespersons for those who cannot address their own healthcare concerns.

MEASUREMENT CRITERIA

Measurement criteria are key indicators of competent practice for each standard. For a standard to be met, all the listed measurement criteria must be met.

Standards should remain stable over time, as they reflect the philosophical values of the profession. Measurement criteria, however, can be revised more frequently to incorporate advancements in scientific knowledge and expectations for nursing practice. Additional measurement criteria that are applicable only to advanced practice registered nurses are included for select standards of practice and professional performance.

Words such as *appropriate* and *possible* are sometimes used because a document like this one cannot account for all situations that the public health nurse may encounter in practice. The registered nurse will need to exercise judgment based on education and experience in determining what is appropriate or possible for a population or situation. Further direction may be available from documents such as guidelines for practice or agency standards, policies, procedures, and protocols.

Standard 1. Assessment

The public health nurse collects comprehensive data pertinent to the health status of populations.

Measurement Criteria:

The public health nurse:

- Collects multi-source data related to the health of the public at large or of a specific population.
- Uses models and principles of epidemiology, demography, and biometry, as well as social, behavioral, and physical sciences to structure data collection.
- Sets assessment priorities based on urgency of need or risk in geographic areas or in populations.
- Conducts an assessment based on criteria that aim to capture the population assets and needs,

values and beliefs, resources, and relevant environmental factors.

- Analyzes data using problem-solving techniques and models from nursing, public health, and other disciplines.
- Interprets data to identify trends and deviations from expected health patterns in the population.
- Documents assessment data in terms that are understandable to all involved in the process.
- Applies ethical, legal, and privacy guidelines and policies to the collection, maintenance, use, and dissemination of data and information.

Additional Measurement Criteria for the Advanced Practice Public Health Nurse:

The advanced practice public health nurse:

- Gathers data from multiple, interdisciplinary sources using appropriate methods to augment or verify population-focused data.
- Partners with populations, health professionals, and other stakeholders to attach meaning to collected data.
- Synthesizes complex, multi-source data gathered through the assessment process.
- Consults with the public health nurse, the population, the interdisciplinary team, and other stakeholders in the design, management, and evaluation of the data system that focuses on population assets, needs, and concerns.

Standard 2. Population Diagnosis and Priorities

The public health nurse analyses the assessment data to determine the population diagnoses and priorities.

Measurement Criteria:

The public health nurse:

- Derives the population diagnoses and priorities based on assessment data such as: input from the population, data related to access and use of health services, factors contributing to health promotion and disease prevention, existing or potential harmful exposures, and basic nursing and public health-related sciences.

- Validates the diagnoses or concerns with the population; local, state, and federal public heath agencies and organizations; and available health data and statistics as applicable.
- Documents diagnoses or concerns in a manner that facilitates population involvement in the determination of the plan and its expected outcomes.

Additional Measurement Criteria for the Advanced Practice Public Health Nurse:

The advanced practice public health nurse:

- Organizes complex data and information obtained during sociocultural, demographic, health status and health risk, geographic, environmental, and other nursing and public heath diagnostic processes to identify population health assets, needs, and risks.
- Systematically analyzes relevant population data, scientific principles, and events in the environment in formulating differential diagnoses and in setting priorities.

Standard 3. Outcomes Identification

The public health nurse identifies expected outcomes for a plan that is based on population diagnoses and priorities.

Measurement Criteria:

The public health nurse:

- Involves the population and other professionals, organizations, and stakeholders in formulating expected outcomes.
- Derives culturally relevant expected outcomes from the diagnoses.
- Considers population values and beliefs, health literacy, risks, benefits, costs, current social policies, current scientific evidence, and expertise when formulating priorities and expected outcomes.
- Incorporates knowledge of environmental factors and events, available resources, time estimates, and ethical, legal, and privacy considerations in defining expected outcomes.

⊕ Develops outcomes that provide continuity in meeting population needs and concerns and enhancing assets.

⊕ Modifies expected outcomes based on changes in population needs or concerns and the availability of resources.

⊕ Documents expected outcomes as measurable objectives using language that is understandable to all involved entities.

⊕ Applies nursing and public health competencies when measuring effective practice in a community or a population.

Additional Measurement Criteria for the Advanced Practice Public Health Nurse:

The advanced practice public health nurse:

⊕ Assures that professional partners are involved in identifying expected outcomes that incorporate scientific evidence and are achievable through implementation of evidence-based practices.

⊕ Assures that measurable outcomes include such factors as cost-effectiveness, satisfaction of stakeholders, the population, and organization, continuity and consistency of services, and resolution of health concerns.

Standard 4. Planning

The public health nurse develops a plan that reflects best practices by identifying strategies, action plans, and alternatives to attain expected outcomes.

Measurement Criteria:

The public health nurse:

⊕ Assists with the development of population-focused plans for health-related services or programs based on an assessment and prioritization of health assets, needs, risks, and concerns.

⊕ Incorporates evidence-based approaches for promotion, improvement, and restoration of health; prevention of illness, injury, or disease; and emergency preparedness and response that address the identified assets, needs, and concerns.

⊕ Provides for continuity within and across programs and services.

⊕ Establishes plans that reflect cultural competence, educational and learning principles, and priorities that address the population needs.

⊕ Ensures participation of the identified population, health professionals, coalitions, organizations, and other stakeholders in determining roles within the planning processes.

⊕ Applies current standards, statutes, regulations, and policies in the planning process.

⊕ Integrates current and emerging trends and research in nursing and public health-related fields in the planning process.

⊕ Considers the economic impacts of the plan on the population and organizations.

⊕ Documents the plan using language that is culturally sensitive and at an appropriate reading level to be understood by all participants.

⊕ Uses standardized terminology to document the plan.

Additional Measurement Criteria for the Advanced Practice Public Health Nurse:

The advanced practice public health nurse:

⊕ Applies assessment, implementation, and evaluation strategies in the plan to reflect current evidence, including data, research, literature, and expert nursing and public health knowledge.

⊕ Designs appropriate strategies and alternatives with community and professional partners to meet the complex needs of at-risk populations.

⊕ Incorporates population values and beliefs with community and professional partners in the planning process.

⊕ Leads other public health nurses and the multi-sector team in the use of principles of planning for population-focused programs and services.

⊕ Contributes to the development and continuous improvement of organizational systems that support the planning process.

⊕ Participates in the integration of human, fiscal, material, scientific, and population resources to enhance and complete the planning process for programs or services.

⊕ Assures that the current standards, statutes, regulations, and policies are considered in the planning process.

Standard 5. Implementation

The public health nurse implements the identified plan by partnering with others.

Measurement Criteria:

The public health nurse:

- ⊕ Implements the identified plan in a safe and timely manner in collaboration with the multi-sector team.
- ⊕ Applies evidence-based strategies and activities, including opportunities for coalition building and advocacy, in a plan that is specific to the population assets, needs, and concerns.
- ⊕ Incorporates systems and population resources in implementing the plan.
- ⊕ Monitors implementation of the plan, including processes and resource utilization.
- ⊕ Documents implementation of the plan, including modifications.

Additional Measurement Criteria for the Advanced Practice Public Health Nurse:

The advanced practice public health nurse:

- ⊕ Interprets surveillance data related to the plan and population health status.
- ⊕ Incorporates new knowledge and strategies into action plans to enhance implementation.
- ⊕ Modifies the plan based on new knowledge, appropriate health behavior change theory, population response, or other relevant factors to achieve expected outcomes.
- ⊕ Advocates for bringing needed resources to the community and for the population to implement the plan.
- ⊕ Fosters new collaborative relationships with nursing colleagues, other professionals, community or population representatives, and other stakeholders to implement the plan through strategies such as coalition building.
- ⊕ Promotes organizations, community coalitions, and systems that support the plan.

Standard 5a. Coordination

The public health nurse coordinates programs, services, and other activities to implement the identified plan.

Measurement Criteria:

The public health nurse:

- ⊕ Promotes policies, programs, and services for the attainment of expected outcomes.
- ⊕ Conducts surveillance, case finding, and reporting functions with health professionals and other stakeholders.
- ⊕ Connects populations with needed services.
- ⊕ Documents the coordination and required reporting.

Additional Measurement Criteria for the Advanced Practice Public Health Nurse:

The advanced practice public health nurse:

- ⊕ Provides leadership for delivery of integrated programs, services, and public policy implementation.
- ⊕ Synthesizes data and information to initiate system, community, and environmental resource allocation that support the delivery of programs and services.

Standard 5b. Health Education and Health Promotion

The public health nurse employs multiple strategies to promote health, prevent disease, and ensure a safe environment for populations.

Measurement Criteria:

The public health nurse:

- ⊕ Includes appropriate health education in the implementation of programs and services for populations.

- Selects teaching and learning methods appropriate to the health literacy of the population and their identified objectives.
- Presents culturally and age-appropriate health promotion, disease prevention, and environmental safety information and educational materials to the population.
- Collects feedback from participants to determine program and service effectiveness and recommended changes.

Additional Measurement Criteria for the Advanced Practice Public Health Nurse:

The advanced practice public health nurse:

- Provides leadership to nursing and other health professionals in planning evidence-based educational programs and services based on assessments.
- Designs health information and programs based on health behavior, learning theories and principles, and research evidence.
- Modifies existing programs based on feedback from participants, providers, health professionals, and other stakeholders.
- Develops health information resources that are culturally and age-appropriate to the population.

Standard 5c. Consultation

The public health nurse provides consultation to various community groups and officials to facilitate the implementation of programs and services.

Measurement Criteria:

The public health nurse:

- Confers with community organizations and groups to facilitate participation in programs and services.
- Provides testimony and professional opinion on programs and service delivery to at-risk populations.
- Communicates effectively using a variety of media with constituent groups during consultation.
- Documents the scope and effectiveness of consultation activities provided to community populations.

Additional Measurement Criteria for the Advanced Practice Public Health Nurse:

The advanced practice public health nurse:

- Synthesizes data from federal, state, local, and other sources with theoretical frameworks and evidence, to provide expert consultation on program and service implementation.
- Provides expert testimony at the federal, state, and local levels on program and service delivery to at-risk populations.
- Communicates information during consultation toward a positive influence on the provision of programs and services to populations.
- Generates proposals and reports in support of needed programs and services.

Standard 5d. Regulatory Activities

The public health nurse identifies, interprets, and implements public health laws, regulations, and policies.

Measurement Criteria:

The public health nurse:

- Educates affected populations on relevant laws, regulations, and policies.
- Participates in the application of public health laws, regulations, and policies, including monitoring and inspecting regulated entities.
- Collects specific information about situations that are reported to public health officials.
- Assists in addressing non-compliance with laws, regulations, and policies.

Additional Measurement Criteria for the Advanced Practice Public Health Nurse:

The advanced practice public health nurse:

- Collaborates in the revision or development of public health laws, regulations, and policies.
- Designs, with other public health professionals, reporting and compliance systems related to laws, regulations, and policies.
- Monitors reporting and compliance systems for quality and appropriate use of resources.

- Analyzes data from reporting and compliance systems.
- Develops reports for public health officials and other decision makers as required by laws, regulations, and policies.
- Participates in coordinating emergency preparedness and response efforts, including receipt and use of the Strategic National Stockpile.

Standard 6. Evaluation

The public health nurse evaluates the health status of the population.

Measurement Criteria:

The public health nurse:

- Participates in a systematic, ongoing, and criterion-based evaluation of service outcomes with the population and other stakeholders.
- Collects data systematically, applying epidemiological and scientific methods to determine the effectiveness of public health nursing interventions on policies, programs, and services.
- Participates in process and outcome evaluation by monitoring activities in programs or services.
- Applies ongoing assessment data to revise plans, interventions, and activities, as appropriate.
- Documents the results of the evaluation including changes or recommendations to enhance effectiveness of interventions.
- Disseminates the process and outcome evaluation results to the population and other stakeholders in accordance with state and federal laws and regulations, as appropriate.

Additional Measurement Criteria for the Advanced Practice Public Health Nurse:

The advanced practice public health nurse:

- Designs an evaluation plan with other public health experts, and with representatives from the population and from stakeholders.
- Modifies the evaluation plan for policies, programs, or services, as appropriate.
- Evaluates the effectiveness of the plan in relationship to expected and unexpected outcomes.

- Synthesizes the results of the evaluation analyses to determine the effect of the plan on populations, organizations, and other stakeholder groups.
- Applies the results of the evaluation analyses to recommend or make process or outcomes changes in policies, programs, or services, as appropriate.

STANDARDS OF PROFESSIONAL PERFORMANCE

Standard 7. Quality of Practice

The public health nurse systematically enhances the quality and effectiveness of nursing practice.

Measurement Criteria:

The public health nurse:

- Demonstrates quality through the application of the nursing process in a responsible, accountable, and ethical manner.
- Implements new knowledge and performance improvement activities to initiate changes in public health nursing practice and in the delivery of care to populations.
- Incorporates creativity and innovation in activities to improve the quality of nursing practice.
- Participates in the development, implementation, and evaluation of procedures and guidelines to improve the quality of practice.
- Participates in the scope of the performance improvement activities as appropriate to the nurse's position, education, and practice environment. Such activities may include:

  Identifying aspects of practice important for quality monitoring.

  Employing evidence-based indicators to monitor the quality and effectiveness of nursing practice.

  Collecting data to monitor public health nursing practice, including availability, accessibility, acceptability, quality, and effectiveness of policies, programs, and services.

  Monitoring indicators of quality and effectiveness of policies, programs, and services.

  Analyzing the data to identify opportunities for improving nursing practice.

Formulating recommendations to improve nursing practice or outcomes.

Implementing activities to enhance the quality of nursing practice.

Participating with the population and other professionals, organizations, and stakeholders in the evaluation of policies, programs, and services.

Assessing professional performance factors related to population safety, accessibility to services, program effectiveness, and cost-benefit options.

Analyzing organization and program processes and systems to remove or decrease barriers and to enhance assets.

⊕ Documents the delivery of programs and services in ways that reflect the quality measures.

⊕ Obtains and maintains professional certification, if available, in the area of expertise.

Additional Measurement Criteria for the Advanced Practice Public Health Nurse:

The advanced practice public health nurse:

⊕ Designs performance improvement initiatives related to policies, programs, and services based on existing evidence.

⊕ Implements initiatives to evaluate the need for change.

⊕ Evaluates the practice environment and quality of nursing care rendered in relation to existing evidence-based information.

⊕ Identifies opportunities for the generation and use of research to enhance the evidence base for public health nursing practice.

Standard 8. Education

The public health nurse attains knowledge and competency that reflects current nursing and public health practice.

Measurement Criteria:

The public health nurse:

⊕ Participates in ongoing educational activities to maintain and enhance the knowledge and skills necessary to promote the health of the population.

⊕ Seeks experiences to develop and maintain competence in the skills needed to implement policies, programs, and services for populations.

⊕ Identifies learning needs based on nursing and public health knowledge, the various roles the nurse may assume, and the changing needs of the population.

⊕ Identifies changes in the statutory requirements for the practice of nursing and public health.

⊕ Maintains professional records that provide evidence of competency and lifelong learning.

⊕ Seeks experiences and formal and independent learning activities to maintain and develop clinical and professional skills and knowledge.

Additional Measurement Criteria for the Advanced Practice Public Health Nurse:

The advanced practice public health nurse:

⊕ Uses current research findings and other evidence to expand nursing and public health knowledge, enhance role performance, and increase knowledge of professional issues.

Standard 9. Professional Practice Evaluation

The public health nurse evaluates one's own nursing practice in relation to professional practice standards and guidelines, relevant statutes, rules, and regulations.

Measurement Criteria:

The public health nurse:

⊕ Implements age-appropriate population-focused policies, programs, and services in a culturally and ethnically sensitive manner.

⊕ Engages in self-evaluation of practice on a regular basis, identifying areas of strength as well as areas in which professional development would be beneficial.

⊕ Seeks feedback regarding one's own practice from community and professional partners and other peers.

⊕ Implements plans for accomplishing goals in one's own work plan.

⊕ Integrates the knowledge of current practice standards, guidelines, statutes, rules, and regulations into one's own work plans.

⊕ Provides rationale for professional practice beliefs, decisions, and actions as part of the evaluation process.

⊕ Applies knowledge of current practice standards, guidelines, statutes, certification, and regulation in self-evaluation and peer review.

Additional Measurement Criteria for the Advanced Practice Public Health Nurse:

The advanced practice public health nurse:

⊕ Engages in a formal systematic process seeking feedback regarding one's own practice from peers, professional colleagues, community and professional organizations, and stakeholders.

⊕ Analyzes practice in relation to advanced certification requirements as appropriate.

Standard 10. Collegiality and Professional Relationships

The public health nurse establishes collegial partnerships while interacting with representatives of the population, organizations, and health and human services professionals, and contributes to the professional development of peers, students, colleagues, and others.

Measurement Criteria:

The public health nurse:

⊕ Shares knowledge and skills with peers, students, colleagues, and others.

⊕ Interacts with peers, students, colleagues, and others to enhance professional nursing or public health practice and role performance of self and others.

⊕ Mentors other public health nurses, colleagues, students, and others as appropriate.

⊕ Maintains compassionate and caring relationships with professional colleagues and other stakeholders involved in population health.

⊕ Contributes to an environment that fosters ongoing educational experiences for colleagues, healthcare professionals, and the population.

⊕ Contributes to a supportive, healthy, and safe work environment.

Additional Measurement Criteria for the Advanced Practice Public Health Nurse:

The advanced practice public health nurse:

⊕ Models expert practice to multi-sector team members and the population.

⊕ Designs mentoring policies and programs for public health nurses and other colleagues.

⊕ Participates in activities that contribute to the development of the advanced practice nursing role in public health.

Standard 11. Collaboration

The public health nurse collaborates with representatives of the population, organizations, and health and human service professionals in providing for and promoting the health of the population.

Measurement Criteria:

The public health nurse:

⊕ Communicates with various constituencies in the community to gather information and develop partnerships and coalitions to address population-focused health concerns.

⊕ Partners with individuals, groups, and community-based organizations in the assessment, planning, implementing, and evaluation of population-focused policies, programs, and services.

⊕ Articulates nursing and public health knowledge and skills to the interdisciplinary team, administrators, policy makers, and other multi-sector partners.

⊕ Partners with other disciplines in teaching, program development and implementation, evaluation, research, and public policy advocacy.

⊕ Contributes to the multi-sector team in implementing public health regulatory requirements such as case identification, program management, and mandatory reporting.

⊕ Partners with key individuals, groups, coalitions, and organizations to effect change in public health policies, programs, and services to generate positive outcomes.

⊕ Documents collaborative interactions and processes related to policies, programs, and services.

Additional Measurement Criteria for the Advanced Practice Public Health Nurse:

The advanced practice public health nurse:

⊕ Develops alliances and coalitions with community organizations to address public health policies, programs, and services.

⊕ Initiates collaborative efforts across constituencies in the population.

⊕ Designs educational, administrative, research, and public policy programs to promote the health of the population.

⊕ Develops systems for documentation and accountability in nursing and public health nursing practice, including compliance with regulatory requirements.

Standard 12. Ethics

The public health nurse integrates ethical provisions in all areas of practice.

Measurement Criteria:

The public health nurse:

⊕ Applies *Code of Ethics for Nurses with Interpretive Statements* (ANA, 2001) and *Principles of the Ethical Practice of Public Health* (Public Health Leadership Society, 2002) to guide public health nursing practice.

⊕ Delivers programs and services in a manner that preserves, protects, and promotes the autonomy, dignity, and rights of the population or community as well as individuals.

⊕ Applies ethical standards in advocating for health and social policy.

⊕ Maintains, individual confidentiality within legal and regulatory parameters.

⊕ Assists populations, communities, and individuals in developing skills for self-advocacy.

⊕ Maintains professional relationships and boundaries with individuals and groups within the

population while delivering public health services and programs.

⊕ Demonstrates a commitment to fostering an environment and conditions in which healthy lifestyles may be practiced by self, colleagues, and identified populations.

⊕ Contributes to resolving social and environmental issues and barriers to healthy living conditions.

⊕ Contributes to resolving ethical issues involving colleagues, community groups, systems, and other stakeholders.

⊕ Reports activities that are illegal, inconsistent with accepted standards of practice, or reflective of impaired practice.

Additional Measurement Criteria for the Advanced Practice Public Health Nurse:

The advanced practice public health nurse:

⊕ Informs populations and communities of the risks, benefits, and outcomes of policies, programs, and services.

⊕ Informs administrators or others of the risks, benefits, and outcomes of policies, programs, and services, and related decisions that affect the delivery of health-related services.

⊕ Partners with multi-sector teams to address ethical risks, benefits, and outcomes of policies, programs, and services.

⊕ Promotes solutions to social and environmental issues and barriers to healthy living conditions.

Standard 13. Research

The public health nurse integrates research findings into practice.

Measurement Criteria:

The Public health nurse:

⊕ Utilizes the best available evidence, including research findings, to guide practice, policy, and service delivery decisions.

⊕ Actively participates in research activities at various levels appropriate to one's own level of education and position. Such activities may include:

Identifying community and professional

opportunities suitable for nursing and public health research.

Participating in data collection.

Participating in agency-, organization-, or population-focused research committees or programs.

Sharing research activities and findings with peers and others.

Implementing research protocols.

Critically analyzing and interpreting research for application to population-focused practice.

Applying nursing and public health research findings in the development of policies, programs, and services for populations.

Incorporating research as a basis for learning.

⊕ Actively involves communities, populations, organizations, and other stakeholder groups in a participatory research process.

Additional Measurement Criteria for the Advanced Practice Public Health Nurse:

The advanced practice public health nurse:

⊕ Contributes to nursing knowledge by conducting or synthesizing research that discovers, examines, and evaluates knowledge, theories, models, criteria, and creative approaches to improve healthcare practice and outcomes.

⊕ Formally disseminates research findings through consultation, presentations, publications, and the use of other media.

Standard 14. Resource Utilization

The public health nurse considers factors related to safety, effectiveness, cost, and impact on practice and on the population in the planning and delivery of nursing and public health programs, policies, and services.

Measurement Criteria:

The public health nurse:

⊕ Evaluates factors such as safety, effectiveness, availability, cost and benefits, efficiencies, and impact on practice and on the population, when choosing practice options that would result in the same expected outcome.

⊕ Assists representatives of specific populations and other stakeholders in identifying and securing appropriate and available services to address health-related needs.

⊕ Assigns or delegates tasks taking into consideration the concerns of the population, potential for harm, complexity of the task, and predictability of the outcomes.

⊕ Helps the population to become informed about the options, costs, risks, and benefits of policies, programs, and services.

Additional Measurement Criteria for the Advanced Practice Public Health Nurse:

The advanced practice public health nurse:

⊕ Utilizes organizational and community resources to formulate multi-sector plans for policies, programs, and services.

⊕ Develops innovative approaches to community and public health concerns that include effective resource utilization and improvement of quality.

⊕ Develops evaluation strategies to demonstrate cost effectiveness and efficiency factors associated with nursing and public health practice and outcomes.

Standard 15. Leadership

The public health nurse provides leadership in nursing and public health.

Measurement Criteria:

The public health nurse:

⊕ Engages in multi-sector team development and coalition building, including other professionals, the population, and stakeholders.

⊕ Promotes healthy community and work environments at local, regional, national, and international levels.

⊕ Articulates the mission, goals, action plan, and outcome measures of nursing and public health programs and services to other professionals and the population.

⊕ Advocates for opportunities for continuous, life-long learning for self and others.

- Teaches peers, stakeholders, and others in the population to succeed through mentoring and other strategies.
- Exhibits creativity and flexibility through times of change.
- Fosters a culture where systems are monitored and evaluated to improve the quality of policies, programs, and services for populations.
- Coordinates programs and services across various community settings and among the multi-sector team.
- Serves in leadership roles in the work setting, in the community, and with the population.
- Promotes advancement of public health and nursing through participation in professional organizations.
- Functions as a public health team leader in emergency preparedness and response situations, delegating tasks as delineated in standardized protocols.

Additional Measurement Criteria for the Advanced Practice Public Health Nurse:

The advanced practice public health nurse:

- Advocates with decision-makers to influence public health policies, programs, and services to promote healthy populations.
- Provides direction to enhance the effectiveness of policies, programs, and services provided by the multi-sector team.
- Initiates and revises protocols or guidelines to reflect evidence-based practice, to reflect accepted changes in program and service delivery, or to address emerging problems in the population.
- Promotes communication of information and advancement of nursing and public health through writing, publishing, and presentations for professional or lay audiences.
- Demonstrates innovative approaches to public health and nursing practice to improve health outcomes for populations.
- Organizes formal plans in response to public health emergencies for populations.

Standard 16. Advocacy

The public health nurse advocates to protect the health, safety, and rights of the population.

Measurement Criteria:

The public health nurse:

- Incorporates the identified needs of the population in policy development and program or service planning.
- Integrates advocacy into the implementation of policies, programs, and services for the population.
- Evaluates the effectiveness of advocating for the population when assessing the expected outcomes.
- Includes confidentiality, ethical, legal, privacy, and professional guidelines in policy development and other issues.
- Demonstrates skill in advocating before providers and stakeholders on behalf of the population.
- Strives to resolve conflicting expectations from populations, providers, and other stakeholders to ensure the safety and to guard the best interest of the population and to preserve the professional integrity of the nurse.

Additional Measurement Criteria for the Advanced Practice Public Health Nurse:

The advanced practice public health nurse:

- Demonstrates skill in advocating before public representatives and decision-makers on behalf of the populations, programs, and services.
- Designs materials for the advocacy process that are based on the needs of the populations, programs, and services.
- Exhibits fiscal responsibility and integrity in the policy development process.
- Serves as an expert for peers, populations, providers, and other stakeholders in promoting and implementing public health policies.

GLOSSARY

Advocacy. The act of pleading or arguing in favor of a cause, idea, or policy on someone else's behalf, with the object of developing the community, system, individual, or family's capacity to plead their own cause or act on their own behalf.

Assessment. The regular and systematic collection, analysis, and dissemination of information on the health of the community or population, including statistics on health status, community health needs, and epidemiological and other studies of health problems.

Assurance. Assuring that services necessary to achieve agreed-upon goals are provided by encouraging actions by other entities (private or public), by requiring such action through regulation, or by providing services directly.

Coalition building. The process by which parties (individuals, organizations, or groups) come together to form a temporary alliance or union to work together for a common purpose and to enhance each other's capacity for mutual benefit and common purpose.

Collaboration. Work with another person or group to achieve some end.

Community. A set of persons in interaction, being and experiencing together, who may or may not share a sense of place or belonging, and who act intentionally for a common purpose. A community is different from the group of people who constitute it and can interact with other entities as a unit.

Community-based organizations. Private nonprofit organizations or other types of groups that work within a community for the improvement of some aspect of that community.

Cultural competence. A set of congruent behaviors, attitudes, and policies that come together in a system or agency or among professionals and enable the system, agency, or professionals to work effectively in cross-cultural settings.

Cultural diversity. The coexistence of different ethnic, gender, racial, and socioeconomic groups.

Determinants of health. Social, economic, and healthcare factors that affect health and well-being independently or in conjunction with each other at the population or community level. Comprehensive factors involve relevant social, economic, environmental, behavioral, political, health, and healthcare indicators that describe the essential features of a social structure and system and the processes through which change occurs.

Ecological model. A model of health that emphasizes the linkages and relationships among multiple factors (or determinants) affecting health.

Environmental health. Those aspects of human health, including quality of life, that are determined by physical, chemical, biological, social, and psychological processes in the environment. It also refers to the theory and practice of assessing, correcting, controlling, or preventing those factors in the environment that can adversely affect the health of the present and future generations.

Epidemiology. The study of the distribution of determinants and antecedents of health and disease in human populations. The ultimate goal is to identify the underlying causes of a disease and then to apply those findings to disease prevention and health promotion.

Evidence. Verifiable knowledge on which belief is based.

Evidence-based practice. An approach to public healthcare practice in which the public health nurse is aware of the evidence in support of one's clinical practice, and the strength of that evidence.

Health status (of a population). The level of illness or wellness of a population at a designated time.

Interdisciplinary team. A group of individuals who rely on each other's overlapping skills and discipline-based knowledge to achieve synergistic effects where outcomes are enhanced and more comprehensive than the simple aggregation of individual members' efforts.

Multi-sector team. A partnership of community organizations and groups representing a variety of viewpoints and perspectives which impact public health issues.

Outcomes. Long-term objectives that define optimal, measurable future levels of health status, maximum acceptable levels of disease, injury, or dysfunction, or prevalence of risk factors.

Partnership. A relationship in which two or more people or groups operate together to achieve a common goal.

Performance improvement. A process that considers the organizational context, describes desired performance, identifies gaps between desired and actual performance, identifies root causes, selects interventions to close the gaps, and measures changes in performance with the goal of achieving desired results or outcomes.

Policy development. Applying comprehensive public health scientific knowledge for decision-making. Policy development includes a systematic course of action to establish priorities, determine effective strategies and interventions, and use community resources, including regulation and law, to achieve the community's goals.

Population. Those living in a specific geographic area (e.g., a neighborhood, community, city, or county) or those in a particular group (e.g., racial, ethnic, age) who experience a disproportionate burden of poor health outcomes.

Population-focused. An approach to health care that operates at the population level of the ecological model.

Priorities. A ranking or ordering of diagnoses, strategies, or activities that identifies those that are most important or that should be addressed first.

Social justice. The principle that all persons are entitled to have their basic human needs met, regardless of differences in economic status, class, gender, race, ethnicity, citizenship, religion, age, sexual orientation, disability, or health. This includes the eradication of poverty and illiteracy, the establishment of sound environmental policy, and equality of opportunity for healthy personal and social development.

Stakeholder. A person or organization that has a legitimate interest in what a public health entity does.

Standard. An authoritative statement, defined and promoted by the profession, by which the quality of practice, service, or education can be evaluated.

Strategic National Stockpile. Large quantities of medicines, antidotes, and medical supples needed to respond to a wide range of circumstances where supplies of critical medical items in any jurisdiction would be rapidly depleted; the stockpile is managed by the Centers for Disease Control and Prevention (CDC).

Surveillance. The systematic collection, analysis, interpretation, and dissemination of data to assist in the planning, implementation, and evaluation of public health interventions and programs.

REFERENCES

American Nurses Association (ANA). (1973). *Standards of nursing practice*. Washington, DC: American Nurses Publishing. (Also available as appendix in ANA 2004a.)

American Nurses Association (ANA). (1986). *Standards of community nursing practice*. Washington, DC: American Nurses Publishing.

American Nurses Association (ANA). (1999). *Scope and standards of public health nursing*. Washington, DC: American Nurses Publishing.

American Nurses Association (ANA). (2001). *Code of ethics for nurses with interpretive statements*. Washington, DC: American Nurses Publishing.

American Nurses Association (ANA). (2003). *Nursing's social policy statement, 2nd edition*. Washington, DC: Nursesbooks.org.

American Nurses Association (ANA). (2004a). *Nursing: Scope and standards of practice*. Silver Spring, MD: Nursesbooks.org.

American Nurses Association (ANA). (2004b). *Scope and standards for nurse administrators, 2nd edition*. Silver Spring, MD: Nursesbooks.org.

American Public Health Association (APHA). Public Health Nursing Section (PHNS). (1996). *The definition and role of public health nursing*. Retrieved August 23, 2005, from http://www.csuchico.edu/horst/about/definition.html.

American Public Health Association (APHA). Public Health Nursing Section (PHNS). (2006). *Environmental health principles and recommendations for public health nursing*. Washington, DC: APHA

Association of Community Health Nursing Educators (ACHNE). (2000). *Essentials of baccalaureate nursing education for entry level community health nursing practice*. Latham, NY: ACHNE.

Association of Community Health Nursing Educators (ACHNE). (2003). *Essentials of master's level nursing education for advanced community/public health nursing practice*. Latham, NY: ACHNE.

Centers for Disease Control and Prevention (CDC). (2001). *National public health performance standards*. Retrieved August 23, 2005, from http://www.cdc.gov/od/ocphp/nphpsp/TheInstruments.htm.

Council on Linkages Between Academia and Public Health Practice. (2001). *Core competencies for public health professionals*. Retrieved August 23, 2005, from http://www.phf.org/competencies.htm.

Department of Health and Human Services (HHS). (2000). *Healthy people 2010, 2nd edition*. Washington, DC: U.S. Government Printing Office.

Institute of Medicine (IOM). (1988). *The future of public health*. Washington, DC: National Academy Press.

Institute of Medicine (IOM). (1995). *Nursing, health, and the environment*. Washington, DC: National Academy Press.

Institute of Medicine (IOM). (2003a). *The future of the public's health in the twenty-first century*. Washington, DC: National Academy Press.

Institute of Medicine (IOM). (2003b). *Who will keep the public healthy?* Washington, DC: National Academy Press.

Public Health Leadership Society. (2002). *Principles of the ethical practice of public health, version 2.2*. Retrieved August 23, 2005, from http://www.phls.org.

Quad Council of Public Health Nursing Organizations. (2004). Public health nursing competencies. *Public Health Nursing, 21*(5), 443–452.

Quad Council of Public Health Nursing Organizations & American Nurses Association. (1999). *Scope and standards of public health nursing practice*. Washington, DC: American Nurses Publishing.

Tickner, J. (2002). Precaution and preventive public health policy. *Policy Health Reports, 117*, 493–497.

Tickner, J., and Raffensberger, C. (1998). *The precautionary principle in action: A handbook, 1st edition*. Retrieved August 16, 2006, from http://www.sehn.org/rtfdocs/handbook-rtf.rtf.

Note. From American Nurses Association (2006). *Public Health Nursing: Scope and Standards of Practice*. Silver Spring, MD: Nursesbooks.org

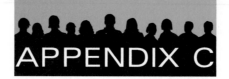

APPENDIX C

American Public Health Association Principles on Public Health and Human Rights (2000)

1. All human beings are equal in dignity and rights.

2. All human beings are entitled to the enjoyment of all human rights without discrimination.

3. The realization of the highest standard of health requires respect for all human rights, which are indivisible, interdependent, and interrelated.

4. An essential dimension of human rights is the right to health, including conditions that promote and safeguard health, and access to culturally acceptable health care.

5. Human rights must not be sacrificed to achieve public health goals, except in extraordinary circumstances, in accordance with the requirements of internationally recognized human rights standards.

6. The active collaboration of public health and human rights workers is a necessary and invaluable means of advancing their common purposes and values (APHA, 2000).

Note. From American Public Health Association (APHA) (2000). *Principles on Public Health and Human Rights.* Washington, DC: Author.

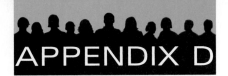

Determinants of Health

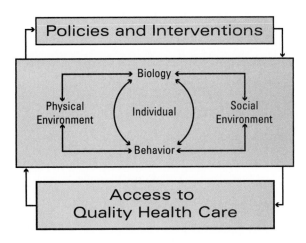

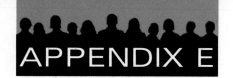

APPENDIX E

Healthy People 2010 Goals

Goal 1: Increase Quality and Years of Healthy Life

Goal 2: Eliminate Health Disparities

FOCUS AREA 1 Access to Quality Health Services

Goal: Improve access to comprehensive, high-quality health care services.

Clinical Preventive Care

1-1   Increase the proportion of persons with health insurance.

1-2   (Developmental) Increase the proportion of insured persons with coverage for clinical preventive services.

1-3   Increase the proportion of persons appropriately counseled about health behaviors.

Primary Care

1-4   Increase the proportion of persons who have a specific source of ongoing care.

1-5   Increase the proportion of persons with a usual primary care provider.

1-6   Reduce the proportion of families that experience difficulties or delays in obtaining health care or do not receive needed care for one or more family members.

1-7   (Developmental) Increase the proportion of schools of medicine, schools of nursing, and other health professional training schools whose basic curriculum for health care providers includes the core competencies in health promotion and disease prevention.

1-8   In the health professions, allied and associated health profession fields, and the nursing field, increase the proportion of all degrees awarded to members of underrepresented racial and ethnic groups.

1-9   Reduce hospitalization rates for three ambulatory-care-sensitive conditions—pediatric asthma, uncontrolled diabetes, and immunization-preventable pneumonia and influenza.

Emergency Services

1-10   (Developmental) Reduce the proportion of persons who delay or have difficulty in getting emergency medical care.

1-11   (Developmental) Increase the proportion of persons who have access to rapidly responding prehospital emergency medical services.

1-12   Establish a single toll-free telephone number for access to poison control centers on a 24-hour basis throughout the United States.

1-13   Increase the number of Tribes, States, and the District of Columbia with trauma care systems that maximize survival and functional outcomes of trauma patients and help prevent injuries from occurring.

1-14   Increase the number of States and the District of Columbia that have implemented guidelines for prehospital and hospital pediatric care.

Long-Term Care and Rehabilitative Services

1-15   (Developmental) Increase the proportion of persons with long-term care needs who have access to the continuum of long-term care services

1-16   Reduce the proportion of nursing home residents with a current diagnosis of pressure ulcers.

FOCUS AREA 2 Arthritis, Osteoporosis, and Chronic Back Conditions

Goal: Prevent illness and disability related to arthritis and other rheumatic conditions, osteoporosis, and chronic back conditions.

Arthritis and Other Rheumatic Conditions

2-1   (Developmental) Increase the mean number of days without severe pain among adults who have chronic joint symptoms.

2-2   Reduce the proportion of adults with chronic joint symptoms who experience a limitation in activity due to arthritis.

2-3   Reduce the proportion of all adults with chronic joint symptoms who have difficulty in performing two or more personal care activities, thereby preserving independence.

2-4   (Developmental) Increase the proportion of adults aged 18 years and older with arthritis who seek help in coping if they experience personal and emotional problems.

2-5   Increase the employment rate among adults with arthritis in the working-aged population.

2-6   (Developmental) Eliminate racial disparities in the rate of total knee replacements.

2-7   (Developmental) Increase the proportion of adults who have seen a health care provider for their chronic joint symptoms.

2-8   (Developmental) Increase the proportion of persons with arthritis who have had effective, evidence-based arthritis education as an integral part of the management of their condition.

Osteoporosis

2-9   Reduce the proportion of adults with osteoporosis.

2-10   Reduce the proportion of adults who are hospitalized for vertebral fractures associated with osteoporosis.

Chronic Back Conditions

2-11   Reduce activity limitation due to chronic back conditions.

FOCUS AREA 3 Cancer

Goal: Reduce the number of new cancer cases as well as the illness, disability, and death caused by cancer.

3-1	Reduce the overall cancer death rate.
3-2	Reduce the lung cancer death rate.
3-3	Reduce the breast cancer death rate.
3-4	Reduce the death rate from cancer of the uterine cervix.
3-5	Reduce the colorectal cancer death rate.
3-6	Reduce the oropharyngeal cancer death rate.
3-7	Reduce the prostate cancer death rate.
3-8	Reduce the rate of melanoma cancer deaths.
3-9	Increase the proportion of persons who use at least one of the following protective measures that may reduce the risk of skin cancer: avoid the sun between 10 A.M. and 4 P.M., wear sun-protective clothing when exposed to sunlight, use sunscreen with a sun-protective factor (SPF) of 15 or higher, and avoid artificial sources of ultraviolet light.
3-10	Increase the proportion of physicians and dentists who counsel their at-risk patients about tobacco use cessation, physical activity, and cancer screening.
3-11	Increase the proportion of women who receive a Pap test.
3-12	Increase the proportion of adults who receive a colorectal cancer screening examination.
3-13	Increase the proportion of women aged 40 years and older who have received a mammogram within the preceding 2 years.
3-14	Increase the number of States that have a statewide population-based cancer registry that captures case information on at least 95 percent of the expected number of reportable cancers.
3-15	Increase the proportion of cancer survivors who are living 5 years or longer after diagnosis.

FOCUS AREA 4 Chronic Kidney Disease

Goal: Reduce new cases of chronic kidney disease and its complications, disability, death, and economic costs.

4-1	Reduce the rate of new cases of end-stage renal disease (ESRD).
4-2	Reduce deaths from cardiovascular disease in persons with chronic kidney failure.
4-3	Increase the proportion of treated chronic kidney failure patients who have received counseling on nutrition, treatment choices, and cardiovascular care 12 months before the start of renal replacement therapy.
4-4	Increase the proportion of new hemodialysis patients who use arteriovenous fistulas as the primary mode of vascular access.
4-5	Increase the proportion of dialysis patients registered on the waiting list for transplantation.
4-6	Increase the proportion of patients with treated chronic kidney failure who receive a transplant within 3 years of registration on the waiting list.
4-7	Reduce kidney failure due to diabetes.
4-8	(Developmental) Increase the proportion of persons with type 1 or type 2 diabetes and proteinuria who receive recommended medical therapy to reduce progression to chronic renal insufficiency.

FOCUS AREA 5 Diabetes

Goal: Through prevention programs, reduce the disease and economic burden of diabetes, and improve the quality of life for all persons who have or are at risk for diabetes.

5-1	Increase the proportion of persons with diabetes who receive formal diabetes education.
5-2	Prevent diabetes.
5-3	Reduce the overall rate of diabetes that is clinically diagnosed.
5-4	Increase the proportion of adults with diabetes whose condition has been diagnosed.
5-5	Reduce the diabetes death rate.
5-6	Reduce diabetes-related deaths among persons with diabetes.
5-7	Reduce deaths from cardiovascular disease in persons with diabetes.
5-8	(Developmental) Decrease the proportion of pregnant women with gestational diabetes.
5-9	(Developmental) Reduce the frequency of foot ulcers in persons with diabetes.
5-10	Reduce the rate of lower extremity amputations in persons with diabetes.
5-11	(Developmental) Increase the proportion of persons with diabetes who obtain an annual urinary microalbumin measurement.
5-12	Increase the proportion of adults with diabetes who have a glycosylated hemoglobin measurement at least once a year.
5-13	Increase the proportion of adults with diabetes who have an annual dilated eye examination.
5-14	Increase the proportion of adults with diabetes who have at least an annual foot examination.
5-15	Increase the proportion of persons with diabetes who have at least an annual dental examination.
5-16	Increase the proportion of adults with diabetes who take aspirin at least 15 times per month.
5-17	Increase the proportion of adults with diabetes who perform self-blood-glucose-monitoring at least once daily.

FOCUS AREA 6 Disability and Secondary Conditions

Goal: Promote the health of people with disabilities, prevent secondary conditions, and eliminate disparities between people with and without disabilities in the U.S. population.

6-1   Include in the core of all relevant Healthy People 2010 surveillance instruments a standardized set of questions that identify "people with disabilities."

6-2   Reduce the proportion of children and adolescents with disabilities who are reported to be sad, unhappy, or depressed.

6-3   Reduce the proportion of adults with disabilities who report feelings such as sadness, unhappiness, or depression that prevent them from being active.

6-4   Increase the proportion of adults with disabilities who participate in social activities.

6-5   Increase the proportion of adults with disabilities reporting sufficient emotional support.

6-6   Increase the proportion of adults with disabilities reporting satisfaction with life.

6-7   Reduce the number of people with disabilities in congregate care facilities, consistent with permanency planning principles.

6-8   Eliminate disparities in employment rates between working-aged adults with and without disabilities.

6-9   Increase the proportion of children and youth with disabilities who spend at least 80 percent of their time in regular education programs.

6-10   (Developmental) Increase the proportion of health and wellness and treatment programs and facilities that provide full access for people with disabilities.

6-11   (Developmental) Reduce the proportion of people with disabilities who report not having the assistive devices and technology needed.

6-12   (Developmental) Reduce the proportion of people with disabilities reporting environmental barriers to participation in home, school, work, or community activities.

6-13   Increase the number of Tribes, States, and the District of Columbia that have public health surveillance and health promotion programs for people with disabilities and caregivers.

FOCUS AREA 7 Educational and Community-Based Programs

Goal: Increase the quality, availability, and effectiveness of educational and
community-based programs designed to prevent disease and improve health and quality of life.

School Setting

7-1   Increase high school completion.

7-2   Increase the proportion of middle, junior high, and senior high schools that provide school health education
to prevent health problems in the following areas: unintentional injury; violence; suicide; tobacco use and
addiction; alcohol and other drug use; unintended pregnancy, HIV/AIDS, and STD infection; unhealthy
dietary patterns; inadequate physical activity; and environmental health.

7-3   Increase the proportion of college and university students who receive information from their institution on
each of the six priority health-risk behavior areas.

7-4   Increase the proportion of the Nation's elementary, middle, junior high, and senior high schools that have a
nurse-to-student ratio of at least 1:750.

Worksite Setting

7-5   Increase the proportion of worksites that offer a comprehensive employee health promotion program to
their employees.

7-6   Increase the proportion of employees who participate in employer-sponsored health promotion activities.

Health Care Setting

7-7   (Developmental) Increase the proportion of health care organizations that provide patient and family
education.

7-8   (Developmental) Increase the proportion of patients who report that they are satisfied with the patient
education they receive from their health care organization.

7-9   (Developmental) Increase the proportion of hospitals and managed care organizations that provide
community disease prevention and health promotion activities that address the priority health needs
identified by their community.

Community Setting and Select Populations

7-10   (Developmental) Increase the proportion of Tribal and local health service areas or jurisdictions that have
established a community health promotion program that addresses multiple Healthy People 2010 focus areas.

7-11   Increase the proportion of local health departments that have established culturally appropriate and
linguistically competent community health promotion and disease prevention programs.

7-12   Increase the proportion of older adults who have participated during the preceding year in at least one
organized health promotion activity.

FOCUS AREA 8 Environmental Health

Goal: Promote health for all through a healthy environment.

Outdoor Air Quality

8-1 Reduce the proportion of persons exposed to air that does not meet the U.S. Environmental Protection Agency's health-based standards for harmful air pollutants.

8-2 Increase use of alternative modes of transportation to reduce motor vehicle emissions and improve the Nation's air quality.

8-3 Improve the Nation's air quality by increasing the use of cleaner alternative fuels.

8-4 Reduce air toxic emissions to decrease the risk of adverse health effects caused by airborne toxics.

Water Quality

8-5 Increase the proportion of persons served by community water systems who receive a supply of drinking water that meets the regulations of the Safe Drinking Water Act.

8-6 Reduce waterborne disease outbreaks arising from water intended for drinking among persons served by community water systems.

8-7 Reduce per capita domestic water withdrawals.

8-8 (Developmental) Increase the proportion of assessed rivers, lakes, and estuaries that are safe for fishing and recreational purposes.

8-9 (Developmental) Reduce the number of beach closings that result from the presence of harmful bacteria.

8-10 (Developmental) Reduce the potential human exposure to persistent chemicals by decreasing fish contaminant levels.

Toxics and Waste

8-11 Eliminate elevated blood lead levels in children.

8-12 Minimize the risks to human health and the environment posed by hazardous sites.

8-13 Reduce pesticide exposures that result in visits to a health care facility.

8-14 (Developmental) Reduce the amount of toxic pollutants released, disposed of, treated, or used for energy recovery.

8-15 Increase recycling of municipal solid waste.

Healthy Homes and Healthy Communities

8-16 Reduce indoor allergen levels.

8-17 (Developmental) Increase the number of office buildings that are managed using good indoor air quality practices.

8-18 Increase the proportion of persons who live in homes tested for radon concentrations.

8-19 Increase the number of new homes constructed to be radon resistant.

8-20 (Developmental) Increase the proportion of the Nation's primary and secondary schools that have official school policies ensuring the safety of students and staff from environmental hazards, such as chemicals in special classrooms, poor indoor air quality, asbestos, and exposure to pesticides.

8-21 (Developmental) Ensure that State health departments establish training, plans, and protocols and conduct annual multi-institutional exercises to prepare for response to natural and technological disasters.

8-22 Increase the proportion of persons living in pre-1950s housing that has been tested for the presence of lead-based paint.

8-23 Reduce the proportion of occupied housing units that are substandard.   *(continues)*

FOCUS AREA 8 Environmental Health (cont'd)

Goal: Promote health for all through a healthy environment.

Infrastructure and Surveillance

8-24   Reduce exposure to pesticides as measured by urine concentrations of metabolites.

8-25   (Developmental) Reduce exposure of the population to pesticides, heavy metals, and other toxic chemicals, as measured by blood and urine concentrations of the substances or their metabolites.

8-26   (Developmental) Improve the quality, utility, awareness, and use of existing information systems for environmental health.

8-27   Increase or maintain the number of Territories, Tribes, and States, and the District of Columbia that monitor diseases or conditions that can be caused by exposure to environmental hazards.

8-28   (Developmental) Increase the number of local health departments or agencies that use data from surveillance of environmental risk factors as part of their vector control programs.

Global Environmental Health

8-29   Reduce the global burden of disease due to poor water quality, sanitation, and personal and domestic hygiene.

8-30   Increase the proportion of the population in the U.S.-Mexico border region that has adequate drinking water and sanitation facilities.

FOCUS AREA 9 Family Planning

Goal: Improve pregnancy planning and spacing and prevent unintended pregnancy

9-1   Increase the proportion of pregnancies that are intended.

9-2   Reduce the proportion of births occurring within 24 months of a previous birth.

9-3   Increase the proportion of females at risk of unintended pregnancy (and their partners) who use contraception.

9-4   Reduce the proportion of females experiencing pregnancy despite use of a reversible contraceptive method.

9-5   (Developmental) Increase the proportion of health care providers who provide emergency contraception.

9-6   (Developmental) Increase male involvement in pregnancy prevention and family planning efforts.

9-7   Reduce pregnancies among adolescent females.

9-8   Increase the proportion of adolescents who have never engaged in sexual intercourse before age 15 years.

9-9   Increase the proportion of adolescents who have never engaged in sexual intercourse.

9-10   Increase the proportion of sexually active, unmarried adolescents aged 15 to 17 years who use contraception that both effectively prevents pregnancy and provides barrier protection against disease.

9-11   Increase the proportion of young adults who have received formal instruction before turning age 18 years on reproductive health issues, including all of the following topics: birth control methods, safer sex to prevent HIV, prevention of sexually transmitted diseases, and abstinence.

9-12   Reduce the proportion of married couples whose ability to conceive or maintain a pregnancy is impaired.

9-13   (Developmental) Increase the proportion of health insurance policies that cover contraceptive supplies and services.

FOCUS AREA 10 Food Safety

Goal: Reduce foodborne illnesses.

10-1   Reduce infections caused by key foodborne pathogens.

10-2   Reduce outbreaks of infections caused by key foodborne bacteria.

10-3   Prevent an increase in the proportion of isolates of *Salmonella* species from humans and from animals at slaughter that are resistant to antimicrobial drugs.

10-4   (Developmental) Reduce deaths from anaphylaxis caused by food allergies.

10-5   Increase the proportion of consumers who follow key food safety practices.

10-6   (Developmental) Improve food employee behaviors and food preparation practices that directly relate to foodborne illnesses in retail food establishments.

10-7   (Developmental) Reduce human exposure to organophosphate pesticides from food.

FOCUS AREA 11 Health Communication

Goal: Use communication strategically to improve health.

11-1   Increase the proportion of households with access to the Internet at home.

11-2   (Developmental) Improve the health literacy of persons with inadequate or marginal literacy skills.

11-3   (Developmental) Increase the proportion of health communication activities that include research and evaluation.

11-4   (Developmental) Increase the proportion of health-related World Wide Web sites that disclose information that can be used to assess the quality of the site.

11-5   (Developmental) Increase the number of centers for excellence that seek to advance the research and practice of health communication.

11-6   (Developmental) Increase the proportion of persons who report that their health care providers have satisfactory communication skills.

FOCUS AREA 12 Heart Disease and Stroke

Goal: Improve cardiovascular health and quality of life through the prevention, detection, and treatment of risk factors; early identification and treatment of heart attacks and strokes; and prevention of recurrent cardiovascular events.

Heart Disease

12-1   Reduce coronary heart disease deaths.

12-2   (Developmental) Increase the proportion of adults aged 20 years and older who are aware of the early warning symptoms and signs of a heart attack and the importance of accessing rapid emergency care by calling 911.

12-3   (Developmental) Increase the proportion of eligible patients with heart attacks who receive artery-opening therapy within an hour of symptom onset.

12-4   (Developmental) Increase the proportion of adults aged 20 years and older who call 911 and administer cardiopulmonary resuscitation (CPR) when they witness an out-of-hospital cardiac arrest.

12-5   (Developmental) Increase the proportion of eligible persons with witnessed out-of-hospital cardiac arrest who receive their first therapeutic electrical shock within 6 minutes after collapse recognition.

12-6   Reduce hospitalizations of older adults with congestive heart failure as the principal diagnosis.

Stroke

12-7   Reduce stroke deaths.

12-8   (Developmental) Increase the proportion of adults who are aware of the early warning symptoms and signs of a stroke.

Blood Pressure

12-9   Reduce the proportion of adults with high blood pressure.

12-10   Increase the proportion of adults with high blood pressure whose blood pressure is under control.

12-11   Increase the proportion of adults with high blood pressure who are taking action (for example, losing weight, increasing physical activity, or reducing sodium intake) to help control their blood pressure.

12-12   Increase the proportion of adults who have had their blood pressure measured within the preceding 2 years and can state whether their blood pressure was normal or high.

Cholesterol

12-13   Reduce the mean total blood cholesterol levels among adults.

12-14   Reduce the proportion of adults with high total blood cholesterol levels.

12-15   Increase the proportion of adults who have had their blood cholesterol checked within the preceding 5 years.

12-16   (Developmental) Increase the proportion of persons with coronary heart disease who have their LDL-cholesterol level treated to a goal of less than or equal to 100 mg/dL.

FOCUS AREA 13 HIV

Goal: Prevent HIV infection and its related illness and death.

13-1   Reduce AIDS among adolescents and adults.

13-2   Reduce the number of new AIDS cases among adolescent and adult men who have sex with men.

13-3   Reduce the number of new AIDS cases among females and males who inject drugs.

13-4   Reduce the number of new AIDS cases among adolescent and adult men who have sex with men and inject drugs.

13-5   (Developmental) Reduce the number of cases of HIV infection among adolescents and adults.

13-6   Increase the proportion of sexually active persons who use condoms.

13-7   (Developmental) Increase the number of HIV-positive persons who know their serostatus.

13-8   Increase the proportion of substance abuse treatment facilities that offer HIV/AIDS education, counseling, and support.

13-9   (Developmental) Increase the number of State prison systems that provide comprehensive HIV/AIDS, sexually transmitted diseases, and tuberculosis (TB) education.

13-10   (Developmental) Increase the proportion of inmates in State prison systems who receive voluntary HIV counseling and testing during incarceration.

13-11   Increase the proportion of adults with tuberculosis (TB) who have been tested for HIV.

13-12   (Developmental) Increase the proportion of adults in publicly funded HIV counseling and testing sites who are screened for common bacterial sexually transmitted diseases (STDs) (chlamydia, gonorrhea, and syphilis) and are immunized against hepatitis B virus.

13-13   Increase the proportion of HIV-infected adolescents and adults who receive testing, treatment, and prophylaxis consistent with current Public Health Service treatment guidelines.

13-14   Reduce deaths from HIV infection.

13-15   (Developmental) Extend the interval of time between an initial diagnosis of HIV infection and AIDS diagnosis in order to increase years of life of an individual infected with HIV.

13-16   (Developmental) Increase years of life of an HIV-infected person by extending the interval of time between an AIDS diagnosis and death.

13-17   (Developmental) Reduce new cases of perinatally acquired HIV infection.

FOCUS AREA 14 Immunization and Infectious Diseases

Goal: Prevent disease, disability, and death from infectious diseases, including vaccine-preventable diseases.

Diseases Preventable Through Universal Vaccination

14-1   Reduce or eliminate indigenous cases of vaccine-preventable diseases.

14-2   Reduce chronic hepatitis B virus infections in infants and young children (perinatal infections).

14-3   Reduce hepatitis B.

14-4   Reduce bacterial meningitis in young children.

14-5   Reduce invasive pneumococcal infections.

Diseases Preventable Through Targeted Vaccination

14-6   Reduce hepatitis A.

14-7   Reduce meningococcal disease.

14-8   Reduce Lyme disease.

Infectious Diseases and Emerging Antimicrobial Resistance

14-9   Reduce hepatitis C.

14-10   (Developmental) Increase the proportion of persons with chronic hepatitis C infection identified by State and local health departments.

14-11   Reduce tuberculosis.

14-12   Increase the proportion of all tuberculosis patients who complete curative therapy within 12 months.

14-13   Increase the proportion of contacts and other high-risk persons with latent tuberculosis infection who complete a course of treatment.

14-14   Reduce the average time for a laboratory to confirm and report tuberculosis cases.

14-15   (Developmental) Increase the proportion of international travelers who receive recommended preventive services when traveling in areas of risk for select infectious diseases: hepatitis A, malaria, and typhoid.

14-16   Reduce invasive early onset group B streptococcal disease.

14-17   Reduce hospitalizations caused by peptic ulcer disease in the United States.

14-18   Reduce the number of courses of antibiotics for ear infections for young children.

14-19   Reduce the number of courses of antibiotics prescribed for the sole diagnosis of the common cold.

14-20   Reduce hospital-acquired infections in intensive care unit patients.

14-21   Reduce antimicrobial use among intensive care unit patients.

Vaccination Coverage and Strategies

14-22   Achieve and maintain effective vaccination coverage levels for universally recommended vaccines among young children.

14-23   Maintain vaccination coverage levels for children in licensed day care facilities and children in kindergarten through the first grade.

14-24   Increase the proportion of young children and adolescents who receive all vaccines that have been recommended for universal administration for at least 5 years.

14-25   Increase the proportion of providers who have measured the vaccination coverage levels among children in their practice population within the past 2 years.

14-26   Increase the proportion of children who participate in fully operational population-based immunization registries.

14-27   Increase routine vaccination coverage levels for adolescents.

14-28   Increase hepatitis B vaccine coverage among high-risk groups.

14-29   Increase the proportion of adults who are vaccinated annually against influenza and ever vaccinated against pneumococcal disease.

Vaccine Safety

14-30   Reduce vaccine-associated adverse events.

14-31   Increase the number of persons under active surveillance for vaccine safety via large linked databases.

FOCUS AREA 15 Injury and Violence Prevention

Goal: Reduce injuries, disabilities, and deaths due to unintentional injuries and violence.

Injury Prevention

15-1	Reduce hospitalization for nonfatal head injuries.
15-2	Reduce hospitalization for nonfatal spinal cord injuries.
15-3	Reduce firearm-related deaths.
15-4	Reduce the proportion of persons living in homes with firearms that are loaded and unlocked.
15-5	Reduce nonfatal firearm-related injuries.
15-6	(Developmental) Extend State-level child fatality review of deaths due to external causes for children aged 14 years and under.
15-7	Reduce nonfatal poisonings.
15-8	Reduce deaths caused by poisonings.
15-9	Reduce deaths caused by suffocation.
15-10	Increase the number of States and the District of Columbia with statewide emergency department surveillance systems that collect data on external causes of injury.
15-11	Increase the number of States and the District of Columbia that collect data on external causes of injury through hospital discharge data systems.
15-12	Reduce hospital emergency department visits caused by injuries.

Unintentional Injury Prevention

15-13	Reduce deaths caused by unintentional injuries.
15-14	(Developmental) Reduce nonfatal unintentional injuries.
15-15	Reduce deaths caused by motor vehicle crashes.
15-16	Reduce pedestrian deaths on public roads.
15-17	Reduce nonfatal injuries caused by motor vehicle crashes.
15-18	Reduce nonfatal pedestrian injuries on public roads.
15-19	Increase use of safety belts.
15-20	Increase use of child restraints.
15-21	Increase the proportion of motorcyclists using helmets.
15-22	Increase the number of States and the District of Columbia that have adopted a graduated driver licensing model law.
15-23	(Developmental) Increase use of helmets by bicyclists.
15-24	Increase the number of States and the District of Columbia with laws requiring bicycle helmets for bicycle riders.
15-25	Reduce residential fire deaths.
15-26	Increase functioning residential smoke alarms.
15-27	Reduce deaths from falls.
15-28	Reduce hip fractures among older adults.
15-29	Reduce drownings.
15-30	Reduce hospital emergency department visits for nonfatal dog bite injuries.
15-31	(Developmental) Increase the proportion of public and private schools that require use of appropriate head, face, eye, and mouth protection for students participating in school-sponsored physical activities.

(continues)

FOCUS AREA 15 Injury and Violence Prevention (cont'd)

Goal: Reduce injuries, disabilities, and deaths due to unintentional injuries and violence.

Violence and Abuse Prevention

15-32	Reduce homicides.
15-33	Reduce maltreatment and maltreatment fatalities of children.
15-34	Reduce the rate of physical assault by current or former intimate partners.
15-35	Reduce the annual rate of rape or attempted rape.
15-36	Reduce sexual assault other than rape.
15-37	Reduce physical assaults.
15-38	Reduce physical fighting among adolescents.
15-39	Reduce weapon carrying by adolescents on school property.

FOCUS AREA 16 Maternal, Infant, and Child Health

Goal: Improve the health and well-being of women, infants, children, and families.

Fetal, Infant, Child, and Adolescent Deaths

16-1   Reduce fetal and infant deaths.

16-2   Reduce the rate of child deaths.

16-3   Reduce deaths of adolescents and young adults.

Maternal Deaths and Illnesses

16-4   Reduce maternal deaths.

16-5   Reduce maternal illness and complications due to pregnancy.

Prenatal Care

16-6   Increase the proportion of pregnant women who receive early and adequate prenatal care.

16-7   (Developmental) Increase the proportion of pregnant women who attend a series of prepared childbirth classes.

Obstetrical Care

16-8   Increase the proportion of very low birth weight (VLBW) infants born at level III hospitals or subspecialty perinatal centers.

16-9   Reduce cesarean births among low-risk (full-term, singleton, vertex presentation) women.

Risk Factors

16-10   Reduce low birth weight (LBW) and very low birth weight (VLBW).

16-11   Reduce preterm births.

16-12   (Developmental) Increase the proportion of mothers who achieve a recommended weight gain during their pregnancies.

16-13   Increase the percentage of healthy full-term infants who are put down to sleep on their backs.

Developmental Disabilities and Neural Tube Defects

16-14   Reduce the occurrence of developmental disabilities.

16-15   Reduce the occurrence of spina bifida and other neural tube defects (NTDs).

16-16   Increase the proportion of pregnancies begun with an optimum folic acid level.

Prenatal Substance Exposure

16-17   Increase abstinence from alcohol, cigarettes, and illicit drugs among pregnant women.

16-18   (Developmental) Reduce the occurrence of fetal alcohol syndrome (FAS).

Breastfeeding, Newborn Screening, and Service Systems

16-19   Increase the proportion of mothers who breastfeed their babies.

16-20   (Developmental) Ensure appropriate newborn bloodspot screening, followup testing, and referral to services.

16-21   (Developmental) Reduce hospitalization for life-threatening sepsis among children aged 4 years and under with sickling hemoglobinopathies.

16-22   (Developmental) Increase the proportion of children with special health care needs who have access to a medical home.

16-23   Increase the proportion of Territories and States that have service systems for children with special health care needs.

FOCUS AREA 17 Medical Product Safety

Goal: Ensure the safe and effective use of medical products.

17-1   (Developmental) Increase the proportion of health care organizations that are linked in an integrated system that monitors and reports adverse events.

17-2   (Developmental) Increase the use of linked, automated systems to share information.

17-3   (Developmental) Increase the proportion of primary care providers, pharmacists, and other health care professionals who routinely review with their patients aged 65 years and older and patients with chronic illnesses or disabilities all new prescribed and over-the-counter medicines.

17-4   (Developmental) Increase the proportion of patients receiving information that meets guidelines for usefulness when their new prescriptions are dispensed.

17-5   Increase the proportion of patients who receive verbal counseling from prescribers and pharmacists on the appropriate use and potential risks of medications.

17-6   Increase the proportion of persons who donate blood, and in so doing ensure an adequate supply of safe blood.

FOCUS AREA 18 Mental Health and Mental Illness

Goal: Improve mental health and ensure access to appropriate, quality mental health services.

Mental Health Status Improvement

18-1   Reduce the suicide rate.

18-2   Reduce the rate of suicide attempts by adolescents.

18-3   Reduce the proportion of homeless adults who have serious mental illness (SMI).

18-4   Increase the proportion of persons with serious mental illness (SMI) who are employed.

18-5   (Developmental) Reduce the relapse rates for persons with eating disorders including anorexia nervosa and bulimia nervosa.

Treatment Expansion

18-6   (Developmental) Increase the number of persons seen in primary health care who receive mental health screening and assessment.

18-7   (Developmental) Increase the proportion of children with mental health problems who receive treatment.

18-8   (Developmental) Increase the proportion of juvenile justice facilities that screen new admissions for mental health problems.

18-9   Increase the proportion of adults with mental disorders who receive treatment.

18-10   (Developmental) Increase the proportion of persons with co-occurring substance abuse and mental disorders who receive treatment for both disorders.

18-11   (Developmental) Increase the proportion of local governments with community-based jail diversion programs for adults with serious mental illness (SMI).

State Activities

18-12   Increase the number of States and the District of Columbia that track consumers' satisfaction with the mental health services they receive.

18-13   (Developmental) Increase the number of States, Territories, and the District of Columbia with an operational mental health plan that addresses cultural competence.

18-14   Increase the number of States, Territories, and the District of Columbia with an operational mental health plan that addresses mental health crisis interventions, ongoing screening, and treatment services for elderly persons.

FOCUS AREA 19 Nutrition and Overweight

Goal: Promote health and reduce chronic disease associated with diet and weight.

Weight Status and Growth

19-1   Increase the proportion of adults who are at a healthy weight.

19-2   Reduce the proportion of adults who are obese.

19-3   Reduce the proportion of children and adolescents who are overweight or obese.

19-4   Reduce growth retardation among low-income children under age 5 years.

Food and Nutrient Consumption

19-5   Increase the proportion of persons aged 2 years and older who consume at least two daily servings of fruit.

19-6   Increase the proportion of persons aged 2 years and older who consume at least three daily servings of vegetables, with at least one-third being dark green or orange vegetables.

19-7   Increase the proportion of persons aged 2 years and older who consume at least six daily servings of grain products, with at least three being whole grains.

19-8   Increase the proportion of persons aged 2 years and older who consume less than 10 percent of calories from saturated fat.

19-9   Increase the proportion of persons aged 2 years and older who consume no more than 30 percent of calories from total fat.

19-10   Increase the proportion of persons aged 2 years and older who consume 2,400 mg or less of sodium daily.

19-11   Increase the proportion of persons aged 2 years and older who meet dietary recommendations for calcium.

Iron Deficiency and Anemia

19-12   Reduce iron deficiency among young children and females of childbearing age.

19-13   Reduce anemia among low-income pregnant females in their third trimester.

19-14   (Developmental) Reduce iron deficiency among pregnant females.

Schools, Worksites, and Nutrition Counseling

19-15   (Developmental) Increase the proportion of children and adolescents aged 6 to 19 years whose intake of meals and snacks at school contributes to good overall dietary quality.

19-16   Increase the proportion of worksites that offer nutrition or weight management classes or counseling.

19-17   Increase the proportion of physician office visits made by patients with a diagnosis of cardiovascular disease, diabetes, or hyperlipidemia that include counseling or education related to diet and nutrition.

Food Security

19-18   Increase food security among U.S. households and in so doing reduce hunger.

FOCUS AREA 20 Occupational Safety and Health

Goal: Promote the health and safety of people at work through prevention and early intervention.

20-1	Reduce deaths from work-related injuries.
20-2	Reduce work-related injuries resulting in medical treatment, lost time from work, or restricted work activity.
20-3	Reduce the rate of injury and illness cases involving days away from work due to overexertion or repetitive motion.
20-4	Reduce pneumoconiosis deaths.
20-5	Reduce deaths from work-related homicides.
20-6	Reduce work-related assaults.
20-7	Reduce the number of persons who have elevated blood lead concentrations from work exposures.
20-8	Reduce occupational skin diseases or disorders among full-time workers.
20-9	Increase the proportion of worksites employing 50 or more persons that provide programs to prevent or reduce employee stress.
20-10	Reduce occupational needlestick injuries among health care workers.
20-11	(Developmental) Reduce new cases of work-related, noise-induced hearing loss.

FOCUS AREA 21 Oral Health

Goal: Prevent and control oral and craniofacial diseases, conditions, and injuries and improve access to related services.

21-1	Reduce the proportion of children and adolescents who have dental caries experience in their primary or permanent teeth.
21-2	Reduce the proportion of children, adolescents, and adults with untreated dental decay.
21-3	Increase the proportion of adults who have never had a permanent tooth extracted because of dental caries or periodontal disease.
21-4	Reduce the proportion of older adults who have had all their natural teeth extracted.
21-5	Reduce periodontal disease.
21-6	Increase the proportion of oral and pharyngeal cancers detected at the earliest stage.
21-7	Increase the proportion of adults who, in the past 12 months, report having had an examination to detect oral and pharyngeal cancers.
21-8	Increase the proportion of children who have received dental sealants on their molar teeth.
21-9	Increase the proportion of the U.S. population served by community water systems with optimally fluoridated water.
21-10	Increase the proportion of children and adults who use the oral health care system each year.
21-11	Increase the proportion of long-term care residents who use the oral health care system each year.
21-12	Increase the proportion of low-income children and adolescents who received any preventive dental service during the past year.
21-13	(Developmental) Increase the proportion of school-based health centers with an oral health component.
21-14	Increase the proportion of local health departments and community-based health centers, including community, migrant, and homeless health centers, that have an oral health component.

(continues)

FOCUS AREA 21 Oral Health (cont'd)

Goal: Prevent and control oral and craniofacial diseases, conditions, and injuries and improve access to related services.

21-15   Increase the number of States and the District of Columbia that have a system for recording and referring infants and children with cleft lips, cleft palates, and other craniofacial anomalies to craniofacial anomaly rehabilitative teams.

21-16   Increase the number of States and the District of Columbia that have an oral and craniofacial health surveillance system.

21-17   (Developmental) Increase the number of Tribal, State (including the District of Columbia), and local health agencies that serve jurisdictions of 250,000 or more persons that have in place an effective public dental health program directed by a dental professional with public health training.

FOCUS AREA 22 Physical Fitness and Activity

Goal: Improve health, fitness, and quality of life through daily physical activity.

Physical Activity in Adults

22-1   Reduce the proportion of adults who engage in no leisure-time physical activity.

22-2   Increase the proportion of adults who engage regularly, preferably daily, in moderate physical activity for at least 30 minutes per day.

22-3   Increase the proportion of adults who engage in vigorous physical activity that promotes the development and maintenance of cardiorespiratory fitness 3 or more days per week for 20 or more minutes per occasion.

Muscular Strength/Endurance and Flexibility

22-4   Increase the proportion of adults who perform physical activities that enhance and maintain muscular strength and endurance.

22-5   Increase the proportion of adults who perform physical activities that enhance and maintain flexibility.

Physical Activity in Children and Adolescents

22-6   Increase the proportion of adolescents who engage in moderate physical activity for at least 30 minutes on 5 or more of the previous 7 days.

22-7   Increase the proportion of adolescents who engage in vigorous physical activity that promotes cardiorespiratory fitness 3 or more days per week for 20 or more minutes per occasion.

22-8   Increase the proportion of the Nation's public and private schools that require daily physical education for all students.

22-9   Increase the proportion of adolescents who participate in daily school physical education.

22-10   Increase the proportion of adolescents who spend at least 50 percent of school physical education class time being physically active.

22-11   Increase the proportion of adolescents who view television 2 or fewer hours on a school day.

Access

22-12   (Developmental) Increase the proportion of the Nation's public and private schools that provide access to their physical activity spaces and facilities for all persons outside of normal school hours (that is, before and after the school day, on weekends, and during summer and other vacations).

22-13   Increase the proportion of worksites offering employer-sponsored physical activity and fitness programs.

22-14   Increase the proportion of trips made by walking.

22-15   Increase the proportion of trips made by bicycling.

FOCUS AREA 23 Public Health Infrastructure

Goal: Ensure that Federal, Tribal, State, and local health agencies have the infrastructure to provide essential public health services effectively.

Data and Information Systems

23-1   (Developmental) Increase the proportion of Tribal, State, and local public health agencies that provide Internet and e-mail access for at least 75 percent of their employees and that teach employees to use the Internet and other electronic information systems to apply data and information to public health practice.

23-2   (Developmental) Increase the proportion of Federal, Tribal, State, and local health agencies that have made information available to the public in the past year on the Leading Health Indicators, Health Status Indicators, and Priority Data Needs.

23-3   Increase the proportion of all major national, State, and local health data systems that use geocoding to promote nationwide use of geographic information systems (GIS) at all levels.

23-4   Increase the proportion of population-based Healthy People 2010 objectives for which national data are available for all population groups identified for the objective.

23-5   (Developmental) Increase the proportion of Leading Health Indicators, Health Status Indicators, and Priority Data Needs for which data—especially for select populations—are available at the Tribal, State, and local levels.

23-6   Increase the proportion of Healthy People 2010 objectives that are tracked regularly at the national level.

23-7   Increase the proportion of Healthy People 2010 objectives for which national data are released within 1 year of the end of data collection.

Workforce

23-8   (Developmental) Increase the proportion of Federal, Tribal, State, and local agencies that incorporate specific competencies in the essential public health services into personnel systems.

23-9   (Developmental) Increase the proportion of schools for public health workers that integrate into their curricula-specific content to develop competency in the essential public health services.

23-10   (Developmental) Increase the proportion of Federal, Tribal, State, and local public health agencies that provide continuing education to develop competency in essential public health services for their employees.

Public Health Organizations

23-11   (Developmental) Increase the proportion of State and local public health agencies that meet national performance standards for essential public health services.

23-12   Increase the proportion of Tribes, States, and the District of Columbia that have a health improvement plan and increase the proportion of local jurisdictions that have a health improvement plan linked with their State plan.

23-13   (Developmental) Increase the proportion of Tribal, State, and local health agencies that provide or assure comprehensive laboratory services to support essential public health services.

23-14   (Developmental) Increase the proportion of Tribal, State, and local public health agencies that provide or assure comprehensive epidemiology services to support essential public health services.

23-15   (Developmental) Increase the proportion of Federal, Tribal, State, and local jurisdictions that review and evaluate the extent to which their statutes, ordinances, and bylaws assure the delivery of essential public health services.

Resources

23-16   (Developmental) Increase the proportion of Federal, Tribal, State, and local public health agencies that gather accurate data on public health expenditures, categorized by essential public health service.

Prevention Research

23-17   (Developmental) Increase the proportion of Federal, Tribal, State, and local public health agencies that conduct or collaborate on population-based prevention research.

FOCUS AREA 24 Respiratory Diseases

Goal: Promote respiratory health through better prevention, detection, treatment, and education efforts.

Asthma

24-1	Reduce asthma deaths.
24-2	Reduce hospitalizations for asthma.
24-3	Reduce hospital emergency department visits for asthma.
24-4	Reduce activity limitations among persons with asthma.
24-5	(Developmental) Reduce the number of school or work days missed by persons with asthma due to asthma.
24-6	Increase the proportion of persons with asthma who receive formal patient education, including information about community and self-help resources, as an essential part of the management of their condition.
24-7	(Developmental) Increase the proportion of persons with asthma who receive appropriate asthma care according to the NAEPP Guidelines.
24-8	(Developmental) Establish in at least 25 States a surveillance system for tracking asthma death, illness, disability, impact of occupational and environmental factors on asthma, access to medical care, and asthma management.

Chronic Obstructive Pulmonary Disease

24-9	Reduce the proportion of adults whose activity is limited due to chronic lung and breathing problems.
24-10	Reduce deaths from chronic obstructive pulmonary disease (COPD) among adults.

Obstructive Sleep Apnea

24-11	(Developmental) Increase the proportion of persons with symptoms of obstructive sleep apnea whose condition is medically managed.
24-12	(Developmental) Reduce the proportion of vehicular crashes caused by persons with excessive sleepiness.

FOCUS AREA 25 Sexually Transmitted Diseases

Goal: Promote responsible sexual behaviors, strengthen community capacity, and increase access to quality services to prevent sexually transmitted diseases (STDs) and their complications.

Bacterial STD Illness and Disability

25-1 Reduce the proportion of adolescents and young adults with *Chlamydia trachomatis* infections.

25-2 Reduce gonorrhea.

25-3 Eliminate sustained domestic transmission of primary and secondary syphilis.

Viral STD Illness and Disability

25-4 Reduce the proportion of adults with genital herpes infection.

25-5 (Developmental) Reduce the proportion of persons with human papillomavirus (HPV) infection.

STD Complications Affecting Females

25-6 Reduce the proportion of females who have ever required treatment for pelvic inflammatory disease (PID).

25-7 Reduce the proportion of childless females with fertility problems who have had a sexually transmitted disease or who have required treatment for pelvic inflammatory disease (PID).

25-8 (Developmental) Reduce HIV infections in adolescent and young adult females aged 13 to 24 years that are associated with heterosexual contact.

STD Complications Affecting the Fetus and Newborn

25-9 Reduce congenital syphilis.

25-10 (Developmental) Reduce neonatal consequences from maternal sexually transmitted diseases, including chlamydial pneumonia, gonococcal and chlamydial ophthalmia neonatorum, laryngeal papillomatosis (from human papillomavirus infection), neonatal herpes, and preterm birth and low birth weight associated with bacterial vaginosis.

Personal Behaviors

25-11 Increase the proportion of adolescents who abstain from sexual intercourse or use condoms if currently sexually active.

25-12 (Developmental) Increase the number of positive messages related to responsible sexual behavior during weekday and nightly prime-time television programming.

Community Protection Infrastructure

25-13 Increase the proportion of Tribal, State, and local sexually transmitted disease programs that routinely offer hepatitis B vaccines to all STD clients.

25-14 (Developmental) Increase the proportion of youth detention facilities and adult city or county jails that screen for common bacterial sexually transmitted diseases within 24 hours of admission and treat STDs (when necessary) before persons are released.

25-15 (Developmental) Increase the proportion of all local health departments that have contracts with managed care providers for the treatment of nonplan partners of patients with bacterial sexually transmitted diseases (gonorrhea, syphilis, and chlamydia).

Personal Health Services

25-16 (Developmental) Increase the proportion of sexually active females aged 25 years and under who are screened annually for genital chlamydia infections.

25-17 (Developmental) Increase the proportion of pregnant females screened for sexually transmitted diseases (including HIV infection and bacterial vaginosis) during prenatal health care visits, according to recognized standards.

25-18 Increase the proportion of primary care providers who treat patients with sexually transmitted diseases and who manage cases according to recognized standards.

25-19 (Developmental) Increase the proportion of all sexually transmitted disease clinic patients who are being treated for bacterial STDs (chlamydia, gonorrhea, and syphilis) and who are offered provider referral services for their sex partners.

FOCUS AREA 26 Substance Abuse

Goal: Reduce substance abuse to protect the health, safety, and quality of life for all, especially children.

Adverse Consequences of Substance Use and Abuse

26-1   Reduce deaths and injuries caused by alcohol- and drug-related motor vehicle crashes.

26-2   Reduce cirrhosis deaths.

26-3   Reduce drug-induced deaths.

26-4   Reduce drug-related hospital emergency department visits.

26-5   (Developmental) Reduce alcohol-related hospital emergency department visits.

26-6   Reduce the proportion of adolescents who report that they rode, during the previous 30 days, with a driver who had been drinking alcohol.

26-7   (Developmental) Reduce intentional injuries resulting from alcohol- and illicit drug-related violence.

26-8   (Developmental) Reduce the cost of lost productivity in the workplace due to alcohol and drug use.

Substance Use and Abuse

26-9   Increase the age and proportion of adolescents who remain alcohol and drug free.

26-10   Reduce past-month use of illicit substances.

26-11   Reduce the proportion of persons engaging in binge drinking of alcoholic beverages.

26-12   Reduce average annual alcohol consumption.

26-13   Reduce the proportion of adults who exceed guidelines for low-risk drinking.

26-14   Reduce steroid use among adolescents.

26-15   Reduce the proportion of adolescents who use inhalants.

Risk of Substance Use and Abuse

26-16   Increase the proportion of adolescents who disapprove of substance abuse.

26-17   Increase the proportion of adolescents who perceive great risk associated with substance abuse.

Treatment for Substance Abuse

26-18   (Developmental) Reduce the treatment gap for illicit drugs in the general population.

26-19   (Developmental) Increase the proportion of inmates receiving substance abuse treatment in correctional institutions.

26-20   Increase the number of admissions to substance abuse treatment for injection drug use.

26-21   (Developmental) Reduce the treatment gap for alcohol problems.

State and Local Efforts

26-22   (Developmental) Increase the proportion of patients who are referred for followup care for alcohol problems, drug problems, or suicide attempts after diagnosis or treatment for one of these conditions in a hospital emergency department.

26-23   (Developmental) Increase the number of communities using partnerships or coalition models to conduct comprehensive substance abuse prevention efforts.

26-24   Extend administrative license revocation laws, or programs of equal effectiveness, for persons who drive under the influence of intoxicants.

26-25   Extend legal requirements for maximum blood alcohol concentration levels of 0.08 percent for motor vehicle drivers aged 21 years and older.

FOCUS AREA 27 Tobacco Use

Goal: Reduce illness, disability, and death related to tobacco use and exposure to secondhand smoke.

Tobacco Use in Population Groups

27-1   Reduce tobacco use by adults.

27-2   Reduce tobacco use by adolescents.

27-3   (Developmental) Reduce the initiation of tobacco use among children and adolescents.

27-4   Increase the average age of first use of tobacco products by adolescents and young adults.

Cessation and Treatment

27-5   Increase smoking cessation attempts by adult smokers.

27-6   Increase smoking cessation during pregnancy.

27-7   Increase tobacco use cessation attempts by adolescent smokers.

27-8   Increase insurance coverage of evidence-based treatment for nicotine dependency.

Exposure to Secondhand Smoke

27-9   Reduce the proportion of children who are regularly exposed to tobacco smoke at home.

27-10   Reduce the proportion of nonsmokers exposed to environmental tobacco smoke.

27-11   Increase smoke-free and tobacco-free environments in schools, including all school facilities, property, vehicles, and school events.

27-12   Increase the proportion of worksites with formal smoking policies that prohibit smoking or limit it to separately ventilated areas.

27-13   Establish laws on smoke-free indoor air that prohibit smoking or limit it to separately ventilated areas in public places and worksites.

Social and Environmental Changes

27-14   Reduce the illegal sales rate to minors through enforcement of laws prohibiting the sale of tobacco products to minors.

27-15   Increase the number of States and the District of Columbia that suspend or revoke State retail licenses for violations of laws prohibiting the sale of tobacco to minors.

27-16   (Developmental) Eliminate tobacco advertising and promotions that influence adolescents and young adults.

27-17   Increase adolescents' disapproval of smoking.

27-18   (Developmental) Increase the number of Tribes, Territories, and States and the District of Columbia with comprehensive, evidence-based tobacco control programs.

27-19   Eliminate laws that preempt stronger tobacco control laws.

27-20   (Developmental) Reduce the toxicity of tobacco products by establishing a regulatory structure to monitor toxicity.

27-21   Increase the average Federal and State tax on tobacco products.

FOCUS AREA 28 Vision and Hearing

Goal: Improve the visual and hearing health of the Nation through prevention, early detection, treatment, and rehabilitation.

Vision

28-1   (Developmental) Increase the proportion of persons who have a dilated eye examination at appropriate intervals.

28-2   (Developmental) Increase the proportion of preschool children aged 5 years and under who receive vision screening.

28-3   (Developmental) Reduce uncorrected visual impairment due to refractive errors.

28-4   Reduce blindness and visual impairment in children and adolescents aged 17 years and under.

28-5   (Developmental) Reduce visual impairment due to diabetic retinopathy.

28-6   (Developmental) Reduce visual impairment due to glaucoma.

28-7   (Developmental) Reduce visual impairment due to cataract.

28-8   (Developmental) Reduce occupational eye injury.

28-9   (Developmental) Increase the use of appropriate personal protective eyewear in recreational activities and hazardous situations around the home.

28-10   (Developmental) Increase vision rehabilitation.

Hearing

28-11   (Developmental) Increase the proportion of newborns who are screened for hearing loss by age 1 month, have audiologic evaluation by age 3 months, and are enrolled in appropriate intervention services by age 6 months.

28-12   Reduce otitis media in children and adolescents.

28-13   (Developmental) Increase access by persons who have hearing impairments to hearing rehabilitation services and adaptive devices, including hearing aids, cochlear implants, or tactile or other assistive or augmentative devices.

28-14   (Developmental) Increase the proportion of persons who have had a hearing examination on schedule.

28-15   (Developmental) Increase the number of persons who are referred by their primary care physician for hearing evaluation and treatment.

28-16   (Developmental) Increase the use of appropriate ear protection devices, equipment, and practices.

28-17   (Developmental) Reduce noise-induced hearing loss in children and adolescents aged 17 years and under.

28-18   (Developmental) Reduce adult hearing loss in the noise-exposed public.

U.S. Department of Health and Human Services. (2000). Healthy People 2010: Understanding and Improving Health (2nd ed.). Washington, DC: U.S. Government Printing Office.

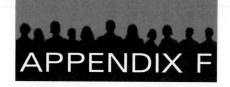

APPENDIX F

Professional Associations, Organizations, and Institutes

Academy for Health Services Research and Health Policy
Focuses on health services research and health policy. http://www.academyhealth.org

Agency for Health Care Research and Quality
Provides information on health care quality, cost, access, and outcomes. http://www.ahrq.org

American Association of Colleges of Nursing
Web site provides information relevant to nursing in colleges and universities. http://www.aacn.nche.edu

American Heart Association (AHA)
Provides information on programs, news, and legislation related to cardiovascular health. http://www.amhrt.org

American Nurses Association (ANA)
Official Web site for the ANA. http://www.nursingworld.org

American Public Health Association (APHA)
Official Web site for the organization. http://www.apha.org

American Social Health Association
Advocacy organization for various social issues. http://www.ashastd.org

Association of State and Territorial Health Officials
Web site represents the state and territorial public health agencies, U.S. territories, and District of Columbia with a mission to formulate and influence policy to promote health and prevent disease. http://www.astho.org

Brookings Institute
Provides health care issues publications. http://www.brook.edu

Center for the Advancement of Health
Translates evidence-based research on health, health care, prevention, and chronic disease management, emphasizing social, behavioral, and economic factors. http://www.cfah.org

Centers for Disease Control and Prevention (CDC)
Provides information on diseases in the United States and worldwide. http://www.cdc.gov

Child Protection Services (CPS), U.S. Department of State
Link to information, laws, agencies, and services for national and international protection of children. http://travel.state.gov

Department of Veterans Affairs
Official Web site of information for veterans. http://www.va.gov

Division of Nursing, Bureau of Health Professions, Health Resources, and Services Administration
Provides nursing leadership in various areas. http://www.bhpr.hrsa.gov/nursing

Environmental Protection Agency (EPA)
Provides information related to environmental issues. http://www.epa.gov

Families USA
National nonprofit organization whose focus is affordable and long-term care for U.S. citizens. http://www.familiesusa.org

FirstGov
Web site for U.S. government information and services. http://www.firstgov.gov/

Food and Drug Administration (FDA)
Official Web site for regulating food, drug, medical devices, biologics, animal feed and drugs, cosmetics, radiation-emitting products, and combination products (e.g., drug-device, drug-biologic, and device-biologic). http://www.fda.gov

Health Insurance Association of America
An association representing private health insurance companies. http://www.hiaa.org

Health Resources and Services Administration (HRSA)
Web site for health resources and improving access to health care for medically underserved, isolated, or medically vulnerable populations. http://www.hrsa.gov

Healthy People 2010
Official Web site for information on the Healthy People objectives. http://www.healthypeople.gov/Publication/HealthyCommunities2001/default.htm

Healthy People in Healthy Communities
A guide for community planning using Healthy People 2010 objectives. http://healthypeople.gov

Heritage Foundation
An educational and research think tank that promotes conservative public policies. http://www.heritage.org

Institute for Children's Health Policy
Provides information on polices related to the health of children. http://www.ichp.edu

Institute of Medicine (IOM)
Official Web site for this institute. http://www.iom.edu

International Council of Nurses (ICN)
International Web site for nurses. http://www.icn.org

INurse
Web site that links to multiple nursing associations. http://www.iNurse.com

Medicare
Official Web site for information about the Medicare program. http://www.medicare.gov

National Black Nurses' Association (NBNA)
Official Web site for NBNA. http://www.nbna.org

National Center for Health Statistics (NCHS)
Nation's principal health statistics agency to compile statistics that guide actions and policies to improve the nation's health. http://www.cdc.gov/nchs

National Center on Elder Abuse (NCEA)
A resource on elder abuse, neglect, and exploitation overseen by the U.S. Administration on Aging. http://www.elderabusecenter.org/default.cfm

National Coalition on Healthcare
A coalition focused on health care issues. http://www.nchc.org

National Council Against Health Fraud
A not-for-profit agency focused on fraud in health care. http://www.ncahf.org

National Council of State Boards of Nursing
Web site that links with various Boards of Nursing. http://www.ncsbn.org

National Indian Health Board (NIHB)
Official site representing and advocating for tribal governments with respect to policy, information, resources, and visibility of Indian health issues. http://www.nihb.org

National Institute of Nursing Research (NINR)
Branch of nursing within NIH. http://www.nih.gov/ninr

National Institute for Occupational Safety and Health (NIOSH)
Official Web site for information on occupational health. http://www.cdc.gov/niosh

National League for Nursing
Provides information on nursing education. http://www.nin.org

Occupational Health and Safety Administration (OSHA)
Provides information on occupational health and safety issues. http://www.osha.com

Office on Violence Against Women (OVW)
Official Web site handles legal and policy issues regarding violence against women for the U.S. Department of Justice. http://www.usdoj.gov/ovw

Pan American Health Organization
Web site to the regional office for the WHO in the Americas. http://www.paho.org

Partners in Information Access for the Public Health Workforce
Collaborative Web site of U.S. government agencies, public health organizations, and health sciences libraries to assist the public health workforce find and use Internet information. http://www.phpartners.org

Project Hope
Provides international assistance such as education, health care, and more. http://www.projhope.org

Public Health Foundation (PHF) http://www.phf.org
Resource for research, training, and technical assistance to manage and improve performance, understand and use data, and strengthen the public health workforce. http://www.phf.org

Public Health Service Act
Web site contains reference to Title 42 United States Code. http://www.fda.gov/opacom/laws/phsvcact/phsvcact.htm

Rand Institute
Nonprofit institute that conducts health related policy research. http://www.rand.org

Sigma Theta Tau International
International honorary society of nursing. http://www.nursingsociety.org

U.S. Department of Health and Human Services
Provides information on the health status of Americans. http://www.dhhs.gov

Wellness Councils of America (WELCOA)
Resource for worksite wellness programs. http://www.welcoa.org

World Health Organization (WHO)
Official Web site for the international organization. http://www.who.int

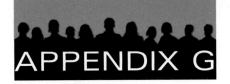

Abbreviations

AAN	American Academy of Nursing
AAOHN	American Association of Occupational Health Nurses
AARP	American Association of Retired Persons
ACE	American College of Endocrinology
ACHNE	Association of Community Health Nurse Educators
ACS	American Cancer Society
ADA	American Diabetes Association
AFDC	Aid to Families with Dependent Children
AHA	American Heart Association
AHP	Accountable Health Plan
AHRQ	Agency for Healthcare Research and Quality
AIDS	acquired immunodeficiency syndrome
ALA	American Lung Association
AMA	American Medical Association
ANA	American Nurses Association
APA	American Psychological Association
APHA	American Public Health Association
ARC	American Red Cross
ARS	acute radiation syndrome
ASTDN	Association of State and Territorial Directors of Nursing
AVERT	Association of Volunteer Emergency Response Teams
BBA	Balanced Budget Act
BBTD	baby bottle tooth decay
BMI	body mass index
BNE	Boards of Nurse Examiners
BRFSS	Behavioral Risk Factor Surveillance System
CASA	Center on Addiction and Substance Abuse
CBA	cost-benefit analysis
CBPR	community-based participatory research
CCA	cost-consequence analysis
CCMC	Committee on Costs of Medical Care
CDC	Centers for Disease Control and Prevention
CEA	cost-effectiveness analysis
CFC	chlorofluorocarbon
CHAMPUS	Civilian Health and Medical Program of the Uniformed Services
CHC	community health center
CHESS	Comprehensive Health Enhancement Support System
CHIP	Community Hypertension Intervention Project
CHIS	Consumer Health Internet Support System
CHPP	Community-based Homelessness Prevention Program
CMA	cost-minimization analysis
CMS	Centers for Medicare & Medicaid Services
COL	Council on Linkages Between Academia and Public Health Practice
CPS	Child Protective Services
CSAP	Center for Substance Abuse Prevention
CSR	Communicable Diseases Surveillance and Response
CUA	cost-utility analysis
DASH	Dietary Approaches to Stop Hypertension
DHHS	Department of Health and Human Services
DHS	Department of Homeland Security
DOE	Department of Energy

DRG	diagnosis-related group
DVA	Department of Veterans' Affairs
EBP	evidence-based practice
EHCY	Education of Homeless Children and Youth
EPA	Environmental Protection Agency
EPZ	emergency planning zone
ERA	Equal Rights Amendment
ERRNIE	Environmental Risk Reduction through Nursing Intervention and Education
ETS	environmental tobacco smoke
FAS	fetal alcohol syndrome
FBI	Federal Bureau of Investigation
FDA	Food and Drug Administration
FEMA	Federal Emergency Management Agency
FNP	family nurse practitioner
FNS	Frontier Nursing Service
FOIA	Freedom of Information Act
FQHC	federally qualified health centers
GDP	gross domestic product
GIS	Geographic Information System
GLBT	gay, lesbian, bisexual, and transgender
GNP	gross national product
GPRA	Government Performance and Results Act
HAN	Health Alert Network
HBM	Health Belief Model
HBV	hepatitis B virus
HCH	Health Care for the Homeless
HFA	Healthy Families America
HIPC	Health Insurance Purchasing Cooperatives
HIV	human immunodeficiency virus
HMO	health maintenance organization
HOPWA	Housing Opportunities for Persons with AIDS
HPLP II	Health Promoting Lifestyle Profile II
HPM	Health Promotion Model
HPSA	Health Professional Shortage Area
HRA	health risk appraisal

HRSA	Health Resources and Services Administration
HSPD	Homeland Security Presidential Declaration
HSV	herpes simplex virus
HUD	Housing and Urban Development
ICESCR	International Covenant on Economic, Social, and Cultural Rights
ICN	International Council of Nurses
ICS	incident command structure
IFG	impaired fasting glucose
IHS	Indian Health Service
IMF	International Monetary Fund
IOM	Institute of Medicine
IPM	integrated pest management
IRB	Institutional Review Board
JC	Joint Commission
JCAHO	Joint Commission on Accreditation of Healthcare Organizations
LST	Life Skills Training
MADD	Mothers Against Drunk Driving
MCO	managed care organization
MDG	Millennium Development Goals
MDR-TB	multidrug-resistant tuberculosis
MSA	medical savings account
MUA	Medically Underserved Area
NACCHO	National Association of City and County Health Officials Nurses
NAFTA	North American Free Trade Agreement
NASA	National Aeronautics and Space Administration
NASN	National Association of School Nurses
NBNA	National Black Nurses Association
NCCDPHP	National Center for Chronic Disease Prevention and Health Promotion
NCEP	National Cholesterol Education Program
NCFH	National Center for Farmworker Health
NCH	National Coalition for the Homeless
NCHS	National Center for Health Statistics
NCHV	National Coalition for Homeless Veterans

NCI	National Cancer Institute	OJJDP	Office of Juvenile Justice and Delinquency Prevention
NCIPC	National Center for Injury Prevention and Control	OMH	Office of Minority Health
NCMHD	National Centers for Minority Health and Health Disparities	OPHS	Office of Public Health and Science
		ORHP	Office of Rural Health Policy
NEDSS	National Electronic Disease Surveillance System	OSHA	Occupational Safety and Health Administration
NFP	Nurse-Family Partnership	PAHO	Pan American Health Organization
NHANES	National Health and Nutrition Examination Survey	PAR	participatory action research
		PBT	persistent bioaccumulative toxics
NHIS	National Health Interview Survey	PCA	Prevent Child Abuse America
NHLBI	National Heart, Lung, and Blood Institute	PCP	primary care provider
NHSC	National Health Service Corps	PHC	primary health care
NIAAA	National Institute on Alcohol Abuse and Alcoholism	PHDSC	Public Health Data Standards Consortium
		PHIN	Public Health Information Network
NIDA	National Institute on Drug Abuse	PHM	People's Health Movement
NIH	National Institutes of Health	PHN	Public Health Nursing
NIMBY	not in my back yard	PHS	Public Health Service
NIMH	National Institute of Mental Health	PPO	preferred provider organization
NIMS	National Incident Management System	PTSD	posttraumatic stress disorder
NINR	National Institute of Nursing Research	PVC	polyvinyl chloride
NIOSH	National Institute for Occupational Safety and Health	QALY	quality adjusted life year
		RCT	randomized clinical trial
NLM	National Library of Medicine	RDD	Radiological Dispersal Device
NNIS	National Nosocomial Infection Surveillance	REALM	Rapid Estimate of Adult Literacy in Medicine
NOC	Nursing Outcomes Classification	RHC	rural health clinic
NOPHN	National Organization of Public Health Nurses	RICHS	Rural Information Center Health Service
NPHPSP	National Public Health Performance Standards Program	SAMHSA	Substance Abuse and Mental Health Services Administration
NPL	National Priorities List (hazardous waste Superfund priorities)	SARS	severe acute respiratory syndrome
		SCHIP	State Child Health Plan
NRC	Nuclear Regulatory Commission	SCT	Social Cognitive Theory
NRHA	National Rural Health Association	SEER	Surveillance Epidemiology and End Results
NRP	National Response Plan		
OASIS	Outcome and Assessment Information Set	SES	socioeconomic status
OBRA	Omnibus Reconciliation Act	SHS	secondhand smoke
ODPHP	Office of Disease Prevention and Health Promotion	SIDS	sudden infant death syndrome
		SNS	Strategic National Stockpile
OGTT	oral glucose tolerance test	SSI	Supplemental Security Income

TANF	Temporary Assistance to Needy Families	USDCESA	U.S. Department of Commerce Economics and Statistics Administration
TARU	Technical Advisory Response Unit	USDHHS	United States Department of Health and Human Services
TEFRA	Tax Equity and Fiscal Responsibility Act	USMBHC	United States-Mexico Border Health Commission
TIP	Treatment Improvement Protocol		
TPB	Theory of Planned Behavior	USPSTF	U.S. Preventive Services Task Force
TRI	Toxic Release Inventory	VARK	Visual, Aural, Read/write, and Kinesthetic
TTM	Transtheoretical Model	VMI	vendor managed inventory
UDHR	Universal Declaration of Human Rights	VOC	volatile organic compound
UN	United Nations	WHCP	Women's Healthcare Partnership
UNAIDS	Joint United Nations Program on HIV/AIDS	WHO	World Health Organization
		WIC	Women, Infants, and Children
UNHCR	United Nations High Commissioner for Refugees	WSF	World Social Forum
		WTO	World Trade Organization
UNICEF	United Nations Children's Fund	YRBS	Youth Risk Behavioral Survey
USAMRIID	U.S. Army Medical Research Institute of Infectious Diseases		

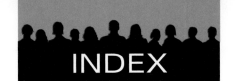

INDEX

Note: figures, illustrations, photographs, sidebars, and tables are indicated by an italicized page locator.

A

AARP (American Association of Retired Persons), 497
Abortion, 484, *484*
Abuse, 329–36, *331, 484. See also* Violence and injuries
Acanthosis nigricans, 454–56
Acceptability, standards of, 318
Access to health care. *See also* Health care
  barriers to, *176,* 464–65, 517–18, 520–21, 563
  health insurance and, 641
  Healthy People 2010 on, 112
  in United States, 135–46
  by vulnerable populations, 512–13, 543–44, 562–63, 574–75
Accountability, 647
Accountable health plans, 143–44
Acculturation, 557–59, *558. See also culture-related entries;* Immigration
Achievements in public health, *28,* 279
ACHNE (Association of Community Health Nursing Educators), 20, 39, 74, 373, 392
Acquired immunity, 413
Acquired immunodeficiency syndrome (AIDS). *See* HIV/AIDS
Acquired Property Sales for Homeless Providers Programs, 582
Active immunity, 413. *See also* Immunizations
Acute care *versus* preventive nursing services, 59
Acute illnesses, 16, 446, 578, *601*
Acute radiation syndrome, 621
Acyclovir, 430
Adaph Judaeus, *372*
Adaptation, 223. *See also* Roy's Adaptation Model
Adaptive health, 254
Addams, Jane, 10–11, 21
Addiction, nicotine, 594. *See also* Substance abuse; Tobacco use
Administration, 346–48
Adolescents
  deaths of, 483–84
  health education and, 488–89
  health of, *486*
  homeless, 576–78
  obesity and, 486–88
  sexual activity and pregnancies of, *484,* 484–86, *558*
  substance abuse and, *262,* 594, 597–600, *598, 600*
Adult day health centers, 71
Adult learners, 283

Advanced practice nurses, 64, 68, *310,* 650
Advocacy. *See* Political activism
Affective domains, 283, 286, *288, 294*
African Americans. *See also* Demographic categories; Racial and ethnic health disparities
  definition of, *531*
  ethics and, *374*
  illnesses and, *243, 381,* 382, 453–54
  as nurses, 13–14, 19–20
  social changes and, 10 (*See also* Civil rights)
African ethics, *374*
Age, health and, 93–96, *94, 95,* 107–12, *113. See also* Adolescents; Aging; Children; Demographic categories; Infant mortality; Older adults; Perinatal health disparities
Age-adjusted rates, 93–96
Ageism, 499, *500*
Agency for Children and Families, 333
Agency for Healthcare Research and Quality, 333
Agency for Toxic Substances and Disease Registry, 212
Agency leadership, 646
Agenda setting, political, 120–21
Agent-host-environment epidemiological triangle, 410
Agents
  bacterial, 616
  biological, 411, 433, *434*
  blood, 622
  chemical, *435*
  choking, 622
  nerve, 621
  vesicant or blistering, 622
  viral, 616
Aging. *See also* Older adults
  myths of, *500*
  physiological changes and, 501–4
  policies on, *316*
  premature, 578
  theories of, 497, *498*
Agricultural Disability Awareness and Risk Education Model, *295*
Agricultural production, 206, *295. See also* Migrant farmworkers
AHA (American Heart Association), 90, 458
AIDS (acquired immunodeficiency syndrome). *See* HIV/AIDS
Aid to Families with Dependent Children, 140
Airborne pathogens, 427. *See also* Infectious diseases
Air pollution, 204–6, *205. See also* Indoor air quality
Airs, Waters, and Places, 3
Ajzen's Theory of Planned Behavior, 257–58

Alaskan Natives, *531. See also* Demographic categories; Racial and ethnic health disparities
Alcohol consumption, 592–93. *See also* Substance abuse
Allocation of resources. *See* Resource allocation
Allocative efficiency, 156–57
Alzheimer's disease, 466
American Academy of Nursing, 174
American Academy of Pediatrics, 334
American Association of Blood Banks, *409,* 422
American Association of Occupational Health Nurses, 70
American Association of Retired Persons (AARP), 497
American College of Endocrinology, 453
American Diabetes Association, 90, 452–53
American Heart Association (AHA), 90, 458
American Journal of Nursing, 14
American Medical Association, 138
American Medical Society, 135
American Nurses Association (ANA)
  on environmental health, 211, 213
  on ethics, 366, 371, 373
  founding of, 13
  on health promotion, 255, 334
  integration of, 19
  on nontherapeutic antibiotics, 206
  on nursing shortages, *561*
  on older adults, 496–97
  on parish nursing, 68
  participation in Quad Council, 20
  political activism and, 14, 124
  on product labeling, 201
  on public health nursing competencies, 39, 392
  on workplace hazards, 208
American Public Health Association (APHA)
  on disaster preparedness, *69, 626*
  on environmental health, 209, 213
  establishment of, 119
  on ethics, 373, 377
  on health and human rights, 178, 363, *363*
  on national system of health care, 146
  participation in Quad Council, 20
  policy statements by, 643
  political activism and, 121, 124, *128*
  on public health nursing competencies, 39, 392
American Red Cross, 14, 16–17, 412, 513, 611
American Translators Association, 564
American Union Against Militarism, 11
ANA. *See* American Nurses Association (ANA)
Analyses
  cost-benefit, *161,* 162–65, 268, 309, 353
  cost-consequence, 309
  cost-effectiveness, 165–66, 309–12, *310*
  cost-minimization, 308–9

Analyses, *continued*
    cost-utility, 309
    economic, 154, 308–12, *311 (See also cost
        analyses entries)*
    power level, 99
    of strengths, weaknesses, opportunities and
        threats (SWOT), *305,* 305–6
Analytical Assessment Skills, 392, *393–94*
Ancient civilizations, sanitation in, 3
Anderson, E. T., *222,* 229
Anderson, R. M., 536–39, 541
Andragogy, 283
Andrews, Janice, 11, 21
Annie E. Casey Foundation, 333
Anthrax. *See* Bioterrorism
Antibiotics, 28, 206, 641
Antibodies
    infectious diseases and, 409, 422–23,
        428–29
    as protective agent, 411, 413, 431
Antigenicity, 411
Antimicrobial drugs, 422, 431
Antiretroviral drugs, 429, *431,* 641
Antiserums, 413
Anti-Sweatshop and Fair Trade
    Campaigns, 181
APHA. *See* American Public Health
    Association (APHA)
Aristotle, 368, 370
Asian ethics, *375–76*
Asians, *531. See also* Demographic categories;
    Racial and ethnic health disparities
Assessment core function, 29, 43–44, 647
Assessment Initiative project, *227*
Assessments. *See also* Evaluation process
    disaster preparedness and, 629
    of elder health, 499–504
    of environmental health, *43,* 190–208, *192*
    evaluations and, 314, 318
    of health communication programs, 266
    of homelessness, 583
    of learners, 284–86
    nursing, 241
    periodic, 312
    of populations, 221, *227,* 537, 541, 543
    of reading levels, 290
Assimilation, of immigrants, 557
Association for Gerontology in Higher
    Education, 496
Association of Collegiate Schools of
    Nursing, 18
Association of Community Health Nursing
    Educators (ACHNE), 20, 39, 74,
    373, 392
Association of State and Territorial Directors
    of Nursing (ASTDN), 20, 39, 72,
    373, 392
Association of State and Territorial Health
    Officers, 643, 650
Assurance, disaster preparedness and, 629

Assurance core function, 30, 45–46, 647
ASTDN (Association of State and Territorial
    Directors of Nursing), 20, 39, 72,
    373, 392
Asthma, 202, 487
Atherosclerosis, 454, 458–59
Atherosclerosis Risk in Communities
    study, 454
Authority rules, 369
Authorization-appropriations process, 122
Autonomy, 366
Avilla, Margaret, *17*
Awareness, definition of, 41
AZT (Zidovudine), 422

B

Baby bottle tooth decay, 518
Baccalaureate-preparation, 39–41, 48–49, 74,
    514. *See also* Education
Back to Sleep Campaign, 545
Bacterial agents, 616
Balanced Budget Act, 522
Bantu Philosophy (Tempels), *374*
Barrier protection, 422
Barriers to health care, *176,* 517–18,
    520–21, 563
Behavior. *See also* Health behaviors
    elder health and, *502*
    health education objectives and, 287, 289
    high-risk adolescent, 483
    organizational, 157–58
    responsible sexual, 108–9, 539
    substance abuse and, 593
Behavioral models of health promotion,
    256–60
Behavioral Risk Factor Surveillance System
    (BRFSS), 89, 96, 100–101, 450
Beliefs, 256–63, 283–84, 287, 290–91, 308.
    See also Ethics; Morality; Values
Bellamy, Carol, 173
Benchmarks, 394
Beneficence, 367–68, *375*
Benefits *versus* costs, *161,* 162–65, 268,
    309, 353
Bentham, Jeremy, 365
Best Practices Initiative, 653
Best practices processes, 652–53
bettermanagement.com, 353
Beyond Pesticides, 202
Bill of Rights, U.S., 362
Bills, in legislative process, 121–22
Biocrime, *436. See also* Bioterrorism
Bioethics, 360, 364–65, 381–82
Biological agents, 411, 433, *434*
Biological exposures, 190, 208
Biological theories of aging, 497, *498*
Biological toxins, 616
Biological weapons, 616, *617–19,* 620–21.
    See also Bioterrorism

Biosphenol A exposure, *196*
Bioterrorism. *See also* Biological weapons;
    Disaster preparedness; Emergency
    preparedness; Terrorism
    core competencies on, 628–29
    drill, *73*
    emergency preparedness for, 408, 432–34
    preparation for and response to, *46, 69, 619*
    types of, 432–34, *434, 435*
    in U.S., *436, 622*
Blacks (African Americans). *See* African
    Americans
Blanchard, K., 350
Blind study, 98
Blistering or vesicant agents, 622
Blood agents, 622
Blood-borne pathogens, 428
Blood pressure, *70,* 461, 461–62
Bloom's Taxonomy of Educational Objectives,
    283, *288*
Blue Cross/Blue Shield, 137
Boards of Nurse Examiners, 123
Boards of nursing, 123
Body mass index (BMI), 450–51, *451,* 486
Bolshevism, 12
Book of Wisesaws (Harburton), 344
Border communities, *175*
Botvin's LifeSkills Training (LST) Program,
    599, *600*
Bound energy, 223
Brainard, Annie, *The Evolution of Public Health
    Nursing,* 9
Breastfeeding, 164, 190, 193, 208
Breckenridge, Mary, 513–14
Brewster, Mary, 8, 58, 119
BRFSS (Behavioral Risk Factor Surveillance
    System), 89, 96, 100–101, 450
Bright Futures, 481–82
Bringing America Home Act, 585
Brominated flame retardants, *197*
Brown, C., 31
Brown County Health Support Clinic, *523*
Brownfield sites, 203, 206
Bubonic plague, 6
Budget cuts, *128,* 626. *See also* Funding
Budgeting, 351–52
Buhler-Wilkerson, K., 7, 9, 391–92
Bureau of Health Professions, 41
Bureau of Primary Health Care, *63,* 64
Bush, George W., *128,* 142
Business plans, 351–52

C

California Adolescent Health Collaborative, *486*
California Healthy Cities project, *335*
Canada, 144, 327, *369,* 554
Cancer
    age and, 93–96, *94, 95*
    cervical, 429–30, 533

health disparities and, 532–33
liver, 97
testicular, *246*
vaginal, 96–97, 430
Capacity building, 48–50, 650–51, *652*
Capital budgets, 352
Carbon monoxide, 200, *205*
Cardiovascular disease, 457–62
  age and, 93
  diabetes and, 456
  health disparities and, 532
  health promotion and, *243, 247, 248, 652*
  overweight, obesity and, 452, 460, 487
  risk factors for, *243,* 459–62, *464, 532*
  study on, 97–98
  in women, 457–58
Cardiovascular system, aging and, 502
Care coordination programs, 485–86
Care ethics, 370
Caregivers, *307,* 465, 498–99
Case-control studies, 96–97
Case management, *65,* 352–53, 584
Case reports, definition of, 88
Case series, definition of, 88
Case Western Reserve University, 514
Cash budgets, 352
Casuistry, 371
Catastrophic health insurance, 162
Catholic ethics, *372*
Causality, 398–99
Causes of death, *449, 457, 458, 458,* 481–83
CBPR (community-based participatory
  research), 37, *39,* 541, 544, *642*
CDC. *See* Centers for Disease Control and
  Prevention (CDC)
Census Bureau. *See* U.S. Census Bureau
Center for Faith-Based & Community
  Initiatives, 68
Center for Occupational and Environmental
  Health, 208
Center for Substance Abuse Prevention, 328
Center for Substance Abuse Treatment, 319
Centers for Disease Control and Prevention
  (CDC)
  on bioterrorism, 432–33, *619*
  on chronic illnesses, *450*
  on community assessments, *227, 229*
  disaster preparedness and, 622, 626, *626*
  on environmental health, 189, *190,* 212
  on epidemiology, 87, 89, 100–101
  on ethics, 377
  on health disparities, 532, 541, *545, 642*
  on health promotion, 327, 328
  on health risk appraisals, *242*
  on infectious diseases, *409,* 426, 438, 616
  model of public health system, 33, *35,*
    35–37
  on overweight and obesity, 450, 486
  on program evaluation, 315
  on program management, 353

on public health, 32, 47
  on school health programs, 489
  on tobacco use, 261
Central Iowa Shelter and Services, *584*
Central obesity, 460
Certification programs. *See* Education
Certified organic food, *207*
Cervical cancer, 429–30, 533
Chadwick, Edwin, "Report into the Sanitary
  Conditions of the Labouring Population
  of Great Britain," 7
Chain of transmission of infectious diseases,
  410–11, *411*
Channels of health communication, 264–69
Charleston Heart Study, 454
Chemical agents, *435*
Chemical exposures
  advocacy on, 209–10
  assessing, 190–208
  communication about, 210–11
  environmental health and, 189–215
  mixtures in, 194
  policies on, 211–12
  public health and, 212–15
  reporting on, *190*
  sources and effects of, *195–97*
  vulnerable populations and, 208–9
Chemical weapons, 621–22
Chemoprophylaxis, 422
Chicago Southeast Diabetes Community
  Action Coalition, *642*
Chickenpox, 620
Child abuse prevention, 329–36, *331*
Child labor, 11
Child Protective Services, 334
Children. *See also* Adolescents; School
  community
  deaths of, 481–83 (*See also* Infant
    mortality)
  environmental exposures and, *198,* 199,
    208–9, *230, 268*
  health care spending and, *483*
  health education and, 488–89
  health insurance for, 140, 162
  health of, 31, 61–63, 107, 489–90, *537*
  homeless, 576–81
  migrant, *520*
  overweight and obesity in, 450–51, 486–88
  substance abuse and, 592–94, 595,
    597–600
  type 2 diabetes in, 451, *454*
Children's Bureau, 11
Children's Environmental Health
  Network, 210
Choking agents, 622
Cholera epidemics, 4, 87
Cholesterol, 90, 460
Christianity, ethics and, 364, *372–73*
"Chronic Disease Prevention and Health
  Promotion" appropriations bill, *450*

Chronic illnesses. *See also* Cardiovascular
  disease; Diabetes
  acute illnesses *versus,* 16
  aging population and, 448–50
  caregivers and, 465
  contextual risk factors for, 462–65
  definition of, 446
  demographic categories of, 463–65
  environment and, 463–65
  epidemiology and, 87
  homelessness and, 574, 578
  immigration and, 558
  impact of, 446, *447–48*
  obesity and, 450–56
  prevalence of, 448–56
  resource allocation and, 464–65
  in rural populations, 516
  substance abuse and, 592–93, 594–95
  trajectory of, 466–67
Chronic inflammatory states, 456
Churches. *See* Faith-based organizations;
  Religion; Religious orders
CityNet Healthy Cities, 329
Civilian Health and Medical Program of the
  Uniformed Services, 143
Civil rights, 11, 585–86
Clark, E. G., *Preventive Medicine for the
  Doctor in His Community,* 413–14
Clean Air Act, 204, 212
Cleaning products, 202
Clinical health, 254
Clinical Practice Guidelines, *401*
Clinton, William (Bill), 143–44, 209
Clothing, protective, 422
Coalition building, 651. *See also* Collaborative
  partnerships
Cobb and Elder Model, 120–21
Cochrane Data Base and Library, *401*
Code for Nurses, 366, 371, 373
Code of Ethics for Nurses, 21, 373
Code of Federal Regulations, 612
Code of Hammurabi, 364
Cognators, 223
Cognitive domain, 283, 286, *288, 294*
Cognitive theorists, 282
Cohort studies, 97–98
COL (Council on Linkages Between Academia
  and Public Health Practices), 37, 628, 648
Cold blisters, 430
Collaborative partnerships
  on aging policies, *316*
  capacity building and, 50, 651, *652*
  disaster preparedness and, 628
  environmental health and, 641–42
  faith-based organizations and, 68
  on health communication, 264
  on health education, 280–82, 289, *295*
  on health policies, 128, *643*
  on health promotion, 255, 327–28, *330,*
    334, 336, *643, 652*

Collaborative partnerships, *continued*
    on Healthy People 2010 initiatives, 105
    on homelessness, 585
    immigrant health care and, 564–65
    to improve health, 644
    nursing and philanthropy, *15*
    participants in, 33, *35*, 35–37
    participatory action research and, 541,
        544, *642*
    peer learning and, 652
    private and public sectors in, *36*, 37,
        123, *645*
    program evaluation and, 314, 317–19
    public engagement and, 354
    public health nursing and, 43–47
    on racial and ethnic health disparities, 541,
        543–44, *545*
    reliance on, 61
    in rural health care settings, 519, 522, *523*
    skills needed to build, 44
    of Turning Point, *38*
Collectivism, 244
Columbia University, 643
Committee for the Study of the Future of
    Public Health, 28–32
Committee on Costs of Medical Care, 135
Common vehicle transmission, 412
Commonwealth Fund Report, 532–33, 538
Communalism principles, *375*
Communicable diseases. *See* Infectious diseases
Communicable Diseases Surveillance and
    Response program, 625
Communication. *See* Health communication
    programs; Risk communication
Communism, 12, 18
Communities. *See also other community-related*
        entries
    assessing (*See* Community assessments)
    border, *175*
    collaboration in (*See* Collaborative
        partnerships)
    culture of, 348, 353
    effects of disasters on, 624–25
    health education in, 280–82, 289
    health program evaluation in, 91
    health promotion in, 325–37, 650–51
    immigrant health and, 559
    leadership in, 646
Community-As-Partner Model, 221–22,
    222, 229
Community assessments, 221–35
    cultural diversity and, 232, *234*, 234–35
    description of, 221
    disaster relief and, 625
    of environmental health risks, 203–7
    epidemiology and, 88–89
    health education and, 284
    health promotion and, 328
    of homelessness, 583
    methods for, 227–32, *231*

models, 221–27, *224–26*, 235
    of needs, 181, *230*, 231–32, *232*, *233*
    of parish needs, *229*
Community-Based Homelessness Prevention
    Program, 584–85
Community-Based Nurse-Midwifery Education
    Program, 514
Community-based participatory research
    (CBPR), 37, *39*, 541, 544, *642*
Community core, 221–22, 229
Community health centers (CHC), 64–65,
    136, *140*
Community intervention trials, 99
Community-level outcomes, *649*
Community subsystems, 221–22, 229
Community wellness center programs, *563*.
    See also Community health centers
Comparative justice, 368
Compendium of Culturally Competent Initiatives
    in Healthcare, 544
Competencies, *214–15*, 235, 392, 544. *See*
    also Core competencies; Skills
Competencies for Providing Essential Public
    Health Services, 648
Competency-based practice, 648–49
Competition, managed, 143–44
Comprehensive Health Enhancement Support
    System, 292
Computer literacy, 292. *See also* Technology
Concept mapping, 306
Condylomata acuminata, 429–30
Confidentiality, of health risk appraisals,
    244, 245
Consequences
    analysis of costs *versus*, 309
    of public health programs, 313
Consolidated Health Centers, 575
Constitution, U.S., 12, 123, 361, 362
Consumer Health Internet Support System, 292
Consumer products, 201, 211, 213
Contact notification, 415, 422
Contagious illnesses. *See* Infectious diseases
Content validity, *649*
Contextual risk factors, 462–65
Contextual stimuli, 223
Contraception, 422, 485
Control groups, 96, 193, *310*, *313*, 395
Control subjects, 89
Convenience samples, 89
Coordinated School Health Programs, 489, *489*
Copayments, insurance, 137, 139
Coping mechanisms, 223
Coping with Disasters: A Guidebook to
    Psychological Disasters, 624
Core competencies
    advocacy and, 127–28
    on bioterrorism, 628–29
    development of, 37, 39
    domains of, *39*, 41–42, 648–49
    as practice standards, 40–42

Core Competencies of Public Health, 39
Core functions, 29–32, 43–47
Core Public Health Worker Competencies for
    Emergency Preparedness and
    Response, 648
Cornish, E., 644–45
Coronary heart disease, 458–62, *532. See also*
    Cardiovascular disease
Correctional facilities, 71, 422
Correlational research design, 398
Cost-benefit analyses, *161*, 162–65, 268,
    309, 353
Cost-consequence analyses, 309
Cost-effectiveness analyses, 165–66,
    309–12, *310*
Cost-minimization analyses, 308–9
Costs
    of hand hygiene regimens, *156*
    of health behavior changes, 268
    of health care, 90–91, 135–45, *242*, 449,
        457, *483*
    of health promotion programs, 328–29
    of intervention, 163–66, *310*, 311
    of mental health screening and
        treatment, *311*
    minimizing, 155–57, 158–60, 308–9
    opportunity, 154, 155, 463–65
    of prescription drugs, 641
    revenues *versus*, 158
    of tobacco use, 595
Cost-utility analyses, 309
Council on Linkages Between Academia and
    Public Health Practices (COL), 37,
    628, 648
Cover the Uninsured Week, 641
C-reactive protein, 456
Creation of Civil Rights Protection for the
    Homeless, 586
Crimes, hate, 575
Crisis assistance, 584
Critical Path Method, 353
Critical thinking, 393–95
Cross-sectional studies, 96
Cultural barriers, 64, 67, 517–18. *See also*
    Language barriers
Cultural competence, 235, 544
Cultural diversity. *See also* Demographic
        categories; Racial and ethnic health
        disparities
    community assessments and, 232, *234*,
        234–35
    ethics and, 371, *372–73*, *374–76*
    health education and, 281–82,
        290–91, 292
    health indicators and, 107–12
    health risk appraisals and, 244
    Healthy People 2010 objectives
        and, *113*
    immigrant health and, 557
    management and, 355

Culture. *See also* Acculturation
  community, 348, 353
  elder health and, 497
  organizational, 346–47
  of rural populations, 516, 519
Culture brokers, 564
Cyber-terrorism, 614

D

Data
  assessment core function and, 29
  for community assessments, 221–27,
    232, 234
  disease surveillance, 99–101, 625
  dissemination of, 47–48
  epidemiologic, 88–96, *89*, 96–99, 99–101,
    241–49
  on health disparities, 532
  health education and, 284, 293–95
  on health in U.S., 189
  for health promotion programs, 328,
    329–30
  on homelessness, 584
  on immunizations, 414
  infectious diseases and, 423, 426
  public health nurses' role with, 45–46
  public health programs and, 305–7, 315,
    317–19
  secondary, 229
Databases, 401, *401*
Dating violence, *484*
Davidson, P. L., 536–39, 541
Death. *See also* Mortality rates
  causes of, *449, 457,* 458, *458,* 481–83
  child, 4, 481–83, 534–36, *535, 536*
  maternal, 479–81
  preventable, 592, 594
Debt repayment, foreign, 177
Decision making
  cost-effectiveness analyses and, 165–66
  economic, 154–55, 157–58, *307,*
    308–12, *311*
  ethics and, *369,* 378–80
  evaluation and, 313–14, 319
  uncertainty and, 154–55, 162–63
Decision trees, 306
Declaration of Alma-Ata, 362
Declaration of Independence, U.S., 362
Deductibles, insurance, 137, 142
Definition of Public Health Nursing, 21, 39
Delinquency, lead and, *198, 199*
Demographic categories. *See also* Cultural
    diversity; Racial and ethnic health
    disparities
  cardiovascular disease and, *464*
  of caregivers, 498–99
  chronic illnesses and, 463–65
  diabetes and, *533*
  epidemiological data and, 96

health education and, 281–82, 292
high blood pressure and, *461,* 461–62
of homeless population, 573, 576–83
insulin resistance and, 453–54
of migrant farmworkers, 517
obesity and, 450–52
older adults and, 496
prenatal care and, 479–81
of public health nurses, 650
of rural health care providers, 519, *520*
of rural populations, 512, 515–16
substance abuse and, 598–99
of tobacco users, 594, 596
of U.S. population, 530, *530*
Dental health, 518
Deontology, 365–66
Departments of government. *See U.S.
    department entries*
Descriptive research design, 398
Developmental and Reproductive Toxicology
    (DART), 208
Diabetes
  cardiovascular disease and, 456
  in children, 451
  demographics of, *533*
  health disparities in, *642*
  mortality rates from, *532, 533*
  overweight, obesity and, 452–53, 487
  screening for, 90, 452–53, *454*
Diabetes Research Group, 545
Diagnoses, 422–23, 629
Diagnosis-related groups, 136
Diamond, Dickson, 624
Diet, 462, 487, 539. *See also* Nutrition;
    Overweight and obesity
Dietary Approaches to Stop Hypertension, 462
Diffusion of Innovations Theory, 319
Dioxin exposure, *197*
Directly observed treatments, 422
Disabled workers, insurance for, 141–43
Disaster preparedness, 611–30. *See also*
    Emergency preparedness
  disaster life cycle and, 627, *627*
  disaster response and management,
    627–28, *628*
  disasters, effects of, 623–25
  disasters, types of, 611–14
  public health preparedness and, 628–30
  Strategic National Stockpile and, 626–27
  weapons of mass destruction and, 614–23
Discount rates, 159–60, 310–11
Discrimination, 19, *381,* 381–82. *See also*
    Civil rights; Racial and ethnic health
    disparities; Racism
Diseases. *See also* Acute illnesses; Chronic
    illnesses; Infectious diseases
  discrimination and, *381,* 381–82
  emerging, 407, 408–9, *409,* 611
  environment and, 3, 9, 189, 193, 204
  eradication and elimination of, 408, 616

management of, 448
natural history of, 409–10, *410, 415*
prevention of, 58–59, 640
trajectory of, 466–67
Disease surveillance, 32, 99–101, 435,
  625–26
Disease theories, *4,* 7
Dissemination, research, 653. *See also* Health
  communication programs
Distributive justice, 368
District nursing, 8
Division of labor in health care, 17–18, 20–21
Dock, Lavinia, 14, 18, 19
Domestic terrorism, 612, 614
Domestic violence, 580–81
Domiciliary Care for Homeless Veterans, 582
Dose-response curve, 193, *194*
Dreher, M.C., 21
Drinking water, safety of, 200, *200,* 203–4
Droplet nuclei, 427
Drugs. *See also* Substance abuse
  antibiotics, 28, 206, 641
  antimicrobial, 422, 431
  antiretroviral, 429, *431,* 641
  disaster preparedness and, *46,* 626
  dose-response curve for, 193, *194*
  penicillin, 430
  prescription, 142, 640–41
  randomized clinical trials and, 98
  resistance to, 407–8, 410, 423, 427–28,
    431, 641
  testing of, 98
Due care, 367
Dula, Annette, 371
Dust, lead-based paint, 197–98
Dyslipidemia, 460–61

E

E. coli (Escherichia coli), 424
Early Head Start/Head Start, 334, 335
Easley, Michael F., 62
Ecological model of health, 29, *29*
Ecological models of health promotion,
  261–63
Economic justice, 585
Economics
  decision making and, 154–55, 157–58,
    307, 308–12, *311*
  globalization of, 176, 179–81
  in public health, 154–68, 308–12
Edelstein, Ruth Greenberg, 18
Education. *See also* Health education
    programs; Learning; School community;
    Teaching
  competency-based, 648–49
  homelessness and, 577, *577,* 580,
    581, 586
  in management, 350–51
  on midwifery, 514

Education, *continued*
  nursing shortages and, 48–49, 166–68
  political competence and, *175*
  positive health behaviors and, 159–60
  professionalism and, 19
  research and, 392, *393–94*
  standards for, 12–14, 39–43, 74, 643
  substance abuse and, 593–94
Education, public, 210–11. *See also* Health
    communication programs; Health
    education programs; Health promotion
Education of Homeless Children and
    Youth, 586
Effectiveness *versus* costs analyses,
    309–12, *310*
Efficiency, 156–57
Egypt, sanitation in, 3
Elder, C. D., 120–21
Elderly people. *See* Older adults
Elder wellness clinics, *222*
E-learning, 291–92. *See also* Learning
Elimination of diseases, 408
Elisa test, 429
Emergency operations centers, *73*
Emergency preparedness. *See also* Disaster
    preparedness
  activities for, *48*
  bioterrorism and, 408, 432–34
  core competencies and, 648
  cost-effectiveness of, 165
  for infectious diseases, *69, 437*
  management and, 355
  public health and, *46,* 50
Emerging diseases, 407, 408–9, *409,* 611
*Emerging Infections: Microbial Threats to
    Health in the United States,* 407
Emigration. *See* Immigration
Emotional readiness, 286
Employees. *See* Occupational health settings;
    Workforce
"Ending Chronic Homelessness: Strategies for
    Action," 583–84
Energy, bound, 223
Energy Theory, Helvie's, 223, 227
England. *See* Great Britain
Enthoven, Alain, 143
Entry, modes of, 411
Envirofacts Web site, 193, 213
EnviroMap, 193
Environment. *See also* Environmental health
  chronic illnesses and, 463–65
  disease and, 3, 9, 189, 193, 204
  health and, *17,* 189–216, 221–27, 500,
    556, 559
  Healthy People 2010 on, 110
  infectious disease transmission and, 411–12
  racial and ethnic health disparities and,
    537–38, 543
  safety in, and health promotion, 325
Environmental epidemiology, 193

Environmental health, 189–216, 221–27
  advocacy for, 209–10
  assessing (*See* Environmental health
    assessments)
  challenges, 189–90
  definition of, 110, 189
  health trends and, 641–42
  infrastructure, 212–13
  justice and, 209
  as local service priority, 31
  nursing and, 213, *214–15*
Environmental health assessments, 190–208
  in community, 203–7
  in homes, *191,* 194–95, 197–201
  I Prepare assessment tool for, *192*
  in occupational settings, 193, 207–8
  public engagement for, *43*
  in schools, 201–3
Environmentalist organizations, 209–10
Environmental justice, 209, 641–42
Environmental Justice Executive Order, 209
Environmental Protection Agency (EPA)
  on air pollution, 204, *205*
  on community exposure, 193
  on drinking water, 200
  on environmental risks, 213
  on indoor air quality, 202
  on noise pollution, 203
  on point source pollutants, 204
  as regulatory agency, 212
  on risk communication, *438*
  on soil contamination, 206
Environmental Risk Reduction through
    Nursing Intervention and Education
    project, *482*
Environmental Task Force (of APHA), 209
Environmental tobacco smoke, 595
Epidemics. *See also* Pandemics
  cholera, 4, 87
  HIV/AIDS (*See* HIV/AIDS)
  influenza (*See* Influenza)
  obesity, 450–56
  polio, *15,* 28
  SARS, 28, 73, 431–32
  smallpox (*See* Smallpox)
Epidemiological data, 88–96, *89, 96*–101,
    241–49
Epidemiological triangle, 410–13, *411*
Epidemiologic Triangle Model, 87,
    222–23, 410
Epidemiology
  definition of, 87
  environmental, 193
  models of, 87–88, 222–23, 410
  in public health nursing, 88–91
  rates in, 91–96, 287
  research and, 393–95
  studies of, 96–99
Epi Response Team, *48*
Equal Rights Amendment, 18

Eradication of diseases, 408, 616
Essential services, 32–37, 43–47, 346,
    346, 648
Essential services model, 37
*Essentials of Baccalaureate Nursing Education
    for Entry Level Community Health
    Practice,* 74
Ethical, legal, and social issues (ELSI)
    programs, 382. *See also* Ethics; Social
    justice
Ethics. *See also* Human rights; Morality
  care, 370
  costs and, 309
  cross-cultural, 371, *372–73, 374–76*
  decision making and, *369,* 378–80
  definition of, 360
  feminist, 370, 371
  genetics, genomics, and, 382–83, 643
  global HIV/AIDS and, 380–82
  health promotion and, 269–71
  history of, in public health, 360–61
  moral rules and, 366, 368–70
  nursing and, 371, 373, 377–78
  principles of, 366–68
  public health and, 364–71, *369*
  randomized clinical trials and, 98–99
  research and, 395
  social justice and, 21, 378
  theories of, 365–66, 370–71
  virtue, 370–71
Ethnic density, 559
Ethnic groups, *113, 531. See also* Cultural
    diversity; Race
Ethnicity, 531, *531, 598,* 598–99. *See also*
    Cultural diversity; Race
Eudaemonistic health, 254
European Union, 212, 327
Euthanasia, 361
Evaluation process
  for community health programs, 91
  decision making and, 313–14, 319
  disaster preparedness and, 630
  health communication and, 265
  of health disparity initiatives, 543
  of health education programs, 293–95, *294*
  of health promotion programs, *335*
  program management and, 353
  public health nurses' role in, 45–47
  of public health programs, 307, 312–19,
    313, 315
  of public health system quality, 46
  research and, 399
Evidence-based practices
  chronic illnesses and, 446
  of health promotion, 328, 335
  maternal-child health and, 489–90
  public health programs and, *307,* 319,
    651–52
  research and, 401
  in rural health care, *522*

Evolution of Public Health Nursing, The (Brainard), 9
Exercise. *See* Physical activity
Exit, modes of, 411
Experiential readiness, 286
Experimental research designs, 399
Experimental study, 98
Expert panel reviews, 653
Explosive/incendiary devices, 623
External evaluators, of public health programs, 313–17
Externalities, 160–62, 310–11
External management, 354–55

F

Face-to-face interviews, 229–30
Faith-based organizations, 68, *113. See also* Religious orders
False positives, 90
Families
    caregivers in, *307,* 465, 498–99
    homeless, 579–80
    substance abuse and, 597, 599
Farm Safety Attitude Instrument, *295*
Fasting glucose, 452–53
Fate and transport of pollutants, 204–5
Fat intake, 462
FBI (Federal Bureau of Investigation), 612, 614
FDA. *See* U.S. Food and Drug Administration
Federal Aviation Administration, 212
Federal Drug Administration, 98
Federal Education Rights and Property Act, 581
Federal Emergency Management Agency (FEMA), 623, 627
Federal government. *See also* United States; *U.S. department entries*
    collaborative efforts of, *36*
    on environmental health, 212
    environmental justice and, 209
    funding by, 64–65, 67–68, 140–41, 144
    health obligations of, 30
    health promotion programs and, 334, 336
    on homelessness, 583–86
    on immigrant health care, 563
    practice settings in, 60
    rural health care and, 514–15, *515*
Federally qualified health centers, 67
Fee-for-service direct care, 20–21, 137
FEMA (Federal Emergency Management Agency), 623, 627
Feminist ethics, 370, 371
Feminist issues, 18. *See also* Suffrage; Women
Fetal alcohol syndrome, 481, 592
Fetal deaths, 481. *See also* Prenatal care
Fever blisters, 430
Fifth Discipline, The (Senge), 347
Filtration of water, 200

Financing of public health. *See* Funding of public health
Fiscal management, 351–52
"Five Keys to Safer Food," 424, *424*
Fixed costs, 155–56
Flame retardants, *197*
Flesch-Kincaid Formula, 290
Fletcher, Joseph, *Morals and Medicine,* 364
Flu. *See* Influenza
Focal stimuli, 223
Focus groups, 230–31, *231,* 397–98, 524, *563*
FOIA (Freedom of Information Act), 201, *201,* 213
Folic acid, *480,* 481, 545
Folic Acid Campaign, 545
Food-borne diseases, 423–24, *436,* 622
Food Quality Protection Act, 194, 212
Formal agenda items, 120–21
Formal justice, 368
Formative evaluations, 293, 318
For-profit organizations, 157–59
Forum on Microbial Threats, 407
Framework for Planning and Implementing Practical Program Evaluation, 315
Framingham study, 97–98
Frances Payne Bolton School of Nursing, 514
Francois-Xavier Bagnoud Center for Health and Human Rights, 178
Frank, Johann Peter, 6
Franklin, Benjamin, 344
Franklin, Martha, 14
Fraser, M., 31
Freddie Mac Corporation, 332
Freedom of Information Act (FOIA), 201, *201,* 213
Free health clinics, 136. *See also* Health centers
Frontier communities, 640. *See also* Rural health care
Frontier Nursing Service, 513–14
Frontier School of Midwifery and Family Nursing, 514
Fuel oil, 204
Funding of health care, 136–45
Funding of public health
    changes to, 16–17, 21
    disaster preparedness and, *626*
    by federal government, 59, 64–65, 67–68, 140–41
    fiscal management and, 351–52
    by foundations, 36
    health promotion and, 334, 336
    history of, 10–11
    infrastructure and, 73
    by local governments, 10
    by philanthropists, 8, 10, 58–59
    public health capacity and, 50
    by religious orders, 10
    by state governments, 145
Future of Public Health, The, 28–32, 61

Future orientation, 355–56
Futures thinking, 644–46, *645*

G

Galton, Francis, 361
Gaming, 645
Gardasil, 430
Gasoline, 199, 204
Gastrointestinal system, aging and, 502–3
Gay, lesbian, bisexual and transgender lifestyle, 576–77
Gender, Healthy People 2010 objectives and, *113*
Generalist public health nurses, 39–40, 44–47
Genetics
    cardiovascular disease and, *464*
    ethics and, 382–83, 643
    health trends and, 642–43
    overweight, obesity and, 486–87
    screening programs, *381,* 382–83
Genital herpes, 430
Genomics, ethics and, 382–83. *See also* Genetics
Geographic Information System (GIS) technology, 584, 645
Germany, 6, 135, 360–62
Germ theory, 7–8
Germ warfare. *See* Bioterrorism
Gerontological Society of America, 496
Getting to Outcomes, 328
Get Up and Go Test, 504, *507*
Gilligan, Carol, *In a Different Voice: Psychological Theory and Women's Development,* 370
GIS (Geographic Information System) technology, 584, 645
Global chemical policies, 212
Global Fund against AIDS, Tuberculosis and Malaria, *431*
Global health, 173–81
Global Influenza Preparedness Plan, 436, *437*
Globalization
    definition of, 173
    of economics, 176, 179–81
    effect on public health, 354–55
    infectious diseases and, 407–9, 431–32
Global migration patterns, 554–56. *See also* Immigration
Global North/South, 177
Global warming, 207
Glucose tolerance, 452–53
Goals. *See also* Objectives
    of health education, 286–91, *288,* 293–95
    of public health programs, 33, 305, 306–7
    visioning process and, 646
Gobineau, Joseph-Arthur de, 361
Gonorrhea, 430–31
Gottry, S., *The On-Time, On-Target Manager,* 350

Government-formal agenda setting, 120
Government Performance and Results Act, 313
Governments, 21, 29–32, 59–63, 160, 177–81. *See also* Federal government; Local governments; Political activism; Public policies; State governments; *specific countries*
Graduate Education for Advance Practice in Community Public Health Nursing, 74
Great Britain, 6–7, 139, 364
Great Depression, 16
Green Guidelines for Health Care, 210
Grembowski, D., 91
Guide to Clinical Preventive Services, 653
Guide to Community Preventive Services, 653

H

Hajat, A., 31
Hall, J., 241
Hancock, Trevor, 327
Hand hygiene regimens, *156*
Harburton, H. C., *Book of Wisesaws*, 344
Harm, inflicting, 366–67
Harris Poll, 144
Harvard University, 178
Hate crimes, 575
Hazard Communication Standard, 213
HCH (Health Care for the Homeless) program, 65, 585
Head lice, *349*
Health. *See also other health-related entries*
    definition of, 254, 326
    effects of disasters on, 623–24
    environment and (*See* Environmental health)
    global, 173–81
    holistic concepts of, 254–55
    homelessness and, 574–75, 578
    as human right, 177–79, 254, 362
    poverty and, 10, 378, *586*
    protection of, 255
    trends in, 639–43
Health Alert Network, 47–48
Health and Retirement Study, *136*
Health and Social Justice: Politics, Ideology, and Inequity in the Distribution of Disease (Hofrichter), 348
Health assessments. *See* Assessments
Health behaviors
    acculturation and, *558*
    chronic illnesses and, 446
    ethics and, 269–71
    health communication and, 263–69
    health education and, 282–95, *285, 287, 295*
    health promotion and, 256–63
    homeless population and, *582*
    immigration and, 558
    positive, 159–60, 241–49
    racial and ethnic health disparities and, 538–39, 544–45

rural health clinics and, *66*
substance abuse and, 592, 597–600
Health Belief Model, 256–57, *260, 427*
Health care
    access to (*See* Access to health care)
    barriers to, *176,* 464–65, 517–18, 520–21, 563
    costs of, 90–91, 135–45, *242,* 449, 457, *483*
    disparities in, 530 (*See also* Health disparities)
    division of labor in, 17–18, 20–21
    funding of, 136–45
    for immigrants, 562–65
    justice, 585
    management, 343–56
    privatization of, 177–78
    single payer system of, 144–45
    specialization of, 16, 18, 20–21
    system, history of, 135–36
Health Care for the Homeless (HCH) program, 65, 585
Health Care for the Homeless Veterans Program, 582
Health Care Without Harm, 210
Health centers, 62–68, *63,* 347, *516, 523, 524. See also* Wellness clinics
Health communication programs
    assessment process and, 44
    health education and, 280–81, *281*
    on lead poisoning, *268*
    models of, 263–69, *264*
    on program evaluation findings, 317–19
    risk communication and, 210–11, 435, *438*
    target populations of, 264–69
Health disparities
    definition of, 112, 530
    in diabetes, *642*
    environmental health and, 641–42
    perinatal, 534–36, 557–58, 592–93, 595
    racial and ethnic (*See* Racial and ethnic health disparities)
    tobacco-related, 595–96
    trends in, 639–40
Health education programs. *See also* Health communication programs; Health promotion
    adolescent sexual health and, 485
    beliefs, values and, 283–84, 287, 290–91
    community assessments and, 284
    cultural diversity and, 281–82, 290–91, 292
    data for, 284, 293–95
    definition of, 279
    on effects of poverty, *586*
    health behaviors and, 282–95, *285, 287, 295*
    health communication and, 280–81, *281*
    Healthy People 2010 objectives and, 279–82, *280*

implementation of, 291–93
needs assessments and, 279–81, 284
objectives of, 286–91, *288,* 293–95
racial and ethnic health disparities and, 544
in schools, 61–63, 488–89
"Health for All," 176–77, 179
Health Forum and Voluntary Hospital Association, Inc., 327
Healthier People Health Risk Appraisal 4.0, *248*
Health indicators, 106–12, *345,* 515–16
Health initiatives. *See* Healthy Cities Model for Health Promotion; Healthy People 2010; Turning Point
Health insurance. *See also* Uninsured people
    access to health care and, 641
    catastrophic, 162
    community health centers and, 64
    copayments, 137, 139
    deductibles, 137, 142
    economics and, 162–63
    homeless population and, 574–75
    immigrant health and, 563
    insurance-based care, 136–43
    lack of, *136, 138, 140*
    national, 135
    nurse practitioners and, 68
    preapprovals, 137
    premiums, 137–38, 142, 144, 163
    purchasing cooperatives, 143–44
    racial and ethnic health disparities and, 543
Health literacy, 289–90, *291,* 488, 544
Health Maintenance Organization Act, 138
Health Maintenance Organizations (HMO), 139, 142
Health outcomes. *See* Outcomes
Health policies. *See also* Policies
    definition of, 119
    health promotion and, 326–27, *336*
    management and, 354
    politics and, 119–21
    public health nurse leadership in, *123, 145,* 643
    in rural health care, 522, 524
Health professional shortage areas (HPSA), 512–13, *513. See also* Shortages of nurses
Health-promoting behavior. *See* Health behaviors; Health promotion
Health-Promoting Lifestyle Profile II, *582*
Health promotion, 255–63. *See also* Healthy Cities Model for Health Promotion
    capacity building and, 650–51
    cardiovascular disease and, *243, 247, 248, 652*
    choosing appropriate programs for, 328–36
    community development and, 325–37, *329–30*
    definition of, 255
    ethics and, 269–71

funding of, 334, 336
health communication programs and, 263–69
health risk appraisals and, *242, 247*
health trends and, 640
history of, 58–59
homeless population and, *575, 582*
immigrant health and, 564
models of, 255–63, *258, 259, 260*
in occupational health settings, *242, 247, 248, 271*
for older adults, *259,* 504–7, *505–6*
program evaluation, *335*
racial and ethnic health disparities and, 544–45
Health Promotion Glossary, 254
Health Promotion Model, Pender's, 227, *228, 243, 257, 258, 259*
Health Resources and Services Administration (HRSA)
on community assessments, 229
on education, 41
on health disparities, 112, 530
on health literacy, *291*
Migrant Health Program, 67
on rural health care, 512, 514–15, *521*
Health risk appraisals, 241–49. *See also* Screenings, health
cultural diversity and, 244
effectiveness of, 243–44
guidelines for use of, 244, *245*
history of, 241–42
in occupational settings, *242, 247, 248*
public health nursing and, 246–47, *249*
target populations of, 244–46
Health screenings. *See* Screenings, health
Health Self-Determination Index, *502*
Health services pyramid, 32, *32*
Health threats, 348, *348, 349,* 407. *See also* Bioterrorism; SWOT analysis
Health trends, 639–43
Healthy Cities Model for Health Promotion, 37, 325–28, *326, 329–30,* 651
Healthy Families America (HFA), *331,* 332–36, 485–86
Healthy Families Indiana, 332–33, 336
Healthy Families Indiana Training and Technical Assistance Project (HFIT&TAP), 332–34
Healthy People: The Surgeon General's Report on Health Promotion and Disease Prevention, 105, 255
Healthy People 2000: National Health Promotion and Disease Prevention Objectives, 105
Healthy People 2010
on access to health care, 112–13
on adolescent pregnancy, 484
on cardiovascular disease, *247*
community assessments and, 227

on cultural diversity, *113*
on definition of health, 254
on diabetes, 533, *533*
on elder health, 500
focus areas of, *105*
on health disparities, 530, 532, 537
on health education, 279–82, *280, 291,* 488
on health risk appraisals, 246
on infectious diseases, 414, 427
leading health indicators of, *345*
on LPHA, 32
on maternal-child health, 479, 481, 490
as national health initiative, 36
on nutrition, 539
objectives of, 105–13
on overweight and obesity, 486, 539
on physical activity, 107, 539
on public health infrastructure, 345–46
research and, 395–96
on rural health care, 519–21
on sexually transmitted diseases, 539
on substance abuse, 107–8, 539, 592, 594, 595
on violence and injuries, 109–10
Healthy People Consortium, 105
Healthy public policies, 119. *See also* Health policies; Public policies
Hearing loss, 503–4, *519*
Heart disease. *See* Cardiovascular disease
Heide, Wilma Scott, 18
Helvie's Energy Theory, 223, 227
Henry County Health Communities, *329–30*
Henry Street Settlement
services provided by, 135, 330
structure of, 7, 9–11, 58, 67, 135
Hepatitis, viral, 428–29
Herd immunity, 413
Heredity. *See* Genetics
Herpes simplex virus types 1 and 2, 430
HFA (Healthy Families America), *331,* 332–36
HFIT&TAP (Healthy Families Indiana Training and Technical Assistance Project), 332–34
HHS. *See* U.S. Department of Health and Human Services (HHS)
High blood pressure, *70, 461,* 461–62. *See also* Hypertension
High-sensitivity C-reactive protein, 456
Hippocratic Oath, The, 364
Hispanic, *531. See also* Demographic categories; Racial and ethnic health disparities
History of Public Health (Rosen), 3
HIV/AIDS
drug treatments for, 429, *431,* 641
emergence of, 408–9, *409*
ethics and, 380–82
human rights *versus* public health and, 363, 381–82
public health and, 28

quality of life and, *106*
race/ethnicity and, 533–34, *534*
sexual behavior and, 108
as sexually transmitted disease, 429
vaccines for, 414
HIV (human immunodeficiency virus). *See* HIV/AIDS
HMOs (Health Maintenance Organizations), 139, 142
Hofrichter, Richard, *Health and Social Justice: Politics, Ideology, and Inequity in the Distribution of Disease,* 348
Holistic care, 67–68, 254–55, 326, *376,* 564
Home health care agencies, 126, 135–36. *See also* Home visiting; Visiting nurse associations
Homeless clinics, 65, *585*
Homelessness, 573–86
definition of, 573
demographics of, 573, 576–83, *580*
health and, 574–75, *575, 578*
health behaviors and, *582*
health promotion and, *575, 582*
policies and programs on, 577–86
shelters and, *584*
Homeless Persons' Survival Act, 583
Homes, health risks in, *191,* 194–95, 197–201
Home visiting. *See also* Home health care agencies; Visiting nurse associations
child abuse prevention and, 330–36, *331*
maternal-child health and, 480–81, 485–86, *537*
as practice setting, 70–71
Hospital Insurance Trust Fund, 141
Hospital Library Service Bureau, 13
Hospitals, 15–16, 141, *167,* 210, 426
Hospital *versus* public health nurses, 13, 15–16, 126
Host-Agent Reservoir Model, 87
Hosts, of infectious diseases, 413
Housing, 7, 9, *9,* 181. *See also* Homelessness; Homes, health risks in
Housing justice, 585
Housing Opportunities for Persons with AIDS, 585
Howe, Julia, 14
HPSA (health professional shortage areas), 512–13, *513. See also* Shortages of nurses
HPV (human papillomavirus), 429–30
HRSA. *See* Health Resources and Services Administration (HRSA)
Hull House, 10–11
Human genome, 382
Human immunodeficiency virus (HIV). *See* HIV/AIDS
Human papillomavirus (HPV), 429–30
Human rights, 177–79, 254, 361–63, 381–82, 556. *See also* Ethics

Human trafficking, 562
Hypercholesterolemia screening, 90
Hyperglycemia, 452–53
Hyperinsulinemia, 453–54, 456
Hypertension, 452, 461–62, *523. See also*
    High blood pressure; Stress

I

IAQ/Tools for Schools, 202
ICN (International Council of Nurses), *174,*
    371, 373, 650
Identity mode, 223, *225*
IMF (International Monetary Fund), 177, 180
Immigration, 554–65
    among nurses, *561*
    health care for immigrants, 562–65
    health issues and, 556–61
    infectious diseases and, 413, 431, 561, 563
    migrant farmworkers and, 518
    patterns of, 554–56
    policies, 555–56
    political activism about, *175*
    public health and, 6–7, 10
Immigration and Naturalization Service, 555
Immune globulins, 413
Immunity, types of, 413
Immunizations. *See also* Vaccinations
    health trends and, 640–41
    Healthy People 2010 on, 110, 112
    for older adults, 504
    as preventive health care, 32, 414
    schedules for, *416–21,* 482–83
    travel and, 431–32
Immunocompromised people, 209, 426. *See
    also* HIV/AIDS
Impoverishment, spousal, 143
*In a Different Voice: Psychological Theory and
    Women's Development* (Gilligan), 370
Incendiary/explosive devices, 623
Incidence rates, 92
Incident command structure, 628
Income, of nurses, 75, 166–68
India, sanitation in, 3
Indiana Department of Child Services, 333
Indiana Public Health Association, *329*
Indiana University School of Nursing, 327,
    329, 332, 334
Indigenous peoples ethics, *376*
Individualism, 244, 269–71, 283–84
Individuals and families
    case management and, 352–53
    core competencies and, 42
    effects of disasters on, 623–24
    health promotion and, 325
    societal needs *versus,* 360–61, 365, 366,
        374–76
Indoor air quality, 201–2
Industrial nurses, 69
Industrial organization, 157

Industrial Revolution, 4, 6–7, 10
Infant mortality, 4, 481, 534–36, *535, 536*
Infectious diseases, 407–39
    common, 423–31
    emergence of, 407–9, 611
    epidemiology and, 87
    genetic diseases *versus,* 383
    in global community, 407–9, 431–32
    immigration and, 413, 431, 561, 563
    as local service priorities, 31
    prevention of, 413–15, *415,* 422–23, *425*
    program management for, 435–36
    public health and, 6, 28
    resources on, 436, 438
    transmission of, 409–13, *411, 412*
Infectivity, 411
Influenza
    as infectious disease, 428
    pandemics, 50, 428, 436, *437*
    public health and, 28
    vaccines, *63,* 110–12, *111,* 160, 504
Informatics, 648–49
Information Age, 291
Information/communication systems capacity,
    47–48
Infrastructure
    of environmental health, 212–13
    of health promotion programs, 334
    of public health, 47–50, 73, 212–13,
        345–46
Ingram, H., 120
Initiative on the Study and Implementation of
    Systems, *643*
Injury prevention, 504, 506–7. *See also*
    Unintentional injuries; Violence and
    injuries
Innovation, 319, 644
Innovators, 223
Institute for Johns Hopkins Nursing, 350–51
Institute for the Future, *645*
Institute for Viral Precautions, 616
Institute of Medicine (IOM)
    on education, 74
    on environmental health, 213, *214–15*
    on ethics, *374*
    on evidence-based programs, 328
    on health disparities, 530, 538, 539–41
    on health literacy, *291*
    on infectious diseases, 407
    influence of, 28–32, 37
    on partnerships, 61
    on public health, 360, 647
    on rural health, 519
Institutional agenda items, 120–21
Institutional racism, 13–14
Institutional Review Board, 395
Insulin resistance, 453–54, *455*
Insulin Resistance Atherosclerosis Study,
    453–54
Insurance, health. *See* Health insurance

Insurance-based health care, 136–43
Intangibles, 310, 312
Integrated pest management (IPM), 202, *203*
Integration
    of American Nurses Association, 19
    of immigrants, 557
    of information technology, 649
Integrations systems biology, 641
Integrative Model for Community Health
    Promotion, *262,* 262–63
Integumentary systems, 503
Interdependence mode, 223, *226*
Interdisciplinary teams, 72, 325. *See also*
    Collaborative partnerships
Intergenerational transmission, 597
Internal evaluators, of public health
    programs, 314
Internal management, 348–54
International Association of Bioethics, 365
International Bill of Human Rights, 362
International Code of Nursing Ethics, 367
International Conference on Healthy Cities and
    Communities, 327
International Conference on Primary Health
    Care, 362
International Covenant on Civil and Political
    Rights, 362
International Covenant on Economic, Social
    and Cultural Rights, 362
International Council of Nurses (ICN), *174,*
    371, 373, 650
International Debt Coalitions, 181
International Health Regulations, 432
International Monetary Fund (IMF), 177, 180
International SOS, *432*
International terrorism, 614. *See also*
    Terrorism
Internet, health education and, 292–93, *293.
    See also* Technology
Interpreters, *140,* 210, 564. *See also* Language
    barriers; Linguistic competence
Interventions
    costs of, 163–66, *310, 311*
    model, 40, *42,* 71–72
    preventive health care and, 160
    strategies for, *230*
Interviews, 229–31, 396–98, *439. See also*
    Focus groups; Media
IOM. *See* Institute of Medicine (IOM)
Ionizing radiation, 190
IPM (integrated pest management), 202, *203*
I Prepare assessment tool, *192*
Islamic ethics, *373*
Isolation, infectious diseases and, 6, 616

J

Jemmott, Loretta Sweet, *397*
Jenner, Edward, 6, 414
Jewish ethics, *372*

Johnson, S., *The One Minute Manager*, 350
Joint Committee on National Health Education
    Standards, 289
Jonsen, Albert, 371
Journaling, 350
Justice, 209, 368, *375*, 585. *See also* Social
    justice

K

Kaiser Family Foundation, 538
Kant, Immanuel, 366
Kantian Theories, 365–66
Kasenene, Peter, *374*
Kass, N. E., 379
Kellogg Foundation, 36
Kinetic energy, 223
Kingdon Model, 120
Knowledge, 41, 96. *See also* Education;
    Learning
Knowles, M. S., 283
Kohlberg, Lawrence, 370
Kolb's Learning Style Inventory, 284–85, *286*
Ku Klux Klan, 11
Kyoto Protocols, 207, 212

L

Labeling, 201, 206, *207*, 213
Labor, child, 11
Labor market, 166–68
Language barriers, 64, 67, 642. *See also*
    Linguistic competence; Translators
Latinos, *531, 558. See also* Demographic
    categories; Racial and ethnic health
    disparities
Laws, 45, 121–22, 124–26, 361. *See also*
    Legal authorities
Leadership roles
    defining, 347
    on health policies, 121, *123*, 128
    on health promotion, 328, 333–36
    management and, 343, 346–48
    multilevel approach to, 646–47
    in public health, 30, 44–45, 50, 333–36
    in rural areas, *521*
Lead exposure, 195, *195*, 197–99, *198, 205,*
    230, 268
Leading health indicators, 106–12, *345*
Learning. *See also* Education; Health education
    programs; Knowledge; Teaching
    assessments of, 284–86
    definition of, 282–83
    e-learning, 291–92
    peer, 652–53
    styles, 284–85, *286*
Leavell, H. R., *Preventive Medicine for the*
    Doctor in His Community, 413–14
Legal authorities, 6, 124–26. *See also* Laws
Legal responsibilities, 126–27

Legal rights, 361. *See also* Human rights
Legislative process, 121–22. *See also* Laws
Leprosy, 6
Liability laws, 124–25
Lice, head, *349*
Life expectancy, 28, 279
Life satisfaction, 159
Lifestyle, 446, 538–39, 576–77, 592, 640. *See*
    also Health behaviors
Linguistic competence, 544. *See also*
    Interpreters; Language barriers
Literacy
    computer, 292 (*See also* Technology)
    health, 289–90, *291*, 488, 544
Literature. *See* Publications
Litigation. *See* Legal authorities; Legal
    responsibilities; Malpractice; Negligence;
    Tort laws
Liver cancer, 97
Lobbyists, 123–24, 522, 524. *See also*
    Political activism
Local governments
    collaborative partnerships and, 37
    disaster preparedness and, 628
    environmental health and, 212–13
    on health education, 488
    health promotion and, 326–27
    public health and, 10, 31
Local public health agencies (LPHA), 31, *31,*
    60–61
Logic model, for program evaluation, 315,
    317–18
Longest's public policy, *123*
Long-term care facilities, 135, 143
Long-term objectives, 286
Los Angeles County Public Health Nursing
    Department, *17*, 72–73
Low birth weight, 481, 534–36, *535,*
    536, 595
LPHA (local public health agencies), *31,*
    31–32, 60–61
LST (Botvin's LifeSkills Training) Program,
    599, *600*
Lyme disease, 424–25, *425*

M

MADD (Mothers Against Drunk Driving),
    121–22
Mahler, Halfdan, 177–78
"Making a Difference: Research Affecting
    Practice," 396
Making Health Communication Programs
    Work, 264
Malaria, 87, 425–26
Malpractice, 125–27
Maltreatment, child. *See* Child abuse
    prevention
Mammography, *260*
Managed care organizations, *145*

Managed care plans, 138–39, 141, 142
Managed competition, 143–44
Management
    administration and, 346–48
    case, *65*, 352–53, 584
    of chronic illnesses, 448
    definition of, 343
    external, 354–55
    fiscal, 351–52
    health care, 343–56
    internal, 348–54
    keys to improvement, 355
    leadership and, 343, 346–48
    outcomes, 652
    performance, 647
    personnel, 350–51
    program, 353–54, 435–36
Mandates, government, 160
Manganese exposure, *196*
Man-made disasters, 611, *613*
Mann, Jonathan, 178, 363, 381–82
Maori people, *376*
Mapping, concept, 306
Marginal benefits, 155, 161, *161*
Marginalization, of immigrants, 557
Marijuana use, 593–94. *See also* Substance
    abuse
Marketing, social, 266–69, *270*
Marketing mix, 269
Massachusetts Health Insurance
    Company, 137
Massachusetts Medical Society, 144
Material Data Safety Sheets (MSDS), *192*, 213
Maternal health, 479–81, *480*, 489–90, *537*
McCarthyism (Joseph McCarthy), 18
McFarlane, J., *222, 229*
McKinney, Stewart B., 583
McKinney-Vento Homeless Assistance Act,
    577, 581, 583, 585. *See also* Stewart B.
    McKinney Homeless Assistance Act
Measles, 28
Media, 204–5, 436, *439*, 623
Medicaid
    community health centers and, 64
    establishment of, 135–36, 139
    funding of, *128*, 139–41
    home health care and, 70
    prenatal care under, *141*
    rural health care and, 65, 66, 514
Medical Ethics (Percival), 364
Medical expenses. *See* Costs, of health care
Medicalization of public health, 20–21
Medically underserved areas, 512
Medical savings accounts, 138
Medicare
    community health centers and, 64
    establishment of, 135–36, 139
    funding of, 141–43
    home health care and, 70
    homeless population and, 578

Medicare, *continued*
  preventive services and, 142, *161*
  rural health care and, 65, 66, 514, 522
Medicare Prescription Drug Improvement and
    Modernization Act, 142
Medication/medicine. *See* Drugs
Medigap policy, 142
Men, homeless, 578
Mental health
  cost of screening and treatment, *311*
  effects of disasters on, 624
  Healthy People 2010 on, 109
  of homeless population, 576
  immigration and, 558, 559, 562
  of older adults, 501
  overweight, obesity and, 487
  racial and ethnic health disparities and, 544
  in rural populations, 516, *523*
  substance abuse and, 504, 593, *601*
Mental health centers, 71
Mentoring, 44–47, 350
Mercury exposure, *195, 205*
Metabolic syndrome, 452–53
Methyl tertiary butyl ether (MTBE), 204
Metropolitan areas, 512
Metropolitan Life Insurance Company, 14,
    16–17
Mexico, 517–18, 554–55
Miasma theory, 3–4
Microbial threats, 407
Middle Ages, public health in, 3, 6
Middle-range nursing theories, 446
Midwifery, 514. *See also* Pregnancy
Migrant farmworkers, 516–18, *520*, 555, 560
Migrant health centers, 66–67, 136, 514
Migration patterns, global, 554–56. *See also*
    Immigration
Military. *See* Service personnel
Mill, John Stuart, "On Liberty," 269
Millennium Development Goals, 179
Mine Safety and Health Administration, 207
Minimization of costs, 155–57, 158–60,
    308–9
Minnesota Department of Health, 74
Minnesota Senior Health Options, *313*
Minnesota Wheel Intervention Model, 40, *42,*
    71–72
Minorities. *See* Cultural diversity; Demographic
    categories; Racial and ethnic health
    disparities; *specific minority groups*
Mission for Homeless Persons, *585*
Mission of public health, 29, 647
Mission statement clarification, 304–5, *305*
Mobilization. *See* Political activism
Models. *See also* Theories
  Agricultural Disability Awareness and Risk
    Education Model, *295*
  community assessment, 221–27
  ecological model of health, 29, *29*
  epidemiologic, 87–88, 222–23, 410

of health communication programs, 263–
    69, *264*
of health promotion, 255–63, *258, 259,*
    260, 262
Healthy Cities, 37, 325–28, *326,*
    329–30, 651
Host-Agent Reservoir Model, 87
of infectious disease transmission, 409–13
Minnesota Wheel Intervention Model, 40,
    42, 71–72
nurse-managed models of care, 524
Person-Place-Time Model, 87–88
PRECEDE-PROCEED Model, 266–69,
    267, 318
program logic, 315
Public Health Ethical Decision-Making
    Model, 379–80
Public Health Nurse Practice, 629–30
of public health nursing practice, 71–73
of public health program evaluation, 315,
    317–19
of public health system, 33, *35,* 35–37
of public policy, 120–21
Purnell Model, 235
school and health model program, 62
systems thinking, *643*
Transtheoretical Model of Behavioral
    Change, 259–60, *260, 295, 490*
Model State Emergency Health Power Act, 616
Modes of entry/exit, 411
Modifiable risk factors, 459–62, 545–46
Mold growth, 202
Monasteries, sanitation in, 3
Monitoring, on-going, 312
Monitoring the Future, 594
Montgomery Ward, 137
Moore, Mary Lou, *397*
Morality, 360, 361, 364, 366, 368–70. *See*
    also Beliefs; Ethics; Human rights; Values
Morals and Medicine (Fletcher), 364
Morbidity rates
  chronic illnesses and, 446, 448
  community assessments and, 229
  epidemiology and, 93
  racial and ethnic health disparities and,
    531–36, *535, 536*
Mortality rates. *See also* Death
  cardiovascular disease and, *458, 532*
  chronic illnesses and, 446, 448
  community assessments and, 229
  diabetes and, *532,* 533
  epidemiology and, 93
  health disparities and, 639
  racial and ethnic health disparities and,
    531–36, *535, 536*
Mothers Against Drunk Driving (MADD),
    121–22
Motivation, 159, 166–67, 256–63,
    283–86, *502*
Motor vehicle accidents, 481–83, 593

MSDS (Material Data Safety Sheets), *192,* 213
MTBE (methyl tertiary butyl ether), 204
Multidisciplinary teams. *See* Collaborative
    partnerships
Multidrug-resistant TB, 427–28, 517
Multinational corporations, 177–78
Multiple sclerosis, 466
Musculoskeletal system, aging and, 503
Muslim ethics, *373*
Myocardial infarction. *See* Cardiovascular
    disease

N

NACCHO (National Association of City and
    County Health Officials), 31, 32, *43,* 643
NACGN (National Association of Colored
    Graduate Nurses), 14, 19
National Adult Literacy Survey, 290
National Advisory Committee on Rural Health
    and Human Services, 514–15
National Agricultural Workers Survey, 67, 517
National Ambient Air Quality Standards,
    204, *205*
National Assessment of Adult Literacy, 290
National Association of Children's Hospitals
    and Related Institutions, 334
National Association of City and County
    Health Officials (NACCHO), 31, 32,
    43, 643
National Association of Clinical Nurse
    Specialists, 496
National Association of Colored Graduate
    Nurses (NACGN), 14, 19
National Association of Counties, 334
National Association of Directors of Nursing
    Administration in Long Term Care, 497
National Association of Nursing Alumnae,
    13, 14
National Association of School-Based Health
    Centers, 63
National Association of School Nurses, 489
National Black Nurses Association, 19
National Cancer Institute, 101, 263, *643*
National Center for Environmental Health,
    43, 212
National Center for Farmworker Health, 514
National Center for Health Statistics (NCHS),
    100, 532
National Center for Injury Prevention and
    Control, 109
National Cholesterol Educational Panel,
    452–53, 460
National Coalition for the Homeless (NCH),
    573, 575–76, 585–86
National Commission for the Protection of
    Human Subjects of Biomedical and
    Behavioral Research, 371
National Commission on Nurse-Midwifery
    Education, 514

National Conference of Gerontological Nurse Practitioners, 496–97
National Electronic Disease Surveillance System (NEDSS), 47–48, 625
National 5-A-Day for Better Health Program, 539
National Gerontological Nursing Association, 496–97
National Health and Nutrition Examination Survey, 100, 189–90, 451, 539
National Health Care for the Homeless Council, 576
National health insurance, 135, 146
National Health Interview Survey, 100
National Health Service Corps, 512, 514, 521
National Housing Trust Fund, 585
National Incident Management System, 628
National Institute for Occupational Safety and Health (NIOSH), 212, 518
National Institute of Environmental Health Sciences, 212
National Institute of Mental Health, 109
National Institute of Nursing Research, 124, 395–96, 396
National Institutes of Health, 212, 229, 333, 382, 395
National League of Nursing Education, 18
National Library of Medicine, 191, 193, 201, 208
National Nosocomial Infection Surveillance system, 426
National Nursing Centers Consortium, 68
National Oceanic Atmospheric Administration Weather Radio, 623
National Organization of Public Health Nurses (NOPHN), 13, 14, 18
National Priorities List, 206
National Public Health Leadership Development Network, 50
National Public Health Performance Standards Program (NPHPSP), 46, 47
National Response Plan, 627–28
National Rural Health Association, 521
National Rural Recruitment and Retention Network, 515
National Safety Council, 519
National Science and Technology Council Committee on Environment and Natural Resources, 623
National Smallpox Vaccination Program, 69
National Standards for Culturally and Linguistically Appropriate Health Services in Health Care, 544
National Survey on Drug Use and Health, 108
Nation's Health, The, 285
Native Americans, 31, 531. See also Demographic categories; Racial and ethnic health disparities

Native Hawaiians, 531. See also Demographic categories; Racial and ethnic health disparities
Natural disasters, 73, 611, 612
Natural immunity, 413
Nazis, medical ethics and, 360–62
NCEP (National Cholesterol Educational Panel), 452–53, 460
NCH (National Coalition for the Homeless), 573, 575–76, 585–86
NCHS (National Center for Health Statistics), 100, 532
NEDSS (National Electronic Disease Surveillance System), 47–48, 625
Needle exchange programs, 422, 429
Needleman, Herbert, 198
Needs
    assessing (See Needs assessments)
    individual versus societal, 360–61, 365, 366, 374–76
    parish, 229
Needs assessments
    in community, 181, 230, 231–32, 232, 233
    health communication and, 264
    health education and, 279–81, 284
    health promotion and, 328–36
    immigrant health and, 564
    public health programs and, 306–8
Negative externalities, 161–62
Negative valences, 256
Negligence, 125–27
Negotiation skills, 44
Neighborhood health centers. See Community health centers (CHC)
Neighborhood Health Councils, 231
Nerve agents, 621
Neuman, Betty, 221
Neural tube defects, 480, 481
Neurobehavioral functions, 198
Neurological system, aging and, 503
Neutral valences, 256
New Castle Healthy Cities, 329–30
News releases and conferences, 439. See also Media
New York City, 12, 58
New York State Nurses Association, 628
Nicotine & Tobacco Research, 285
Nightingale, Florence, 7, 8, 213, 255
Nineteenth Amendment, 12
NIOSH (National Institute for Occupational Safety and Health), 212, 518
Nitrous dioxide, 205
No Child Left Behind Act, 577
NOC (Nursing Outcomes Classification) scheme, 399–400, 649
Noise pollution, 203
Noncomparative justice, 368
Nongovernmental community agencies, 63–71
Nongovernmental-systematic agenda setting, 120

Noninsurance-based models of health care, 143–45
Nonionizing radiation, 190
Nonmaleficence, 366–67, 375
Nonmetropolitan areas, 512. See also Rural health care
Nonmodifiable risk factors, 459, 464
Nonparametric data, 294, 294
Non-point source pollutants, 204
Nontherapeutic antibiotics, 206
NOPHN (National Organization of Public Health Nurses), 13, 14, 18
Normative ethics, 364
Nosocomial infections, 426
Not-for-profit organizations, 157–59
"Not in My Back Yard" on homeless shelters, 584
NPHPSP (National Public Health Performance Standards Program), 46, 47
Nuclear/radiological weapons, 621
Nurse-Family Partnership, 331–32
Nurse Home Visiting Program, 486
Nurse-managed health centers
    community needs and, 347
    establishing, 63
    as practice setting, 67–68
    in rural areas, 516, 523, 524
Nurse-managed models of care, 524
Nurse Manager Academy, 350–51
Nurse Practice Act, 123, 124
Nurses. See also Shortages of nurses
    advanced practice nurses, 64, 68, 310, 650
    African American, 13–14, 19–20
    generalist public health nurses, 39–40, 44–47
    in hospitals versus public health, 13, 15–16, 126
    industrial nurses, 69
    nurse practitioners, 64, 68, 145
    occupational health nurses, 69–70, 70, 97
    public health nurse managers, 343–56
    registered nurses, 167
    school nurses, 16, 58–59, 61–63
    specialist public health nurses, 40, 43–47
    visiting nurses, 7–8, 58, 401
Nurses Settlement, 9, 58
Nursing. See also Public health nursing
    assessments, 241
    district, 8
    history of, 6, 15
    practice, regulation of, 123
    process, 304, 393–95
    professionalization of, 13, 19
    sensitivity, 649
    theories, 446
Nursing, Health and Environment, 213, 214–15
Nursing homes, 135, 143
Nursing Leadership Forum Training programs, 350

Nursing Outcomes Classification (NOC) scheme, 399–400, *649*
Nursing Research, 241
Nutrition, 486–88, 504, 539. *See also* Diet; Overweight and obesity
Nutritionists, 17

O

Oath of Asaph, 372
Obesity. *See* Overweight and obesity
Objectives
    of health education, 286–91, *288,* 293–95
    of Healthy People 2010, 105–13
    maximizing, 158–60
    organizational, 157–58
    of program evaluation, 312–13, 318–19
    of public health programs, 305, 306–7
OBRA (Omnibus Reconciliation Act), 126, 141
Occupational Health and Safety Act, 207
Occupational Health and Safety Administration (OSHA), 203, 207, 212
Occupational health nurses, 69–70, *70,* 97
Occupational health settings
    environmental health risks in, 193, 207–8
    hazards for health care workers in, 210
    health promotion in, *242, 247, 248, 271*
    health risk appraisals in, *243, 247, 248*
    immigration and, 560–61
    migrant farmworkers and, 518
    potential liabilities in, 126–27
    as practice setting, 68–70, *70*
    rural work settings as, 206, *295, 516, 519*
    screenings in, 422
    tobacco use in, *345*
    travel and health risks in, *432*
    unsafe working conditions in, 11
    vaccinations in, *427*
Odds ratios, 97. *See also* Health risk appraisals; Risk communication
Office of Juvenile Justice and Delinquency Prevention, 328, 332
Office of Rural Health Policy, 515, *521*
Older adults. *See also* Aging
    chronic illnesses and, 448–50
    culture and health of, 497
    demographics of, 496
    environmental health and, 204, 209
    family caregivers for, 498–99
    health assessments of, 499–504
    health education and, 292
    health insurance for, 141–43
    health promotion and, *259,* 504–7, *505–6*
    health research on, *502*
    homelessness among, 578–79, *580*
    public health programs and, *313*
    rural nursing program for, 312–19
    substance abuse and, 504, 593, *601*
    transitional care for, *310*

Older Americans Act Amendments of 2000, *316*
Omaha System, 400–401
Omnibus Reconciliation Act (OBRA), 126, 141
One Minute Manager, The (Blanchard and Johnson), 350
On-going monitoring, 312
"On Liberty" (Mill), 269
On-Time, On-Target Manager, The (Blanchard and Gottry), 350
Opportunities. *See* SWOT analysis
Opportunity costs, 154, 155, 463–65
Oregon, bioterrorism in, *436, 622*
Oregon Healthy Start, *331*
Organic farming, 206, *207*
Organizational and systems capacity, 50
Organizational behavior and objectives, 57–58
Organizations, public health, 346–54
Orientation, future, 355–56
OSHA (Occupational Health and Safety Administration), 203, 207, 212
Osteoporosis, 503
Ottawa Charter for Health Promotion, 119, 255, 362
Outcome and Assessment Information Set, 126
Outcomes
    community-level, *649*
    evaluation of, 293–95, *294*
    expectancies, 257, 261
    home visiting and, *537*
    identification, 306, 629
    management, 652
    racial and ethnic health disparities and, 536–37
    research and, 399–401
Outputs, of public health programs, 313
Overweight and obesity
    cardiovascular disease and, 452, 460, 487
    in children and adolescents, 450–51, 486–88
    chronic illnesses and, 450–56, 486–87
    health promotion and, *271*
    Healthy People 2010 on, 107
    prevalence of, *451*
    racial and ethnic health disparities and, 539
Ozone, *205*

P

Pacific Islanders, *531. See also* Demographic categories; Racial and ethnic health disparities
Pacifism, 11
Pan American Health Organization, 326
Pandemics. *See also* Epidemics
    HIV/AIDS, 380–82, 429
    influenza, 50, 428, 436, *437*
Parametric data, 294, *294*
Parasitic diseases, 426

Parents as Teachers, 335
Parish nursing program, *229. See also* Religious orders
Participatory action research, 37, *39,* 541, 544, *642*
Participatory development, 326
Particulate matter, *205*
Partnerships, public health. *See* Collaborative partnerships
Passive immunity, 413
Paternalism, 367–68
Pathogenesis, 410, *410, 415*
Pathogenicity, 411
Pathogenic organisms, 190, 206, 407, 422–23, 427–28. *See also* Infectious diseases
Patient Self-Determination Act, 126
PCA (Prevent Child Abuse) America, 332–36
PCB exposure, *196*
Pedagogy, 283
Peer learning, 652–53
Pender's Health Promotion Model, 227, *228, 243, 257, 258, 259*
Penicillin, 430
People's Health Assembly, 177
People's Health Charter, 177, 179
People's Health Movement (PHM), 178, 181
Perceptions, 221–22, 229, 256–63, 264. *See also* Perspectives
PERC exposure, *197*
Percival, Thomas, *Medical Ethics,* 364
Performance management, 647
Performance measures, 647
Performance standards, 647
Perinatal health disparities, 534–36, 557–58, 592–93, 595
Periodic assessments, 312
Persistence of pollutants, 190
Persistent, bioaccumulative, and toxic chemicals, 204
Persistent Organic Pollutants Treaty, 212
Personal development, 349–50, 646
Personal Responsibility and Work Opportunities Act, 140, 563
Personnel management, 350–51. *See also* Management
Person-Place-Time Model, 87–88
Person-to-person transmission, 412
Perspectives, 175, 313–14, 646–47. *See also* Perceptions
Pesticides, 189–90, *192,* 194, 201–2, 204–8
Petition for rulemaking, 122
Pew Internet and American Life Project, 292
Pharmaceuticals, testing standards for, 211
Philanthropists, 7–8, 10, *15,* 58–59
PHM (People's Health Movement), 178, 181
PHS (Public Health Service). *See* U.S. Public Health Service
Physical activity
    cardiovascular disease and, 462
    Healthy People 2010 on, 107, 539

HIV and, *106*
older adults and, 503, 504
overweight, obesity and, 487–88
promoting, *490*
racial and ethnic health disparities and, 539
women and, *463*
Physical hazards, 208
Physical mode, 223, *224*
Physicians for Social Responsibility, 210
Physiological changes, aging and, 501–4
PKU (phenylketonuria) screening, 382–83
Plague, bubonic, 6
Planning
disaster preparedness and, 629
futures thinking and, 644
public health programs, 304–8, *305*
Plato, 370
Pneumococcal diseases vaccines, 110, 112, 504
Pneumonia, 428
Point source pollutants, 203–4
Policies. *See also* Health policies
on aging, *316*
on chemical exposures, 212
on genetic research, 643
on homelessness, 574–76, 577–86
immigration, 555–56
Medigap, 142
on racial and ethnic health disparities, 539–41, *540*
Policy development core function, 30, 44–45, 647
Policy streams, 120
Polio epidemics, *15*, 28
Political activism
environmental health and, 209–10
global health and, 176–81
health policies and, 119–21
on homelessness, 583
on immigration issues, *175*
nurses and, 121–26, *125*, 127–28, 643
nursing shortages and, *174*
of rural public health nurses, 522, 524
understanding of, *175*
women and, 12
Political streams, 120
Polling, 644
Pollution, 189–216, *192*. *See also* *environment-related entries*
Population. *See also* Target populations; Vulnerable populations
assessments, 221, *227*, 537, 541, 543 (*See also* Community assessments)
epidemiological data and, 94–96
health, 263–69
movement of, 554–55 (*See also* Immigration)
school-aged, 599–600, *600* (*See also* Adolescents; Children; Young adults)
segmentation of, 267

Population-focused service delivery
chronic illnesses and, 467
core competencies and, 42
Intervention Wheel and, 71–72
LPHA and, 32
maternal-child health and, 490
nurse-managed health centers and, 68
program management and, 353–54
public health nursing and, 40
Positive externalities, 160–61, *161*
Positive health behaviors, 159–60, 241–49. *See also* Health behaviors
Positive valences, 256
Postpartum depression, 480–81
Postpartum Depression Checklist, 480
Posttraumatic stress disorders, 561–62, 581–82, 624
Potential energy, 223
Poverty
health and, 10, 378, 560–61, *586*
homelessness and, 573–74, 578, 579–80, 582, *586*
sanitation and, 4
theories on, 6, 7
Power level analyses, 99
Practical normative ethics, 364
Practice settings
examples of, *59, 61–63, 65, 67, 73*
in government agencies, 59–63
history of, 58–59
legal responsibilities in, 126–27
in nongovernmental community agencies, 63–71
Practice standards, 40–42. *See also Scope and Standards entries*
Preapprovals, insurance, 137
Precautionary Principle, 211
PRECEDE-PROCEED Model, 266–69, *267*, 318
Preferences, 154–55
Preferred provider organizations, 139
Pregnancy, 108, 479–81, *480, 484,* 484–86. *See also* Midwifery; Perinatal health disparities; Prenatal care
Premature aging, 578
Premiums, insurance, 137–38, 142, 144, 163
Prenatal care
demographic categories and, 479–81
environmental exposures and, 208
health education and, *287*
at Henry Street Settlement, 135
maternal health and, 479–80, *480*
in Medicaid managed care programs, *141*
substance abuse and, 592–93, 595
Prepathogenesis, 410, *410, 415*
Prescription drugs. *See* Drugs
Pre-start up planning, 304–6
Prevalence rates, 92, *287*
Preventable deaths, 592, 594
Prevent Child Abuse (PCA) America, 332–36

Preventive health care
acute care *versus*, 59
chronic illnesses and, 446
cost-effectiveness of, 309–12, *310*
disaster preparedness and, 625
disease prevention and, 58–59, 640
disease surveillance as, 32
focus on, 16
health risk appraisals as, 241–49
immunizations as, 32, 414
individual investment in, 159–60
infectious diseases and, 413–15, *415*, 422–23, *425*
lack of insurance and, *136*
life expectancy and, 28
Medicare and, 142, *161*
nurse-managed health centers and, 67–68
older adults and, 504–7
racial and ethnic health disparities and, 545–46
substance abuse and, 344, *345, 597,* 599–600
value of, 11, 344, *344*
Preventive Medicine for the Doctor in His Community (Leavell and Clark), 413–14
Primary care centers, 64, 65
Primary care providers, 139
Primary care services, 67–68
Primary health care, definition of, 64
Primary prevention, 414–15, 422, 545
Principles. *See* Beliefs; Ethics; Morality; Values
Principles for Environmental Health Nursing Practice, 213
Principles of the Ethical Practice of Public Health, 377, *377*
Principles on Public Health and Human Rights, 363, *363*
Prisons. *See* Correctional facilities
Private insurance, 136–39. *See also* Health insurance
Privatization of health care, 177–78
Problem identification, 305, *305*
Problem solving, 394–95, 651
Problem streams, 120
Procedural rules, 369–70
Process evaluation, 265, 293. *See also* Evaluation process
Professional development, 349–50
Professionalization of nursing, 13, 19
Professional leadership, 646
Proficiency, definition of, 41
Profits, 155–57, 159
Program development, 304–19
definition of, 304
economic analyses of, 308–12
evaluation, 307, 312–19, *313, 315*
on homelessness, 577–86
planning and, 304–8, *305*
target populations of, 305, 306–8, 319
Program Evaluation Review Technique, 353

Program logic model, 315
Program management, 353–54, 435–36
Project Public Health Ready, 50
Promoting Health/Preventing Disease: Objectives for the Nation, 105, 255
Prospective cohort design, 97
Prospective payment system, 137
Protease inhibitors, 429
Protective clothing, 422
Proteomics, 641
Protestant ethics, *372*
Protocol for Assessing Community Excellence in Environmental Health, *43*
Psychological health, 254. *See also* Mental health
Psychological theories of aging, 497, *498*
Psychomotor domain, 283, 286, *288, 294*
Psychosocial issues, 487. *See also* Mental health
Publications
    on environmental health, 642
    on living with chronic illnesses, 446, *447–48*
    on racial and ethnic health disparities, 539–41, *540*
Public engagement, *43,* 354. *See also* Participatory action research
Public health. *See also other public health-related entries*
    achievements in, *28,* 279
    definition of, 3, 29, 360
    history of, 3–7, *4, 5*
    infrastructure of, 47–50, 73, 212–13, 345–46
    mission of, 29, 647
    preparedness, 628–30 (*See also* Disaster preparedness; Emergency preparedness)
    programs (*See* Program development)
    systems, 33, *35,* 35–37, 46, 646–47
Public Health Code of Ethics Committee, 377
Public Health Data Standards Consortium, 47
Public Health Ethical Decision-Making Model, 379–80
Public Health Functions Steering Committee, 32, *33,* 346
Public Health in America, 32–33, *34*
Public Health Information Network, 625
Public Health Interventions: Application for Public Health Nursing Practice, 74
Public Health Leadership Society, 377
Public Health Nurse Practice Model, 629–30
Public health nursing. *See also* Nurses; Nursing
    definition of, 40
    demographic categories of, 650
    expansion of, 176
    future of, 639–53
    guiding principles for, *392*
    history of, 6, 7–22
    models of practice, 71–73, 629–30
    tenets of, 40, *40, 41,* 127
    tools of, 11

Public Health Nursing Competencies, 21. *See also* Competencies
Public Health Nursing Scope and Standards. See also Scope and Standards entries
    on advocacy, 127
    on ethics, 373, 377
    on focus of public health nursing, *20,* 21, 59, 344
    on public health nursing competencies, 39
Public health organizations, 346–47, 348–54
Public Health Response Team, *48*
Public Health Security and Bioterrorism Preparedness and Response Act (PL 107–188), *46*
Public Health Service Act, 64
Public Health Training Center Network, 41
Public insurance, 136, 139–43. *See also* Health insurance; Medicaid; Medicare
Public policies, 119, 120–21, 354. *See also* Health policies; Policies
Public sector. *See* Governments
Pulmonary system, aging and, 502
Purnell Model, 235

Q

Quad Council of Public Health Nursing Organization
    on advocacy, 127–28
    on educational requirements, 74
    establishment of, 20
    on ethics, 373
    on management, 344
    on public health nursing competencies, 39, 41, 392, 648
Qualitative research design, 396–98, *398*
Quality adjusted life year (QALY), 165–66, 309
Quality assurance, 393–95
Quality improvements, in public health nursing, 647
Quality of life, *106*
Quantitative research design, 398–99, *400*
Quarantines, 616
Quasi-experimental research designs, 399
Questionnaires, community assessment, 229
Quinlan, Karen Ann, 364

R

Race, 107–12, *113,* 531, *531*
Racial and Ethnic Approaches to Community Health 2010 Risk Factor Survey, 539, *545, 642*
Racial and ethnic health disparities, 530–46
    definition of, 530–31
    factors influencing, 536–39
    immigration and, 556, 557–58
    morbidity and mortality trends in, 531–36, *535, 536*
    policies, reports and publications on, 539–41, *540*

    strategies to reduce, 541–46, *542, 545*
    tobacco use and, 538, 595–96
    trends in, 639
Racism, 10, 13–14, 559
Radiological Dispersal Device, 621
Radiological exposures, 190, 208
Radiological/nuclear weapons, 621
Radon, *191,* 193, 199–200, *482*
Rajneeshees (followers of Bhagwan Shree Rajneesh), *436, 622*
RAND, 328
Random House Dictionary of the English Language, 343
Randomization, in epidemiological studies, 96
Randomized clinical trials, 98–99
Randomized control trials, 395
Random samples, 89
Rapid Estimate of Adult Literacy in Medicine, 290
Rates, epidemiological, 91–96, 287. *See also* Morbidity rates; Mortality rates
Rathbone, William, 8
Readiness, learner, 285–86
Reading levels, assessment of, 290
Reasoning, economic, 155–68
Recharge in Minutes (Zoglio), 350
Recreational water, safety of, 203–4
Recruitment strategies, 49, 66, 74, 521–22, 650
Red Cross, 14, 16–17, 412, 513, 611
Refugee Protection Act, 555
Refugees, 555–56, 561–62. *See also* Immigration
Registered nurses, *167*
Registered Nurses Association of Ontario, *401*
Registration, Evaluation, and Authorization of Chemicals program, 212
Regulations, public health, 45, 123
Regulators, 223
Regulatory process, 122–24, 212–13. *See also* Environmental Protection Agency
Reisch, Michael, 11, 21
Relational autonomy, 366
Relative risk, 98
Relief workers, 624
Religion, ethics and, 364, *372–73*
Religious orders, 6, 10, 135. *See also* Faith-based organizations
Ren-Zong Qui, *375*
"Report into the Sanitary Conditions of the Labouring Population of Great Britain" (Chadwick), 7
Reports. *See* Publications
Reproductive system, aging and, 503
REPROTOX, 208
Rescue workers, 624
Research
    databases on, *401*
    dissemination, 653
    evidence-based practice and, 401

future of public health nursing and, 651–53
on living with chronic illnesses, 446,
    447–48
on older adults, *502*
outcomes, 399–401
participatory action, 37, *39*, 541, 544, *642*
priorities, 395–96
problem solving and, 394–95
prominent figures in, 391–92, *397*
public health and, 46–47, 391–401
in rural health care, *522*, *524*
types of studies, 396–99
Reservation wages, 166
Reservoirs of agents, 411
Residual stimuli, 223
Resilience, 559
Resolutions, of public health associations, 643
Resource allocation
    capacity building and, 651
    chronic diseases and, 464–65
    disaster relief and, 625
    economic analyses and, 154, 164–65, 312
    efficiency and, 156–57
    ethics and, 367, 368
Respect, *20, 21,* 289. *See also* Cultural
    diversity
Respiratory infections, 426–28. *See also*
    Asthma; Influenza; Tuberculosis (TB)
Responsible sexual behavior, 108–9, 539. *See*
    also Contraception; Sexual activity
Results, defining, 647. *See also* Outcomes
Retention strategies, *49,* 521–22, 650
Retrospective cohort design, 97
Retrospective payment system, 137
Return on investment, of preventive health
    care, 159–60
Revenues *versus* costs, 158. *See also other cost-*
    related entries
Reverby, Susan, 12, 19, 21
Rewards of public health nursing, 75
Risk communication, 210–11, 435, *438*
Risk factors. *See also* Health risk appraisals
    assessing, *192,* 192–94
    for cardiovascular disease, *243,*
        459–62, *464*
    categories of, *242*
    child health and, 481–83
    contextual, for chronic illnesses, 462–65
    geography, environment and, 348, *348*
    homelessness and, 576–83
    identification of, 222, 306
    incidence rates and, 92
    modifiable, 459–62, 545–46
    of pregnancy, 479–81, *480*
    relative, 98
Risk markers, *456*
RNPMHU (Rural Nurse Practitioner Mobile
    Health Unit), 312–19
Robbins, L., 241
Robert Wood Johnson Foundation, 36, 327

Robinson, Mary, 8
Rocky Mountain spotted fever, 425
Rogers, Lina, 61
Role function mode, 223, *225*
Role-performance health, 254
Roman Catholic ethics, *372*
Romans, sanitation and, 3
Ronald McDonald House Charities, 332
Roosevelt, Eleanor, 178
Roosevelt, Franklin D., 135
Rosen, G., *History of Public Health,* 3–4
Rothman, N. L., *397*
Roy's Adaptation Model, 223, *224–26*
Rules, 122, 366, 368–70
Rural, definition of, 512–13
Rural health care
    access to adequate, 512–13
    American Red Cross and, 14
    federal initiatives in, 514–15, *515*
    health policies and, 522, 524
    history of, 513–15, *514*
    nurse-managed clinics and, *523*
    for older adults, 312–19
    public health nursing and, 518–22, *520,*
        521, 640
    radon exposure and, *482*
    research in, *522, 524*
    rural populations and, 515–16, *517*
    technology and, 519, 640
Rural health clinics, 65–66, *66,* 514
Rural Health Clinic Services Act, 65,
    512–13, 514
Rural Healthy People, A Companion Document
    to Healthy People 2010, 512
Rural Information Center Health Service, 515
Rural Nurse Practitioner Mobile Health Unit
    (RNPMHU), 312–19
Rural Nursing Service, 513
Rural Voices Program, *521*

S

Safe Drinking Water Act, 200, 212
Safety. *See also* Risk factors; Violence and
    injuries
    child health and, 481–82
    environment and, 325
    homelessness and, 579
    in occupational health settings, 11
    older adults and, 500
    of water, 200, *200,* 203–4
Safety net providers, 67–68
Salaries, 75, 166–68
Salmonellosis, 424, *436, 622*
Samples, convenience/random, 89
Sanitation, 3, 7, 8
SARS (severe acute respiratory syndrome), 28,
    73, 431–32
Scarcity of resources, 154. *See also* Resource
    allocation

Scenario development, 644–46, *645*
Schiff, Jacob, 10
Schneider and Ingram Model, 120
School-aged populations, 599–600, *600. See*
    also Adolescents; Children; Young adults
School and health model program, 62
School-based health centers, 62, *127*
"School-Based Health Centers: A Blue Print for
    Health Learners," 63
School community. *See also* Education
    diabetes education in, *454*
    environmental health in, 201–3
    head lice in, *349*
    health education in, 61–63, 488–89
    liability issues in, 127
    locations of, 202–3
    nurses in, 16, 58–59, 61–63
    nutrition in, 487–88
    physical activity in, 487–88
    practice settings in, 61–63, *62*
    standards of health within, 45
    substance abuse prevention in, 599–600
    vaccinations and, 160, 413
School Health Policies and Programs
    Study, 488
Schoor, Lizbeth, 332
Scope and Standards of Gerontological Nursing
    Practice, 497
Scope and Standards of Nursing, 20, 255. *See*
    also Public Health Nursing Scope and
    Standards
Screenings, health
    for acanthosis nigricans, 454–56
    blood pressure, 70, 462
    for cholesterol, 90
    for chronic inflammatory states, 456
    for diabetes, 90, 452, 453, *454*
    epidemiology and, 89–91
    genetic, *381,* 382–83
    homeless population and, *575*
    for hypercholesterolemia, 90
    immigration and, 556, 563
    for infectious diseases, 422
    for insulin resistance, 453–54
    for metabolic syndrome, 452–53
    older adults and, 504, *505–6*
    racial and ethnic health disparities and,
        543–44, *545*
    for substance abuse, 596–97
Secondary data, 229
Secondary prevention, 422–23, 545–46
Secondhand smoke exposure, *196,* 595
Segmentation of population, 267
Self-determination, 269–71, 283–84, 366
Self-efficacy, 257, 260, 261, 263
Senge, P.M., *The Fifth Discipline,* 347
Senior centers, 71
Senior citizens. *See* Older adults
Seniors ALIVE program, *259*
Sensitivity of screening, 90

Sensitivity ratios, *649*

Separation, of immigrants, 557

Service-learning experiences, 522

Service personnel, 31, 143, 241. *See also* Veterans

Severe acute respiratory syndrome (SARS), 28, 73, 431–32

Sexual activity
  of adolescents, *484,* 484–86, *558*
  of homeless population, 577
  older adults and, 503, 504
  responsibility and, 108–9, 539

Sexually transmitted diseases (STDs), 108, 485, 539, 577

Sexually transmitted infections, 429–31

Sexual orientation, 576–77

Sexual violence, 562, 577

Shellman, J., *222*

Sheppard-Towner Act, 12, 135

Shortages of nurses
  auxiliary workers and, 17
  effect in public health sector, 48–50, 650
  funding and, 73
  global, 174, *174*
  immigration and, *561*
  recruitment strategies and, 49, 66, 74, 521–22, 650
  retention strategies and, *49,* 521–22, 650
  rural health care and, 640
  surveys on, *167*

Short-term objectives, 286

Sickle cell diseases, *381,* 382

Simulations, 645

Single payer system of health care, 144–45

Skills, 44, 343, 392, *393–94,* 646. *See also* Competencies

Sleep apnea, 487

Sliding fee scales, 64, 158

Smallpox
  as infectious disease, 408, 616, *620,* 620–21
  vaccinations for, *59, 69*

Smell, sense of, 504

Smith, Carol E., *397*

SMOG Readability Formula, 290

Smoking. *See* Tobacco use

Snow, John, 4, 87

SNS (Strategic National Stockpile), *46, 626–27*

Social Cognitive Theory, 261

Social construction, 120

Social Darwinism, 7, 361

Social duties, 367

Social ecological model of health promotion, 325. *See also* Healthy Cities Model for Health Promotion

Social health, 254

Social insurance, 135

Social justice, 3, 21–22, 177, 378. *See also* Justice

Social learning model of health promotion, 325

Social marketing, 266–69, *270*

Social medicine, 135

Social practices, human rights and, 361

Social reforms, 11–13, 18, 21–22. *See also* Civil rights; Suffrage

Social Security, 578

Social Security Act, 139

Social support
  for caregivers, *307*
  HIV and, *106*
  homelessness and, 581–82
  immigrant health and, 559–60, *560*
  of older adults, 500–501

Social workers, 17, 21

Societal *versus* individual needs, 360–61, 365, 366, *374–76*

Society for Public Health Education, 279

Society of Medical Interpreters, 564

Society of Prospective Medicine, 244, *245*

Socioeconomic level, 463–65, 639. *See also* Poverty

Socioenvironmental conditions, 556. *See also environment-related entries*

Sociological theories of aging, 497, *498*

Soil contamination, 204, 206

Solvents exposure, *197*

Somatization, 562

Specialist public health nurses, 40, 43–47

Specialization of health care, 16, 18, 20–21

Special Outreach and Benefits Assistance, 582

Specificity of screening, 90

Spencer, Herbert, 361

Spider Web Pamphlet, 12

Spiritual health, 254

Spousal impoverishment, 143

SSI (Supplemental Security Income), 140, *483*

Stabilizers, 223

Stakeholders, *305,* 305–8, 313–15, 317

Standardized information and data, 48

Standard population, 94–96

Standards of acceptability, 318

State Child Health Plan, 140

State Children's Health Insurance Program, 162–63

State governments
  on chronic illness programs, *450*
  collaborative partnerships and, *36,* 37
  disaster preparedness and, 628
  environmental health and, 212–13
  environmental justice and, 209
  funding for public health nurses, 145
  on health education, 488
  health promotion programs and, 334
  on immigrant health care, 563
  Medicaid funding from, 140–41
  practice settings in, 60–61
  public health core responsibilities of, 31

"Statement on Smallpox Vaccination and Emergency Preparedness," *69*

Staupers, Mabel, 19

STD (sexually transmitted diseases), 108, 485, 539, 577

Stereotypes, 380, 499, *500*

Stewart B. McKinney Homeless Assistance Act, 573. *See also* McKinney-Vento Homeless Assistance Act

Stimuli, 223

Stockholm Convention, 205, 212

Strategic National Stockpile (SNS), *46,* 626–27

Strengths. *See* SWOT analysis

Stress, 516, 557, 558–59, 624. *See also* Hypertension

Strokes, *307, 532. See also* Cardiovascular disease

Structural Model of Health Behavior, 262–63

Stuart, Peggy, *580*

Substance abuse, 592–601
  adolescent health and, 483
  alcohol use and, 592–93
  case study of, *601*
  Healthy People 2010 on, 108, 539, 592, 594, 595
  homelessness and, 577
  marijuana use and, 593–94
  maternal-child health and, 480
  in older adults, 504, 593, *601*
  populations at risk for, 597–600
  prevention, 595, *597,* 599–600, *600*
  racial and ethnic health disparities and, 538–39
  tobacco use and, 594–97 (*See also* Tobacco use)

Substance Abuse and Mental Health Services Administration, 332

Substantive rules, 369

Suffrage, *11,* 11–12, 14

Sulfur dioxide, *205*

Summative evaluations, 318

Superfund sites, 206

Supplemental Security Income (SSI), 140, *483*

Supply and demand, 154, *154, 161*

Supportive Housing for Persons with Disabilities, 585

Support services, 351. *See also* Social support

Surveillance, disease, 32, 99–101, 435, 625–26

Surveillance, Epidemiology, and End Results, 101

Surveillance data, 99–101, 625

Surveys
  Behavioral Risk Factor Surveillance Survey, 100–101
  community assessments and, 227, 229
  National Adult Literacy Survey, 290
  National Agricultural Workers Survey, 67, 517
  National Health and Nutrition Examination Survey, 100, 189–90, 451, 539
  National Health Interview Survey, 100
  National Survey on Drug Use and Health, 108

Racial and Ethnic Approaches to Community Health 2010 Risk Factor Survey, 539, *545*, *642*
on shortages of nurses, *167*
Youth Risk Behavior Survey, *63*, 89, 96
Survival sex, 577
Sustainability, of community-based programs, 332
SWOT (strengths, weaknesses, opportunities and threats) analysis, *305*, 305–6
Syphilis, 6, 430
Systemic agenda items, 120–21
Systems capacity, 48–50
Systems planning perspectives, 646–47
Systems thinking, *643*

T

TANF (Temporary Assistance to Needy Families), 140, *483*
Tangwa, Godfrey, *374–75*
Tapu, laws of, *376*
Target populations
health communication and, 264–69
of health education, 279–82, 284–95, 291
health risk appraisals and, 244–46
of needs assessments, 231
of public health programs, 305, 306–8, 319
of research, 396–97
TARU (Technical Advisory Response Unit), 626–27
Task Force on Community Preventive Services, 653
Taste, sense of, 504
Tax Equity and Fiscal Responsibility Act (TEFRA), 137, 142
Taxes, 161–62
Taxonomy of Educational Objectives, 283, *288*
TB. *See* Tuberculosis (TB)
Teaching, 283. *See also* Education; Health education programs; Learning; School community
Team building skills, 44. *See also* Collaborative partnerships
Team leadership, 646
Technical Advisory Response Unit (TARU), 626–27
Technical efficiency, 156–57
Technological disasters, 611, *613*. *See also* Cyber-terrorism
Technology. *See also* Cyber-terrorism
disease management and, 448
health education and, 284, 291–93, *293*
health risk appraisals and, 244
information, 648–49
medical advancements through, 639
medical ethics and, 364
rural health care and, 519, 640
Teenagers. *See* Adolescents; Young adults

TEFRA (Tax Equity and Fiscal Responsibility Act), 137, 142
Telephone interviews, 229–30
Tempels, Placied, *Bantu Philosophy*, *374*
Temperature, sensitivity to, 504
Temporary Assistance to Needy Families (TANF), 140, *483*
Tenement housing, 7, 9, *9*
Terminology, educational, 287, *288*
Terrorism, 73, 611–14, *614–15*. *See also* Bioterrorism; Disaster preparedness; Emergency preparedness
Tertiary prevention, 423, 545–46
Testicular cancer, *246*
Tetrachloroethylene exposure, *197*
Theories. *See also* Models
of aging, 497, *498*
Ajzen's Theory of Planned Behavior, 257–58
Diffusion of Innovations Theory, 319
disease theories, 4, 7
of ethics, 365–66, 370–71
germ theory, 7–8
Helvie's Energy Theory, 223, 227
miasma theory, 3–4
middle-range nursing theories, 446
on poverty, 6, 7
Theory of Planned Behavior, 257–58
Theory of Uncertainty, 446
value-expectancy theories, 256, 286
Thinking
critical, 393–95
futures, 644–46, *645*
systems, *643*
Third party payer, 137–43, *145*
Threats, health, 348, *348*, *349*, 407. *See also* Bioterrorism; SWOT analysis
Time, value of, 164, 167
Timelines, on public health, 4, 5
Title V (homelessness federal task force), 583
Tobacco Control Program, 261
Tobacco use
cardiovascular disease and, 459–60
community assessments and, *226*
exposure to smoke, *196*, 595
health education and, *285*
health promotion and, 261, *262*
Healthy People 2010 on, 107–8
as negative externality, 161–62
preventive health care and, 344, *345*, 597
racial and ethnic health disparities and, 538, 595–96
strategies to control, *643*
substance abuse and, 594–97
Tort laws, 124–25
Torture, 562
Toulmin, Stephen, 371
Town and Country Nursing Service, 513
Toxicity, 192
Toxicogenomics, 641

Toxicology, 193
Toxic Release Inventory, 213
Toxic Shock Syndrome, 92
Toxins, biological, 616
ToxNet Program, 191
Transitional care, *310*
Translational research, 653
Translators, *140*, 210, 564. *See also* Language barriers; Linguistic competence
Transmission
of infectious diseases, 409–13, *411*, *412*
intergenerational, 597
Transnationalism, 554
Transtheoretical Model of Behavioral Change, 259–60, *260*, *295*, 490
Travel, and infectious diseases, 413, 431–32, *432*
Treating Tobacco Use and Dependence Clinical Practice Guideline, *596*, 596–97
Treatment Improvement Protocols, 319
Treatments, 181, 395, 422, 423, 596–97
Treaty of Waitanga, *376*
Trends, public health, 639–43, 650
Triadic reciprocal determinism, 261
Tri Care, 143
Triglycerides, 460
Trust, 519, 579
Tuberculosis (TB)
funding for, 50
as infectious disease, 426–28
in vulnerable populations, 222–23, 517, 561, *575*
Turning Point, *36*, 36–37, *38*, 647
Tuskegee study, *374*
Type 2 diabetes, 451–53, *454*, 456–57, 487, 533

U

UDHR (Universal Declaration of Human Rights), 178–79, 362, 365, 556
Uncertainty, 154–55, 159, 162–63, 446
Underground storage tanks, 204
Unequal Treatment: Confronting Racial and Ethnic Disparities in Healthcare, *374*, 539–41
UNICEF (United Nations Children's Fund), 176–77, 179
Uninsured people, 138, 140, 162–63, 515–17, 521. *See also* Health insurance
Unintentional injuries, 481–83, 504, 506–7. *See also* Violence and injuries
Unionization of nurses, 19
United Nations
Commission on the Status of Women, 178
Covenant on Civil and Political Rights, 179
Covenant on Economic, Social, and Cultural Rights, 179
on global health, 179, 180
on global migration patterns, 554

United Nations, *continued*
on human rights, 178, 362, 556
on human trafficking, 562
Programme on HIV/AIDS, 380
on refugees, 555
on toxic chemicals, 205
United States. *See also main entries for each
subject below*
access to health care in, 135–46
adolescent pregnancy in, 484
aging policies in, *316*
aging population in, 448–50
cardiovascular disease in, *457,* 457–62, *458*
causes of death in, *449*
chemical policies of, 211
chronic illnesses in, 463–65, 466–67
data on health in, 189
demographics of population in,
530, *530*
disaster preparedness in, 625
financing health care in, 136–45
on global health, 179–80
on global warming, 207
health insurance in, 137–43
Healthy Cities models in, 327 (*See also*
Healthy Families America; Healthy
Families Indiana)
high blood pressure in, *461,* 461–62
HIV/AIDS in, 408–9
homelessness in, 573–86
immigrants in, 10, 554–65
leadership in, 347
literacy in, 290
medical ethics in, 364
migrant farmworkers in, 517
obesity in, 450–56, *451*
prenatal care in, 479
public health nursing in, 7–8, 174
terrorism in, *436,* 612, 614, *622*
United States-Mexico Border Health
Commission, 555
Universal coverage, 144–45
Universal Declaration of Human Rights
(UDHR), 178–79, 362, 365, 556
University of Iowa, 399
Urgent Relief for the Homeless Act,
577, 583
Urinary system, aging and, 503
U.S. Bill of Rights, 362
U.S. Census Bureau
on community assessments, 229
on definition of rural, 512
on epidemiologic data, 100
on immigration, 554
on older adults, 496
on racial/ethnic definitions, *531*
on U.S. demographics, 530
U.S. Constitution, 12, 123, 361, 362
U.S. Declaration of Independence, 362
U.S. Department of Agriculture, 212

U.S. Department of Energy, 212, 382
U.S. Department of Health and Human
Services (HHS). *See also* Healthy People
2010
on best practices, 653
on disaster preparedness, 627
on environmental health, 212
on health disparities, 532, 541
on health literacy, 289
on health promotion, 327
on homelessness, 583–84
Public Health Service and, 60
U.S. Department of Homeland Security,
433–34, 614
U.S. Department of Transportation, 212
U.S. Department of Veterans Affairs, 581, 582
U.S. Food and Drug Administration
(FDA), 212
U.S. Geological Survey, 204
U.S. Joint Committee on Health Education
Terminology, 279
U.S. Nuclear Regulatory Commission, 621
U.S. Office of Management and Budget,
512, 531
U.S. Office of Refugee Resettlement, 554
U.S. Office of the Assistant Secretary for
Health Panel on Cost Effectiveness in
Health and Medicine, 309, 311
U.S. Public Health Service
on health promotion, 255, 256
on immigrant health care, 563
participants in, 60
on tobacco use, *596,* 596–97
Tuskegee study by, *374*
Utilitarianism, 365
Utility, 159, 309, 365
Utilization of health services, *313*

V

Vaccinations. *See also* Immunizations
administering, *59,* 67
development of, 28
HIV, 414
HPV, 430
influenza, *63,* 110–12, *111,* 160, 504
pneumococcal diseases, 110, 112, 504
school-required, 160, 413
smallpox, *59, 69,* 616, 620–21
Vaginal cancer, 88, 96–97, 430
Valences, 256
Validity, of health risk appraisals, 243
Value-expectancy theories, 256, 286
Values. *See also* Beliefs; Ethics; Morality
definition of, 360
health behaviors and, 256–63
health education and, 283–84, 287,
290–91
public health program development
and, 308

Van Leeuwenhoek, Anthony, 4
Variable costs, 155–56
VARK (Visual, Aural, Read/write, and
Kinesthetic) Inventory, 285
VA (Veterans Affairs), 581, 582
Vector-borne diseases, 424–26
Vector transmission, 412
Venereal warts, 429–30
Vermont Marble Company, 69
Vesicant or blistering agents, 622
Veterans, homeless, 581–83
Veterans Benefits Assistance, 582
Violence and injuries. *See also* Abuse;
Unintentional injuries
in dating relationships, *484*
domestic, 580–81
Healthy People 2010 on, 109–10
homelessness and, 575–76, 577–78,
580–81
immigrant health and, 562
substance abuse and, 593
Viral agents, 616
Viral hepatitis, 428–29
Virtue ethics, 370–71
Virulence, 411
Vision changes, 503
Visioning, 645–46
Visiting Nurse Association of Omaha,
Nebraska, 401
Visiting nurse associations, 7–8, 58, 401. *See
also* Home health care agencies; Home
visiting
Vital force principle, *374–75*
Volatile organic compounds, 200, 202, 204
Vulnerable populations. *See also specific types
of vulnerable populations (e.g., children,
older adults, refugees, etc.)*
access to health care by, 512–13
community health centers serving, 136
definition of, 573
environmental health and, 208–9
substance abuse in, 597–600

W

W. K. Kellogg Foundation, 327, *329*
Wages, 75, 166–68
Wald, Lillian, *9*
as advocate of national health
insurance, 135
as founder of public health nursing, 8–12, 58
health policies and, 119
home visiting by, 330
research and, 391–92, *392*
respect for, *20,* 21
on rural public health nursing, 14, 513
on school nursing, 61
Walking, *463. See also* Physical activity
War, 11
Wasco-Sherman Public Health Department, *622*

Water, safety of, 200, *200*, 203–4
Water-borne diseases, 423–24
Watershed, 200
Weaknesses. *See* SWOT analysis
Weapons of mass destruction. *See also*
    Bioterrorism; Terrorism
  awareness training, *61*
  biological weapons, 616, *617–19*,
    620–21
  chemical weapons, 621–22
  disaster preparedness and, 614–23
  incendiary/explosive devices, 623
  nuclear/radiological weapons, 621
  terrorism and, *614–15*
Weathering effect, 538
Weight. *See* Low birth weight; Overweight and
    obesity
Weiss, C. H., 91
Well-child visits, *67. See also* Children,
    health of
Wellness clinics, *140, 222, 563*
Westberg, Granger, 68
Western Blot test, 429
West Nile virus, 73
White (Caucasian), *531. See also* Demographic
    categories; Racial and ethnic health
    disparities
White House Conference on Aging, *316,*
    496–97
*Who Will Keep the Public Health? Educating
    Public Health Professionals for the 21st
    Century,* 74
WHO (World Health Organization). *See*
    World Health Organization (WHO)

WIC (Women, Infants, and Children), 164,
    268, 490
Windshield surveys, 227, 229
Women. *See also feminist entries;* Maternal
    health
  cardiovascular disease in, 457–58
  HIV/AIDS and, 380–81, 533–34
  homeless, 578–79, 580–81, *582*
  nursing role of, 6, 7
  physical activity and, *463*
  political activism of, 10–12, *11,* 14
  treatment and counseling of, 181
Women, Infants, and Children (WIC), 164,
    268, 490
Women's Health Care Partnership, *145*
Women's Peace Party, 11
Wood, Mary Morris, 513
Workforce, 37, 48–50, 73–74, *640,* 647–50.
    See also Nurses; Occupational health
    settings; Shortages of nurses
Working Group on National Disaster
    Information Systems, 623
Working poor, 138, 515. *See also* Poverty
Workplaces. *See* Occupational health settings
Worksite Community Health Promotion/Risk
    Reduction Project, *242*
World Bank, 177, 180–81
World Health Assembly, Thirtieth, 254
World Health Organization (WHO)
  on chronic illnesses, *466*
  on definition of health, 254
  on disaster preparedness, 625
  on environmental health, 110
  on global health, 176–77, 179

on health as human right, 362
on health education, 279, *291*
on health promotion, 255, 327, 651
on healthy public policy, 119
on HIV/AIDS, 409
on infectious diseases, 407–8, 412, 424,
    426, 431, *431,* 436–38, *437*
on insulin resistance, 453
on media communication, *439*
on smallpox, 616
on tobacco use, 595
on tuberculosis, 517
World Medical Association, 364
World Social Forum, 179, 181
World Trade Organization, 177, 180

X

Xenophobia, 559

Y

Young adults, deaths of, 483–84
Youth. *See* Adolescents; Children
Youth Risk Behavior Survey, *63,* 89, 96

Z

Zero-base budgets, 352, *352*
Zero to Three, 334
Zidovudine (AZT), 422
Zoglio, S., *Recharge in Minutes,* 350
Zoning, 213